Kim Moller
1081 Fleming   by W. WI
                    High school
773-5564

Second Edition / ADDISON-WESLEY'S
NURSING
EXAMINATION
REVIEW

Second Edition ADDISON-WESLEY'S NURSING EXAMINATION REVIEW

Sally L. Lagerquist, Editor

CONTRIBUTING AUTHORS

Irene M. Bobak, R.N., M.N., M.S.N.
San Francisco State University, San Francisco

Sandra Forrest Fritz, R.N., M.N.
University of California, Los Angeles

Sally L. Lagerquist, R.N., M.S.
University of California, San Francisco

Mary Jane Sauvé, R.N., M.S.
Doctoral Candidate, University of California, San Francisco

Special collaborators in Unit 2, Mental Health Nursing and Coping Behaviors

Williamina Rose, R.N., M.S.
Montana State University, Bozman
and
Ralph Matteoli, R.N., M.S.
San Francisco State University, San Francisco

Special contributors

Questions and rationale for Unit 6,
Ethical and Legal Aspects of Nursing:
Judy Massong, R.N., J.D.
Director of Government Relations
Washington State Nurses Association

Sample comprehensive integrated case studies:
Lois A. Fenner Giles, R.N., M.S.N.
University of Maryland, Baltimore

Addison-Wesley Publishing Company
Medical/Nursing Division
Menlo Park, California • Reading, Massachusetts • London
Amsterdam • Don Mills, Ontario • Sydney

To Lagie, Elana, and Kalen

Plus qu' hier
Moins que demain

With untold appreciation for your patience, endurance, and gentleness when they were needed most, the second time around.

Sally

Sponsoring Editor: Pat Franklin Waldo
Production Editor: Susan Harrington
Copyeditor: Amy Klatzkin
Interior and Cover Designer: John Edeen
Cover photo: Lee Youngblood
Product Manager: Deborah Collins-Stephens

Library of Congress Cataloging in Publication Data
Main entry under title:

Addison-Wesley's nursing examination review:

   Bibliography: p.
   Includes index.
   1. Nursing—Outlines, syllabi, etc.   2. Nursing—Examinations, questions, etc.   I. Lagerquist, Sally L.
[DNLM: 1. Nursing—Examination questions.   WY   18   A227]
RT52.A3   1982   610.73′076   81-20532
ISBN 0-201-14190-6   AACR2

ISBN 0-201-14190-6
EFGHIJKLM-MU-8987654

The authors and publishers have exerted every effort to ensure that drug selection and dosages set forth in this text are in accord with current recommendations and practice at the time of publication. However, in view of ongoing research, changes in government regulations, and the constant flow of information relating to drug therapy and drug reactions, the reader is urged to check the package insert for each drug for any change in indications of dosage and for added warnings and precautions. This is particularly important where the recommended agent is a new and/or infrequently employed drug.

Addison-Wesley Publishing Company
Medical/Nursing Division
2725 Sand Hill Road
Menlo Park, California 94025

About the Authors

Sally L. Lagerquist is founder and president of Review for Nurses, Inc., of San Francisco, and author of *R.N. State Board Examination Practice Questions and Answers,* published by Review for Nurses Tapes, Inc. She is presently lecturer on test-taking techniques at workshops held nationwide for graduating senior nursing students. She is also a Marriage, Family, and Child counselor, and a member of Sigma Theta Tau Society. She received her R.N. and M.S. degrees from the University of California at San Francisco.

Irene M. Bobak is a professor of nursing at San Francisco State University and a maternity nurse practitioner. In addition to *Addison-Wesley's Nursing Examination Review,* she has co-authored another textbook, on maternity nursing. She is a member of the California Perinatal Association, the Nurses Association of the American College of Obstetricians and Gynecologists, and Sigma Theta Tau Society. She received her M.N. from Case Western Reserve University and her M.S.N. from the University of California at San Francisco.

Sandra Forrest Fritz is presently engaged in private practice with Consultants in Pediatrics in Southern California. She is guest lecturer for pediatrics courses at the University of California at Los Angeles and also teaches continuing education and extension courses there. She is a frequent contributor to various nursing magazines and a member of Sigma Theta Tau Society. She received her R.N. and B.S. from the University of Oregon and her M.N. from the University of California at Los Angeles.

Mary Jane Sauvé, in addition to lecturing and writing for other books besides *Addison-Wesley's Nursing Examination Review,* is presently a clinical research specialist in cardiology and a doctoral candidate at the University of California at San Francisco. She is also a member of Sigma Theta Tau Society. She received her B.S.N. at Loyola University of Chicago and her M.S. at the University of California at San Francisco.

Preface

Addison-Wesley's Nursing Examination Review has been substantially revised and restructured in its second edition to meet the needs of students preparing to take the latest NCLEX–R.N. Licensure Examination. *Addison-Wesley's Nursing Examination Review* follows the *nursing process* format both in the content outline section and in the more than 1200 practice test questions and answers. Distinguished by its easy-to-read outlines with *complete* and *comprehensive* coverage, this text maintains the strong features that have made the first edition a favorite among students.

Information on the Latest Licensure Exam

We have provided a special section with a clear and complete description of the latest National Council Licensure Examination and how to study for it. This book also answers the 40 most commonly asked questions regarding the NCLEX–R.N., for example:

"How is the new NCLEX–R.N. different from the previous one?"
"Is the new exam supposed to be harder in 1982?"

For answers to these questions, see page 6 in the Orientation unit.

NCLEX–R.N. Simulated Questions

The second edition of *Addison-Wesley's Nursing Examination Review* now contains over 1000 NCLEX–R.N. simulated questions with rationales for *all* answers. We have included effective test-taking strategies and do-it-yourself relaxation techniques to help you score higher. You will also find easy-to-use self-test sheets for every question section in *Addison-Wesley's Nursing Examination Review*.

We have also, in the second edition, added a new unit: "Sample Comprehensive Integrated Case Studies," with 240 questions and answers with detailed rationale.

All the questions and answers in this book were prepared to test your ability to *apply the nursing process* as well as your knowledge of nursing content. *To assist you and your instructor in evaluating your strengths and weaknesses in applying the nursing process, we have included a unique coding of each question in Units 2, 3, 4, and 5 to the step(s) in the nursing process to which it applies.* This will help you identify questions that focus on specific nursing behaviors, and will guide you to areas where you need further study.

Orientation

This section discusses the mechanics and the format of the latest National Council Licensure Examination as well as test-taking strategies and relaxation techniques that we recommend to alleviate test anxiety. The Orientation section also contains advice to foreign-educated nurses who are preparing to take the licensure examination. Please refer to this section before beginning your review for pointers on how best to use *Addison-Wesley's Nursing Examination Review* as a guide to study.

Content Scope and Sequence

The content in *Addison-Wesley's Nursing Examination Review* stresses the *nursing process*: assessment, analysis, planning, implementation, and evaluation.

The content follows a life-cycle format, and each unit has special features to ensure thorough review and to help you recall and retain essential content in these areas:

Unit 1 Growth and Development through the Life Span

This unit provides the temporal framework for the conditions of human health and disease discussed in the rest of the book. Special care has been taken to include the appropriate nursing interventions when discussing the problems of life-cycle development, body image disturbance, and human sexuality.

Unit 2 Mental Health Nursing and Coping Behaviors

This unit highlights the most commonly observed disorders in the mental health field, with the emphasis on *assessment, analysis* of data, and *nursing interventions* based on the therapeutic use of self as the cornerstone of a helping process. Nursing actions are listed in priority whenever possible. Hence, the *nursing-process framework* is followed throughout.

Categorization of disorders has been modified according to the revised Diagnostic and Statistical Manual (DSM III) of the American Psychiatric Association (1980 edition).

Unit 3 Nursing Care during the Reproductive Years

This unit reflects pertinent current theoretical bases and their nursing applications. The chapter is divided into four parts: (a) Basic issues, (b) Normal pregnancy, (c) Complications of childbearing and the high-risk neonate, and (d) Reproductive-system disorders of women and men. New material has been added on the preconception period and there is more detailed discussion of drugs, health assessment, patient counseling, diabetes and effects on pregnancy, assessment and prevention of premature labor, and the pregnant adolescent. Some of these changes were necessary to keep current with the proposed changes in the R.N. Licensure Examination.

Unit 4 Nursing Care of Children and Families

This unit presents a review of basic pediatric concepts and entities with which the nurse should be familiar. The unit's scope has been extended to include more preventive health concepts and well-child topics for nurse-client counseling. We have also expanded the unit's disease coverage to include congenital heart diseases, Down's syndrome, osteomyelitis, oncology, scoliosis, and herpes simplex. Additionally, the special concerns for each age group have been expanded to include sex education and psychosocial behavior problems.

Unit 5 Nursing Care of the Acutely or Chronically Ill Adult

This unit focuses on the broad concepts and skills needed to apply the *nursing process* to the care of the adult patient. The unit opens (Section I) with a discussion of stress and adaptation, which provides a format for collecting data and identifying nursing problems. Section II includes a discussion of common medical problems to help the student identify these problems and provide a rationale for nursing interventions. Section III discusses common surgical problems and emergency procedures to promote an understanding of the principles and concepts of care that can be applied to the broad spectrum of patients undergoing the same or similar surgical interventions.

Unit 6 Ethical/Legal Aspects of Nursing

This section contains a brief overview answering 25 of the most frequently asked questions. Ethical and legal issues are of concern to all practicing nurses, and this overview will help you focus on essential information.

Unit 7 Cultural Diversity in Nursing Practice

This unit was developed to help the student develop a sensitivity to the cultural aspects of client care. Such a sensitivity can only be fostered by a committed openness to diversity and by a willingness to learn about the background, values, beliefs, and particular health concerns of various groups.

Appendices

No other review book has such extensive coverage of valuable information in summary chart and tabular format; this includes information on diets, common drugs, intravenous therapy, oxygen therapy, and more—*all listing nursing implications.*

Sample Comprehensive Integrated Case Studies

These will help you evaluate your proficiency in integrating nursing content with the nursing process via simulated case situations (six case studies with 240 additional questions).

This book provides *test blanks* for all questions following the units as well as for the "Sample Comprehensive Integrated Case Studies." In addition, this book provides duplicates of these test blanks with the correct responses filled in to facilitate quick self-checking.

We have compiled the *index* with students' needs in mind. The index is comprehensive to assist in locating any and all material for quick review.

Key Feature Recap

No other review book helps students to review with such thoroughness and confidence for the R.N. exam. Here are a few of the special features to help you successfully prepare to pass the exams:

- At last, a special section with a clear and comprehensive *description of the latest R.N. Licensure Examination* and how to study for it
- Unique *coding of all questions by nursing process* steps to help you identify questions that focus on specific behaviors of the nursing process
- New unit of comprehensive *integrated* sample cases with 240 questions and detailed rationale for all answers
- Over 1000 R.N. Licensure Examination simulated situation questions with rationale for *all* answers; compare the thoroughness of these answers with those in other books
- Content follows a life-cycle format that stresses the *nursing process*—assessment, analysis, planning, implementation, and evaluation
- Over 125 charts, illustrations, and tables screened for easy reading and quick reference

- Effective test-taking strategies and relaxation techniques to help you score high
- Valuable advice to foreign-educated nurses preparing to take the licensure examination

This book was prepared by authors who have extensive experience in successfully helping over 19,000 students review for the State Boards at Review for Nurses, Inc. nationwide courses. The author-editor is a widely known lecturer at these reviews and is president of Review for Nurses, Inc., a company that has offered more than 100 review sessions since 1976.

Question and answer books are not enough for a thorough review. You need to review nursing content to make sure you know what makes an answer correct. *Addison-Wesley's Nursing Examination Review, Second Edition*, is the *one* review book you'll need to score higher on the latest National Council Licensure Examination.

Acknowledgements

We are gratified by the manner in which we were able to work together on this challenging venture. Without mutual support, cooperation, and assistance, this book could not have been completed.

We are grateful also to Valerie Weller and Cynthia Ignacio, who had the formidable task of clearing through our tangle of handwritten pages and of transforming them into a typewritten manuscript. Our appreciation also extends to the following reviewers: Albert Aliciene, Rita Bakan, Judy Brusich, Lucille Davis, Sharon Guthrie, Carolyn Kaiser, Ann Macdonald, Eileen Massura, Judy McAulay, Karen Miller, Louise Timmer, and Sheila Zerr.

The task of writing this book has been considerably lightened by the enthusiasm, encouragement, and good counsel of Addison-Wesley's Medical/Nursing editorial staff.

Sally L. Lagerquist
Irene M. Bobak
Sandra Forrest Fritz
Mary Jane Sauvé

Brief Contents

Detailed Contents

List of Tables and Figures

TABLES

FIGURES

Second Edition / ADDISON-WESLEY'S
NURSING
EXAMINATION
REVIEW

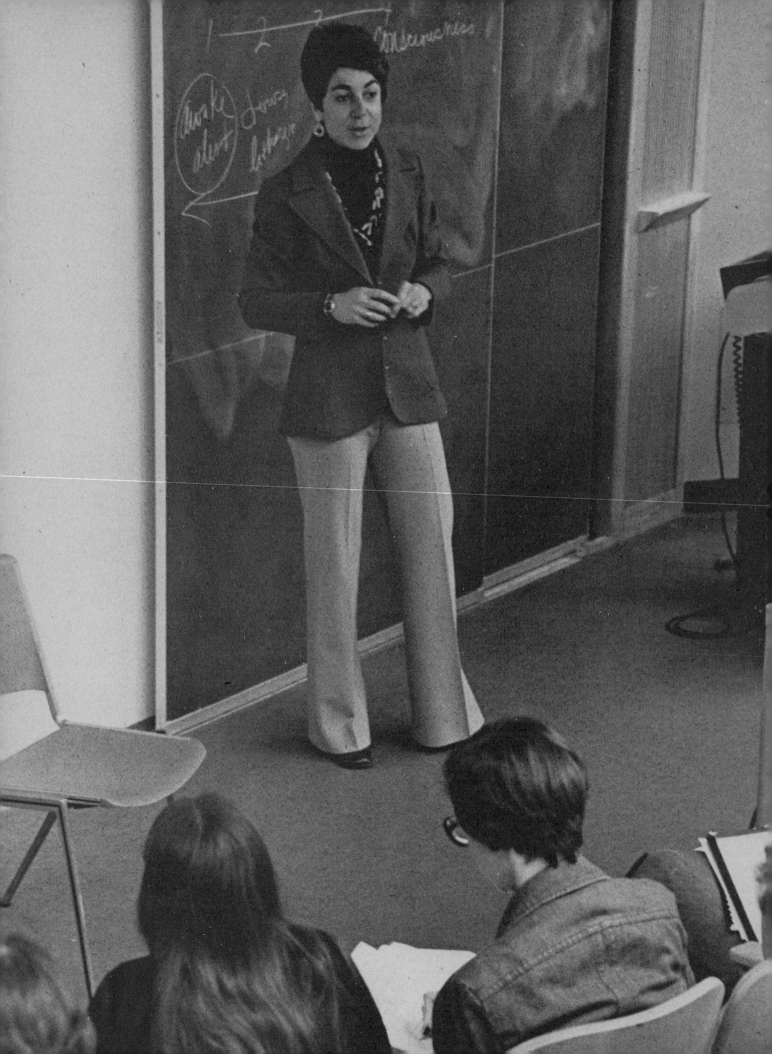

Orientation

HOW TO USE THIS REVIEW BOOK AS A STUDY GUIDE

Although nursing students may know that they are academically prepared to take the National Council Licensure Examination (NCLEX–R.N.), many find that reviewing nursing content for the licensure examination itself presents special concerns about *what* and *how* to study.

Some typical concerns about *what to study* are reflected in the following questions:

- Since there will be about 480 questions on the exam, how does one select what is the most important content for review? How does one narrow the focus of study and distinguish the relevant from the nonrelevant material?
- What areas should be emphasized?
- How detailed should the review be?
- How does one know what areas to review most?
- Should basic sciences, such as anatomy, physiology, microbiology, and nutrition, be included in the study?

Concerns relating to *how to study* include:

- How does one make the best use of limited review time to go over content that may be in lecture and clinical notes compiled during two to four years of schooling?
- Is it best to review from all the major textbooks used in nursing school?
- Should material be memorized, or should one study from broad principles and concepts?

We have written this nursing review book with the *general* intent of assisting nurses in identifying what they need to study in a format designed to use their study time effectively, productively, and efficiently while preparing for the examination.

Each contributing author has selected content and developed a style of presentation that has been tested by thousands of nursing students attending review courses coordinated by the editor in various cities throughout the United States. *Addison-Wesley's Nursing Examination Review* is the result of this study. This review book can be used in a variety of ways: (a) as a starting point for review of essential content specifically aimed at NCLEX or Canadian exam preparation, (b) as an end point of studying for the examinations, (c) as an anxiety reduction tool, (d) as a general guide and refresher for nurses not presently in practice, and (e) as a guide for graduates of foreign nursing schools.

As a starting point
This text can be used in early review when a longer study period is needed to *fill in gaps* of knowledge. One cannot remember what one does not know or understand. A lengthy review before the exam allows students time to rework and organize notes accumulated during two to four years of basic nursing education. In addition, an early review allows time for *self-evaluation*. We have provided questions and answers to help students identify areas requiring further study and to help them *integrate* unfamiliar material with what they already know.

As an end point

This text can also be used for a *quick* review (a) to *promote retention* and *recall* and (b) to aid in determining *nursing actions* appropriate to specific health situations. During the time immediately preceding the examination, the main objective might be to *strengthen previous learning* by refreshing the memory. Or a brief overview may serve to *draw together* the isolated points under key concepts and principles in a way that shows their relationships and relative importance.

As an anxiety reduction tool

In some students, anxiety related to taking examinations in general may reach such levels that it causes students to be unproductive in study and to function at a lower level during the actual examination. Sections of this text are directed toward this problem and provide simple, *practical approaches to general anxiety* reduction. For anxiety specifically related to unknown aspects of the licensure examination itself, the section on the *structure, format, and mechanics of the R.N. examination* might bring relief through its focus on basic examination information.

For anxiety related to lack of confidence or skill in test-taking "know-how," the special section on *test-taking techniques may be helpful*.

As a general study guide and as a refresher for nurses not presently in practice

Many student nurses will find this review book useful as a general study guide throughout their education as they prepare patient care plans and study for midterm and final exams. It will help them put information into perspective as they learn it. And nurses who have not been in practice for several years will find it a useful reference tool and review device.

As a guide for graduates of foreign nursing schools

Nurses who are foreign educated can use this book to serve their special needs:

1. To check their experiences, skills, and knowledge for *equivalency* to those of nursing candidates from U.S. programs, in terms of their ability to deliver effective and safe health care as determined by U.S. standards of practice.
2. To identify cultural differences in perception of patient needs, nursing responses and actions.
3. To learn the necessary requirements in the various states for application to take the RN licensure exam.
4. To learn what the structure and format of the exam is like.
5. To learn how to prepare for the exam, including what books to read.
6. To practice taking tests made up of multiple choice questions.
7. To assess the level of language difficulty in reading the exam.

If you are a foreign-educated nurse and wish to compare your preparation to that of U.S.-educated nurses, you will find that the practice questions with detailed answers that are included at the end of each major content unit can serve as an effective self-assessment guide. If you find that you need further in-depth study after taking the practice test questions and reviewing the essential content presented in outline format throughout the book, you may wish to seek assistance from review courses or self-paced review on audiocassette tapes. A list of suggested references is also provided at the end of each unit to guide you in selecting textbooks frequently used in the United States. In addition, *Appendix D* may help you review drugs used in the U.S. that may be called by other names outside the U.S.

Cultural differences may be one cause of incorrect answers stemming from your different perception of clients' needs or nursing action. *Appendix G,* on Patients' Rights, contains useful information that may reflect cultural differences in belief systems directly related to health care. In addition, Unit 6 contains the code of ethics and standards of nursing practice and legal aspects that pertain to nursing *in the U.S.* We suggest that the foreign-educated nurse become familiar with these sections in order to determine what is *emphasized* in this country, as well as Appendix I, to learn what is considered to be *safe and effective care in the U.S.*

To assist the nurse in making contact with Boards of Registered Nursing, *Appendix H* contains a directory of addresses to write for information about each state's specific requirements for application to take the RN licensing exam.

The Orientation unit is designed to help the foreign-educated nurse know what to expect during the two-day exam, what the exam structure and format will be like, what content will be covered, and how it will be scored. It will also help him or her learn how to study for the test, how to take a multiple choice test and how to reduce test-taking anxiety.

If you are not familiar with or proficient in taking exams with multiple choice questions, the more than 1000 sample test questions in this book will provide you with sufficient practice for taking such a test. In addition, if after reading this unit you feel that additional assistance in test-taking techniques or anxiety reduction approaches might be useful, refer to the suggested references and audiocassette tapes listed at the end of the unit.

If you are concerned about your ability to read and comprehend English as it might be used in the exam, first check yourself by looking at the exam questions in this book. The terms used here are those used in the health care field and are considered to be those a nurse needs to know and use. If the vocabulary is different from yours or is difficult, consult local colleges for courses in *English as a second language (ESL courses)*.

Where to begin

In using this review book to prepare for the licensure examination, the nurse must:

1. Be prepared mentally.
   a. Know the purpose of the examination.
   b. Know the purpose of reviewing.
   c. Anticipate what is to come.
   d. Decide on a good study method—set a study goal before beginning a particular subject area (number of pages, for example); plan the length of the review period by the amount of material to be covered, not by the clock.
2. Plan the work to be done.
   a. Select one subject at a time for review, and establish and follow a sequence for review of each subject.
      (1) Using the perforated answer sheets at the back of the book, answer the practice questions following the outline of the selected subject area. (Set a time limit, as pacing is important.)
      (2) Compare your answers with those provided as a means of evaluating areas of competence.
   b. Identify those subjects that will require additional concentrated study in this review book as well as in basic textbooks.
   c. Study the review text outlines, noting headings, subheadings, and *italics* and **bold face** type for emphasis on relative importance.
   d. Study the content presented in the appendices, which contain much information presented in synthesized format to facilitate memorization, understanding, and application.
   e. Repeat the self-evaluation process by taking the test again.
   f. Look up the answers for the correct response to the multiple choice questions and read the

rationale for *why* it was the correct response. (These explanations serve to correct as well as reinforce. Understanding the underlying principles also serves as an aid in applying the same principles to questions that may be phrased differently on the actual examination.)
   g. If necessary, refer to the annotated bibliography for other basic textbooks to relearn aspects of anatomy, physiology, nutrition, or basic nursing procedures that are unclear.

While reviewing

1. Scan the outline for main ideas and topics.
   a. Do not try to remember verbatim what is on each page.
   b. Paraphrase or explain this material to another person.
2. Refer to basic textbooks for details and illustrations as necessary to recall specific information related to basic sciences.
3. Integrate reading with experience.
   a. Think of examples that illustrate the key concepts and principles.
   b. Make meaningful associations.
   c. Look for implications for nursing actions as concepts are reviewed.
4. Take notes on the review outline—use stars and arrows, underscore, and write comments in margins, such as "most important" and "memorize," to reinforce relative importance of points of information.

After reviewing

1. Repeat the self-evaluation process as often as necessary to gain mastery of content essential to safe nursing practice.
2. Continue to refer to major textbooks to fill in gaps where greater detail or in-depth comprehension is required.
3. Look for patterns in your selection of responses to the multiple-choice practice questions—identify sources of difficulty in choosing the most appropriate answers.

KEY POINTS TO RECALL FOR BETTER STUDY

1. *Schedule*—study time should be scheduled so that review begins close to the time at which it will be used. Retention is much better following a well-

spaced review. It may be helpful to group material into small learning segments. Study goals should be set before beginning each period of study (number of pages, for example).

2. *Overlearn*—many students have better retention of material after they have reorganized and relearned it.

3. *Rephrase and explain*—try to rephrase material in your own words or explain it to another person. Reinforce learning through repetition and usage.

4. *Decide on order of importance*—organize study time in terms of importance and familiarity.

5. *Use mechanical memory aids*—mnemonic (memory) devices simplify recall, for example, "On Old Olympus's Towering Top a Finn and German Viewed Some Hops." The first letter in each word identifies the first letter of a cranial nerve.

6. *Association*—associate new material with related concepts and principles from past experience.

7. *Original learning*—if an unfamiliar topic is presented, do more than review. Seek out sources of additional information such as those given in the bibliographies.

8. *Make notes*—look for key words, phrases, and sentences in the outlined review material and mark them for later reference.

9. *Definitions*—look up unfamiliar terms in a dictionary or the glossary of a basic text.

10. *Additional study*—refer to other textbook references for more detailed information.

11. *Distractors*—keep a pad of paper on hand to jot down extraneous thoughts; get them out of the mind and on to the paper.

THE MECHANICS OF THE NATIONAL COUNCIL LICENSURE EXAMINATIONS FOR REGISTERED NURSES (NCLEX–R.N.)

Frequently candidates for the nursing licensing examination have many questions about the structure and format of the test itself and the rules and regulations concerning the examination procedure.

As an aid to reducing apprehension and time spent on speculation, this chapter is intended to provide information that candidates commonly seek. The information in this section was verified as correct at the time that it was compiled from a survey of responses by each state's board of nursing registration, as well as from literature distributed by the National Council of State Boards of Nursing, Inc., and the National League for Nursing. If you have further questions, contact the board of nursing in your state.

1. *What is required for admission to the examination center?* In some states a 2- by 2-inch or 3- by 3-inch head and shoulders photo of the candidate must be attached to the admission card. The photo must be a recent likeness of the candidate for positive identification. In some states, only those holding these admission cards and photos will be admitted to the examination room. Exceptions: Washington, Oregon, and Alaska.

2. *Can I bring any material into the examination room?* No, do *not* take any study materials, including books, notes, or cameras, into the examination building. You may be asked to place your personal belongings (purses, books, etc.) on tables provided.

3. *Is there assigned seating?* Yes, in some states. At the examination, each table will be identified with a number corresponding to the numbers assigned on admittance slips. The proctor will check your admittance slip and personal I.D. as you enter the examination room each time. You need to find your assigned seat.

4. *Can I bring my own pencil to blacken the circles?* Yes, in some states you need to provide your own No. 2 pencil; plan to bring two to three *sharpened* No. 2 pencils with erasers. Blacken the circle corresponding to the answer you have chosen.

5. *What do I do when I finish the test?* You must turn in the test booklet to the proctor before leaving the exam room.

6. *Where do the exam questions come from?* The individual state boards nominate item writers who represent various regions and types of nursing programs to the National Council of State Boards of Nursing, which selects persons meeting the criteria for item-writing to write questions for the State Board Test Pool Examination. The state boards administer the exam under the control of the National Council of State Boards of Nursing, Inc. The new test writing service is the California Test Bureau.

7. *Are there any questions with which I may not have had previous experience in my basic nursing program?* Most of the questions are about clients with conditions familiar to you and are representative of common health problems on a national basis. Some questions may relate to nursing problems with which you may not have had prior experience. Their purpose is to test your ability to *apply*

knowledge of specific principles from the physical, biologic, and social sciences to *new* situations.

8. *Will there be questions on nutrition and diet therapy, pharmacology, nursing fundamentals, and communicable diseases?* Yes, in addition to questions related to major health areas, the tests will include questions from such areas as nutrition and diet therapy, pharmacology, fundamentals of nursing, communicable-disease nursing, psychosocial aspects of nursing, natural and behavioral sciences, legal aspects, and ethical responsibilities.

9. *How many questions does the total test contain?* 480 questions. The exam is divided into four two-hour parts, with approximately 120 questions in each part.

10. *Are all of the questions multiple choice?* Yes.

11. *How many choices are included?* Four.

12. *Do some questions have more than one answer?* No, only *one* of the four suggested alternatives is the *best* answer. Mark only *one* answer to each question.

13. *What will happen if I mark more than one response to a question?* You will not receive any credit for that question.

14. *Is it advisable to guess when I do not know the answer?* Answer those questions to which you *think* you know the right answer, although you may not be sure. Do not use wild guessing, as this might lower your score. Leaving a large number of questions blank, however, may also adversely affect your score.

15. *Will I get partial credit for selecting the next-to-the-best answer?* No.

16. *May I make marks in the test booklet?* Yes, you may make marks in the test booklet.

17. *What is the passing score?* At the time of this writing, the suggested passing score is 1600. There will be *one* score for the total exam.

18. *How is the exam scored?* It is scored by machine. Standardization and conversion tables are used to convert raw scores into standard scores. If normative scoring will be used, one standard deviation (400) below the mean (2000) is the recommended passing score (1600). However, *criterion referencing* may be used in place of normative scoring. Please consult your local Board of Registered Nursing for further information.

19. *How much time is usually allowed for each part?* For the first day: two test booklets, each two hours long. For the second day: two additional test booklets, each two hours long, plus, in July 1982, an additional one-hour test booklet (No. 5) used to field test future test questions, but that does not count toward the final score. Starting in February 1983, booklet No. 5 will not be used; instead experimental questions will be integrated in each of the four exam booklets (as few as ten questions).

20. *Is there time for lunch?* Yes, 1 to 1½ hours; with a 15-minute afternoon break, until February 1983.

21. *What if I need to leave my seat during a test?* You must have permission from the examiner or a designee. Without this permission, your papers will not be counted if you leave. You may be accompanied by a proctor.

22. *How often is the exam given?* Twice a year, on the same date in every state. The scheduled dates for NCLEX–R.N. are as follows:

1982	February 2–3	July 13–14
1983	February 1–2	July 12–13
1984	February 7–8	July 10–11
1985	February 5–6	July 16–17
1986	February 4–5	July 15–16
1987	February 3–4	July 14–15
1988	February 2–3	July 12–13
1989	February 14–15	July 11–12
1990	February 6–7	July 10–11
1991	February 5–6	July 9–10

23. *Do I have to repeat the entire exam if I do not pass only one or two parts?* Yes.

24. *Can the exam be retaken before results from the previous exam are known?* No.

25. *How many times can the exam be repeated?* Unlimited within two to three years in 16 states; other states have limits and may require remedial work. Currently, many states require that an applicant pass in no more than three writings within an 18-month period. However, each state can set its own limits. Examples—Arkansas: no limits. Hawaii: maximum of two retakes within three years. Illinois: no more than two years may elapse between writings. Maryland: after three trials, must complete state-approved nursing course. Massachusetts: must pass in two-year period. Michigan: maximum of two retakes, then enrollment in approved nursing education program. North Carolina: no more than three writings. North Dakota: six writings in three years. Ohio: unlimited number of times to repeat. Pennsylvania: unlimited number of times, unlimited number of years. South Dakota: up to five times in three years; then must return to school for remedial assistance. Tennessee: no limits. Please check with the individual State Board of

Nursing for the most current information (see Appendix H) for addresses and phone numbers.

26. *Does the exam fee have to be paid each time the test is repeated by an applicant?* It varies from state to state. In some states, if it is within one year from the first sitting, there is no additional fee. In most states, a new fee is required.

27. *Do diploma graduates take the same test as associate or baccalaureate degree graduates?* Yes.

28. *Do the different states have different exams?* All states as well as Guam and the Virgin Islands use the examination from the National Council Licensure Examination. However, each state decides on the minimum passing score.

29. *When will the exam results be known?* It varies from six to eight weeks to two to four months, with an average time span of 50 days.

30. *Who grants the nursing license?* The state board of nursing for which you wrote the exam.

31. *Will every candidate have the same exam booklet at a given location?* No, it is anticipated that, starting in February 1983, there may be as many as 30 different test forms distributed at a given time to the candidates.

32. *How is the new test different from the previous one?* Prior to 1982, the exam tested for nursing abilities in ten categories and was divided into five subject areas. The new test plan beginning in July, 1982 focuses on *nursing behaviors:* assessment, analysis, planning, implementation, and evaluation.
It will be *one comprehensive exam* divided equally into four parts, with only *one score* (not five as formerly). The questions will test mainly for *application* of knowledge of a given situation, not merely recall of facts.

33. *Is the exam supposed to be harder in 1982?* No. The range of the level of complexity will be the same.

34. *Why was the test changed rather than updated?* The implied framework of the former test which utilized the five headings (medical, surgical, obstetrical, pediatric and psychiatric nursing), was criticized as following the medical model rather than a nursing model.
Also, new information became available from a project that was designed to provide a data base to study the validity of the licensing exam. Eleven thousand critical incidents in practice were collected and analyzed. These were events in which a nurse did or did not do something that influenced the client's well-being. The events reflected current nursing practice for providing safe and effective care and were used as a resource for the new exam. See Appendix I, Critical Requirements for Safe/Effective Nursing Practice.

35. *How is the exam constructed?* The Examination Committee of the National Council of State Boards of Nursing (12 members selected from 53 Boards of Registered Nursing, representing all regions of the U.S.) prepare the test *plan*. The plan is approved by delegates of the National Council (who represent the boards of nursing). States take turns submitting names of item writers (each state nominates every fourth year). Board of Directors of the National Council select item writers on the basis of their credentials and expertise in a particular area of nursing, types of nursing program, and region of the U.S. Item writers may be faculty, clinical nurse specialists, or beginning practitioners.
Item writers meet as a group for a week to be instructed by staff of the test service on how to write questions. At this time, reference books are not used to write common clinical situations and series of questions, to insure that the language of any *particular* textbook is *not* used. *After* the questions are written, current nursing journals and textbooks are checked to validate correctness of the answers.
After the exam questions are written, they are sent to the Boards of Nursing for suggestions for revision and their recommendation whether to revise, accept, or reject questions and to rate priority. Up to this point, each question has been reviewed by item writers composed of faculty and clinical specialists, test service staff, members of the 12 participating State Boards of Nursing, and by members of the Executive Committee of the National Council of State Boards of Nursing.
These questions are then put into booklet form and field tested as an experimental test at the actual licensure exam. The scores on this test do *not* affect the passing score. Information attained by this nationwide field test serves to eliminate questions that may be unclear, vague, confusing, ambiguous, irrelevant, or not equally applicable to all regions of the United States.

36. *What is the purpose of the licensure exam?* To test for competencies needed by a newly-licensed nurse to perform his or her work safely and effectively, as reported in a study by Jacobs that reflects nursing practice today. See Appendix I, *Critical Requirements for Safe/Effective Nursing Practice* and the ANA Standards of Practice.

37. *What will the new exam cover? Nursing behaviors*

applied to client situations will be selected from all stages in the *life cycle* as well as *common* health problems drawn from the major health areas and based on current morbidity studies. Most of the items (80%) on a given test will test for the ability to *apply* knowledge (principles, ideas, theories) and *analyze* data (break information down into elements or parts, set priorities, and see relationships between ideas); others will test for recall and comprehension.*

38. *What is the new test plan?* Table O–1 is a *sample* of how items *may* be selected for testing behaviors in accordance with the established test plan; the *nursing process* is the basis for this test plan.†

39. *What categories of nursing knowledge are included in this exam?* (Comments in parentheses indicate how and where this book covers this content.)*
    1. Normal growth and development (see Unit 1).
    2. Basic human needs (see Unit 2).
    3. Individual coping mechanisms (see Unit 2).
    4. Actual or potential health problems (see Units 2, 3, 4, and 5).
    5. Effect of age, sex, culture, ethnicity, and/or religion on health needs (see Unit 7).
    6. Ways by which nursing can assist individuals to maintain health and cope with health problems (see nursing goals/implementation and nursing intervention sections in each unit of this book).

40. *What other concepts relevant to nursing practice are integrated throughout the exam?**
    1. Management.
    2. Accountability (see Unit 6).
    3. Life cycle (see the Table of Contents to see how

*Source: A new licensing exam for nurses. 1980. (*American Journal of Nursing,* April), pp. 723–725
†Source: National Council of the State Boards of Nursing

the conceptual framework of this book is organized by life cycle).
    4. Client environment. (There is continuous reference throughout this book related to protection from harm against airborne irritants, cold, and heat; identification of environmental discomforts such as noise, odors, dust, and poor ventilation; elimination of potential *safety hazards;* maintenance of environmental order; and *cleanliness.*)

41. *What weight will be given to the questions?* About 55%–65% of the test items will focus on situations where *both the client and the nurse* share in the decision-making process (e.g., the nurse and a hospitalized patient who is admitted for specific, diagnostic or therapeutic treatment or convalescent situations where client is able to exercise some control in performing selected activities of daily living in order to improve health or maintain life).† Some 20%–30% of the test items will focus on situations where the locus of decision-making is centered on the *nurse*—for example, emergency situations in which a client is unable to participate in decisions about his physical and/or psychological condition (e.g., when the client is comatose or in an acute phase of substance abuse, or when the client is an acutely ill child, acutely ill psychotic client, premature infant, or in a postanesthesia period).†

About 10%–20% of the test items will focus on situations where the locus of decision-making is centered in the *client*—for example, supportive, rehabilitation and educational situations—where the client needs guidance to prevent disease but is able to take care of his own health needs independently. These clients present situations in which a nurse can provide education to promote

TABLE O–1. *Sample nursing behaviors and situations to be tested in any one of the four test booklets (based on 120 questions in each booklet)*

Systems to be tested‡	Behaviors					
	Assessment	Analysis	Planning	Implementation	Evaluation	Total
Locus of decision: nurse	6	6	6	6	6	30
Locus of decision: shared	14	14	14	14	14	70
Locus of decision: client	4	4	4	4	4	20
Total number of test items per test booklet (sample)	24	24	24	24	24	120

‡See No. 41 above for description of terms.

TABLE O–2. *Exam "weight" given to various nursing behaviors*

Nursing behaviors tested	Percentage of test items based on specific behaviors
Assessment	15%–25%
Analysis	15%–25%
Planning	15%–25%
Implementation	15%–25%
Evaluation	15%–25%

health and provide an environment for growth. (Examples of such clients and situations are normal pregnant women, families with normal newborns, independent geriatric clients, healthy clients, and clients with stable but chronic conditions who do *not* require therapeutic measures).

Table O–2 shows the weight given on the exam to various *nursing behaviors.*†

42. *What is the expected range of scores?* Eight hundred to almost 3200.

HOW TO PREPARE FOR AND SCORE HIGHER ON EXAMS

The psychology of test-taking

Many nursing students know the nursing material they are being tested on and can demonstrate their nursing skills in practice but do not know how to prepare themselves for, take, and pass the examination.

It is not just a matter of taking exams but of *knowing how* to take them, making educated guesses, and utilizing the allotted time in the most productive way. You must learn to use strategy and judgement in answering questions when you are not sure of the right answer. This chapter will discuss practical strategies for eliminating wrong answers and for increasing your chances of selecting the best ones.

1. *The first hunch is usually a good one.* Pay attention to your intuition, which may indicate which answer "feels" best.

2. *If you cannot decide between two choices, make a note of the numbers of the two choices about which you are not sure.* This will narrow down your focus when you come back to this question. Leave the question; do not spend much time on the ones in doubt. When you have completed the test, go back and spend more time on those with which you had trouble.

3. *Answer the easy ones first.* This is a basic rule of exam-taking. Too often examinees focus on one question for ten minutes, for example, instead of going on to answer 20 additional questions during this time. The main purpose is to answer correctly as many questions as possible.

4. *Be wise about the timing.* Divide your time. For example, if you have 120 questions and 2 hours for the test, aim for an average of 1 question per minute. Keep working! Do not lose time looking back at your answers.

5. *Use care and caution when using electronically scored booklets.* You will receive an exam booklet containing the test questions that will be electronically scored. It is essential that you use the special No. 2 pencil required by the examiners. This pencil contains lead that the electrical grading impulse will pick up. If you need to erase, erase completely. A trace of lead in the wrong space might throw out the answer. Be especially cautious in placing your answers by the correct question number. If you leave out a question, make sure that you skip that number on the answer sheet. Otherwise, all the other answers may be out of sequence and result in wrong answers by accident. It might be helpful to say to yourself as you answer each question, "Choice No. 4 to question No. 3," to make sure that the right answer goes with each question.

6. *Stay the entire time allotted.* If you complete the section early, check your answers. On a second look (after you have completed the entire section), you may find something that you are now sure you marked in error the first time. Also, look for and erase stray marks. If you were undecided between two possible answers on any questions, use left-over time to reconsider those questions.

7. *It is better not to guess wildly.* Prior to the date of your exam, check with the literature put out by your local nursing state board as to whether or not they still deduct wrong answers from correct ones. If this is still the current practice, it is safer not to guess, for if the question is left blank, there will be no wrong answer to deduct.

8. *On the morning of the exam, avoid excessive oral intake of products that act as diuretics for you.* If you know that coffee, beer, or cigarettes, for example, increase urgency and frequency, it is best to limit their intake. Undue physiologic discomforts can distract your focus from the exam at hand.

9. *Increase your oral intake of foods high in glucose and protein.* These foods reportedly have been helpful to some examinees for keeping up their blood-sugar level. This may enable greater con-

centration and problem-solving ability at the times when you most need to function at a high level.

10. *Prior to examination days, avoid eating exotic or highly seasoned foods to which your system may not be accustomed.* Avoid possible gastrointestinal distress when you least need it!

11. *Using hard candy or something similar* during the test may help relieve the discomfort of a dry mouth related to a state of anxiety. However, some states may not allow anything on the table except the exam booklet, the answer sheet, and pencils.

12. *Wear comfortable clothes that you have worn before.* The day of the exam is not a good time to wear new clothes and footwear that may prove to be constricting, binding, or uncomfortable, especially at the waistline and shoulder seams.

13. Anxiety states can bring about rapid increases and decreases in body temperature. *Wear clothing that can be shed or added on.* For example, you might wear a sweater that can be put on when you feel chilled or removed when your body temperature fluctuates again.

14. *Women need to be prepared for early, irregular, and unanticipated onset of menses on exam day, a time of stress.*

15. Exam jitters can elicit anxietylike reactions, both physiologic and emotional. Since anxiety tends to be contagious, *try to limit your contacts with those who are either also experiencing exam-related anxiety or who elicit those feelings in you.*

16. *The night before the exam is a good time to engage in a pleasurable activity* as a means of anxiety reduction. The exam involves many hours of endurance for sitting, thinking, and reacting. Give yourself a chance for restful, not energy- or emotion-draining, activities in the days before the exam.

17. *Get an early start* on the day you take the examination to avoid raising your anxiety level before the actual exam starts. Allow yourself time for delays in traffic and in public transportation or for finding a parking place. Even allow for a dead battery, flooded engine, flat tire, or bus breakdown. If you are unfamiliar with the city in which you will take the exam, find the examination building the day before.

18. *Try a relaxation process* (see pp. 11–13) if anxiety reaches an uncomfortable level that cannot be channeled into the service of learning.

19. When you arrive home after the exam, *jot down content areas that were unfamiliar to you.* This may serve as a key focus for review.

20. If your anxiety level is high *after* the exam because you did not answer every question, remember that *you do not need to get all the answers right to pass.* The exam is not designed for obtaining perfect scores. Achieving the highest score on the NCLEX–R.N. will not earn you a gold star on your license or a differently designated license.

21. Aim to do as well as you can but avoid the same competitive pressures and strivings to attain an "A" grade that you might have previously experienced in working for school or college grades. Good luck!

Purpose of memorization

You'll need to memorize some items before you can rapidly assess or apply that knowledge to a particular situation; for example, you need to be able to recall the standard and lethal doses of a drug before deciding to administer it. Items you should memorize include, but are not limited to:

1. Names of common drugs.
2. Lethal and therapeutic doses.
3. Lab norms and values.
4. Growth and development norms.
5. Foods high or low in iron, protein, sodium, potassium, or carbohydrates.
6. Conversion formulas.
7. Anatomical names.
8. List of cranial nerves and their innervations.

How to memorize: the strategy of memory training

1. Before you work on training your mind to remember, you must *want* to remember the material.
2. You cannot memorize what you do not understand; therefore *know* your material.
3. Visualize what you want to memorize; picture it; draw a picture.
4. Use the familiar to provide vivid mental pictures, to peg the unfamiliar.
   a. When needing to remember a *sequence,* use your body to turn material into a picture. Draw a person, then list the first item to be memorized on top of the head, the next item on the forehead, and so on for nose, mouth, neck, chest, abdomen, thighs, knees and feet.
   b. Use what you already know to tie in with what you want to remember; make it memorable.
   c. Use as "pegs" the unexpected, the exaggerated. Weird imagery is easiest to recall.
5. Use the blank paper technique—
   a. Place a large blank sheet on the wall.
   b. After you have studied, draw on the blank paper what you remember.

c. When you have drawn all that you can recall, check with the book and study what you did correctly and incorrectly.

d. Take another sheet and do it again. Purpose: to reinforce what you already know and work with what you want to remember.

6. Make up and use mnemonic devices to help you remember the important elements.

7. Repetitively explain the material you want to memorize to another person.

8. Saturate your environment with the material you want to memorize.

    a. Purpose: to overcome the mind's tendency to ignore.

    b. Tape facts, formulas, concepts on walls.

9. Above all, feel confident in your ability to memorize!

Strategies in answering questions

If you can intelligently eliminate false answers, you can reduce a four-answer question to a two-answer one to make your chances as good as those in the true-false type of question; that is, odds will favor your guessing half of the answers correctly.

We think that the following pointers will assist you to narrow down your choices intelligently.

1. *Always, all, never, none.* Answers that include global words such as these should be viewed with caution because they imply that there are no exceptions. There are very few instances in which a correct answer is that absolute. Any suggested answer such as—

Nurses should exercise caution in interviewing alcoholics because:
(1) Alcoholics *always* exaggerate.
(2) Alcoholics are *never* consistent.

—should be looked at with care because any exception will make that a false response. A more reasonable answer to the preceding might be "Alcoholics may not be reliable historians."

2. *Broad, most comprehensive answers.* Choose the answer that includes all of the others, which is referred to here as the "umbrella effect." For example, in answering the question—

A main nursing function in group therapy is to:
(1) Help patients give and receive feedback in the group.
(2) Encourage patients to bring up their concerns.
(3) Facilitate group interaction among the members.
(4) Remind patients to address their comments to the group.

—No. 3 is the best choice because all other choices go under it.

3. Test how *reasonable* the answer is by posing a specific situation to yourself. For example, the question might read, "The best approach when interviewing children who have irrational fears is to: (1) help them analyze why they feel this way." Ask yourself if it is reasonable to use Freudian analysis with 2-year-old children.

4. *Focus on the patient.* Usually the reason for doing something with a patient is *not* to preserve the good reputation of the doctor, hospital, or nurse, or to enforce rules. Wrong choices would focus on enlisting the patient's cooperation for the purpose of fulfilling orders or because it is the rule. On seeing a patient out of bed against orders, instead of just saying, "It's against doctor's orders for you to get up," you might better respond by focusing on how the patient is reacting to the restriction on his mobility, by saying, for example, "I can see that you want to get up and that it is upsetting to you to be in bed now. Let me help you get back to bed safely and see what I can do for you."

5. *Eliminate any answer that takes for granted that anyone is unworthy or ignorant.* For example, in the question, "The patient should not be told the full extent of her condition because": a poor response would be, "she would not understand."

6. *Look for the answer that may be different from the others.* For example, if all choices but one are stated in milligrams and that one reads, "1 gm," that choice may be a distractor. In that case, you can narrow your selection to the other choices.

7. Read the question carefully to see if a *negative verb* is used. If the question asks, "Which of the following are *not* applicable," be sure to gear your thinking accordingly. You may want to underline a key word like "not" as you read the questions.

8. *Do not look for a pattern* in the answers shaded under a given numbered choice. If you have already shaded four successive answers under choice three for each of the four questions, do not be reluctant to shade choice three for the fifth question in a row if you think that it is the correct response.

9. *Look for the choices that you know are either correct or incorrect.* You can save time and narrow your selection by using this strategy.

10. In eliminating potentially wrong answers, remember to look for examples of what has been included in the *nontherapeutic response* list in Unit 2, Mental Health Nursing and Coping Behaviors.

11. Wrong choices tend to be either *very brief* in response or *very long and involved.*

12. Better choices to select are those responses that (a) focus on *feelings,* "How did that make you feel?" (b) *reflect* the patient's comments, "You say that made you angry," (c) communicate *acceptance* of the patient by the nurse rather than criticism or a value judgment, (d) *acknowledge* the patient, "I see that you are wincing," and (e) stay in the *here-and-now,* "What will help now?" Examples of better choices can be found in the *therapeutic responses* list in Unit 2, Mental Health Nursing and Coping Behaviors.

13. Look for the *average, acceptable, safe, common, "garden variety"* responses, not the "exception to the rule," esoteric, and controversial responses.

14. Eliminate the response that may be the best for a *physician* to make. Look for an *RN role-appropriate* response; for example, *psychiatrists analyze* the past, and *nurses* in general focus on *present* feelings and situations.

15. *Look for similarities and groupings* in responses and the one-of-a-kind key idea in multiple-choice responses. For example:

At which activity would it be important to protect the patient who is on phenothiazines from the side effects of this drug?
(1) Sunday church services.
(2) A twilight concert.
(3) A midday movie in the theater.
(4) A luncheon picnic on the hospital grounds.

Choices No. 1, 2, and 3 all involve indoor activities. Choice No. 4 involves outdoor exposure during the height of the sun's rays. Patients need to be protected against photosensitivity and burns when on phenothiazines.

16. Be sure to note if the question asks for what is the *first* or *initial* response to be made or action to be taken by the nurse. The choices listed may all be correct, but in this situation selecting the response with the *highest priority* is important.

17. When you do not know the specific facts called for in the question, use your *skills of reasoning;* for example, when an answer involves amounts or time (mainly numbers) and you do not know the answer and cannot find any basis for reasoning (all else being equal), avoid the extreme responses (the highest or lowest numerical values).

18. *Give special attention to questions in which each word counts.* The purpose of this type of question may not only be to test your knowledge, but also to see if you can read accurately and look for the main point. In such questions, each answer may be a profusion of words, but there may be one or two words that make the critical difference.

19. All else being equal, select the response that you best *understand.* Long-winded statements are likely to be included as distractors and may be a lot of words signifying little or nothing, such as "criteria involved in implementing conceptual referents for standardizing protocol."

20. *Apply skim-reading techniques.* Read the descriptive case quickly. Pick out *key* words (write them down, if that is helpful to you). Translate, into *your own* words, the gist of what is asked in the question. You might close your eyes at this point and see if the answer "pops" into mind. *Then,* skim the choices of answers, looking for that response that corresponds to what first came into your mind. Key ideas or themes to look for in responses have been covered in this section (that is, look for a "feeling" response, acceptance, acknowledgment of the patient, and reflection, for example).

HOW TO REDUCE ANXIETY

Most people have untapped inner resources for achieving relaxation and tension release in stressful situations (such as during an examination) when they need to function at their highest potential.

In anxiety-producing settings whenever you feel overwhelmed or blocked, a fantasy experience can be of help in mastering the rising anxiety by promoting a feeling of calm, detached awareness and a sense of deeper personal coping resources. Through the fantasy you can gain access to a zone of tranquility in the center of your being. Guided imagery often carries with it feelings of serenity, warmth, and comfort. The goal of this discussion is to help you experience a self-guided approach to reducing your anxiety level to one that is compatible with learning and high performance.

Fantasy experiences are, of course, highly individual. Techniques that may help one person experience serenity may frustrate another. Try out the self-guided experiences suggested here, make up your own, and select ones that are best for you. There are endless possibilities for fantasy journeys. The best approach is to work with whatever fantasy occurs to you at the moment. The ideas for a journey presented here are meant to be a springboard for variation of your own.

A fantasy will be more effective if you take as comfortable a physical position as possible, with eyes closed and attention focused on the inner experience. Get in touch with physical sensations, your pattern and rate of breathing, your heart beat, and pressure points of your body as it comes in contact with the chair and floor.

When you take a fantasy journey by yourself, it is important for you to read over the instructions several times so that you will be able to recall the over-all structure of the fantasy. *Then,* close your eyes and take your trip without concern for following the instructions in detail.

Instructions

Sit comfortably in a chair. Shut your eyes and chase your thoughts for a minute; go where your thoughts go.

Then, let the words go. Become aware of how you *feel,* here and now, not how you would like to feel.

Shift your awareness to your feet. Do not move them. Become aware of what they are doing.

Spend 20 to 30 seconds focusing progressively on different parts of your body. Relax each part in turn:

Relax each of your toes; the tops of your feet; the arch of each foot; the insteps, balls, and heels; your ankles, calves, knees, thighs, and buttocks. Become aware of how your body is contacting the chair in which you are sitting. Let go of your abdominal and chest muscles; relax your back. Release the tension in your shoulders, arms, elbows, forearms, wrists, hands, and each finger in turn; relax the muscles in your throat, lips, and cheeks. Wrinkle your nose; relax your eyelids and eyebrows (first one and then the other); relax the muscles in your forehead and top and back of your head. Relax your whole body.

Concentrate on your breathing: become aware of how you breathe. Allow yourself to inhale and exhale in your usual way. Become aware of the depth of your breathing. Are you expanding the lungs all the way? Or, are you breathing shallowly? Increase your depth of breathing. Now focus on the rate at which you are breathing. See if you can slow the rate down. When you breathe in, can you feel an inflow of energy that fills your entire body?

Now concentrate on the sounds in the room.
Focus on how you feel right now.
Slowly open your eyes.

Progressive relaxation

Relaxation approaches are used in a variety of anxiety states whenever stress interferes with the ability to function.

Progressive relaxation training was originated in 1929 by Dr. Edmund Jacobson. It is a technique for attaining self-control over skeletal muscles in order to induce low-level tonus in the major muscle groups. The approach involves learning systematically and sequentially to tense and relax various muscle groups throughout the body.

The *objectives* of this approach are to soothe nerves, combat hypertonus in muscles, and substitute relaxing activities for stressful ones in order to feel comfortable in and more alert to the internal and external environments.

The *theory* behind this method takes as its basis the idea that muscular relaxation and anxiety states produce directly opposite physiologic effects and thus cannot coexist. In other words, it is not possible to be tense in any body part that is completely relaxed.

The *physiologic changes* during relaxation include decreased oxygen consumption, decreased carbon dioxide elimination, and decreased respiratory rate.

The basic factors vital to eliciting a relaxation response include:

1. *Quiet setting*—eliminate unnecessary internal and external stimuli.
2. *Passive, "let-it-happen" attitude*—empty your mind of thoughts and distractions.
3. *Comfortable position*—sit or recline in one position for 20 minutes or so.
4. *Constant stimulus on which to focus*—a repetitive sound, constant gaze on an object or image, or attention to one's own breathing pattern.

Relaxation training is a procedure that can be defined, specified, and memorized until you can go through the exercises mechanically. If you regularly practice relaxation, you will be able to cope more effectively with difficult situations by reaping the physiologic and psychologic benefits of a balanced and relaxed state.

Suggestions for additional experiential vignettes

• Imagine yourself leaving the room. In your mind's eye go through the city and over the fields. Come to a meadow covered with fresh, new grass and flowers. Look out on the meadow and focus on what you see, hear, smell, and feel. Walk through the meadow. See the length and greenness of the grass; see the brilliance and feel the warmth of the sunlight.

• For a more expansive feeling, visualize a mountain in the distance. Fantasize going to the country and slowly ascending a mountain. Walk through a forest.

Climb to the top until at last you reach a height where you can see forever. Experience your awareness.

• Focus on a memory of a beautiful place you have been to, enjoyed, and would like to enjoy again. Be there; experience it.

• Imagine that you are floating on your back down a river. It may help at first to breathe deeply and feel yourself sinking. Visualize that you are coming out on a gentle river that is slowly winding its way through a beautiful forest. The sun is out and the rays feel warm on your skin. You pass trees and meadows of beautiful flowers. Smell the grass and flowers. Hear the birds. Look up in the blue sky; see the lazy tufts of clouds floating by. Leave the river and walk across the meadow. Enjoy the grass around your ankles. Come to a large tree. . . .

Fill in the rest of the trip—what do you see now? Where do you want to go from here?

Sally L. Lagerquist

SUGGESTED REFERENCES

Alexander, A. B.: Relaxation training script, modified Jacobsonian method, Denver, 1972, Children's Asthma Research Hospital.

Benson, H.: The relaxation response, New York, 1975, William Morrow and Co.

Benson, H., et al.: The relaxation response, *Psychiatry,* 37:37–46, February 1974.

———: Your innate assets for combatting stress, *Harvard Business Review,* 52:49–60, July–August 1974.

Bernstein, D. A., and Borkovec, T. D.: *Progressive relaxation training,* Champaign, Illinois, 1973, Research Press.

Fuller, G.: Relaxation approaches for nurses, R. N. Tapes, Inc. Audiocassette tape available from R. N. Tapes, Inc., 1400 Coleman Ave., Santa Clara, Calif. 95050.

Helm, P.: Strategies for success on nursing exams, R. N. Tapes, Inc. Audiocassette tape with booklet available from R. N. Tapes, Inc., 1400 Coleman Ave., Santa Clara, Calif. 95050.

Jacobson, E.: *Progressive relaxation,* ed. 3, Chicago, 1974, University of Chicago Press.

———: *You must relax,* ed. 4, New York, 1957, McGraw-Hill Book Co.

Lagerquist, S.: Effective test-taking techniques, R. N. Tapes, Inc. Audiocassette tape available from R. N. Tapes, Inc., 1400 Coleman Ave., Santa Clara, Calif. 95050.

Martin, I. C. A.: Relaxation on record, *Lancet,* 2:1340, December 20, 1969.

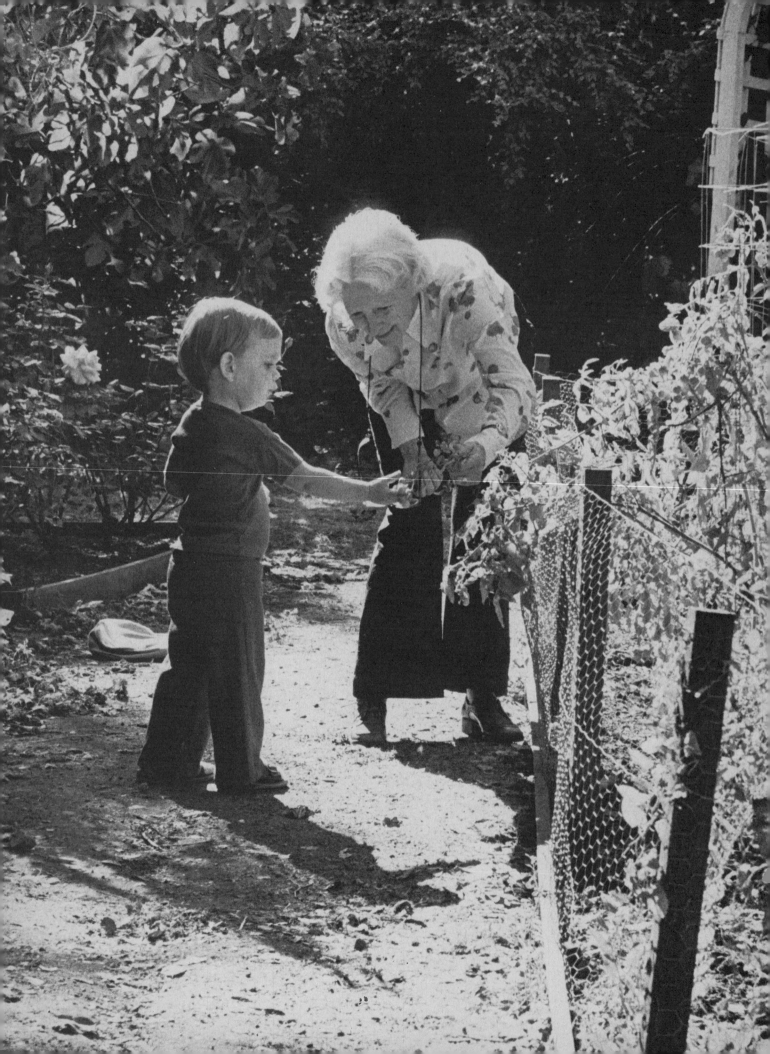

Unit 1 / GROWTH AND DEVELOPMENT THROUGH THE LIFE SPAN

Introduction

The purpose of this unit is to provide the temporal framework for the conditions of human health and disease discussed in the rest of this book. The effects of biologic time have been divided into three major areas: (a) general biophysical and psychosocial changes from adolescence through the middle years to the elderly period; (b) the development and disruptions of body image; and (c) the problems and issues of human sexuality. In addition, general principles of health teaching, which is vital to the nurse in assisting normal development and helping patient and clients care for their own health, are included in this unit.

The framework outlined here underlies, and should be integrated with, the more specific problems and issues described in the subsequent units; therefore, no review questions are included here. It is assumed that the student will apply the information from this unit, when appropriate, in answering questions later on.

Special care has been taken to include the appropriate nursing interventions when discussing the problems of life cycle development, body image disturbance, and human sexuality.

Because Unit 4 contains a detailed discussion of the childhood and adolescent years, the emphasis in Part A in this unit will be on the critical developmental eras of the *adult* years, middle age and senescence.

Part A begins with a brief summary of the *adolescent age span* to serve as a transition between childhood and adulthood before turning its focus to the adult age span.

Table 1–2 at the end of Part A serves as a summary of growth and development by comparing four important *theories* that concern the entire life span.

Sally Lagerquist

Part A | LIFE CYCLE

ADOLESCENCE

Adolescence is the period of time when a person becomes physically and psychologically mature. (A detailed discussion of childhood may be found in Unit 4, Nursing Care of Children and Families.)

1. Biophysical assessment
A. Appear poorly coordinated, as skeleton grows more rapidly than musculature; changes in proportion.
B. Feel tired until heart and lungs develop to take care of increased growth needs; may feel weak and exhausted for psychosocial reasons as well.
C. Male:
 1. Maturing process takes over two years (between ages 14 and 18).
 2. Facial hair appears.
 3. Voice changes.
 4. Penis and testes enlarge.
D. Female:
 1. Maturing process takes over six months (between ages 12 and 14).
 2. Onset of menarche.
 3. Maturing breasts.
 4. Maximum height reached around age 16.
E. Vital signs:
 1. Decreased pulse rate.
 2. Increased BP, which then levels off.

2. Needs as nursing goals
A. *Nutrition:* increase calories, protein, calcium, vitamin D.
B. *Rest, sleep:* up to ten hours per day.
C. *Sexual education:* information about VD, reproduction, contraception.

3. Psychologic tasks as nursing goals
A. Achieving emotional independence from parents and other adults.
B. Developing stable self-concept that recognizes both strengths and weaknesses.
C. Accepting one's physique and masculine/feminine identity.
D. Developing effective new relations with peers of both sexes.
E. Selecting and preparing for an occupation.

F. Developing intellectual skills.
G. Acquiring values and ethics in harmony with socially responsible behavior.

4. Common health problems
A. Obesity.
B. Acne due to increased secretions from apocrine glands.
C. Vehicle accidents.
D. Pregnancy.
E. Venereal disease (VD).
F. Gastric indigestion and acidity.
G. Substance abuse.
H. Suicide.

THE MIDDLE YEARS—AGES 40 TO 65

1. Assessment: biophysical changes
A. Illness and mortality patterns:
 1. Out of 100 men and women, 64–68 have one or more chronic conditions.
 2. Deaths—
  a. One in four from heart attacks.
  b. One in six from strokes (under age 65).
  c. Increase in deaths from diabetes, emphysema, lung cancer.
B. Skeletomuscular and neuromuscular:
 1. Increased muscle atrophy due to gradual loss of muscle function.
 2. Impaired heat and cold sensation due to nerve conduction inefficiency.
 3. Gradual erosion of articular cartilage due to repeated trauma and decreasing regenerative capacities.
 4. Progressive decrease in bone density. Increased incidence of fractures and osteoarthritis.
 5. Decreased REM sleep.
C. Cardiovascular:
 1. Decreased cardiac output and decreased glomerular filtration rate by 30% between 30 and 70 years of age.
 2. Decreased peripheral circulation.
 3. Increased peripheral resistance.
D. Gastrointestinal: decreased esophageal and gastric motility.
E. Respiratory:
 1. 40% decrease in vital lung capacity.
 2. 50% decrease in maximum breathing capacity.
F. Metabolic:
 1. 50% decrease in basal metabolic rate leads to weight gain.

2. Redistribution of adipose tissue to the abdomen in men, to the midline in women.
G. Endocrine (hormonal) changes in men:
   1. *Climacteric* (andropause)—change of life in men when sexual activity decreases.
   2. *Physical* symptoms—
      a. Fatigue and insomnia.
      b. Headaches.
      c. Psychosomatic (gastrointestinal, respiratory, urinary, cardiac, anorexic).
      d. Integumentary—
         (1) Gray hair.
         (2) Facial crease lines.
      e. Eyes and ears—diminishing hearing and visual acuity.
      f. Energy quickly expended and slowly recovered.
   3. *Psychological* symptoms—
      a. Increased moodiness, impatience, worry.
      b. Inability to make decisions.
      c. Self-doubt.
      d. Depression (guilt, worthlessness, suicidal thoughts).
   4. *Sociocultural* problems—
      a. Reacting to reaching career plateau with decreasing advancement opportunities and difficulty in switching jobs.
      b. Economic pressure to prepare for retirement.
      c. Coping with illness in peers (cancer, heart disease).
      d. Increased demands from mate.
      e. Caring for aging parents.
      f. Changes in sexual life.
H. Endocrine (hormonal) changes in women:
   1. *Menopause*—cessation of menstruation and reproductive capability.
   2. *Physical* symptoms—
      a. Vasomotor instability (hot flashes, numbness and tingling, cold hands and feet, heart palpitations, headache).
      b. Menstrual irregularities.
      c. Atrophic vaginitis due to estrogen insufficiency.
      d. Osteoporosis due to absence of estrogens.
      e. Coronary atherosclerosis, increased incidence after age 50.
      f. Decreased skin and muscle strength due to decreased skin elasticity and decreased estrogen levels.
      g. Diminished hearing and visual acuity.

   3. *Psychological* symptoms*—
      a. Emotional lability.
      b. Insomnia.
      c. Fatigue.
      d. Depression as reaction to loss of procreativity and threat to image of femininity; may go through grief process.
      e. High degree of anxiety.
   4. *Sociocultural* problems**—
      a. Perceived loss of femininity and motherhood role.
      b. Loss of source of self-esteem based on youth and femininity.
      c. Readjustment to couple role as opposed to parenting role.

2. **Assessment: psychosocial changes for men and women**
A. *Role changes* due to:
   1. "Empty nest" and end of child-rearing when last offspring leaves home.
   2. Aging and ailing parents; need to adjust to aging parents by being "parent" to them, as well as increased emphasis on role as offspring once again.
   3. Increased leisure time and how to use it.
   4. Becoming "in-laws" and grandparents.
   5. Increased competition from younger coworkers on the job may lead to greater stress, tension, loss of self-esteem.
   6. Changes in relationship with mate; less emphasis on being a coparent; see mate once again as a person, not a role.
B. *Changes in body image:*
   1. Adjustment to signs of aging: gray, thinning hair; wrinkles, obesity.
   2. Coping with chronic illness.
C. *Changes in home environment*—anxiety with decision-making about geographically moving to warmer climate, smaller home, etc.
D. *Value system changes:*
   1. Work ethic is challenged.
   2. Rethink values about extramarital sex and sexual expressions.
   3. Consciousness-raising in women.
   4. Choosing "second career."

---

*Changes may vary according to the individual. Most recent data indicate that women may *not* experience many of these psychosocial problems. For many, menopause is a *positive* experience.
**See above.

E. *Changes in social network:*
1. Parents' physical and mental capacities may slowly disintegrate, exhibiting regression and dependency, and demanding attention.
2. Diminishing social network as friends and peers begin to die.
3. Establishing and maintaining an economic standard of living, with plans for retirement activities.
4. Couples needing to reestablish their relationship with each other.
5. Anticipating and adjusting to widowhood.
F. *Developmental tasks*—turn from being other-oriented to self-oriented.
1. Increase self-esteem through greater self-awareness.
   a. Develop love relationship with significant person.
   b. Assess own assets and limitations.
2. Separate from own parents and children and become a more secure, independent adult by making independent decisions.
3. Review own values.
   a. Confront existing values.
   b. Change or reinforce existing values.
4. Recognize the aging process and initiate plans for the future to incorporate aging.
   a. Plan retirement.
   b. Develop new activities and sources of enjoyment.

3. *Nursing goals/implementation*—major goal: assist with readjustments needed in life style and habits.
A. *Diet*—goal: reduce risks of heart attack, hypertension, diabetes, and renal failure.
1. Assess 24-hour family diet patterns.
2. *Reduce* intake of calories, quantity, saturated fats and cholesterol, between-meal snacks.
3. *Increase* foods high in vitamins A and C, iron, water consumption.
4. Dietary counseling—discourage fast weight reduction diets; discuss techniques of low-calorie food preparation; provide specific examples of polyunsaturated oils.
B. *Activity level*—goal: increase circulation, relaxation, strength, and coordination.
1. Assess amount of sedentary activity, which can predispose to increased muscle atrophy, stress, insomnia, joint pain, infections, or weight gain.
2. Encourage moderate, well-paced, indoor and outdoor recreation and physical fitness program.

C. *Drug and tobacco use:*
1. Behavior modification, psychotherapy, and/or group self-help may be tried to discourage use of sedatives and tranquilizers, sleeping pills, or depressants as attempts to cope with increasing stresses and anxieties; decreased REM and deep sleep may result from use of sleeping medications and depressants.
2. Conduct health teaching regarding effects of smoking (increased risk of emphysema, heart attacks, night blindness; lung, oral, and throat cancer).
D. *Preventive care:*
1. Understand role of heredity, sex, race, and age in predisposing to certain diseases.
   a. *Heredity:* for example, heart, diabetes, cancer.
   b. *Sex:* for example, premenopausal women less prone to heart attacks than men of same age.
   c. *Race:* for example, hypertension twice as high among Black Americans than among Whites.
   d. *Age:* for example, 60-year-old more prone to chronic illness than 50-year-old.
2. Decrease susceptibility to certain diseases by minimizing or eliminating risk factors in life style, such as obesity, lack of exercise.
3. Encourage routine preventive exams, including: medical history and physical assessment of body systems; vital signs, blood and urine tests, EKG, sigmoidoscopy; examination of thyroid, mouth, throat, skin; examination of prostate gland for men; examination of breasts, pelvis, cervix for women; updating immunizations; routine dental, vision, and hearing examinations.
E. *Health maintenance and promotion:*
1. Provide anticipatory guidance about the changes of life.
2. Supplement knowledge with education about menopausal body changes, causes of symptoms and feelings.
3. Recognize when person needs help in coping with menopause or aging or middle-years' crises.

THE ELDERLY—OVER AGE 65

The aging process is insidious, bringing about changes in *all* body systems. Table 1–1 summarizes the main

TABLE 1–1.   *The aging process*

Physical changes	Assessment of physiologic condition	Pathology (cause)	Implication for health care interventions
Hair	Baldness, thinning, graying.	Atrophy: hair follicle. Genetic, hormonal, racial.	Observe for negative or positive response.
Skin/cutaneous tissue	Wrinkles.	Prolonged sun exposure; loss of adipose and elastic fiber.	Decreased cold tolerance results in increased need for protection from exposure to cold.
	Ecchymoses.	Capillary fragility (vitamin deficiency).	Add vitamins C and K to diet.
	Dryness and itchiness.	Deterioration of nerve fibers and sensory endings.	Avoid soap; keep skin lubricated.
	Pale, blotchy.	↓ Air exposure; ↓ capillaries.	Need outdoor exercise.
	↓ Perspiration.	Sweat gland atrophy.	Less bathing.
	Pressure sores, epidermal fissures.	Subcutaneous tissue atrophy.	Pad bony prominences.
Nails	Brittle and thick.	↓ Blood supply.	Good hygiene and nail care.
Body temperature	Lowered (35 C).	↓ BMR.	Note: 37.5 C can represent fever.
	Cold intolerance.	Poor shiver reflex.	Avoid prolonged cold exposure.
	Heat intolerance.	Sluggish sweating and circulatory mechanisms.	Avoid heat exposure.
Skeletal	Height loss.	Calcification of vertebral ossification. Disc atrophy of vertebrae.	Pay attention to posture.
	Flexed posture.	Muscle weakness.	Proper body alignment in bed, chair, and ambulation.
	Prone to fractures.	Osteoporosis.	Female hormones may be given.
	Diminished weight bearing.	Increased bone brittleness. Decreased bone density.	Check environment for hazards; prevent falls.
	Stiff joints.	Inactivity.	Regular exercise.
	Ankylosis.	Degenerative changes. Cartilaginous joint ossification.	
	Contractures.	Fibrocartilaginous atrophy.	Positioning.
	Paralysis.	CVA.	Passive exercises.
Muscles	Reduction in speed, power, sustained effort.	Decrease in muscle fibers. Muscle atrophy.	Exercise with rest periods.

(Continued)

TABLE 1–1.   *(Continued)*

Physical changes	Assessment of physiologic condition	Pathology (cause)	Implication for health care interventions
Vision	Loss of acuity.	Retinal atrophy: cataracts due to lens opacity. Genetic.	Discuss surgical removal.
	Loss of dark accommodation.	Ciliary muscle.	Avoid night driving.
	Loss of peripheral vision.	Corneal degeneration. Arteriosclerosis.	Alertness to dangers of slowed reaction time.
	Difficulty in color discrimination.	Decreased blood supply to the retina (retinal sclerosis).	Assess problem with red–yellow stop lights.
	Slow blink reflex.	Poor muscle tone.	Protect from foreign objects in eyes.
	Shrunken appearance around the eyes.	Loss of orbital fat.	Assess problems with self-image.
	Blindness.	Diabetes.	Provide safe, secure, familiar environment.
Hearing	Greater (L) ear loss.	Change of nerve tissue and atrophy of inner ear.	Face person directly. Speak slowly and clearly.
	Higher tone loss.	Thickening of ear drum.	Speak in low voice.
Taste/smell	Loss of sense of taste and smell.	Reduced buds in tongue. Atrophy of olfactory bulb.	Problem with food disinterest.
Balance	Decreased.	Lack of sensory perception.	Prevent falls and accidents.
Pain perception	Decreased tactile discrimination. Increased pain tolerance (raised pain threshold).	Tendon reflex atrophy.	May be burned and not realize. Cautious use of heating pads.
Voice	High-pitched. Restricted in range.	Laryngeal muscle atrophy. Hardening and decreased elasticity of laryngeal cartilages. Slackening of vocal cords.	Difficulty with talking loudly. Cannot sing.
	Slower, slurred dysphagia.	Central nervous system changes (CVA).	Speech therapy. Give more time to speak.
Respiratory	Suceptible to infection.	Mucous secretions collect readily due to decreased action of cilia.	Need expectorants. Postural drainage. Encourage to deep breathe and cough.
	Dyspnea/apnea.	Oxygen debt in muscles.	Avoid strenuous activity.
	Smaller volume of air.	Decreased chest size.	Deep breathing.
	Impaired ventilation, diffusion, pulmonary circulation.	Thickened membrane, alveoli, and capillaries.	Isometric exercises for diaphragm and intercostals.
	Decreased cough capacity.	Weak expiratory muscles.	Avoid sprays, dust.

TABLE 1–1. *(Continued)*

Physical change	Assessment of physiologic condition	Pathology (cause)	Implication for health care interventions
	Limited mobility.	Increased volume of residual air after expiration.	Avoid restrictive clothing.
Nervous system	Increased susceptibility to shock.	Neuron pigmentation.	
	Decreased reaction time.	Decreased conduction speed of nerve fibers. Decreased muscle tone from decreased activity.	Teach regarding the danger of excessively cautious driving.
	Hard to arouse from sleep.	Change in sensory nerve endings.	Problem with fire detection; get smoke detector for home.
	Behavioral changes: narrow interests; confused, rigid, diminished memory.	Atrophy: brain surface, bulk, cells.	Give more time, simple directions. Encourage social activity.
Circulation	Increased shortness of breath on exertion.	Valves hard, less pliable. Decreased pumping action.	Avoid strenuous exercise.
	Pooling of blood in systemic veins (edema).	Decreased filling and emptying of valves. Changes in coronary arteries.	Wear supportive hose. Raise feet.
	Pain on exertion in calf muscles (impaired tissue nourishment and removal of tissue waste).	Thickening of artery walls. Increased calcium deposits in muscular layer.	Limited walking.
	Increased systolic and diastolic pressure.	Decreased elasticity of systemic arteries (artery elongation).	Treat for hypertension.
	Dizziness.	Decreased blood supply to the brain due to decreased arterial elasticity.	Encourage slow rising.
Digestion and elimination	Disinterest in food.	Stomatitis. Vitamin B_{12} deficiency.	Provide adequate nutrition. Provide attractive social eating environment with enough time.
	Deficiencies in diet: meat, fresh fruit or vegetables.	Poorly fitting dentures or difficult mastication due to poor teeth.	Appropriate, regular dental care.
	Diminished peristalsis (constipation).	Muscle atrophy. Decreased fluid intake, roughage, exercise, fat.	Regulate bowels. Correct diet. Increase activity. Remove impaction.
	Protein and fat digestion altered.	Decrease in digestive enzymes (lipase, ptyalin, trypsin).	Avoid highly spiced or fried foods.
	Delayed gastric emptying.	Mucosal lining atrophy. Achlorhydria.	

(Continued)

TABLE 1-1.   *(Continued)*

Physical change	Assessment of physiologic condition	Pathology (cause)	Implication for health care interventions
	Incontinence, polyuria, nocturia.	Male: enlarged prostate. Female: weak or atrophic muscles or urethral.	May need surgery.
		Decreased bladder capacity.	Nightlight for nocturia; unobstructed pathway.
	Urinary stasis, frequency.	Decreased bladder emptying.	Observe for bladder infection.
	Retention, pain, infection.	Decreased blood flow to the kidney.	Keep intake/output records.
		Decreased filtration. Atrophy of collecting tubules and interstitial fibrosis.	Bladder training to regulate output.
Sexual organs	Men: gradually decreased sperm production.	Degenerative gonadal changes.	Decreased fertility.
	Women: cessation of menses complete.	Decreased ovarian hormones.	Discuss menopausal problems.
	Breast atrophy.	Decreased adipose tissue.	Discuss cosmetic measures.
	Painful intercourse.	Decreased vaginal secretions.	Need lubricant.

physical changes, with emphasis on assessment, cause, and implications for health care and nursing interventions.

1. Psychosocial development

A. *Developmental tasks:*
   1. Finding satisfactory physical *living arrangements* (adequate heating, lighting, safety).
   2. Adjusting to decreasing physical *strength and health.*
   3. Adjusting to *retirement* and decreased income.
   4. Adjusting to living *alone.*
   5. Establishing satisfying relationships with grandchildren, if any.
   6. Facing *bereavement* and widowhood.
   7. Keeping interest in people *outside* of the family and people of one's own age group.
   8. Finding *meaning in life,* ways to keep active, and a comfortable daily routine.
   9. Learning to live in the *present* with losses, to account for the *past,* and to face the *future,* which includes death.
   10. Maintaining *independence;* need praise and *recognition* for accomplishments, *respect* for ideas,

thinking, decisions, waning abilities, values, and standards.

B. *Needs of elderly: nursing goals/implementation*—correlate with physical changes and psychologic adjustments.
   1. *Protection* from fires, burns, and accidents due to failing memory, decreased pain and heat perception, limited vision, slowed reflexes, brittle bones. Need: handrails, nonskid rugs and bath surfaces, good lighting, woolen socks when cold rather than heating devices.
   2. *Nutrition*—need: smaller servings with fewer calories; high protein, moderate carbohydrate, low fat; proper dentures; company for meals.
   3. *Elimination:* problems with constipation and nocturia. Need: roughage, exercise, fluid intake (except at night), prostatic surgery, vaginal surgery for cystocele and rectocele.
   4. *Exercise and rest*—need: regular, moderate exercise program with rest periods; sleep for shorter intervals, more frequently.
   5. *Hygiene*—use skin lubricant; avoid daily bathing; protect bony prominences and skin folds; remove excessive facial hair in women.

6. *Sex*—increased need for physical contact and expression of affection.
7. *Health promotion*—check for glaucoma, cataracts, denture fit, hearing, and vision.
8. *Social needs and interaction*—physical and social immobility may result in enforced social isolation, reinforcing depression and excessive self-preoccupation. Encourage out-of-house activities, reaching out to others (especially to children), establishing new relationships, and maintaining contact with long-term friends.

SUMMARY OF FOUR PSYCHOSOCIAL DEVELOPMENTAL THEORIES (TABLE 1–2)

TABLE 1–2. *Summary of theories of psychosocial development throughout the life cycle*

Freud	Sullivan	Erikson	Piaget
EMPHASIS ON:			
Pathology.	Pathology.	Both health and illness.	*Normal* children.
Anxiety.	Anxiety.		*No* emphasis on ego, anxiety, identity, libido.
Unconscious, uncontrollable drives.	Unconscious, uncontrollable drives.	Problems are manageable and can be solved.	Cognitive development.
Ego or self-system needing defense.	Ego or self-system needing defense.	Need to integrate individual and society.	Tasks can be accomplished through learning process.
PATHOLOGICAL DEVELOPMENT INFLUENCED BY:			
Early feelings. Repressed experiences in unconscious mind.	Unconscious mind *and* interpersonal relationships.	Ego, anxiety, identity, libido concepts *combined* with social forces.	Individual differences and social influences on the mind.
CHANGE POSSIBLE WITH:			
Understanding content and meaning of unconscious.	Improved IPR and understanding basic good-bad transformations.	Integration of attitudes, libido, and social roles for strong ego identity.	Socialization process to facilitate cognitive development.
AGE GROUP:			
First five years of life.	Adolescence.	Middle age, old age.	Middle childhood years.
FOCUS ON:			
Emotional development.	Emotional and interpersonal development.	Emotional, interpersonal, spiritual.	Cognitive skills.
Psychosexual aspects.	Psychosocial aspects.	Psychosocial aspects.	Cognitive, interactive aspects.
CAUSE OF CONFLICTS AND PROBLEMS:			
Oral, anal, genital stage problems (especially unresolved Oedipal/castration conflicts).	Threats to self-system. Disturbed communication process; 7 stages not complete.	Unresolved conflicts, crises in 8 successive life cycle stages.	Faulty adaptation between individual and environment for intellectual development.
PROGNOSIS:			
Few changes possible after age 5.	Change usually possible with improved IPR.	Change not only possible but *expected* throughout life.	Little change in adult cognitive structure after middle adolescence.
Sexual problems as basis for disturbed behavior.	Sexual problems are only one type of faulty IPR affecting behavior.	Sexual identity as one of many problems solved by interaction of desire and social process.	Sex as a variable in learning (age, IQ).

Part B / BODY IMAGE

DEVELOPMENT OF BODY IMAGE

1. **Definition**—"Mental picture of body's appearance; an interrelated phenomenon which includes the surface, depth, internal and postural picture of the body, as well as the attitudes, emotions, and personality reactions of the individual in relation to his body as an object in space, apart from all others"* (Table 1–3).

2. **Operational definition****
A. Body image is created by social interaction.
   1. Approval is given for "normal" and "proper" appearance, gestures, posture, etc.
   2. Behavioral and physical deviations from normality are not given approval.
   3. Body image is formed by the person's response to the approval and disapproval by others.
   4. Person's values, attitudes, and feelings about self are continuously evolving and are unconsciously integrated.
B. Self-image, identity, personality, sense of self, and body image are interdependent.
C. Behavior is determined by body image.

3. **General behavior**—person with problems of body image.
A. Analysis of data—concepts related to body image:
   1. Image of self changes with *changing posture* (walking, sitting, gestures).
   2. *Mental picture of self* may not correspond with the actual body; subject to continuous revision.
   3. The degree to which people like themselves (good self-concept) is directly related to how well defined they perceive their body image to be.
      a. *Vague, indefinite, or distorted body image* correlates with the following personality traits:
         (1) Sad, empty, hollow feelings.
         (2) Mistrustful of others; poor peer relations.
         (3) Low motivation.
         (4) Shame, doubt, sense of inferiority, poor self-concept.
         (5) Inability to tolerate stress.
      b. *Integrated body image* correlates with following personality traits:
         (1) Happy, good self-concept.
         (2) Good peer relations.
         (3) Sense of initiative, industry, autonomy, identity.
         (4) Able to complete tasks.
         (5) Assertive.
         (6) Academically competent; high achievement.
         (7) Able to cope with stress.
4. Child's concept of body image can indicate degree of *ego strength* and personality integration; vague, distorted self-concept may indicate schizophrenic processes.
5. *Successful* completion of various developmental phases determines body concept and degree of *body boundary definiteness* (see Table 1–3).
6. *Physical changes* of height, weight, and body build lead to changes in perception of body appearance and of how body is used.
7. Success in *using* one's body (motor ability) influences the value one places upon self (self-evaluation).
8. *Secondary sex characteristics* are significant aspects of body image (too much, too little, too early, too late, in the wrong place, may lead to disturbed body image).
   a. Sexual differences in body image are in part related to differences in anatomical structure and body function, as well as to contrasts in life styles and cultural roles.
9. Different *cultures and families* value bodily traits and bodily deviations differently.
10. Different *body parts* (for example, hair, nose, face, stature, shoulders, etc.) do not have same significance; therefore there is variability in degree of threat, personality integrity, and coping behavior.
11. *Attitudes* concerning the self will influence and be influenced by person's physical appearance and ability. Society has developed stereotyped ideas regarding outer body structure (body physique) and inner personalities (temperament).
    a. *Endomorph*—talkative, sympathetic, good natured, trusting, dependent, lazy, fat.

---

*From Kolb, L.: "Disturbances in body image," American handbook of psychiatry, S. Arieti, New York, 1959, Basic Books, pp. 749–769.
**From Norris, C.: "Body image," Behavioral concepts and nursing intervention, ed. 2, C. Carlson and B. Blackwell, Philadelphia, 1978, J. B. Lippincott Co., p. 6.

TABLE 1–3.   *Body image development through life cycle*

Age group	Development of body image	Developmental disturbances in body image
Infant and toddler	Becomes aware of body boundaries and separateness of own external body from others through sensory stimulation. Exploration of external body parts; handling and controlling the environment and body through play, bathing, and eating. Experiences are painful, shameful, fearful, and pleasurable. Feeling of doubt or power in mastery of motor skills and striving for autonomy. Learning who one is in relation to the world.	*Infant:* Inadequate somatosensory stimulation → impaired ego development, increased anxiety level, poor foundation for reality testing. Continues to see external objects as extension of self → unrealistic, *distorted* perceptions of significant persons, inability to form normal attachments to others (possessive, engulfing, autistic, withdrawn). *Toddler:* If body fails to meet parental expectations → shameful, self-deprecating feelings. Failure to master environment and control own body → helplessness, inadequacy, and doubt.
Preschool and school-age	Praise, blame, derogation, or criticism for body, its part or use (pleasure, pain, doubt, or guilt). Exploration of genitals—discovery of anatomical differences between sexes with joy, pride, or shame. Beginning of sexual identity. Differentiates self as a body and self as a mind. Beginning of self-concept; of self as male or female. Learning mastery of the body (to *do,* to protect *self,* to protect *others*) and environment (run, skip, skate, swim); feelings of pleasure, competence, worth, or inadequacy.	*Preschool:* Distortion of body image of genital area due to conflict over pleasure versus punishment. If body build does not conform to sex-typed expectations and sex role identification → body image confusion. *School-age:* Physical impairments (speech, poor vision, poor hearing) → feelings of inadequacy and inferiority. Overly self-conscious about, and excessive focus on, body changes in puberty.
Adolescent	Physical self is of more concern than at any other time except old age. Forced body awareness due to physical changes (new senses, proportions, features); feelings of pleasure, power, confidence, or helplessness, pain, inadequacy, doubt, and guilt. Adult body proportions emerge. Anxiety over ideal self versus emerging/emerged physical self; body is compared competitively with same-sex peers. Use of body (its values and attitudes) to relate with opposite sex. Body image crucial for self-concept formation, status achievement, and adequate social relations.	Growth and changes may produce distorted self view → overemphasis on defects with compensations; inflated ideas of body ability, beauty, perfection; preoccupation with body appearance or body processes, females more likely than males to see body fatter than it is; egocentrism.

(Continued)

TABLE 1–3. *(Continued)*

Age group	Development of body image	Developmental disturbances in body image
	Physical changes need to be integrated into evolving body image (strong, competent, powerful, or weak and helpless).	
Early adulthood	Learns to accept own body without undue preoccupation with its functions or control of these functions.	
	Stability of body image.	
Middle age	New challenges due to differential rates of aging in various body parts.	Less dependable, less likable body → regression to adolescent behavior and dress due to denial of aging, defeat, depression, self-pity, egocentrism due to fear of loss of sexual identity, withdrawal to early old age.
	Body not functioning as well; unresolved fears, misconceptions, and experiences in relation to body image persist and become recognized.	Females more likely to judge themselves uglier than do males or younger and older females.
Old age	Accelerated physical decline with influence on self-concept and life style.	
	Can accept self and personality as a whole; continued emphasis on physical self, with increased emphasis on inner, emotional self.	Ill health → fear of invalidism, hypochondriasis. Denial related to feelings of threatened incapacity and fear of declining functions.
		Despair over loss of beauty, strength, and youthfulness, with self-disgust about body → projection of criticism onto others.
		Regression.
		Isolation (separation of affect and thought) leads to less intense response to death, disease, aging.
		Compartmentalization (focus on one thing at a time) causes narrowing of consciousness, resistance, rigidity, repetitiveness.
		Resurgence of egocentrism.

  b. *Mesomorph*—adventuresome, self-reliant, strong, tall.
  c. *Ectomorph*—thin, tense and nervous, suspicious, stubborn, pessimistic, quiet.
12. Person with a *firm ego boundary or body image* is more likely to be independent, striving, goal-oriented, influential.
  a. Under stress, may develop skin and muscle disease.
13. Person with *poorly integrated body image and weak ego boundary* is more likely to be passive, less goal-oriented, less influential, more prone to external pressures.
  a. Under stress, may develop heart and GI diseases.
14. Any situation, *illness,* or *injury* that causes a change in body image is a crisis, and the person will go through the phases of crisis in an attempt to reintegrate the body image (Table 1–4).
B. Analysis of data—body image may be affected by:
  1. *Obvious* loss of a major body part—amputation of an extremity, hair, teeth, eye, breast.

2. Surgical procedures in which the relationship of body parts is *visibly* disturbed—colostomy, ileostomy, gastrostomy, ureteroenterostomy.

3. Surgical procedures in which the loss of body parts is *not* visible to others—hysterectomy, lung, gallbladder, stomach.

4. Repair procedures (plastic surgery) that *do not* reconstruct body image as assumed—rhinoplasty, plastic surgery to correct large ears, breasts.

5. *Changes in body size and proportion*—obesity, emaciation, acromegaly, gigantism, pregnancy.

6. Other changes in *external body* surface—hirsutism in women, mammary glands in men.

7. Skin *color* changes—chronic dermatitis, Addison's disease.

8. Skin *texture* changes—scars, thyroid disease, excoriative dermatitis.

9. *Crippling* changes in bones, joints, muscles—arthritis, multiple sclerosis, Parkinson's.

10. Failure of a body part to *function*—quadriplegia, paraplegia, CVA.

11. Distorted ideas of structure, function, and significance stemming from *symbolism* of disease seen in terms of *life and death* when heart or lungs are afflicted—heart attacks, asthmatic attacks, pneumonia.

12. *Side effects* of drug therapy—moon face, hirsutism, striated skin, changes in body contours.

13. *Violent attacks* against the body—incest, rape, shooting, knifing, battering.

14. *Mental, emotional disorders*—schizophrenia with depersonalization, somatic delusions, and hallucinations about the body; anorexia nervosa, hypochondriasis; hysteria, malingering.

15. *Diseases requiring isolation* may convey attitude that body is undesirable, unacceptable—tuberculosis, malodorous conditions (for example, gangrene, cancer).

16. *Women's movement and sexual revolution*—use of body for pleasure, not just procreation, sexual freedom, wide range of normality in sex practices, legalized abortion.

17. *Medical technology*—organ transplants, lifesaving but scar-producing burn treatment, alive but hopeless, alive but debilitated with chronic illnesses.

4. *Nursing goals/implementation:*
A. Support strengths despite presence of handicaps.
B. Assist patient to look at self in totality rather than focus on limitations.

C. Provide perceptual feedback, for example, touch, describe, look at scar.
D. Provide kinesthetic feedback to paralyzed part, for example, "I am raising your leg."
E. Teach patient and family about expected changes in functioning.
F. Encourage expression of feelings.

BODY IMAGE DISTURBANCE

1. *Definition*—A body image disturbance arises when a person is unable to accept the body as is and to adapt to it; a conflict develops between the body as it actually is and the body that is pictured mentally; that is, the ideal self (Table 1–4).

2. *Types of body image distortions*
A. Sensation of *size change* due to obesity, pregnancy, weight loss.
B. Feelings of being *dirty*—may be imaginary due to hallucinogenic drugs, psychoses.
C. Dual change of body *structure and function* due to trauma, amputation, stroke, etc.
D. Progressive *deformities* due to chronic illness, burns, arthritis.
E. Loss of body boundaries and *depersonalization* due to sensory deprivation such as blindness, immobility, fatigue, stress, anesthesia. May also be due to psychoses or hallucinogenic drugs.

3. *Body image disturbance caused by amputation*
A. Assessment:
1. Loss of self-esteem; feelings of helplessness, worthlessness, shame, and guilt.
2. Fear of abandonment may lead to appeals to sympathy by exhibiting helplessness and vulnerability.
3. Feelings of castration (loss of self) and symbolic death; loss of wholeness.
4. Existence of phantom pain in most patients.
5. Passivity, lack of responsibility for use of disabled body parts.
B. Nursing goals/implementation:
1. Avoid stereotyping person as being less competent now than previously.
2. Foster independence; encourage self-care.
3. Help person to set realistic short- and long-term goals.
4. Assist family to work through their feelings; to accept person as she presents herself; to set realistic goals and limitations.

TABLE 1–4.   *Four phases of body image crisis*

Phase	Assessment	Nursing goals/interventions
Acute shock	Anxiety, numbness, helplessness.	Provide sustained support, be available to listen, express interest and concern.
		Person may need time and privacy, not talk.
Denial	Retreat from reality; fantasy about the wholeness and capability of the body; euphoria; rationalization; refusal to participate in self-care.	Accept denial without reinforcing it. Avoid arguing and overloading with reality. Gradually raise questions, reply with doubt to convey unrealistic ideas.
		Follow patient's suggestions for personal-care routine to help increase feelings of adequacy and to decrease helplessness.
Acknowledgement of reality	Grief over loss of valued body part, function, or role; depression, apathy; agitation, bitterness; physical symptoms (insomnia, anorexia, nausea, crying) serve as outlet for feeling; redefinition of body structure and function, with implications for change in life style; acceptance of and cooperation with realistic goals for care and treatment; preoccupation with body functions.	Expect and accept displacement onto nurse of anger, resentment, projection of patient's inadequacy.
		Examine own behavior to see if patient's remarks may be justified.
		Simply listen if this is the only way the patient can handle feelings at this time.
		Offer sustained, nonjudgemental listening without being defensive or taking remarks personally.
		Help dispel anger by encouraging its ventilation.
		Encourage self-care activities.
		Support family members as they cope with changes in patient's health or body image, role changes, treatment plans.
Resolution and adaptation	Perceive crisis in new light; increased mastery leads to increased self-worth; can look at, feel, and ask questions regarding altered body part; tests others' reactions to changed body; repetitive talk on painful topic of changed self; concentration on *normal* functions in order to increase sense of control.	Teaching and counseling by same nurse in warm, supportive relationship.
		Assess level of knowledge; begin at that level.
		Consider motivational state.
		Provide gradual, nontechnical medical information and specific facts.
		Repeat instructions frequently, patiently, consistently.
		Support sense of mastery in self-care; draw on inner resources.
		Do not discourage dependence while gradually encouraging independence.
		Focus on necessary adaptations of life style due to realistic limitations.
		Provide follow-up care via referral to community resources after patient is discharged.

5. Acknowledge phantom pain. Assure person that this is a normal experience.

4. Body image disturbance in CVA (stroke)
A. Assessment:
  1. Feelings of shame (personal, private, self-judgement of failure) due to loss of bowel and bladder control, speech function.
  2. Body image boundaries disrupted; contact with environment is hindered by wheelchair; may result in personality deterioration due to diminished number of sensory experiences.
    a. Lose orientation to body sphere; feel confused, trapped in own body.
B. Nursing goals/implementation:
  1. Reduce frustration and infantilism due to communication problems by—
    a. Rewarding all speech efforts.
    b. Listening to all nonverbal cues.
    c. Restating verbalizations to see if correct meaning is understood.
    d. Speaking slowly, using two- to three-word sentences.
  2. Assist reintegration of body parts and function; help regain awareness of paralyzed side by—
    a. Tactile stimulation.
    b. Verbal reminders of existence of affected parts.
    c. Direct visual contact via mirrors and grooming.
    d. Use of safety features like the Posey belt.

5. Body image disturbance in myocardial infarction (MI)
A. Emotional problems (such as anxiety, depression, sleep disturbance, fear of another MI) during convalescence can seriously hamper rehabilitation. The adaptation and convalescence is influenced by the multiple symbolic meanings of the heart, for example:
  1. Seat of emotions (love, pride, fear, sadness).
  2. Center of the body (one-of-a-kind organ).
  3. Life itself (can no longer rely on the heart; failure of the heart means failure of life).
B. Assessment of effects of MI:
  1. *Changes in life style*—eating, smoking, drinking; activities, employment, sex.
  2. *Overly cautious and restrictive attitude* may result in boredom, weakness, insomnia, exaggerated dependency.
  3. *Family members* may be anxious and overprotective.
  4. *Role reversal;* loss of incentive for work.
  5. *Family conflicts* over activity and diet, dependency-independency issues.
  6. Use of *self-destructive* behavior; denial of MI.
  7. *Job and social pressure* to "slow down"; may lose job, be reassigned, forced into early retirement; "has-been" social status.
C. Nursing goals/implementation:
  1. Prevent "cardiac cripple" by shaping person's and family's attitude toward damaged organ.
    a. Instill optimism.
    b. Encourage *productive* living rather than inactivity.
  2. Set up a physical and mental activity program with patient and mate.
  3. Provide anticipatory guidance regarding expected weakness, fear, uncertainty.
  4. Do health teaching regarding nature of coronary disease, interpretation of medical regime, effect on sexual behavior.

6. Obesity and body image
A. *Definition:* Body weight exceeding 20% above the norm for person's age, sex, and height constitutes obesity.
B. Assessment of characteristics:
  1. One out of three under 30 years of age is more than 10% overweight.
  2. Increased risks of CVA, MI.
  3. Feelings of self-hate, self-derogation, failure, helplessness; tendency to avoid shopping for clothes and to avoid mirror reflections.
  4. Viewed by others as ugly, repulsive, lacking in willpower, weak, unwilling to change, neurotic.
  5. Most successful weight loss is quickly and repetitively followed by failure, that is, weight gain.
  6. Discrepancy develops between actual body size (real self) and person's concept of it (ideal self).
  7. Although a faulty adaptation, obesity may serve as a "protection against more severe illness; it represents an effort to function better, be powerful, stay well, or be less sick," according to Hilde Bruch.
  8. The *problem* may *not* be difficulty in losing weight; reducing may *not* be the appropriate *cure*.
  9. Obese persons usually eat in response to outer environment (for example, food odor, time of day, food availability, degree of stress, anger), *not inner* environment (hunger, increased gastric motility).

TABLE 1–5. *Sexual behavior through the life cycle*

Age	Development of sexual behavior
First 18 months	Major source of pleasure from touch and oral exploration.
18 months to 3 years	Pleasurable and sexual feelings are associated with genitals (acts of urination and defecation). Masturbation without fantasy or eroticism.
Age 3 to 6 years	Resolution of Oedipal and Electra complexes; foundation for heterosexual relationships; masturbation with curiosity about genitals of opposite sex.
Age 6 to 11 years	Peer relations with same sex; onset of sex play; morality and sexual attitudes taught and learned; phase of sexual tranquility.
Age 12 to 18 years (adolescence)	Onset of puberty with biologic development of secondary sex characteristics; menstruation and ejaculation occur. Frequent masturbation. Intense anxiety and guilt may occur over heterosexual or homosexual behavior (petting, coitus, masturbation, VD, pregnancy, genital size).
Age 18 to 23 years (early adulthood)	Maximum interpersonal and intrapsychic self-consciousness about sexuality. Issues: premarital coitus, sexual freedom. Anxiety about: sexual competency, genital size, impotence, fear of pregnancy, rejection.
Age 23 to 30 years	Focus on sexual activity in coupling and parenthood; mutual masturbation.
Age 31 to 45 years (middle adulthood)	For females—peak sexuality without new sexual experiences. Conflict regarding extramarital sex may increase.

PURPOSE OF INTERCOURSE

Need for body contact.

Physical expression of trust, love, and affection.

Reaffirmation of self-concept as sexually desirable and sexually competent due to worry about effects of aging.

SEXUAL DYSFUNCTIONS

Men: impotence, premature ejaculation, decreasing libido.

Women: intermittent lack of orgasmic response, vaginismus, dyspareunia.

For either or both: changes or divergences in degree of sexual interest.

CAUSES OF SEXUAL DYSFUNCTION

Overindulgence in food or drink.

Preoccupation with career and economic pursuits.

Mental or physical fatigue.

Boredom with monotony of relationship.

Drug dependency: alcohol, tobacco, certain medications.

Fear of failure.

Chronic illness: Diabetes, alcoholism → peripheral neuropathy → impotence. (Smoking and drinking may result in decreased testosterone production); excessive smoking → vascular constriction → decreased libido; spinal-cord injuries.

Self-devaluation due to accumulation of role function losses, sexual self-image, and body image.

Past history of lack of sexual enjoyment in younger years.

TABLE 1–5. *(Continued)*

Age	Development of sexual behavior
	CAUSES OF SEXUAL DYSFUNCTION Belief in myths regarding "shoulds and should nots" of frequency, variations, and enjoyment. Widowhood: inhibition and loyalty to deceased.
Age 46–60 years (later adulthood)	Menopause occurs. Little or no fear of pregnancy; evidence of sexual activity differences in male and female: women may have increased pleasure, men take longer to reach orgasm; may prefer less strenuous mutual masturbation.
Over age 60 years (old age)	Activity depends on earlier sexual attitude. May suffer guilt and shame when engaging in sex. Can have active and enjoyable sex life with continuing sex needs. Age is not a barrier provided there is opportunity for sexual activity with a partner or for sublimated activities. Women in this age group outnumber men; single women outnumber men by an even larger margin.

10. Experience less pleasure in physical activity; less active than others.
11. All obese people are *not* the same.
    a. In *obese newborns and infants,* there is an increased *number* of adipocytes via *hyperplastic* process.
    b. In *obese adults,* there may be increased body fat deposits, resulting in increased *size* of adipocytes via *hypertrophic* process.
    c. When an *obese infant becomes an obese adult,* the result may be an increased *number* of cells available for fat *storage.*
12. Loss of control of own body or eating behavior.

C. Analysis: contributing factors
    1. Genetic.
    2. Thermodynamic.
    3. Endocrine.
    4. Neuroregulatory.
    5. Biochemical factors in metabolism.
    6. Ethnic and family practices.
    7. Psychological.
        a. Compensation for feelings of helplessness and inadequacy.
        b. Maternal overprotection; overfed and forcefed, especially formula-fed infants.
        c. Food offered and used to solve anxiety, frustration, anger, and rage can lead to difficulty in differentiating between hunger and other needs.
        d. Food offered instead of love as a child.
    8. Social factors.
        a. Food easily available.
        b. Use of motorized transportation and labor-saving devices.
        c. Refined carbohydrates.
        d. Social aspects of eating.
        e. Restaurant meals high in salt, sugar content.

D. Nursing goals/implementation:
    1. Encourage *prevention* of life-long body image problems.
        a. Support *breastfeeding,* where infant determines quantity consumed, not mother; work through her feelings against breastfeeding (fear of intimacy, dependence, feelings of repulsion, concern about confinement, and inability to produce enough milk).
        b. Help mothers *not to overfeed* the baby if formula-fed: suggest water between feedings; do not start solids until 6 months old or 14 pounds; do not enrich the prescribed formula.
        c. Help mothers *differentiate* between hunger and other infant cries; help her to try out different responses to the expressed needs other than offering food.
    2. Use *case findings* of obese infants, young children, and adolescents.
    3. Promote awareness of certain *stressful* periods

that can produce maladaptive responses such as obesity—for example, puberty, postnuptial, postpartum, menopause.

4. Alleviate guilt and reduce the stigma of being obese.
5. Assess current eating patterns.
6. Identify person's need to eat, and relate the need to preceding events, hopes, fears, or feelings.
7. Assist in drawing up a meal plan for slow, steady weight loss.
8. Support eating five small meals a day.
9. Employ behavior modification techniques.
10. Encourage outside interests not related to food or eating.

Part C / HUMAN SEXUALITY

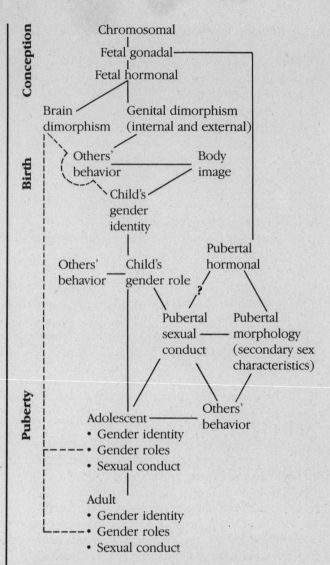

SCOPE OF HUMAN SEXUALITY

Human sexuality refers to all the characteristics of an individual (social, personal, and emotional) that are manifest in his or her relationship with others and that reflect gender-genital orientation.

1. Components of sexual system

A. *Biological sexuality*—refers to chromosomes, hormones, primary and secondary sex characteristics, and anatomical structure.

B. *Sexual identity*—based on own feelings and perceptions of how well traits correspond with own feelings and concepts of maleness and femaleness; also includes gender identity.

C. *Gender identity*—a sense of masculinity and femininity shaped by biological, environmental, and intrapsychic forces as well as cultural traditions and education.

D. *Sex role behavior*—includes components of both sexual identity and gender identity (Figure 1–1). Aim: sexual fulfillment through masturbation, heterosexual, and/or homosexual experiences. Selection of behavior is influenced by: personal value system and sexual, gender, and biological identity. Gender identity and roles are learned and constantly reinforced by input and feedback regarding social expectations and demands (Table 1–6).

FIGURE 1–1. Influencing factors in development of gender identity, role, and conduct.
Based on J. Money and A. Erhardt, *Man woman/boy girl* © 1973 The Johns Hopkins University Press.

2. Human sexual response cycle

A. *Excitement phase*—stimulus leads to increased sexual tension.
B. *Plateau phase*—intensification of sexual tension.
C. *Orgasm phase*—release of sexual tension, with dissipation of muscle tension (myotonia) and vasocongestion (engorgement of blood vessels).
D. *Resolution phase:*
   1. Men—involution, reversal of previous phases leads to refractory period.

2. Women—may start another sex response cycle.

3. Concepts and principles of human sexual response
A. Human sexual response involves not only the genitals, but the total body.
B. Factors in early prenatal and childhood period influence gender identity, gender role, sex typing, and sexual responses in later life.
C. Cultural and personally subjective variables influence ways of sexual expression and perception of what is satisfying.
D. Healthy sexual expressions vary widely.
E. Requirements for human sexual response:
  1. Intact central and peripheral nervous system to provide *sensory* perception, *motor* reaction.
  2. Intact circulatory system to produce *vasocongestive* response.
  3. Desirable and interested partner, if sex outlet involves mutuality.
  4. *Freedom* from guilt, anxiety, misconceptions, and interfering conditioned responses.
  5. Acceptable physical *setting*, usually private.

SEXUAL-HEALTH COUNSELING— GENERAL ISSUES

1. Issues in sexual practices with implications for counseling
A. *Sex education*—need to provide accurate and complete information on all aspects of sexuality to all people.
B. *Sexual-health care*—should be part of total health care planning for all.
C. *Sexual orientation*—need to avoid discrimination based on sexual orientation (such as homosexuality); the right to satisfying, nonexploitative relationship with others regardless of gender.
D. *Sex and the law*—sex between consenting adults not a legal concern.
E. *Explicit sexual material* (pornography)—can be useful in fulfilling various needs in life, as in quadriplegia.
F. *Masturbation*—a natural behavior in all ages that can fulfill a variety of needs. (See section on masturbation, page 38.)
G. Availability of *contraception* for minors—the right of access to medical contraceptive care should be available to all ages.
H. *Abortion*—confidentiality for minors.

I. *Treatment for VD*—naming of partners as part of VD control.
J. *Sex and the elderly*—need opportunity for sexual expression; need privacy when in communal living setting.
K. *Sex and the disabled*—need to have possible means available for rewarding sexual expressions.

2. Sexual myths *
A. *Myth:* Ignorance is bliss.
   Fact: What you don't know *can* hurt you (note the high frequency of VD and abortions); myths can perpetuate fears and misinformation such as:
   1. Masturbation causes mental illness.
   2. Women don't or shouldn't have orgasms.
   3. Tampons cause VD.
   4. Plastic wrap works better than condoms.
   5. Coca-Cola is an effective douche.
   Fact: Lack of knowledge during initial experiences may result in fear and set precedence for future sexual reactions.
B. *Myths:* The planned sex act is not okay and somewhat immoral for "nice" girls. If a woman gets pregnant it is her own fault. Contraceptives are solely a woman's responsibility.
   Fact: Sex and contraception are the prerogative and responsibility of both partners.
C. *Myth:* A good relationship is a harmonious relationship, free of conflict and disagreement (which are signs of rejection and incompatibility).
   Fact: Conflict can induce growth in self-understanding and in understanding of others.
D. *Myth:* Sexual deviance (such as homosexuality) is a sign of personality disturbance.
   Fact: No single sexual behavior is the most desirable, effective, or satisfactory. Personal sexual choice is a fundamental right.
E. *Myth:* A woman's sexual needs and gratification should be secondary to her partner's; a woman's role is to satisfy others.
   Fact: A woman has as much right to sexual freedom and experience as a man.
F. *Myth:* Menopause is an affliction signifying the end of sex.

*From Sedgwick, R.: "Myths in human sexuality: a social-psychological perspective," *Nursing Clinics of North America*, 10(3): 539–550, September 1975.

Fact: Many women do not suffer through menopause, and many report renewed sexual interest.

G. *Myth:* Sexual activity past 60 years of age is not essential.

   Fact: Sexual activity is therapeutic:
   1. Affirms identity.
   2. Provides communication.
   3. Provides companionship.
   4. Meets intimacy needs.

H. *Myth:* The sex drive of the woman decreases in postmenopausal period.

   Fact: The strength of the sex drive becomes greater as androgen overcomes the inhibitory action of estrogen.

I. *Myth:* Men over age 60 cannot achieve an erection.

   Fact: According to Masters and Johnson, the major difference between the aging male and the younger man is the duration of each phase of the sexual cycle. The older male is slower in achieving an erection.

J. *Myth:* Regular sexual activity cannot help the aging person's loss of function.

   Fact: Research is revealing that "disuse atrophy" may lead to loss of sexual capacity. Regular sexual activity helps preserve sexual function.

3. Basic principles of sexual-health counseling

A. There is no universal consensus about what are acceptable values in human sexuality. Each social group has very definite values regarding sex.

B. Counselors need to examine own feelings, attitudes, values, biases, knowledge base.

C. Help reduce fear, guilt, ignorance.

D. Offer guidance and education rather than indoctrination or pressure to conform.

E. Each person needs to be helped to make personal choices regarding sexual conduct.

4. Counseling in sexual health

A. General considerations:
   1. Create atmosphere of *trust and acceptance* for objective, nonjudgemental dialogue.
   2. Use *language* related to sexual behavior that is mutually comfortable and understood between client and nurse.
      a. Use alternate terms for definitions.
      b. Determine exact meaning of words and phrases, since sexual words and expressions have different meanings to people with different backgrounds and experiences.
   3. *Desensitize* own stress reaction to the emotional component of taboo topics.
      a. Increase awareness of own sexual values, biases, prejudices, stereotypes, and fears.
      b. Avoid overreacting, underreacting.
   4. Become sensitively aware of *interrelationships* between sexual needs, fears, and behaviors and other aspects of living.
   5. Begin with *commonly* discussed areas (such as menstruation) and progress to discussion of individual sexual experiences (such as masturbation). Move from areas where there is less voluntary control (noctural emissions) to more responsibility and voluntary behavior (premature ejaculation).
   6. Offer *educational information* to dispel fears, myths; give tacit permission to explore sensitive areas.
   7. Bring into awareness possibly *repressed* feelings of guilt, anger, denial, and suppressed sexual feelings.
   8. Explore possible *alternatives* of sexual expression.
   9. Determine *interrelationship* between mental, social, physical, and sexual well-being.

B. *Assessment parameters:*
   1. Self-awareness of body image, values, and attitudes toward human sexuality; comfort with own sexuality.
   2. Ability to identify sex problems on basis of own satisfaction or dissatisfaction.
   3. Developmental history, sex education, family relationships, cultural and ethnic values, and available support resources.
   4. Type and frequency of sexual behavior.
   5. Nature and quality of sex relations with others.
   6. Attitude toward and satisfaction with sexual activity.
   7. Expectations and goals.
   See Table 1–6 as a guideline in conducting an assessment interview.

C. *Nursing goals/implementation:*
   1. *Long-term goals:*
      a. Increase knowledge of reproductive system and types of sex behavior.
      b. Promote positive view of body and sex needs.
      c. Integrate sex needs into self-identity.
      d. Develop adaptive and satisfying patterns of sexual expression.

TABLE 1–6. *Suggested format for assessment interview*

Interview step	Rationale
1. Open the discussion of sexual matters subtly with an open-ended question. "People with your illness or stresses often experience other difficulties, sometimes with sexual functioning."	This gentle opening lets the client know that other people have difficulties, too. It gives the client permission to talk with the nurse about sexual matters without labeling these matters as problems.
2. Follow up with another open-ended question about the client's current status. "Has your illness or stresses made any difference in what it's like for you to be a wife or husband (lover, boy friend, girl friend, sexual partner)?"	The phrasing of this question enables the client to acknowledge a problem without admitting a shortcoming.
3. If the client speaks of having a dysfunction, ask about its effect. "How does this affect you?" or "How do you feel about it?"	This indicates that the nurse is willing to explore sexual matters more completely.
4. Ask about the severity and duration of the dysfunction. "Is it always difficult to control your ejaculation?" "Tell me when you first noticed this."	These questions are directed at identifying the specific problem.
5. Ask about the effects on the client's sexual partner. "Has this affected your relationship with your partner?"	This question is directed toward exploring the interactional aspects of the identified problem.
6. Ask what the client has already done to alleviate the situation. "Have you made any adjustments in your sexual activity?"	This question yields data that will help the nurse to formulate an intervention plan.
7. Ask the client if and how he or she would like the situation changed. "How would you like to change the situation to make it more satisfying?"	This question conveys the negotiated nature of the therapeutic relationship, in which the client's own goals play an important part.

Source: Wilson, H. S. and Kneisl, C. R. 1979. *Psychiatric nursing.* Addison-Wesley. Adapted from M. P. Whitley and D. Willingham, "Adding a sexual assessment to the health interview," *Journal of Psychiatric Nursing and Mental Health Services,* Vol. 16, No. 4, April 1978, pp. 17–27.

e. Understand effects of physical illness on sexual performance.
2. *Primary sexual health interventions—*
   a. Goals: minimize stress factors, strengthen sexual integrity.
   b. Provide education to uninformed or misinformed.
   c. Identify stress factors (myths, stereotypes, negative parental attitudes).
3. *Secondary sexual health interventions:* identify sexual problems early and refer for treatment (Table 1–7).
4. *Tertiary sexual health interventions—*
   a. Reduce impairment or dysfunction from acute sex problem or chronic unresolved one.
   b. Evaluate how client's goals were achieved in terms of positive thoughts, feelings, and satisfying sexual behaviors.

TABLE 1–7. *A comparison of different types of sex therapy modalities*

Parameters	Psychoanalysis	Psychotherapy	Behavioral therapy	Masters and Johnson's approach
Client population	Individuals, couples	Individuals, couples, groups, families	Individuals, couples, groups	Individuals, couples
Therapist activity	*Passive*—challenges defenses; gives no personal response	*Active*—strengthens functional coping style; guides in developing new styles for expressing sexuality	*Directive*—creates or role models new ways of thinking, feeling, and behaving intrapersonally and interpersonally	*Authoritative*—educates, teaches, identifies, clarifies, verifies sexual responses
Frequency and duration	1 to 5 times a week for 1 to 3 years	1 to 3 times a week for 6 months to 3 years	1 to 3 times a week for 3 to 6 months	1 to 3 times a week for 6 months to 2 years
Major therapeutic process	Transference, ventilation, catharsis, reality testing	Reality testing, ventilation, catharsis	Reinforcement, conditioning, relaxation	Education, practice, change
Goals	Resolution of sexual conflict through restructuring whole personality	Developing insight into a specific sexual dysfunction or concern through exploration of personality traits, communication, trust, spontaneity	Relief of specific sexual symptom through modification of thinking, feeling, behaving	Maximum sexual enjoyment through education, practice, change

Source: Constantino, Rose Eva Bana: Role of the nurse in sex health intervention. In Stuart, G. W., and Sundeen, S. J.: Principles and practice of psychiatric nursing, St. Louis, 1979, The C.V. Mosby Co.

SEXUAL HEALTH COUNSELING— SPECIFIC SITUATIONS

Rape

1. **Definition**—forcible perpetration of an act of sexual intercourse on the body of an unwilling person.

2. **Assessment**
A. *Signs of physical trauma*—physical findings of entry.
B. *Symptoms of physical trauma*—verbatim statements regarding type of sexual attack.
C. *Signs of emotional trauma*—tears, hyperventilation, extreme anxiety, withdrawal, self-blame, anger, embarrassment, fears, sleeping and eating disturbances, desire for revenge.
D. *Symptoms of emotional trauma*—statements regarding method of force used and threats made.
E. *Phases of response to rape*—

1. *Acute response:* volatility, disorganization, disbelief, shock, incoherence, agitated motor activity, nightmares, phobias (crowds, being alone, sex).
2. *Outward coping:* denial and suppression of anxiety and fear (silent rape syndrome), feelings appear controlled.
3. *Integration and resolution:* confronts anger with attacker; realistic perspective.

3. **Nursing goals/implementation** in counseling rape victims. Figure 1–2 is a summary of self-care decisions a victim faces the first night following a sexual assault. Figure 1–3 is a list of rights to which the rape victim is entitled.
A. Overall goals:
1. Acknowledge feelings.
2. Face feelings.
3. Resolve feelings.
4. Maintain and restore self-respect, dignity, integrity, and self-determination.

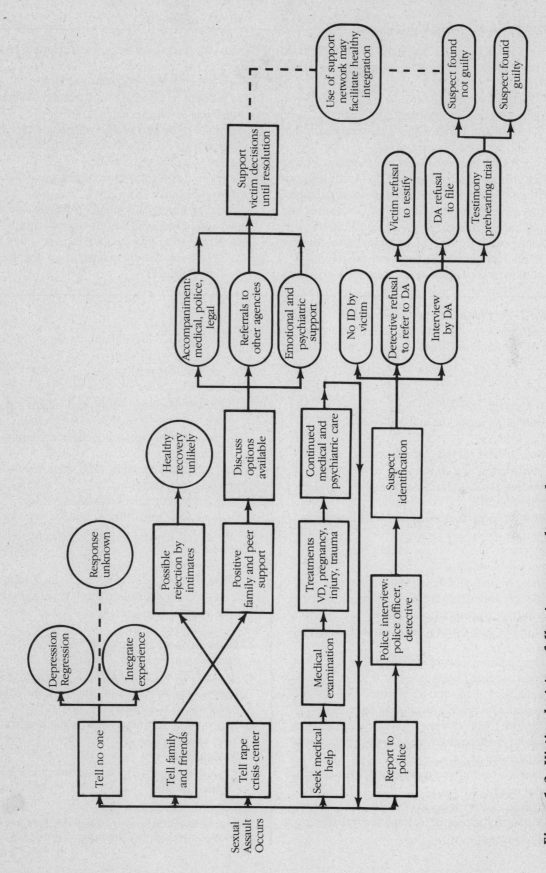

Figure 1–2. Victim decisions following a sexual assault.
From the Rape Crisis Services of the YWCA of Greater Harrisburg, Harrisburg, PA.

1. To transportation to a hospital when incapacitated
2. To emergency room care with privacy and confidentiality
3. To be carefully listened to and treated as a human being with respect, courtesy, and dignity
4. To have an advocate of choice accompany her through the treatment process
5. To accurate collection and preservation of evidence in an objective record that includes signs and symptoms of physical and emotional trauma
6. To receive clear explanations of procedures and medication in language she can understand
7. To know what treatment is recommended, for what reasons, and who will administer the treatment
8. To know any possible risks, side effects, or alternatives to proposed treatment, including all drugs prescribed
9. To ask for another physician or nurse
10. To consent to or refuse any treatment even when her life is in serious danger
11. To refuse to be part of any research or experiment
12. To reasonable complaint and to leave a care facility against the physician's advice
13. To receive an explanation of and understand any papers she agrees to sign
14. To be informed of continuing health care needs after discharge from the emergency room, hospital, physician's office, or care facility
15. To receive a clear explanation of the bill and review of charges

FIGURE 1–3. Patient's rights handout.
Adapted from Pittsburgh Action Against Rape: Patient's rights handout, 1976–1977 and from Westmorland Alliance Against Rape: Patient's rights, 1978.

B. Work-through issues:
  1. Handle legal matters and police contacts.
  2. Clarify facts.
  3. Get medical attention, if needed.
  4. Notify family and friends.
  5. Understand emotional reaction.
  6. Attend to practical concerns.
  7. Evaluate need for psychiatric consultations.
C. Acute phase:
  1. Decrease victim's stress, anxiety, fear.
  2. Seek medical care.
  3. Increase self-confidence and self-esteem.
  4. Identify and accept feelings and needs (to be in control, cared about, to achieve).
  5. Reorient perceptions, feelings, and statements about self.
  6. Help resume normal life style.
D. Outward coping phase:
  1. Remain available and supportive.
  2. Reflect words, feelings, and thoughts.
  3. Explore real problems.
  4. Explore alternatives regarding contraception, legal issues.
  5. Evaluate response of family and friends to victim and rape.
E. Integration and resolution phase:
  1. Assist exploration of feelings (anger) regarding attacker.
  2. Explore feelings (guilt and shame) regarding self.
  3. Assist in making own decisions regarding health care.
G. Maintain confidentiality and neutrality—facilitate person's own decision.
H. Search for alternatives to advice-giving.
I. Evaluate long-term effects of rape.

Masturbation

1. Definition—act of achieving sexual arousal and orgasm through manual or mechanical stimulation of the sex organs.

2. Characteristics of masturbation
A. Can be an interpersonal as well as a solitary activity.
B. "It is a healthy and appropriate sexual activity, playing an important role in ultimate consolidation of one's sexual identity."*
C. Accompanied by fantasies that are important for:
  1. Physically disabled.
  2. Fatigued.
  3. Compensation for unreachable goals and unfulfilled wishes.

---

*Marcus, I. M., and Francis, J. J.: Masturbation from infancy to senescence, New York, 1975, International Universities Press.

4. Rehearsal for future sexual relations.
5. Absence or impersonal action of partner.
D. Can help release tension harmlessly.

3. Concepts and principles related to masturbation

A. Staff's feelings and reactions influence their responses to client and affect continuation of masturbation (that is, negative staff actions increase client's frustration, which increases masturbation).
B. Masturbation is normal and universal; *not* physically or psychologically harmful in itself.
C. Pleasurable genital sensations important for increasing *self-pride,* finding *gratification* in *own* body, increasing sense of *personal value* of being lovable, helping to *prepare for adult* sexual role.
D. Excessive masturbation—some needs not being met through interpersonal relations; may use behavior to *avoid* interpersonal relations.

4. Long-term goals

A. Gain insight into *preference* for masturbation.
B. Relieve accompanying guilt, worry, self-devaluation (Figure 1–4).

5. Short-term goals

A. Clarify myths regarding masturbation.
B. Help client see masturbation as an acceptable sexual activity for individuals of all ages.
C. Set limits on masturbation in inappropriate settings.

6. Nursing interventions

A. Examine, control nurse's own negative feelings; show respect.
B. *Avoid* reinforcement of guilt and self-devaluation; scorn; threats, punishment, anger, alarm reaction; use of masturbation for rebellion in power struggle between staff and patient.

C. *Identify* patient's or client's unmet needs; consider purpose served by masturbation (may be useful behavior).
D. *Examine* pattern in which behavior occurs.
E. Intervene when degree of functioning is *impaired* in other daily life activities.
1. Remain calm, accepting, but nonsanctioning.
2. Promptly help clarify client's or patient's feelings, thoughts, at stressful time.
3. Review precipitating events.
4. Be a neutral "sounding board"; avoid evasiveness.
5. If unable to handle situation, find someone who can.
F. For patients who masturbate at *inappropriate* times or in inappropriate places:
1. Give special attention when they are not masturbating.
2. Encourage new interests and activities, but not immediately after observing masturbation.
3. Keep patients distracted, occupied with interesting activities.

7. Desired results

A. Acknowledgement of function of own sexual organs.
B. Sexually satisfying experience.
C. View of sexuality as pleasurable and wholesome.
D. Sex organs as acceptable, enjoyable, and valued part of body image.
E. Aid in maintaining and restoring self-image as fully functioning person.

Problems of conception

1. Infertility—for additional information, see Unit 3/ Nursing Care During the Reproductive Years.

A. *Assessment:*

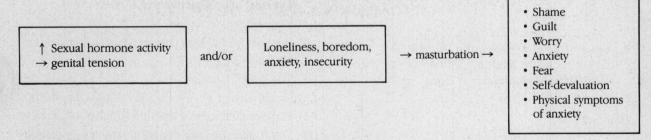

FIGURE 1–4. *Operationalization of behavioral concept—masturbation*

1. Alteration of self-concept due to doubt of own sexual potency and fertility.
2. Possible factors related to infertility; do work-up of both partners.

B. *Nursing goals/implementation:*
 1. Support feelings, frustrations, threatened masculine/feminine identity.
 2. Explore religious-cultural issues.
 3. If cause of infertility is found, help couple explore alternatives.
  a. Remaining childless.
  b. Adoption.
  c. Artificial insemination—AIH (Artificial insemination by husband) or AID (Artificial insemination by donor).
  d. Foster parents.

2. **Contraception**—see Unit 3/Nursing Care During the Reproductive Years.

3. **Therapeutic abortion**—for additional information, see Unit 3/Nursing Care During the Reproductive Years.

A. *Assessment parameters:*
 1. Religious factors—limitations and open options.
 2. Potential effect on woman and family—closeness or disunity.
 3. Support system—expectant father, extended family, peer group, social network.

B. *Nursing goals/implementation:*
 1. Explore all open options; leave out nurse's personal beliefs, opinions, and feelings.
 2. Include expectant father and significant family or peers.
 3. Define problem areas (refer for counseling).
 4. Support decision; accept and respect client's choice.
 5. Give information about procedure, effects on future conceptions, and sex relations.
 6. Counsel to prevent future unwanted pregnancies.

4. **Venereal diseases**—see Unit 3/Nursing Care During the Reproductive Years and Unit 4/Nursing Care of Children and Families.

Homosexuality

1. **Definition**—alternate sexual behavior, applied to sexual relations between persons of the same sex.

2. **Theories regarding causes**
A. Hereditary tendencies.
B. Imbalance of sex hormones.
C. Environmental influences and conditioning factors, related to learning and psychodynamic theories.
 1. Defense against unsatisfying relationship with father.
 2. Unsatisfactory and threatening early relationships with opposite sex.
 3. Oedipal attachment to parent.
 4. Seductive parent (incest).
 5. Castration fear.
 6. Labeling and guilt leading to sexual acting out.
 7. Faulty sex education.

3. **Nursing goals/implementation**
A. Nurse needs to work through own negative attitudes.
B. Accept and respect life style of gay (male homosexual) or lesbian (female homosexual) client.
C. Assess and treat for possible venereal disease and hepatitis.

Sex and the disabled person

1. **Assessment parameters**
A. Previous level of sex functioning and conflict.
B. Client's view of sex activity (self and mutual pleasure, tension release, procreation, control).
C. Cultural environment (influence on body image).
D. Degree of acceptance of illness.
E. Support system (partner, family, support group).
F. Body image and self-esteem.
G. Outlook on future.

2. **Nursing goals/implementation**
A. Approach with nonjudgemental attitude.
B. Elicit concerns about current physical state and perceptions of changes in sexuality.
C. Observe nonverbal clues of concern.
D. Identify genital assets.
E. Support client and partner during adjustment to current state.
F. Teach self-help skills.
G. Teach partner to care for client's physical needs.
H. Explore culturally acceptable sublimation activities.
I. Teach alternate sex behaviors and acceptable sublimation (touching, for example).
J. Promote adjustment to body image change.

Inappropriate sexual behavior

1. Situational examples—public exhibitions of sexual behaviors that are offensive to others; making sexual advances to other clients, patients, or staff.

2. Assessment and interventions
A. Contributory factors:
 1. Acting out angry and hostile feelings.
 2. Lack of awareness of hospital and agency rules regarding acceptable public behavior.
 3. Variation in cultural interpretations of what is acceptable public behavior.
 4. Reaction to unintended seductiveness of nurse's attire, posture, tone, or choice of terminology.
B. Nursing goals/implementation:
 1. Maintain calm, nonjudgemental attitude.
 2. Set firm limits on unacceptable behavior.
 3. Encourage verbalization of feelings rather than unaccceptable physical expression.
 4. Reinforce appropriate behavior.
 5. Provide constructive diversional activity for clients or patients.

Sexual abuse of children

For more information, see Unit 4/Nursing Care of Children and Families.

1. Assessment: characteristic behaviors
A. Relationship of offender to victim: many filling paternal role: uncle, grandfather, cousins with repeated, unquestioned access to the child.
B. Methods of pressuring victim into sexual activity: offering material goods, misrepresenting moral standards ("it's okay"), exploiting need for human contact and warmth.
C. Method of pressuring victim to secrecy in order to conceal the act is inducing fear: of punishment, of not being believed, of rejection, of being blamed for the activity, of abandonment.
D. Disclosure of sexual activity via:
 1. Direct visual or verbal confrontation and observation by others.
 2. Verbalization of act by victim.
 3. Visible clues: excess money and candy, new clothes, pictures, notes.
 4. Signs and symptoms: bed-wetting, excessive bathing, tears, avoiding school, somatic distress (GI and urinary tract pains).

2. Nursing goals/implementation
A. Encourage child to verbalize feelings about incident to dispel tension built up by secrecy.
B. Ask child to draw a picture of what happened.
C. Observe for symptoms over a period of time:
 1. Phobic reactions when see or hear offender's name.
 2. Sleep pattern changes, recurrent dreams, nightmares.
D. Look for silent reaction to being an accessory to sex (that is, child keeping burden of the secret activity within self); help deal with unresolved issues.

Part D | HEALTH-TEACHING

GENERAL PRINCIPLES OF HEALTH-TEACHING

One key nursing function is to promote and restore health. This involves teaching patients or clients new psychomotor skills, general knowledge, coping attitudes, and social skills related to health and illness (such as proper diet, exercises, colostomy care, wound care, insulin injections, urine-testing, etc.). The teaching function of the nurse is vital in assisting normal development and helping patients and clients meet health-related needs.

1. Purpose of health-teaching
A. *General goal:* motivate health-oriented behavior.
B. Nursing interventions:
 1. Fill in gaps in information.
 2. Clarify misinformation.
 3. Teach necessary skills.
 4. Modify attitudes.

2. Educational theories—on which effective health teaching is based.
A. *Motivation theory:*
 1. Health-oriented behavior is determined by the degree to which person sees health problem as *threatening*, with *serious consequences, high probability of occurrence*, and *belief in availability of effective course of action.*
 2. Non-health-related motives may *supersede* health-related motives.

3. Health-related motives may not always give rise to health-related behavior, and vice versa.
4. Motivation may be influenced by:
   a. *Phases of adaptation* to crisis (poor motivation in early phase).
   b. *Anxiety and awareness of need* to learn. (Mild anxiety is highly motivating.)
   c. *Mutual* versus externally imposed goal-setting.
   d. Perceived *meaningfulness* of information and material. (If within client's frame of reference, both meaningfulness and motivation increase.)

B. *Theory of planned change:*
   1. *Unfreeze* present level of behavior—develop awareness of problem.
   2. Establish *need* for change and relationship of trust and respect.
   3. *Move* toward change—examine alternatives, develop intentions into real efforts.
   4. *Freeze* on a new level—generalize behavior, stabilize change.

C. Elements of *learning theory:*
   1. *Drive* must be present, based on experiencing uncertainty, frustration, concern, or curiosity; understand hierarchy of needs.
   2. *Response* is a learned behavior that is elicited when associated stimulus is present.
   3. *Reward and reinforcement* are necessary for response (behavior) to occur and remain.
   4. *Extinction of response,* that is, elimination of undesirable behavior, can be attained through conditioning.
   5. Learning proceeds from learner's perception of the whole as important, to a progressive differentiation of components to clarify the original whole.
   6. After introduction of new material, there is a period of floundering when assimilation and insight occur.
   7. Memorization is the easiest level of learning, but least effective in changing behavior.
   8. Understanding involves the incorporation of generalizations and specific facts.
   9. Content, terminology, pacing, and spacing of learning needs to correspond to learner's capabilities, maturity level, feelings, attitudes, and experiences.
   10. Decreased visual and auditory perception leads to decreased readiness to learn.
   11. Successful learning leads to more successes in learning.
   12. Feedback increases learning.
   13. Teaching and learning should take place in the area where targeted activity normally occurs.
   14. Priorities for learning are dependent on client's physical and psychologic status.
   15. Learning flourishes when client feels respected, accepted by enthusiastic nurse; learning occurs best when differing value systems are accepted.
   16. Learning is a two-way process between learner and teacher; defensive behavior in either makes both activities difficult, if not impossible.

3. *Analysis of factors influencing learning*
A. Internal:
   1. Anxiety.
   2. Physical condition.
   3. Age.
   4. Motivation.
   5. Education.
   6. Experience.
   7. Senses (sight, hearing, touch).
   8. Values.
   9. Comprehension.
B. External:
   1. Physical environment (heat, light, noise, comfort).
   2. Timing, duration, interval.
   3. Teaching methods and aids.
   4. Content, vocabulary.

4. *Concepts and principles of health-teaching*
A. *Teaching methods* need to be:
   1. Compatible with the three domains of learning—
      a. *Cognitive* (knowledge, concepts): use written and audiovisual materials, discussion.
      b. *Psychomotor* (skills): use demonstrations, illustrations, role models.
      c. *Affective* (attitudes): use discussions, maintain atmosphere conducive to change; use role models.
   2. Appropriate to educational material.
   3. Related to learner's abilities and perceptions.
   4. Related to objectives of teaching.
B. *Teaching guidelines* to use with clients:
   1. Select conducive environment and best timing for activity.
   2. Assess the client's needs, interests, perceptions, motivations, and readiness for learning.
   3. State purpose and realistic goals of planned teaching/learning activity.

4. Actually involve the client by giving him or her the opportunity to *do, react, experience,* and *ask questions.*
5. Make sure that the client views the activity as useful and worthwhile and that it is within the client's grasp.
6. Use comprehensible terminology.
7. Proceed from the *known to the unknown,* from *specific to general* information.
8. Provide opportunity for client to see results and progress.
9. Give feedback and positive reinforcement.
10. Provide opportunities to achieve success.
11. Offer repeated practice in *real-life* situations.
12. Space and distribute learning sessions over a period of time.
13. Evaluate results.

SUGGESTED REFERENCES

LIFE CYCLE

Diekelman, N., et al.: "The middle years," *American Journal of Nursing,* 75(6): 994–1024, June 1975.

Kaluger, G., and Kaluger, M.: *Human development: the span of life,* St. Louis, Missouri, 1974, The C. V. Mosby Co.

Murray, R., et al.: *Nursing assessment and health promotion through the life span,* Englewood Cliffs, New Jersey, 1975, Prentice-Hall, Inc.

Smith, D., and Bierman, E.: *The biologic ages of man, from conception through old age,* Philadelphia, 1973, W. B. Saunders Co.

Sutterley, D. C., and Ferraro-Donnelly, G.: *Perspectives in human development: nursing throughout the life cycle,* Philadelphia, 1973, J. B. Lippincott Co.

HEALTH-TEACHING

Murray, R., and Zentner, J.: "Guidelines for more effective health teaching," *Nursing '76,* 6(2): 44–53, February 1976.

Redman, B.: *The process of patient teaching in nursing,* St. Louis, Missouri, 1976, The C. V. Mosby Co.

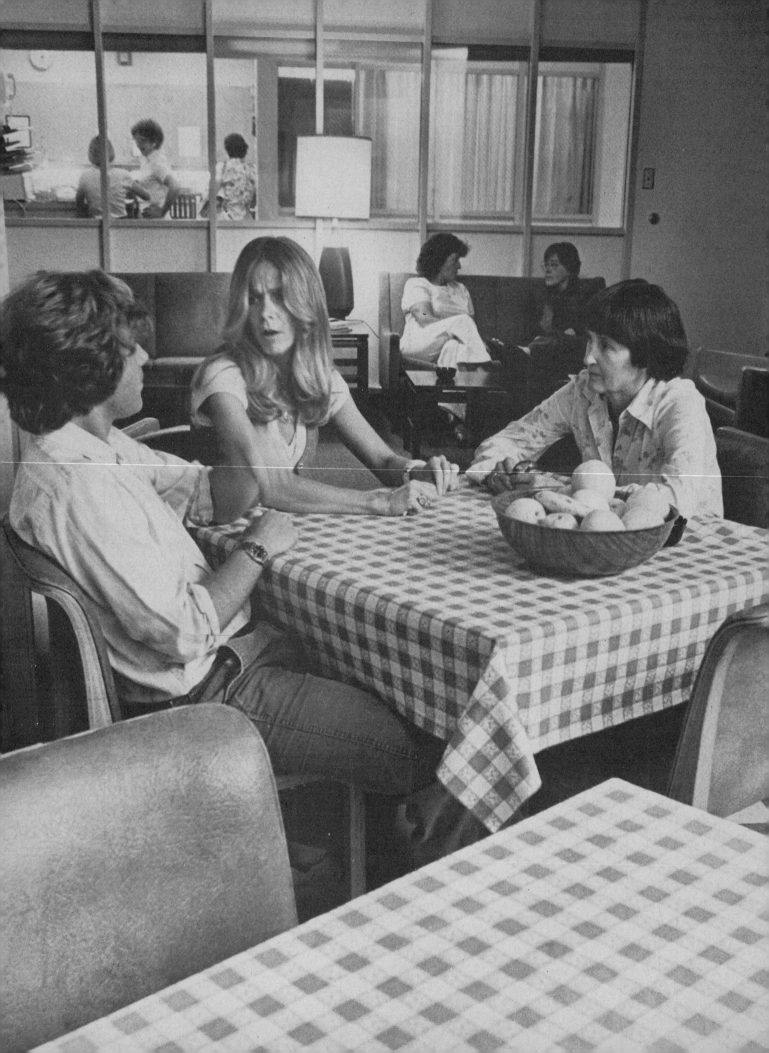

Unit 2 / MENTAL HEALTH NURSING AND COPING BEHAVIORS

Introduction

The chief *objective* of this unit is to highlight the most commonly observed disorders in the mental health field. The emphasis is on (a) main points for *assessment,* (b) *analysis* of data based on underlying *basic concepts and general principles* drawn from a psychodynamic and interpersonal theoretical framework, and (c) *nursing interventions* based on the therapeutic use of self as the cornerstone of a helping process. Nursing actions are listed in *priority* whenever possible. Hence the *nursing-process framework* is followed throughout. Note that "planning" and "implementation" behaviors (long- and short-term *goals,* with *priority* of actions) are covered under "nursing interventions." Evaluation of results is not listed separately, as this step of the nursing process is circular and relates back to "assessment" and "goals."

I recognize that the categorization of psychiatric-emotional disorders can be complex and controversial. For purposes of clarity and simplicity, an attempt has been made here to capsulize many theoretical principles and component skills of the helping process that these disorders have in *common.* The term "client" has replaced "patient" to reflect the interpersonal rather than medical model of psychiatric nursing. The diagnostic categorization of disorders is included here to update the reader in current terminology in the mental health field.

The underlying organizational framework for this chapter is based on the concept of *anxiety* as a common denominator for the disorders—an umbrella under which most behaviors and syndromes can be grouped.

Categorization of disorders has been modified according to the revised Diagnostic and Statistical Manual (DSM III) of the American Psychiatric Association (1980 edition).

In addition, a special section is included on organic mental disorders; mental health of the child, the adolescent, and the aged; and current developments in treatment modalities—for example, crisis intervention, milieu therapy, behavior modification, activity therapy, group and family therapy, electroconvulsive therapy, and psychopharmacology.

This unit also includes *definitions* of frequently used and/or misunderstood terms in the mental health field, as well as examples of the most common *therapeutic and nontherapeutic nurse-client responses.* Changes in this unit for the second edition include revised and updated sections on suicide, alcoholism, death and dying (throughout the life cycle), substance abuse, and family therapy. New material is included on *major theoretical models, mental status assessment, interviewing techniques, psychiatric emergencies,* and the 12 *most common general problematic behaviors* (denial, confusion and disorientation, immobility, anger, hostility, combativeness, demandingness, dependence, manipulation, noncooperation, pain, sensory disturbance). Additional tables and figures facilitate review of essential material. Question and answer sections have been expanded to include *twice* the number of questions, with more detailed answers explaining reasons for the best answers and discussing why the other options can be eliminated.

Sally L. Lagerquist

Part A / ORGANIZATIONAL FRAMEWORK

MAJOR THEORETICAL MODELS

1. Medical/biologic model (Kraepelin)
A. Assumptions: disturbances seen as diagnosable diseases with classifiable symptoms (or syndromes) that have a characteristic course, prognosis, and treatment.
B. Focus on diagnostic categories, e.g.:
1. Neurosis (anxiety, dissociative, phobias).
2. Psychosis (schizophrenia, affective).
3. Psychophysiologic.
4. Personality disorders.
C. Caused by organic conditions such as:
1. Arrested mental development (Down's syndrome).
2. Vascular (cerebral arteriosclerosis).
3. Infectious (meningitis, tertiary syphilis).
4. Metabolic (hepatic and renal failure, COPD).
5. Drug-induced (alcoholism, LSD).
6. Neoplasm (cancer of the brain).
7. Traumatic (blow on head).
8. Endocrine (thyroid disease).

2. Psychodynamic model (Freud)
A. Assumptions and key ideas:
1. No human behavior is accidental; each psychic event is determined by preceding ones.
2. Unconscious mental processes occur with very great frequency and significance.
3. Psychoanalysis is used to uncover childhood trauma, which leads to conflict, which then can lead to repressed feelings.
4. Psychoanalytic methods are used: therapeutic alliance, transference, regression, dream association, catharsis.
B. Freud—shifted from classification of behavior to understanding and explaining in psychologic terms, and changing behavior under constructed conditions.
1. Structure of the mind: id, ego, superego, unconscious, preconscious, conscious.
2. Stages of psychosexual development (Table 2–1).
3. Coping mechanisms. (Refer to sections on coping mechanisms and glossary in this unit.)

3. Psychosocial development model (Erikson, Maslow, Piaget, Duvall)
A. Erik Erikson—Eight Stages of Man (1963):
1. Psychosocial development—interplay of biology with social factors, encompassing total life span from birth to death in progressive developmental tasks.
2. Stages of life cycle—life consists of a series of developmental phases (Table 2–2): (See also Table 1–2, Unit 1, for comparison summary, and Table 4–1, Unit 4.)
   a. Universal sequence of biologic, social, psychologic events.
   b. Each person experiences a series of normative conflicts and crisis and thus needs to accomplish specific psychosocial tasks.
   c. Two opposing energies (positive and negative forces) coexist and need to be synthesized.
   d. How each age-specific task is accomplished influences the developmental progress of the next phase and the ability to deal with life.
B. Abraham Maslow—Hierarchy of Needs (1962):
1. Beliefs regarding emotional health based on comprehensive, multidisciplinary approach to human problems, involving all aspects of functioning.
   a. Premise: cannot understand mental illness without prior knowledge of mental health.

TABLE 2–1. Freud's stages of psychosexual development		
Stage	*Age*	*Behaviors*
Oral	Birth–1 year	Dependency and oral gratification.
Anal	1–3 years	Creativity, stinginess, cruelty.
Phallic or oedipal	3–6 years	Sexual, aggressive feelings.
Latency	6–12 years	Reactivation of pregenital impulses.
Genital	12–18 years	Displacement of pregenital impulses.

TABLE 2–2. *Erikson's stages of life cycle (See also Tables 1–2 and 4–1)*

Age and stage of development	Conflict areas needing resolution	Evaluation: result of resolution/nonresolution
Infancy (birth–18 months)	Trust	Shows affection, gratification, recognition, hopefulness; trusts self and others; begins to tolerate frustrations.
	Mistrust	Withdrawn, alienated.
Early childhood (18 months–3 years)	Autonomy	Cooperative, self-controlled, self-expressive, can delay gratification.
	Shame and doubt	Exaggerated self-restraint; defiance; compulsiveness; overly compliant.
Late childhood (3–5 years)	Initiative	Realistic goals; can evaluate self; explorative; imitates adult, shows imagination; tests reality; anticipates roles.
	Guilt	Self-imposed restrictions and denial.
School age (6–12 years)	Industry	Sense of duty; social and school competencies; persevering in real tasks.
	Inferiority	School and social drop-out; social loner; incompetent.
Adolescence (12–20 years)	Identity	Has ideologic commitments, self-actualizing; sense of self; experiments with roles; experiences sexual polarizations.
	Role diffusion	Ambivalent, confused, indecisive; may act out (antisocial acts).
Young adulthood (18–25 years)	Intimacy	Makes commitments to love and work relationships; able to sustain mutual love relationships.
	Isolation	Superficial, impersonal, biased.
Adulthood (25–65 years)	Generativity	Productive, creative, procreative, concerned for others.
	Stagnation	Self-indulgent.

TABLE 2–2. *(Continued)*

Age and stage of development	Conflict areas needing resolution	Evaluation: result of resolution/nonresolution
Late adulthood (65 years–death)	Integrity	Appreciates past, present, and future; self-acceptance of own contribution to others, of own self-worth, and of changes in life style and cycle; can face "not being."
	Despair	Preoccupied with loss of hope, of purpose; contemptuous.

b. Focus: positive aspects of human behavior (e.g., contentment, joy, happiness).

2. Hierarchy of Needs: as each stage is mastered, the next stage becomes dominant (Figure 2–1).

3. *Characteristics of optimal mental health*—keep in mind that wellness is on a continuum with cultural variations.

   a. *Self-esteem:* entails self-confidence and self-acceptance.

   b. *Self-knowledge:* involves accurate self-perception of strengths and limitations.

   c. *Satisfying interpersonal relationships:* able to meet reciprocal emotional needs through collaboration rather than exploitation or power struggles or jealousy; able to make full commitments in close relationship.

   d. *Environmental mastery:* can adapt, change, and solve problems effectively; can make decisions, choose from alternatives, and predict consequences. Actions are conscious, not impulsive.

   e. *Stress management:* can delay seeking gratification and relief; does not blame or dwell on past; assumes self-responsibility; either modifies own expectations, seeks substitutes, or withdraws from stressful situation when cannot reduce stress.

C. *Jean Piaget—Cognitive/Intellectual Development* (1963):

1. Assumptions—child development steered by interaction of environmental and genetic influences; therefore focus is on environmental and social forces (Table 2–3). (See also Table 1–2, Unit 1, for comparison with other theories, and Table 4–2, Unit 4.)

2. Key concepts:

   a. *Assimilation*—process of acquiring new knowledge, skills, and insights by using what they already know and have.

   b. *Accommodation*—adjust to change by solving heretofore unsolvable problems because of newly assimilated knowledge.

   c. *Adaptation*—coping process to handle environmental demands.

D. *E. M. Duvall—Family Development* (1971).

1. Developmental tasks are family-oriented, presented in eight categories throughout the life cycle:

   a. Married couple.

   b. Child-bearing years.

   c. Preschool-age years.

   d. School-age years.

   e. Teenage years.

   f. Families as launching centers.

   g. Middle-aged parents.

   h. Aging family members.

4. Community mental health model (Gerald Kaplan)

A. Levels of prevention:

1. *Primary prevention*—lower the risk of mental illness and increase capacity to resist contributory influences by providing anticipatory guidance and maximizing strengths.

2. *Secondary prevention*—decrease disability by shortening its duration and reducing its severity through detection of early warning signs and effective intervention following case-finding.

3. *Crisis intervention*—(see pp. 113–114).

4. *Tertiary prevention*—avoid permanent disorder through rehabilitation.

5. Behavioral model (Pavlov, Watson, Wolpe, and Skinner)

A. Assumptions:

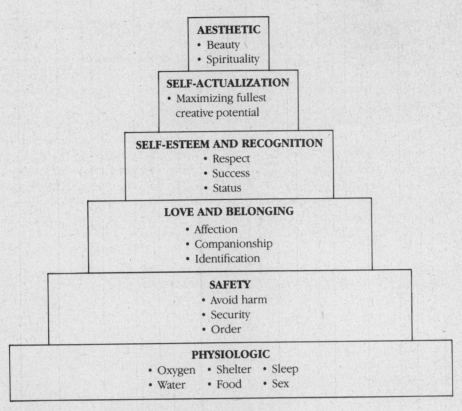

FIGURE 2–1. Maslow's hierarchy of needs.

TABLE 2–3. *Piaget's age-specific developmental levels (See also Tables 1–2 and 4–2)*

Age	Stage	Abilities
Infant–2 years	Sensorimotor	Pre-verbal; uses all senses; coordinates simple motor actions.
2–4 years	Preconceptual	Can use language; egocentric; imitation in play, parallel play.
4–7 years	Intuitive	Asks questions; can use symbols and associate subjects with concepts.
7–12 years	Concrete	Sees relationships, aware of viewpoints; understands causal effect; can make conclusions; solves concrete problems.
12 years and on	Formal operational thought	Abstract and conceptual thinking; can check out ideas, thoughts, and beliefs; lives in present and nonpresent; can use formal logic and scientific reasoning.

1. Roots in neurophysiology.
2. Stimulus-response learning can be *conditioned* through *reinforcement*.
3. Behavior is what one does.
4. Behavior is observable, describable, predictable, and controllable.
5. Classification of mental disease is clinically useless, only provides legal labels.

B. Aim: change *observable* behavior. There is *no underlying* cause, *no internal* motive.

6. **Comparison of models**—Table 2–4 compares three models of *therapeutic intervention* based on crisis, psychotherapy, and medical models.

MENTAL STATUS ASSESSMENT

1. **Components of mental status exam**
A. *Appearance*—appropriate dress, grooming, facial expression, stereotyped movements, mannerisms, rigidity.
B. *Behavior*—anxiety level, congruency with situation, cooperativeness, openness, hostility, reaction to interview, consistency.
C. *Speech characteristics*—relevancy, coherency, meaning, repetitiveness, qualitative (*what* is said), quantitative (*how much* is said), abnormalities, inflections, affectations, congruency with level of education, impediments, tone quality.

TABLE 2–4. *Comparison of crisis, psychotherapy, and medical institutional models*

Characteristic	Crisis intervention model	Psychotherapy model	Medical institutional model
People served	Individuals and families in crisis or precrisis states	Those who wish to correct neurotic personality or behavior patterns	People with serious mental or emotional breakdowns
Service goals	Growth promotion; personal and social integration	Working through of unconscious conflicts; reconstruction of behavior and personality patterns; personal and social growth	Control adjustment; recovery from acute disturbance
Service methods	Social and environmental manipulation; focus on feelings and problem solving; may use medication to promote goals; decision counseling	Introspection; catharsis; interpretation; free association; use of additional techniques depending on philosophy and training of therapist	Medication; behavior modification; electric shock; group activities; use of additional techniques depending on philosophy of institution
Activity of workers	Active/direct (depends on functional level of client)	Exploratory; nondirective; interpretive	Direct, noninvolved; or indirect
Length of service	Short—usually six or fewer sessions	Usually long-term	Short or long (depends on degree of disability and approach of psychiatrist); high repeat rate
Beliefs about people	Social—people are capable of growth and self-control	Individualistic or social (depends on philosophy of therapist)	Individualistic—social aspect secondary; institution and order often more important than people
Attitudes toward service	Flexible, any hour	Emphasis on wisdom of therapist and fifty-minute hour; flexibility varies with individual therapist	Scheduled; staff attitudes may become rigid and institutionalized

Source: Adapted from L. A. Hoff, *People in crisis: understanding and helping* (Menlo Park, Calif.: Addison-Wesley Publishing Co., 1978), pp. 54–55.

D. *Mood*—appropriateness, intensity, suicidal/homicidal ideation or plans, duration, swings.

E. *Thought content*—delusions, hallucinations, obsessive ideas, phobic ideas, themes, areas of concern, self-concept.

F. *Thought processes*—organization and association of ideas, coherence, ability to abstract and understand symbols.

G. *Sensorium:*
1. Orientation for person, time and place, situation.
2. Memory—immediate, rote, remote, and recent.
3. Attention and concentration—susceptibility to a distraction.
4. Information and intelligence—account of general knowledge, history, and reasoning powers.
5. Comprehension—concrete and abstract.
6. Stage of consciousness—alert/awake, somnolent, lethargic, delirious, stuporous, comatose.

H. *Insight and judgement:*
1. Extent to which client sees self as having problems, needing treatment.
2. Awareness of intrapsychic nature of own difficulties.
3. Soundness of judgement.

2. Individual assessment
A. Consider the following in Figure 2–2:
1. Physical and intellectual factors.
2. Socioeconomic factors.
3. Personal values and goals.
4. Adaptive functioning and response to present involvement.
5. Developmental factors.

B. Figure 2–3 provides a sample of a mental health assessment form for clinical use.

3. Interviewing
A. *Definition:* a goal-directed method of communicating facts, feelings, and meanings.
1. For interviewing to be effective, interaction between two persons involved must be effective.

B. *Nine principles for verbal interaction:*
1. *Client's initiative* begins the discussion.
2. *Indirect approach,* moving from the periphery to the core.
3. *Open-ended* statements, using incomplete forms of statements such as "You were saying...." to prompt rather than close off an exchange.
4. *Minimal verbal activity* in order not to obstruct thought process and client's responses.
5. *Spontaneity,* rather than fixed interview topics, may bring out much more relevant data.

6. *Facilitate expression of feelings* to help assess events and reactions by asking, for example, "What was that like for you?"
7. *Focus on emotional areas* about which client may be in conflict, as noted by repetitive themes.
8. *Pick up cues, clues and signals from client,* such as facial expressions and gestures, behavior, emphatic tones, and flushed face.
9. *Introduce material related to content* already brought up by client; do not bring in a tangential focus from "left field."

C. *Purpose and goals of interviewing:*
1. *Initiate and maintain a positive nurse-client relationship,* which can decrease symptoms, lessen demands and move client toward optimum health when nurse demonstrates understanding and sharing of client's concerns.
2. *Determine client's view of nurse's role* in order to utilize it or change it.
3. *Collect information on emotional crisis* to plan goals and approaches in order to increase effectiveness of nursing interventions.
4. *Identify and resolve crisis;* the act of eliciting cause or antecedent event may in itself be therapeutic.
5. *Channel feelings directly* by exploring interrelated events, feelings, and behaviors in order to discourage displacement of feelings onto somatic and behavioral symptoms.
6. *Channel communication* and transfer significant information to the physician and other team members.
7. *Prepare for health-teaching* in order to help the client function as effectively as possible.

THE THERAPEUTIC NURSING PROCESS

A *therapeutic nursing process* involves an interaction between the nurse and client in which the nurse offers a series of planned, goal-directed activities that are useful to a particular client in relieving discomfort, promoting growth, and satisfying interpersonal relationships.

1. Characteristics of therapeutic nursing
A. Movement from first contact through final outcome:
1. Eight general phases occur in a typical unfolding of a natural process of problem-solving.
2. Stages are not always in the same sequence.
3. Not all stages are present in a relationship.

The individual assessment should consider the following factors:

Physical and intellectual

1. Presence of physical illness and/or disability
2. Appearance and energy level
3. Current and potential levels of intellectual functioning
4. How client sees personal world, translates events around self; client's perceptual abilities
5. Cause and effect reasoning, ability to focus

Socioeconomic factors

1. Economic factors—level of income, adequacy of subsistence; how this affects lifestyle, sense of adequacy, self-worth
2. Employment and attitudes about it
3. Racial, cultural, and ethnic identification; sense of identity and belonging
4. Religious identification and link to significant value systems, norms, and practices

Personal values and goals

1. Presence or absence of congruence between values and their expression in action; meaning of values to individual
2. Congruence between individual's values and goals and the immediate systems with which client interacts
3. Congruence between individual's values and assessor's values; meaning of this for intervention process

Adaptive functioning and response to present involvement

1. Manner in which individual presents self to others—grooming, appearance, posture
2. Emotional tone and change or constancy of levels
3. Style of communication—verbal and nonverbal; ability to express appropriate emotion, follow train of thought; factors of dissonance, confusion, uncertainty
4. Symptoms or symptomatic behavior
5. Quality of relationship individual seeks to establish—direction, purposes, and uses of such relationships for individual
6. Perception of self
7. Social roles that are assumed or ascribed; competence in fulfilling these roles
8. Relational behavior
   a. Capacity for intimacy
   b. Dependence-independence balance
   c. Power and control conflicts
   d. Exploitiveness
   e. Openness

Developmental factors

1. Role performance equated with life stage
2. How developmental experiences have been interpreted and used
3. How individual has dealt with past conflicts, tasks, and problems
4. Uniqueness of present problem in life experience

FIGURE 2–2. Individual assessment. *Source:* Holly S. Wilson and Carol Ren Kneisl, *Psychiatric Nursing.* (Menlo Park, Calif.: Addison-Wesley Publishing Co., 1979), pp. 89–90. Adapted from the problem-solving model of Compton and Galaway, *Social Work Processes.* The Dorsey Press, 1975.

B. Phases*
1. *Beginning* the relationship. *Goal:* build trust (Table 2–5).
2. *Formulating* and clarifying a problem and concern. *Goal:* clarify patient's statements.
3. *Setting a contract* or working agreement. *Goal:* decide on terms of the relationship.
4. *Building* the relationship. *Goal:* increase depth of relationship and degree of commitment.
5. *Exploring* goals and solutions, gathering data, expressing feelings. *Goals:* (a) maintain and enhance relationship (trust and safety), (b) explore blocks to goal, (c) expand self-awareness, and (d) learn skills necessary to reach goal.
6. *Developing action plan. Goals:* (a) clarify feelings, (b) focus on and choose between alternate courses of action, and (c) practice new skills.
7. *Working through* conflicts or disturbing feelings. *Goals:* (a) channel earlier discussions into specific course of action and (b) work through unresolved feelings (Table 2–6).
8. *Ending* the relationship. *Goals:* (a) evaluation of goal attainment and (b) leave-taking (Table 2–7).

---

*Lawrence M. Brammer, *The helping relationship: process and skills,* © 1973, p. 55. Reprinted by permission of Prentice-Hall, Inc., Englewood Cliffs, N.J.

MENTAL HEALTH ASSESSMENT

Identifying Data

Date of Admission 12/5/77

Date of Interview 12/7/77

NAME Fred C. Carlton SOCIAL SECURITY NUMBER 462-60-8910

SEX M AGE 52 BIRTHDATE 12/7/24 RACE/CULTURE Caucasian

MARITAL STATUS M RELIGION Presby EDUCATIONAL BACKGROUND 3 yrs college

OCCUPATION Regional Exec.- lge oil company FINANCIAL STATUS $45,000+/yr.

DIAGNOSIS A-L (massive) M.I. ALLERGIES NKA

CHIEF COMPLAINT (IN QUOTES) "I really can't believe this is happening to me."

1. Physical Appearance (a brief description including height, weight, bodily functions, energy level, sleep patterns, and dress)
   5'8", 182 lbs. ment. c/o constipation 3 day duration, c/o fatigue, weakness c̄ minimal exertion (i.e. from bed → bathrm) sleep's during night + naps during day, hospitalization wearing PJ's gown, refused to change x 2 days.

2. Motor Ability (posture, gait, gestures)
   Slumped shoulders, walks slowly c̄ hesitation. Rubs forehead + chin c̄ hand frequently while talking.

3. Sensory Ability (see, hear, touch, taste, smell)
   Intact - pulls away when touched.

4. Level of Consciousness

   Responsive to:
	(check)
Verbal stimuli	✓
Touch	✓
Noxious stimuli	
Unresponsive	

5. Orientation
Person	✓	Place	✓	Time	✓

6. Memory
   | Recent | ✓ | Past | ✓ |

7. Intelligence (cite supporting data)
   Bright, 3 years college - responds c̄ executive positive c̄ his corporation. Excellent vocabulary.

8. Fund of Information
   General good

   About illness (state specifics) Limited - "I usually feel fine, now it is hard to imagine my heart is in as bad shape as they say..."

9. Judgment/Insight (cite supporting data)
   Realizes poor judgment relating to personal welfare can't (they work long hrs, smoke 2 ppd.) thought limited about illness (i.e. MI). Questions need to provide changes in lifestyle.

10. Thought Process
Logical	✓	Coherent	✓	Relevant	✓

    Unusual patterns (cite supporting data) none noted.

11. Speech Pattern (speech, comprehensiveness, spontaneity)
    Lacks spontaneity - slightly slow, responses terse. Poor eye contact. slow- won't have heart attack."

12. Ideation (cite supporting data) history upon health "I've always been till health slow- won't have a heart attack."
    Self-destructive/suicidal
    denies suicide plan.
    Suspicious/paranoid

13. Affect (cite supporting data) depressive, nonverbal: slumped shoulders, unshaven, poor eye contact at times. Verbal: repeatedly mentions things he has from old. he will have to give up - i.e. smoking, coffee, work habits...

14. Family and Significant Others
    A. Position in family oldest child + only son in family of origin
    B. Others in family wife, one married son
    C. Living arrangements large house in upper-middle class neighborhood
    D. Role/roles in family breadwinner, husband, father
    E. Significant others work colleague
    F. Other support systems none mentioned
    G. Interactional ability Adequate, wife states wants input into he defers all decisions to him.

15. Addictive/Coping Habits and Amounts (positive and negative)
    A. Smoking ✓ Amount 2 pk/d x 28 yrs.
    B. Alcohol ✓ Amount 1-2 cocktail Frequency every night
    C. Medications (list all: over the counter, legal, illegal)
       Colace - 10-12 tabs taken throughout the day Amount

    D. Food intake overindulges Amount by lunch + dinner When ↑ caloric, fatty foods ↑ increasing intake in particular
    E. Other Coffee intake 7-8 cups/day, immersed in work routine and responsibilities.

16. Sexual Functioning data is inadequate, throughout past several years sexual activity "I guess that is something that I'll have to give up."

17. Need Level safety

18. Developmental Level
    Currently functioning at 6-12 y.o. level - Erikson "industry vs insecurity"

19. Coping Devices and Defense Mechanisms (assess for effectiveness, usefulness, and appropriateness)
    Coping devices: in past- making typing mechanisms: currently on ETOH, smbg + + attempts effective denial and regression. and useful in past, now not as appropriate

20. Assets, Resources, Interests
    Financially secure, nearby retirement would ↓ to family, opportunities; intelligent, good rapport with doctors and nursing staff

21. Impression/Nursing Diagnoses
    Impression: 52 y.o. M., 11 day post massive M.I., regarding to getting changes in lifestyle, and altered body image c̄ a moderate depression evidenced typically - nonverbal - wishes to see. Many of past coping skills inappropriate to predict health status.
    Nsg Dx: ① Moderate depression related to current changes in body image (↑ insecurity, ↑ dependence) attested in dangers lifestyle (quit, stop smoking, alter work habits.)
    ② Knowledge deficit re inappropriate of "good coping devices (↑ work, smoking, ETOH, etc)

    Recorder Jann Logsdon Date 12/7/77

    Developed by Janis Reynolds and Jann Logsdon. 1977. Revised. 1978.

TABLE 2–5. *Summary of beginning (orientation) phase*

Objective	Therapeutic tasks	Approaches

Establishment of contact in the form of a working relationship with the client	Clarification of purpose of relationship, role of nurse, and responsibilities of client	Educative
		  Provide information regarding purpose, roles, and responsibilities
		
		  Address misconceptions, fantasies, and fears regarding relationship and/or nurse

	Addressing of client suffering	Use facilitative characteristics, especially empathic understanding Avoid premature reassurance (allow trust to evolve) Be explicit about who has access to client's revelations (degree of confidentiality)
	Negotiation of therapeutic contract (client's definition of personal goals for treatment and nurse's professional responsibilities)	Encourage delineation of goals that 1. Are specific 2. Address behavioral patterns 3. Designate degree of change necessary for client self-satisfaction Determine place, duration and time of meeting Consider optional referral sources

Source: Holly S. Wilson and Carol Ren Kneisl, *Psychiatric Nursing* (Menlo Park, Calif.: Addison-Wesley Publishing Co., 1979), p. 139.

TABLE 2–6. *Summary of middle (working) phase*

Objectives	Therapeutic tasks	Approaches
Maintenance and analysis of contact Consists of: Mutual determination of dynamics of client's behavior patterns, especially those considered dysfunctional	Identification and detailed exploration of important behavior patterns	Explore behavior pattern in depth, including origin, causes, operation, and effect of pattern (intrapersonally and interpersonally) Separate environmental factors (familial, political, economic, cultural) from intrapersonal factors Link elements of one behavior pattern to other patterns as appropriate, for a gradual unfolding of central life patterns
	Analysis of client's mode of conflict resolution	Encourage detailed exploration of how client reacts to reduce anxiety associated with conflict Increase awareness of defenses employed to ward off anxiety awakened by such exploration

TABLE 2–6. *(Continued)*

Objectives	Therapeutic tasks	Approaches
	Facilitation of client self-assessment of growth-producing and growth-inhibiting behavior patterns	Encourage client to assert own needs when external environmental conditions (group, agency, institution) are an inhibiting force.
Institution of behavioral change, especially in dysfunctional behavior patterns	Address forces that inhibit desired change (problematic thoughts, feelings, and behaviors)	Assist client in challenging client's personal resistance to change
		Use problem-solving strategies, active decision making, and personal accountability
		Encourage client to assert own needs when external environmental conditions (group, agency, institution) are an inhibiting force.
	Create an atmosphere offering permission for active experimentation to test and assess effectiveness of new behaviors	Allow freedom to make and assess mistakes and blunders
		Avoid parental judgment of any behavioral experimentation—encourage client self-assessment instead
	Facilitate development of coping skills to deal with anxiety associated with behavioral change	Address, rather than avoid, anxiety and its manifestations
		Strengthen existing growth-promoting coping skills, especially regarding unalterable conditions (e.g., terminal illness, physical deformity, loss of significant other by death)
		Encourage development of new coping skills and their application to actual life experiences

Source: Holly S. Wilson and Carol Ren Kneisl, *Psychiatric Nursing* (Menlo Park, Calif.: Addison-Wesley Publishing Co., 1979), p. 142.

2. Therapeutic nurse-client interactions

A. Planning and goals:

1. Demonstrate unconditional *acceptance,* interest, concern, and respect.
2. Develop trust—be consistent and congruent.
3. Make frequent contacts with the client.
4. Be honest and direct, authentic and spontaneous.
5. Offer support, security, and empathy, not sympathy.
6. Focus comments on concerns of client (client-centered), not self (social responses). *Refocus* when client changes subject.
7. Encourage expression of feelings; focus on feelings and here-and-now behavior.
8. Give attention to a client who complains.
9. Give information at client's level of understanding, at appropriate time and place.
10. Use open-ended questions; ask "how," "what," "where," "who," and "when" questions; avoid "why" questions; avoid questions that can be answered by "yes" or "no."
11. Use feedback or reflective listening.
12. Maintain hope, but avoid false reassurances, clichés, and pat responses.
13. Avoid verbalizing value judgements, giving personal opinions, or moralizing.
14. Do not change the subject unless the client is redundant or focusing on physical illness.

TABLE 2–7.   *Summary of end (resolution) phase*

Objective	Therapeutic tasks	Approaches
Termination of contact in a mutually planned, satisfying manner	Assist client evaluation of therapeutic contract and of psychotherapeutic experience in general	Encourage client's appraisal of personal therapeutic goals (motivation, effort, progress, outcome)
		Provide appropriate feedback regarding appraisal of goals
		Underline client's assets and therapeutic gains
		Underline areas for further therapeutic work
	Encourage transference of dependence to other support systems	Encourage client to develop reliance on others in client's immediate environment (spouse, relative, employer, neighbor, friend) for empathic, emotional support
	Participate in explicit therapeutic goodbye with client	Be alert to surfacing of any behavior arising on termination (repression, regression, acting out, anger, withdrawal, acceptance, etc.)
		Assist client in working through feelings associated with these behaviors
		Anticipate own reaction to separation and share in a manner that does not burden client
		Allow "time" and "space" for termination; the longer the duration of the one-to-one relationship, the more time is needed for the resolution phase

Source: Holly S. Wilson and Carol Ren Kneisl, *Psychiatric Nursing* (Menlo Park, Calif.: Addison-Wesley Publishing Co., 1979), p. 144.

15. Point out reality; help the client leave "inner world."
16. Set limits on behavior when client is acting out unacceptable behavior that is self-destructive or harmful to others.
17. Assist clients in arriving at their own decisions by demonstrating problem-solving or involving them in the process.
18. Do not talk if it is not indicated.
19. Approach, sit, or walk with agitated clients; stay with the person who is upset.
20. Focus on nonverbal communication.
21. Remember the psyche has a soma! Do not neglect appropriate physical symptoms.

B. Examples of **therapeutic** responses as interventions:
1. Being *silent*—being able to sit in silence with a person can connote acceptance and acknowledgement that the person has the right to silence. (Dangers: the nurse may wrongly give the client the impression that there is a lack of interest, or the nurse may discourage verbalization if acceptance of this behavior is prolonged.)
2. *Using nonverbal communication*—nodding head, moving closer to the client, and leaning forward, for example; use as a way to encourage client to speak.

3. Give encouragement to continue with *open-ended leads*—nurse's responses: "Then what?" "Go on," "For instance," "Tell me more," "Talk about that."

4. *Accepting, acknowledging*—nurse's responses: "I hear your anger," or "I see that you are sitting in the corner."

5. *Commenting on nonverbal behavior* of client—nurse's responses: "I notice that you are swinging your leg," "I see that you are tapping your foot," or "I notice that you are wetting your lips." Client may respond with, "So what?" If she does, the nurse needs to reply why he commented, for example, "It is distracting," "I am giving the nonverbal behavior meaning," "Swinging your leg makes it difficult for me to concentrate on what you are saying," or "I think when people tap their feet it means they are impatient. Are you impatient?"

6. Encouraging clients to *notice with their senses* what is going on—nurse's response: "What did you see (or hear)?" or "What did you notice?"

7. Encouraging *recall and description* of details of a particular experience—nurse's response: "Give me an example," "Please describe the experience further," "Tell me more," or "What did you say then?"

8. *Giving feedback by reflecting, restating, and paraphrasing* feelings and content—
   Client: I cried when he didn't come to see me.
   Nurse: You cried. You were expecting him to come and he didn't?

9. *Picking up on latent content* (what is implied)—nurse's response: "You were disappointed. I think it may have hurt when he didn't come."

10. *Focusing, pinpointing,* asking "what" questions—
    Client: They didn't come.
    Nurse: Who are 'they'?
    Client: [Rambling.]
    Nurse: Tell it to me in a sentence or two. What is your main point? What would you say is your main concern?

11. *Clarifying*—nurse's response: "What do you mean by 'they'?" "What caused this?" or "I didn't understand. Please say it again."

12. *Focusing on reality* by expressing doubt on "unreal" perceptions—
    Client: Run! There are giant ants flying around after us.
    Nurse: That is unusual. I don't see giant ants flying.

13. *Focusing on feelings,* encouraging client to be aware of and describe personal feelings—
    Client: Worms are in my head.
    Nurse: That must be a frightening feeling. What did you feel at that time? Tell me about that feeling.

14. Helping client to *sort and classify impressions, make speculations, abstract* and *generalize* by making connections, seeing common elements and similarities, making comparisons, and placing events in logical sequence—nurse's responses: "What are the common elements in what you just told me?" "How is this similar to," "What happened just before?" or "What is the connection between this and."

15. *Pointing out discrepancies* between thoughts, feelings, and actions—nurse's response: "You say you were feeling sad when she yelled at you; yet you laughed. Your feelings and actions do not seem to fit together."

16. *Checking perceptions* and *seeking agreement* on how the issue is seen, *checking out* with the client to see if the message sent is the same one that was received—nurse's response: "Let me restate what I heard you say," "Are you saying that," "Did I hear you correctly?" "Is this what you mean?" or "It seems that you were saying."

17. *Encouraging client to consider alternatives*—nurse's response: "What else could you say?" or "Instead of hitting him, what else might you do?"

18. *Planning a course of action*—nurse's response: "Now that we have talked about your on-the-job activities and you have thought of several choices, which are you going to try out?" or "What would you do next time?"

19. *Imparting information*—give additional data as new input to help client; for example, state facts and reality-based data that client may not have.

20. *Summing up*—nurse's response: "Today we have talked about your feelings toward your boss, how you express your anger, and about your fear of being rejected by your family."

21. *Encouraging client to appraise and evaluate* the experience or outcome—nurse's response: "How did it turn out?" "What was it like?" "What was your part in it?" "What difference did it make?" or "How will this help you later?"

C. Examples of **nontherapeutic** responses:

1. *Changing the subject, tangential response,* moves away from problem and/or focuses on inciden-

tal, superficial content—
Client: I hate you.
Nurse: Would you like to take your shower now?
Suggested responses: reflect, "You hate me; tell me about this," or "You hate me; what does hate mean to you?"
Client: I want to kill myself today.
Nurse: Isn't today the day your mother is supposed to come?
Suggested responses: (a) give open-ended lead, (b) give feedback, "I hear you saying today that you want to kill yourself," or (c) clarifying, "Tell me more about this feeling of wanting to kill yourself".

2. *Moralizing:* saying with approval or disapproval that the person's behavior is good or bad, right or wrong; *arguing* with stated belief of person; directly opposing the person—
Nurse: That's good. It's wrong to shoot yourself.
Client: I have nothing to live for.
Nurse: You certainly do have a lot!
Suggested response: similar to those in No. 1.

3. *Agreeing with client's autistic inventions—*
Client: The eggs are flying saucers.
Nurse: Yes, I see. Go on.
Suggested response: use clarifying response first, "I don't understand," and then, depending on client's response, use either *accepting, acknowledging; focusing on reality,* or *focusing on feelings.*

4. *Agreeing with client's negative view of self—*
Client: I have made a mess of my life.
Nurse: Yes, you have.
Suggested response: use clarifying response about "mess of my life"—"Give me an example of one time where you feel you messed up in your life."

5. *Complimenting, flattering—*
Client: I have made a mess of my life.
Nurse: How could you? You are such an attractive, intelligent, generous person.
Suggested response: same as that in No. 4.

6. *Giving opinions and advice* concerning client's life situation—examples of poor responses include: "In my opinion," "I think you should," or "Why not?"
Suggested response: (a) encourage the client to consider alternatives ("What else do you think you could try?"); (b) encourage the client to appraise and

evaluate for him/herself ("What is it like for you?").

7. *Seeking agreement* from client with nurse's personal opinion—examples of poor responses include: "I think ... don't you?" and "Isn't that right?"
Suggested responses: (a) it is best to keep personal opinion to oneself and only to give information that would aid the client's orientation to reality; (b) if you give an opinion as a *model* of orienting to reality, ask client to *state his/her* opinion ("My opinion is this .... What is your opinion?").

8. *Probing* and/or *offering premature solutions and interpretations;* jumping to conclusions—
Client: I can't find a job.
Nurse: You could go to an employment agency.
Client: I'd rather not talk about it.
Nurse: What are you unconsciously doing when you say that? What you really mean is ....
Client: I don't want to live alone.
Nurse: Are you afraid of starting to drink again?
Suggested responses: use responses that seek clarification and elicit more data.

9. *Changing client's words* without prior validation—
Client: I am *not feeling well* today.
Nurse: What makes you feel so *depressed?*
Suggested response: "In what way are you not feeling well?" Use the same language as the client.

10. *Following vague content* as if understood or *using vague global* pronouns, adverbs, and adjectives—
Client: *People* are so *unfair.*
Nurse: I know what you mean.
Suggested response: clarify vague referents such as "people" and "unfair."
Client: I feel sad.
Nurse: *Everyone feels that way* at one time or another.
Suggested response: "What are you sad about?"

11. *Questioning on different topics without waiting for a reply—*
Client: [Remains silent.]
Nurse: What makes you so silent? Are you angry? Would you like to be alone?
Suggested response: choose one of the above and wait for a response before asking the next question.

12. *Ignoring client's questions or comments*—
   Client: Am I crazy, nurse?
   Nurse: [Walking away as if he did not hear her.]
   Suggested responses: "I can't understand what makes you bring this up at this time," or "Tell me what makes you bring this up at this time." Ignoring questions or comments usually implies that the nurse is feeling uncomfortable. It is important not to "run away" from the client.

13. *Closing off exploration* with questions that can be answered by "yes" or "no"—
   Client: I'll never get better.
   Nurse: Is something making you feel that way?
   Suggested response: "What makes you feel that way?" Use open-ended questions that start with *what, who, when, where,* etc.

14. *Using clichés* or stereotyped expressions—
   Client: The doctor took away my weekend pass.
   Nurse: The doctor is only doing what's best for you. Doctor knows best. [Comment: also an example of moralizing.]
   Suggested response: "Tell me what happened when the doctor took away your weekend pass."

15. *Overloading:* giving too much information at one time—
   Nurse: Hello, I'm Mr. Brown. I'm a nurse here. I'll be here today, but I'm off tomorrow. Ms. Anderson will assign you another nurse tomorrow. This unit has five RNs, three LVNs, and students from three nursing schools who will all be taking care of you at some time.
   Suggested response: "Hello, I'm Mr. Brown, your nurse today." Keep your initial orienting information simple and brief.

16. *Underloading:* not giving enough information so that meaning is not clear; withholding information—
   Client: What are visiting hours like here?
   Nurse: They are flexible and liberal.
   Suggested response: "They are flexible and liberal, from 10 A.M. to 12 noon and from 6 to 8 P.M." Use specific terms and give specific information.

17. *Saying no without saying no*—
   Client: Can we go for a walk soon?
   Nurse: We'll see.

Perhaps.
Maybe.
Later.
   Suggested response: "I will check the schedule in the nursing office and let you know within an hour." Vague, ambiguous responses can be seen as "putting the client off." It is best to be clear, specific, and direct.

18. *Using double-bind communication;* sending conflicting messages that do not have "mutual fit" or are incongruent—
   Nurse [continuing to stay and talk with the client]: It's time for you to rest.
   Suggested response: "It's time for you to rest and for me to leave [proceeding to leave]."

19. *Protecting;* defending someone else while talking with client; implying client has no right to personal opinions and feelings—
   Client: This hospital is no good. No one cares here.
   Nurse: This is an excellent hospital. All the staff were chosen for their warmth and concern for people.
   Suggested response: focus on feeling tone or clarifying information.

20. *Asking "why" questions* implies that the person has immediate conscious awareness of the reasons for his/her feelings and behaviors—examples of this include: "Why don't you?" "Why did you do that?" or "Why do you feel this way?"
   Suggested response: ask clarifying questions like "how," "what," etc.

21. *Coercion;* using the interaction between people to force someone to do *your* will, with the implication that if they don't "do it for your sake," you won't love them or stay with them—
   Client: I refuse to talk with him.
   Nurse: *Do it for my sake,* before it's too late.
   Suggested response: "Something keeps you from wanting to talk with him?"

22. Focusing on *negative* feelings, thoughts, actions—
   Client: I can't sleep; I can't eat; I can't think; I can't do anything.
   Nurse: How long have you not been sleeping, eating, or thinking well?
   Suggested response: "What *do* you do?"

23. *Rejecting* client's behavior or ideas—
   Client: Let's talk about incest.
   Nurse: Incest is a bad thing to talk about; I don't want to.

Suggested response: "What do you want to say about incest?"

24. *Accusing, belittling—*
    Client: I've had to wait five minutes for you to change my dressing.
    Nurse: Don't be so demanding. Don't you see that I have several people who need me?
    Suggested response: "It must have been hard to wait for me to come when you wanted it to be right away."

25. *Evading a response* by asking a question in return—
    Client: I want to know your opinion, nurse. Am I crazy?
    Nurse: Do you think you are crazy?
    Suggested response: "I don't know. What do you mean by crazy?"

26. *Circumstantiality;* communicating in such a way that the main point is only reached after many side comments, details, and additions—
    Client: Will you go out on a date with me?
    Nurse: I work every evening. On my day off I usually go out of town. I have a steady boyfriend. Besides that, I am a nurse and you are a client. Thank you for asking me, but no, I will not date you.
    Suggested response: abbreviate your response to: "Thank you for asking me, but no, I will not date you."

27. *Making assumptions* without checking them out—
    Client: [Standing in the kitchen by the sink, peeling onions, with tears in her eyes.]
    Nurse: What's making you so sad?
    Client: I'm not sad. Peeling onions always makes my eyes water.
    Suggested response: use simple acknowledgment and acceptance initially, such as "I notice you have tears in your eyes."

28. *Giving false fear reassurance—*
    Client: I'm scared.
    Nurse: Don't worry; everything will be all right. There's nothing to be afraid of.
    Suggested response: "I'd like to hear about what you're afraid of, so that together we can see what could be done to help you." Open the way for clarification and exploration and offer yourself as a helping person—not someone with magic answers.

ANXIETY

Anxiety is a subjective warning of danger in which the specific nature of the danger is usually not known. It occurs when a person faces a new, unknown, or untried situation. Anxiety is also felt when a person perceives threat in terms of past experiences. It is a general concept underlying most disease states. In its milder form, anxiety can contribute to learning and is necessary for problem-solving. In its severe form, anxiety can impede a client's treatment and recovery. The general feelings elicited on all levels of anxiety are nervousness, tension, and apprehension.

It is essential that nurses recognize their own sources of anxiety and behavior in response to anxiety, as well as help clients recognize the manifestations of anxiety in themselves.

1. Assessment of anxiety
A. *Physiologic* manifestations:
   1. Increased heart rate and palpitations.
   2. Increased rate and depth of respiration.
   3. Increased urinary frequency and diarrhea.
   4. Dry mouth.
   5. Decreased appetite.
   6. Cold sweat and pale appearance.
   7. Increased menstrual flow.
   8. Increased or decreased body temperature.
   9. Increased or decreased blood pressure.
   10. Dilated pupils.
B. *Behavioral* manifestations—stages of anxiety:
   1. *Mild anxiety—*
      a. Increased perception (visual and auditory).
      b. Increased awareness of meanings and relationships.
      c. Increased alertness (notice more).
      d. Ability to utilize problem-solving process.
   2. *Moderate anxiety—*
      a. Selective inattention (for example, may not hear someone talking).
      b. Decreased perceptual field.
      c. Concentration on relevant data; "tunnel vision."
      d. Muscular tension, perspiration, GI discomfort.
   3. *Severe anxiety—*
      a. Focus on many fragmented details.
      b. Physical and emotional discomfort (headache, nausea, dizziness, dread, horror, trembling).
      c. Not aware of total environment.
      d. Automatic behavior aimed at getting immediate relief instead of problem-solving.

e. Poor recall.

f. Inability to see connections between details.

g. Drastically reduced awareness.

4. *Panic state of anxiety*—

a. Increased speed of scatter; does not notice what goes on.

b. Increased distortion and exaggeration of details.

c. Feeling of terror.

d. Dissociation (hallucinations, loss of reality, and little memory).

e. Inability to cope with any problems; no self-control.

2. Concepts and principles of anxiety

A. *Causes of anxiety:*

1. Threats to biologic well-being (food, drink, pain, and fever, for example).

2. Threats to self-esteem—

a. Unmet wishes or expectations.

b. Unmet needs for prestige and status.

c. Inability to cope with environment.

d. Not utilizing own full potential.

e. Alienation.

f. Value conflicts.

g. Anticipated disapproval from a significant other.

h. Guilt.

B. *Reactions to anxiety:*

1. *Fight*—

a. Aggression.

b. Hostility, derogation, belittling.

c. Anger.

2. *Flight*—

a. Withdrawal.

b. Depression.

3. *Somatization* (psychosomatic disorders).

4. *Learning,* searching for causes of anxiety, and identifying behavior.

3. Nursing interventions in anxiety

A. *Moderate to severe anxiety:*

1. Provide motor outlet for tension energy, such as working at a simple, concrete task, walking, crying, or talking.

2. Help clients *recognize* their anxieties by talking about how they are behaving and exploring their underlying feelings.

3. Help the clients *gain insight* into their anxieties by helping them to understand how their behavior has been an expression of anxiety and to recognize the threat that lies behind this anxiety.

4. Help the clients *cope* with the threat behind their anxieties by reevaluating the threats and learning new ways to deal with them.

B. *Panic state:*

1. Give simple, clear, concise directions.

2. Avoid decision-making by client.

3. Stay with the client; walk.

4. Avoid touching.

5. Do not isolate.

6. Do not try to reason with client as he is irrational and cannot cooperate.

7. Allow client to seek motor outlets.

8. Encourage activity that requires no thought.

COPING MECHANISMS

Coping mechanisms (ego defense mechanisms or mental mechanisms) consist of all the *coping* means used by individuals to seek relief from emotional conflict and to ward off excessive anxiety.

1. Definitions *

blocking a disturbance in the rate of speech when a person's thoughts and speech are proceeding at an average rate but are very suddenly and completely interrupted, perhaps even in the middle of a sentence. The gap may last several seconds up to a minute. Blocking is often a part of the thought disorder found in schizophrenic disorders.

compensation making up for real or imagined handicap, limitation, or lack of gratification in one area of personality by overemphasis in another area to counter the effects of failure, frustration, and limitation; for example, the blind compensate by increased sensitivity in hearing; the unpopular student compensates by becoming an outstanding scholar; small men compensate for short stature by demanding a great deal of attention and respect; a nurse who does not have manual dexterity decides to go into psychiatric nursing.

confabulating filling in gaps of memory by inventing what appear to be suitable memories as replacements. This symptom may occur in various organic psychoses but is most often seen in Korsakoff's syndrome (deterioration due to alcohol) and in organic mental disorders.

conversion psychologic difficulties are translated into physical symptoms *without conscious* will or knowledge; for example, pain and immobility on moving your writing arm the day of the exam.

---

*From Kalkman, M.: Psychiatric nursing, ed. 3, New York, 1967, © McGraw-Hill Book Company, pp. 88–93.

denial   an intolerable thought, wish, need, or reality factor is disowned automatically; for example, a student, when told of a failing grade, acts as if he never heard of such a possibility.

displacement   transferring the emotional component from one idea, object, or situation to another more acceptable one. Displacement occurs because these are painful or dangerous feelings that cannot be expressed toward the original object; for example, kicking the dog after a bad day at school or work; anger with clinical instructor gets transferred to classmate who was late to meet you for lunch.

dissociation   splitting off or separation of different elements of the mind from each other. There can be separation of ideas, concepts, emotions, or experiences from the rest of the mind. Dissociated material is deeply repressed and becomes encapsulated and inaccessible to the rest of the mind. This usually occurs as a result of some very painful experience, for example, split of affect from idea in anxiety disorders and schizophrenics.

fixation   a state in which personality development is arrested in one or more aspects at a level short of maturity.

idealization   overestimation of some admired aspect or attribute of another person.

ideas of reference   fixed, false ideas and interpretations of external events as though they had direct reference to self.

identification   the wish to be like another person; situation in which qualities of another are unconsciously transferred to oneself; for example, boy identifies with his father and learns to become a man; a woman may fear she will die in childbirth because her mother did; a student adopts attitudes and behavior of her favorite teacher.

introjection   incorporation into the personality, without assimilation, of emotionally charged impulses or objects; a quality or an attribute of another person is taken into and made part of self; for example, a girl in love introjects the personality of her lover into herself—his ideas become hers, his tastes and wishes are hers; this is also seen in severe depression following death of someone close—patient may assume many of deceased's characteristics; similarly, working in a psychiatric unit with a suicidal person brings out depression in the nurse.

isolation   temporary or long-term splitting off of certain feelings or ideas from others; separating emotional and intellectual content; for example, talking emotionlessly about a traumatic accident.

projection   attributes and transfers own feelings, attitudes, impulses, wishes, or thoughts to another person or object in the environment, especially when ideas or impulses are too painful to be acknowledged as belonging to oneself; for example, in hallucinations and delusions by alcoholics; or, "I flunked the course because the teacher doesn't know how to teach," and "I hate him" reversed into "He hates me," or a student impatiently accusing an instructor of being intolerant.

rationalization   justification of behavior by formulating a logical, socially approved reason for past, present, or proposed behavior. Commonly used, conscious or unconscious, with false or real reason. For example, upon losing a class election, a student states she really did not want all the extra work and is glad she lost.

reaction formation   going to the opposite extreme from what one wishes to do or is afraid one might do; for example, being overly concerned with cleanliness when one wishes to be messy, being an overly protective mother through fear of own hostility to child, or showing great concern for a person whom you dislike, going out of your way to do special favors.

regression   when individuals fail to solve a problem with the usual methods at their command, they may resort to modes of behavior that they have outgrown but that proved themselves successful at an earlier stage of development; retracing developmental steps; going back to earlier interests or modes of gratification. For example, a senior nursing student about to graduate becomes dependent on his clinical instructor for directions.

repression   involuntary exclusion of painful and unacceptable thoughts and impulses from awareness. *Forgetting* these things solves the situation by not solving it; for example, by not remembering what was on the difficult exam after it was over.

sublimation   channeling a destructive or instinctual impulse that cannot be realized into a *socially acceptable*, practical, and less dangerous outlet, with some relation to the original impulse for emotional satisfaction to be obtained; for example, sublimation of sexual energy in other creative activities (art, music, or literature) or hostility and aggression into sports or business competition; or an infertile person putting all energies into pediatric nursing.

substitution   when individuals cannot have what they wish and accept something else in its place for symbolic satisfaction, for example, pin-up pictures in absence of sexual object, or a person who failed an RN exam signing up for an LVN exam.

suppression a deliberate process of blocking from the conscious mind thoughts, feelings, acts, and impulses that are undesirable, for example, "I don't want to talk about it," "Don't mention his name to me," or "I'll think about it some other time"; or willfully deciding to refuse to think about or discuss disappointment with exam results.

symbolism sign language that stands for many related ideas and feelings, conscious and unconscious. Used extensively by children, primitive peoples, and psychotic patients. There is meaning attached to this sign language that makes it very important to the individual. For example, a student wears dark, somber clothing to the exam site.

undoing a coping mechanism against anxiety, usually unconscious, designed to negate or neutralize a previous act; for example, Lady Macbeth's attempt to wash her hands (of guilt) after the murder. A repetitious, symbolic acting out in reverse of an unacceptable act already completed.

2. Characteristics of coping mechanisms

A. Coping mechanisms are utilized to some degree by everyone occasionally; they are normal processes by which the ego reestablishes equilibrium unless used to extreme degree, in which case they interfere with maintenance of self-integrity.
B. Much overlapping:
   1. Same behavior can be explained by more than one mechanism.
   2. May be used in combination—e.g., isolation and repression, denial and projection.
C. Common defense mechanisms compatible with mental well-being:
   1. Compensation.
   2. Compromise.
   3. Identification.
   4. Rationalization.
   5. Sublimation.
   6. Substitution.
D. Typical coping mechanisms in:
   1. *Paranoids*—denial, projection.
   2. *Dissociative disorders*—denial, repression.
   3. *Obsessive-compulsives*—displacement, reaction-formation, isolation, denial, repression.
   4. *Phobias*—displacement, rationalization, repression.
   5. *Conversion disorders*—symbolization, dissociation, repression, isolation, denial.
   6. *Depression*—displacement.
   7. *Manic-depressives*—reaction-formation, denial, projection, introjection.
   8. *Schizophrenics*—symbolization, repression, dissociation, denial, fantasy, regression, projection.
   9. *Organic disorders*—regression.

3. Concepts and principles related to coping mechanisms

A. Unconscious process—coping mechanisms are used as a substitute for more effective problem-solving behavior.
B. *Main functions*—increase *self-esteem;* decrease, inhibit, minimize, alleviate, avoid, or eliminate anxiety; maintain feelings of personal worth and adequacy and soften failures; *protect the ego; increase security.*
C. *Drawbacks*—involve high degree of self-deception and reality distortion; may be maladaptive because they superficially eliminate or disguise conflicts, leaving conflicts unresolved but still influencing behavior.

4. Nursing interventions with coping mechanisms

A. Accept coping mechanisms as normal, but not when overused.
B. Look beyond the behavior to the need that is expressed by the use of the coping mechanism.
C. Discuss alternative coping mechanisms that may be more compatible with mental health.
D. Assist the person to translate defensive thinking into nondefensive, direct thinking; a problem-solving approach to conflicts minimizes the need to use coping mechanisms.

COMMON BEHAVIORAL PROBLEMS

1. Anger

A. Definition: feelings of resentment in response to anxiety when threat is perceived; need to discharge tension of anger.
B. *Analyze source of stress of anger* (stressors):
   1. *Biologic stressors*—instinctual drives (Lorenz, on aggressive instincts, and Freud), endocrine imbalances, seizures, tumors, hunger, fatigue.
   2. *Psychologic stressors*—frustration leads to aggression; real or imagined threatened loss of self-esteem; conflict, lack of control; anger as a learned, reinforced response.

3. *Socio-cultural stressors*—crowding, personal space intrusion, role-modeling of abusive behavior by significant others and by media personalities.
C. Assess *degree of anger and frequency*.
  1. Scope of anger ranges on a continuum from everyday mild annoyance → frustration from interference with goal accomplishment → assertiveness (behavior used to deal with anger effectively) → anger related to helplessness and powerlessness that may interfere with functioning → rage and fury, when coping means are depleted or not developed.
D. Assess *mode of expression of anger:*
  1. *Covert,* passive expression of anger: being overly nice; body language with little or no eye contact, arms close to body, soft voice, little gesturing; sarcasm through humor; sublimation through art and music; projection onto others; denying and pushing anger out of awareness; psychosomatic illness in response to internalized anger, e.g., headache.
  2. *Overt,* active expression of anger: physical activity to work off excess physical energy associated with biologic response (e.g., hitting punching bag, taking a walk); aggression, assertiveness.
E. *Assess physiologic behaviors*—result of secretion of epinephrine and sympathetic nervous system stimulation preparing for fight-flight.
  1. *Cardiovascular* response: increased blood pressure and pulse, increased free fatty acid in blood.
  2. *Gastrointestinal* response: increased nausea, salivation, decreased peristalsis.
  3. *Genito-urinary* response: urinary frequency.
  4. *Neuromuscular* response: increased alertness, increased muscle tension and deep tendon reflexes, ECG changes.
F. *Positive functions of anger:*
  1. Energizes behavior.
  2. Protects positive image.
  3. Provides ego defense during high anxiety.
  4. Gives greater control over situation.
  5. Alerts to need for coping.
  6. A sign of a healthy relationship.
G. *Interventions*—long-term goals: constructive use of angry energy to accomplish tasks and motivate growth.
  1. Promote self-awareness and problem-solving abilities. Encourage and assist client to:
    a. Accept self as a person with a right to experience angry feelings.
    b. Explore reasons for anger.

c. Describe situations where anger was experienced.
d. Discuss appropriate alternatives for expressing anger (including assertiveness training).
e. Decide on one feasible solution.
f. Act on solution.
g. Evaluate effectiveness.
  2. Limit-setting and control of violence:
    a. Clearly state expectations and consequences of acts.
    b. Teach client to assume responsibility for behavior.
    c. Enforce consequences.
    d. Explore reasons and meaning of negative behavior.
    e. Explore other ways to express feelings and provide activities that allow appropriate expression of anger.

2. Combative-aggressive behavior
A. *Definition:* acting out feelings of frustration, anger, anxiety, etc., through physical or verbal behavior.
B. *Analysis—causes:*
  1. Frustration as response to breakdown of self-control coping mechanisms.
  2. Acting out used as customary response to anger.
  3. Confusion.
  4. Physical restraints, such as when postoperative patient discovers wrist restraints.
  5. Fear of intimacy, intrusion of emotional and physical space.
  6. Feelings of helplessness, inadequacy.
C. *Assessment*—recognize precombative behavior:
  1. Demanding, fist-clenching.
  2. Boisterous, loud.
  3. Vulgar, profane.
  4. Limited attention span.
  5. Sarcastic, taunting, verbal threats.
  6. Restless, agitated, elated.
  7. Frowning.
D. *Interventions:*
  1. *Long-term goal*—channel aggression—help person express feelings rather than act them out.
  2. *Immediate goal*—prevent injury to self and others.
    a. Calmly call for assistance; do not try to handle alone.
    b. Approach cautiously, with eye contact, observing client's personal space.
    c. Protect against self-injury and injury to

others; be aware of your position in relation to the weapon, door, escape route.

   d. Minimize stimuli to control the environment—clear the area, close doors, turn off TV so person can hear you.

   e. Divert attention from the act; engage in talk and lead away from others.

   f. Assess triggering cause.

   g. Identify immediate problem.

   h. Focus on remedy for immediate problem.

   i. Choose one calm, quieting individual to interact with person; nonauthoritarian, nonthreatening.

   j. Maintain verbal contact to keep communication open; offer empathetic ear but be firm and consistent in setting limits on dangerous behavior.

   k. Negotiate, but don't make false promises or argue.

   l. Restraints may be necessary as a last resort.

   m. Place person in quiet room so he/she can calm down.

3. Demanding behavior

A. *Definition:* a strong and persistent struggle to obtain satisfaction of self-oriented needs (such as control, self-esteem) or relief from anxiety.

B. *Analysis—causes:*
1. Feelings of helplessness and hopelessness.
2. Feelings of powerlessness and fear.
3. A way of coping with anxiety.

C. *Assessment:*
1. Attention-seeking behavior.
2. Multiple requests.
3. Frequency of questions.
4. Lack of reasonableness; irrationality of request.

D. *Interventions:*
1. *Long-term goal*—teach and encourage appropriate methods to gain attention.
   a. Control own irritation; assess reasons for own annoyance.
   b. Confront with behavior; discuss reasons for behavior.
   c. Anticipate and meet client's needs; set time to discuss requests.
   d. Ignore negative attention-seeking and reinforce appropriate requests for attention.
   e. Make plans with entire staff to set limits.
   f. Set up contractual arrangement for brief, frequent, regular, uninterrupted attention.

4. Denial of illness

A. *Definition:* an attempt or refusal to acknowledge some anxiety-provoking aspect of oneself or external reality.

B. *Analysis—causes:*
1. Untenable wishes, needs, ideas, deeds, or reality factors.
2. Inability to accept changes in body image or role perception.
3. Under intense stress and anxiety.

C. *Assessment:*
1. Observe for coping mechanisms such as dissociation, repression, selective inattention, suppression, displacement of concern to another person.
2. Note behaviors that may indicate denial of diagnosis—
   a. Failure to follow treatment plan.
   b. Missed appointment.
   c. Refusal of medication.
   d. Inappropriate cheerfulness.
   e. Ignoring symptoms.
   f. Use of humor.
   g. Use of second or third person in reference to illness.
   h. Flight into wellness, overactivity.
3. Use of earliest and most primitive defense by closing eyes, turning head away to separate from what is unpleasant and anxiety-provoking.
4. While observing fantasy play of children, note where they blot out unpleasant reality.
5. Note *range* of denial: *explicit* verbal denial of obvious facts, disowning or *ignoring* aspects or *minimizing* by understatement.
6. Be aware of situations such as long-term physical disability that make people more prone to denial of anger. Denial of illness protects the ego from overwhelming anxiety.

D. *Interventions:*
1. *Long-term goal*—understand needs met by denial.
2. *Short-term goal*—avoid reinforcing denial patterns.
   a. Recognize behavioral cues of denial of some reality aspect; be aware of level of awareness and degree to which reality is excluded.
   b. Determine if denial interferes with treatment.
   c. Support moves toward greater reality orientation.
   d. Determine person's stress tolerance.

e. Supportively help person discuss events leading to, and feelings about, hospitalization.

5. Dependence

A. *Definition:* reliance on other people to meet basic needs, usually for love and affection, security and protection, and support and guidance.

B. *Analysis—causes:*
1. Low self-esteem.
2. Feelings of helplessness and hopelessness.
3. Holding a belief that one's own actions cannot affect life situations.

C. *Assessment:*
1. Excessive need for advice and answers to problems.
2. Lack of confidence in own decision-making ability and lack of confidence in self-sufficiency.
3. Clinging, too trusting behavior.
4. Gestures, facial expressions, body posture, recurrent themes conveying "I'm helpless."

D. *Interventions:*
1. *Long-term goal*—increase self-esteem, confidence in own abilities.
2. *Short-term goals*—provide activities that promote independence.
   a. *Limit-setting*—clear, firm, consistent; acknowledge when demands are made; accept client but refuse to respond to demands.
   b. *Break cycle* of: nurse avoids client when he/she is clinging and demanding → client's anxiety increases → demands for attention increase → frustration and avoidance on nurse's part increase.
   c. *Give attention* before demand exists.
   d. Use behavior modification approaches—
      (1) Reward appropriate behavior (such as making decisions, helping others, caring for own needs) with attention and praise.
      (2) Give no response to attention-seeking, dependent, infantile behavior; goal is to increase incidence of mature behavior as client realizes little gratification from dependent behavior.
   e. *Avoid secondary gains* of being cared for, which impede progress toward above goals.
   f. Assist in developing *ability to control* panic by responding less to client's high anxiety level.
   g. Help client develop ways to seek gratification other than excessive turning to others.
   h. Resist urge to act like a parent when client becomes helpless, demanding, and attention-seeking.
   i. *Promote decision-making* by not giving advice.
   j. *Encourage accountability* for own feelings, thoughts, and behaviors.
      (1) Help identify feelings through nonverbal cues, thoughts, recurrent themes.
      (2) Convey expectations that client does have opinions and feelings to share.
      (3) Role model how to express feelings.
   k. *Reinforce self-esteem* and ability to work out problems independently. (Consistently ask: "How do you feel about. . . ." "What do you think?")
   l. Teach family ways of interacting to enforce less dependency.

6. Manipulation

A. Definition: process of playing upon and using others by unfair, insidious means to serve own purpose without regard for others' needs; may take many forms; occurs consciously, unconsciously to some extent, in all interpersonal relations.

B. Operational definition (Figure 2–4):
1. Conflicting needs, goals exist between client and other person (e.g., nurse).
2. Other person perceives need as unacceptable, unreasonable.
3. Other person refuses to accept client's need.
4. Client's tension increases and he begins to relate to others as objects.
5. Client increases attempts to influence others to fulfill his need.
   a. Appears unaware of others' needs.
   b. Exhibits excessive dependency, helplessness, demands.
   c. Sets others at odds (especially staff).
   d. Rationalizes, gives logical reasons.
   e. Uses deception, false promises, insincerity.
   f. Questions and defies nurse's authority and competence.
6. Nurse feels powerless and angry at having been used.

C. *Analysis—contributing causes:*
1. Mistrust and contemptuous view of others' motivations.
2. Life experience of rejection, deception.
3. Low anxiety tolerance.

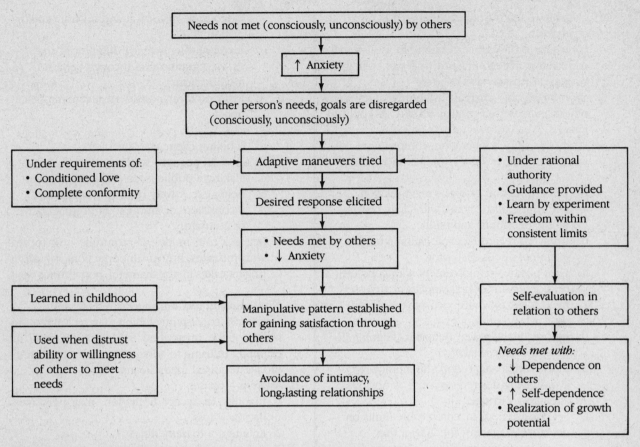

FIGURE 2–4. *Operationalization of concept–manipulation.*

4. Inability to cope with tension.
5. Unmet dependency needs.
6. Need to avoid anxiety when cannot obtain gratification.
7. Need to obtain something that is forbidden, or need for instant gratification.
8. Attempt to put something over on another when no real advantage exists.
9. Intolerance of intimacy, maneuvering effectively to keep others at a safe distance in order to dilute the relationship by withdrawing and frustrating others or distracting attention away from self.
10. Attempt to demand attention, approval, disapproval.
D. Assessment:
1. Acts out sexually, physically.
2. Dawdles, always last minute.
3. Uses insincere flattery; expects special favors, privileges.
4. Exploits generosity and fears of others.
5. Feels no guilt.

6. Plays staff against one another.
7. Tests limits set.
8. Finds weaknesses in others.
9. Makes excessive, unreasonable, unnecessary demands for staff time.
10. Pretends to be helpless, lonely, distraught, tearful.
11. Can't distinguish betwen truth and falsehood.
12. Plays on sympathy or guilt.
13. Offers many excuses, lacks insight.
14. Pursues unpleasant issues without genuine regard or feelings for individuals involved.
15. Intimidates, derogates, threatens, bargains, cajoles, violates rules to obtain reactions or privileges.
16. Betrays information.
17. Uses communication as a medium for manipulation; as verbal, nonverbal means to get others to cooperate, to behave in certain way, to get something from another for own use.
18. May be coercive, illogical, or skillfully deceptive.

19. Unable to learn from experience.
E. *Interventions:*
  1. *Long-term goal*—define relationship as a mutual experience in learning and trust rather than a struggle for power and control.
  2. *Short-term goal*—increase awareness of self and others; increase self-control; learn to accept limitations.
  3. Promote use of cooperation, compromise, collaboration, rather than exploitation or deception.
  4. Decrease level and extent of manipulation.
    a. Set firm, realistic goals, with clear, consistent expectations and limits.
    b. Confront regarding exploitation attempts; examine, discuss behavior.
    c. Give positive reinforcement with concrete reinforcers for nonmanipulation, to lessen need for exploitative, deceptive, and self-destructive behaviors.
    d. Ignore "wooden-leg" behavior (feigning illness to evoke sympathy).
    e. Allow verbal anger; don't be intimidated; avoid giving desired response to obvious attempts to irritate.
    f. Set consistent, firm, enforceable limits on *destructive,* aggressive behavior that impinges on others' health, rights, and interests, and on excessive dependency; give reasons when can't meet requests.
    g. Keep staff informed of rules and reasons; obtain staff *consensus.*
    h. Enforce *direct* communication; encourage openness about *real* needs, feelings.
    i. Do not accept gifts, favors, flattery, or other guises of manipulation.
  5. Increase responsibility for self-control of actions.
    a. Decide who (client, nurse) is responsible for what.
    b. Provide opportunities for success to increase self-esteem, experiencing acceptance by others.
    c. Evaluate actions, *not* verbal behavior; point out the difference between talk and action.
    d. Support efforts to be responsible.
    e. Assist client to increase emotional repertoire; explore alternative ways of relating interpersonally.
    f. Avoid submission to control based on fear of punishment, retaliation, loss of affection.
  6. Facilitate awareness of, and responsibility for, manipulative behavior and its effects on others.
    a. Reflect back client's behavior.

    b. Discourage distortion and misuse of information.
    c. Increase tolerance for differences and delayed gratification through behavior modification.
    d. Insist on clear, consistent staff communication.
  7. Avoid—
    a. Labeling client as a "problem."
    b. Hostile, negative attitude.
    c. Making a public issue of client's behavior.
    d. Being excessively rigid or permissive, inconsistent or ambiguous, argumentative or accusatory.
  8. Act as a role model; demonstrate how to deal with mistakes, human imperfections, by admitting mistakes in nonshameful, nonvirtuous ways.

7. Noncompliant and uncooperative behavior
A. *Definition:* consistently failing to meet the requirements of the prescribed treatment regimen; for example, refusing to adhere to dietary restrictions or take required medications.
B. *Analysis—causes:*
  1. Inability to accept limitation; may perceive a limit as a loss.
  2. An attempt to *deny* illness.
  3. *Acting* out of anger and frustration.
  4. Inability to accept dependence (rebellious counterdependence).
C. *Assessment:*
  1. Refuses to participate in routine or planned activities.
  2. Refuses medication.
  3. Violates rules, ignores limits, and abuses privileges.
D. *Interventions:*
  1. *General goal:* reduce need to act out by nonadherence.
    a. Take preventive action—be alert to signs of noncompliance, such as intent to leave against medical advice.
    b. Explore feelings and reasons for lack of cooperation.
    c. Assess and allay fears in client in reassuring manner.
    d. Provide adequate information about, and reasons for, rules and procedures.
    e. Avoid threats or physical restraints; maintain calm composure.
    f. Demonstrate tact and firmness when confronting violations.
    g. Offer alternatives.

h. Firmly insist on cooperation in selective important activities, but not all activities.

8. Hostility

A. *Definition:* a feeling of intense anger or an attitude of antagonism or animosity, with the destructive component of intent to inflict harm and pain to another or to self; may involve hate, anger, rage, aggression, regression.

B. *Operational definition:*
1. Past experience of frustration, loss of self-esteem, unmet needs for status, prestige or love.
2. Present expectations of self and others not met.
3. Feelings of humiliation, inadequacy, emotional pain, and conflict.
4. Anxiety experienced and converted into hostility, which can be:
   a. Repressed, with result of becoming withdrawn.
   b. Disowned to the point of overreaction with extreme compliance.
   c. Overtly exhibited: verbal, nonverbal.

C. *Analysis—causes:*
1. A learned means of dealing with the anxiety of an interpersonal threat.
2. A reaction to loss of self-esteem and power.
3. Intense frustration, insecurity, and/or apprehension.

D. *Analysis—situations with high potential for hostility:*
1. Enforced illness and hospitalization cause anxiety, which may be expressed as hostility.
2. Dependency feelings related to acceptance of illness may result in hostility as a coping mechanism.
3. Certain illnesses or physical disabilities may be conducive to hostility.
   a. Preoperative cancer patient may displace hostility onto staff and family.
   b. Postoperatively, if diagnosis is terminal, the family may displace hostility onto nurse.
   c. Anger, hostility is a stage of dying the person may experience.
   d. Amputee may focus frustration on others due to dependency and jealousy.
   e. Patients on hemodialysis are prone to helplessness, which may be displaced as hostility.

E. Assessment:
1. Fault-finding, scapegoating, sarcasm, derision.
2. Arguing, swearing, abusiveness, verbal threatening.
3. Deceptive sweetness, joking at others' expense, gossiping.
4. Physical abusiveness, violence, murder, vindictiveness.

F. *Concepts and principles* (Figure 2–5):
1. Aggression and violence are two outward expressions of hostility.
2. Hostility is often unconscious, automatic response.
3. Hostile wishes and impulses may be underlying motives for many actions.
4. Perceptions may be distorted by hostile outlook.
5. Continuum: from extreme politeness to externalization as murderous rage or homicide; or internalization as depression or suicide.
6. Hostility also seen as a defense *against* depression as well as a *cause* of it.
7. Hostility may be repressed, dissociated, or expressed covertly or overtly.
8. Normal hostility may come from justifiable fear of real danger; irrational hostility stems from anxiety.
9. Developmental roots of hostility—
   a. *In infants:* look away, push away, physically move away from threat; give defiant look. Role-modeling by parents.
   b. *Three-year-olds:* replace overt hostility with protective shyness, retreat, and withdrawal. Feel weak, inadequate in face of powerful person against whom cannot openly ventilate hostility.
   c. Frustrated or unmet needs for status, prestige, or power serve as a basis for *adult* hostility.

G. *Interventions:*
1. *Long-term goal:* help alter response to fear, inadequacy, frustration, threat.
2. *Short-term goal:* express and explore feelings of hostility without injury to self or others.
   a. Remain calm, nonthreatening; endure verbal abuse in unconcerned manner; speak quietly.
   b. Protect from self-harm, acting out.
   c. Discourage hostile behavior while showing acceptance of client.
   d. Offer support to express feelings of frustration, anger, and fear constructively, safely, and appropriately.
   e. Explore hostile feelings without fear of retaliation, disapproval.
   f. *Avoid* arguing, advice-giving, reacting with hostility, punitiveness, fault-finding.
   g. *Avoid* joking, teasing, which can be misinterpreted.

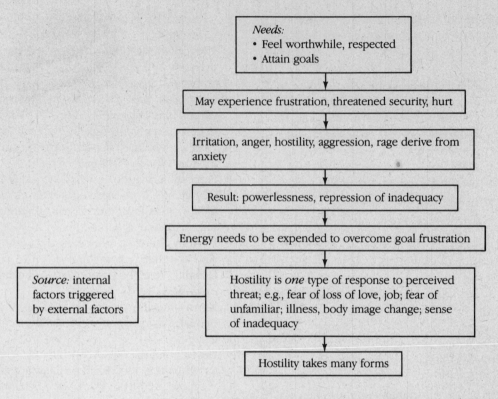

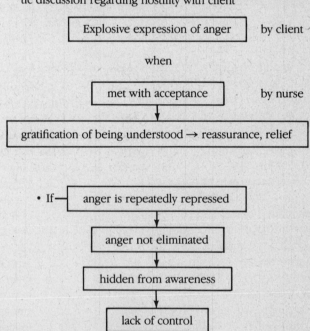

FIGURE 2–5. The concept of hostility operationalized.

h. *Avoid* words like "anger," "hostility"; use client's words ("upset," "irritated").

i. Do not minimize problem or give client reassurance or hasty, general conclusions.

j. Do not stop verbal expression of anger unless detrimental.

k. Respond matter-of-factly to attention-seeking behavior, not defensively.

l. *Avoid* physical contact; allow client to set pace in "closeness."

m. Look for clues to antecedent events and focus *directly* on those areas; *do not evade* or ignore.

n. Constantly focus on *here and now* and affective component, rather than content, of message.

o. Reconstruct what happened and why, discuss client's reactions; seek observations, *not* inferences.

p. Learn how client would like to be treated.

q. Look for ways to help client relate better without defensiveness, *when ready*.

r. Plan to channel feelings into *motor* outlets (occupational and recreational therapy, physical activity, games, debates).

s. Explain procedures beforehand; approach frequently.

t. Withdraw attention, set limits, when acting out.

9. Confusion/disorientation

A. *Definition:* loss of reality orientation as to person, time, place, events, ideas.

B. *Analysis—causes:*

1. *Physical*—metabolic (uremia, diabetes, hepatic dysfunction), cardiac arrhythmias, congestive heart failure; anemia, massive blood loss with low hemoglobin; organic brain disease; nutritional deficiency; pain; sleep disturbance; drugs (antidepressants, tranquilizers, sedatives, antihypertensives, diuretics).

2. *Unfamiliar environment*—unfamiliar routine and people; procedures that threaten body image; noisy equipment.

3. *Loss of sensory acuity* from partial or incomplete reception of orienting stimuli or information.

4. *Disability in screening out* irrelevant and excessive sensory input.

5. *Memory impairment.*

C. *Assessment*—note unusual behavior:

1. Picking, stroking movements in the air, or on clothing and linens.

2. Frequent crying or laughing.

3. Alternating periods of confusion and lucidity (for example, confused at night, when alone in the dark).

4. Fluctuating mood, actions, rationality (argumentative, combative, withdrawn).

5. Increasingly restless, fearful, leading to insomnia, nightmares.

6. Acts bewildered; trouble identifying familiar people.

7. Preoccupied; irritable when interrupted.

8. Lack of response to questions; problem with concentration and setting realistic priorities.

9. Sensitivity to noise and light.

10. Unrealistic perception of time, place, and situation.

11. Nurse no longer seen as supportive, but as threatening.

D. *Interventions:*

1. Check *physical signs;* for example, vital signs, neurologic status, fluid and electrolyte balance, and blood urea nitrogen.

2. Be calm, make contact to *reorient to reality*—

a. Avoid startling if person is alone, in the dark, sedated.

b. Make sure person can see, hear, and talk to you—turn off TV; put on client's glasses, hearing aids, dentures; turn on light.

c. Call by name, clearly and distinctly.

d. Approach cautiously, close to eye level.

e. Keep your hands visible; for example, on bed.

3. *Take care of immediate problem;* for example, disconnected IV tube or catheter.

a. Give instructions slowly and distinctly; avoid threatening tone and comments.

b. Stay with person until reoriented.

c. Put side rails up.

4. Use conversation to *reduce* confusion—

a. Use simple, concrete phrases; language person can understand; repeat as needed.

b. Avoid shouting, arguing, false promises, use of medical abbreviations (for example, NPO).

c. Give more time to concentrate on what you said.

d. Focus on reality-oriented topics or objects in the environment.

5. *Prevent confusion by establishing a reality-oriented relationship*—

a. Introduce self by name.

b. Jointly establish routines to prevent

confusion from unpredictable changes and variations. Determine client's usual routine; attempt to incorporate this to lessen disruption in life style.

   c. Explain what to expect in understandable words—where client is and why, what will happen, noises and activities client will hear and see, people client will meet, tests and procedures client will have.

   d. Find out what meaning hospitalization has to client; reduce anxiety related to feelings of apprehension and helplessness.

   e. Spend as much time as possible with client.

6. *Maintain orientation by providing nonthreatening environment:*
   a. Assign to room near nurse's station.
   b. Surround with familiar objects from home (for example, photos).
   c. Provide clock, calendar, and radio.
   d. Have flexible visiting hours.
   e. Open curtain for natural light.
   f. Keep glasses, dentures, hearing aids nearby.
   g. Check client often, especially at night.
   h. Avoid using intercom to answer calls.
   i. Avoid low-pitched conversation.

7. *Take care of other needs:*
   a. Promote sleep according to usual habits and patterns in order to *prevent sleep deprivation.*
   b. Avoid sedatives, which may lead to or increase confusion.
   c. Promote independent functions, self-help activities, to *maintain dignity.*
   d. Encourage *nutritional* adequacy; incorporate familiar foods, ethnic preferences.
   e. Maintain *routine;* avoid being late with meals, medication, or procedures.
   f. Have *realistic expectations.*
   g. *Discover hidden fears.*
     (1) Do not assume confused behavior is unrelated to reality.
     (2) Look for clues to meaning from client's background, occupation.
   h. *Provide support to family:*
     (1) Encourage expression of feelings; avoid being judgemental.
     (2) Explain possible causes of confusion.
     (3) Reassure that it is common.
     (4) Teach how to react to confused behavior.
     (5) Check what worked in previous situations.

10. *Immobility*

A. Definition: "prescribed or unavoidable restriction of movement in any area of person's life" (Carnevali, 1970).

B. Analysis—types of immobility:
  1. *Physical*—physical restriction due to limitation in movement or physiologic processes (e.g., breathing).
  2. *Intellectual*—lack of action due to lack of knowledge (e.g., mental retardation, brain damage).
  3. *Emotional*—immobilized when highly stressed (e.g., after loss of loved person or diagnosis of terminal illness).
  4. *Social*—decreased social interaction due to separation from family when hospitalized, or when alone, as in aged.

C. Assessment of *physical* effects of immobility:
  1. Cardiovascular—
    a. Orthostatic hypotension.
    b. Increased cardiac load.
    c. Thrombus formation.
  2. Gastrointestinal—
    a. Anorexia.
    b. Diarrhea.
    c. Constipation.
  3. Metabolic—
    a. Tissue atrophy and protein catabolism.
    b. BMR reduced.
    c. Fluid-electrolyte imbalances.
  4. Musculoskeletal—
    a. Demineralization (osteoporosis).
    b. Contractures and atrophy.
    c. Skin breakdown.
  5. Respiratory—
    a. Decreased respiratory movement.
    b. Accumulation of secretions in respiratory tract.
    c. O_2/CO_2 ratio imbalance.
  6. Urinary—
    a. Calculi.
    b. Bladder distention.
    c. Incontinence.
    d. Infection.
    e. Frequency.

D. Assessment of *psychologic/social* effects of immobility:
  1. Decreased motivation to learn; decreased retention.
  2. Decreased problem-solving abilities.
  3. Diminished drives; hunger and emotions (result: apathy, withdrawal, aggression).
  4. Changes in body image, self-concept.

5. Exaggerated emotional reactions, inappropriate to situation or person.
6. Deterioration of time perception.
7. Fear, anxiety, worthlessness related to change in role activities, e.g., when no longer employed.

E. *Interventions*—general goal: prevent physical, psychologic hazards.
   1. Prevent *physical hazards* of decreased mobility. Apply nursing measures to promote venous flow, muscle strength, endurance, joint mobility, skin integrity.
   2. Assess and counteract *psychological* impact of immobility (e.g., feelings of helplessness, hopelessness, powerlessness).
   3. Help maintain accurate sensory processing to prevent and lessen *sensory disturbances*. (See section on sensory disturbances.)
   4. Help adapt to *altered body image* due to increased dependency, sensory deprivation, and changes in status and power which accompany immobility. (See section on body image.)
   5. Offer counseling when sexual expression is impaired. (See section on sex.)

11. Pain

A. *Characteristics of pain:*
   1. Highly unpleasant.
   2. Personal, cannot be shared.
   3. Can occupy thinking, change one's life.
   4. May be a sign of health problem.
   5. Usually accompanied by other sensations such as pressure, heat, or cold.
   6. May be *acute, chronic, intractable.*

B. *Analysis—types of pain:*
   1. *Superficial somatic tissues*—skin, subcutaneous or fibrous tissue, ligaments have pain receptors and thus pain is localized.
   2. *Deep somatic tissues and viscera*—may be diffuse and radiating pain because do not have direct connection with sensory-discriminative system.
   3. *Neurogenic pain*—results from damage to peripheral or central nervous system; any sensation perceived as pain due to abnormal processing of afferent impulses or paroxysmal activity.
   4. *Psychogenic pain*—due to fantasies and need for injury or punishment (called conversion).

C. *Analysis—components of pain experience:*
   1. *Stimuli*—sources: chemical, ischemic, mechanical trauma, extremes of heat/cold.
   2. *Perception*—viewed with fear by children, can be altered by level of consciousness, interpreted and influenced by previous and current experience, is more severe when alone at night or immobilized.
   3. *Response*—variations in physiologic, cultural, and learned responses; anxiety is created; pain seen as justified punishment; pain as means for attention-getting.

D. *Assessment:*
   1. *Site*—medial, lateral, proximal, distal.
   2. *Strength:*
      a. Certain tissues are more sensitive.
      b. Change in intensity.
      c. Based on expectations.
      d. Affected by distraction or concentration, state of consciousness.
      e. Described as slight, medium, severe, excruciating.
   3. *Time/duration*—onset, duration, recurrence, interval, last occurrence.
   4. *Quality*—aching, burning, crushing, dull, piercing, shifting, throbbing, tingling.
   5. *Antecedent factors*—physical exertion, eating, extreme temperatures, physical and emotional stressors (fear, for example).
   6. *Previous experience*—influences reaction to pain.
   7. *Nonverbal clues*—clenching teeth, grimacing, splinting of body parts, body position, knees drawn up, involuntary reflex movements, tossing/turning, rhythmic rubbing movements, voice pitch and speed, eyes shut.
   8. *Verbal clues*—moaning, groaning, crying.
   9. *Behavioral clues*—demanding, worried, irritable, restless, difficult to distract, sleepless.
   10. *Physical clues*—breathing irregularities, abdominal distention, skin color changes, skin temperature changes, excessive salivation, perspiration.

E. Concepts and principles:
   1. Pain may serve biologic purpose of protection from actual or threatened injury and threat to life.
   2. Pain tends to:
      a. Enforce preoccupation with self and body.
      b. Lead to anticipation of more pain.
      c. Limit awareness, involvement with environment.
   3. Reaction may be autonomic, skeletal-muscular, psychic.
   4. Cerebral cortex—*not* able to sustain more than a certain amount of circuit activity at a given time; *is* able to react *selectively* to stimuli.

5. Modification of pain perception possible by:
   a. Providing interesting diversion.
   b. Providing information, which affects patient's understanding of pain.
   c. Giving hypnotics, ataractics, or analgesics during or prior to pain.
   d. Reassurance, supportive care.
6. Pain perception (intensity), reaction, and action are affected by emotional state, nature of thinking process and past experience.

F. Interventions:
   1. *Long-term goals—*
      a. Relieve pain source.
      b. Decrease stimulation of pain receptors.
      c. Block pain pathway.
      d. Find alternative coping mechanism.
   2. *Short-term goals—*
      a. Provide immediate pain relief.
      b. Take measures to prevent pain.
      c. Determine meaning of pain to person.
   3. Determine cause and try nursing comfort measures before giving drugs.
      a. *Environmental factors:* noise, light, odors, motion.
      b. *Physiologic needs:* elimination, hunger, thirst, fatigue, circulatory impairment, muscle tension, ventilation, pressure on nerves.
      c. *Emotional:* fear of unknown, helplessness, loneliness (especially at night).
   4. Determine pain reactions; explore meaning of "pain" (how much, when, how long, where, why, what it feels like).
   5. Relieve anger, anxiety, boredom, loneliness.
   6. Report sudden, severe, new pain; pain not relieved by medications or comfort measures; pain associated with casts or traction.
   7. *Remove pain stimulus.*
      a. Administer pain medication (e.g., antispasmodic) at appropriate time intervals; do not withhold due to overestimated danger of addiction.
      b. Apply heat (to relieve ischemia).
      c. Change activity (e.g., restrict activity in cardiac pain).
      d. Change, loosen dressing.
      e. Comfort (e.g., smooth wrinkled sheets, change wet dressing).
      f. Give food (e.g., for ulcer).
   8. *Reduce pain receptor reaction.*
      a. Ointment (use as coating).
      b. Local anesthetics.
   c. Padding (of bony prominences).
   9. *Block pain impulse transmission.* Assist with medical/surgical interventions to block pain impulse transmission.
      a. Injection of local anesthetic into nerve (e.g., dental).
      b. Chordotomy—sever anterolateral spinal cord nerve tracts.
      c. Electrical stimulation—transcutaneous (skin surface), percutaneous (peripheral nerve).
      d. Peripheral nerve implant—electrode to major sensory nerve.
      e. Dorsal column stimulator—electrode to dorsal column.
   10. *Alter pain perception* by raising pain threshold.
      a. By *distraction,* e.g., TV (cerebral cortical activity blocks impulses from thalamus).
      b. By *analgesics*—give *prior* to occurrence of severe pain.
      c. By *hypnosis*—assess appropriateness for use for psychogenic pain and for anesthesia; need to be open to suggestion.
      d. *Acupuncture*—assess emotional readiness and belief in it.
   11. *Alter interpretation and response to pain.*
      a. Administer narcotics—result: no longer see pain as disturbing.
      b. Administer hypnotics—result: change perception and decrease reaction.
      c. Help patient obtain interpersonal satisfaction from ways other than attention received when in pain.

12. Sensory disturbance

A. *Types of sensory disturbance:*
   1. *Sensory deprivation*—amount of stimuli less than required, such as isolation in bed or room, deafness, stroke victim.
   2. *Sensory overload*—receive more stimuli than can tolerate, for example, bright lights, noise, strange machinery, barrage of visitors.
   3. *Sensory deficit*—impairment in functioning of sensory or perceptual processes, for example, blindness, changes in tactile perceptions.
B. *Assessment*—based on awareness of behavioral changes:
   1. *Sensory deprivation*—boredom, daydreaming, increasing sleep, thought slowness, inactivity, thought disorganization, hallucinations.
   2. *Sensory overload*—same as above, plus restlessness and agitation, confusion.

3. *Sensory deficit*—may not be able to distinguish sounds, odors, and tastes or differentiate tactile sensations.
C. Interventions:
   1. *Prevention* of sensory disturbance involves education of parents during child's growth and development regarding tactile, auditory and visual stimulation.
      a. Hold, talk, and play with infant when awake.
      b. Provide bright toys with different designs for children to hold.
      c. Change environment.
      d. Provide music and auditory stimuli.
      e. Give foods with variety of textures, tastes, colors.
   2. *Management of existing* sensory disturbances in *acute sensory deprivation:*
      a. Increase interaction with staff.
      b. Use TV.
      c. Provide touch.
      d. Help clients choose menus that have aromas, varied tastes, temperatures, colors, textures.
      e. Use light cologne or after-shave lotion, bath powder.
   3. *Sensory overload:*
      a. Restrict number of visitors and length of stay.
      b. Reduce noise and lights.
      c. Reduce newness by establishing and following routine.
      d. Organize care to provide for extended rest periods with minimal input.
   4. *Sensory deficits:*
      a. Report observations about hearing, vision.
      b. May imply need for new glasses, medical diagnoses, or therapy.

PSYCHIATRIC EMERGENCIES *

1. **Definition**—sudden onset (days or weeks, not years) of unusual (for that individual), disordered (without pattern or purpose), or socially inappropriate behavior caused by emotional or physiologic situation. For example: suicidal feelings or attempts, overdose, acute psychotic reaction, acute alcoholism, acute anxiety.

2. *General assessment*
A. The presence of great distress without reasonable

---

*Adapted from Aguilera, Donna, *Review of Psychiatric Nursing,* C. V. Mosby, 1977.

explanation; *extreme* degree of behavior in comparison with antecedent event:
   1. *Fear*—related to a particular person, activity, or place.
   2. *Anxiety*—fearful feeling without any obvious reason, not specifically related to a particular person, activity, or place (for example, adolescent turmoil).
   3. *Depression*—continuous pessimism, easily moved to tears, hopelessness, and isolation (for example, student depression around exam time, middle-aged depression, elderly hopelessness).
   4. *Mania*—unrealistic optimism.
   5. *Anger*—many events seen as deliberate insults.
   6. *Confusion*—diminished awareness of who and where one is; memory loss.
   7. *Loss of reality contact*—hallucinations or delusion (as in acute psychosis).
   8. *Withdrawal*—neglect or giving away of belongings and neglect of appearance; loss of interest in activities; apathy.
B. Assessment of degree of seriousness:
   1. *Life-threatening emergencies*—violent toward self or others (for example, suicidal, homicidal).
   2. *Serious emergencies*—confused and unable to care for or protect self from dangerous situations (as in substance abuse).
   3. *Potentially serious emergencies*—anxious and in pain; disorganized behavior; can become worse or better (as in grief reaction).
C. *General nursing goals and interventions:*
   1. Remove from stressful situation and persons.
   2. Engage in dialogue at a nonthreatening distance to offer help.
   3. Use calm, slow, deliberate approach to relieve stress and disorganization.
   4. Explain what will be done about the problem and the likely outcome.
   5. Avoid using force, threat, or counterthreat.
   6. Use confident, firm, reasonable approach.
   7. Encourage client to relate.
   8. Elicit details.
   9. Encourage ventilation of feelings without interruption.
   10. Accept distortions of reality without arguing.
   11. Give form and structure to the conversation.
   12. Contact significant others to gain information and to be with client, including previous therapist.
   13. Treat emergency as temporary and readily resolved.

14. Check every half hour if cannot remain with client.

3. Categories of psychiatric emergencies

A. *Acute nonpsychotic reactions,* such as acute anxiety attack or panic reaction (see section on *Anxiety* for symptoms).

   1. *Assessment* includes differentiating hyperventilation that is anxiety-connected from asthma, angina, and heart disease.

   2. *Interventions* in hyperventilation syndrome:

      a. *Goal*—prevent paresthesia, tetanic contractions, disturbance in awareness; reassure client vital organs are not impaired.

      b. Increase CO_2 in lungs by rebreathing from paper bag.

      c. Demonstrate how to slow breathing rate.

      d. Minimize secondary gains; avoid reinforcing behavior.

B. *Delirium or acute brain syndromes*—conditions produced by changes in the cerebral chemistry or tissue by metabolic toxins, direct trauma to the brain, drug effects, and/or withdrawal.

   1. General assessment: emotional lability, memory defects, loss of judgement, disorientation.

   2. *Acute alcohol intoxication* (see *Alcohol dependence*).

      a. *Assessment*—signs of head and other injury (past and recent).

      b. *Intervention*—

         (1) Observe, monitor vital signs.

         (2) Prevent aspiration of vomitus.

         (3) Place in quiet area of emergency room.

         (4) Speak and handle calmly.

         (5) Give medication: Thorazine, Valium, to control agitation.

   3. *Hallucinogenic drug intoxication*—LSD, mescaline, amphetamines, cocaine, scopolamine, and belladonna.

      a. *Assessment:*

         (1) Perceptual and cognitive distortions (for example, feels heart stopped beating).

         (2) Anxiety (apprehension → panic).

         (3) Subjective feelings: omnipotence → worthlessness.

         (4) Interrelationship of dose, potency, setting, expectations, and experiences of user.

         (5) Eyes: red—marijuana; dilated—LSD, mescaline, belladonna; constricted—heroin and derivatives.

      b. *Interventions—"talk down":*

         (1) Establish verbal contact, attempt to have client verbally express what is being experienced.

         (2) Environment—few people, normal lights, calm, supportive.

         (3) Allay fears.

         (4) Encourage to keep eyes open.

         (5) Focus on inanimate objects in room as a bridge to reality contact.

         (6) Use simple, concrete, repetitive statements.

         (7) Repetitively orient to time, place, and temporary nature.

         (8) Do not moralize, challenge beliefs, or probe into life style.

         (9) Emphasize confidentiality.

      c. *Interventions—medication (minor tranquilizer—Valium, Librium):*

         (1) Allay anxiety.

         (2) Reduce aggressive behavior.

         (3) Reduce suicidal potential; check client every half hour.

         (4) Avoid anticholinergic crisis (precipitated by use of phenothiazines, belladonna, and scopolamine ingestion) with 2–4 mg IM or PO of physostigmine salicylate.

      d. *Interventions—hospitalization:* if hallucinations, delusions last more than 12 to 18 hours; if client has been injecting amphetamines for extended time; if client is paranoid and depressed.

   4. *Acute delirium*—seen in postoperative electrolyte imbalance, systemic infections, renal and hepatic failure, oversedation, metastatic cancer.

      a. *Assessment:*

         (1) Disorientation regarding time, at night.

         (2) Hallucinations, delusions, illusions.

         (3) Alterations in mood.

         (4) Increased emotional lability.

         (5) Agitation.

         (6) Lack of cooperation.

         (7) Withdrawal.

         (8) Sleep pattern reversal.

         (9) Alterations in food intake.

      b. *Interventions:*

         (1) Identify and remove toxic substance.

         (2) Reality orientation—well-lit room; constant attendance to inform repetitively of place and time and to protect from injury to self and others.

         (3) Simplify environment.

(4) Avoid excessive medication and restraints; use low-dose phenothiazines; do not give barbiturates or sedatives (these increase agitation, confusion, disorientation).

C. *Acute psychotic reactions*—disorders of mood or thinking characterized by hallucinations, delusions, excessive euphoria (mania), or depression.

1. *Acute schizophrenic reaction* (see *Schizophrenia*).
   a. *Assessment:*
      (1) Auditory hallucinations and delusions.
      (2) Violent, assaultive, suicidal behavior directed by auditory hallucinations.
      (3) Assault, withdrawal, and panic related to paranoid delusions of persecution; fear of harm.
      (4) Disturbance in mental status (associative thought disorder).
      (5) History of previous hospitalization, no illicit drug ingestion, use of major tranquilizers and recently going off them.
   b. *Interventions* (see *Hallucinations, delusions,* Unit 2).
      (1) Hospitalization.
      (2) Medication—phenothiazines.
      (3) Avoid physical restraints or laying on hands when fears and delusions of sexual attack exist.
      (4) Allow client to diffuse anger and intensity of panic through talk.
      (5) Use simple, concrete terms, avoid figures of speech or content subject to multiple interpretations.
      (6) Do not agree with reality distortions; point out to client that his/her thoughts are difficult for you to understand but that you are willing to listen.

2. *Manic reaction.*
   a. *Assessment:*
      (1) History of depression requiring antidepressants.
      (2) Thought disorder (flight of ideas, delusions of grandeur).
      (3) Affect (elated, irritable, irrational anger).
      (4) Speech (loud, pressured).
      (5) Behavior (rapid, erratic, chaotic).
   b. *Interventions:*
      (1) Hospitalization to protect from injury to self and others.

(2) Medication: lithium carbonate
(3) Same as for acute schizophrenic reaction, *except do not encourage talk,* as need to decrease stimulation.

3. *Homicidal or assaultive reaction*—seen in acutely drug-intoxicated, delirious, paranoid, acutely excited manic, or acute anxiety-panic conditions.
   a. *Assessment*—history of obvious antisocial behavior, paranoid psychosis, previous violence, sexual conflict, rivalry, substance abuse, recent moodiness, and withdrawal.
   b. *Interventions:*
      (1) May need group of people to help physically restrain person with a weapon.
      (2) Allow person to "save face" in giving up weapon.
      (3) Separate from intended victims.
      (4) Approach: calm, unhurried; *one person* to offer support and reassurance; use clear, unambiguous statements.
      (5) Immediate and rapid admission procedures.
      (6) Observe for suicidal behavior which may follow homicidal attempt.

4. *Suicidal reaction*—seen in anxiety attacks, substance intoxication, toxic delirium, schizophrenic auditory hallucinations, and psychotic depressive reactions.
   a. *Assessment of risk regarding statistical probability of suicide*—composite picture: over-45-year-old male, unemployed, divorced, living alone, depressed (weight loss, somatic delusions, sleep disturbance, preoccupied with suicide), history of substance abuse and suicide within family.
   b. *Interventions:*
      (1) Medical—gastric lavage for overdose; respiratory and vascular support; repair inflicted wound.
      (2) Take suicide precautions.
      (3) Decide whether to hospitalize or discharge to home care with responsible person.

Part B / DISORDERS

MAJOR AFFECTIVE DISORDERS: DEPRESSION

The term depression is used to describe morbid sadness, dejection, or melancholy. Severe depression should be distinguished from grief, which is realistic and proportionate to what has been lost.

1. General assessment of depression

A. *Physical*—early-morning awakening, *insomnia* at night, increased need for sleep during the day, fatigue, constipation, *anorexia,* loss of sexual interest, *psychomotor retardation,* physical complaints, amenorrhea.

B. *Psychologic*—inability to remember, decreased *concentration,* slowing or blocking of thought, all-or-nothing thinking, *less interest* and involvement with external world and own appearance, feeling worse at certain times of day or after any sleep, difficulty in enjoying activities, monotonous voice, repetitive discussions, inability to make decisions due to ambivalence, impaired coping with "practical problems."

C. *Emotional*—loss of self-esteem, feelings of *hopelessness* and *worthlessness,* shame and self-derogation due to guilt, *irritability,* despair and *futility* (leading to *suicidal* thoughts), alienation, *helplessness,* passivity, avoidance, *inertia,* powerlessness, denied anger; uncooperative, tense, crying, demanding, and *dependent* behavior.

2. Differentiation between reactive and endogenous depression

A. *Reactive depression without melancholia (external factors present):*
   1. *Precipitating event*—easy to identify, for example, death of a loved one.
   2. *Symptom cluster*—precipitating event, difficulty getting to sleep at night, feeling *worse* as day progresses, and weight loss of less than 10 lb.
   3. *Response to environment*—responds to environmental stimuli.

B. *Endogenous depression* or depression with psychotic features (internal factors):
   1. *Precipitating event*—precipitant may *not* be evident; history shows no clear-cut event.
   2. *Symptom cluster*—retardation of thought and action, substantial weight loss (over 10 lb), feeling of depression came on gradually, feeling worse in morning but *better* as day progresses, and feelings of worthlessness.
   3. *Response to environment*—does *not* respond to environmental stimuli.
   4. Family history of depression.
   5. May be biochemical disturbance.

C. Table 2–8 summarizes the main points of difference between two types of major depression.

TABLE 2–8. *Differentiation between two types of major depression.*

Criteria	Major depression without melancholia	Major depression with psychotic features
Intensity	Down but marginally managing to meet commitments	Totally devastated
		Marked motor retardation or agitation
Severity of ego impairment	Difficulty concentrating, unable to follow directions, ruminating over the past	Delusional and severely impaired judgment
Regression	Regressed to being whiny and self-pitying	Unable to get out of bed for weeks and must be fed by others
Precipitating factors	Identifiable factor such as a loss	Absence of any specific precipitating factors
Social class	Middle or upper class	The poor, lower and working classes
Sex/race	Men in most cultures	Women (especially at the menopausal stage of life and at any phase in the childbirth experience); old people; ethnic minorities

Source: Holly S. Wilson and Carol Ren Kneisl, *Psychiatric Nursing* (Menlo Park, Calif.: Addison-Wesley Publishing Co., 1979), p. 310 (modified according to DSM III).

3. Concepts and principles related to depression

A. Self-limiting—most depressions are self-limiting disturbances, making it important to look for a change in functioning and behavior.

B. Theories of cause of depression:
1. Aggression turned inward.
2. Response to separation or object loss.
3. Genetic and/or neurochemical basis (Table 2–9).

C. Need to distinguish between normal sadness or grief and depression; anxiety and depression; and schizophrenia and depression.

D. Depression is manifested by a disturbance in *affect* (mood), *thought processes* and *content, behavior,* and *self-concept.*

E. Normal concern and appropriate cheerfulness will help in reactive depression. This attitude makes the depressed person with psychotic features more depressed.

4. Nursing interventions in depression

A. Promote sleep and food intake—take nursing measures to ensure the *physical* well-being of the client.

B. Provide steady company to assess suicidal tendencies and to diminish feelings of loneliness and alienation; build trust in a one-to-one relationship.

C. Interact with clients on a nonverbal level if that is their immediate mode of communication; this will promote feelings of being recognized, accepted, and understood.

D. Focus on *today,* not the past or too far into the future.

E. Reassure that present state is temporary and that they will be protected and helped.

F. Make the environment nonchallenging and non-threatening.
1. Use a kind, firm attitude with warmth.
2. See that client has favorite foods; respond to other wishes and likes.
3. Protect from overstimulation and coercion.

G. Postpone client's decision-making and resumption of duties.
1. Allow more time than usual to complete activity (dressing, eating) or thought process and speech.
2. Structure the environment for clients to help them reestablish a set schedule and predictable routine during ambivalence and problems with decisions.

H. Provide nonintellectual activities (for instance, sanding wood)—avoid chess and crossword puzzles, for example, as thinking capacity at this time tends to be circular.

I. Encourage outlets for anger that may be underlying the depression; as clients become more verbal with their anger and recognize the origin and results of

TABLE 2–9. *Analysis: factors related to the development of depressive reactions*

Biological	Psychological	Cognitive	Sociocultural
Possible genetic influence	Dependency	Narrow, negative perspective called "cognitive triad": view of self, world, and the future	Social situations that contribute to feelings of powerlessness and low self-esteem:
Hormonal influence (drop in estrogen and progesterone)	Low self-esteem		
	Powerlessness	Draws conclusions on inadequate or contradictory evidence	1. Status of minority groups
Biochemical activities of monoamine oxidase (MAO) and catecholamines (high levels)	Ambivalence		2. Status of women in male-oriented professional and business culture
	Guilt	Overgeneralizes from one instance	
		Focuses on a single detail rather than on the whole	3. Role loss such as loss of mother role in empty nest phase
		Distortion of long-range consequences, hence bad judgment	4. Being the object of cultural stereotypes (e.g., blacks, aged, Jews)

Source: Holly S. Wilson and Carol Ren Kneisl, *Psychiatric Nursing* (Menlo Park, Calif.: Addison-Wesley Publishing Co., 1979), p. 311.

anger, help them resolve their feelings—allow clients to complain and be *demanding* in initial phases of depression.

J. Discourage redundancy in speech and thought—redirect focus from a monologue of painful recounts to an appraisal of more neutral or positive attributes and aspects of situations.

K. Encourage clients to assess their goals, unrealistic expectations, and perfectionist tendencies—may need to change their goals or give up some goals that are incompatible with abilities and external situations.

L. Assist clients to recapture what was lost through substitution of goals, sublimation, or relinquishment of unrealistic goals—reanchor clients' self-respect to other aspects of their existence; help them free themselves from *dependency* on one person or single event or idea.

M. Indicate that success is possible and not hopeless.
1. Explore what steps clients have taken to achieve goals and suggest new or alternate ones.
2. Set small, immediate goals to help attain mastery.
3. Recognize their efforts to mobilize themselves.
4. Provide positive reinforcement for clients through exposure to activities in which they can experience a sense of success, achievement, and completion to build their self-esteem and self-confidence.
5. Help clients experience pleasure; help them start good relationships in social setting.

N. *Long-term goal:* to encourage interest in external surroundings, outside of self.
1. Encourage purposeful activities.
2. Let clients advance to activities at their own pace (graded-task assignments).

MAJOR AFFECTIVE DISORDERS: BIPOLAR DISORDERS

Bipolar disorders (previously called manic-depressive illness) are major emotional illnesses characterized by mood swings, alternating from depression to elation, with periods of relative normality between episodes. Most persons experience a single episode of manic or depressed type; some have recurrent depression or recurrent mania or mixed. There is increasing evidence that a biochemical disturbance may exist, and that most individuals with manic episodes eventually develop depressive episodes.

1. *Assessment of bipolar disorders*
A. Manic and depressed types are opposite sides of the same coin.
1. Both are disturbances of mood and self-esteem.
2. Both have underlying aggression and hostility.
3. Both are intense.
4. Both are self-limited in duration.

B. *Depression*—mild to severe psychomotor *retardation* of movement and speech; preoccupation with *suicide;* feelings of doom and self-degradation; *delusions* of guilt and unworthiness; concern about money and sin, *anorexia* with weight loss, *constipation,* and *insomnia;* may become mute, immobile, and *stuporous.*

C. *Acute manic reaction*—escalating mild hypomania to acute and irrational delirium state; exhibitionistic and boisterous acting out behavior and dress; rapid speech with rhyming, punning, *flight of ideas,* and *delusions* of grandeur; sarcastic and witty; much physical energy; demanding and attempting to control; does not attend to personal care, food, or sleep; increased sex activity; full of pranks; quarrelsome, haughty, arrogant, and aggressive. May engage in activities not exhibited previously, for example, large-scale spending of money.

D. Incidence—most prevalent in women 18 to 35 years of age.

E. Prognosis—good, but recurrence is common.

2. *Concepts and principles related to bipolar disorder*
A. The psychodynamics of manic and depressive episodes are related to hostility and guilt.

B. The struggle between the unconscious impulses and moral conscience produces feelings of *hostility, guilt,* and *anxiety.*

C. To relieve the internal discomfort of these reactions, the person *projects* long-retained hostile feelings onto others or onto objects in the environment during *manic* phase; during *depressive* phase, hostility and guilt are *introjected* toward self.

D. Demands, irritability, sarcasm, profanity, destructiveness, and threats are signs of the projection of hostility; guilt is handled through persecutory delusions and accusations.

E. Feelings of inferiority and fear of rejection are handled by being gay and amusing.

F. Both phases, though appearing distinctly different, have the same objective: to gain attention, approval, and emotional support. These objectives and behaviors are unconsciously determined by the client; this behavior may be either biochemically determined or *both* biochemically and unconsciously determined.

3. Nursing interventions in bipolar disorders
A. *Manic:*
   1. Reduce outside stimuli or remove to quieter area. Give lithium carbonate.
   2. Prevent physical dangers stemming from suicide and exhaustion—promote rest, sleep, and intake of nourishment; use suicide precautions.
   3. Provide high-calorie beverages, finger foods within sight and reach.
   4. Attend to client's personal care.
   5. Absorb with understanding and without reproach behaviors such as talkativeness, provocativeness, criticism, sarcasm, dominance, profanity, and dramatic actions.
      a. Allow, postpone, or partially fulfill demands and freedom of expression *within limits* of ordinary social rules, comfort, and safety of client and others.
      b. Do not cut off manic stream of talk, as this increases anxiety and need for release of hostility.
   6. Constructively utilize excessive energies with activities that do not call for concentration or follow-through.
      a. Outdoor walks, gardening, putting, and ball-tossing are therapeutic.
      b. Exciting, disturbing, and highly competitive activities should be avoided.
      c. Creative occupational therapy activities promote release of hostile impulses, as does creative writing.
B. *Depressed:*
   1. Take routine suicide precautions.
   2. Give attention to physical needs for food and sleep and to hygiene needs.
   3. Prepare warm baths and hot beverages to aid sleep.
   4. Initiate frequent contacts; do not allow long periods of silence to develop or client to remain withdrawn.
   5. Use a kind, understanding, but emotionally neutral approach.
   6. Allow dependency in severe depressive phase; since dependency is one of the underlying concerns with depressive persons, if nurses allow dependency to occur as an initial response, they must plan for resolution of the dependency toward them as an example for the client's other dependent relationships.
   7. Slowly repeat simple, direct information.
   8. Assist in daily decision-making until client regains self-confidence.
   9. Select mild exercise and diversionary activities instead of stimulating exercise and competitive games, as they may overtax physical and emotional endurance and lead to feelings of inadequacy and frustration.
   10. Give antidepressive drugs.

MAJOR DEPRESSION WITH MELANCHOLIA

Major depression with melancholia occurs during the menopausal, climacteric, or involutional period of life. (This used to be called involutional melancholia or psychosis.)

1. Assessment
A. Occurs in women of menopausal age (40 to 55 years) and men (50 to 65 years).
B. *No* prior history of affective psychosis.
C. Premorbid personality—meticulous, worrisome, rigid, and overconscientious.
D. Onset—slow with increase in *hypochondriasis,* leading to *delusions* about body function, *pessimism,* irritability, and nihilistic thoughts.
E. Main symptoms—*agitation,* restless activity, fear and apprehension, ideas of reference, *depression,* self-reproach and *guilt* over wrongdoing and sin, delusions of unworthiness.
F. High suicide potential.

2. Concepts and principles
A. The depression is a response to a real or fancied loss of loved ones, possessions, health and vigor, or sexual attractiveness.
B. The loss results in anger; the anger is turned upon the self.
C. It is a reactive psychosis in which the symptoms are exaggerated reactions to a change in life style and body function—physical limitations and social restrictions associated with aging process.

3. Nursing interventions
A. Prevention of suicide is first priority.
B. Look after physical needs for food, sleep, and protection from self-destruction.

C. Respond to clients' need to be understood, helped, and supported when feeling alone and hopeless.

D. Be prepared to absorb hostile, clinging, demanding behavior.

E. Guide client from repetitious complaints and self-accusations by encouraging client to note normal and cheerful features of surrounding environment; avoid "persuading" client out of self-accusatory ideas, as this may increase guilt and prolong depression.

F. Encourage interest in simple craft activity.

SUICIDE—A "CRY FOR HELP"

1. Assessment of suicide *

A. Ten factors to predict potential suicide and assess risk:

1. *Age and sex*—teenage, older age; more women make attempts; more men complete suicide act. Highest risk: older women rather than young boys; older men rather than young girls.

2. *Recent stress*—family problems: death, divorce, separation, alienation; financial pressures; loss of job; loss of status; failing grades.

3. *Clues to suicide:*

   a. *Verbal clues*—
      (1) Direct: "I am going to shoot myself."
      (2) Indirect: "It's more than I can bear."
      (3) Coded: "This is the last time you'll see me." "I want you to have my coin collection."

   b. *Behavioral clues*—
      (1) Direct: trial run with pills or razor, for example.
      (2) Indirect: sudden lifting of depression, buying a casket, giving away cherished belongings, putting affairs in order, writing a will.

   c. *Syndromes*—
      (1) *Dependent-dissatisfied:* emotionally dependent but dislikes dependent state, irritable, helpless.
      (2) *Depressed:* detachment from life; feels life is a burden; hopelessness, futility.
      (3) *Disoriented:* delusions or hallucinations, confusion, delirium tremens, organic brain syndromes.

---

*Copyright May 1965, the American Journal of Nursing Company. Reproduced with permission from the American Journal of Nursing, Vol. 65, No. 5.

      (4) *Willful-defiant:* active need to direct and control environment and life situation, with low frustration tolerance and rigid set, rage, shame.

4. *Suicidal plan*—the more details about method, timing, and place, the higher the risk.

5. *Previous suicidal behavior*—history of prior attempt increases risk.

6. *Medical status*—chronic ailments, terminal illness, and pain increase suicidal risk.

7. *Communication*—the more withdrawn and apathetic, the greater potential for suicide, unless extreme psychomotor retardation is present.

8. *Style of life*—high risks include substance abusers, those with sexual-identity conflicts, unstable relationships (personal and job-related).

9. *Alcohol*—can reinforce helpless and hopeless feelings; may be lethal if used with barbiturates; can decrease inhibitions, result in impulsive behavior.

10. *Resources*—the fewer the resources, the higher the suicide potential. Examples of resources: family, friends, colleagues, religion, pets, meaningful recreational outlets, satisfying employment.

B. Eight out of ten suicide attempts give verbal and behavioral warnings as listed above.

C. Suicidal thoughts are usually time-limited and do not last forever. Early assessment of behavioral and verbal clues is important.

D. Suicidal tendencies are not inherited, but learned from family and other interpersonal relationships.

E. Assess styles of communicating and stress reactions of significant others.

F. Assess needs commonly communicated by individuals who are suicidal:

1. To trust.
2. To be accepted.
3. To bolster self-esteem.
4. To "fit in" with groups.
5. To experience success and interrupt the failure syndrome.
6. To expand capacity for pleasure.
7. To increase autonomy and sense of self-mastery.
8. To work out an acceptable sexual identity.

G. Suicide occurs in all races and socioeconomic groups.

2. Concepts and principles related to suicide

A. *Based on social theory:*

1. Suicidal tendency is a result of *collective social*

forces, rather than isolated individual motives (Durkheim's *Le Suicide*).
   a. Common factor: increased *alienation* between person and social group; psychologic isolation, called "anomie," when links between groups are weakened.
   b. "Egoistic" suicide: results from lack of integration of individual with others.
   c. "Altruistic" suicide: results from insufficient individualization.
   d. *Implication:* increase group cohesiveness and mutual interdependence, making group more coherent and consistent in fulfilling needs of each member.
2. *Based on symbolic interaction theory:*
   a. Person evaluates self according to *others' assessment.*
   b. Thus, suicide stems from *social rejection* and disrupted social relations.
   c. Perceived failure in relationships with others may be inaccurate, but seen as real by the individual.
   d. *Implication:* need to recognize difference in perception of alienation between own viewpoint and others'.
3. *Based on field theory:*
   a. The individual's *internal* needs, drives, and impulses as well as *external* social environment are part of the "field" of forces determining behavior.
   b. Certain social conditions determine whether suicide will take place: when future seen as hopeless, suicide is considered an alternative; lack of response and hopeful assurance from others.
   c. *Implication* for suicide prevention: awareness of and response to "cry-for-help" messages.
B. *Based on psychoanalytic theory:*
1. Suicide stems mainly from the individual, with external events only as precipitants.
2. There is a strong life urge in people.
3. *Universal death* instinct always present (Freud).
4. Person may be balancing life wishes and death wishes.
   a. When self-preservation instincts are diminished, death instincts may find direct outlet via suicide.
5. When *love* instinct is frustrated, *hate* impulse takes over (Menninger).
   a. Desire to kill → desire to be killed → desire to kill oneself.

   b. Suicide may be an act of extreme hostility, manipulation, and revenge to elicit guilt and remorse in significant others.
   c. Suicide may also be act of self-punishment to handle own guilt or to control fate.
C. *Based on synthesis of social and psychoanalytic theories:*
1. Suicide is seen as *running away* from an intolerable situation in order to interrupt it, rather than *running to* something more desirable.
2. Process *defined in operational terms* involves:
   a. Despair over inability to cope.
   b. Inability to feel hope or adequacy.
   c. Frustration with others when others cannot fill needs.
   d. Rage and aggression experienced toward significant other is turned inward.
   e. Psychic blow acts as precipitant.
   f. Life seen as harder to cope with, with no chance of improvement in life situation.
   g. *Implication:* persons who experience suicidal impulses can gain a certain amount of control over these impulses through the support they gain from meaningful relationships with others.
D. *Based on crisis theory (Dublin):*
1. Concept of emotional disequilibrium—
   a. Everyone at some point in life is in a crisis, with temporary inability to solve problems or to master the crisis.
   b. Usual coping mechanisms do not function.
   c. Person unable to relate to others.
   d. Person consciously and unconsciously searches for useful coping techniques, with suicide as one of various solutions.
   e. With inadequate communication of needs and isolation, suicide is possible.
E. *Based on the view that suicide is an individual's personal reaction and decision, a final response to own situation:*
1. *Process* of anger turned inwards → self-inflicted, destructive action.
2. *Definition* of concept in operational steps:
   a. Frustration of individual needs → anger.
   b. Anger turned inward → feelings of guilt, despair, depression, incompetence, hopelessness, and exhaustion.
   c. Stress felt and perceived as unbearable and overwhelming.
   d. Attempt to communicate hopelessness and defeat to others.
   e. Others do not provide hope.

f. Sudden change in behavior, as noted when depression appears to lift, may indicate *danger*, as person has more energy to act on his suicidal thoughts and feelings.

g. Decision to end life → plan of action → self-induced, self-destructive behavior.

3. May be pseudo-suicide attempts where there is not an actual or realistic desire to achieve finality of death. Intentions or causes may be:
   a. "Cry for help," where nonlethal attempt notifies others of deeper intentions.
   b. Desire to manipulate others.
   c. Need for attention and pity.
   d. Self-punishment.
   e. Symbol of utter frustration.
   f. Wish to punish others.
   g. Misuse of alcohol and other drugs.

4. Other reasons for self-destruction, where the individual *gives his life* rather than takes it, include:
   a. Strong parental love that can overcome fear and instinct of self-preservation to save child's life.
   b. "Sacrificial death" during war, such as kamikaze pilots in WW II.
   c. Submission to death for religious beliefs (martyrdom).

3. Nursing interventions in suicidal behavior

A. *Long-term goals:*
   1. Increase client's self-reliance.
   2. Help client achieve more realistic and positive feelings of self-esteem, self-respect, acceptance by others, and sense of belonging.
   3. Help client experience success, interrupt failure pattern, and expand views about pleasure.

B. *Short-term goals:*
   1. Provide protection from self-destruction until clients are able to assume this responsibility themselves.
   2. Allow outward and constructive expression of hostile and aggressive feelings.
   3. Provide for physical needs.

C. *General approaches:*
   1. *Observe* closely at all times to assess suicide potential.
   2. Be *available*.
      a. Demonstrate concern for client as a person.
      b. Be sensitive, warm, and consistent.
      c. Listen with empathy.

d. Avoid imposing your own feelings of reality on client.
e. Avoid extremes in your own mood when with client (especially exaggerated cheerfulness).

3. *Focus directly* on client's self-destructive ideas.
   a. Reduce alienation and immobilization by discussing this "taboo" topic.
   b. Acknowledge suicidal threats with calmness and without reproach—do not ignore or minimize threat.
   c. Find out details about suicide plan and reduce environmental hazards.
   d. Help client verbalize aggressive, hostile, and hopeless feelings.
   e. Explore death fantasies—try to take "romance" out of death.

4. Acknowledge that suicide is one of several *alternatives*.

5. *Make a contract* and structure a plan of alternatives for coping when next confronted with the need to commit suicide (for example, the client could call someone, express feeling of anger outwardly, or ask for help).

6. Point out client's *self-responsibility* for suicidal act.
   a. Avoid manipulation by client who says, "You are responsible for stopping me from killing myself."
   b. Emphasize protection against self-destruction rather than punishment.

7. *Support* the part of the client that wants to live.
   a. Focus on ambivalence.
   b. Emphasize meaningful past relationships and events.
   c. Look for reasons left for wanting to live. Elicit what is meaningful to the client at the moment.
   d. Point out effect of client's death on others.

8. *Remove sources of stress*.
   a. Decrease uncomfortable feelings of *alienation* by initiating one-to-one interactions.
   b. Make all *decisions* in severe depression.
   c. Progressively let client make simple decisions: what to eat, what to watch on TV, etc.

9. *Provide hope*.
   a. Let client know that problems are not insoluble and can be solved with help.
   b. Bring in new resources for help.

   c. Talk about likely changes in client's life.

   d. Review past effective coping behaviors.

10. *Provide with opportunity to be useful.*

   a. Reduce self-centeredness and brooding by planning diversional activities within the client's capabilities.

11. *Involve as many people as possible.*

   a. Gradually bring in others, for instance, other therapists, friends, staff, clergy, family, co-workers.

   b. Prevent staff "burn-out," found when only one nurse is working with suicidal client.

CONCEPT OF DEATH THROUGHOUT THE LIFE CYCLE

1. Ages 1 to 3

A. No concept per se, but experiences separation anxiety and abandonment any time significant other disappears from view over a period of time.

B. Coping means: fear, resentment, anger, aggression, regression, withdrawal.

C. *Nursing interventions:* help the family:

   1. Facilitate the transfer of affectional ties to another nurturing adult.

   2. Decrease separation anxiety.

   3. Provide stable environment.

2. Ages 3 to 5

A. Least anxious about death.

B. Denial of death as regular and final process.

C. Death is separation, being alone.

D. Death is sleep and sleep is death.

E. "Death" is part of vocabulary; seen as real, gradual, temporary, not permanent.

F. Dead person is seen as alive but in altered form, that is, lacks movement.

G. There are degrees of death.

H. Death means not being here anymore.

I. Living and lifeless are not yet distinguished.

J. Illness and death seen as punishment for "badness"; fear and guilt about sexual and aggressive impulses.

K. Death happens, but only to others.

L. *Nursing interventions* (in addition to those above):

   1. Encourage play for expression of feelings.

   2. Encourage verbal expression of feelings using children's books.

   3. Model appropriate grieving behavior.

   4. Protect child from overstimulation by hysterical adult reactions.

5. Clearly state what death is—death is final, no breathing, eating, awakening—and that death is *not* sleep.

6. Check child at night and provide support through holding and staying with child.

7. Allow a choice of attending the funeral and, if child decides to attend, describe what will take place.

3. Ages 5 to 10

A. Death is cessation of life.

B. Death seen as definitive, universal, inevitable, irreversible.

C. Death occurs to all living things, including self.

D. Death is distant from self (an eventuality).

E. Believe death occurs by accident, happens only to the very old or very sick.

F. Death is personified (as a separate person) in fantasies and magical thinking.

G. Death anxiety handled by nightmares, rituals, and superstitions (related to fear of darkness and sleeping alone because death is an external person, like a skeleton, who comes and takes people away at night).

H. Dissolution of bodily life seen as a perceptible result.

I. Fear of body mutilation.

J. *Nursing interventions* (in addition to those above):

   1. Allow to experience the loss of pets, friends, and family members.

   2. Help child talk it out and experience the appropriate emotional reactions.

   3. Understand need for increase in play, especially competitive play.

   4. Involve child in funeral preparation and rituals.

   5. Understand and accept regressive or protest behaviors.

   6. Rechannel protest behaviors into constructive outlets.

4. Adolescence

A. Death seen as permanent; corporal life stops; body decomposes.

B. Do not fear death, but concerned with how to live now.

C. Experience anger, frustration, and despair over lack of future, lack of fulfillment of adult roles.

D. Openly ask difficult, honest, direct questions.

E. Anger at healthy peers.

F. Conflict between developing body versus deteriorating body, independent identity versus dependency.

G. *Nursing interventions* (in addition to those above):
1. Facilitate full expression of grief.
2. Help let out feelings, especially through creative and esthetic pursuits.
3. Encourage participation in funeral ritual.
4. Encourage full use of peer group support system.

5. Young adulthood
A. Death seen as unwelcome intrusion, interruption of what might have been.
B. Reaction: rage, frustration, disappointment.
C. *Nursing interventions:* all of those above, especially peer group support.

6. Middle age
A. Concerned with consequences of own death and that of significant others.
B. Death seen as disruption of involvement, responsibility, and obligations.
C. End of plans, projects, experiences.
D. Death is pain.
E. *Nursing interventions* (in addition to those above): assess need for counseling when also in midlife crisis.

7. Old age
A. Philosophic rationalizations: death as inevitable, final process of life, when "time runs out."
B. Religious view: death represents only the dissolution of life and is a doorway to a new life (a preparatory stage for another life).
C. Time of rest and peace, supreme refuge from turmoil of life.
D. *Nursing interventions* (in addition to those above):
1. Help person prepare for own death by helping with funeral prearrangements, wills, and sharing of mementos.
2. Facilitate life review and reinforce positive aspects.
3. Provide care and comfort.
4. Be present at death.

DEATH AND DYING

Too often the process of death has had such frightening aspects that people have suffered alone. Today there has been a vast change in attitudes; death and dying are no longer taboo topics. There is a growing realization that we need to accept death as a natural process. Elisabeth Kübler-Ross has written extensively on the process of dying, describing the stages of *denial* ("not me!"), *anger* ("why me?"), *bargaining* ("Yes me—but"), depression ("yes, me"), and *acceptance* ("my time is close now, it's all right"), with implications for the helping person.

1. Assessment of death and dying
A. *Physical:*
1. Observable deterioration of physical and mental capacities—person is unable to fulfill physiologic needs, such as eating and elimination.
2. Circulatory collapse (blood pressure and pulse).
3. Renal or hepatic failure.
4. Respiratory decline.
B. *Psychosocial:*
1. Fear of death is signaled by agitation, restlessness, and sleep disturbances at night.
2. Anger, agitation, blaming.
3. Morbid self-pity with feelings of defeat and failure.
4. Depression and withdrawal.
5. Introspectiveness and calm acceptance of the inevitable.

2. Concepts and principles related to death and dying
A. Persons may know or suspect they are dying and may want to talk about it; often they look for someone to share their fears and the process of dying.
B. Fear of death can be reduced by helping clients feel that they are not alone.
C. The dying need the opportunity to live their final experiences to the fullest, in their own way.
D. People who are dying remain more or less the same as they were during life; their approaches to death are consistent with their approaches to life.
E. Dying persons' need to review their lives may be a purposeful attempt to reconcile themselves to what "was" and "what could have been."
F. *Four tasks* facing a dying person are (a) reviewing life, (b) coping with physical symptoms in the end-stage of life, (c) making a transition from known to unknown state, and (d) reacting to separation from loved ones.
G. *Three ways* of facing death are (a) quiet acceptance with inner strength and peace of mind, (b) restlessness, impatience, anger, and hostility, and (c) depression, withdrawal, and fearfulness.
H. Crying and tears are an important aspect of the grief process.
I. There are many *blocks* to providing a helping relationship with the dying and bereaved:

1. Nurses' unwillingness to share the process of dying—minimizing their contacts and blocking out their own feelings.
2. Forgetting that a dying person may be feeling lonely, abandoned, and afraid of dying.
3. Reacting with irritation and hostility to the person's frequent calls.
4. Nurses' failure to seek help and support from team members when feeling afraid, uneasy, and frustrated in caring for a dying person.
5. Not allowing client to talk about death and dying.
6. Nurses' use of technical language or social chit-chat as a defense against their own anxieties.

3. Nursing interventions in death and dying

A. *Long-term goal:* foster environment where person and family can experience dying with dignity.

B. *Short-term goals:*
   1. Express feelings (person and family).
   2. Support person and family.
   3. Minimize physical discomfort.

C. Explore your own feelings about death and dying with team members; form support groups.

D. Be aware of the normal grief process:
   1. Allow person and family to do the work of grief and mourning.
   2. Allow crying and mood swings, anger, demands.
   3. Permit yourself to cry.

E. Allow person to express feelings, fears, and concerns.
   1. Avoid pat answers to questions seeking "why."
   2. Pick up symbolic communication.

F. Provide care and comfort with relief from pain; do not isolate person.

G. Stay physically close.
   1. Use touch.
   2. Be available to form a consistent relationship.

H. Reduce isolation and abandonment by assigning person to room in which it is less likely to occur and by allowing flexible visiting hours.

I. Keep activities in room as near normal and constant as possible.

J. Speak in audible tones, not whispers.

K. Be alert to cues when person needs to be alone (disengagement process).

L. Leave room for hope.

M. Help person die with peace of mind by lending support and providing opportunities to express anger, pain, and fears to someone who will accept him and not censor his verbalization.

GRIEF

Grief is a typical reaction to the loss of a source of psychologic gratification. It is a syndrome with somatic and psychologic symptoms that diminish when grief is resolved. Grief processes have been extensively described by Erich Lindemann and George Engle.*

1. Assessment: characteristic stages of grief responses

A. *Shock and disbelief:*
   1. Denial of reality. ("No, it can't be.")
   2. Stunned, numb feeling.
   3. Feelings of loss, helplessness, impotence.
   4. Intellectual acceptance.

B. *Developing awareness:*
   1. Anguish about loss.
      a. Somatic distress.
      b. Feelings of emptiness.
   2. Anger and hostility toward person or circumstances held responsible.
   3. Guilt feelings—may lead to self-destructive actions.
   4. Tears (inwardly, alone, or inability to cry).

C. *Restitution:*
   1. Funeral rituals are an aid to grief resolution by emphasizing the reality of death.
   2. Expression and sharing of feelings by gathered family and friends are a source of acknowledgement of grief and support for the bereaved.

D. *Resolving the loss:*
   1. Increase dependency on others as an attempt to deal with painful void.
   2. More aware of own bodily sensations—may be identical with symptoms of the deceased.
   3. Complete preoccupation with thoughts and memories of the dead person.

E. *Idealization:*
   1. All hostile and negative feelings about the dead are repressed.
   2. Mourner may assume qualities and attributes of the dead.
   3. Gradual lessening of preoccupation with the dead; reinvesting in others.

F. *Outcome* (takes one year or more)—can remember comfortably and realistically both pleasurable and disappointing aspects of the lost relationship.

---

*Engle, G.: Grief and grieving, Am J Nurs 9(64):93–98, September 1964.

2. Concepts and principles related to grief
A. Cause of grief: reaction to loss (real or imaginary, actual or pending).
B. Symptomatology and course: predictable and observable (Table 2–10).
C. Healing process can be interrupted.
D. Grief is universal.
E. Grief is a self-limiting process.

F. Grief responses may vary in degree and kind (for example, absence of grief, delayed grief, and unresolved grief).
G. People go through stages similar to stages of death described by Elisabeth Kübler-Ross.
H. Many factors influence "successful" outcome of grieving process:
  1. The more dependent the person on the lost

TABLE 2–10. *Symptomatology of grieving*

Symptom classification	Characteristics
1. Somatic distress	Occurs in waves lasting from twenty minutes to one hour
	Deep, sighing respirations most common when discussing grief
	Lack of strength
	Loss of appetite and sense of taste
	Tightness in throat
	Choking sensation accompanied by shortness of breath
2. Preoccupation with image of deceased	Similar to daydreaming
	May mistake others for deceased person
	May be oblivious to surroundings
	Slight sense of unreality
	Fear that he or she is becoming "insane"
3. Feelings of guilt	Accuses self of negligence
	Exaggerates existence and importance of negative thoughts, feelings, and actions toward deceased
	Views self as having failed deceased—"If I had only . . ."
4. Feelings of hostility	Irritability, anger, and loss of warmth toward others
	May attempt to handle feelings of hostility in formalized and stiff manner of social interaction
5. Loss of patterns of conduct	Inability to initiate or maintain organized patterns of activity
	Restlessness, with aimless movements
	Loss of zest—tasks and activities are carried on as though with great effort
	Activities formerly carried on in company of deceased have lost their significance
	May become strongly dependent on whoever stimulates him or her to activity

Source: Holly S. Wilson and Carol Ren Kneisl, *Psychiatric Nursing* (Menlo Park, Calif.: Addison-Wesley Publishing Co., 1979), p. 247.

relationship, the greater the difficulty in resolving the loss.
2. A child has greater difficulty resolving loss.
3. A person with few meaningful relationships also has greater difficulty.
4. The more losses the person has had in the past, the more affected that person will be, as losses tend to be cumulative.
5. The more sudden the loss, the greater the difficulty in resolving it.
6. The more ambivalence (love-hate feelings, with guilt) there was toward the dead, the more difficult the resolution.
7. Loss of a child is harder to resolve than loss of an older person.

3. Nursing interventions in grief
A. *Apply crisis theory and interventions.*
B. *Demonstrate respect* for cultural, religious, and social mourning customs.
C. *Utilize knowledge of the stages of grief* to anticipate reactions and facilitate the grief process.
   1. Anticipate and permit expression of different manifestations of shock, disbelief, and denial.
      a. News of impending death is best communicated to a family group (rather than an individual) in a private setting.
      b. Let mourners see the dead/dying to help them accept reality.
   2. Accept anger and rage as a common response to coping with guilt and helplessness.
      a. Be aware of potential suicide by the bereaved.
      b. Permit crying.
   3. Promote hospital policy that allows gathering of friends and family in a private setting.
   4. Allow dependency on staff while person is attempting to resolve loss.
   5. Respond to somatic complaints.
   6. Permit reminiscence.
   7. Begin to encourage new interests and social relations with others by the end of the idealization stage.
   8. Encourage mourner to relate accounts connected with the lost relationship that reflect positive and negative feelings and remembrances.

SCHIZOPHRENIC DISORDERS

Schizophrenia is a group of interrelated symptoms with a number of common features involving disorders of *mood, thought, content, feelings, perception,* and *behavior.* The term means "splitting of the mind," alluding to the discrepancy between the content of *thought processes* and their emotional expression; this should *not* be confused with "multiple personality" (dissociative reaction).

Half of the clients in mental hospitals are diagnosed as schizophrenics; many more live in the community. The onset of symptoms for this disorder generally occurs between 15 to 27 years of age. Causes, psychodynamics, and psychopathology are still a matter of controversy.

Note: new categories are used, according to the third edition of the Diagnostic and Statistical Manual of the American Psychiatric Association (DSM III). The categories included in parentheses refer to the previous DSM II listing where they are equivalent to or have been subsumed by DSM III listings.

1. Common subtypes of schizophrenia (without clear-cut differentiation)

schizotypal personality disorder (simple type) insidious disinvolvement with environment; apathetic, indifferent to others.

disorganized type (hebephrenic) disordered thinking ("word salad"), inappropriate affect, regressive behavior, incoherent speech, preoccupied and withdrawn.

catatonic type (stupor and excitement phases) disorder of muscle tension, with rigidity, waxy flexibility, posturing, mutism, violent rage outbursts, and frenzied activity.

paranoid type disturbed perceptions leading to disturbance in thought content of persecutory, grandiose, or hostile nature; projection is key mechanism, with religion a common preoccupation.

brief reactive psychoses (acute undifferentiated) a sudden onset, brief confusion, excitement, depression, or fear, with ideas of reference.

borderline personality disorder (latent type) clear symptoms of schizophrenia, with no history; also called "borderline."

residual continued difficulty in thinking, mood, perception, and behavior after schizophrenic episode.

infantile autism (childhood) symptoms before puberty, characterized by autism, withdrawal, and failure to develop separate ego identity from mother.

undifferentiated type (chronic undifferentiated) unclassifiable schizophrenic-like disturbance with mixed symptoms.

2. Assessment of schizophrenic disorders

A. Eugene Bleuler described four classic and primary symptoms as the "four A's":

1. *Associative looseness*—impairment of logical thought progression, resulting in confused, bizarre, and abrupt thinking.
   a. *Neologisms*—making up new words or condensing words into one.
2. *Affect*—exaggerated, apathetic, blunt, flat, inappropriate, inconsistent feeling tone that is communicated through face and body posture.
3. *Ambivalence*—simultaneously conflicting feelings or attitudes toward person or object.
   a. Stormy outbursts.
   b. Poor, weak interpersonal relations.
4. *Autism*—withdrawal from external world; preoccupation with fantasies and idiosyncratic thoughts.
   a. *Delusions*—false, fixed beliefs, not corrected by logic; a defense against intolerable feeling. The two most common delusions are:
      (1) *Delusions of grandeur*—conviction in a belief related to being famous, important, or wealthy.
      (2) *Delusions of persecution*—belief that thoughts, moods, or actions are controlled or influenced by strange forces or by others.
   b. *Hallucinations*—false sensory impressions without observable external stimuli.
      (1) Auditory—affecting hearing (hears voices).
      (2) Visual—affecting vision (sees snakes).
      (3) Tactile—affecting touch (feels electric charges in body).
      (4) Olfactory—affecting smell (smells rotting flesh).
      (5) Gustatory—affecting taste (food tastes like poison).
   c. *Ideas of reference*—clients interpret cues in the environment as having reference to them. Ideas symbolize guilt, insecurity, and alienation; may become delusions, if severe.
   d. *Depersonalization*—feelings of strangeness and unreality about self or environment or both; difficulty in differentiating boundaries between self and environment.
B. Negativism and hostility.
C. *Catatonic stupor*—marked decrease in involvement with environment and in spontaneous movements.

D. *Catatonic excitement*—purposeful and stereotyped motor behavior.
E. *Regression*—extreme withdrawal and social isolation, as in hebephrenia.

3. Concepts and principles related to schizophrenic disorders

A. General:

1. Symbolic language used expresses schizophrenic's life, pain, and progress toward health; all symbols used have meaning.
2. Physical care provides media for relationship; nurturance may be initial focus.
3. Consistency, reliability, and empathic understanding build trust.
4. *Denial, regression,* and *projection* are key defense mechanisms.
5. Felt anxiety gives rise to distorted thinking.
6. Attempts to engage in verbal communication may result in tension, apprehensiveness, and defensiveness.
7. Person rejects real world of painful experiences and creates fantasy world through illness.

B. *Withdrawal:*

1. Withdrawal from and resistance to forming relationships are attempts to reduce anxiety related to:
   a. Loss of ability to experience satisfying human relationships.
   b. Fear of rejection.
   c. Lack of self-confidence.
   d. Protection and restraint against potential destructiveness of *hostile* impulses (toward self and others).
2. *Ambivalence* results from need for approaching a relationship and need for avoiding it.
   a. Cannot tolerate swift emotional or physical closeness.
   b. Needs more time than usual to establish a relationship; time to test sincerity and interest of nurse.
3. Avoidance of client by others, especially staff, will reinforce withdrawal to create problem of mutual withdrawal and fear.

C. *Hallucinations:*

1. It is possible to replace hallucinations with satisfying interactions.
2. Person can relearn to focus attention on real things and people.
3. Hallucinations originate during extreme emotional stress when unable to cope.
4. Hallucinations are very real to client.

5. Client will react as the situation is perceived, regardless of reality or consensus.
6. Concrete experiences, not argument or confrontation, will correct sensory distortion.
7. Hallucinations are substitutes for human relations.
8. Purposes served by or expressed in falsification of reality:
   a. Reflection of problem in inner life.
   b. Statement of criticism, censure, self-punishment.
   c. Promotion of self-esteem.
   d. Satisfaction of instinctual strivings.
   e. Projection of unacceptable unconscious content in disguised form.
9. Perceptions *not* as *totally* disturbed as they seem.
10. Clients attempt to restructure reality through hallucinations to protect remaining ego integrity.
11. Hallucinations may result from a variety of psychologic and biologic conditions (extreme fatigue, drugs, pyrexia, and organic brain disease, for example).
12. Hallucinating persons need to feel free to describe their perceptions if they are to be understood by the nurse.

4. Nursing interventions in schizophrenic disorders

A. *General:*
1. Set short-range goals, realistic to client's levels of functioning.
2. Use nonverbal level of communication to demonstrate concern, caring, and warmth, as clients often distrust words.
3. Set climate for free expression of feelings in whatever mode, without fear of retaliation, ridicule, or rejection.
4. Seek clients out in their own fantasy worlds.
5. Try to understand meaning of symbolic language; help them communicate less symbolically.
6. Provide distance, as clients need to feel safe and to observe nurses for sources of threat or promises of security.
7. Help clients tolerate nurses' presence and learn to trust nurses enough to move out of isolation and share painful and often unacceptable (to clients) feelings and thoughts.
8. Anticipate and accept negativism; do not personalize.
9. Avoid joking, abstract terms, and figures of speech when client's thinking is literal.

10. Give antipsychotic medications.

B. *Withdrawn behavior:*
1. *Long-term goal:* develop satisfying interpersonal relationships.
2. *Short-term goal:* help client feel safe in one-to-one relationship.
3. Seek clients out at every chance and establish some bond.
   a. Stay with them, in silence.
   b. Initiate talk when they are ready.
   c. Draw out, but do not demand, response.
   d. Do *not* avoid the clients.
4. Use simple language, specific words.
5. Use an object or activity as medium for relationship; initiate activity.
6. Focus on everyday experiences.
7. Delay decision-making.
8. Accept one-sided conversation, with silence from the client; avoid pressuring to respond.
9. Accept the client's outward attempts to respond and inappropriate social behavior without remarks or disdain; teach social skills.
10. Avoid making demands on client or exposing client to failure.
11. Protect from aggressive persons and from impulsive attacks on themselves and others.
12. Attend to nutrition, elimination, exercise, hygiene, and signs of physical illness.
13. Add structure to the day; tell them, "This is your 9 A.M. medication."

C. *Hallucinations:*
1. *Long-term goal:* establish satisfying relationships with *real* persons.
2. *Short-term goal:* interrupt *pattern* of hallucinations.
3. Provide a structured environment with routine activities. Use *real* objects to keep client's interest or to stimulate new interest (in painting or crafts, for example).
4. Protect against injury to themselves and others resulting from "voices."
5. Short, frequent contacts initially, increasing social interaction gradually (one person → small groups).
6. Ask person to describe experiences as hallucinations occur.
7. Respond to anything real the clients say, for example, with acknowledgement or reflection. Focus more on *feelings,* not on delusional, hallucinatory content.
8. Distract clients' attention to something real when they hallucinate.
9. Avoid direct confrontation that voices are com-

ing from clients themselves; do not argue, but listen.

10. Clarify who "they" are—
    a. Use personal pronouns, avoiding universal and global pronouns.
    b. Nurse's own language needs to be clear and unambivalent.
11. Use one sentence, ask only one question, at a time.
12. Encourage consensual validation. Point out that experience is not shared by you; voice doubt.

D. *Delusions* (see *Nursing interventions in paranoid disorders,* Unit 2).

PARANOID DISORDERS

Paranoid disorders have a concrete and pervasive delusional system, usually persecutory. *Projection* is a chief coping mechanism of this disorder.

1. Assessment of paranoid disorders
A. Chronically suspicious, distrustful (think "people are out to get me.").
B. Distant, but not withdrawn.
C. Poor insight; blame others.
D. Misinterpret and distort reality.
E. Difficulty in admitting own errors; take pride in intelligence and in being correct (superiority).
F. Maintain false persecutory belief despite evidence or proof (may refuse food and medicine and insist they are poisoned).
G. Literal thinking.
H. Dominating and provocative.
I. Hypercritical and intolerant of others; *hostile,* quarrelsome, and aggressive.
J. Very sensitive in perceiving minor injustices, errors, and contradictions.
K. Evasive.

2. Concepts and principles related to paranoid disorders
A. Delusions are attempts to cope with stresses and problems.
B. May be a means of allegorical or symbolic communication and of testing others for their trustworthiness.
C. Interactions with others and activities interrupt delusional thinking.
D. To establish a rational therapeutic relationship, gross distortions, misorientation, misinterpretation, and misidentification need to be overcome.

E. Delusional people have extreme need to maintain self-esteem.
F. False beliefs cannot be changed without first changing experiences.
G. A delusion is held because it performs a function.
H. When people who are experiencing delusions become at ease and comfortable with people, delusions will not be needed.
I. Delusions are misjudgements of reality based on a series of mental mechanisms: (a) *denial,* followed by (b) *projection* and (c) *rationalization.*
J. There is a kernel of truth in delusions.
K. Behind the anger and suspicion in a paranoid, there is a lonely, terrified person feeling vulnerable due to feelings of inadequacy.

3. Nursing interventions in paranoid disorders
A. *Long-term goals:* gain clear, correct perceptions and interpretations through corrective experiences.
B. *Short-term goals:*
    1. Help client recognize distortions, misinterpretations.
    2. Help client feel safe in exploring reality.
C. Help clients learn to trust *themselves;* help them develop self-confidence and ego assets through positive reinforcement.
D. Help them *trust others.*
    1. Be consistent and honest at all times.
    2. Do not whisper, act secretive, or laugh with others in their presence when they cannot hear what is said.
    3. Do not mix medicines with food.
    4. Keep promises.
    5. Let them know ahead of time what they can expect from others.
    6. Give reasons and careful, complete, and repetitive explanations.
    7. Ask permission to contact others.
    8. Consult clients first about all decisions concerning them.
E. Help them *test reality.*
    1. Present and repeat reality of the situation.
    2. Do not confirm or approve distortions.
    3. Help them accept responsibility for their own behavior rather than project.
    4. Divert them from delusions to reality-centered focus.
    5. Let them know when behavior does not seem appropriate.
    6. Assume nothing and leave no room for assumptions.

7. Structure time and activities to limit delusional thought, behavior.
8. Set limit for *not* discussing delusional content.
9. Look for underlying needs expressed in delusional content.

F. Provide *outlets* for anger and aggressive drives.
1. Listen matter-of-factly to angry outbursts.
2. Accept rebuffs and abusive talk as symptoms.
3. Do not argue, disagree, or debate.
4. Allow expression of negative feelings without fear of punishment.

G. Provide *successful group experience*.
1. Avoid competitive sports involving close physical contact.
2. Give recognition to skills and work well done.
3. Utilize managerial talents.
4. Respect their intellect and engage them in activities with others requiring intellect (chess, puzzles, and Scrabble, for example).

H. Limit physical contact.

PERSONALITY DISORDERS

A personality disorder, also referred to as *character disorders* or *antisocial, sociopathic,* or *psychopathic personality,* is a syndrome in which the person's inner difficulties are revealed by a pattern of living that seeks *immediate gratification of impulses* and instinctual needs without regard for society's laws, mores, and customs and *without censorship* of personal conscience.

1. Assessment of personality disorders
A. Display disorder of *behavior* rather than of *feelings* or thoughts.
B. Usually violate laws, mores, and customs.
C. Seek immediate gratification of impulses and instinctual needs without regard for society's rules.
D. Do not tolerate frustration.
E. Do not appear to profit from experience; repeat same punishable or antisocial behavior.
F. Have poor interpersonal relationships, although they are usually very charming, bright, and intelligent.
G. Exhibit poor judgement; may have intellectual, but not emotional, insight to guide judgements.
H. May have a history of drug abuse and/or habituation.
I. Use manipulative behavior patterns in treatment setting (see *Manipulation,* Unit 2):
1. Demand and control.

2. Pressure and coerce.
3. Violate rules, routines, procedures.
4. Request special privileges.
5. Betray confidences and lie.
6. Ingratiate.
7. Threaten.
8. Monopolize conversation.

2. Concepts and principles related to personality disorders
A. One defense against severe anxiety is "acting out" or dealing with distressful feelings or issues through action.
B. Faulty or arrested emotional development in the preoedipal period has interfered with development of adequate social control or superego.
C. Since there is a malfunctioning or weakened superego, there is little internal demand and therefore no tension between ego and superego to evoke guilt feelings.
D. The defect is not intellectual; persons show lack of moral responsibility, inability to control emotions and impulses, and deficiency in normal feeling responses.
E. Pleasure principle is dominant.
F. The initial stage of treatment is most crucial; the treatment situation is very threatening because it mobilizes their anxiety, and they end treatment abruptly.
1. The key underlying emotion is fear of closeness, with threat of exploitation, control, and abandonment.

3. Nursing interventions in personality disorders
A. *Long-term goal:* help person accept responsibility and consequences of own actions.
B. *Short-term goal:* minimize manipulation and acting out.
C. Set fair, firm, consistent limits and follow through on consequences of behavior; let clients know what they can expect from staff and what the unit's regulations are, as well as the consequences of violations. Be explicit.
D. Avoid letting staff be played against one another by a particular client; staff should present a unified approach.
E. Nurses should control their own feelings of anger and defensiveness aroused by any person's manipulative behavior.
F. Change focus when clients persist in raising inappropriate subjects (such as personal life of a nurse).

G. Encourage expression of feelings as an alternative to acting out.

H. Aid clients in realizing and accepting responsibility for their own actions and social responsibility to others.

I. Use group therapy as a means of peer control and multiple feedback about behavior.

SUBSTANCE USE DISORDERS (PREVIOUSLY CALLED DRUG DEPENDENCE, ADDICTION)

Substance dependence is a state of chronic or recurrent intoxication from the use of a drug and is characterized by *habituation* (psychological need to take the drug), *tolerance* (requires increase in dose to obtain desired effect), and *physical dependency* (withdrawal symptoms occur when abstain).

Only in recent years has substance abuse been viewed as an illness rather than a moral delinquency or criminal behavior. The disorders are very complex and little understood. There are physiologic, psychologic, and social aspects to their causality, dynamics, symptoms, and treatment, where personality disorder has a major part.

Physiologic aspects—current unproven theories include "allergic" reaction to alcohol, disturbance in metabolism, genetic susceptibility to dependency, and hypofunction of adrenal cortex. There are *organic effects* of chronic excessive use.

Psychologic aspects—disrupted parent-child relationship and family dynamics; deleterious effect on ego-function.

Social and cultural aspects—local customs and attitudes vary about what is excessive.

ALCOHOL DEPENDENCE (PREVIOUSLY CALLED ALCOHOL ADDICTION)

Alcohol dependence is a chronic disorder in which the individual is unable, for physical or psychologic reasons, or both, to refrain from frequent consumption of alcohol in quantities that produce intoxication and disrupt health and ability to perform daily functions.

1. Assessment of alcohol dependence (alcohol addiction)

A. Vicious cycle—(a) low tolerance for coping with frustration, tension, guilt, resentment, (b) alcohol for relief, (c) new problems created by drinking, (d) new anxieties, and (e) more drinking.

B. Coping mechanisms used: *denial, rationalization, projection.*

C. For symptoms associated with alcohol withdrawal, see Figure 2–6.

D. *Complications of abuse and dependence (alcoholism):*

1. *Alcohol withdrawal delirium (delirium tremens—DTs)*—result of nutritional deficiencies and toxins; requires sedation and constant watchfulness against unintentional suicide and convulsions.

 a. *Impending* signs relate to *central nervous system*—marked nervousness and restlessness, increased irritability, gross tremors of hands, face, lips; weakness; also *cardiovascular*—increased blood pressure, tachycardia, diaphoresis; *depression; gastrointestinal*—nausea, vomiting, anorexia.

 b. *Actual*—serious symptoms of mental confusion, convulsions, hallucinations (visual, auditory, tactile). Without cure, 15% to 20% may die.

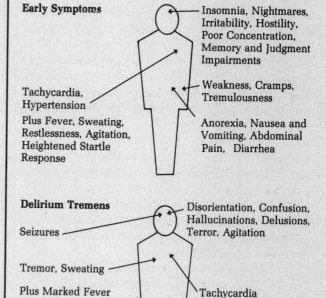

FIGURE 2–6. Symptoms associated with alcohol withdrawal. *Source:* Holly S. Wilson and Carol Ren Kneisl, *Psychiatric Nursing* (Menlo Park, Calif.: Addison-Wesley Publishing Co., 1979), p. 605.

2. *Alcohol amnestic disorder (Korsakoff's syndrome)*—degenerative neuritis:
   a. Impaired thoughts.
   b. Confusion.
   c. Loss of sense of time and place.
   d. Use of confabulation to fill in memory gaps.
3. *Wernicke's syndrome*—a *thiamine* deficiency producing alcohol-related delirium. A neurologic disease manifested by confusion, ataxia, eye movement abnormalities, and memory impairment. Other problems include:
   a. Disturbed vision.
   b. Mind-wandering.
   c. Stupor and coma.
4. *Polyneuropathy*—sensory and motor nerve endings are involved, causing pain, itching, and loss of limb control.
5. *Others*—*gastritis, esophageal varices, cirrhosis, pancreatitis, diabetes,* pneumonia, REM sleep deprivation, *malnutrition.*

2. Concepts and principles related to alcohol dependence (alcohol addiction)

A. Alcohol affects cerebral cortical functions:
   1. Memory.
   2. Judgement.
   3. Reasoning.
B. Alcohol is a depressant:
   1. Relaxes the individual.
   2. Lessens use of repression of unconscious conflict.
   3. Releases inhibitions, hostility, and primitive drives.
C. Drinking represents a tension-reducing device and a relief from feelings of insecurity.
   1. Strength of drinking habit equals degree of anxiety and frustration intolerance.
D. Alcohol abuse and dependence (alcoholism) is a symptom rather than a disease.
E. The spouse of the alcoholic often unconsciously contributes to the drinking behavior because of own emotional needs (co-alcoholic).
F. Underlying fear and anxiety, associated with inner conflict, motivate the alcoholic to drink.
G. Alcoholics can never be cured to drink normally; cure is to be a "sober alcoholic," with total abstinence.
H. Intoxication occurs with a blood alcohol level of 0.15% or above. Signs of intoxication are:
   1. Incoordination.
   2. Slurred speech.
   3. Dulled perception.
I. Tolerance occurs with alcohol dependence. Increasing amounts of alcohol must be consumed in order to obtain the desired effect.

3. Nursing interventions in alcohol dependence

A. *Detoxification phase:*
   1. *Administer adequate sedation* to control anxiety, insomnia, agitation, tremors.
   2. *Administer anticonvulsants* to prevent withdrawal seizures.
   3. *Control nausea and vomiting* to avoid massive GI bleeding or rupture of esophageal varices.
   4. *Assess fluid and electrolyte balance* for dehydration (may need IV fluids) or overhydration (may need a diuretic).
   5. *Reestablish proper nutrition:* high protein, carbohydrate, vitamins C and B complex.
   6. *Provide calm, safe environment:* bedrest with rails, well-lit room to reduce illusions; constant supervision and reassurance about fears and hallucinations; assess depression for suicide potential.
B. *Recovery-rehabilitation phase:* encourage participation in group activities; avoid sympathy when clients tend to rationalize their behavior and seek special privileges—use acceptance and a nonjudgemental, consistent, firm, but kind approach; avoid scorn, contempt, and moralizing or punitive and rejecting behaviors, as they may reinforce feelings of worthlessness, self-contempt, hopelessness, and low self-esteem.
C. *Problem behaviors:*
   1. *Manipulative*—be firm and consistent; avoid "bid for sympathy."
   2. *Demanding*—set limits.
   3. *Acting out*—set limits, enforce rules and regulations, strengthen impulse control and ability to delay gratification.
   4. *Dependency*—place responsibility on client; avoid advice-giving.
   5. *Superficiality*—help client make realistic self-appraisals and expectations in lieu of grandiose promises and trite verbalizations; encourage formation of lasting interpersonal relationships.
D. *Common reactions among staff:*
   1. Disappointment—instead, set realistic goals, take one step at a time.
   2. Moral judgement—instead, support each other.
   3. Hostility—instead, offer support to each other when feeling frustrations from lack of results.
E. Refer clients from hospital to community resources

for follow-up treatment with social, economic, and psychologic problems, as well as to self-help groups, in order to reduce "revolving-door" situation in which clients come in, are treated, go out, and come in again the next night.

1. *Alcoholics Anonymous (AA)*—a self-help group of addicted drinkers who confront, instruct, and support fellow drinkers in their efforts to stay sober one day at a time through fellowship and acceptance.

2. *Alanon*—support group for *family* of alcoholic. *Alateen*—support group for teenagers when parent is alcoholic.

3. *Antabuse*—drug that produces intense headache, severe flushing, extreme nausea, vomiting, palpitations, hypotension, dyspnea, and blurred vision when alcohol is consumed while person is taking this drug.

4. *Aversion therapy*—clients are subjected to revulsion-producing or pain-inducing stimuli at the same time they take a drink, to establish alcohol-rejection behavior.

5. *Group psychotherapy*—the goals of group psychotherapy are for the client to give up alcohol as a tension reliever, identify cause of stress, build different means for coping with stress, and accept drinking as a serious symptom.

ABUSE OF OTHER NON-ALCOHOLIC SUBSTANCES

Substance dependence (drug addiction) is an overpowering desire or need to continue taking a natural or synthetic drug having habit-forming properties, producing tolerance and subsequent need to increase dose. Psychologic and sometimes physical dependency results.

1. Assessment: abuse of nonalcoholic substances

A. Affects both sexes and all levels of educational, social, and economic status.

B. Effects:
1. Contentment-inducing.
2. Hallucinogenic.
3. Tension-reducing.

C. Person may resort to illegal means to obtain money for ever-increasing drug consumption or to obtain the drug itself.

D. Overdose (OD) may result when purity of drug is altered or when, after a period of abstinence, individual goes back to former high dose.

E. Other commonly abused substances:

1. Sedatives (barbiturates)—may result in poor concentration, irritability, mood swings, slurred speech, tremor, staggering gait, suicide.

2. Stimulants (amphetamines)—may result in loud, irritable behavior; tremulousness; persecutory delusions.

3. Hypnotics—prolonged use may lead to dependency; causes same signs as barbiturates.

4. Hallucinogens (LSD, marijuana, STP, peyote)—produce euphoria, relaxation, perceptual impairment, feelings of omnipotence, "bad trip," "flashbacks," suicide.

5. Narcotics (heroin, morphine, Demerol)—used by "snorting," "skin-popping," and "mainlining"; may lead to abscesses and hepatitis.

F. *Withdrawal symptoms (narcotics)*—begins within 12 hours of last dose, peaks in 24 to 36 hours, subsides in 72 hours, and disappears in 5 to 6 days.
1. Pupil dilatation.
2. Muscle twitches and tremors.
3. Goose flesh.
4. Lacrimation.
5. Rhinorrhea.
6. Sneezing.
7. Profuse sweating.
8. Potential for fever.
9. Vomiting.
10. Dehydration.
11. Abdominal distress.
12. Rapid weight loss.

G. *Withdrawal syndrome (barbiturates)*—may be gradual or abrupt ("cold turkey"); latter is dangerous or life-threatening; should be hospitalized.
1. *Gradual* withdrawal reaction:
   a. Postural hypotension.
   b. Tachycardia.
   c. Elevated temperature.
   d. Insomnia.
   e. Tremors.
   f. Agitation.
2. *Abrupt* withdrawal from barbiturates:
   a. Apprehension.
   b. Weakness.
   c. Tremors.
   d. Postural hypotension.
   e. Twitching.
   f. Anorexia.
   g. *Grand mal seizures.*
   h. *Psychosis.*

H. Differences between alcohol (alcoholism) and other abused substances:
1. Opium and its derivatives are obtained by illegal

means, making it a legal and criminal problem as well as a medical and social problem; not so with alcohol abuse and dependency.

2. Opium and its derivatives inhibit aggression, whereas alcohol releases it.

3. As long as they are on large enough doses to avoid withdrawal symptoms, abusers of narcotics, sedatives, and hypnotics are comfortable and function well, whereas chronically intoxicated alcoholics cannot function normally.

4. Direct physiologic effects of long-term opioid abuse and dependence are much less critical than those in chronic alcohol dependence.

2. **Concepts and principles related to opioid dependence**

A. Three interacting key factors give rise to opioid dependence—*psychopathology* of the individual; frustrating *environment;* and *availability* of powerful, addicting, and temporarily satisfying drug.

B. According to conditioning principles, substance abuse and dependence proceed in *several phases:*
   1. Use of opiates for relief from daily tensions and discomforts or anticipated withdrawal symptoms.
   2. Habit is reinforced with each relief by drug use.
   3. Development of dependency—opiate has less and less efficiency in reducing tensions.
   4. Dependency is further reinforced as addict fails to maintain adequate drug intake—increase in frequency and duration of periods of tension and discomfort.

3. **Nursing interventions in substance abuse**

A. Generally the same as those used to treat antisocial personality and alcohol abuse and dependence.

B. *Participation in group therapy—goals:* peer pressure, support, and identification.

C. *Assist with medical treatment:*
   1. *Detoxification* (or dechemicalization).
   2. *Withdrawal*—may be gradual or abrupt ("cold turkey").
   3. *Methadone*—person must have been dependent at least two years and have failed at other methods of withdrawal before admission to program of readdiction by methadone.
      a. *Characteristics:*
         (1) Synthetic.
         (2) Appeases desire for opiates without producing euphoria of narcotics.
         (3) Given by mouth.
         (4) Distributed under federal control (*Narcotic Addict Rehabilitation Act*).

         (5) Given with urinary surveillance.
      b. *Advantages:*
         (1) Prevents opiate withdrawal reaction.
         (2) Tolerance not built up.
         (3) Person remains out of prison.
         (4) Lessens perceived need for heroin or morphine.

D. Refer to halfway houses and group living (Daytop, for example).

E. Support employment as therapy (work training).

F. Expand client's range of interests to relieve characteristic boredom and stimulus hunger.
   1. Provide structured environment and planned routine.
   2. Provide educational therapy (academic and vocational).
   3. Arrange activities to include current events discussion groups, lectures, drama, music, and art appreciation.

G. Achieve role of *stabilizer and supportive* authoritative figure; this can be achieved through frequent, regular contacts with the same client.

DISORDERS PREVIOUSLY CATEGORIZED AS NEUROTIC

An anxiety disorder is a mild to moderately severe functional disorder of personality in which repressed inner conflicts between drives and fears manifest themselves in behavior patterns, including generalized anxiety, and phobic, obsessive-compulsive disorders. Other related disorders are dissociative, conversion, and hypochondriasis.

In the second edition of the Diagnostic and Statistical Manual of the American Psychiatric Association (DSM II), disorders in which the chief characteristic was anxiety, whether "felt or expressed directly" or "controlled unconsciously and automatically by conversion, displacement, and various other psychological mechanisms," were grouped together as neuroses. In contrast, in the 1980 edition of the Diagnostic and Statistical Manual (DSM III), the disorders in which anxiety is expressed directly are grouped together in the class of *anxiety disorders*. The other DSM III neuroses are distributed among other classes, such as somatoform disorders and dissociative disorders.

1. **Assessment of anxiety and other related disorders**

A. Use of behavior to avoid tense situations.

B. Are frightened, suggestive.

C. Are prone to minor physical complaints (for exam-

ple, fatigue, headaches, and indigestion) and are reluctant to admit recovery from physical illnesses.
D. Have attitude of martyrdom.
E. Often feel helpless, insecure, inferior, inadequate.
F. Use *repression, displacement, and symbolism* as key coping mechanisms.

2. Concepts and principles of anxiety and related disorders

A. Behavior may be an attempt to "bind" anxiety: to *fix* it in some particular area (hypochondriasis) or to *displace* it from the rest of personality (phobic, conversion, and dissociative disorders—amnesia, fugue, multiple personalities; obsessive-compulsive disorders).
B. Purpose of symptoms:
1. To intensify *repression* as a defense.
2. To exhibit some repressed content in *symbolic* form.
C. Analysis—behavioral dynamics:
1. Hypochondriasis (now classified as a somatoform disorder)—
   a. *Regression,* such as dependency, missing school or work.
   b. Oral-stage behaviors.
2. Phobic disorders (now considered a subcategory of anxiety disorders)—
   a. *Displacement* (symbolism of sexual conflict).
   b. Phallic-stage disorders.
   c. Conversion of conflict into avoidable external situations.
3. Conversion disorders (now classified as somatoform disorders)—
   a. Prevents acting out repressed desires.
   b. Inspires distorted expression of what is repressed.
   c. Regresses to Oedipal stage (primal scene, sexual conflict).
   d. Converts conflict into somatic symptoms, which prevents acting on repressed wish.
4. Dissociative disorders (previously called dissociative hysteria)—
   a. Repression (forgetting, becoming another identity, geographically removed by fugue).
   b. Converts conflict into physical or mental flight to prevent acting out the repressed.
5. Obsessive-compulsive disorder (now considered a subcategory of anxiety disorders)—
   a. Undoing (hostile or aggressive impulses).
   b. Anal-stage rigidity.
   c. Overdeveloped superego.
   d. Conversion of conflict into elaborate

retreats to deal with the repressed.
D. Analysis: specific patterns—
1. Anxiety disorders—
   a. *Generalized anxiety disorders:*
      (1) "Free-floating," unknown fears.
      (2) Suffer from guilt feelings, unknown cause.
      (3) Feelings of impending doom.
      (4) Disturbed emotional feeling: worry and high-level apprehension continuously present.
      (5) Dependent.
   b. *Phobic disorders:*
      (1) Irrational, abnormal fears; for example, acrophobia, hydrophobia, claustrophobia, and agoraphobia; fear out of proportion to actual danger.
      (2) Anxiety is displaced from original source and projected onto symbolic source.
   c. *Obsessive-compulsive disorders:*
      (1) Obsessive—persistent, irrational *idea;* for example, death, murder, or suicide.
      (2) Compulsive—bizarre, incomprehensible, repetitive *actions.*
      (3) Cannot be banished by will.
      (4) Comes into consciousness inappropriately; clients themselves do not understand irrational idea or action.
      (5) Behavior can be almost disabling and controlling of others.
      (6) Usually a *symbolic,* indirect way of resolving anxiety or repressed desire.
2. *Dissociative disorders*—extreme *repression* of painful reality.
   a. Amnesia—loss of memory for names, addresses, and past personal experience.
   b. Fugue—physical flight.
   c. Multiple personality:
      (1) Two or more distinct personalities develop that alternate into consciousness.
      (2) Conflicting motives exist at same time; satisfied only by *repressing* consciousness of one set while gratifying another.
3. *Somatoform disorders*—
   a. *Conversion disorders*—
      (1) Emotional distress converted to body disturbance, for example, paralysis or blindness.
      (2) Involves no actual biologic, cellular, or structural changes.

(3) Symptoms are result of an *unconscious* process.

(4) *Not* deliberate faking (malingering).

(5) Symptoms occasionally or usually disappear under hypnosis.

b. *Hypochondriasis:*

(1) Overawareness of body activities and concern with body functions; self-centered.

(2) Enjoyment gained from recounting past illnesses and operations in great detail; secondary gains occur.

(3) Eager to try quack cure-alls; read all medical literature.

(4) History of numerous medical visits.

c. See discussion of disorders with somatic complaints.

3. Nursing interventions in anxiety and related disorders

A. Attitude of acceptance and recognition of the person's worth is especially important, even though staff experience frustration.

B. Clients who are *fearful* and *anxious* (phobic and anxiety disorders):

1. Fulfill needs as promptly as possible; listen to and stay with them.

2. Eliminate need for clients to make decisions or to be in competitive situations.

3. Promote rest; decrease environmental stimuli.

4. Never force contact with feared object or situation.

C. Clients who are *ritualistic* (obsessive-compulsive disorders):

1. Accept rituals permissively (excessive hand-washing, for example); stopping ritual will increase anxiety.

2. Avoid criticism or "punishment," making demands, or showing impatience with client.

3. Allow extra time for slowness and client's need for precision.

4. Protect from rejection by others.

5. Protect from self-inflicted harmful acts.

6. Engage in nursing therapy after the ritual is over, when client is most comfortable.

7. Redirect client's actions into substitute outlets.

D. Clients who have *dissociative* and *conversion disorders:*

1. Remove clients from immediate environment to reduce pressures.

2. Divert attention to topics other than physical complaints.

3. Avoid pity and oversolicitous approach to client's "illnesses."

4. Avoid leaving clients isolated; encourage socialization.

E. Clients who have *hypochondriasis:*

1. Offer empathy without sentimentality.

2. Avoid sternness; use good-natured firmness.

3. Restore client's energy.

4. Encourage sense of humor and proper evaluation of nonessentials.

5. Provide instruction in hobbies, profitable activities, and recreation to occupy interest and decrease time for hypochondriacal thoughts.

ANOREXIA NERVOSA

Anorexia nervosa is an eating disorder, usually seen in adolescence, where a person is underweight and emaciated and refuses to eat. It can result in death due to irreversible metabolic processes.

1. Assessment of anorexia nervosa

A. Body image disturbance—delusional, obsessive (for example, doesn't see self as thin and is bewildered by others' concern).

B. Usually preoccupied with food, yet dreads gaining too much weight. Ambivalence: avoids food, hoards food.

C. Feels ineffectual, with low sex drive. Repudiation of sexuality.

D. Pregnancy fears, including misconceptions of oral impregnation through food.

E. Self-punitive behavior leading to starvation.

2. Concepts and principles related to anorexia nervosa

A. *Not* due to lack of appetite or problem with appetite center in hypothalamus.

B. Normal stomach hunger is *repressed, denied, depersonalized;* no conscious awareness of hunger sensation.

3. Nursing interventions in anorexia nervosa

A. Help reestablish connections between body sensations (hunger) and responses (eating).

1. Use stimulus-response conditioning methods to set up eating regime (see *Behavior modification,* Unit 2).

B. Monitor physiologic signs and symptoms (amenorrhea, constipation, hypoproteinemia, hypoglycemia, anemia, secondary sexual-organ atrophy, hypothermia, hypotension).

1. Weigh regularly.

2. Give one-to-one supervision during and thirty minutes after mealtime to prevent attempts to vomit food.

OTHER DISORDERS IN WHICH PSYCHOLOGIC FACTORS AFFECT PHYSICAL CONDITIONS

This group of disorders occurs in various organs and systems, whereby emotions are expressed by their effect on body organs.

1. Assessment of physiologic factors
A. Persistent psychologic factors may produce structural *organic* changes resulting in *chronic diseases,* which may be *life-threatening* if untreated.
B. All body systems are affected:
   1. Skin (pruritus and dermatitis, for example).
   2. Musculoskeletal (*backache,* muscle cramps, and rheumatism, for example).
   3. Respiratory (*asthma,* hiccups, and hay fever, for example).
   4. Gastrointestinal (ulcers, ulcerative colitis, irritable colon, heartburn, constipation, and diarrhea, for example).
   5. Cardiovascular (paroxysmal tachycardia, *migraines,* palpitations, and hypertension, for example).
   6. Genitourinary (dysuria and *dysmenorrhea,* for example).
   7. Endocrine (hyperthyroidism, for example).
   8. Nervous system (general fatigue, anorexia, and exhaustion, for example).

2. Concepts and principles related to psychologic factors affecting physical conditions
A. Majority of organs involved are usually under control of *autonomic* nervous system.
B. Coping mechanisms:
   1. *Repression or suppression* of unpleasant emotional experiences.
   2. *Introjection*—illness seen as punishment.
   3. *Projection*—others blamed for illness.
   4. *Conversion*—physical symptoms rather than underlying emotional stresses are emphasized.
C. Often exhibit the following underlying needs in excess:
   1. Dependency.
   2. Attention.
   3. Love.
   4. Success.
   5. Recognition.
   6. Security.
D. Need to distinguish between:
   1. *Malingering*—deliberate *conscious* faking of illness to avoid an uncomfortable situation.
   2. *Conversion disorder*—affecting *sensory* systems that are usually under *voluntary* control; generally *non-life-threatening;* symptoms are symbolic solution to anxiety; *no* demonstrable *organic* pathology.
   3. *Psychologic factors affecting physical condition*—under *autonomic* nervous system control; structural *organic* changes; may be life-threatening.
E. A decrease in emotional security tends to produce an increase in symptoms.
F. When treatment is confined to physical symptoms, emotional problems are not usually relieved.

3. Nursing interventions in disorders in which psychologic factors affect physical conditions
A. *Long-term goal:* release of feelings through verbalization.
B. *Short-term goals:*
   1. Take care of physical problems during acute phase.
   2. Remove from anxiety-producing stimuli.
C. Prompt attention in meeting clients' basic needs, to gratify appropriate need for dependency, attention, and security.
D. Do not say, "There is nothing wrong with you," because emotions do in fact cause somatic disabilities.
E. Maintain an attitude of respect and concern; the clients' pains and worries are very real and upsetting to them; do not belittle the symptoms.
F. Treat organic problems as necessary but without undue emphasis (that is, do not reinforce preoccupation with bodily complaints).
G. Help clients express their feelings, especially anger, hostility, guilt, resentment, and humiliation, which may be related to such issues as sexual difficulties, family problems, religious conflicts, and job difficulties.
   1. Help clients recognize that when stress and anxiety are not released through some channel, such as verbal expression, the body will release the tension through "organ language."
   2. Teach clients more effective ways of responding to stressful life situations.
H. Provide outlets for release of tensions and diversions from preoccupation with physical complaints.

1. Provide social and recreational activities to decrease time for preoccupation with illness.
2. Encourage clients to use physical and intellectual capabilities in constructive ways.

I. Protect clients from disturbing stimuli; help the healing process in the acute phase of illnesses (myocardial infarct, for example).

J. Help clients feel in control of situations and be as independent as possible.

K. Be supportive; assist clients to bear painful feelings through a helping relationship.
1. Teach the family supportive relationships.
2. Encourage expression of conflicts.

ORGANIC MENTAL DISORDERS (ORGANIC BRAIN SYNDROMES)

Organic mental disorders are those in which organic changes and neuropathology *can* be demonstrated, for example, tumors, syphilis, cerebral arteriosclerosis. Organic mental disorders have in the past been classified by *acute* and *chronic* forms, psychotic and nonpsychotic situations, and specific syndromes such as Alzheimer's disease, Pick's disease, senile brain disease, cerebral arteriosclerosis (now called *infarct dementia*), and presenile disease. A number of these syndromes characteristically occur in the elderly.

1. Assessment of organic mental disorders
A. *Most common areas of difficulty* for the person with an organic mental disorder can be grouped under the mnemonic term *JOCAM: J*—judgement, *O*—orientation, *C*—confabulation, *A*—affect, and *M*—memory.
1. *Judgement:* impaired, resulting in socially inappropriate behavior (such as hypersexuality toward inappropriate objects).
2. *Orientation:* confused, disoriented; perceptual disturbances (for example, illusions, misidentification of other persons and objects; misperception to make unfamiliar more familiar; *visual, tactile, and auditory* hallucinations may appear as images and voices or disorganized light and sound patterns). *Paranoid delusions* of persecution.
3. *Confabulation:* common use of this defense mechanism in order to fill in memory gaps with invented stories.
4. *Affect:* mood changes and unstable emotions; quarrelsome, with outbursts of morbid anger (as in cerebral arteriosclerosis); tearful; withdrawn from social contact; *depression* is a frequent reaction to loss of physical and social function.
5. *Memory:* impaired, especially for names and *recent* events; may compensate by confabulating and by using *circumstantiality* and *tangential* speaking patterns.

B. *Other areas of difficulty:*
1. *Seizures* (in Alzheimer's disease and cerebral arteriosclerosis, for example).
2. *Intellectual capacities diminished.*
a. Difficulty with abstract thought.
b. Compensatory mechanism is to stay with familiar topics; repetition.
c. Short concentration periods.
3. *Personality changes:*
a. Loss of ego flexibility; adoption of more rigid attitudes.
b. Ritualism in daily activities.
c. Hoarding.
d. Somatic preoccupations (hypochondriases).
e. Restlessness.

2. Concepts and principles related to organic mental disorders
A. Course may be progressive, with steady deterioration.
B. Alternate pathways and compensatory mechanisms may develop to show a clinical picture of remissions and exacerbations.
C. Etiologic factors: aging, substance-induced.
D. DSM III lists nine different syndromes:
1. Intoxication.
2. Withdrawal.
3. Delirium.
4. Dementia.
5. Amnestic syndromes (Alzheimer's disease).
6. Delusional.
7. Hallucinosis.
8. Affective syndromes.
9. Personality syndrome.

3. Nursing interventions in organic mental disorders— also see interventions in *Confusion/disorientation,* Unit 2.
A. *Long-term goal:* minimize regression related to memory impairment.
B. *Short-term goal:* provide structure and consistency to increase security.
C. Make brief, frequent contacts, as attention span is short.
D. Allow clients time to talk and to complete projects.

E. Stimulate associative patterns to improve recall (repeat, summarize, and focus).
F. Allow clients to review their lives and focus on the past.
G. Utilize concrete questions in interviewing.
H. Reinforce reality-oriented comments.
I. Keep environment the same as much as possible (same room and placement of furniture, for example); *routine* is important to diminish stress.
J. Recognize the importance of compensatory mechanisms (confabulation, for example) to increase self-esteem; build psychological reserve.
K. Give recognition for each accomplishment.
L. Use recreational and physical therapy.

MENTAL AND EMOTIONAL DISORDERS IN CHILDREN AND ADOLESCENTS

Children have certain developmental tasks to master in the various stages of development (for example, learning to trust, control primary instincts, and resolve basic social roles; see Unit 4, Nursing Care of Children and Families).

1. Assessment of selected disorders
A. Infantile autism (previously called childhood schizophrenia):
   1. Disturbance in how perceptual information is processed; normal abilities present.
      a. Behave as though they cannot hear, see, etc.
      b. Do not react to external stimulus.
      c. Mute or echolalic.
   2. Lack of self-awareness as a unified whole—may not relate bodily needs or parts as extension of themselves.
   3. Severe difficulty in communicating with others—may be mute and isolated.
   4. Bizarre postures and gestures (headbanging, rocking back and forth).
   5. Disturbances in learning.
   6. Etiology is unknown.
   7. Prognosis depends on severity of symptoms and age of onset.
B. Characteristics of *brain injury:*
   1. Hyperactivity.
   2. Explosive outbursts.
   3. Distractibility.
   4. Impulsiveness.
   5. Perceptual difficulties (visual distortions, such as figure-ground distortion and mirror-reading; body-image problems; difficulty in telling left from right).
   6. Receptive or expressive language problems.
C. *Enuresis*—related to feelings of insecurity due to unmet needs of attention and affection; important to preserve their self-esteem.
D. *School phobias*—anxiety about school is accompanied by physical distress. Usually observed with fear of leaving home, rejection by mother, fear of loss of mother, or history of separation from mother in early years.
E. *Behavior disorders*—include lying, stealing, running away, truancy, substance abuse, sexual delinquency, vandalism, and fire-setting; chief motivating force is either overt or covert hostility; history of disturbed parent-child relations.

2. Concepts and principles related to mental and emotional disorders in children and adolescents
A. Most emotional disorders of children are related to family dynamics and the place the child occupies in the family group.
B. Children must be understood and treated within the context of their *families.*
C. Many disorders are related to the phases of development through which the children are passing. (Erik Erikson's developmental tasks for children are trust, autonomy, initiative, industry, identity, and intimacy.)
D. Table 2–11 summarizes age-related key disturbances, lists main symptoms and causes, and highlights medical and nursing interventions.
E. Children are not miniature adults; they have special needs.
F. Play and food are important media to make contact with children and help them release emotions in socially acceptable forms, prepare them for traumatic events, and develop skills.
G. Children who are physically or emotionally ill regress, giving up previously useful habits.
H. Adolescents have special problems relating to need for *control* versus need to *rebel; dependency* versus *independency;* and search for *identity* and *self-realization.*
I. They often *act out* their underlying feelings of insecurity, rejection, deprivation, and low self-esteem.
J. Strong feelings may be evoked in nurses working with children; these feelings should be expressed, and each nurse should be supported by team members.

TABLE 2–11. *Emotional disturbances in children*

Stage	Disturbance	Assessment: symptoms or characteristics	Analysis: etiology	Interventions
Oral	Feeding disturbances	Refusal of food.	Rigid feeding schedule. *Psychological* stress. Incompatible formula. *Physiological:* pyloric stenosis.	Pediatric evaluation, especially if infant is not gaining weight or is losing weight. Rule out physiological etiology or incompatible formula. Evaluate *feeding style* of caretaker. Is baby on demand feeding? Is caretaker sensitive to infant's needs or communications about holding, hunger, or satiation?
		Colic. Crying is usually confined to one part of day and starts after a feeding. Commonly lasts from first to third month.	Sharp intestinal pains caused by gas, possibly due to periodic tension in infant's immature nervous system.	Reassure parents and give them information about condition. *Hot water bottle, rocking, rubbing back, pacifier* may soothe infant.
	Sleeping disturbances	Infant resists being put down for sleep or going to sleep.	Infant wants parental attention. Can be a pattern formed during period of colic or other illness. Emotional disturbance related to anxiety.	If attention-getting strategy, parental lack of response for few nights usually breaks pattern. If emotional disturbance is suspected, evaluation of *infant-caretaker interaction* and possible psychotherapeutic intervention.
	Failure to thrive (see also Unit 4)	Infant does not grow or develop over a period of time.	*Psychologically* inadequate caretaking. *Physiological:* heart, kidneys, central nervous system (CNS).	*Hospitalization* is essential. Evaluation of physiological functioning, especially heart, kidneys, and CNS. *Nurturing* plan for infant, using specifically assigned personnel and the caretaker parent. If the infant grows and

(Continued)

TABLE 2–11.   *(Continued)*

Stage	Disturbance	Assessment: symptoms or characteristics	Analysis: etiology	Interventions
Oral (cont.)				develops with nurturing, thus confirming problems of parenting as causative factor, psychotherapeutic and child protective interventions are necessary.
	Severe disturbances	*Autistic psychosis:* Very early onset; lack of response to others; bizarre, repetitive behavior; normal to above normal intelligence; failure to develop language or use communicative speech. Autism is one of the most severe and debilitating psychiatric disturbances.	Etiology is uncertain. The autistic child is thought to be regressed to, or fixated at, the earliest developmental stage before the child differentiates "me" from "not me." A "nature versus nurture" controversy exists over the causative factors. These are variously thought to be: 1. *Environment only:* Infant is tabula rasa and all disturbance is directly attributable to the environment (primarily the parenting). 2. *Heredity only:* For genetic, biochemical, or other predetermined reasons, some infants will be psychotic regardless of the environment. 3. *Combination of environment and heredity* plus *the interaction between them:*	The severely disturbed child requires intensive psychotherapy and often milieu therapy available in residential or day care programs. Therapy is usually indicated for parents also. Nurses can work on a *primary level* of *prevention* by assessing parenting skills of prospective parents and teaching them these skills. On a *secondary level* of *prevention,* psychiatric nurses can be knowledgeable about and teach others the early signs of childhood psychosis, making appropriate referrals. The earlier the intervention, the better the prognosis. On a *tertiary level* of *prevention,* Nurses work with severely disturbed children and their families in child guidance clinics and residential and day care settings.

TABLE 2–11. *(Continued)*

Stage	Disturbance	Assessment: symptoms or characteristics	Analysis: etiology	Interventions
Oral (cont.)			A susceptible infant, less than optimal parenting, and negative interaction between parent and infant will combine to produce disturbance.	
		Symbiotic psychosis: Identified later than autistic type, usually between two and five years. These children seem to be unable to function independently of the care-giving parent. A situational stress such as hospitalization of parent or child or entry into school may precipitate a psychotic break in the child.	The child progresses beyond the self-absorbed autistic stage to form an object relationship with another (usually the mother). Having progressed to this stage, the child then fails to differentiate his or her own identity from that of the mother. The same "nature versus nurture" controversy exists with respect to the origin of symbiotic psychosis.	
Anal	Disturbances related to toilet training	*Constipation*	If diet is not at fault, child may be withholding due to one or two painful, hard bowel movements. *Psychological* causation occurs when child withholds from parents to express anger, opposition, or passage through a very independent developmental stage.	Evaluate *diet* and consistency of stools. Fecal softener can be prescribed if necessary. In all cases, help parent avoid making an issue of constipation with the child. Enemas are *contraindicated.* If child is withholding, work with parents around not forcing rigid toilet training on child. Most children are more cooperative about *toilet training* at eighteen to twenty-four months.

(Continued)

TABLE 2–11.   *(Continued)*

Stage	Disturbance	Assessment: symptoms or characteristics	Analysis: etiology	Interventions
Anal (cont.)		*Encopresis* (soiling)	Rarely physiological. Encopresis is the child's expression of anger or hostility. It is usually directed toward the parent the child is experiencing conflict with.	Medical evaluation, then assessment and intervention in the child-parent relationship. Therapy for child (and possibly for parent) may be indicated.
		Enuresis. Ordinarily refers to wetting while asleep (nocturnal enuresis), though some enuretic children wet themselves during the day also. Enuresis is a *symptom,* not a diagnosis or disease entity.	The child under four years old is usually not considered enuretic but is included in this section because bladder training is part of toilet training. Etiology is uncertain. Causative factors are thought to be *faulty toilet training* (especially if child wets during the day also) or *psychological stress. Physiologic* etiology, such as genitourinary (GU) tract infections or CNS disease, is rare.	Many approaches have been tried with varying degrees of success. These include Trofand, *fluid restriction, behavioral intervention* (in which a buzzer wakes the child when the child starts to wet), and psychotherapy. Educating parents in *bladder training* techniques and attitudes can help solve the problem on a primary level. It is important when working with enuretic children or their parents to devise ways to help the child overcome feelings of shame and guilt. These feelings are often exacerbated by well-meaning, but misguided parents.
	Excessive rebelliousness	Frequent temper tantrums, fighting, destruction of toys and other objects, consistent oppositional behavior.	This should not be confused with expression of negativism normal at around two, which is a necessary (though trying) developmental stage. Excessive rebelliousness usually indicates a *frightened* child.	Inconsistency in handling the child, the setting of rigid limits, or the parents' refusal or inability to set limits can all create insecurity and fear in the child. The nurse should offer parent counseling if necessary. When working with the child, the nurse needs to be receptive

TABLE 2–11.   *(Continued)*

Stage	Disturbance	Assessment: symptoms or characteristics	Analysis: etiology	Interventions
Anal (cont.)				and sympathetic while establishing and maintaining firm limits.
	Excessive conformity	Lack of spontaneity, anxious desire always to please all adult authority figures, timidity, refusal to assert own needs, passivity.	These children have established very rigid control in an attempt to handle fears. Harsh *toilet training* can produce an overcompliant child. These children need help as much as overrebellious children, but they get it less frequently because their behavior is not a "problem"—that is, it is not difficult for parents to tolerate.	Excessive conformity can lead to compulsive, ritualistic, or obsessive behavior later. The nurse needs to be able to identify these children, then work with the child and parents to encourage *self-expression* in the child. Psychotherapy may be necessary to help the child deal with repressed anger.
Oedipal	Excessive fears	Child will be frightened even in nonthreatening situations. *Nightmares and other sleep disturbances* occur. Usually, child will be very "clingy" with parents in an attempt to gain reassurance.	*Anxiety* is the causative factor. Anxiety can be induced by many things, such as parental failure to set appropriate limits, *physical or psychological abuse, illness,* and fear of *mutilation.* Imaginary worries are common at this age, so a four-year-old who is suddenly afraid of the dark, or dogs, or fire engines is not necessarily suffering from excessive fears.	If possible, identify and deal with the factors that are producing the anxiety. Offer child calm reassurance. *Night-light and open doors* can help allay night fears, but counsel parents that it is unwise to allow the child to sleep with the parents. This may make the child feel that the Oedipal retaliation has succeeded. With the hospitalized child, the nurse needs to be aware of and work with the mutilation fears common at this age. Fears around certain procedures (like injections) can often be resolved by helping the child *play out fears.*

(Continued)

TABLE 2–11.   *(Continued)*

Stage	Disturbance	Assessment: symptoms or characteristics	Analysis: etiology	Interventions
Oedipal (cont.)	Excessive masturbation	Touching and fondling of genitals excessively, sometimes in a preoccupied or absent-minded manner.	Exploration and stimulation of the genital area is *normal* and common in this age group. However, if it is compulsive, the behavior is a signal that the child is *insecure.* Occasionally, it is related to a *specific fear.* For example, a boy viewing a baby sister's genitals may have castration fears. These can be dealt with directly.	*Assess* the child's masturbating activity. When does it occur and why? Then help the child develop other *strategies* for coping with anxiety. *Answer questions about sexuality* in an open manner. Counsel parents that *threats and shaming are contraindicated,* and help parents deal with *their* feelings about masturbation.
	Regression	Resumption of activities (such as *thumb sucking, soiling and wetting, baby talk)* characteristic of earlier developmental levels.	Child is attempting to regain a more comfortable previous level of development in response to a *threatening* situation (such as a new baby), or in response to difficulty resolving Oedipal *conflicts.*	Counsel parents not to make an issue of behavior. Offer child emotional support and acceptance, though not approval of regressive behavior.
	Stuttering	Articulation difficulty characterized by many stops and repetitions in speech pattern.	Stuttering usually occurs when the affected child feels *anxious, frustrated, insecure,* or *excited.* The origins of stuttering are not understood. It is *common around two to three years* and is not a cause for concern at that time.	Speech therapy is usually indicated. Psychotherapy may also be indicated, if stuttering is an expression of anxiety and conflict.
Latency	Hyperactivity and hyperkinesis	Both hyperactivity and hyperkinesis are occasionally observed in school children; characterized by a *short attention* span, restlessness, distractibility, and *impulsivity.*	An *organic disturbance* of the *CNS,* of uncertain origin, is thought to be the basis of *hyperkinesis.* Because the primary symptom—difficulty with attention span—is the same as that presented by the hyperactive child, the	For the hyperkinetic child, psychopharmaceutical intervention— usually *Ritalin*—is most often employed. Psychotherapy and special education classes may also be indicated. Ritalin is also frequently prescribed for the

TABLE 2–11.   *(Continued)*

Stage	Disturbance	Assessment: symptoms or characteristics	Analysis: etiology	Interventions
Latency (cont.)			hyperactive child is frequently and incorrectly labeled hyperkinetic. In reality the hyperactive child is attempting to *control* anxiety through *reducement* and *can* attend when interested or relaxed. Some psychologists speculate that hyperactive children do not fit smoothly into their environment, but the problem may be with the environment rather than the child. In other words, the school situation requires a high degree of conformity. The child who does not fit the mold is *not* necessarily emotionally disturbed.	hyperactive child—which raises the issue of whether an individual should be medicated to fit more smoothly into the environment. Therapy can help the hyperactive child *decrease anxiety* and *increase self-esteem,* thus reducing the symptoms.
	Withdrawal	Reduced body movement and verbalization, lack of close relationships, *detachment,* timidity, and seclusiveness.	Withdrawal is defensive behavior through which the child controls anxiety by *reducing contact* with the outer world. Like the overcompliant child, the withdrawn child is frequently not identified as needing help, because this behavior is not a "problem."	Offer *positive reinforcement* when the child is more active. Techniques designed to help these children *assert* themselves and *experience success* at certain tasks can be helpful. Occasionally, parents of the withdrawn child are extremely over-protective. In this case the nurse needs to work with the parents also. Therapy may be useful to work through anxiety and provide the child with the chance to form a *trusting* relationship with another.

(Continued)

TABLE 2–11.   *(Continued)*

Stage	Disturbance	Assessment: symptoms or characteristics	Analysis: etiology	Interventions
Latency (cont.)	Psychophysiological symptoms	The child experiences physical symptoms (such as vomiting, headaches, eczema, asthma, colitis) with no apparent physiologic cause.	*Conversion* of anxiety into physical symptoms.	After medical evaluation has established lack of physiological etiology, psychotherapy is usually indicated. Family therapy may be treatment of choice, since *dysfunctional interpersonal family dynamics* are common in these cases. The nurse can also provide the child with a healthy interpersonal relationship. Nurses are frequently in a position to talk to parents and teachers about the importance of mental health counseling for children with physical symptoms.
	School "phobia"	Sudden and seemingly inexplicable fear of going to school. These children often don't know what it is they fear at school. Frequently occurs *after an illness* and absence from school.	Not actually a phobia, but an *acute anxiety reaction related to separation* from home.	If the child is allowed to stay home, the dread of returning to school usually increases. The child and parent should have psychiatric intervention quickly (before the problem becomes worse) to help the child separate from the parent.
	Learning disabilities	Failure or difficulty in learning at school.	Emotional disorder can cause school failure. It can also result from school failure and the attendant feelings of *inferiority, discouragement,* and loss of confidence. Learning disabilities may be caused by many factors or	A comprehensive evaluation is essential. Ideally, this would include assessments by a pediatric neurologist, a mental health worker such as a psychiatric nurse or psychiatrist, a learning disabilities teacher specialist, and

TABLE 2–11.   *(Continued)*

Stage	Disturbance	Assessment: symptoms or characteristics	Analysis: etiology	Interventions
Latency (cont.)			combinations of factors. These include *anxiety, poor sensory or sensorimotor integration, dyslexia, and receptive aphasia.*	possibly an occupational therapist trained to work with sensory integration. Treatment is then based on the specific problem or problems.
	Behavior problems	Behavior that is nonproductive; that is repeated in spite of threats, punishments, or rational argument; and that usually leads to punishment. Persistent *stealing and truancy* are examples.	*Conflicts* are expressed and communicated through behavior rather than verbally. Child knows what he or she is doing but is unaware of the underlying motivations for the problem behavior.	Counseling or therapy for the child by a child psychiatric nurse or other mental health worker can allow the child to resolve the basic conflict, thus making the problem behavior unnecessary.

Source: Holly S. Wilson and Carol Ren Kneisl, *Psychiatric Nursing* (Menlo Park, Calif.: Addison-Wesley Publishing Co., 1979), pp. 489–495.

3. Nursing interventions in mental and emotional disorders in children and adolescents
A. *General goals:* corrective behavior—behavior modification.
B. Help children gain self-awareness.
C. Provide structured environment to orient children to reality.
D. Impose limits on destructive behavior toward themselves or others without rejecting the children.
  1. *Prevent* destructive behavior.
  2. *Stop* destructive behavior.
  3. *Redirect* nongrowth behavior into constructive channels.
E. Be consistent.
F. Meet developmental and dependency needs.
G. Recognize and encourage each child's strengths, growth behavior, and reverse regression.
H. Help these children reach the next step in social growth and development scale.
I. Use play and projective media to aid children in working out feelings and conflicts and in making contact.
J. Offer support to parents and strengthen the parent-child relationship.

MENTAL HEALTH PROBLEMS OF THE AGED

In general, problems affecting the elderly are *similar* to those affecting persons of any age. This section will highlight the *differences* from the viewpoint of etiology, frequency, and prognosis.

1. Assessment
A. *Assessment: psychologic characteristics of the aged:*
  1. Increasingly *dependent* on others, not only for physical needs, but also for emotional security.
  2. Concerns focus more and more *inward* with narrowed outside interests.
    a. Decreased emotional energy for concern with social problems unless these issues affect them.
    b. Tendency to reminisce.
  3. May appear selfish and unsympathetic.
  4. Sources of pleasure and gratification are more childlike; *food, warmth, and affection,* for example.
    a. Tangible and frequent evidence of affection is important (letters, cards, and visits, for example).

b. May hoard articles.

5. Fears of being unloved or forgotten.

6. Attention span and memory are short; may be forgetful and accuse others of stealing.

7. Deprivation of any kind is not tolerated:
   a. Easily frustrated.
   b. Change is poorly tolerated; need to have favorite chairs and established daily routine, for example.

8. Main *fears* in the aged include fear of dependency, chronic illness, loneliness, and boredom and fear of being deserted by those close to them.

9. Nocturnal delirium may be due to problems with night vision and inability to perceive spatial location.

2. Analysis

A. Psychiatric problems in aging:

1. *Loneliness*—related to loss of mate, diminishing circle of friends and family through death and geographical separation, decline in physical energy, loss of work (retirement), sharp loss of income, and loss of a life-long life style.

2. *Insomnia*—pattern of sleep changes in significant ways: disappearance of deep sleep, frequent awakening, daytime sleeping.

3. *Hypochondriasis*—anxiety may shift from concern with finances, job, or social prestige to concern about own bodily function.

4. *Depression*—common problem in the aging, with a high suicide rate; partly because of bodily changes which influence the self-concept, the older persons may direct their hostility toward themselves and therefore may be subject to feelings of depression and loneliness.

5. *Senility*—four early symptoms:
   a. Change in attention span.
   b. Memory loss for recent events and names.
   c. Altered intellectual capacity.
   d. Diminished ability to respond to others.

B. *Successful aging:*

1. Being able to *perceive* signs of aging and limitations resulting from the aging process.

2. *Redefining* life in terms of effects on social and physical aspects of living.

3. Seeking *alternatives* for meeting needs and finding sources of pleasure.

4. Adopting a *different outlook* about self-worth.

5. *Reintegrating* values with goals of life.

C. Causative factors of mental disorder in the aged:

1. Nutritional problems and physical ill health related to acute and chronic illness:

a. Cardiovascular diseases (heart failure, stroke, hypertension).
b. Respiratory infection.
c. Cancer.
d. Alcohol dependence and abuse.

2. Decreased physical capacity.

3. Problems related to loss, grief, and bereavement.

4. Retirement.

5. Social isolation.

6. Financial problems (reduced incomes).

7. Environmental *change* (moving within a community or from home to institution).

8. Attitudes toward condition and circumstances.

3. Concepts and principles related to mental health problems of the aged

A. The elderly *do* have a capacity for growth and change.

B. Human beings, regardless of their age, need a sense of future and hope for things to come.

C. An inalienable right of all individuals should be to make or participate in all decisions concerning themselves and their possessions as long as they can.

D. Physical disability due to the aging process may enforce dependency, which may be unacceptable to elderly patients and may evoke feelings of anger and ambivalence.

E. In an attempt to reduce feelings of loss, elderly patients may cling to concrete things that most represent, in a *symbolic* sense, all that has been significant to them.

F. As memory diminishes, *familiar objects* in the environment and *familiar routines* are important in helping to keep the clients oriented and in contact with reality.

G. Familiarity of environment brings security; routines bring a sense of security about what is to happen.

H. If individuals feel unwanted, they may tell stories about their earlier achievements.

I. Many of the traits in the elderly result from the cumulative effect of past experiences of frustrations and the present awareness of limitations rather than from any primary consequences of physiologic deficit.

4. Nursing interventions in mental health problems of the aged

A. *Long-term goal:* help reduce hopelessness and helplessness.

B. *Short-term goal:* focus on ego assets.

C. Help elderly *preserve* what facet of life they can and/or *regain* that which has already been lost.
   1. Help minimize regression as much as possible.
   2. Help retain their adult status.
   3. Help preserve their self-image as useful individuals.
   4. Identify and preserve their abilities to perform, emphasizing what they *can* do.
D. Attempt to prevent loss of dignity and loss of worth—address them by titles, not "Gramps."
E. Be sensitive to concrete things they may want to keep.
F. Use touch to reduce feelings of alienation and loneliness.
G. Provide sensory experiences for those with visual problems:
   1. Let them touch objects of various textures and consistencies.
   2. Encourage heightened use of remaining senses to make up for those that are diminished or lost.
H. Allow them to reminisce, to reduce depression and feelings of isolation.
I. Avoid changes in surroundings or routine.
J. Use simple, unhurried conversation:
   1. Protect from rush and excitement.
   2. Allow extra time to organize their thoughts.
K. Help them keep track of time (for example, by marking off days on a calendar).

Part C / TREATMENT MODES

CRISIS INTERVENTION

Crisis intervention is a type of brief psychiatric treatment in which individuals and/or their families are helped in their efforts to forestall the process of mental decompensation in reaction to severe emotional stress by direct and immediate supportive approaches.

1. **Definition of crisis**—Sudden event in one's life that disturbs homeostasis, during which usual coping mechanisms cannot resolve the problem. Types of crisis:
A. *Developmental* (internal): see Erik Erikson's eight stages of developmental crises anticipated in the development of the infant, child, adolescent, and adult.
B. *Coincidental* (external): occurs at any time; for example, loss of job, loss of income, death of significant person, illness, hospitalization, etc.

2. **Characteristics of crisis intervention**
A. Acute, sudden onset related to a stressful precipitating event of which individual is aware but which immobilizes previous coping abilities.
B. Responsive to brief therapy with focus on immediate problem.
C. Focus shifted from the psyche in the individual to the *individual in the environment;* deemphasis on intrapsychic aspects.
D. Crisis period is time-limited (usually up to six weeks).

3. **Concepts and principles related to crisis intervention**
A. Crises are turning points where changes in behavior patterns and life styles can occur; individuals in crisis are most amenable to altering old and unsuccessful coping mechanisms and are most likely to learn new and more functional behaviors.
B. Social milieu and its structure are contributing factors in both the development of psychiatric symptoms and eventual recovery from them.
C. If crisis is handled effectively, the person's mental stability will be maintained; individual may return to a precrisis state or better.
D. If crisis is not handled effectively, individual may progress to a worse state with exacerbations of earlier conflicts; future crises may not be handled well.
E. There are a number of universal developmental crisis periods (maturational crises) in every individual's life.
F. Each person tries to maintain equilibrium through use of adaptive behaviors.
G. When individuals face a problem they cannot solve, tension, anxiety, narrowed perception, and disorganized functioning occur.
H. Immediate relief of symptoms produced by crisis is more urgent than exploring their cause.

4. **Nursing interventions in crises**
A. Goals:
   1. Avoid hospitalization.
   2. Return to precrisis level and preserve ability to function.
   3. Assist in problem-solving, with *here-and-now* focus.
B. Assess the crisis:
   1. Identify stressful *precipitating* events: duration, problems created, and degree of significance.
   2. Assess *suicidal and homicidal risk*.

3. Assess amount of *disruption* in individual's life and effect on significant others.
4. Assess *current coping skills,* strengths, and general level of functioning.

C. Plan the intervention:
   1. Consider *past coping* mechanisms.
   2. Propose *alternatives* and untried coping methods.

D. Intervention approach:
   1. Help client relate the crisis event to current feelings.
   2. Encourage expression of all feelings related to disruption.
   3. Explore past coping skills and reinforce adaptive ones.
   4. Use all means available in social network to take care of client's immediate needs (significant others, law enforcement agencies, housing, welfare, employment, medical, and school, for example).
   5. Set limits.

MILIEU THERAPY

Milieu therapy consists of treatment by means of controlled modification of the client's environment to promote positive living experiences.

1. Characteristics of milieu therapy

A. Absence of serious conflict among personnel.
B. Opportunity to discuss interpersonal relationships in the unit among clients and between clients and staff (decreased social distance between staff and clients).
C. Friendly, warm, trusting, secure, supportive, comforting atmosphere throughout the unit.
D. Maximum of individualization in dealing with clients, especially regarding treatment and privileges in accordance with clients' needs.
E. Opportunity for clients to take responsibility for themselves and for the welfare of the unit in gradual steps.
   1. Client government.
   2. Client-planned and client-directed social activities.
F. An optimistic attitude about prognosis of illness.
G. Attention to comfort, food, and daily living needs; help with resolving difficulties related to tasks of daily living.
H. Program of carefully selected resocialization activities to prevent regression.

I. Opportunity to live through and test out situations in a realistic way by providing a setting that is a microcosm of the larger outside world.

2. Concepts and principles related to milieu therapy

A. Everything that happens to clients from the time they are admitted to the hospital or treatment setting has a potential that is either therapeutic or antitherapeutic.
   1. Not only the therapists, but all who come in contact with the clients in the treatment setting, are important to the clients' recovery.
   2. Emphasis is on the social, economic, and cultural dimension, the interpersonal climate, as well as the physical environment.
B. Clients have the right, privilege, and responsibility to make decisions about daily living activities in the treatment setting.

3. Nursing interventions in milieu therapy

A. *New structured relationships*—allow clients to develop new abilities and use past skills; support them through new experiences as needed; help build liaisons with others; set limits; help clients modify destructive behavior; encourage group solutions to daily living problems.
B. *Managerial*—inform clients about expectations; preserve orderliness of events.
C. *Environmental manipulation*—regulate the outside environment to alter daily surroundings.
   1. Geographically move clients to units more conducive to their needs.
   2. Work with families, clergy, employers, etc.
   3. Control visitors for the benefit of the client.
D. Team approach uses the milieu to meet each client's needs.

BEHAVIOR MODIFICATION

Behavior modification is a therapeutic approach involving the application of learning principles to change maladaptive behavior.

1. Definitions

conditioned avoidance   (also *aversion therapy*) a technique whereby there is a purposeful and systematic production of strongly unpleasant responses in situations to which the client has been previously attracted but now wishes to avoid.
desensitization   frequent exposure in small, but

gradually increasing, doses of anxiety-evoking stimuli until undesirable behavior disappears or is lessened (as in phobias).

token economy desired behavior is reinforced by rewards, such as candy, money, and verbal approval as tokens.

operant conditioning a method designed to elicit and reinforce desirable behavior (especially useful in mental retardation).

positive reinforcement giving rewards to elicit or strengthen selected behavior or behaviors.

2. Objectives and process of treatment in behavior modification

A. Emphasis is on changing unacceptable, overt, and observable behavior to that which is acceptable; emphasis is on changed way of *acting* first, not of thinking.

B. Mental health team determines behavior to change and treatment plan to use.

C. Therapy is based on the knowledge and application of *learning* principles, that is, *stimulus-response,* the unlearning or *extinction* of undesirable behavior, and the *reinforcement* of desirable behavior.

D. Therapist identifies what events are important in the life history of the client and arranges situations in which the client is therapeutically confronted with them.

E. Two primary aspects of behavior modification:
   1. Eliminate unwanted behavior by *punishment* (negative reinforcement) and *ignoring* (withholding positive reinforcement).
   2. Create acceptable new responses to an environmental stimulus by *positive* reinforcement.

3. Assumptions of behavioral therapy

A. Behavior is what an organism does.

B. Behavior can be observed, described, and recorded.

C. It is possible to predict under what conditions the same behavior may recur.

D. Undesirable social behavior is not a symptom of mental illness, but is behavior that can be modified.

E. Undesirable behaviors are learned disorders that relate to acute anxiety in a given situation.

F. Maladaptive behavior is learned in the same way as adaptive behavior.

G. People tend to behave in ways that "pay off."

H. Three ways in which behavior can be reinforced:
   1. Positive reinforcer (adding something pleasurable).
   2. Negative reinforcer (removing something unpleasant).
   3. Adverse stimuli (punishing).

I. If an undesired behavior is ignored, it will extinguish.

J. Learning process is the same for all; therefore, all conditions (except organic) are accepted for treatment.

4. Nursing interventions in behavior modification

A. Find out what is a "reward" for the person.

B. Break the goal down into small successive steps.

C. Maintain close and continuous observation of the selected behavior or behaviors.

D. Be consistent with on-the-spot, immediate intervention and correction of undesirable behavior.

E. Record focused observations of behavior frequently.

F. Participate in close teamwork with the entire staff.

G. Evaluate procedures and results continuously.

ACTIVITY THERAPY

Activity therapy consists of a variety of recreational and vocational activities (RT, recreational therapy; OT, occupational therapy; and music, art, and dance therapy) designed to test and examine social skills and serve as adjunctive therapies.

1. Characteristics of activity therapy

A. Usually planned and coordinated by other team members, the recreational therapists or music therapists, for example.

B. Goals:
   1. Encourage socialization in community and social activities.
   2. Increase self-esteem.
   3. Teach new skills, help clients find new hobbies.
   4. Provide pleasurable activities.
   5. Free and/or strengthen physical and creative abilities.
   6. Offer graded series of experiences, from passive spectator role and vicarious experiences to more direct and active experiences.
   7. Help clients release tensions and express feelings.

2. Concepts and principles related to activity therapy

A. Socialization counters the regressive aspects of illness.

B. Activities need to be selected for specific psychosocial reasons to achieve specific effects.

C. Nonverbal means of expression as an additional

behavioral outlet add a new dimension to treatment.

D. Sublimation of sexual drives is possible through activities.

3. Nursing interventions in activity therapy

A. Encourage, support, and cooperate in client's participation in activities planned by the adjunct therapists.

B. Share knowledge of client's illness, talents, interests, and abilities with others on the team.

GROUP THERAPY

Group therapy is a treatment modality in which two or more clients and one or more therapists interact in a helping process to bring about relief in emotional difficulties, increase self-esteem and insight, and improve behavior in relations with others (Table 2–12).

1. General group aims

A. Provide opportunity for self-expression of ideas and feelings.

B. Provide a setting for a variety of relationships through group interaction.

C. Explore current behavioral patterns with others and observe dynamics.

D. Provide peer and therapist support and source of strength for the individuals to modify present behavior and try out new behaviors; made possible through development of identity and group identification.

E. Provide on-the-spot, multiple feedback (that is, incorporate others' reactions to behavior), as well as give feedback to others.

F. Resolve dynamics and provide insight.

2. Concepts and principles related to group therapy

A. People's problems usually occur in a social setting, thus they can best be evaluated and corrected in a social setting (see Table 2–13 for summary of curative factors).

B. Not all are amenable to group therapies, for example:
1. Brain-damaged.
2. Acutely suicidal.
3. Acutely psychotic.
4. Persons with very passive-dependent behavioral patterns.
5. Acutely manic.

C. It is best to match group members for *complementarity in behaviors* (verbal with nonverbal, with-

drawn with outgoing) but for *similarity in problems* (obesity, predischarge group, cancer patients, prenatal group) to facilitate empathy in the sharing of experiences and to heighten intragroup identification and cohesiveness.

D. Feelings of *acceptance,* belonging, respect, and comfort develop in the group and facilitate change and health.

E. In a group, members can *test reality* by giving and receiving *feedback.*

F. Patients have a chance to experience in the group that they are not alone (concept of *universality*).

G. Expression and *ventilation* of strong emotional feelings (anger, anxiety, fear, and guilt) in the safe setting of a group is an important aspect of the group process aimed at health and change.

H. The group setting and the *interactions* of its members may provide corrective emotional experiences for its members.
1. A key mechanism operating in groups is *transference* (strong emotional attachment of one member to another member, to the therapist, and/or to the entire group).

I. To the degree that people modify their behavior through corrective experiences and identification with others rather than through personal-insight analysis, group therapy may be of special advantage over individual therapy in that the possible number of interactions is greater in the group and the patterns of behavior are more readily observable.

J. There is a higher client-to-staff ratio, and it is thus less expensive.

3. Nursing interventions in group setting

A. Nurses have different roles and functions in the group, depending on the type of group, its size, its aims, and the stage in the group's life cycle.
1. The multifaceted roles may include:
   a. Catalyst.
   b. Transference object.
   c. Clarifier.
   d. Interpreter of "here-and-now."
   e. Role model and resource person.
   f. Supporter.

B. During the *first session,* explain the purpose of the group, go over the "contract" (structure, format, and goals of sessions), and facilitate introductions of group members.

C. In *subsequent* sessions, promote greater group cohesiveness:
1. Focus on *group concerns* and group process rather than on intrapsychic dynamics of individuals.

TABLE 2–12.   *Differences in characteristics of types of groups*

Characteristic	Task groups	Self-awareness/ growth groups	Therapy groups	Social groups
Purpose, goals	Performance of specific job or task explicitly agreed on by all members at initiation of group. Member participation is determined by task.	Development or use of interpersonal strengths. Broad objectives, such as to study group process, communication patterns, or problem solving are usually apparent at initiation of group.	Clearly defined: to do the work of therapy. Individual works toward self-understanding, more satisfactory ways of relating, handling stress, and so on.	Recreation, relaxation, and comfort promoted through mutual pleasure and enjoyment among friends and acquaintances in a social situation, such as a party at someone's home.
Shared aim	To achieve group's task goal.	To improve functioning of group one returns to (job, family, community) through translation of one's own interpersonal strengths or To improve perception of members.	To improve perception of members and to improve individual health.	To experience fun, companionship, and satisfying relationships with friends.
Format	Defined at outset by leader and/or members. Method is specific to task to be performed.	Specific format, if any, and methods defined throughout group process by all members and leader/ trainer. Lack of agenda and structure may produce some difficulty.	Defined by therapist within context of some psychotherapeutic orientation. Definition is apparent through implementation of therapeutic principles.	Usually spontaneous. May be defined by members in case of planned recreational activities.
Focus	Completion of specific task.	Interpersonal concerns around current situations.	Member-centered. Past experiences may be just as relevant as current concerns depending on therapist's orientation.	Member-centered toward enjoyment and mutual meeting of needs.

(Continued)

TABLE 2–12. *(Continued)*

Characteristic	Task groups	Self-awareness/ growth groups	Therapy groups	Social groups
Role of leader	To establish exchange of information among members and direct group toward task accomplishment, adhering to agenda.	To establish group interaction at emotional level among group members, and to serve as resource person guiding group by calling attention to certain events or processes and facilitating problem solving, mutual understanding, communication.	To establish group interaction between self and individual members and among group members. To facilitate members' interactions in work of therapy.	To meet basic requirements for social companionship, providing place, planning activity, preparing food, drink, etc.
Title of leader	Usually called chairperson.	Usually called trainer.	Usually called therapist.	Usually called host or hostess.
How leader differs from members	Chairperson identifies specific task, clarifies communication, and assists in expressing opinions and offering solutions.	Trainer differs from members by having superior skills in specialized area (understanding and facilitating group process). Trainer's superiority diminishes as group continues and members learn and implement similar skills.	Therapist differs from members by having superior skills in specialized area (group psychotherapy). Therapist never truly becomes member but may at times take on members' roles.	Host or hostess is member of group and works toward own as well as others' pleasure and enjoyment.
Requirements of leader	Qualified back-ground and expertise in area of task emphasis. Must be accepted by members as an appropriate leader.	Sufficient preparation, experience, and skill to maintain effective control of interpersonal tensions.	Sufficient preparation and skill to undertake psychotherapy within context of situation.	Willingness to take steps to initiate social interaction.
Orientation of group work	Reality-oriented in terms of adhering to explicit work goal. If group deviates into interpersonal realm, task is not accomplished most efficiently.	Reality testing with here-and-now emphasis. Assumption is that members can correct inefficient patterns of relating and communicating with each other. Members learn group process experientially through participation and involvement.	Oriented toward having members gain insight as basis for changing patterns of behavior toward health.	Oriented toward having fun, seeking pleasure and relaxation, releasing tension.

TABLE 2–12. *(Continued)*

Characteristic	Task groups	Self-awareness/ growth groups	Therapy groups	Social groups
Selection of members	Selection made possibly in terms of individual's functional role, not usually in terms of personal characteristics, often in terms of employment status.	Selection criteria range from simply expressed desire to become more self-aware to mixture of criteria based on personality characteristics— Fundamental Interpersonal Relationship Orientation (FIRO) scales, defenses, behavior patterns, etc.	Selection usually based on extensive consideration of constellation of personalities, behaviors, and needs and identification of group therapy as treatment of choice.	Selection based on considerations of friendship or social obligation. Host or hostess chooses whom to invite.
Title of members	Known as committee members.	May be called trainees.	Known as clients or, in some settings, patients.	Known as guests.
Interviewing of prospective members	Usually not interviewed before entry into group.	May or may not be interviewed and/or requested to complete questionnaires on personal data and personality characteristics before entry into group.	Extensive selection interview(s) required before entry into group.	Not interviewed. Usually known through prior social acquaintance.
Length of group life	Target date usually set in advance.	Tends to be short-term, with target date set in advance.	Usually not set. Termination date usually determined mutually by therapist and members.	May be set in advance or spontaneously determined.

Source: Holly S. Wilson and Carol Ren Kneisl, *Psychiatric Nursing* (Menlo Park, Calif.: Addison-Wesley Publishing Co., 1979), pp. 437–438.

2. Demonstrate nonjudgemental acceptance of behaviors within the limits of the group contract.
3. Help group members handle their anxiety, especially during the initial phase.
4. Encourage silent members to interact at their level of comfort.
5. Encourage members to interact verbally without dominating the group discussion.
6. Keep the focus of discussion on related themes; *set limits and interpret group rules.*
7. Facilitate sharing and *communication* between members.
8. Provide *support* to members as they attempt to work through anxiety-provoking ideas and feelings.
9. Set the expectation that the members are to take responsibility for carrying the group discussion and exploring issues on their own.

D. *Termination phase:*
1. Make early preparation for group termination

TABLE 2–13. *Curative factors of group therapy*

Factor	Definition
Instilling of hope	Imbuing the client with optimism for the success of the group therapy experience
Universality	Disconfirming the client's sense of aloneness or uniqueness in misery or hurt
Imparting of information	Giving didactic instruction, advice, or suggestions
Altruism	Finding that the client can be of importance to others; having something of value to give
Corrective recapitulation of the primary family group	Reviewing and correctively reliving early familial conflicts and growth-inhibiting relationships
Development of socializing techniques	Acquiring sophisticated social skills, such as being attuned to process, resolving conflicts, and being facilitative toward others
Imitative behavior	Trying out bits and pieces of the behavior of others and experimenting with those that fit well
Interpersonal learning	Learning that the client is the author of his or her interpersonal world and moving to alter it
Group cohesiveness	Being attracted to the group and the other members with a sense of "we"-ness rather than "I"-ness
Catharsis	Being able to express feelings
Existential factors	Being able to "be" with others; to be a part of a group

Source: Holly S. Wilson and Carol Ren Kneisl, *Psychiatric Nursing* (Menlo Park, Calif.: Addison-Wesley Publishing Co., 1979), p. 468.

(end point should be announced at the first meeting).

2. Anticipate common reactions from group members to separation anxiety and help each member to work through these reactions:
   a. Anger
   b. Acting out.
   c. Regressive behavior.
   d. Repression.
   e. Feelings of abandonment.
   f. Sadness.

FAMILY THERAPY

Family therapy is a process, method, and technique of psychotherapy in which the focus is not on an individual but on the total family as an interactional system.

1. **Developmental tasks of North American family (Duvall, 1971)**
   A. *Physical maintenance*—provide food, shelter, clothing, health care.
   B. *Resource allocation*—(physical and emotional) allocate material goods, space, and facilities; give affection, respect, and authority.
   C. *Division of labor*—decide who earns money, manages household, cares for family.
   D. *Socialization*—guidelines to control food intake, elimination, sleep, sexual drives, and aggression.
   E. *Reproduction, recruitment, release of family members*—give birth to, or adopt, children; rear children; incorporate in-laws, friends, etc.
   F. *Maintenance of order*—ensure conformity to norms.
   G. *Placement of members in larger society*—interaction in school, community, etc.
   H. *Maintenance of motivation and morale*—reward achievements, develop philosophy for living; create rituals and celebrations to develop family loyalty. Show acceptance, encouragement, affection; meet crises of individuals and family.

2. **Basic theoretic concepts related to family therapy**
   A. The ill family member (called the identified patient, or IP), by symptoms, sends a message about the "illness" of the family as a *unit*.
   B. *Family homeostasis* is the means by which families attempt to maintain the status quo.
   C. *Scapegoating* is found in disturbed families and is usually focused on one family member at a time, with the intent to keep the family in line.
   D. Communication and behavior by some family members bring out communication and behavior in other family members.
      1. Mental illness in the IP is almost always accompanied by emotional illness and disturbance in other family members.
      2. Changes occurring in one member will produce changes in another; that is, if the IP improves, another IP may emerge or family may try to place original person back into IP role.
   E. Human communication is a key to emotional stability and instability—to normal and abnormal health.

1. Conjoint family therapy is a communication-centered approach that looks at interactions between family members.
F. *Double bind* is a "damned-if-you-do, damned-if-you-don't" situation; it results in helplessness, insecurity, anxiety, fear, frustration, and rage.
G. *Symbiotic tie* usually occurs between one parent and a child, hampering individual ego development and fostering strong dependence and identification with the parent (usually the mother).
H. Three basic premises of communication:*
   1. One cannot *not* communicate; that is, silence is a form of communication.
   2. Communication is a multilevel phenomenon.
   3. The message sent is not necessarily the same message that is received.
I. *Family assessment* should consider the following factors:
   1. *Family as a social system*
      a. Family as responsive and contributing unit within network of other social units
         (1) Family boundaries—permeability or rigidity
         (2) Nature of input from other social units
         (3) Extent to which family fits into cultural mold and expectations of larger system
         (4) Degree to which family is considered deviant
      b. Roles of family members
         (1) Formal roles and role performance (father, child, etc.)
         (2) Informal roles and role performance (scapegoat, controller, follower, decision maker)
         (3) Degree of family agreement on assignment of roles and their performance
         (4) Interrelationship of various roles—degree of "fit" within total family
      c. Family rules
         (1) Family rules that foster stability and maintenance
         (2) Family rules that foster maladaptation
         (3) Conformity of rules to family's life style
         (4) How rules are modified; respect for difference
      d. Communication network
         (1) How family communicates and provides information to members
         (2) Channels of communication—who speaks to whom

      (3) Quality of messages—clarity or ambiguity
   2. *Developmental stage of family*
      a. Chronological stage of family
      b. Problems and adaptations of transition
      c. Shifts in role responsibility over time
      d. Ways and means of solving problems at earlier stages
   3. *Subsystems operating within family*
      a. Function of family alliances in family stability
      b. Conflict or support of other family subsystems and family as a whole
   4. *Physical and emotional needs*
      a. Level at which family meets essential physical needs
      b. Level at which family meets social and emotional needs
      c. Resources within family to meet physical and emotional needs.
      d. Disparities between individual needs and family's willingness or ability to meet them
   5. *Goals, values, and aspirations*
      a. Extent to which family members' goals and values are articulated and understood by all members
      b. Extent to which family values reflect resignation or compromise
      c. Extent to which family will permit pursuit of individual goals and values
   6. *Socioeconomic factors* (see list under individual assessment, Figure 2–2).

3. Nursing interventions in family therapy
A. Establish a family *contract* (who attends, when, duration of sessions, length of therapy, fee, and other expectations).
B. Encourage family members to identify and clarify own *goals*.
C. *Set ground rules:*
   1. Focus is on the family as a whole unit, not on the IP.
   2. No scapegoating or punishment of members who "reveal all" should be allowed.
   3. Therapists should not align themselves with issues or individual family members.
D. *Use self* to empathetically respond to family's problems; share own emotions openly and directly; function as a role model of interaction.
E. Point out and encourage the family to *clarify* unclear, inefficient, and ambiguous family communication patterns.
F. Identify family *strengths.*

*From Watzlawick, P.: An anthology of human communication, Palo Alto, California, 1964, Science and Behavior Books, Inc.

TABLE 2–14.   *Preventive approaches for family mental health*

Target population	Goals	General approach	Specific examples
1. Families in crisis due to the *loss* of a member (death, desertion, chronic hospitalization).	Provision of flexible support according to the event, how perceived and managed, and the resources and the life style of the surviving family fragment.	Primary and secondary preventive, high-risk and communitywide approaches.	Group meetings in hospital of parents of fatally ill children; expanded emergency room coverage; neighborhood information centers; walk-in clinics for problems of living; some mental health clinics.
2. Families under stress due to a *handicapped* parent (mental illness, retardation, alcoholism, or other chronic disorder).	Identification and support as needed for these families as in 1, above.	Primary and secondary preventive, high-risk approaches for children; tertiary preventive, communitywide approaches for parents.	Public health nurse makes regular home visits to family of alcoholic; family medical clinics; mental-hospital-based services; homemaker services for mentally ill mothers.
3. Families under stress due to *internal imbalance* or disorder (schism, double bind, skew, pseudomutuality, and other types of marital discord).	Assistance either in correcting the imbalance or in minimizing the impact on the children.	Primary or secondary preventive, high-risk approaches for children; secondary or tertiary preventive, communitywide approaches for parents.	Marital counseling; family therapy, parents' groups, individual therapy; legal guardian ad litem for children in divorce actions; legal aid for low-income families through neighborhood law offices.
4. Families under stress as a result of vulnerability to *normal developmental changes* (birth of a child, school entry, puberty, climacterium, retirement).	Sensitivity to the variety of family stresses or crises that may result, leading to earlier recognition and intervention as needed, often via very short-term crisis-oriented therapy.	Primary and secondary preventive, high-risk, communitywide, and milestone approaches.	Many of the above programs, especially neighborhood and/or comprehensive health, mental health, and social welfare services. Awareness of the opportunities for stress and crisis assistance is more important than the specific program setting.
5. Families *living in areas lacking necessary biopsychosocial supplies* (police protection, housing, quality education, etc.), in areas such as urban slums, depressed rural areas, migrant workers' camps, Indian reservations, and housing projects.	Provision of these basic necessities through community development approaches.	Primary, secondary, and tertiary preventive, high-risk approaches.	Community development approaches originating through schools, churches, social agencies, neighborhood service centers, family life educators, mental health centers, etc.

TABLE 2–14.   *(Continued)*

Target population	*Goals*	*General approach*	*Specific examples*
6. Families caught in the cycle of *intergenerational* poverty.	Provision of multiple and flexible opportunities for attaining desired personal, social, and economic goals.	Primary, secondary, and tertiary preventive, high-risk approaches.	Same as in 5; also a variety of antipoverty programs, such as Headstart, Upward Bound, and Job Corps, and agencies such as Mobilization for Youth, and Community Progress, Inc.
7. Disorganized families characterized by *multiple and complex problems* (emotional disorder, social dependence, poverty, chronic physical illness, child neglect or abuse, alcoholism and other addictions) and multiple needs (personal, social, medical, economic).	Use of a problem-centered versus a discipline-centered approach to diagnose the total range of causative factors, identify those most accessible to change, and plan a step-by-step program.	Primary, secondary, and tertiary preventive, high-risk approaches for adults and children.	All programs in this section may be relevant. Again, the point of view or approach is more important than the program. Several additional possibilities include twenty-four-hour emergency homemakers, and other emergency care for children needing substitute parenting.
8. Families with potentially stressful *role handicaps* (childlessness, adoptive parenthood, foster-parenting, working mothers, and student families, such as medical and other graduate students).	Awareness of the potential for stress or crisis so that early recognition and supportive help are available.	Secondary preventive, high-risk, and communitywide approaches.	Groups for adoptive or foster parents, groups for adoptive children; reliable day care centers.

Source: W. M. Bolman, "Preventive Psychiatry for the Family: Theory, Approaches, and Programs," *The American Journal of Psychiatry,* vol. 125:4, pp. 464–65, 1968. Copyright 1968, the American Psychiatric Association. Reprinted by permission.

G. Listen for repetitive interpersonal *themes, patterns,* and attitudes.

H. Attempt to *reduce guilt and blame* (important to neutralize the scapegoat phenomenon).

I. Present possibility of *alternate* roles and rules in family interaction styles.

4. *Preventive community approaches for family mental health*—See Table 2–14.

ELECTROCONVULSIVE THERAPY (ECT)

Electroconvulsive therapy is a physical treatment that induces grand mal convulsions by applying electric current to the head. It is also called electric shock therapy (EST).

1. *Characteristics of electroconvulsive therapy*

A. Usually used in treating depression.

B. Consists of a series of treatments (6 to 25) over a period of time (three times a week, for example).

C. Person is asleep through the procedure and for 20 to 30 minutes afterwards.

D. Convulsion starts with tonic spasm of entire body, followed by series of clonic, jerking motions, especially in extremities.

E. Confusion is present for 30 minutes after treatment.

F. Induces loss of memory for *recent* events.

2. *Proposed views concerning success of electroconvulsive therapy*

A. Posttreatment sleep is the "curative" factor.

B. Shock treatment is seen as punishment, with an accompanying feeling of absolution from guilt.

C. Chemical alteration of thought patterns results in

memory loss, with decrease in redundancy and awareness of painful memories.

3. Nursing interventions in electroconvulsive therapy

A. Always tell the client of the treatment.
B. Inform client about temporary memory loss for recent events after the treatment.
C. *Pretreatment care:*
  1. Take vital signs.
  2. See to client's toileting.
  3. Remove client's dentures, eyeglasses or contact lenses, and jewelry.
  4. NPO for 8 hours beforehand.
  5. Atropine sulfate subcutaneously 30 minutes before treatment to decrease bronchial and tracheal secretions.
  6. Anesthetist gives anesthetic and muscle relaxant IV (succinylcholine chloride, or Anectine) and oxygen for two to three minutes and inserts airway. Often all three are given close together—anesthetic first, followed by another syringe with Anectine and atropine sulfate. Electrodes and treatment must be given within two minutes of injections, as Anectine is very short-acting (two minutes).
D. *During the convulsion* the nurse holds the person in a safe position and in such a way as to avoid dislocation and compression fractures.
E. *Care during recovery stage:*
  1. Take blood pressure and respirations.
  2. Stay until person awakens, responds to questions, and can care for self.
  3. Orient client to time and place and inform that treatment is over.
  4. Offer support to help client feel more secure and relaxed as the confusion and anxiety decrease.

PSYCHOPHARMACOLOGY: COMMON PSYCHOTROPIC DRUGS

1. Antipsychotics

A. Phenothiazines (Compazine, Sparine, Thorazine, Mellaril, Stelazine, Trilafon, Vesprin, Prolixin Enanthate).
  1. *Use*—acute and chronic psychoses; most useful in cases of disorganization of thought or behavior; to decrease panic, fear, and hostility, restlessness, aggression, and withdrawal.
  2. *Side effects:*
    a. Hypersensitivity effects—
      (1) *Blood dyscrasia*—agranulocytosis, leukopenia, granulocytopenia.
      (2) *Skin reactions*—photosensitivity, dermatitis, flushing, blue-gray skin.
      (3) Obstructive *jaundice.*
    b. *Extrapyramidal symptoms (EPS)* affecting voluntary movement and skeletal muscles—
      (1) *Parkinsonism*—tremors, cogwheel rigidity, shuffling gait, pill-rolling, masklike facies, salivation, and difficulty starting muscular movement (dyskinesia).
      (2) *Dystonia*—limb and neck spasms (torticollis), extensive rigidity of back muscles (opisthotonus), oculogyric crisis, speech and swallowing difficulty, and protrusion of tongue.
      (3) *Akathisia*—motor restlessness, pacing, foot-tapping, inner tremulousness, and agitation.
      (4) *Tardive dyskinesia (TD)*—excessive blinking; vermiform tongue movement; coordinate, stereotyped, abnormal, involuntary sucking, chewing, licking, and pursing movements of tongue and mouth; grimacing, blinking, frowning, rocking.
        (a) *Cause*—long-term use of high doses of antipsychotic drugs.
        (b) *Predisposing factors*—age, women, OBS, history of ECT or use of tricyclics or antiParkinson drugs.
    c. *Potentiates* central nervous system depressants.
    d. *Orthostatic hypotension.*
    e. *Anticholinergic effects* (atropinelike)—dry mouth, stuffy nose, blurred vision, urinary retention, and constipation.
    f. Ocular changes (lens and corneal opacity).
B. Butyrophenones (Haldol, Innovar, Serenace)—side effects the same as those listed for phenothiazines, but less orthostatic hypotension.
C. Thioxanthenes (Taractan, Navane)—chemically related to phenothiazines, with similar therapeutic effects.
D. Nursing interventions:
  1. Anticipate, observe for, and check for side effects.
    a. Protect the person's skin from sunburn when outside.
    b. Take BP and have person lie down for 30 minutes, especially after an injection, for hypotension.

c. Watch for signs of sore throat, fever, malaise.

2. Teach client of the danger of drug potentiation with alcohol or sleeping pills.

3. Advise about driving or occupations where blurred vision may be a problem.

2. Antidepressants

A. Tricyclic (Tofranil, Elavil, Triavil, Aventyl, Vivactil, Sinequan)—effective in one to three weeks.
1. *Use*—elevate mood in depression, increase physical activity and mental alertness; may bring relief of symptoms of depression so that client can attend individual or group therapy.
2. *Side effects:*
   a. *Behavioral*—activation of latent schizophrenia, hypomania, suicide attempts.
   b. *Central nervous system* (CNS)—tremors, ataxia, jitteriness.
   c. *Autonomic nervous system* (ANS)—dry mouth, aggravation of glaucoma, constipation, urinary retention, edema, paralysis, EKG changes (flattened T waves; arrhythmia severe in overdose).

B. Monoamine-oxidase inhibitors (MAOI)—Nardil, Marplan, Parnate, Marsilid, Eutonyl, Niamid.
1. *Side effects:*
   a. *Behavioral*—may activate latent schizophrenia, mania, excitement.
   b. *CNS*—tremors; *hypertensive crisis* (avoid cheese, coke, caffeine, wine, beer, yeast, chocolate, chicken liver, or other substances high in tyramine or pressor amine; for example, amphetamines, and cold and hay fever medication); *intracerebral hemorrhage; hyperpyrexia.*
   c. *ANS*—dry mouth, aggravation of glaucoma, bowel and bladder control problems; edema, paralysis, EKG changes (arrhythmia severe in overdose).
   d. *Allergic* hepatocellular jaundice.

C. *Nursing interventions:*
1. Anticipate, observe, and check for side effects.
2. Teach danger of MAOIs and ingestion of certain foods and drugs.
3. Advise about long time lag (two to four weeks) in tricyclics before effect is felt by client.

3. Antianxiety

A. Librium:
1. *Used in* alcoholism, tension, and irrational fears; has muscle relaxant and anticonvulsant properties.

2. *Side effects*—drowsiness, motor uncoordination, confusion, skin eruptions, edema, menstrual irregularities, constipation, extrapyramidal symptoms, and blurred vision.
3. *Nursing interventions* focus on precautions, as drug may:
   a. Be habituating (causing withdrawal convulsions; therefore gradual withdrawal necessary).
   b. Potentiate CNS depressants.
   c. Have adverse effect on pregnancy.
   d. Be dangerous for those with suicidal tendencies.

B. Valium (diazepam):
1. *Use*—muscle relaxant; *not* used in psychotics.
2. *Side effects*—same as those for Librium, plus double or blurred vision, difficult speech, headache, hypotension, incontinence, tremor, and urinary retention.
3. *Precautions*—same as those for Librium; also may cause liver damage.
4. *Nursing interventions:*
   a. Anticipate, observe, and check for side effects, especially depression and suicidal risk.
   b. Teach client about sedative effects, potentiation of other drugs and alcohol, and problem of habituation.

4. Antimanic

A. Lithium—effect occurs one to three weeks after first dose.
1. *Use*—acute manic attack and prevention of recurrence of cyclic manic-depressive episodes.
2. *Side effects*—levels up to 1.6 mEq/liter may cause tremors, nausea and vomiting, diarrhea, polyuria, polydipsia; levels above 2 mEq/liter may cause motor weakness, headache, edema, and lethargy; *signs of severe toxicity:* neurologic; for example, twitching, marked drowsiness, slurred speech, athetotic movements, convulsions, delirium, stupor, coma.
3. *Precautions*—cautious use with persons on *diuretics;* those with disturbed *electrolytes* (sweating, dehydrated, and postoperative persons), with *thyroid* problems, on *low-salt* diets, with congestive *heart* failure, and with impaired *renal* function. Risk of suicide.
4. *Dosage—therapeutic* level 0.8–1.6 mEq/liter; dose for maintenance 300–1500 mEq/day; *toxic* level > 2.0 mEq/liter; blood sample drawn in

acute phase 10–14 hours after last dose, taken tid.

B. *Nursing interventions:*
1. Anticipate, observe, and check for signs and symptoms of toxicity.
2. Caution client to continue with usual dietary salt intake.
3. Report fever right away.
4. Monitor effect (therapeutic and toxic) through blood samples taken:
   a. Every two to three days until 1.6 mEq/liter is reached.
   b. Once a week while in hospital.
   c. Every two to three months to maintain blood levels under 1 mEq/liter.
5. Advise client of seven- to ten-day lag time for effect.

5. **AntiParkinson agents**—used to counteract extrapyramidal reactions.

A. Artane:
1. *Side effects*—dry mouth, blurred vision, dizziness, nausea, constipation, drowsiness, urinary hesitancy or retention, pupil dilation, headache, and weakness.
2. *Precautions*—cautious use with cardiac, liver, or kidney disease, glaucoma, or obstructive gastrointestinal-genitourinary disease.

B. Cogentin:
1. *Side effects*—same as those for Artane, plus—
   a. Effect on *body temperature* may result in life-threatening state.
   b. *Gastrointestinal distress.*
   c. *Inability to concentrate,* memory difficulties, and mild confusion (often mistaken for senility).
   d. May lead to toxic psychotic reactions.
   e. *Subjective sensations*—light or heavy feelings in legs, numbness and tingling of extremities, light-headedness or tightness of head, and giddiness.

C. *Nursing interventions:*
1. Prevent constipation through diet.
2. Observe for toxic psychotic reaction.
3. Relieve GI distress by giving after or with meals.

GLOSSARY

affect feeling or mood communicated through the face and body posture. Can be blunted, blocked, flat, inappropriate, or displaced.

ambivalence contradictory (positive and negative) emotions, desires, or attitudes coexisting toward an object or person (for example, love-hate relationship).

amnesia loss of memory due to physical or emotional trauma.

anxiety state of uneasiness or response to a vague, unspecific danger cued by a threat to some value that the individual holds essential to existence (or by a threat of loss of control); the danger may be real or imagined. Physiologic manifestations are increased pulse, respiration, and perspiration, with feeling of "butterflies."

autism self-preoccupation and absorption in fantasy as found with schizophrenia, with a complete exclusion of reality and loss of interest in and appreciation of others.

catatonia type of schizophrenia characterized by muscular rigidity, alternating with excitability.

compulsion an insistent, repetitive, intrusive, and unwanted urge to perform an act that is contrary to ordinary conscious wishes or standards.

conflict emotional struggle resulting from opposing demands and drives of the id, ego, and superego.

coping mechanism device used to ward off anxiety or uncomfortable thoughts and feelings; an activity of the ego that operates outside of awareness to hold impulses in check which might cause conflict (repression and regression, for example).

cyclothymia alterations in moods of elation and sadness, with mood swings out of proportion to apparent stimuli.

delusion a false fixed belief, idea, or group of ideas that are contrary to what is thought of as real and that cannot be changed by logic; arise out of the individual's needs and are maintained in spite of evidence or facts (grandeur and persecution, for example).

depression morbid sadness or dejection accompanied by feelings of hopelessness, inadequacy, and unworthiness. Distinguished from grief, which is realistic and in proportion to loss.

disorientation loss of awareness of the position of self in relation to time, place, or person.

echolalia automatic repetition of phrases or words heard.

echopraxia automatic repetition of observed movements.

ego the "I," "self," and "person" as distinguished from "others"; that part of the personality, according to Freudian theory, that *mediates* between the primitive, pleasure-seeking, instinctual drives of the id and the self-critical, prohibitive, restraining forces of the superego; that aspect of the psyche that is *conscious* and most in touch with external reality and is directed by the *reality principle*. The part of the personality that has to make the decision. Most of the ego is conscious and represents the *thinking-feeling* part of a person. The *compromises* worked out on an unconscious level help to resolve intrapsychic conflict by keeping thoughts, interpretations, judgements, and behavior practical and efficient.

electroshock electroshock treatment (EST) or electroconvulsive treatment (ECT) is the treatment of certain psychiatric disorders (best suited for depression) by therapeutic administration of regulated electrical impulses to the brain to produce convulsions.

empathy an objective awareness of another's thoughts, feelings, or behavior and their meaning and significance; intellectual identification versus emotional identification (sympathy).

euphoria exaggerated feeling of physical and emotional well-being not related to external events or stimuli.

flight of ideas a thought disorder where one thought moves rapidly to another without reaching a main idea or point, as in manic behavior. The next sentence may be triggered by a word in the previous sentence or by something in the environment.

fugue dissociative state involving amnesia and actual physical flight.

hallucination *false* sensory perception in the absence of an actual external stimulus. May be due to chemicals or inner needs and may occur in any of the five senses. Seen in psychosis and acute and chronic brain disorder.

hypochondriasis state of morbid preoccupation about one's health (somatic concerns).

id psychoanalytic term for that division of the psyche that is unconscious, contains instinctual primitive drives that lead to immediate gratification, and is dominated by the *pleasure principle*. The id wants what it wants when it wants it.

illusion misinterpretation of a real, external sensory stimulus. (A person may see a shadow on the floor and think it is a hole, for example.)

insanity legal term for mental defect or disease that is of sufficient gravity to bring person under special legal restrictions and immunities.

labile unstable and rapidly shifting emotions.

manipulation process of influencing another to meet one's own needs, regardless of the other's needs.

mental retardation term for mental deficiency or deficit in normal development in intelligence that makes intellectual abilities lower than normal for chronologic age. May result from a condition present at birth, from injury during or after birth, or from disease after birth.

narcissism exaggerated self-love with all attention focused on own comfort, pleasure, abilities, appearance, etc.

neologism newly coined word or condensed combination of several words not readily understood by others—found in schizophrenia.

neurosis an older, no longer used term for mild to moderately severe illness in which there is a disorder of feeling or behavior but not gross mental disorganization, delusions, or hallucinations, as in serious psychoses. Typical neurotic reactions include disproportionate anxiety, phobias, and obsessive-compulsive behavior.

obsession persistent, unwanted, and uncontrollable urge or idea that cannot be banished by logic or will.

organic psychosis mental disease resulting from defect, damage, infection, tumor, or other physical cause that can be observed in the body tissues.

paranoid term indicating feelings of suspicion and persecution (one type of schizophrenia).

personality disorder broad category of illnesses in which inner difficulties are revealed not by specific symptoms, but by antisocial behavior.

phobia irrational, persistent, abnormal, morbid, and unrealistic dread of external object or situation displaced from unconscious conflict.

premorbid personality state of an individual's personality before the onset of an illness.

psyche synonymous with mind or the mental and emotional "self."

psychoanalysis theory of human development and behavior, method of research, and form of treatment described by Freud that attributes abnormal behavior to repressions in the unconscious mind. Treatment involves dream interpretation and free association to bring into awareness the origin and effects of unconscious conflicts in order to eliminate or diminish them.

psychodrama a therapeutic approach that involves a structured, dramatized, and directed acting out of emotional problems and troubled interactions by the client in order to gain insight into individual's own difficulties.

psychogenic symptoms or physical disorders caused by emotional or mental factors, as opposed to organic.

psychopath older inexact term for one of a variety of personality disorders in which person has poor impulse control, releasing tension through immediate action without social or moral conscience.

psychosis severe emotional illness characterized by a disorder of thinking, feeling, and action with the following symptoms: loss of contact, denial of reality, bizarre thinking and behavior, perceptual distortion, delusions, hallucinations, and regression.

schizoid form of personality disorder characterized by shyness, introspection, introversion, withdrawal, and aloofness.

schizophrenia severe functional mental illness characterized in general by a disorder in perception, thinking, feeling, behavior, and interpersonal relationships.

sociopathic pertaining to a disorder of behavior in which a person's feelings and behavior are asocial, with impaired judgement and inability to profit from experience; the intellect remains intact. This term is often used interchangeably with "psychopath."

soma term meaning the body or physical aspects.

superego in psychoanalysis, that part of the mind that incorporated the parental or societal values, ethics, and standards. It guides, restrains, criticizes, and punishes. It is unconscious and learned and is sometimes equated with the term *conscience*.

transference unconscious projections of feelings, attitudes, and wishes that were originally associated with early significant others onto persons or events in the present; may be positive or negative transference.

waxy flexibility psychomotor underactivity in which the

individual maintains the posture in which he or she is placed.

word salad   meaningless mixture of phrases and words often seen in schizophrenic behavior. For example, the ridjams frast wolmix.

Questions | MENTAL HEALTH NURSING AND COPING BEHAVIORS

Select the one answer that is best. (Answer blanks are provided at the back of this book.)

1. One therapeutic psychiatric nursing attitude is to be accepting and permissive. To convey this attitude most therapeutically, the nurse might:
   1. Wait for a client to initiate contact.
   2. Let the client make decisions.
   3. Ignore undesirable behavior.
   4. Meet clients at their own levels of functioning.

2. When a client's behavior is considered abnormal, the nurse first needs to:
   1. Ignore the client.
   2. Serve as a role model.
   3. Point out the client's disturbed behavior.
   4. Focus on the feelings communicated by the client's behavior.

3. When a client is in isolation or seclusion, it is essential that:
   1. Restraints be applied.
   2. All the furniture be removed from the isolation room.
   3. A staff member have frequent contacts with the client.
   4. The client be allowed to come out after 4 hours.

4. The major basic function in psychiatric nursing is to:
   1. Plan activity programs for clients.
   2. Maintain a therapeutic environment.
   3. Understand various types of family therapy and psychologic tests and how to interpret them.
   4. Advance the science of psychiatry by initiating research and gathering data for current statistics on emotional illness.

5. When interacting with clients who have autistic thinking and speaking patterns, which of the following is likely to pose the *greatest difficulty* for the nurse?
   1. Showing acceptance for their incomprehensible acts and verbalizations.
   2. Ignoring their bizarre behavior.
   3. Speaking in a way that clients can understand.
   4. Determining which of the clients' needs are being met by their autistic expressions.

6. The client was telling the nurse about her parents' impending divorce. She said, "I couldn't believe that he was going to leave us for someone else." Which would be best for the nurse to reply?
   1. "Was your mother expecting this to happen?"
   2. "Yes, go on."
   3. "Did you cry?"
   4. "I can understand how you must feel."

7. Arnold related angrily to the nurse that his wife says he is selfish. Which would be the most helpful response?
   1. "That's just her opinion."
   2. "I don't think you're that selfish."
   3. "Everybody is a little bit selfish."
   4. "You sound angry—tell me more about what went on."

8. Lynn talks about her daughter who is mentally retarded. "She's really an inspiration to me, do you know what I mean?" Which would be the most appropriate initial comment by the nurse?
   1. "What makes her an inspiration?"
   2. "It seems to be important to you to find something positive about her."
   3. "No, explain more about what you mean."
   4. "Tell me more about her."

9. The mother relates to the nurse, "When my baby had asthma five years ago, I thought he was going to die." What could the nurse say that would be the most appropriate?
   1. "What made you think that he was going to die?"
   2. "What did you do?"
   3. "You thought he was dying?"
   4. "How did you feel then?"

10. One effective way to start an interaction with a client who is silent is to:
    1. Tell the client something about yourself and hope that the client does the same.
    2. Remain silent, waiting for the client to bring up a topic.
    3. Bring up a controversial topic to elicit the client's response.
    4. Introduce a neutral topic, giving the client a broad opening.

11. What might be the most therapeutic response you could make to a student who begins crying on hearing that she failed an exam?
    1. "You'll make it next time."
    2. "Failing an exam is an upsetting thing to happen."
    3. "How close were you to passing?"
    4. "It won't seem so important five years from now."

12. A client tells you that he has something he wants to say to you but does not want you to tell anyone else. As a nurse, you:
1. Agree not to "tell."
2. Refuse to agree to this.
3. Say nothing, allowing him to go on.
4. Let him know that you cannot promise this.

13. Which nursing intervention is effective when clients are severely anxious?
1. Encourage group participation.
2. Give detailed instructions before treatment procedure.
3. Impart information succinctly and concretely.
4. Increase opportunities for decision-making.

14. When a client tells the nurse that she cannot sleep at night because of fear of dying, what would be the best initial response?
1. "Don't worry, you won't die. You're just here for some tests."
2. "Why are you afraid of dying?"
3. "Try to sleep. You need the rest before tomorrow's test."
4. "It must be frightening for you to feel that way. Tell me more about it."

15. Which of the following are common physiologic reactions that occur in response to anxiety?
1. Clammy hands and increased perspiration.
2. Palpitations and pupillary constriction.
3. Diarrhea and vomiting.
4. Pupillary dilation, retention of feces and urine.

16. Which behavior is most characteristic of a panic response?
1. Behavior is goal-directed and aimed at a "flight" response from apparent threat.
2. Behavior is automatic, with poor judgement.
3. The severity of the reaction is not related to the severity of the threat to self-esteem.
4. There is a delayed reaction in perceiving the danger.

17. The most common defense mechanism is:
1. Introjection.
2. Projection.
3. Repression.
4. Rationalization.

18. Paranoid clients tend to use projection. The main purpose of this action is to:
1. Control and manipulate others.
2. Deny reality.
3. Handle feelings and thoughts not acceptable to the ego.
4. Express resentment toward others.

19. Reaction formation can be described as:
1. Finding a socially acceptable outlet for impulses from the id.

2. Adopting the feelings and attitudes of a hero.
3. Keeping unacceptable ideas or feelings from awareness.
4. Adopting a feeling or attitude that is the opposite of the original attitude.

20. Regression is common in physical and emotional illness. Which of the following best explains this mechanism?
1. When faced with frustration, conflict, and/or anxiety, people may need to return to a previous level of functioning where they felt secure and comfortable.
2. Immature behavior has secondary benefits.
3. Childlike behavior is a way of getting away with expressing hostility.
4. Individuals enjoy the sympathy and attention they received as children when they were ill.

21. Fixation can best be understood as:
1. Reversion to an earlier developmental phase.
2. Behavior persisting into later life that was appropriate in an earlier developmental phase.
3. A disturbance in the rate of speech.
4. The wish to be like another and to assume attributes of the other.

22. An angry man channels his hostilities into competitive sports in which there are many opportunities for combat. This can be seen as:
1. Sublimation.
2. Repression.
3. Rationalization.
4. Reaction formation.

23. Repression can be defined as:
1. Selective forgetting and storing unacceptable thoughts, wishes, and impulses in the unconscious mind.
2. Conscious, deliberate forgetting.
3. Transferring to another situation an emotion felt in a previous situation where its expression would not have been acceptable.
4. Unconscious imitating of the manners, behavior, and feelings of another.

24. Mary, a client who attempted suicide recently, remarks to the nurse the next morning, "Let's not think about that now. Maybe I'll feel like thinking about it later." This can be identified as:
1. Blocking.
2. Denial.
3. Suppression.
4. Repression.

25. Repetitive handwashing is often seen when a client is experiencing guilt feelings. This ritualistic behavior can be described as a mechanism whereby the client attaches significance to the act of washing. This is seen as:
1. Symbolism.
2. Fantasy.

3. Isolation.
4. Conversion.

26. The client shouts at the nurse one morning, "Why do you waste your time on me? I'm not sick; I don't need you. Go talk to Mr. Gomez. He's really sick!" This can be identified as:
1. Reaction formation.
2. Denial.
3. Intellectualization.
4. Rationalization.

Mrs. Allen, a 28-year-old woman, is admitted to the psychiatric hospital with symptoms of severe depression. Fourteen months ago, her 9-month-old boy died of crib death. Since then, Mrs. Allen has lost weight, will not eat, spends most of her time immobile, and speaks only in monosyllabic responses. She pays little attention to her appearance.

27. Which one of the following nursing approaches would be best for Mrs. Allen while her symptoms are severe?
1. Allow her time for quiet thought; remain silent.
2. Ask her to join you and the other clients in the TV lounge.
3. State that you would like to go with her for a short walk around the outside grounds, and assist her with her coat.
4. Give her a choice of recreational activities.

28. One afternoon, Mrs. Allen comes to lunch with her hair combed and traces of lipstick. What could a nurse say to reinforce this change in behavior?
1. "What happened? You combed your hair!"
2. "This is the first time I've seen you look so good."
3. "You must be feeling better. You look much better."
4. "I see that your hair is combed and you have lipstick on."

29. Which of the following are important nursing approaches in depression?
1. Providing motor outlets for aggressive, hostile feelings.
2. Protecting against harm to others.
3. Reducing interpersonal contacts.
4. Deemphasizing preoccupation with elimination, nourishment, and sleep.

30. When Mrs. Allen says to the nurse, "I can't talk; I have nothing to say," and continues being silent, what should the nurse do?
1. Say, "All right. You don't have to talk. Let's play cards, instead."
2. Explain that talking is an important sign of getting well and that she is expected to do so.
3. Be silent until Mrs. Allen speaks again.
4. Say, "It may be difficult for you to speak at this time; perhaps you can do so at another time."

31. In working with clients who are depressed, it is essential that the nurse know that depression may stem from:

1. A sense of loss, actual, imaginary, or impending.
2. Revived memories of a painful childhood.
3. A confused sexual identity.
4. An unresolved oedipal conflict.

Mr. Short, a 35-year-old man, is brought to the psychiatric hospital by his wife. His history included periodic episodes of manic behavior, alternating with depression. Questions 32 through 35 refer to this case.

32. Which characteristic is shared by both a client who may be in the depressed phase and one who may be in the manic phase of bipolar affective disorders (manic-depressive reaction)?
1. Suicidal tendency.
2. Underlying hostility.
3. Delusions.
4. Flight of ideas.

33. A nursing-care plan for a hospitalized hyperactive client in manic reaction needs to include:
1. Involvement in a group activity and encouragement to talk.
2. Attention to adequate food and fluid intake.
3. Protection against suicide.
4. Permissive acceptance of bizarre behavior.

34. One evening the nurse sees Mr. Short in the dayroom without any clothes. He is shouting vulgarities and dancing wildly about the room while other clients are watching TV. The best initial response by the nurse at this time would be:
1. "Let's sit down with the others and watch TV; I'll put this blanket over you to keep you warm."
2. "We do not allow this behavior in the hospital. It is embarrassing the other clients."
3. "Please put your clothes on."
4. "Come put your clothes on, Mr. Short. I will help you."

35. When talking with a manic client in the acute phase who has flight of ideas, the nurse primarily needs to:
1. Speak loudly and rapidly to keep the client's attention, as the client is easily distracted.
2. Focus on the feelings conveyed rather than the thoughts expressed.
3. Encourage the client to complete one thought at a time.
4. Allow the client to talk freely.

36. Depression with psychotic features (involutional depression) may be differentiated from other depressive states by:
1. The age period in which it is most likely to occur.
2. Its characteristic symptoms of delusions stemming from suspiciousness.
3. Premorbid personality profile traits of an outgoing person with narrowed interests.
4. The degree of suicidal risk.

37. In caring for a person who is a suicide risk, the most important consideration is:
    1. Maintain constant awareness of the client's where-abouts.
    2. Ignore the client as long as he/she is talking about suicide, because a suicide attempt is unlikely.
    3. Relax vigilance when the client seems to be recovering from depression.
    4. Administer medication.

38. John, a new client admitted *last* night, relates to the nurse in the *morning*, "I was going to kill myself." What is the best initial response by the nurse?
    1. Say nothing. Wait for his next comment.
    2. "What were you going to do this time?"
    3. "Have you felt this way before?"
    4. "You seem upset. I am going to be here with you; perhaps you will want to talk about it."

39. Suicide assessment is clearly indicated for:
    1. Depression with melancholia (involutional melancholia).
    2. Schizophrenic disorders (schizophrenia).
    3. Bipolar affective disorder, manic (manic-depressive, hypomanic phase).
    4. Psychological factors affecting physical condition (psychosomatic disorder).

40. A nurse discovers a 19-year-old man crouched in a corner of the psychiatric unit corridor. There is blood on the floor. He is holding on to a gushing wound on his right wrist and looks pale and frightened. A razor is nearby on the floor. What should the nurse do first?
    1. Sit down on the floor next to the client and, in a quiet, reassuring tone, say "You seem frightened. Can I help?"
    2. Ask the aide to watch the client and run to get the doctor.
    3. Apply pressure on the wrist, saying to the client, "You are hurt. I will help you."
    4. Go back down the hall to get the emergency cart.

41. A 10-year-old boy, diagnosed with acute leukemia, terminal stage, asks the nurse one morning while she is fixing his bed: "I am going to die, aren't I?" What would be the most appropriate response by the nurse?
    1. "No, you're not. You are getting the latest treatment available and you have a very good doctor. Your white count was better yesterday."
    2. "We are all going to die sometime."
    3. "What did the doctor tell you?"
    4. "I don't know. You have a serious illness. Do you have feelings that you want to talk about now?"

42. Ruth, an acutely ill 40-year-old wife and mother hospitalized for treatment of metastatic lung carcinoma, begs the nurse to ask the doctor to give her a pass to attend her son's high school graduation in a city 100 miles from the hospital. "If only I could be free of pain to do just this one thing, then I'll be ready to die," she says. Ruth is:
    1. Being unrealistic and denying the degree of her illness.
    2. Using bargaining as a reaction to death and dying.
    3. Being manipulative to get her way.
    4. Unaware of her diagnosis.

Mrs. Betty Barnes, mother of a 5-year-old girl and an 11-year-old boy and long estranged from her husband, received a letter informing her that her husband had recently died from cancer. Her immediate reaction was stunned silence, followed by expression of anger: "I suppose he didn't have any insurance benefits to leave to the children." Questions 43 through 45 refer to this case.

43. Which of the following indicates that the nurse best understands Mrs. Barnes's reaction?
    1. She is experiencing a normal grief reaction.
    2. Her reaction can best be understood if more was known about the marital relationship and breakup.
    3. The children and the injustice done to them by the father's death are her main concern.
    4. She is not reacting normally to the news.

44. Resolution of grief is most likely to be complicated when:
    1. There are ambivalent feelings for the deceased.
    2. Death was due to a chronic illness.
    3. It is the first loss to be experienced.
    4. Little emotional dependency was attached to the deceased.

45. Mr. Barnes's mother comes to stay with them. Betty notices that her mother-in-law is acting more and more like her deceased son, even complaining of similar physical symptoms that her son had before he died. She is preoccupied solely with thoughts about his positive attributes. You will see signs of grief resolution in Mrs. Barnes when she:
    1. Encourages Betty to remarry.
    2. Is able to talk about both the pleasurable and the painful aspects connected with her son.
    3. Tries to make up for his deficiencies, saying, "He would have wanted me to do this for you."
    4. Is finally able to feel anger with her son and agree with Betty that he had failed them all.

46. The main nursing goal with schizophrenic clients is to:
    1. Set limits on their bizarre behavior.
    2. Establish a trusting, nonthreatening, reality-based relationship.
    3. Quickly establish a warm, close relationship to counteract their aloofness.
    4. Protect them from self-destructive impulses.

47. Symptoms that are characteristic of schizophrenic disorders include:
    1. Symbolization.

2. Depression.

3. Flight of ideas.

4. Confabulation.

48. Jean has been having auditory hallucinations. When the nurse approaches her, Jean whispers, "Did you hear that terrible man? He is scarey!" Which would be the best response for the nurse to make initially?
    1. "What is he saying?"
    2. "I didn't hear anything. What scarey things is he saying?"
    3. "Who is he? Do you know him?"
    4. "I didn't hear a man's voice, but you look scared."

49. In responding to a neologism, it would be best for the nurse to:
    1. Divert the client's attention to an aspect of reality.
    2. State that what the client is saying has not been understood and then divert attention to something that is reality-bound.
    3. Acknowledge that the word has some special meaning for the client.
    4. Try to interpret what the client means.

50. Jean looks at a mirror and cries out, "I look like a bird. My face is no longer me." Which would be the best response by the nurse?
    1. "Which bird?"
    2. "That must be a distressing experience; your face doesn't look different to me."
    3. "Maybe it was the light at that particular time. Would you like to use another mirror?"
    4. "What makes you think that your face looks like a bird?"

A 23-year-old premedical student, Georgia, is admitted to a psychiatric hospital in a withdrawn catatonic state. She was an honor student and very active in student government and had become progressively withdrawn, silent, and mute. For two days prior to admission, she remained seated in one position without moving or speaking. On the ward, she continues to exhibit waxy flexibility as she sits all day.

51. During the initial phase of hospitalization, the nurse's first priority is to:
    1. Watch for edema and cyanosis of the extremities.
    2. Encourage Georgia to discuss her concerns leading to the catatonic state.
    3. Provide a warm, nurturing relationship, with therapeutic use of touch.
    4. Identify the predisposing factors in her illness.

52. Janice, another client on the ward with Georgia, seems preoccupied with her own thoughts as she grins, giggles, grimaces, and frowns. Although she is 28 years old, her behavior seems childish and regressed. She is unkempt, voids on the floor, disrobes, and openly masturbates. The initial nursing care for Janice should be directed toward:

1. Improving her social conduct to meet hospital standards.
2. Controlling her narcissistic impulses.
3. Finding out why she is behaving this way.
4. Showing acceptance of her.

53. Mr. Carlson refuses to eat his meals in the hospital, stating that the food is poisoned. The patient is expressing an example of:
    1. Hallucination.
    2. Illusion.
    3. Delusion.
    4. Negativism.

54. Mr. Carlson cannot find his slippers. During the community meeting, he accuses clients and staff of stealing them during the night. The most therapeutic approach is to:
    1. Listen without reinforcing his belief.
    2. Logically point out that he is jumping to conclusions.
    3. Inject humor to defuse the intensity.
    4. Divert his attention.

55. Clients with symptoms such as Mr. Carlson's use projection. This mechanism is chiefly a way to:
    1. Provoke anger in others.
    2. Control delusional thought.
    3. Handle their own unacceptable feelings.
    4. Manipulate others.

Alice, an attractive, intelligent 15-year-old, has a history of truancy from school, running away from home, and "borrowing" other people's things without their permission. She denies that she steals, rationalizing instead that as long as no one was using the items, she thought it was all right to borrow them. She has been referred by the juvenile court to the local mental health center.

56. Psychodynamically, this behavior may be largely attributed to what developmental defect?
    1. Id.
    2. Ego.
    3. Superego.
    4. Oedipal complex.

57. In interacting with Alice, what would be the most therapeutic approach, consistent with question No. 56?
    1. Reinforce her self-concept as a young woman.
    2. Gratify her inner needs.
    3. Give her opportunities to test reality.
    4. Provide external controls.

58. A new nursing student reports to the unit. He is assigned to take clients for an outing. Alice approaches him and says, "I like you. I'm glad you'll be the one to take us out. My doctor told me that I can go too." Which initial response by the nurse is best?
    1. "Since I am new here and not familiar with unit routine, I will go check with the staff and be back."
    2. "It's a beautiful day, and I'm glad that you have ground privileges now."

3. "When did the doctor tell you that?"

4. "You seem pleased."

59. Alice arouses anxiety and frustration in the staff and tends to intimidate by her manipulative patterns. One morning Alice shouts at the nurse, "Since you won't give me a pass, go away, you fat pig, or I'll hit you." What is the most effective response by the nurse to a client who threatens or derogates?
    1. "You are rude and I don't like it. It makes me not want to talk with you."
    2. "That kind of talk will keep you here longer."
    3. "What did I do wrong?"
    4. "I don't like to hear insults and threats. What is important about getting the pass today?"

Reva Jones, age 38 years and mother of two children, ages 12 and 14, was brought to the emergency ward at the hospital by her husband, Paul. Her diagnosis was alcohol withdrawal (delirium tremens). Questions 60 through 62 refer to this case.

60. On admission, the client is likely to exhibit signs of:
    1. Perceptual disorders.
    2. Impending coma.
    3. Recent alcohol intake.
    4. Depression with mutism.

61. To relate therapeutically with Mrs. Jones, it is important that the nurses base their care on the understanding that alcohol abuse and dependence (alcoholism):
    1. Is hereditary.
    2. Is due to lack of willpower and true remorse.
    3. Results in always breaking promises.
    4. Cannot be cured.

62. A characteristic physiologic consequence of alcohol abuse and dependence (chronic alcoholism) is:
    1. Cardiac arrhythmias.
    2. Convulsive disorder.
    3. Psychomotor hyperactivity.
    4. Cirrhosis of the liver.

63. The signs of heroin withdrawal may include:
    1. Rhinorrhea, sneezing, and high fever.
    2. Pupillary dilation, diaphoresis, and weight loss.
    3. Pupillary constriction, vomiting, and pruritus.
    4. Choreiform movements and frequent lip wetting.

64. Methadone treatment for heroin abuse and dependence (addiction) is likely to:
    1. Produce sedation.
    2. Produce euphoria.
    3. Produce neuritis.
    4. Block the euphoric effect of heroin and eliminate craving.

65. In establishing a therapeutic nursing approach with a client who abuses and is dependent on substances, the nurse primarily needs to:

1. Promote a permissive, accepting environment.
2. Use a straightforward and confronting approach.
3. Meet the client's need for a chemical substitute for the drug.
4. Prevent the client's use of the addictive drug.

Mr. David's behavior has been a source of concern to the staff. He refuses to attend group therapy sessions at 9:00 A.M. because he says he has to wash his hands for at least 45 minutes from 9:00 A.M. until 9:45 A.M. At the team meeting, staff members discuss the problem. They feel it is important for Mr. David to participate in group therapy sessions to learn more successful methods of interaction with others.

66. Which concept does the staff need to keep in mind in planning nursing interventions for this client?
    1. Fears and tensions are often expressed in disguised form through symbolic processes.
    2. Unmet needs are discharged through ritualistic behavior.
    3. Ritualistic behavior makes others uncomfortable.
    4. Depression underlies ritualistic behavior.

67. To help reduce stress and to aid this client in using less maladaptive means of handling stress, the nurse could:
    1. Provide varied activities on the unit, as change in routine can break a ritualistic pattern.
    2. Give him ward assignments that do not require perfection.
    3. Tell him of changes in routine at the last minute to avoid build-up of anxiety.
    4. Provide an activity in which positive accomplishment can occur so he can gain recognition.

68. Which of the following is an example of *limit-setting* as an effective nursing intervention in ritualistic behavior patterns?
    1. "I don't want you to wash your hands so often anymore."
    2. "If you continue to wash your hands so frequently, the skin on your hands will break down."
    3. "You may wash your hands before the group therapy meeting if you wish, but not during group therapy."
    4. "The doctor wrote an order that you are to stop washing your hands so often."

69. Mr. David's repetitive handwashing is probably an attempt to:
    1. Punish himself for guilt feeling.
    2. Control unacceptable impulses or feelings.
    3. Do what the voices tell him to do.
    4. Seek attention from the staff.

In the last five years, Alice Adams has gone to a number of different doctors for nonspecific complaints of chest pains without any conclusive findings of an organic disease process. She has collected all the medical literature on the subject of coronary diseases. Most of her time is spent recounting details of her symptoms. Her latest internist has referred her to the local mental health center's day-treatment facility.

70. When meeting Alice for the first time at the day-treatment center, which approach by the nurse would be best initially?
    1. Encourage the client to describe her physical problems to become familiar with them.
    2. Comment on a neutral topic instead of the usual conversation opener of "How are you today?"
    3. Give the client a simple but direct explanation of the physiologic basis for her symptoms.
    4. Let the client know that you are familiar with her psychogenic problems and guide the discussion to other areas.

71. All of the following goals are important for a client who has the diagnosis of hypochondria. Which would be appropriate for an *initial* nursing goal?
    1. Help the client learn how to live with her functional organic disturbance without using her symptoms to control others.
    2. Assist the client in developing new and varied interests outside of herself in which she can be successful.
    3. Accept the client as a person who is sick and *needs* help.
    4. Help the client see how she uses her illness to avoid looking at or dealing with her problems.

72. To formulate an effective care plan for this client, the nurse *needs* to have an understanding of which of the following psychodynamic principles related to hypochondriasis?
    1. The major fundamental mechanism is regression.
    2. An extensive, prolonged study of her symptoms will be reassuring to the client, as she seeks sympathy, attention, and love.
    3. The symptoms of hypochondriasis are an attempt to adjust to painful life situations or to cope with conflicting sexual, aggressive, or dependent feelings.
    4. The client's symptoms are imaginary and her suffering is faked.

73. What aspect of malingering is not true of conversion disorders?
    1. It is a conscious reaction to stress.
    2. It provides an escape from a difficult situation.
    3. The symptoms occur in organs that usually are under voluntary control.
    4. The symptoms may reduce anxiety.

74. It would not be helpful for the nurse to use logic and reason to assist the client with conversion disorder symptoms (such as paralysis of the arm) in order to remove focus from the client's physical state because:
    1. The client is not in contact with reality and thus is unable to "hear" or understand the nurse.

2. The client may need the symptoms to handle feelings of guilt or aggression.
3. The nature of the client's particular illness makes her suspicious of all medical personnel.
4. Paralysis of the arm has become a habitual response to stress.

75. The most common coping mechanisms utilized in anxiety disorders (psychoneurotic reactions) are:
    1. Repression and symbolism.
    2. Sublimation and regression.
    3. Substitution and displacement.
    4. Reaction formation and rationalization.

76. Which adaptive behavior by a client with anxiety disorders (psychoneurosis) might indicate that he is showing the greatest improvement in his condition?
    1. He recognizes that his behavior is unreasonable.
    2. He agrees to go to occupational therapy and recreational therapy every day.
    3. His symptoms are replaced by expressions of hostility.
    4. He is verbalizing how he feels instead of demonstrating it by pathologic body language.

77. In caring for a client with a psychophysiologic illness, the nurse needs to know that:
    1. The symptoms will go away in time.
    2. The client has an inadequately formed superego.
    3. The client's ability to express emotions appropriately is impaired.
    4. Attention to the physical illness will alleviate the psychologic difficulties.

78. Psychophysiologic disorders differ from anxiety disorders (psychoneurotic) in that the former:
    1. May have long-term reactions.
    2. Bring about secondary benefits.
    3. May be helped by psychotherapy.
    4. Have symptoms that may be life-threatening.

Mr. Simon, a 35-year-old married clerk, had surgery for ulcerative colitis ten days ago. The physical symptoms have abated, but he continues to complain angrily and to be demanding of the nursing staff. He makes numerous requests, such as to open or close the windows, to bring him fresh water, and so on. Questions 79 through 84 refer to this case.

79. What might Mr. Simon's behavior be saying?
    1. "You aren't doing your job."
    2. "I am alone and helpless and need to depend on you to take care of me when I need you."
    3. "Everyone needs attention."
    4. "I'm going to get even with you for thinking I'm a crank by making you work."

80. Mr. Simon's family is ready to make discharge plans jointly with him and the staff. What will have the greatest bearing on his rehabilitation course?

1. The amount of emotional support his family gives him.
2. His wife's interest in, and ability to take care of, his postoperative dietary needs.
3. The family's expectations of him to resume his role in the home.
4. Mrs. Simon's understanding that the course of his illness may have exacerbations and remissions.

81. Mr. Simon's somatoform (psychophysiologic) symptoms will probably show the most improvement when he:
1. Accepts the fact that his physical symptoms have an emotional component.
2. Finds more satisfying ways of expressing feelings through verbalization.
3. Becomes involved in group activities and focuses less on his symptoms.
4. Understands that his current way of reacting to stress is not healthy.

82. One day Mr. Simon became angry with a client who was monopolizing the group therapy meeting. What assessment could be made regarding this noted change in Mr. Simon's behavior that would indicate the nurse's understanding of the dynamics of his somatoform (psychophysiologic) disorder?
1. He is intolerant of others.
2. He has strong competitive drives.
3. He has his own ideas of how the group members should act.
4. He is repressing fewer of his feelings.

83. When Mr. Simon asks his doctor about his prognosis, he becomes alternately depressed and agitated about his impending discharge. Which nursing approach would be best at this time?
1. "You *are* much better than when you first were hospitalized. You have to decide whether you need to be hospitalized longer or whether you are ready to go home."
2. "You seem to have concerns about going home."
3. "What is it about going home that bothers you?"
4. "You seem sad about going home. Would you like to talk about it?"

84. What would be the most realistic statement about Mr. Simon's prognosis after a course of necessary treatment?
1. His symptoms will recur.
2. His ulcerative lesions will heal, but under stress the same symptoms may reappear.
3. It is not possible to prognosticate the future course.
4. Ongoing psychotherapy is going to be essential if he is to be free of symptoms.

85. The main function confabulation serves in clients, especially those with organic mental disorders (organic brain syndromes), is to:

1. Impress others.
2. Protect their self-esteem.
3. Control others by distance maneuvers.
4. Maintain a sense of humor.

86. A key consideration in planning the care of clients with organic mental disorders (organic brain syndrome) is that:
1. They be protected from suicide attempts.
2. Their capacity for physical activity is diminished.
3. Team effort be aimed at increasing their independence.
4. The staff be sympathetic when clients mention their failing abilities.

87. Which of the following most commonly occurs in the clinical picture of organic mental disorders (organic brain syndrome)?
1. Memory loss for events in the distant past.
2. Quarrelsome behavior directly related to the extent of cerebral arteriosclerosis.
3. Increased resistance to change.
4. Insight into one's situation, its probable causes, and its logical consequences.

88. An important part of care for a client with chronic arteriosclerotic brain syndrome would be:
1. Minimizing regression.
2. Correcting memory loss.
3. Rehabilitating toward independent functioning.
4. Preventing further deterioration.

89. One morning Mr. Allen, an 80-year-old client, said to the nurse, "I'm going to the university today to be their guest lecturer on aerodynamics." Which response by the nurse would be most therapeutic?
1. "Do you know that you are in the hospital now?"
2. "Are you saying that you would like to be asked to give a lecture at the university?"
3. "How about watching a movie on television instead?"
4. "It's more important that you don't tire yourself out."

90. In planning an elderly client's schedule, it is most important that the daily activities:
1. Be highly structured.
2. Be changed by the nurse each day to meet the client's needs for variety.
3. Be simplified as much as possible to avoid problems with decision-making.
4. Provide many opportunities for making choices to stimulate the client's involvement and interest.

91. The mental health of the aged client is most directly influenced by:
1. The attitude of relatives in providing for the client's needs.
2. Societal factors such as role change, loss of loved ones, and loss of physical energy.

3. The client's level of education and economic situation.

4. The attitudes the client has toward life circumstances.

92. Which of the following is the *most* common basic need of the aged?
    1. Sexual outlets and security.
    2. Unconditional acceptance by others of their impairments and deficits.
    3. Preservation of self-esteem.
    4. Socialization.

93. Erikson's stages of growth and development characterize the task of old age as:
    1. Ego integrity versus despair.
    2. Autonomy versus shame and doubt.
    3. Trust versus mistrust.
    4. Industry versus inferiority.

94. Mrs. Jacobson, a 90-year-old client who is hard of hearing, tells the same story over and over again to all personnel who come to take care of her in a convalescent home—about the exciting time when her family came out West in a covered wagon. Which of the following statements would not demonstrate understanding of this behavior?
    1. Mrs. Jacobson has better recall for past events than for recent ones.
    2. She enjoys reliving pleasurable aspects of her life, since the present and future are bleak.
    3. Repeating her stories is one way of interacting, to compensate for a two-way conversation that is difficult for her to sustain.
    4. She wants to impress others.

95. Mr. Bell has Alzheimer's disease. One night, at 4 A.M., the nurse finds 88-year-old Mr. Bell in the hallway trying to open the door to the fire escape. Which response by the nurse would probably indicate the most accurate assessment of the situation?
    1. "Mr. Bell, you look confused. Would you like to sit down and talk with me?"
    2. "That door leads to the fire escape. Why do you want to go outside now?"
    3. "This is the fire escape door. Are you looking for the bathroom?"
    4. "Something seems to be bothering you. Let's go back to your room and talk about it."

96. According to Erikson's stages of psychosexual development, puberty and adolescence are characterized by what task?
    1. Identity versus role confusion.
    2. Initiative versus guilt.
    3. Ego integrity versus despair.
    4. Intimacy versus isolation.

97. Johnny, age 10 years, was admitted to the hospital for a tonsillectomy. In the morning, the nurse notes that the bedding is wet. There are several boys his age in the room. Which initial approach would best demonstrate a nurse's understanding of the condition and Johnny's stage of growth and development?
    1. While proceeding to change the wet linens, ask Johnny what sports he likes best, purposefully staying on impersonal topics.
    2. Draw the curtains around his bed while changing the linen, saying, "I know that this must be embarrassing to you."
    3. Say nothing while changing the bed; return at another time when the other boys are not in the room and explain to Johnny the medical-emotional reasons for enuresis.
    4. Sit down on the bed and convey acceptance of him as a person rather than acceptance of his symptoms.

98. A symptom that characteristically differentiates an autistic child from one with Down's syndrome is:
    1. Retardation of activity.
    2. Short attention span.
    3. Difficulty in responding to a nurturing relationship.
    4. Poor academic performance.

99. The main characteristic of crisis includes which of the following:
    1. Unknown cause(s).
    2. Abnormal stresses during growth and development.
    3. Intervention from a therapist is not needed.
    4. Usual coping mechanisms are ineffective.

100. A key characteristic feature of milieu therapy is:
    1. Inclusion of family therapy in the treatment process.
    2. Permissiveness, with lack of rules or structure.
    3. Client-planned, client-led activities.
    4. Staff's nonparticipation in decision-making.

101. A client in a therapeutic community setting approached the nurse one weekend evening, complained of being bored, and requested that some activity be provided. Which response by the nurse would be consistent with a milieu-therapy approach?
    1. "All right. I'm not busy. How about playing cards with me?"
    2. "I'll go ask the head nurse and see if we can come up with something."
    3. "Why don't you ask Mr. Anderson to play cards with you?"
    4. "Let's get the clients and staff together and discuss this."

102. Which of the following are not terms commonly associated with behavior therapy?
    1. Conditioned avoidance and positive reinforcement.
    2. Token economy and desensitization.
    3. Operant conditioning and reciprocal inhibition.
    4. Complementary transaction.

103. In their role in a behavior therapy program, it is essential that nurses:

1. Ask clients about the content of their dreams.
2. Only interact with clients who are verbal.
3. Continuously observe clients' behavior and immediately intervene if necessary.
4. Obtain a detailed account of each client's growth and development.

104. In setting up a successful behavior modification program, it is *not* essential that:
1. There is agreement and support from all personnel involved in daily contact with the clients.
2. Goals be broken down into sequential substeps.
3. The "positive reinforcer" be specifically selected for the individual client.
4. The clients begin with insight into problem behaviors.

105. Which of the following activities would be best for a client with manic behavior?
1. Solitary activity, such as reading.
2. Hammering on metal in a jewelry-making class.
3. Playing chess.
4. Competitive games.

106. Which of the following activities would be best for a client who is depressed?
1. Folding laundry or stapling paper sheets for charts.
2. Playing checkers.
3. Doing a crossword puzzle.
4. Ice skating.

107. The nursing role in group therapy may include all except:
1. Role model and catalyst.
2. Transference object.
3. Participant, observer, and facilitator.
4. Directive.

108. Although each of the following have been proposed as advantages of group therapy over individual therapy as a treatment modality, which is the most relevant from a theoretical point of view?
1. More people can be treated in the same time period.
2. Multiple transference is facilitated in a group setting, and corrective feedback and experiences can be readily provided.
3. Peer group identification occurring in group fosters feelings of relief based on emotional catharsis.
4. Group therapy is less expensive per session to the individual than individual therapy.

109. In family therapy sessions the nurse should:
1. Serve as an arbitrator during disputes.
2. Focus on the person with the presenting problem.
3. Neutralize the scapegoating phenomenon.
4. Use paradoxical communication.

110. Family therapy is the choice mode of therapy in the treatment of:
1. Children and adolescents.
2. Alcoholism.
3. Character disorders.
4. Anxiety disorders (neuroses).

111. Electroconvulsive therapy is ordered as treatment for a client who is depressed. What is the most important item for the nurse to know to plan immediate post-treatment care?
1. The client will not be as depressed as before and therefore will be a high suicide risk.
2. The client needs to be left alone and needs to sleep.
3. The client may look bewildered, be confused, and experience memory loss.
4. The client will be hungry after being NPO and will need nourishment on awakening.

112. The following activities have been planned for Ms. Carson, a client who is mute and autistic. In which of the following activities will it be important for the nursing staff to take precautionary measures for a common side effect of Thorazine (chlorpromazine)?
1. Shopping in an enclosed mall after lunch.
2. Attending the symphony on Wednesday evening.
3. A day at the beach, if the weather permits.
4. A morning at the art museum.

113. Some clients who are on phenothiazines are also given Cogentin. The purpose of this practice is to:
1. Prevent skin reactions.
2. Increase the effectiveness of the phenothiazines.
3. Decrease motor restlessness.
4. Reduce extrapyramidal side effects.

114. Mr. Bill has been on Prolixin, IM, for three years now. He has recently complained of frequent sore throats and malaise. What potentially serious side effect might these symptoms indicate?
1. Agranulocytosis.
2. Akathisia.
3. Dystonia.
4. Dyskinesia.

115. When nialamide (Niamid) or isocarboxazid (Marplan) are administered, what must the nurse know about these drugs?
1. They lower the threshold for seizures.
2. They potentiate the effects of many other drugs and common foods.
3. They decrease muscular contractions.
4. They commonly cause obstructive jaundice.

116. Lithium salts are frequently used to treat manic disorders. What is not a frequent side effect?
1. Slurred speech.
2. Twitching and athetotic movements.
3. Motor weakness.
4. Tardive dyskinesia.

117. Which of the following is the most appropriate in

response to a client who states emphatically, "I hate them"?

1. "I will stay with you as long as you feel this way."
2. "Tell me about your hate."
3. "I understand how you can feel this way."
4. "For whom do you have these feelings?"

118. At 2:30 A.M., a client walked out to the nurse's station complaining that he was choking, suffocating, weakening, and dying. He demanded a cigarette. What is the best response by the nurse?

1. Refuse and tell him it is against the rules.
2. Call the doctor and inform him of the client's request and behavior.
3. Refuse and tell him the cigarettes are locked.
4. Give him a cigarette and stay with him while he smokes.

119. What is the best way to handle psychiatric clients' behavior?

1. Approve their behavior.
2. Maintain consistency of approach.
3. Encourage them not to express negative opinions.
4. Interpret for them the reasons for their behavior.

120. When talking to a psychiatric client for the first time, which concept applies?

1. Hostile behavior from the client indicates that the nurse's initial approach has been inadequate.
2. The client's history needs to be read and discussed with the doctor before talking with the client.
3. The client's physical appearance provides an accurate index of whether he will be receptive to the nurse.
4. The client is a stranger to the nurse and the nurse is a stranger to the client.

121. In a therapeutic environment, rules and regulations:

1. Need to be kept to a minimum.
2. Serve as solutions for commonly occurring problems.
3. Teach clients self-control.
4. Should be rigidly enforced.

122. On which of the following models of treatment is family therapy based?

1. Psychodynamic.
2. Medical.
3. Systems.
4. Behavior modification.

123. Which of the following is the major goal of group therapy?

1. Give the therapist a chance to supply authoritative answers common to group problems.
2. Provide for feedback from several people regarding problems discussed in group.
3. Give the mentally ill opportunity to hear other people's problems.
4. Give the therapist the chance to interact with many patients.

124. The goal of therapy in crisis intervention is to:

1. Restructure the personality.
2. Remove specific symptoms.
3. Remove anxiety.
4. Resolve immediate problems.

125. Focus of treatment in crisis intervention is on the:

1. Present and restoration to usual level of functioning.
2. Past and freeing the unconscious.
3. Past in relation to present.
4. Present and repression of unconscious drives.

Jenny, age 19, is brought to the emergency room because she slashed her wrists. Jenny is in the middle of her first year of college. She has always had many friends and has been popular with both sexes. She has, in the past, done well in school. Two weeks ago her boyfriend "dropped" her. Since then Jenny has had trouble concentrating on her studies and has refused to date other boys.

126. What is the nurse's first concern?

1. Stabilization of physical condition.
2. Determination of antecedent, causal factors relevant to Jenny's wrist-slashing.
3. Reduction of anxiety.
4. Obtaining a detailed nursing history.

127. Three days after her admission, Jenny meets with a crisis intervention therapist. The initial goal of the therapist is to:

1. Determine precipitating event, determine how many people are involved in the incident, and determine how angry Jenny is.
2. Determine if Jenny has an immediate support system, determine what the people in the support system think of Jenny's cutting her wrists, and determine how angry Jenny is.
3. Determine precipitating event, determine if Jenny has an immediate support system, and assess the likelihood of immediate recurrence of suicidal act.
4. Assess likelihood of immediate recurrence of suicidal act.

128. The crisis intervention therapist and physician agree hospitalization is not necessary for Jenny; therefore, a crisis intervention therapist needs to:

1. Wish Jenny luck and terminate the session.
2. Make an appointment for Jenny for tomorrow and give Jenny a telephone number where the therapist can be reached tonight.
3. Make an appointment for Jenny in two weeks, when her wrists might be healed.
4. Tell Jenny to make an appointment when she wants to, at her local mental health clinic.

129. A principle of crisis intervention therapy is that crises:

1. May go on indefinitely.
2. Seldom occur in normal people's lives.
3. Usually are resolved in 4–6 weeks.
4. Are related to deep underlying problems.

130. At the first therapy session with Jenny, what does the therapist need to do?
1. Discourage discussion of Jenny's suicide attempt.
2. Encourage Jenny to dwell on her feelings about how badly she was treated as a child.
3. Encourage Jenny to discuss the suicide attempt in detail.
4. Help Jenny see how her suicide attempt hurt others.

Mr. Rains is a 47-year-old client who has been in a mental hospital for 10 years. His table manners are crude and upset other clients. Questions 131 through 133 refer to this case.

131. Which the following will probably be most therapeutic for Mr. Rains, a client on a behavior modification ward?
1. Accept his table manners without comment.
2. Urge him to eat like the other clients do.
3. Offer him a reward for each improvement in his table manners.
4. Point out to him that his eating habits distress the other clients.

132. It is likely that this approach will be most helpful because it:
1. Protects him from embarrassment about his table manners.
2. Offers him an incentive for improving his behavior.
3. Helps him achieve socially acceptable behavior.
4. Permits him to examine his own behavior without further loss of self-esteem.

133. Behavior can be decreased by:
1. Negative punishment.
2. Positive punishment.
3. Both positive and negative punishment.
4. Severe punishment.

134. What are two major types of precipitating factors in anxiety?
1. Fear of disapproval and shame.
2. Conflicts involving avoidance and pain.
3. Threats to one's biologic integrity and threats to one's self system.
4. A person's poor health and poor financial condition.

135. Physical behaviors associated with anxiety are primarily monitored through what system?
1. Parasympathetic nervous system.
2. Iambic system.
3. Hormonal system.
4. Autonomic nervous system.

136. Psychomotor manifestations of anxiety include:
1. Decreased activity.
2. Increased activity.
3. Increased lability of emotions.
4. Decreased lability of emotions.

137. Anxiety may increase intellectual functioning and is characterized by:
1. Increased perceptual field.
2. Increased ability to concentrate.

3. Decreased perceptual field.
4. Decreased random activity.

138. When working with persons who are anxious, what is the *overall* goal of nursing intervention?
1. Remove anxiety.
2. Develop person's awareness of anxiety.
3. Protect person from anxiety.
4. Develop person's capacity to tolerate mild anxiety and to use it constructively.

139. The best descriptive term applicable to assertive behavior is that it is:
1. Similar to aggressive behavior.
2. An example of destructive use of anger.
3. Obnoxious to others because it is frightening to them.
4. An example of constructive use of anger.

140. The steps in therapeutic nursing intervention with an angry client would be to describe the situation, then:
1. Discuss alternate solutions, decide on several solutions, try the solutions out, and evaluate their effectiveness.
2. Focus on one solution, try the solution out, and evaluate its effectiveness.
3. Outline to the client exactly what to do about the anger.
4. Discuss alternate solutions, decide on one solution, use the solution, evaluate its effectiveness, and continue repeating the process until the client is satisfied.

141. When an aggressive client starts demolishing the recreation room, what is the best response and action by the nurse?
1. Firmly set limits on his behavior.
2. Allow him to continue since he is seeking to express himself.
3. Tell him he is trying to intimidate other clients.
4. Let him know that he doesn't need to express his anger at her by demolishing the recreation room.

142. The expression of hostility is appropriate and useful when the:
1. Energy from anger is utilized to accomplish what needs to be done.
2. Expression intimidates others.
3. Degree of hostility is less than the provocation.
4. Expression of anger dissipates the energy.

143. All of the following nursing interventions with a person who is expressing anger are acceptable *except:*
1. Stating your observations of the expressed anger.
2. Assisting the person to describe the feelings.
3. Helping the person find out what preceded the anger.
4. Helping the person refrain from expressing anger verbally.

Mrs. Dawn, age 28, has been married for three years and has one child. A year ago, while nursing the child, she discovered a lump in her breast. She refused to see a physician or have a biopsy, stating that the lump was cystic thickening as a result of nursing the infant. Questions 144 through 148 refer to this case.

144. Mrs. Dawn's refusal to see a physician about the lump in her breast can be interpreted as:
1. Rationalization.
2. Projection.
3. Sublimation.
4. Denial.

145. Body image is the:
1. Conscious attitude the individual has toward his or her body.
2. Attitude others have about an individual's body.
3. Image the person sees of him/herself in the mirror.
4. Sum of the conscious and unconscious attitudes the person has toward his or her body.

Mrs. Dawn went to a physician for a routine physical. She discovered several lumps and suggested a biopsy and possible radical mastectomy. On biopsy, the tissue was discovered to be malignant, so a radical mastectomy was performed.

146. Immediately following surgery, Mrs. Dawn might display:
1. Signs of grief and grief resolution.
2. Signs of deep depression.
3. Relief that the operation is over.
4. Denial of possibility of carcinoma.

147. Two days after the operation, Mrs. Dawn was crying and saying, "My husband won't love me anymore." This statement might stem from:
1. Mrs. Dawn's deep insecurity about her marriage.
2. Preexisting marital disharmony.
3. Mrs. Dawn's concerns about her body and a resultant change in her beliefs about her own self-worth.
4. A momentary fear about her husband's fidelity.

148. Following Mrs. Dawn's statement in the preceding question, what would be most therapeutic for the nurse to respond at this time?
1. "Of course your husband loves you."
2. "Tell me what has happened that makes you think your husband won't love you anymore."
3. "If you stop crying and fix yourself up, you will look good to your husband."
4. "Do you think your husband won't love you because you have lost a breast?"

Frank Gregg, a 19-year-old male, was an excellent student, president of the freshman class in college, on the freshman football team, and active in his church. Two months ago, while home from college on a visit, he got up one morning and started screaming at his mother, "I am not me. You are controlling me." He grabbed a knife and started chasing his mother. However, before he hurt her, he suddenly stopped

chasing her and went to his room. For two days he did not talk or eat. After two days, his parents had him see a psychiatrist, who had him admitted to the psychiatric hospital.

149. From the above history, you could suspect overcompliance with his parents' expectations for his behavior. Acceptance of the role Frank perceives his parents require could result in:
1. Lack of development of a separate identity.
2. Confusion of his sex role.
3. Successful development of a separate identity.
4. Identification of a weak superego.

150. If Frank had become rebellious in puberty, it could be seen as:
1. Abnormal, because he had always been "good."
2. Normal in early adolescence.
3. A depressive syndrome.
4. An early sign of a psychotic disease process.

151. The nurse establishes a nurse-client relationship with Frank. One of the goals is to help him develop a separate self-identity. One way to do this is to:
1. Call him by a "pet" name frequently.
2. Use "you" and "I" rather than "we."
3. Correct his opinions.
4. Encourage "should" responses.

152. Frank's parents asked the nurse what she thought Frank meant when he said to the mother, "You are controlling me." What would be the best response by the nurse?
1. "He is upset and thinks you are taking charge of him."
2. "He resents always having to be good."
3. "I can't tell you, you will have to ask Frank."
4. "I think you can ask Frank that question. Do you want me to stay with you while you ask Frank?"

Maria Galvez, age 38, is a brilliant research chemist who came into the hospital with a diagnosis of paranoid schizophrenia. Questions 153 through 159 refer to this case.

153. What part of her personality was weak?
1. Id.
2. Ego.
3. Superego.
4. "Not me."

When Maria was in the second grade, she had difficulty with the teacher. She began to misbehave in class. She was taken from the public school and placed in a private school where others in the neighborhood were going. Her grades were not good because she was attempting to make an adjustment to her new peers. Her father severely reprimanded her and forced her to study after school rather than play with other children.

154. At this point, what normal phase of development was Maria deprived of forming?
1. A love relationship with her father.

2. Close relationships with her peers.
3. Heterosexual relationships.
4. A dependency relationship with her father.

155. In college Maria did exceptionally well. Her chemistry professor complimented her and arranged for her to be a lab assistant and to do advanced research. She was very thorough in her work. However, when given constructive criticism she became angry and stalked out of the lab for a few hours. The most theoretically plausible explanation is that she:
1. Knew she was right.
2. Thought the professor was jealous of her.
3. Needed to feel and know that she was perfect.
4. Felt anxiety as a result of a threat to her security and self-image.

156. Recently in the laboratory, when an experiment went wrong, Maria complained of a plot against her and accused the lab assistants of sending signals about her to each other. This is an example of:
1. Delusions of grandeur.
2. Illusion.
3. Ideas of reference.
4. Echolalia.

157. Maria began to refuse to eat her husband's cooking because she thought he was poisoning her. This is an example of:
1. Delusion of persecution.
2. Ideas of reference.
3. Illusion.
4. Hallucination.

158. Maria is diagnosed as paranoid schizophrenic. What implication might this have for the nurse?
1. Let Maria talk about her suspicions without correcting misinformation.
2. Avoid talking to other nurses when Maria can see them but can't hear what is being said.
3. Placate her by agreeing with what she says.
4. Argue with her about her ideas.

159. One day Maria said to the nurse, "That woman over there is a lesbian." What is the best response by the nurse?
1. "Are you afraid she will attack you?"
2. "That woman is not a lesbian."
3. "What did the woman do that makes you think she is a lesbian?"
4. "Then stay away from her."

160. A hallucination is a disorder of:
1. Affect.
2. Memory.
3. Orientation.
4. Perception.

161. Which of the following terms describes the experience of an individual who thought he heard a machine gun when his neighbor's lawnmower backfired as she was mowing the lawn?
1. Delusion.
2. Hallucination.
3. Identification.
4. Illusion.

162. The doctor asked you to activate his client. The client is hallucinating, withdrawn, and negativistic. What might be your best approach with this client?
1. Give him a long explanation of the benefits of activity.
2. Let him know that you need a partner for an activity.
3. Demand that he join a group activity.
4. Mention that his "voices" would want him to participate.

163. While communicating with a withdrawn schizophrenic client, what would be important for the nurse to do at first?
1. Remain silent with the client and not encourage her to talk.
2. Talk with the client as he would to a normal person.
3. Allow the client to do all the talking.
4. Use simple, concrete language in speaking to the client.

164. Which of the following is the best definition of the term schizophrenia?
1. Appearance of more than one distinct set of personality traits in one individual.
2. Apparent splitting of the activities of the mind from the body of one individual.
3. Distortion of normal synthesis of thought, feeling, and activity in one individual.
4. Physical dysfunction of the limbic system from the cerebrum within the brain.

While Marshall Brown was driving the car with his wife in a blizzard one evening, he slid on some ice and hit the edge of a bridge. His wife was killed instantly, and he was admitted to the hospital with severe chest injuries. His wife's family made and carried out the funeral arrangements for his wife. Before the accident, the couple appeared to be happily married. Because Marshall cannot attend the viewing of the body, the funeral, or the burial, you expect that he may later have difficulty with resolution of his grief.

165. Which present situation could forecast his future difficulties?
1. Feelings of anger at the hospital staff for keeping him hospitalized during the funeral.
2. Feelings of anger at himself for having been injured but not killed in the accident.
3. His inability to participate in the cultural rituals of grief, wherein the reality of his wife's death is emphasized.
4. His preoccupation with his own physical distress at this time.

166. As you are giving morning care to Marshall, you are aware that he is in the grief stage of developing awareness of his loss. What behavior might he display at this stage in reaction to his wife's death?
    1. Crying and/or anger.
    2. Appearing dazed and repeatedly saying, "No, it can't be."
    3. Preoccupation with thoughts of how ideal the marriage was.
    4. Responding with a brief complaint about his own physical pain.

Mr. Gonzalez is a 60-year-old, highly successful businessman who, in the last year, has refused to attend to his business, is now refusing to eat because he is too "bad" to eat, and has sat quietly in a chair mumbling to himself. Mr. Gonzalez is diagnosed as having major depression with psychotic features (psychotic depressive). Questions 167 through 171 refer to this case.

167. Mr. Gonzalez says, "I don't cry because my wife can't bear it." This is an example of what?
    1. Suppression.
    2. Undoing.
    3. Repression.
    4. Rationalization.

168. What feeling is most apt to be demonstrated during major depression with psychotic features (psychotic depression)?
    1. Suspicion.
    2. Agitation.
    3. Loneliness.
    4. Worthlessness.

169. According to Freudian theory, Mr. Gonzalez has a:
    1. Strong id.
    2. Driving ego.
    3. Weak superego.
    4. Punitive superego.

170. After Mr. Gonzalez makes a home visit, his wife reports that it was a stressful time. In an interview, Mr. Gonzalez says, "We had a marvelous visit." This is an example of what?
    1. Compensation.
    2. Denial.
    3. Symbolism.
    4. Identification.

171. It would be important for the nurse to implement definite suicide precautions for Mr. Gonzalez if his mood changed suddenly to one of:
    1. Cheerfulness.
    2. Psychomotor retardation.
    3. Agitation.
    4. Hostility.

172. Which of the following characteristics apply to a person

engaged in gradual self-destructive behavior such as obesity, drug addiction, and smoking?
    1. Acceptance of the death wish.
    2. Denial of own eventual death.
    3. Ability to control own behavior.
    4. Ignorance of the consequences of own behavior.

173. Persons engaged in gradual self-destructive behavior:
    1. Believe they can stop this behavior at any time.
    2. Have decreased anxiety when they stop the behavior.
    3. Believe the behavior controls them.
    4. Believe the behavior, in some manner, is "good" for them.

174. Psychologically, which of the following feelings is an antecedent of self-destructive behavior?
    1. Omnipotence.
    2. Grandiosity.
    3. Low self-esteem.
    4. Self-satisfaction.

175. Freudian therapists view self-destructive behavior as the:
    1. Direction of hostile feelings toward self.
    2. Direction of hostile feelings toward others.
    3. Direction of hostile feelings toward an internalized love object.
    4. Internalization of the fear of death.

176. According to Freudian theory, in which phase of development do addicts tend to be fixated?
    1. Anal.
    2. Oedipal.
    3. Oral.
    4. Latent.

177. Self-destructive behavior is determined by:
    1. A variety of factors, with the same factors present in each individual.
    2. Genetic disturbances.
    3. Interpersonal disturbances.
    4. A variety of factors, different for each individual.

Jane Green is a 23-year-old who stands 5 feet high and weighs 180 pounds. She has, since the beginning of her teenage years, become more overweight. Ms. Green has a busy social life with other women in the office where she works as a consultant. However, she does not date and has had few social contacts with males. She went to a physician for a physical and the physician suggested therapy, as there was no physical reason for her obesity problem. Questions 178 through 180 refer to this case.

178. Ms. Green was referred by the physician to the nurse for diet counseling. What action would the nurse take?
    1. Develop a diet, together with the person, that will allow gradual weight loss.
    2. Ask the person to describe her eating patterns.
    3. Support the person's interests in other activities.

4. Put Ms. Green on a faster diet so she will have an immediate weight loss.

179. Ms. Green says to the nurse, "My therapist told me I eat because I didn't get enough love from my mother. What does he mean?" Which statement best describes the theory underlying the therapist's statement? A person overeats because:
    1. She feels she wasn't loved enough as a child, and eating constantly is a way of getting revenge on Mother.
    2. She feels she wasn't loved enough as a child, and eating all she wants demonstrates she has control rather than Mother.
    3. She feels she wasn't loved enough as a child, and food represents an infantile dependency on Mother for love.
    4. Eating pleases Mother and therefore might win more love.

180. Which statement is the best response to "What does he mean?"?
    1. "Tell me what you think the therapist means."
    2. "We are here to deal with your diet, not with your psychological problems."
    3. "You need to ask your therapist."
    4. "What do you think is the connection between not getting enough love and your overeating?"

181. Sexual problems are identified by the:
    1. Nurse, after taking a careful history.
    2. Doctor, on the basis of client's report of satisfaction or dissatisfaction.
    3. Client, on basis of own satisfaction or dissatisfaction, provided rights of others are not being violated.
    4. Legal system, after an act has been perpetrated.

182. In primary sex health intervention, what is the nurse's major task?
    1. Identifying sexual problems.
    2. Referring clients to other health care providers.
    3. Providing therapy for sexual dysfunction.
    4. Providing education to individuals who are uninformed or misinformed about the nature of human sexuality.

183. Which of the following statements is most accurate about masturbation?
    1. It is unhealthy because it prevents a person from acknowledging the function of his or her sexual organs.
    2. It is a healthy and appropriate sexual activity that enables a person to consolidate his or her sexual identity.
    3. It prevents a person from enjoying heterosexual sexual activity.
    4. It is an unhealthy and inappropriate sexual activity that confuses a person's sexual identity.

184. The incidence of rape is:
    1. The slowest-rising violent crime in the U.S. and has the lowest proportion of cases closed by arrest and conviction.
    2. The fastest-rising violent crime in the U.S. and has the lowest proportion of cases closed by arrest and conviction.
    3. The fastest-rising violent crime in the U.S. and has the highest proportion of cases closed by arrest and conviction.
    4. The slowest-rising violent crime in the U.S. and has the highest proportion of cases closed by arrest and conviction.

185. The overall goal in rape counseling is to help the victim:
    1. Forget the incident and repress her feelings in order to be able to carry on with her life.
    2. Accuse the rapist in a court of law.
    3. Accept her part in the rape.
    4. Acknowledge, face, and resolve the reaction she is experiencing.

186. Chronological age:
    1. Is a valid guide for physical maturation.
    2. Facilitates prediction of emotional maturation.
    3. Facilitates prediction of sexual maturation.
    4. Is not a valid guide for physical or emotional maturation.

187. The necessity to intervene with conflicted adolescents is determined by:
    1. The extent of the adolescent conflicts.
    2. The disruptive social behavior.
    3. The seriousness of the sexual identity conflict.
    4. The inability of the adolescent to cope with the many conflicts.

The nurse has been asked to see John Sorenson, age 15, because he is disruptive in the school room. She knows that he has, on occasion, used alcohol and engaged in sexual activities with both males and females. His complaints are that no one will let him do his "own thing."

188. John comes to the first session and sits glaring at the nurse. What is the best response by the nurse?
    1. "I know you are angry, but how does being angry help?"
    2. "Stop being angry and tell me what is wrong."
    3. "I think you are angry because you feel you don't need any help."
    4. "We have to meet because your parents are concerned about you."

189. During the session John says, "I suppose you have to tell my parents everything." What would be the best response by the nurse?
    1. "What are you going to tell me that is so secret that I can't tell your parents?"

2. "If you tell me you are going to do something to hurt yourself I will have to tell your parents, but I will tell you first before I tell them."
3. "Everything you tell me is confidential. I will not tell your parents anything."
4. "Everything you tell me I will need to tell your parents. They have a right to know."

190. During one session John says, "I want you to go tell the teacher I am sick and I am to be allowed to do what I want." This statement best represents:
1. Insight.
2. Manipulation.
3. Dependency.
4. Trust.

191. To the statement, "I want you to go tell the teacher I am sick and I am to be allowed to do what I want," the best response by the nurse would be:
1. "Certainly, you are sick and need some relaxation of rules in the classroom."
2. "I am glad you recognize you are sick."
3. "No, John, you are expected to follow the rules of the classroom."
4. "All teachers are too strict. I agree some rules need to be relaxed."

192. In discussions between parents and adolescents about their relationship, adolescents will benefit because they will be able to:
1. See themselves as the victims.
2. View their parents and themselves realistically.
3. Enlist the therapist's aid as an ally against their parents.
4. See their parents as victims.

Mr. Sundowner is a 52-year-old man who has just been admitted to the general hospital for a possible acute appendicitis. The nurse who admits him notices that he is wearing very thick glasses and a hearing aid. He does not seem to be having any trouble understanding what is being said. The nurse, in her orientation of Mr. Sundowner, tells him that if he goes to surgery, he will wake up in the postoperative recovery room, not in his hospital room. Mr. Sundowner immediately says, "Oh, I will need to have either my glasses or my hearing aid or preferably both with me in the recovery room or I will be confused and upset when I wake up."

193. Mr. Sundowner is trying to tell the nurse that he:
1. Has periods of confusion and may have a psychiatric problem.
2. Is psychologically dependent on his hearing aid and glasses.
3. Needs his hearing aid and/or glasses in order to correctly perceive what is going on around him, and misperception will cause confusion.
4. Needs his hearing aid and/or glasses because he wants to be sure people are taking proper care of him.

194. Which of the following statements by the nurse is the best response to the above situation?
1. "You won't need your glasses or hearing aid. The nurses will take care of you."
2. "I understand. You will be able to cooperate best if you know what is going on, so I will find out how I can arrange to have your glasses and hearing aid available to you in the recovery room."
3. "I understand you might be more cooperative if you have your aid and glasses, but that is just not possible. Rules, you know."
4. "Do you get upset and confused often?"

Answers— Rationale / MENTAL HEALTH NURSING AND COPING BEHAVIORS

1. (4) If a particular client is nonverbal, for example, the nurse should not expect that client to function at a verbal level until ready. In choice No. 1, if the nurse waits for a withdrawn client, for example, to make contact, it may not be helpful. In No. 2, an ambivalent client may need assistance in making decisions. In No. 3, the client's undesirable behavior may be adversely affecting those around.

2. (4) Focusing on feelings is usually the best choice. Ignoring the client is rarely an acceptable intervention (No. 1). Pointing out disturbed behavior and role modeling by the nurse are valid, but *not* as first interventions (Nos. 2 and 3).

3. (3) Frequent contacts at times of stress are important, especially when a client is isolated. The following are not useful because: No. 1, isolation does not automatically imply the use of restraints; No. 2, *all* furniture need not be removed, depending on the institution and the type of behavior exhibited by the client; No. 4, there is no specific time limit, as time depends on individual behavior and the client's individual needs.

4. (2) This is the most neutral answer by process of elimination. No. 1 is mainly the function of a recreational-occupational therapist, although nurses participate. No. 3 is usually filled by psychologists and social workers, and No. 4 is carried out primarily by psychologists or statisticians, although nurses are involved. "Maintenance of a therapeutic environment" fits more readily into a nursing role by virtue of the number of hours per day a nurse spends with the clients on a unit, in

comparison with the number spent by other professionals.

5. (4) Decoding symbolic, autistic expressions calls for skill and sensitivity in understanding latent messages. Answer No. 1 is not a good choice since showing "acceptance" is a basic, initial nursing goal that does not require a complexity of skills. No. 2 points out a nontherapeutic nursing action, which is best not to use at all. No. 3 implies that the nurse use short sentences with clear, concise, unambiguous meaning; this can be accomplished with practice. Nos. 1 and 3 need to be accomplished before No. 4 is possible.

6. (2) Offering a broad opening by giving a general lead is most therapeutic to elicit further description of the client's reaction and to clarify her feelings, which were vaguely stated. No. 1 is a switch of focus from the client to the mother. No. 3 is nontherapeutic because a question that can be answered by a yes or no often closes off further exploration. No. 4 could be a helpful intervention but is premature acknowledgment before feelings have been elaborated.

7. (4) It is important to pick up on a feeling tone and encourage exploration of the feelings and the situation. No. 1 stops exploration of the client's feeling. Nos. 2 and 3 shift the focus away from feelings to content of selfishness.

8. (3) An appropriate direct response to a "you know what I mean" comment is to say you do *not* automatically know what is meant. Nos. 1, 2, and 4 are not the best responses because they shift the focus from the client's experience to the characteristics of the other person.

9. (4) Attempts to focus on encouraging the client to describe feelings are important. Nos. 1 and 2 ask for facts rather than focus on feelings, and No. 3 is an example of reflecting—a therapeutic response, but in this case it only reflects a *thought,* instead of a feeling.

10. (4) This is the least threatening. No. 2 is not good because the nurse *needs* to intervene into a pattern of silence. It is not therapeutic for the focus to be on the *nurse,* as in Nos. 1 and 3, and bringing up a *controversial* topic (such as religion or politics) usually results in an exchange of opinions and arguments.

11. (2) Nos. 1 and 4 focus on "there-and-then" rather than "here-and-now" feelings and events, and No. 3 is irrelevant because the focus is on a *fact* rather than a feeling.

12. (4) Information that is given to you, the nurse, that may interfere with the client's recovery needs to be related to other team members. The following are not the best responses because: No. 1 is withholding information from other staff who are also responsible for care and may interfere with recovery needs; No. 2 is a refusal

that may stop the interaction—a negotiation is needed; No. 3 does not provide a client with the clear feedback needed in order to work through conflict.

13. (3) Brief and specific information *can* be processed during severe anxiety. In severe anxiety, the person cannot respond to the social environment (as in No. 1); giving detailed information results in overload, as the client cannot retain and recall data (as in No. 2). Only directive information that is brief and specific is effective when the client cannot focus on what is happening. Decision-making needs to be postponed until person is less anxious; hence, No. 4 is wrong.

14. (4) Acknowledging a feeling tone is the most therapeutic response and provides a broad opening for the client to elaborate feelings. The following are not the best response because: No. 1 is false reassurance that does not allay feelings; No. 2 is asking a "why" question which is confrontive and may increase anxiety; No. 3 gives advice, which stops exploration of underlying feelings.

15. (1) Common reactions: pupillary dilation, *not* constriction (No. 2); diarrhea, *not* constipation (No. 4). Vomiting is not typical of an anxiety response. (No. 3 is incorrect.) No. 1 is the best choice.

16. (2) In panic, a person is highly suggestible and follows "herd instinct" rather than exercising independent judgement and problem-solving (No. 1). No. 3 is incorrect because the severity of the reaction *is* related to the severity of the threat. The more severe the perceived threat (actual or imaginary), the more intense the reaction to the danger, and not delayed as in No. 4.

17. (4) The first three answers are examples of more *pathogenic* defenses; that is, they predispose or lead to illness.

18. (3) Projection is a coping mechanism. Most coping mechanisms are aimed at either reducing anxiety to the *self* system or maintaining self-esteem. Although answer No. 2 may be correct at times, it is not so in *all* instances of projection. Denial may operate in *some* cases of projection. Nos. 1 and 4 are not good answers because the main focus of coping mechanisms is on *self,* not on others.

19. (4) By definition, No. 1 describes sublimation; No. 2, introjection; and No. 3, repression.

20. (1) It is the most comprehensive, inclusive choice, which may also encompass Nos. 2 and 4. Since regression is a coping mechanism, we know that the key purpose is to increase self-esteem and/or decrease anxiety; therefore, No. 3 does not fit, as expressing hostility does not necessarily increase esteem and/or decrease anxiety.

21. (2) No. 1 describes regression; No. 3, blocking; and No. 4, identification.

22. (1) By definition, this is the release of energy or impulses into socially acceptable outlets.

23. (1) By definition, No. 2 is suppression; No. 3, displacement; and No. 4, identification.

24. (3) By definition, this is the conscious, deliberate effort to avoid talking or thinking about painful, anxiety-producing experiences.

25. (1) Symbolism is the most clearly descriptive mechanism. No. 2, fantasy, is a mental activity; No. 3, isolation, is the exclusion from awareness of a feeling; and No. 4, conversion, is a disruption of motor or sensory functioning.

26. (2) Denial is the mind's way of protecting the self-system from a disturbing reality. No. 1, reaction formation, is an expression of an attitude opposite to unconscious feelings; No. 3, intellectualization, is giving rational reasons without expression of underlying feelings; No. 4, rationalization, is the attempt to make one's behavior look like the result of logical thinking.

27. (3) This will reduce the isolation and withdrawal, while at the same time does not put the burden of decision making on her. She needs a structured routine that is simple. She may not be able to handle close proximity with more than one person at this point, as in No. 2. No. 1 incorrectly allows her to remain isolated; No. 4 is incorrect because she needs a structured routine until she can make decisions for herself.

28. (4) A simple acknowledgment of what the nurse sees is the best response. No. 3 makes an assumption that she feels better if she looks better. Nos. 1 and 2 can be taken as a "put-down."

29. (1) It is important to externalize the anger away from self. No. 2 is incorrect because usually the client is turning anger *inward* toward the self. No. 3 increases sense of isolation. The needs in No. 4 should be taken care of but *not* emphasized, as the depressed client often has somatic delusions.

30. (4) Meet the client at her level of functioning, and provide support and encouragement for a higher level in the near future. No. 1 implies that the nurse agrees that the client has nothing to say. No. 2 does not convey empathy or understanding. No. 3 is incorrect because silences reinforce silence and a sense of isolation.

31. (1) "Loss" is most basic to the development of depression. Nos. 2, 3, and 4 are not essential to development of depression.

32. (2) In the depressed person, anger is turned inward; in the manic, it is noted in sarcasm, demanding behavior, and angry outbursts. Nos. 3 and 4 occur in the manic phase; No. 1 is a particular problem in depressed phase.

33. (2) The manic client may be too busy to eat and sleep. Nos. 1 and 3 are more appropriate for depressed phase; No. 4 is more appropriate for schizophrenia with bizarre behavior. Manic clients exhibit hyperactive behavior.

34. (4) It is a matter-of-fact statement that is direct, while offering assistance and setting limits on inappropriate behavior. The following are not useful because: No. 1 reinforces inappropriate social behavior; No. 2 sets limits but does not state a positive expectation for the client to follow; No. 3 neither offers assistance nor sets limits, which he needs.

35. (2) Often the verbalized ideas are jumbled, but the underlying feelings are discernible and need to be acknowledged. Flight of ideas should be curtailed. Thus, No. 4 is incorrect. The client may not be able to control the internal stimuli to focus on one idea at a time as in No. 3. A louder and more rapid tone by the nurse may only increase the external stimuli for the client, making No. 1 incorrect.

36. (1) Characteristic age of onset is at or following middle age. The following choices are wrong because: No. 2, characteristic delusions are usually *hypochondriacal*; No. 3, premorbid personality traits are *compulsive, inhibited,* frugal, and worrisome; No. 4, *all* depressions have suicidal risks, so this is *not* a differentiating factor.

37. (1) No. 2 is incorrect because all suicidal talk and gestures are to be taken seriously. If the client *talks* about suicide, there *may* be an attempt. No. 3 is incorrect because suicide risk is greater when depression is lifting, requiring greater vigilance. No. 4 is incorrect because medication for depression may take up to two weeks to decrease symptoms and the client needs vigilant surveillance *now*.

38. (4) The client needs to have his feelings acknowledged, with encouragement to discuss feelings, and be reassured about the nurse's presence. The client may interpret the nurse's silence as discomfort in talking about his suicidal feeling and thoughts (No. 1). No. 2 focuses on facts too swiftly without providing an opportunity for the client to express his feelings. Also, No. 2 would be most appropriate in *crisis* intervention when client was *first* admitted, *not* the next morning. No. 3 moves away from focus on here-and-now to focus on the past.

39. (1) Another name for depression with melancholia (involutional melancholia) is depression with psychotic features (involutional depression). Suicide risk is part of all depressions. Nos. 2, 3, and 4 are incorrect because the diagnosis alone does not indicate suicide risk like the diagnosis of depression.

40. (3) In Nos. 1 and 2 the client could suffer extensive

blood loss if the nurse focuses on feelings at this point or leaves him without first attempting to control the bleeding. In choice No. 4, the client is left alone, bleeding, frightened, and with a razor still next to him.

41. (4) An honest, direct answer that focuses on feelings is the best approach. Nos. 1, 2, and 3 stop further exploration of the client's feelings.

42. (2) Refer to Elisabeth Kübler-Ross's emotional stages of death and dying. She is neither being unrealistic (No. 1), manipulative (No. 3), nor unaware of her diagnosis (No. 4).

43. (1) Shock and anger are commonly the primary initial reactions. Choice No. 2 is irrelevant; and No. 3 is a literal, concrete interpretation of Mrs. Barnes's reaction, not aimed at the possible latent feelings. No. 4 is incorrect because it contradicts correct answer No. 1.

44. (1) Reactions to loss tend to be cumulative in effect, in that the more loss experienced in the past, the greater the reaction the next time. Thus, No. 3 is wrong. Reactivation of feelings connected with previous losses by the current loss accounts for the increased intensity of the reaction. Sudden, unexpected death, rather than death due to a chronic illness, as in No. 2, is harder to resolve, and strong, not little, emotional dependency (as in No. 4) also complicates grief resolution.

45. (2) When the mourner can pass through the idealization stage and be more realistic about the positive and negative aspects of the loss, resolution of grief is beginning. Choices Nos. 3 and 4 occur in *earlier* stages of grief. Choice No. 1 could be a sign of denial, an initial grief reaction.

46. (2) A permissive atmosphere is the key, as well as a *slowly* evolving (not quickly evolving, as in No. 3) relationship with room for *distance*. Self-destruction is not a persistent problem requiring major focus for concern, as in No. 4. No. 1 is not the best response because "acceptance" of *bizarre* behavior is more important than setting limits.

47. (1) The schizophrenic tries not to communicate and uses defenses such as *symbolization* to decrease direct communication. No. 2 is characteristic of an affective disorder. No. 3 is characteristic of bipolar disorder (manic-depression). No. 4 is characteristic of organic mental disorder (organic brain syndrome), such as the late stage of alcoholism.

48. (4) This is a reality-based response, as well as one that acknowledges the client's nonverbal reaction. The following are not the best choices because: Nos. 1 and 3 focus on "voice," which reinforces the hallucination, and no doubt is placed; in No. 2 doubt is placed but focus is on "voice" and not on client's feelings.

49. (3) Choice No. 1 is not a *direct* response; No. 2 leaves

out the importance of the meaning of a neologism to the client; and No. 4 is less valid and important than *acknowledgment* of the meaning to the client.

50. (2) This acknowledges the experience and points out reality as the nurse sees it. Nos. 1, 4, and 3 do not focus on the client or attempt to explore feelings.

51. (1) Circulation may be severely impaired in a client with waxy flexibility who tends to remain motionless for hours unless moved. No. 2 is *not* the first priority. "Touch" is not used in this stage, as in choice No. 3. And No. 4 is incorrect because she is *mute* and also because intellectual discussion of predisposing factors ignores the *feelings* of the client.

52. (4) The primary initial focus of the nurse-client relationship is in showing the client through acceptance that it is *the client* one is concerned about, *not* the *symptoms*. Nos. 1 and 2 are incorrect because the focus of *initial* nursing care is on the client, not on meeting hospital standards or controlling impulses. No. 3 is incorrect because it is an attempt to analyze the *why's* of behavior, which is not an appropriate *basic* nursing intervention and certainly *not* an initial aspect of care.

53. (3) This is a false belief developed in response to an emotional need. In No. 1 the situation is *not* a perceptual disorder. In No. 2 the situation is *not* a misperception. In No. 4, while the client refuses meals, the reason for this is a false belief (delusion).

54. (1) Listening is probably the most effective response of the four choices. A key consideration in interacting with clients who are suspicious is to *avoid* the use of logic and argument; thus, No. 2 is incorrect. Humor usually intensifies the anger and suspicion; thus No. 3 is incorrect. Changing the topic, as in No. 4, may serve to reinforce the client's belief in the guilt of others.

55. (3) Definition of projection as a coping mechanism. Nos. 1, 2, and 4 are incorrect because they have nothing to do with the coping mechanism, projection. Coping mechanisms in general function in the service of "self"—that is, they protect the ego and preserve self-esteem in an effort to cope with anxiety; the focus is *not* on *others*, as in Nos. 1 and 4. Mr. Carlson's symptoms of projection do in fact *express* delusional thought, rather than *control* it, contrary to No. 2.

56. (3) This shows a weak sense of moral consciousness. According to Freudian theory, personality disorders stem from a *weak* superego. No. 1 is incorrect, as the id is *strong*. These disorders are *not* characterized by a weak ego, as in No. 2, whereas schizophrenia is. No. 4 is of relevance in sexual-identity difficulties rather than character disorders.

57. (4) A weak superego implies a lack of adequate controls. No. 1 is not relevant, as her *self-identity* as a woman is not a focus here. No. 2 is incorrect because Alice typically gratifies her own inner needs, which is part of the difficulty with a strong id and which requires external controls, such as that in No. 4. No. 3 is incorrect because she is not psychotic but psycho*pathic,* where reality testing is *not* impaired. She *is* aware of reality.

58. (1) Prevent use of manipulative patterns. In Nos. 2, 3, and 4, the nurse needs to seek validation, and these responses indicate acceptance without validation.

59. (4) Let client know without anger how you feel and that you are not intimidated, then help her examine what she is doing and why. No. 1 is incorrect because it points the finger in an angry, accusatory way and labels the client in turn ("*You* are rude"). No. 2 makes the nurse sound like "Big Nurse"—authoritarian and punitive. No. 3 may place the nurse in a position to be intimidated and "kicked" by the client.

60. (1) Frightening visual hallucinations are especially common. No. 2, coma, is usually *not* a consequence of DTs. No. 3 is incorrect because DTs are usually a result of *withdrawal* from alcohol. No. 4 is incorrect because the client will be *agitated* and *rambling* in conversation, not mute and depressed.

61. (4) Arrest of the disease is possible through abstinent behavior, not through change in psychophysiologic response to alcohol. Nos. 1, 2, and 3 are stereotyped statements, not generally or universally accepted.

62. (4) The liver is affected by the direct effect of alcohol and nutritional deficiencies associated with alcohol abuse and dependence (alcoholism). Nos. 1, 2, and 3 are areas not usually affected by alcohol abuse and dependence (alcoholism).

63. (2) Note the eyes: when *on* heroin, the pupils are constricted; during *withdrawal,* they are dilated. Withdrawal does *not* usually include high fever, pupil constriction, or choreiform movements, as in Nos. 1, 3, and 4.

64. (4) Methadone is a synthetic narcotic and has no euphoric effect. Methadone does not produce sedation (No. 1), euphoria (No. 2), or neuritis (No. 3).

65. (2) It is important to provide external support in helping develop the superego. No. 1 may promote manipulative behavior in the client. No. 3 may foster additional dependence. And preventing the client's use of drugs (No. 4) is *not* the primary step in building a nurse–client relationship based on therapeutic communication.

66. (1) Anxiety is generated by group therapy at 9 A.M. The ritualistic behavioral defense of handwashing decreases anxiety by avoiding group therapy. No. 2 is incorrect because *tension,* not unmet needs, is discharged through ritualistic behavior. No. 3 may be true, but it is not essential to planning care. No. 4 is incorrect, as depression is *not* characteristic of ritualism.

67. (4) The opposite of what is stated in the first three choices is true. The client seems to do best when (1) routine activities are set up and anxiety-provoking changes are avoided; (2) perfection-type activities bring satisfaction (cleaning and straightening a linen closet, for example); and (3) he knows ahead of time about changes in routine.

68. (3) This is the best example of setting limits on the behavior. Choices Nos. 1 and 4 may be closely linked to nontherapeutic use of power. Choice No. 2 is more of an example of a punishment approach.

69. (2) A ritual, such as compulsive handwashing, is an attempt to allay anxiety caused by unconscious impulses that are frightening. No. 1 is incorrect because it is the opposite of what the handwashing ritual is intended to do—the ritual is aimed at *absolving* guilt, not *punishing.* No. 3 is related to *psychotic* symptoms and not at all relevant to symptoms of ritualism. No. 4 is incorrect because handwashing is aimed at relief of guilt and self-help to reduce anxiety, *not* at seeking attention from staff.

70. (1) It shows acceptance by listening to the initial account by the client about her physical problems. Neither a superficial focus nor a technical explanation of physical problems (Nos. 2 and 3) conveys acceptance of the client as a person; No. 4 is too abrupt for an initial response.

71. (3) Showing *acceptance* and gaining trust and confidence are usually the key initial nursing goals. You need to show acceptance before *helping* (Nos. 1 and 4) and *assisting* (No. 2). Note the lead verb: *accept* before *help* or *assist.*

72. (3) No. 1 is incorrect because conversion, not regression, is the major coping mechanism, and No. 2 is incorrect because, if a possible cause is identified and treatment relieves the discomfort, the client often develops another symptom. Frequently, clients do not want to be cured of their symptoms because they *need* the symptoms to control the behavior of others or because they do not know how else to get attention. In No. 4, the converse is true.

73. (1) The other choices are all *similarities* between malingering and conversion disorder.

74. (2) This is a better choice than No. 4, which may be true, but is a tangential and irrelevant reason. No. 1 is not correct because the client *is* aware of reality, but may not understand the *cause* for her conversion disorder. No. 3 is more relevant in a *paranoid* reaction.

75. (1) The original source of conflict, pain, and/or guilt is repressed (pushed out of awareness), only to surface in a symbolic way. Nos. 2, 3, and 4 are only partially correct: regression is common, not sublimation; displacement is common, not substitution; reaction formation is common, not rationalization.

76. (4) This answer also incorporates No. 3. Agreement to attend activities (No. 2) does not indicate the *greatest* improvement. The client *already* recognizes that her behavior is irrational but cannot understand the cause or banish the behavior by will, as in No. 1.

77. (3) It is believed at this time that if the client had another acceptable outlet for emotions (such as verbalizing anger, frustration, and disappointments) the emotions would not directly affect the organs. No. 1 is not correct because some disorders may be life-threatening (ulcers, for example). No. 2 is irrelevant; however, in Freudian terms, the opposite would be more true; No. 4 is incorrect in that it is well known that when one physical illness is "cured," another disorder may come to light.

78. (4) All other responses describe the *similarities* between the two forms of disorders.

79. (2) Characteristic underlying needs in psychophysiologic reactions are dependency, attention, and the need for security through trust. Nos. 1 and 4 are incorrect because the clients' complaints are not aimed at blaming others or at seeking vengeance, but at expressing dependency need and seeking security. No. 3 is inappropriate because Mr. Simon is expressing his own need for attention; he is not speaking for everyone.

80. (1) Emotional support is a key need. No. 2 does *not* focus on emotional support. No. 3, role expectation, in itself has *no* bearing. Emotional support of role would. No. 4 would help Mrs. Simon and her own emotional reaction, but not Mr. Simon.

81. (2) All the other choices are correct but can be dovetailed into No. 2.

82. (4) One coping mechanism often seen in psychophysiologic reactions is repression. As the client is better able to handle the anxiety connected with underlying feelings, the need for repression lessens. Nos. 1, 2, and 3 may be the content of his feelings, but do not explain their dynamics: the *reason* he is expressing more feelings.

83. (2) It reflects the client's underlying concerns in the most open-ended manner. No. 1 is incorrect because the *nurse* cannot say how the client is feeling; she is *assuming* here that he *is* better, which is inappropriate. No. 4 only focuses on *one* aspect: *sadness*. What about the *agitation* he *also* expresses? No. 3 is not incorrect, but it is also not the *best* choice because it asks a direct question when a simple acknowledgment (as in No. 2) would be better initially.

84. (3) This answer is the best choice because the other choices seem too certain for a disorder which, although it has a pattern, can be altered if and when the client adopts different outlets for expressing his emotions.

85. (2) Since confabulation is a coping mechanism, the best choice is the one that defines one of the main functions of coping mechanisms—to protect self-esteem. Nos. 1 and 3 are incorrect because they focus on others, not on self. No. 4 is completely irrelevant.

86. (2) An important principle to remember here is that a program of care should not increase physiologic losses by overtaxing the clients' physical capacities. It is important to remember that suicide is the *main* concern of *depression* and not a key concern of organic mental disorder, as in No. 1. Empathy (No. 4) rather than sympathy is a helpful behavior. No. 3, increasing independence, is not realistic; *maintaining* it is.

87. (3) One of the main needs experienced by most elderly clients with organic mental disorders is the need for most things to be the same. The other choices are wrong for the following reasons: there has been no demonstrable evidence of relationship between any behavior symptom and the extent or severity of pathophysiologic condition (No. 2); intellectual *blunting* usually occurs, which interferes with ability to deal with abstract thoughts (No. 4); and memory loss is for *recent* events and names, not those in the distant past, as in No. 1.

88. (1) Memory loss is usually permanent, not corrective; thus, No. 2 is wrong. However, disorientation attributed to loss of memory can be minimized. Clients usually become *more* dependent in the course of illness and deteriorate progressively. Thus, Nos. 3 and 4 are incorrect. Use of regression as a coping response (No. 1) *can* be minimized.

89. (2) This is the best choice. The other choices are not helpful for the following reasons: Nos. 3 and 4 switch the focus and ignore the client's statement; No. 1 is too brusque an attempt to bring client back to reality.

90. (1) Elderly clients feel more secure when they can count on their environment being the same, predictable, and consistent in detail from day to day (hence, structured) to compensate for feelings of loss of the familiar in terms of body functions, social environment, and so on. Nos. 2 and 4 imply change, not routine. No. 3, while correct, is not the *most* important.

91. (4) Although all the other choices are valid and important, the fourth answer encompasses them all and is therefore the most *comprehensive* answer.

92. (3) Self-esteem is *the most basic* psychologic need of *any* age, especially of the elderly. Nos. 1, 2, and 4, while also important, are not the most basic needs.

93. (1) No. 2 relates to toddler; No. 3 to infancy; No. 4 to latency period in childhood.

94. (4) Redundancy is *not* meant to impress others, but is due to *pleasure* gained through focus on the *past* and need to *control* the conversation when memory or hearing deficit is present. Choices No. 1, 2, and 3 *would* demonstrate understanding of this behavior.

95. (3) Nocturnal urination is a most common need, complicated by disorientation related to the client's age, disorder, and unfamiliar environment by night. To sit down (No. 1) or to go back to room and talk (No. 4) does not take care of the possible problem, the need to urinate. Asking a person "why" questions (No. 2) is not helpful and is too literal a response to his behavior.

96. (1) Choice No. 2 refers to preschool age, No. 3 is characteristic of "maturity" in later years of life, and No. 4 refers to young adulthood.

97. (4) The goal is to preserve ego strength through acceptance and respect of him as a person. Choice No. 1 focuses on the tangential and irrelevant; No. 2 makes the problem more obvious to others in the room and makes an assumption without validation about how Johnny must feel; No. 3 is incorrect because it is usually not helpful to give a rational explanation for an emotional difficulty related to enuresis.

98. (3) Most children with Down's are affectionate and enjoy being held and cuddled, whereas the *opposite* is usually the case with an autistic child. All other responses may apply to *both* Down's and autism.

99. (4) A crisis situation is one in which the person's usual means for handling difficulties are not effective at this time, and the situation *may* call for therapeutic intervention. Hence, No. 3 is incorrect. There *is* usually a precipitating event to the crisis, making No. 1 false. No. 2 is also incorrect because stresses occurring during *normal* stages of growth and development may cause a crisis.

100. (3) Clients plan and lead activities rather than staff. Although families and significant others are brought in when needed, *family therapy* is neither a key feature nor an emphasis in milieu therapy. Thus, No. 1 is incorrect. Structured activities based on members' needs, rather than permissiveness (No. 2), is the keynote. Staff do participate *with* (not dominate) clients in discussing plans for activities. Thus, No. 4 is wrong.

101. (4) This calls for joint client-staff planning and decision-making. The other responses are typical of a high degree of direction by the staff, with clients in the passive-dependent role.

102. (4) This term is associated with transactional analysis. Others are examples of behavior modification and are techniques that emphasize overt behavior, *not* unconscious processes.

103. (3) Focus on dreams is part of Freudian analysis; thus, No. 1 is incorrect. Behavior modification is used in the treatment of *mute* clients also; thus, No. 2 is incorrect. The emphasis of behavioral therapy is in the present (No. 3) and not the past developmental history, as in No. 4.

104. (4) A major assumption of behavior therapy is that it *is* possible to change behavior *without* insight. All others are correct.

105. (2) It will provide energy release without the external stimuli and pressure of competitive games (Nos. 3 and 4). Reading usually requires sitting, which a manic client cannot readily do, as in No. 1.

106. (1) An undemanding task that the client could finish would allow a feeling of successful accomplishment. Nos. 2 and 3 require intellectual activity that is usually slowed down during a depressive phase. No. 4 requires a skill that the client may not have, and which the client might experience frustration in learning; also, the client may not have the psychomotor energy for the ice skating.

107. (4) The directive role decreases responsibility and independence in the client. All of the other options are true.

108. (2) Nos. 1 and 4 relate to socioeconomic justification for the advantages of group therapy. No. 3 can be incorporated into No. 2, with No. 2 being the more comprehensive and inclusive response. Multiple transference can be therapeutic from the standpoint of eliciting positive as well as negative feelings, not only by seeing similarities between self and others but also by experiencing differences.

109. (3) A contract early in therapy is essential to make expectations clear, which includes no scapegoating or blaming of one family member by another. The opposites of Nos. 2 and 4 are important to practice. It is crucial that nurses not take sides or try to referee a family fight, as suggested in No. 1.

110. (1) Often children bear the problems in the family. In order to effect change in a child's behavior, change needs also to occur in family dynamics. Alcoholism and character disorders are usually best treated in groups with peers; thus, Nos. 2 and 3 are incorrect. *Behavior modification* (desensitization) is currently the most effective mode of treatment in anxiety disorders (neuroses); thus, No. 4 is incorrect.

111. (3) The client will be in a confused state after treatment and will require siderails and the reassuring presence of a nurse. Nos. 1 and 4 are incorrect because hunger and suicide are *not* immediate posttreatment concerns. No. 2 is incorrect because the client needs *someone* there to help orient him, as he is likely to wake up and be somewhat disoriented.

112. (3) The client needs to be protected against photosensitivity and dermatitis when exposed to the sun; a sunscreen preparation should be applied to exposed parts

of the skin and the client should wear long sleeves and cover-up clothing. Nos. 1, 2, and 4 refer to indoor activities where there is no danger of sunburn.

113. (4) This is the best choice, as it encompasses No. 3. Nos. 1 and 2 are definitely incorrect.

114. (1) Blood dyscrasias often are overlooked when first symptoms of possible adverse drug effects appear in the form of a minor cold. Nos. 2, 3, and 4 refer to extra pyramidal tract symptoms that are not life-threatening.

115. (2) Hypertensive crisis can be precipitated by combining this drug with common cold medications and foods high in tyramine or pressor amines (yogurt, Chianti wine, cheese, coke, and coffee, for example). All other options are incorrect.

116. (4) This effect is seen in clients taking a major tranquilizer. All of the other options are correct.

117. (2) You are asking the client to clarify and further discuss feelings. No. 1 is incorrect because, while staying with client *might* convey acceptance, it does not help him clarify or deal with feelings. No. 3 is incorrect because it cuts off any further response from the client and because it is doubtful that you can understand another person's feelings. No. 4 is incorrect because it is more important to *clarify* the client's feelings than it is to understand the object of hate.

118. (4) The client is anxious and needs someone with him. No. 1 is incorrect because it ignores the client's anxiety and needs. No. 2 is incorrect because it also ignores the client's anxiety and uses the doctor as an excuse to ignore his needs. No. 3 is incorrect because it also ignores the client's anxiety and needs, and gives a poor reason for refusal.

119. (2) Consistency lets clients know consequences of behavior and develops trust. No. 1 is incorrect because you cannot approve all behavior (e.g., destructive behavior). No. 3 is incorrect because it can be therapeutic to express negative opinions. No. 4 is incorrect because interpretation of behavior is not always advisable. Clients may use interpretations of behavior to avoid consequences of behavior or may see them as an excuse not to change behavior.

120. (4) Nurse and client, on initial contact, are strangers, and therefore responses need to be heard and reacted to with little background data and without preconceived ideas. No. 1 is incorrect because at first contact you *do not have enough data* to indicate cause of hostility. No. 2 is incorrect because previous knowledge of the client's history and the doctor's opinions may interfere with the nurse's ability to respond appropriately to a given interaction. No. 3 is incorrect because physical appearance is an easily misinterpreted nonverbal message.

121. (1) If rules and regulations are at a minimum, clients can work out their own solutions. No. 2 is incorrect because imposed solutions do not allow for personal growth. No. 3 is incorrect because adults do not learn self-control from imposed rules but from working out their own rules. No. 4 is incorrect because it is important to teach people to reason and problem solve about rules, rather than to respond rigidly.

122. (3) In family therapy a family is seen as a homeostatic system, and a change in functioning of one family member results in compensatory change in the functioning of other family members. Nos. 1, 2, and 4 are incorrect because they would treat individuals in the family, but not necessarily the interactions between family members.

123. (2) One of the purposes of group therapy is to discover a universality of problems and a diversity of solutions. No. 1 is incorrect because people do not use authoritative answers, and to give authoritative answers lessens learning. No. 3 is incorrect because it is not as complete as No. 2. No. 4 is incorrect because the goal of therapy is to assist clients, not the therapist.

124. (4) The major goal of crisis intervention is to resolve immediate problems. No. 1 is incorrect because restructuring personality is the goal of *psychoanalytic* therapy. Nos. 2 and 3 are incorrect because they are goals of *brief* psychotherapy, and while they may occur in the resolution of immediate problems, they are not the goal.

125. (1) To resolve immediate problems you focus on a person's ability to cope and usual level of functioning. No. 2 is incorrect because it is a *psychoanalytic* focus. Nos. 3 and 4 are incorrect because they are the focus of *brief* psychotherapy.

126. (1) Deal first with the life-saving situation. Nos. 2 and 3 are incorrect because they are done *following* stabilization of physical condition. No. 4 is incorrect because it is not a necessary life-saving concern.

127. (3) It incorporates all information a crisis intervention therapist needs immediately. Nos. 1 and 2 are incorrect because the nurse does not need to know how angry Jenny is at this time. No. 4 is incorrect because it is not as complete an answer as No. 3.

128. (2) On principle, the therapist needs to be immediately available to Jenny. No. 1 is incorrect because it abandons her. No. 3 is incorrect because Jenny needs to deal with the situation immediately. No. 4 is incorrect because Jenny might decide that therapist is not interested in helping her, and she needs immediate assistance.

129. (3) Part of the definition of a crisis is a time span of 4–6 weeks. No. 1 is incorrect because, by definition, crises do not continue indefinitely. No. 2 is incorrect because all people have crises, and having crises does

not determine normality. No. 4 is incorrect because, although crises may be related to deep underlying problems, one of the principles of crisis intervention therapy is to deal with the immediate situation, not the underlying problem.

130. (3) Jenny needs to be aware of her actions and possible ramifications of her actions. No. 1 is incorrect because she needs to discuss her actions. No. 2 is incorrect because the purpose of crisis intervention is to deal with the present problem and situation, *not* the past. No. 4 is incorrect because the focus needs to be on the client, *not* on others.

131. (3) A principle of behavior modification is to reward behavior. No. 1 is incorrect because he is allowed to continue with unacceptable behavior. Nos. 2 and 4 are incorrect because they are not suitable reinforcers. If he could eat like others, he would, and it is doubtful that he is concerned about others' distress.

132. (2) A principle of behavior modification is to reward behavior. Nos. 1, 3, and 4 are not suitable reinforcers for regressed client. See question 131.

133. (3) Research has shown that behavior is decreased by both positive and negative punishment. Nos. 1 and 2 are incorrect because they are not complete answers. No. 4 is incorrect because severe punishment is unacceptable.

134. (3) This is the most inclusive answer. Nos. 1, 2, and 4 are all incorporated in No. 3.

135. (4) Behavior associated with anxiety is primarily monitored through the autonomic nervous system and prepares the body to fight. No. 1 is incorrect because the parasympathetic nervous system acts to conserve bodily responses. Nos. 2 and 3 are incorrect because they are part of the autonomic, and parasympathetic, nervous system.

136. (2) Research shows *increased* activity is a psychomotor manifestation of anxiety; No. 1 is therefore wrong. Nos. 3 and 4 are incorrect because emotion is not a psychomotor manifestation.

137. (3) Research shows that anxiety decreases the perceptual field—No. 1 therefore is incorrect. Research also shows that anxiety decreases the ability to concentrate and increases random activity. Therefore, Nos. 2 and 4 are incorrect.

138. (4) Some anxiety is necessary to learn. No. 2 is incorrect because it is incomplete. Nos. 1 and 3 are incorrect because anxiety is necessary for learning and growth.

139. (4) Assertive behavior is an example of constructive use of anger. No. 2 is therefore incorrect. No. 1 is incorrect because it does not go far enough in describing the relationship between assertive and aggressive behavior. No. 3 is not a good choice because it has not

been substantiated and is an irrelevant answer in this case.

140. (4) It provides the complete steps. No. 1 is incorrect because of the phrase "decide on *several* solutions"; it should be one solution at a time. No. 2 is incorrect because it doesn't include "discuss alternate solutions." No. 3 is incorrect because it does not describe a requested *series* of steps and because *giving* a person one answer is untherapeutic.

141. (1) The nurse needs to set limits to assure safety of client and others. No. 2 is incorrect because he may hurt himself or others. Nos. 3 and 4 are incorrect because they are interpretations that may or may not be correct and they do *not control* his *unsafe* behavior.

142. (1) This is the proper use of anger. No. 2 is incorrect because, while anger can be used to intimidate others, that use creates interpersonal problems. No. 3 is incorrect because in order for hostility to be a good communication mechanism, the degree of hostility must be appropriate to the provocation. No. 4 is incorrect because this expression of anger does not produce positive accomplishment.

143. (4) A person needs to be allowed to express his anger appropriately. Nos. 1, 2, and 3 are incorrect responses because they *are* things you assist a person to do when intervening in anger.

144. (4) Denial is defined as the avoidance of disagreeable realities by ignoring or refusing to recognize them; avoidance implies refusing to take action. No. 1 is incorrect because rationalization involves offering a socially acceptable or logical explanation to justify feelings or behavior. In rationalization, one does not need to take action; one merely offers an explanation. No. 2 is incorrect because projection involves attributing one's thoughts or impulses to others. No. 3 is incorrect because sublimation is the acceptance of a socially approved substitute for a drive that is blocked.

145. (4) This is the most complete description of body image. Nos. 1, 2, and 3 are partial answers and therefore incorrect.

146. (1) It is most likely that grief would be expressed because of object loss. No. 2 is incorrect because deep depression, if it occurs, would be the result of lack of resolution of grief over object loss. No. 3 is incorrect because relief is not part of grief process. No. 4 is incorrect because question asks for immediate response. Denial of carcinoma, if it occurs, would probably occur *later*.

147. (3) A change in body image has made Mrs. Dawn feel unloved and unworthy of love. Nos. 1, 2, and 4 are incorrect because there are no supporting data.

148. (2) This question attempts to get a specific description of what has happened and will allow client to describe grief and feelings of low self-worth because of loss of breast. No. 1 is incorrect because it offers a false reassurance. No. 3 is incorrect because it is a stereotyped response to a female and denies the client's actual loss. No. 4 is incorrect because it is an interpretation which, although possibly true, the client may reject. Resolution of grief, etc., is better achieved if the client can state connection.

149. (1) Overcompliance leads to lack of development of self-identity, one of the major problems in schizophrenia. No. 2 is incorrect because there are no substantiating data. No. 3 is incorrect because it contradicts the correct statement in No. 1. No. 4 is incorrect because he probably has a *strong* superego due to implied "should" system (overcompliance with his parents' expectations of behavior).

150. (2) Rebellion is normal in early adolescence. Theorists partially attribute schizophrenic symptoms to lack of rebellion. Therefore, Nos. 1 and 4 are incorrect. No. 3 is completely irrelevant.

151. (2) Use of "you" and "I" forces him to acknowledge separate identities. No. 1 is incorrect because "pet names" are usually not a person's choice. Frank needs to be called by his real name. No. 3 is incorrect because he has no identity if he can't have his own opinions. No. 4 is incorrect because "should" responses imply others' ideas, not his.

152. (4) The parents need to ask Frank, not nurse, but the nurse should also support the parents and encourage them to interact with Frank. Nos. 1 and 2 are incorrect because they are interpretations that state opinions about Frank without Frank's participation. No. 3 is incorrect because no support is given to the parents.

153. (2) A diagnosis of schizophrenia implies weak ego development. Nos. 1, 3, and 4 are incorrect because a schizophrenic might have strong id, superego, and "not me" components.

154. (2) In second grade a person needs to form close relationship with peers. No. 1 needs to occur earlier than second grade or later in early teen years. No. 3 occurs later. No. 4 is incorrect because her father's actions make her dependent on him rather than on her peers.

155. (4) This is the all-inclusive answer. Nos. 1, 2, and 3 are all parts of No. 4.

156. (3) The meaning of "ideas of reference" is that all that goes on is somehow connected to a person. No. 1 is incorrect because delusions of grandeur mean a person has an exalted opinion of self. No. 2 is incorrect because illusion is a false perceptual experience occurring in response to a stimulus. No. 4 is incorrect because echolalia is a person's automatic repetition of what is said.

157. (1) Maria has ideas that someone (her husband) is out to kill her. No. 2 is incorrect; see question 158. No. 3 is incorrect. (See preceding question.) No. 4 is incorrect because a hallucination is a sensory experience triggered by a person's inner needs, functioning independently of stimulation from the environment.

158. (2) A paranoid schizophrenic is suspicious, so a nurse must make every effort not to engage in behavior Maria can misinterpret. Nos. 1 and 3 are incorrect because a nurse should give her correct information about what she says and not placate her because she will sense the falseness. No. 4 is incorrect because arguing just solidifies her ideas. In a neutral voice, the nurse should give correct information.

159. (3) The nurse should encourage Maria to explain her statement in order to understand the experience Maria is having. No. 1 is incorrect because it is an interpretation that may or may not be true. No. 2 is incorrect because it denies Maria's perception without clarification. No. 4 is incorrect because the nurse agrees with an unsupported statement.

160. (4) Correct by definition.

161. (4) Correct by definition. No. 1 is incorrect because delusion is a fixed idea arising out of person's inner needs and contrary to observed facts. No. 2 is incorrect—see question 160. No. 3 is incorrect because identification is the process of taking another person's attribute.

162. (2) You help him do things by doing something with him. No. 1 is incorrect because the client won't hear a long explanation. No. 3 is incorrect because demanding won't work. He can't join in unless you are with him (as in No. 2). No. 4 is incorrect because you should not produce psychosis in order to motivate a person.

163. (4) Withdrawn schizophrenics tend to think in concrete terms. Therefore, use of simple language enables them to grasp meaning. No. 1 is incorrect because if you remain silent, the client will remain silent. No. 2 is incorrect because if you are not concrete, the client might have trouble understanding some terms in normal conversation. No. 3 is incorrect, as client has difficulty talking.

164. (3) Correct by definition. No. 1 is incorrect, as it is a definition of hysteria. No. 2 is not as complete as No. 3. No. 4 is incorrect because it is not necessarily true.

165. (3) One way to enhance the development of unresolved grief is *not* to participate in activities that demonstrate death. Nos. 1, 2, and 4 may occur, but they are *not* the best predictors of grief resolution difficulties.

166. (3) Correct by definition according to Kübler-Ross grief stages. Hence, Nos. 1, 2, and 4 are incorrect.

167. (4) Rationalization is the process of constructing plausible reasons for one's responses. No. 1, suppression, is the intentional exclusion of material from consciousness. No. 2, undoing, is an act that partially negates a previous one. No. 3, repression, is the involuntary exclusion of painful or conflicting thoughts or feelings from awareness.

168. (4) Feelings of worthlessness or low self-esteem are the underlying problem in depression. Nos. 1, 2, and 3 may occur but are not most apt.

169. (4) The punitive superego enhances feelings of low self-esteem. Nos. 1 and 3 refer primarily to the sociopath, not the depressed person. No. 2 does not characterize any particular disorder.

170. (2) Denial is the act of avoiding disagreeable realities by ignoring them. No. 1 is incorrect because compensation is the process by which a person makes up for a deficiency in self-image by emphasizing an asset. No. 3, symbolism is the use of one mental image to represent another. No. 4 is also incorrect. (See answer to question 161, choice No. 3.)

171. (1) A person who has settled on a plan for suicide will become more cheerful. No. 2 is incorrect because a person who is severely retarded in the psychomotor area cannot carry out a suicide act. Nos. 3 and 4 are incorrect because Mr. Gonzalez is more likely to be hostile and agitated if he does not have a suicide plan. Agitated behavior can also represent the need to "repent" for sins thought to be committed.

172. (2) Persons engaged in self-destructive behavior other than active suicide behavior fantasize they can control their behavior and deny the likelihood of death as a result. Thus Nos. 1, 3, and 4 are incorrect.

173. (1) These persons have not faced up to the idea that they are controlled by their behavior, and this relieves their anxiety. Contrary to No. 2, persons have increased anxiety if they stop the behavior. No. 3 is also incorrect (see question 172). No. 4 is incorrect because these persons know the behavior is bad for them.

174. (3) When feelings of low self-esteem are high, self-destructive behavior reaches its peak. Hence, Nos. 1, 2, and 4 are incorrect.

175. (3) Correct by Freudian theory. Nos. 1, 2, and 4 are incorrect because they are incomplete.

176. (3) Freudian theory says addicts are fixated at the oral phase of development. Hence, Nos. 1, 2, and 4 are incorrect.

177. (4) A variety of factors can cause self-destructive behavior, and these differ for each individual. Hence, Nos. 1, 2, and 3 are not the best choices because, although correct, they are *examples* of a *variety* of factors; No. 4 is more inclusive.

178. (1) The nurse should formulate a diet, in cooperation with the client, that allows for a gradual weight loss, not immediate loss as in No. 4. Nos. 2 and 3 are incorporated in No. 1.

179. (3) This describes the correct relationship between eating, love, and mother in this case. Hence, Nos. 1, 2, and 4 are incorrect.

180. (1) This reply asks for information that the nurse can use. If the client understands the statement, the nurse can support the therapist when focusing on connections between food, love, and mother. If the client does not understand the statement, the nurse can help her get clarification from the therapist. No. 2 alienates the client, and the nurse loses the chance for collaboration with the therapist. No. 3 shuts the client off. No. 4 is incorrect because it is asked before the nurse is sure the client understands the therapist's statement.

181. (3) The *client* determines if a problem exists as long as others' rights are not violated. Neither the nurse, the doctor, nor the legal system identifies sexual problems. Hence, Nos. 1, 2, and 4 are incorrect.

182. (4) Providing information is the primary sex health intervention. Nos. 1 and 2 are secondary health interventions. No. 3 is a tertiary intervention.

183. (2) Masturbation can provide appropriate sexual activity that enables a person to become comfortable with his or her sexual identity. No. 1 is incorrect because masturbation can be healthy. No. 3 is incorrect because masturbation can enhance heterosexual activity. No. 4 is the opposite of correct answer No. 2.

184. (2) This is a statistical fact. The first clause of No. 1 is incorrect; the last clause of No. 3 is incorrect; and both clauses of No. 4 are incorrect.

185. (4) The victim needs to engage in expression of the experience, which will assist her to work through her feelings so that the experience may not interfere in future interpersonal relations. To repress the incident, as in No. 1, would make it continually interfere in her relationships. No. 2 is only done after No. 4 has been accomplished. No. 3 is incorrect because the rape victim has no "part" in the rape.

186. (4) Growth in the individual occurs in spurts, emotionally and physically, and growth patterns differ from person to person. Thus Nos. 1 and 2 are incorrect. No. 3 is incorrect because sexual maturation occurs at different ages for different individuals.

187. (3) No. 3 includes Nos. 1, 2, and 4.

188. (3) The nurse tells him she heard his statement about "not doing his own thing" and states she *thinks* he is angry. No. 1 is incorrect because the nurse states she *knows* he is angry. No. 2 is incorrect because an angry person can't stop being angry on command. No. 4 is incorrect because using the parents puts the nurse on their side.

189. (2) Confidentiality cannot be guaranteed if there is a danger to the client or to others. No. 1 is incorrect because it is a sarcastic response and denies that the client has serious problems. No. 3 contradicts No. 2. No. 4 is incorrect because parents do not have the right to know the content of therapy sessions except in the circumstances described in No. 2.

190. (2) Manipulation is the attempt to control the behavior of others to achieve one's own goals. No. 1, insight, is understanding and using understanding to correct one's behavior. Nos. 3 and 4 are incorrect because, although the client may be trying to con the therapist into believing he needs her to do something for him and he trusts her, the real purpose of the request is manipulation.

191. (3) This response stops the manipulation and suggests John is responsible for his own behavior. Nos. 1, 2, and 4 are incorrect because they indicate the therapist has been conned and manipulated.

192. (2) Part of maturing is learning to view one's parents and oneself realistically. Nos. 1, 3, and 4 are incorrect because they represent the misinformation that creates problems between individuals.

193. (3) A person with limited hearing and sight becomes confused and disturbed. Nos. 1 and 4 are unwarranted assumptions. No. 2 is incorrect because Mr. Sundowner's situation is not psychological dependency but actual sensory need.

194. (2) Mr. Sundowner will be easier to care for if he has aid and glasses. In No. 1, the nurse is denying the client his right to the full information of his senses. No. 3 is incorrect because the nurse has the responsibility to change rules for clearly therapeutic reasons. No. 4 does not respond to the client's needs.

ANNOTATED BIBLIOGRAPHY

American Psychiatric Association: Diagnostic and statistical manual of mental disorders (DSM–III), ed. 3, Washington, D.C., 1980. A systematic descriptive approach to the classification of mental disorders. Provides specific diagnostic criteria. Each disorder is described in the following areas: essential features, associated features, age at onset, course, impairment, complications, predisposing factors, prevalence, and differential diagnosis.

Burgess, A., and Lazare, A.: Psychiatric nursing in the hospital and the community, Englewood Cliffs, N.J., 1976, Prentice-Hall, Inc. The most valuable feature of this book is the simple format and writing style. It is not as comprehensive in scope or theory as Kyes and Hofling, or Kalkman and Davis; however, the intent is to devote a major part of the book to the application of basic concepts to nursing management of clinical syndromes. The art work is effective; key points are enumerated in outline form, key phrases are placed in the margins, and end-of-chapter summaries serve to promote this as a useful book for initial learning and review of major psychiatric conditions.

Haber, J., Leach, A., Schudy, S., and Sideleau, B. F.: Comprehensive psychiatric nursing, New York, 1978, McGraw-Hill Book Co. This excellent book uses an integrated approach throughout the life span in a variety of settings. The focus is on nursing management of clients with a variety of behavioral difficulties; for example, anxiety, fear, frustration, anger, depression, and guilt. The nursing process is continuously stressed, with sections labeled "Nursing Assessment," "Planning and Implementation," "Nursing Intervention," and "Evaluation."

Hays, J. S., and Larson, K. H.: Interacting with patients, New York, 1963, Macmillan, Inc. This is a compendium of process recordings with lists and numerous easy-to-understand examples of therapeutic and nontherapeutic responses for beginning students.

Kalkman, M., and Davis, A.: New dimensions in mental health–psychiatric nursing, ed. 4, New York, 1974, McGraw-Hill Book Co. In addition to chapters on disorders, this text includes chapters concerning group and family therapy, the dying person, and old age. Implications for nursing appear throughout the book.

Kyes, J., and Hofling, C.: Basic psychiatric concepts in nursing, ed. 3, Philadelphia, 1974, J. B. Lippincott Co. This text is a comprehensive reference covering personality development, neuroses, psychoses, character disorders, psychosomatic disorders, emotional disorders of children and adolescents, and treatment modes. It also includes a glossary and quick reference index. It contains a clear description of theory, is illustrated with case examples, and has suggestions for nursing management.

Sundeen, S., and Stuart, G.: Principles and practice of psychiatric nursing, St. Louis, 1979, The C. V. Mosby Co. This comprehensive overview of the field of psychiatric nursing reflects the changing emphasis in psychiatric nursing practice through its use of the nursing process model as a framework. The nursing role is viewed as one that influences health promotion, treatment of disturbances, and rehabilitation. There is an excellent section on the various models of psychiatric care, as well as current treatment modalities. Patient disturbances are seen as adaptive or maladaptive; terminology used emphasizes the concept of stress and stressors, with levels of primary, secondary, and tertiary prevention. A valuable feature is the summary of important points at the end of each chapter.

Topalis, M., and Aguilera, D.: Psychiatric nursing, ed. 7, St. Louis, 1978, The C. V. Mosby Co. Case studies illustrate the major concepts of the practice of psychiatric nursing. Tables of psychotropic medication are included, providing rapid access to recommended dosage, effect, and lethality. The book covers a comprehensive range of complex behavioral theories, yet it is easy to read and understand. This succinct text of useful information is applicable to most nursing situations.

Wilson, H., and Kneisl, C.: Psychiatric nursing, Menlo Park, California, 1979, Addison-Wesley Publishing Co. This is the most inclusive book available in the field of psychiatric nursing. It can be used as an overall reference. It contains the most thorough information, concepts, theories, and ideas relevant to the field of psychiatric nursing. A unique feature is its extensive use of charts and tables. It includes unique chapters on human sexuality, parenting, group dynamics, psychiatric nursing ethics, and alternative therapies.

SUGGESTED REFERENCES

Alcoholism
Estes, E.: "Assessing alcoholic patients," *American Journal of Nursing*, 76(5):785–789, May 1976.

Uffer, L.: "How to recognize and care for the alcoholic patient," *Nursing '77*, 7(10):37–38, October 1977.

Psychiatric Emergencies
Aguilera, D.: *Review of psychiatric nursing*, St. Louis, Missouri, 1977, The C. V. Mosby Co.

Rogerson, K.: "Psychiatric emergencies," *Nursing Clinics of North America*, 8(3):457–466, September 1973.

Psychopharmacology
Newton, M., et al.: "How you can improve the effectiveness of psychotropic drug therapy," *Nursing '78*, 8(7):46–55, July 1978.

Psychosocial Assessment
Snyder, J., and Wilson, M.: "Elements of a psychological assessment," *American Journal of Nursing*, 77(2):235–239, 1977.

Vincent, P., Broad, J., and Dylworth, L.: "Developing a mental health assessment form," *Journal of Nursing Administration*, 6(1):25–28, 1976.

Psychosocial Development
Duvall, E. M.: Marriage and family development, Philadelphia, 1977, J. B. Lippincott Co.

Erikson, E. Childhood and society, New York, 1963, W. W. Norton and Co.

Kalish, R.: The psychology of human behavior, Monterey, California, 1973, Wadsworth, Inc.

Maslow, A.: Motivation and personality, New York, 1970, Harper and Row, Publishers, Inc.

Piaget, J.: Origins of intelligence in children, New York, 1963, W. W. Norton and Co.

Stress and Crisis
Aguilera, D., and Messick, J.: Crisis intervention, St. Louis, Missouri, 1978, The C. V. Mosby Co.

Sedgwick, R.: "Psychological response to stress," *Journal of Psychiatric Nursing and Mental Health Services*, 13(5):20–23, September–October 1975.

Selye, H.: Stress without distress, Ontario, 1974, New American Library of Canada.

General Behavioral Problems
Disturbance in body image
Blaesing, S., Brockhaus, J., Dempsey, M., and Murray, R.: "The development of body image in the child, the adolescent, and adulthood," *Nursing Clinics of North America*, 7(4):597–630, December 1972.

Corbeil, M.: "The nursing process for a patient with a body image disturbance," *Nursing Clinics of North America*, 6(1):155–163, March 1971.

Immobility
Carnevali, D., and Brueckner, S.: "Immobilization—reassessment of a concept," *American Journal of Nursing*, 70(7):1502–1507, July 1970.

Sensory disturbance
Bolin, R., "Sensory deprivation: an overview," *Nursing Forum*, 13(3):240–258, Summer 1974.

Chodil, J., et al.: "The concept of sensory deprivation," *Nursing Clinics of North America*, 5(3):544–548, September 1970.

Pain
McCaffery, M.: Nursing management of the patient with pain, Philadelphia, 1972, J. B. Lippincott Co.

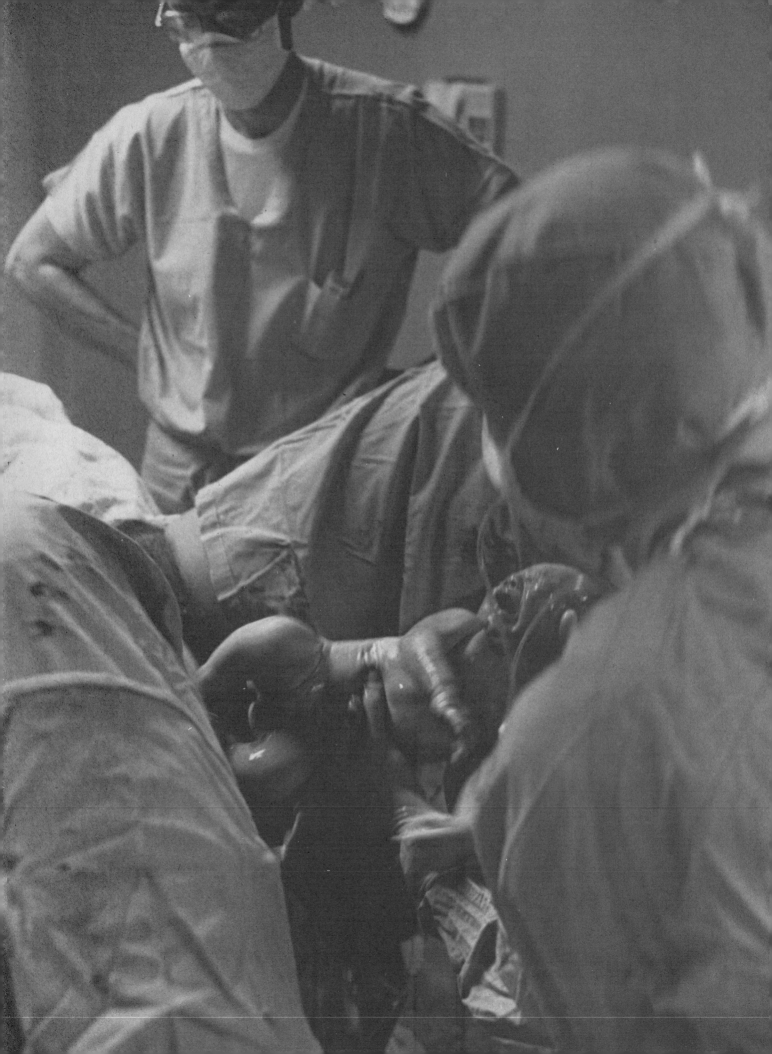

Unit 3 / NURSING CARE DURING THE REPRODUCTIVE YEARS

Introduction

This unit reflects pertinent current theoretical bases (both biophysical and psychosocial) and their nursing applications during the reproductive years. Content is presented in a study outline format, with *numerous charts and tables* wherein it is synthesized and condensed. Related material is grouped for optimum comparison and contrast in order to facilitate review, retention, and recall, using a *nursing process framework.*

Nutrition and pharmacology relevant to the reproductive years are integrated throughout. Key concepts and measures are included where pertinent, but the student is referred to basic textbooks for detailed discussions.

The emphasis on hospital-based practice reflects the *orientation of state board examinations.* Alternatives for birth settings and management, while recognized, are not universally accepted or practiced, and are therefore not covered in detail in this unit.

The unit is divided into four parts:

A. Basic Issues—emergency conditions, their assessment and management; anatomy and physiology of the reproductive tract; genetics and genetic counseling; statistics; legal aspects; trends and options; family planning and decision-making.
B. Normal Pregnancy—fetal development, labor (including when it is the nurse who assists a woman giving birth), puerperium, the normal newborn, the adolescent parent, and the older parent.
C. Complications of childbearing and the high-risk neonate.
D. Reproductive-system disorders of women and men—infections, neoplasms, infertility, and other conditions.

New material has been added in this second edition on the *preconception period* and the *normal newborn.* I have also included a *more detailed discussion of drugs, health assessment, client counseling and education, diabetes and its effects on pregnancy,* and the *assessment* and *prevention of premature labor.* A new section on the *pregnant adolescent* has also been added. Some of these additions were necessary to keep the text current with the rapidly changing area of health science and the *proposed changes in the state board examination.* Many, however, were necessitated by the expanded responsibilities of today's nurse in his or her role as a health professional.

The review questions at the end of this unit are intended for self-evaluation. Questions are constructed in a *format similar to that of the state board examinations.* To reinforce learning, the answer section provides the correct responses along with their *rationales,* which stress the key concepts and principles underlying the best response and detail the flaws in the incorrect responses.

Irene M. Bobak

Part A BASIC ISSUES

EMERGENCY CONDITIONS

The nurse may be called upon to assess and provide initial care for various obstetric and gynecologic problems. The most common emergencies are hemorrhage, hypertension, convulsions, labor complications, neonatal complications, and pelvic pain. In Table 3–1, these emergency conditions and their management are presented.

THE REPRODUCTIVE SYSTEM IN WOMEN

The anatomy and physiology of the reproductive system of the female is presented in a manner to facilitate the nursing process. Lettered entries describe the structure and function of specific tissues and organs. Numbered subentries give examples of *nursing actions to assess* a client's health status and *to plan and implement* health-teaching.

1. External genitalia (vulva or pudendum)
A. *Mons veneris* (name of mons pubis in the female): area over symphysis pubis covered with coarse hair; rounded and soft during childbearing years due to adipose tissue; thins after menopause.
   1. Refer for endocrine study if thin during childbearing years or if hair pattern changes.
   2. Becomes edematous as preeclamptic condition worsens.
B. *Labia majora:* folds of skin, pigmented slightly darker than surrounding skin, sparsely hairy, extending downward from mons to perineum in midline. In nulliparas, they obscure the vagina. Become thinner after menopause.
   1. Normally darken during pregnancy; whitened lesions need to be evaluated for neoplastic changes.
   2. Asymmetry, swelling, excoriations, erythema, other lesions are referred for diagnosis.
C. *Labia minora:* narrow folds of hairless skin, extending from clitoris to fourchette between labia majora and vagina.
   1. Same assessment and action as for labia majora (see above).
D. *Glans clitoris:* short (1–2 cm), sensitive erectile organ fixed just beneath pubic arch and above urinary meatus.
   1. If enlarged, refer for genetic workup; overstimulation during sexual activity is painful.
E. *Vestibule:* ovoid area between labia minora, clitoris, and fourchette. Contains urinary meatus and vagina.
   1. Easily irritated by discharge from infection.
F. *Hymen:* partial, rarely complete, tough, elastic, mucosa-covered fold over vagina.
   1. Assess each female for adequate vaginal opening; assess for gynatresia—imperforate hymen.
G. *Paraurethral (Skene's) glands:* open just posterolaterally immediately inside urethral meatus.
   1. Site of infection, such as gonorrhea. Difficult to treat.
H. *Vulvovaginal (Bartholin's) glands:* located on each side of vaginal wall, open on the vulva; thought to secrete mucus during sexual excitement.
   1. Site of cyst formation, or infection, e.g., gonorrhea.
   2. If enlarged, may impede birth.
I. *Perineal body:* wedge-shaped fibromuscular mass (4 cm × 4 cm) between lower vagina and anal canal. In obstetrics—the perineum.
   1. Stretched and flattened and occasionally lacerated or deliberately incised (episiotomy) during vaginal birth.

2. Internal structures
A. *Ovaries:* two flattened, intraperitoneal pelvic organs measuring 2 cm × 3 cm × 3.5 cm. Attached to uterus by ovarian ligaments. Genetic endowment at birth is 40,000 primordial ova. Function: ovulation of mature eggs and production of steroid sex hormones, estrogen, progesterone, and androgens.
   1. Agenesis (Turner's or streak ovaries): contain no primordial ova so woman is sterile.
   2. All of woman's eggs are present at birth; chromosomal aberrations increase as woman ages.
B. *Fallopian tubes:* extend laterally from the cornu of the uterus for 10 cm. The distal fimbriated ends are bell-shaped. At ovulation, the opening enlarges and the fimbria become turgescent, almost erectile, to facilitate the entrance of the ovum. Fertilization, assisted by tubal enzyme action, takes place in the middle third. Peristaltic and ciliary action move the fertilized egg toward the intrauterine cavity.
   1. During tubal sterilization, fimbriated ends that facilitate retrieval of ovum after ovulation are often removed.
   2. Removal of portion of middle third of tube results in physiologic changes that cannot be

TABLE 3–1. *Emergency conditions*

Assessment/observations	*Possible problem*	*Nursing/medical management*
1. HEMORRHAGE: VAGINAL OR INTRAABDOMINAL		
a. Nonpregnant woman of childbearing age: Take menstrual history—note usual frequency and amount of bleeding to assess excessive or irregular bleeding. (One or more pads soaked in two hours is of concern.) Take coital history—since last normal menstrual period. Do pregnancy test—after assessing menstrual and coital history. Take history of contraceptive method used.	Fibroid or cervical polyp, carcinoma, vaginal ulceration, cervicitis. Excessive menstrual flow or early abortion. Break-through bleeding with oral-contraceptive use. Uterine irritability with IUD.	Refer to physician for diagnosis; save all pads for physician prn. Refer to physician. Change oral contraceptive. Change type of IUD or change to another method.
b. Menopausal woman	At menopause, if no period for 6 months, then return of heavy flow or intermittent flow, R/O cancer with D & C.	Curettage: hormonal—progesterone, IM × 1 day or PO. × 5 days. Menses should start in 2 to 6 days. D & C.
2. DURING PREGNANCY: FIRST TRIMESTER		
a. Cramping—with or without bleeding or passage of tissue.	Abortion (prior to 20 weeks), p. 230. Threatened. Imminent, incomplete, septic.	Bedrest, sedation, avoid coitus—if threatened; bedrest in Trendelenburg, start IV fluids and draw blood for laboratory work: CBC, type/cross-match, electrolytes, platelets, HCG levels.
b. Passage of tissue (products of conception; grapelike vesicles) or brown spotting; fundus is too high for gestational age; blood pressure elevated above baseline.	Hydatidiform mole (trophoblastic disease), p. 231.	Vital signs q 5–15 minutes, prn.
c. Severe pain, shock out of proportion to amount of overt blood; shoulder-strap pain (Kehr's sign), a "referred pain" that indicates intraabdominal bleeding (or rupture of ovarian cyst); amenorrhea of 6–12 weeks.	Ectopic pregnancy, p. 231.	Save all pads or tissue passed by vagina for physician evaluation. No rectal or vaginal examination until physician is present.
d. Malodorous discharge; hyperthermia and chills; tender abdomen.	Septic abortion (self-induced or "criminal").	Take complete history, if possible. Convulsion precautions if hypertensive.
e. Ecchymosis or bleeding—with a history that includes any or all of the following: had symptoms of pregnancy, but they subsided; pregnancy test negative; uterine size diminishing; no FHT.	Missed abortion with possible DIC.	Emotional support for loss of pregnancy (through nurse's manner, tone of voice, touch, use of her name, keep her informed of what is happening). Oxygen, prn.

(Continued)

TABLE 3-1.   *(Continued)*

Assessment/Observations	Possible problem	Nursing/medical management
3. SECOND TRIMESTER		
a. Cramping; passage of products of conception.	Late abortion.	As above.
b. Labor—cervical changes, "show."	Incompetent cervix, p. 231.	As above.
c. Prolonged nausea and vomiting; unexplained hypertension or preeclampsia; passage of dark blood or grapelike vesicles; absent FHTs; fundal height excessive for gestational age; may present to emergency room in shock.	Hydatidiform mole.	As above.
4. THIRD TRIMESTER		
a. Painless, bright-red bleeding; contractions and/or uterine tone usually normal.	Placenta previa, p. 232.	As above; apply fetal monitor; assess for labor: semi- to high-Fowler's position.
b. Abdominal pain and tenderness to touch with increased uterine tone; signs of shock disproportionate to amount of bleeding seen; may have loss of FHTs; associated with hypertension, multiparity, precipitous labor, oxytocin induction.	Abruptio placentae, p. 232.	As above; side-lying position; apply fetal monitor; assess for labor.
c. Retained placenta.	Placenta accreta, p. 218.	Hysterectomy.
5. FOURTH TRIMESTER— PUERPERIUM		
a. Loss of 500 ml of blood or more.	Uterine atony, p. 252.	Massage fundus; express clots, give oxytocic drug; keep bladder empty.
Uterine atony.	Retained placental fragments, p. 252.	Save pads, tissue; report to physician.
Continuous trickling of blood with contracted uterus.	Lacerations, p. 252.	Report to physician.
b. Failure of uterus to involute at 1 fingerbreadth per day after postpartum day one.	Subinvolution, p. 253.	May need D & C; cure infection, if present.
c. Hematoma formation.	Hematoma formation, p. 252.	May need to be evacuated. Blood replacement as needed for any of the conditions above, therefore have typed/cross-matched units on hand.
6. HYPERTENSION: PREGNANCY-INDUCED HYPERTENSION (PIH)— PREECLAMPSIA/ECLAMPSIA		
a. *Preeclampsia/eclampsia:* hypertension first noted after 24 weeks' gestation. Presenting symptoms: headache,	Preeclampsia/eclampsia, p. 233. With increased severity of the disorder, renal failure, circulatory collapse, CVA, coagulation defects	Pharmacologic management of gravida with hypertension, see Table 3–21, p. 235. Convulsion precautions: emergency

TABLE 3-1. *(Continued)*

Assessment/Observations	Possible problem	Nursing/medical management
blurring or double vision, epigastric pain. Signs: hypertension 160/110 mm Hg, proteinuria 3 +, facial and finger edema, oliguria, pulmonary edema, hyperreflexia, eyegrounds show retinal sheen and segmental arteriolar spasm (AV nicking). Woman may first present with convulsions or coma.	(DIC) are possible sequelae. Placenta abruptio is a possible sequela.	drug box or tray at bedside, along with oxygen, suction, padded side rails, someone in constant attendance. Start IV; insert urinary catheter, check reflexes; weigh, if possible, start I & O sheet; note and record effect and any complaints. Order laboratory work: type and cross-match; CBC; platelets, BUN, and creatinine.
b. Convulsions but *no* hypertension, proteinuria, or facial edema.	Other causes of convulsions: CVA, hypertensive encephalopathy, epilepsy, intracranial injury, drug toxicity, diabetic complication.	Convulsion care: keep airway open; oxygen by mask; drugs (diazepam IV), magnesium sulphate (see Table 3–21). Observe for uterine tone and activity; FHR pattern; fetal activity. Assess for labor. Provide emotional support for woman and family.

7. OTHER LABOR COMPLICATIONS

Assessment/Observations	Possible problem	Nursing/medical management
a. Fetal heart rate decelerations (periodic patterns): *Uniform shape;* deceleration begins with onset of uterine contraction and ends with contraction. *Variable shape* ("U," "V") (nonuniform), not necessarily in relation to contractions. *Uniform shape;* usually begins at acme of contraction and continues beyond end of contraction.	FHR decelerations: p. 245. 1. Early: head compression. 2. Variable: cord compression. 3. Late: placental insufficiency (secondary to abrupt circulatory changes).	Maintain side-lying position when she is in bed to maximize perfusion to uterus/placenta/fetus: 1. No treatment. For variable or late deceleration: 2. Side-lying position, oxygen (8–10L/min) by mask; increase rate of IV fluids; stop Pitocin induction, if in progress. 3. Possible cesarean delivery.
b. Hard contractions closer than every 2 minutes, lasting longer than 90 seconds.	Precipitous labor or Pitocin induction, p. 220.	Stop Pitocin induction; notify physician stat; side-lying position, oxygen, increase rate of IV fluids; assess uterus for impending rupture.
c. Rupture of membranes—note station of presenting part at time of rupture (if high, cord has greater chance to prolapse); color; odor; consistency; amount: hydramnios or oligoamnios; time; changes in character of contractions, cervical dilatation, effacement—in addition to FHR.	Ruptured membranes, p. 245.	
1. FHR deceleration.	1. Cord compression, p. 245, with overt or covert prolapse, p. 245.	1. Position: side-lying with hips elevated or knee-chest; or push presenting part away from cervix (with examiner's gloved fingers).

(Continued)

TABLE 3-1. *(Continued)*

Assessment/Observations	Possible problem	Nursing/medical management
2. Green-stained amniotic fluid.	2. Possible fetal hypoxia, p. 245.	2. Notify physician; monitor FHR.
3. Umbilical cord seen in vagina or emerging from vagina.	3. Prolapsed umbilical cord, p. 245	3. As under 1. above.
4. Air hunger, dyspnea, restlessness, and anxiety. Usually follows rupture of membranes.	4. Amniotic fluid embolism, p. 245.	4. Notify physician; keep airway open; oxygen by mask; order lab work for platelets (R/O DIC).
d. Feeling of nausea, "seeing stars," and hypotension.	Hypotension: supine (or vena cava) syndrome; anesthesia.	Side-lying position; oxygen per mask; increase flow rate of IV; notify physician or anesthesiologist.
e. Imminent delivery with no physician or midwife present.	Emergency delivery, p. 217.	See p. 217.
f. Alterations in baseline FHR: 1. Tachycardia (× 10 minutes)—FHR: 160/min or more; 30/min or more over baseline.	Infection, prematurity, anemia, acute hemorrhage, cardiac failure, chemotherapy, maternal tachycardia, hypotension, fetal heart defect.	Diagnostic search for cause, follow with appropriate therapy. Closely monitor, record, report FHR.
2. Bradycardia (× 10 minutes)—FHR: 120–90 bpm (moderate)—usually benign, 70–89 bpm (marked)—fetal acidosis, under 70 bpm—acidosis of rapid onset.	Fetal heart conduction defect or reaction to drugs (caine drugs).	Assess FHR tracings for changes in variability and significant period patterns—if none, no treatment is needed.
8. NEONATAL COMPLICATIONS a. Apgar score of 6 or less.	Depressed neonate in delivery area.	Resuscitative measures: open airway, oxygen, warmth; medicate for drug-induced narcosis.
b. Cardiac arrest.	Asphyxia; narcosis.	Cardiopulmonary resuscitation, p. 218.
c. Lethargy; hypotonia or jitteriness; convulsions; sweating; tachypnea or apneic episodes; shrill, high-pitched cry; feeding difficulty.	Hypoglycemia; injury to CNS, e.g., tumor, bleeding, asphyxia, drug toxicity.	Test for blood sugar, then feed with glucose water per hospital protocol. Assess carefully, record and report: Heart rate, rhythm, location of PMI. Color, activity level. Muscular hypo- or hypertonia. Response to oxygen therapy or change of position.
9. PELVIC PAIN a. History: previous infections; IUD in place; multiple sex partners.	Pelvic inflammatory disease (PID): severe, with high fever and peritonitis, p. 269.	Hospitalization: start vital sign sheet; prepare for monitoring IV fluids with parenteral antibiotics; order repeat culture and sensitivity; prepare for surgery—remember to obtain an "informed consent."
b. Symptoms: bilateral pelvic pain that may begin just after menses ends;	Complications: tuboovarian abscesses, cul-de-sac abscesses.	

TABLE 3-1. *(Continued)*

Assessment/Observations	Possible problem	Nursing/medical management
increased discomfort with coitus and even walking; chills; vomiting (in some cases); vaginal spotting.		
c. Physical examination: fever 39 C (103 F); lower abdominal tenderness with guarding and rebound; pain when cervix is touched; purulent drainage from cervix.	R/O appendicitis (usually unilateral abdominal pain localizing in RLQ and associated with GI upsets).	
d. Laboratory results: leukocytosis, elevated sedimentation rate, usually *Gonococcus* organism is demonstrated, but other microorganisms may be implicated.	R/O ectopic pregnancy (fever, leukocytosis, and purulent vaginal discharge usually not present).	
e. Dull to intense pelvic pain; palpable mass in the ovary.	Ovarian cyst.	Refer to physician for diagnosis and treatment.
f. Acute, one-sided pelvic pain often accompanied by nausea, vomiting.	Torsion of pelvic structures.	If in shock, put in Trendelenburg and start an intravenous infusion; keep NPO; order laboratory studies. Start vital sign sheet.
g. Pain in inner thigh.	Ovarian cyst or paraovarian cyst.	
h. Abdominal tenderness with guarding and rebound.	Pedunculated subserous fibroid. Normal or abnormal fallopian tube.	
i. Laboratory results: leukocytosis with a shift to the left.	R/O appendicitis.	

reversed even if tubes are reanastomosed. These changes are: removal of lining that produces enzymes; and surgical interruption of vascularization in the area, which results in altered production of estrogen and progesterone.

C. *Uterus:* uterus (fundus and corpus) and cervix together look like an inverted pear. The isthmus is the juncture between the corpus and the cervix. It is thick-walled, muscular, and flattened in anteroposterior aspect. The uterus consists of three layers: perimetrium (outer lining), myometrium (muscular layer; see D below), and endometrium (inner lining; see E below).

D. *Myometrium:* three layers of interwoven smooth muscle; thicker in fundus, thinner in isthmus. Outer—hoodlike over fundus. Middle—figure eight (loops go around fallopian tubes); this layer contains the blood vessels. Inner—circles the orifices to fallopian tubes and cervix.

1. Contraction of muscles forms a "living ligature" that compresses blood vessels in early period after delivery.
2. The construction and layered structure of these muscles increase muscle strength and are well suited to pull cervix up and push fetus out.

E. *Endometrium:* responds to estrogen and progesterone; primary site for implantation.
1. Oral hormone contraception alters cyclic changes, thus discouraging implantation.
2. Normal lining requires adequate hormone levels—biopsies done to determine endometrial condition in infertility studies.

F. *Cervix:* "neck of womb" that extends into vagina. Has an anterior and a posterior lip. Nulliparous: rounded, firm, 2–2.5 cm, circular, with centered os. Parous: external os appears as a slit because of lacerations during birth process. Os is usually more open during ovulation. Consistency of cervix (if no infections or lesions): firm like tip of nose when not pregnant; softer like earlobe when pregnant; softest when "ripe" for labor.

1. Self-help: self-exam throughout cycle for consistency and color of cervix, appearance of cervical os, characteristics of mucus. Can be used to—
   a. Achieve pregnancy if ovulation time can be identified.
   b. Prevent conception.
   c. Determine first ovulation while lactating.
   d. Determine ovulatory cycles with approaching menopause.
   e. Determine reestablishment of ovulatory cycles after discontinuing use of oral hormone contraception.
2. Pap smear: cells are taken from squamo-columnar junction, the most frequent site of neoplastic changes.
3. Assessing mucus: amount and characteristics determined by cyclic changes in hormones.
   a. Days 1 to 3 or 5: menses.
   b. Days 4 to 5 or 6: "dry."
   c. Days 6 to 13: increasing levels of estrogen resulting in increasing amounts of mucus that become clearer, more like egg-white, slippery, with stretchability (spinnbarkeit); dries in a fernlike pattern ("fern").
   d. Days 14 (ovulation) to 24 or 25: increasing progesterone levels result in increasing cloudiness, stickiness. Loses spinnbarkeit. Forms amorphous pattern when dried.
   e. Days 26 to 28: rapid fall in ovarian hormones; anterior pituitary begins to secrete FSH.
G. *Vagina:* thin-walled musculofascial tube lined with mucosa. Characterized by transverse rugae during childbearing years. Nulliparous—length, 10 cm; width, 4 cm. Parous—width increases. Vaginal mucosa responds promptly to estrogen and progesterone stimulation. pH: acidotic—3.5 to 6; prevents invasion by pathogens.
1. Steroid sex hormone levels can be assessed from exfoliated mucosal cells (test for fertility).
2. Leukorrhea: usually sign of local disease (moniliasis), but occasionally systemic (chicken pox). Also seen with estrogen deficiency following delivery or menopause.
3. Acidotic environment favors yeast infection.

3. Accessory structures
A. *Mammary glands:* large exocrine glands, each composed of 18 segments embedded in fat and connective tissues. Function: to secrete nourishment for human infant.
   1. Size is no indication of functional capacity.
B. *Nipples:* protrude ½ to ¼ inch; sensitive, erectile; more prominent during pregnancy. Contain openings for from 15 to 20 milk ducts.
   1. Enlargement and darkening in color during pregnancy, returning to prepregnant state after delivery.
   2. These changes may occur in response to oral hormone contraception.
C. *Areolae:* circular, pigmented areas, 1 to 4 inches in diameter, surrounding nipple.
   1. Pinch test reveals if nipple is everted (best suited for breastfeeding) or inverted (less suited).
   2. If inverted, may try nipple-rolling or breast shield during pregnancy to "bring nipple out."

4. Prostaglandins (PG)
A. Fatty acids classified as hormones; produced in most organs, most notably by the endometrium and the prostate; therefore, both menstrual flow and semen are potent sources of PG. Have important roles in many body functions.
   1. Implicated in infertility, dysmenorrhea, hypertensive states (including preeclampsia and eclampsia), and anaphylactic shock.
B. Role in reproduction: ovulation, sloughing of endometrium, cervical changes, tubal and uterine motility, onset of ovulation, onset and maintenance of labor (preterm, term), increasing myometrial response to oxytocic stimulation, and enhancing uterine contractions and cervical dilation.
   1. Utilized for induction of abortion (see Table 3–6 on p. 179) and induction or augmentation of true labor.
   2. Possible side effects: severe nausea and diarrhea.

5. Menstrual cycle
—The cycle, based on a feedback mechanism, is described in Table 3–2 under the following headings: hormone source and target tissue, mechanics of the cycle, and implications for nursing actions.

THE REPRODUCTIVE SYSTEM IN MEN

1. External genitalia
A. *Mons pubis*—pubic hair.
B. *Penis*—organ of copulation and urination.
   1. Shaft—body of penis.
   2. Glans—enlarged end of penis containing many sensitive nerve endings and a urethral meatus at

TABLE 3–2. *The menstrual cycle*

Hormone source and target tissue	Feedback system	Nursing implications
1. HYPOTHALAMUS AND ANTERIOR PITUITARY a. Follicle stimulating hormone (FSH). *Target:* ovary—graafian follicle. b. Luteinizing hormone (LH). *Target:* ovary—ovulation and luteinization of graafian follicles.	During first half of cycle, stimulates maturation of an ovum. During second half of cycle, stimulates ovulation, and the development of the corpus luteum from the graafian follicle.	Function may be altered: circulating high serum levels of estrogen/progesterone due to oral-contraceptive therapy suppress function so that ovum does not mature; neoplastic tissue changes alter function resulting in infertility.
2. OVARY—Graafian follicle (first half of cycle) that progresses into corpus luteum (second half of cycle) a. Estrogen (small amount also produced by adrenal cortex). *Target:* endometrium, cervical mucus glands, hypothalamus and anterior pituitary.	Primary hormone prior to ovulation. Following a resting phase, begins build-up of endometrium by stimulating development of spiral and basal arteries. Cervical mucus changes, see above. Supports passage and survival of sperm. Woman is most fertile immediately following the peak mucus symptom: egg-white consistency, slippery, good spinnbarkeit. Alters patterns of serum proteins, such as clotting factors. Alters carbohydrate metabolism.	Insufficient estrogen cannot begin build-up of endometrium—may be implicated in infertility. Knowledge of characteristic changes of cervical mucus throughout the menstrual cycle is basic to the use of the ovulation (Billings, cervical mucus) method of "natural family planning"; see Table 3–4. Knowledge of effects on serum proteins and carbohydrate metabolism is basic to anticipatory guidance regarding side effects of the pill, e.g., thromboembolism, exposure of prediabetic condition. See Table 3–4.
b. Progesterone. *Target:* endometrium, cervical mucus glands, hypothalamus, and anterior pituitary.	Primary hormone following ovulation. Prepares and stimulates secretion from endometrial glands. Increases basal body temperature (BBT) by 0.5 C. Affects movement of fertilized egg through oviduct. Cervical mucus changes, see above. Acts as a barrier to sperm penetration of cervical canal.	Knowledge of characteristic changes of cervical mucus throughout menstrual cycle is basis of ovulation and temperature (symptothermal) method of "natural family planning." Presence of hormone through cycle (e.g., use of the pill) keeps cervical mucus impervious to sperm.

the tip (usually), covered by the prepuce or fore-skin in the uncircumcized man.

C. *Scrotal sac*—a double sac containing the testes and serving to maintain optimum temperature for spermatogenesis (for example, in cold weather, scrotum is drawn up closer to body).

2. Internal organs

A. *Testes*—two male gonads or testicles; almond-shaped structures normally situated in the scrotum.
1. Supplied by internal spermatic arteries.
2. Descend into scrotum during the seventh or eighth month of gestation via inguinal canal.

3. Leydig's or interstitial cells are stimulated by the pituitary interstitial cell stimulating hormone (ICH) to produce the male sex hormone, testosterone.
4. Sertoli's cells line the one- to three-foot-long seminiferous tubules, where spermatids attach and develop into spermatozoa.
5. Epididymis—20 feet of coiled (convoluted) tubules, situated on top of each testis, that serve as storage places for sperm for the three weeks needed for sperm to mature and become motile.

B. *Canal system:*
1. Seminiferous tubules—one to three feet long.
2. Epididymis—20 feet long.
3. Vas deferens—18 inches long and about the size of a strand of cooked spaghetti.
   a. Storage site for sperm.
   b. Avenue of sperm transport from epididymis to urethra. (Note—vas passes from scrotum *over* pubic bone.)
   c. Vasectomy interrupts sperm transport.
4. Ejaculatory duct—formed where vas deferens and ducts from seminal vesicles join and enter urethra.
5. Urethra—common duct to transport urine or semen.

3. Accessory structures

A. *Seminal vesicles*—two glands, situated just above prostate glands, that produce a thick milky nutrient fluid forming the major constituent of the ejaculate.
B. *Prostate glands*—two glands, *encircling* the urethra just below the bladder, that produce a clear, thin, and slightly alkaline fluid to maintain sperm motility by neutralizing the normal acidity of the urethra.
C. *Bulbourethral* or *Cowper's glands*—two pea-sized glands, located on either side of the urethra below the prostate glands, that secrete a clear viscid (sticky) fluid into the urethra to facilitate passage of semen during ejaculation.

4. Semen—carrier of spermatozoa and secretions from seminal vesicles, prostate, and Cowper's glands.

A. pH 7.35 to 7.50 (slightly alkaline).
B. Amount per ejaculate—about 1 tsp. or 3 to 4 ml.
C. Sperm count—averages 120 million/ml but may vary from 45 to 200 million/ml; infertility is probable with counts at or below 40 million/ml.
D. Sperm deposited close to the cervix may be found within the cervix 90 seconds after ejaculation.

E. Sperm may remain motile within female genital tract for two to three days but may not be capable of fertilization that long.

5. Testicular functioning

A. Puberty—occurs between the ages of 10 and 16; usually on the average of one year later in men than in women.
B. Climacteric—cessation of reproductive (testicular) functioning accompanied by endocrine, somatic, and psychic changes; no specific age in men.
C. Table 3–3 summarizes structures within the female and male reproductive tracts that are analogous or homologous.

TABLE 3–3.   *Analogous structures*

Female	Male
Glans clitoris	Glans penis
Labia majora	Scrotum
Fallopian tubes or oviducts	Vas deferens or sperm ducts
Ovary: sex organ Ova: germ cell or gamete	Testis: sex organ Sperm: germ cell or gamete
Paraurethral (Skene's) glands	Prostatic glands
Vulvovaginal (Bartholin's) glands	Bulbourethral (Cowper's) glands

GENETICS AND GENETIC COUNSELING

1. Goals

A. Provide families with accurate information regarding hereditary disorders, methods of transmission, and risk of occurrence and/or recurrence.
B. Alert health professionals to families within which there is a possibility of a genetic disorder.
C. Decrease numbers of children affected with a hereditary condition through screening and anticipatory guidance regarding family planning.

2. Genes

A. Minute particles of hereditary material that form the blueprints for the patterns and timing of development from conception to old age.

B. Composed of deoxyribonucleic acid (DNA).

C. Arranged in linear order to form chromosomes.

3. Chromosomes

A. Each somatic cell contains 46 pairs (two sets or *diploid* number); 23 from each parent.

B. Each sex cell or gamete (that is, ovum or sperm) contains 23 chromosomes (one set or *haploid* number).
1. Twenty-two are autosomes.
2. One is a sex chromosome (that is, an *X* in each ovum, or an *X* or a *Y* in each sperm).

C. Haploid number (23 chromosomes) is achieved during cell division in gametogenesis. Abnormal cell division is the basis of some disorders, such as Down's syndrome.

D. *Zygote:* a one-celled organism with two sets of chromosomes (46-diploid number) that results from the union of an ovum and a sperm (fertilization).

4. Gene transmission

A. *Dominant* gene: when each gene of a given pair has a different effect, the gene that is expressed is called dominant (for example, dark hair color is dominant over light hair color).

B. *Recessive* gene: both genes of a given pair must have the same effect before it is expressed (for example, inborn errors of metabolism such as PKU, galactosemia, familial cretinism, cystic fibrosis, Tay-Sachs, G6PD).

C. *X-linked.* Defective gene appears on the *X* chromosome.
1. Male neonate: there is only one *X* chromosome, so if a defect occurs on it, it is expressed, as in hemophilia.
2. Female neonate: if defect appears on one *X* chromosome and it is recessive, it will not be expressed, as in a daughter-carrier of hemophilia.
3. If defect on *X* chromosome is dominant, it will be expressed whether neonate is female or male, as in vitamin D–resistant rickets.

D. *Chromosomal aberrations* due to abnormal cell division. Examples of syndromes:
1. Nondisjunction—trisomy 21 or Down's syndrome.
2. Deletion of part of one chromosome 5—cri-du-chat syndrome.
3. Sex chromosome—
   a. Multiples of sex chromosomes—*XXY* females (Klinefelter's).
   b. Monosomy—*XO* (Turner's).

5. Detection

A. Antepartum:
1. History; family tree.
2. Amniocentesis (see p. 246).
3. Ultrasound (see pp. 246, 248).

B. Postpartum:
1. Physical assessment of neonate, including the cry.
2. Biochemical—PKU, galactosemia, T_4.
3. Cytologic—sex chromatin (Barr body).
4. Dermatoglyphics.

6. Management of genetic disorders

A. Medical/nursing assessment to identify the problem.

B. Medical/surgical therapy.
1. Surgical repair: heart defects.
2. Product replacement: thyroid extract for cretinism.
3. Diet modification: low-phenylalanine diet for PKU.
4. Corrective devices: replace missing limbs.
5. Immunologic prevention: $Rh_o(D_u)$ immunoglobulin.
6. Modifications of daily living:
   a. Avoid certain chemicals, in presence of G6PD.
   b. In presence of sickle cell anemia, avoid situations that predispose to decreased oxygen perfusion of tissues.

C. Nursing role:
1. Assess history and physical/anatomic examination to assist in identifying problem.
2. Assist with diagnostic tests and therapies.
3. Counsel parent(s).
   a. Prepare for tests/procedures.
   b. Interpret risks—clarify, reinforce physician's explanations.
   c. Follow-up care: decrease guilt (not all causes are known or preventable); provide support; help them develop coping mechanisms through role-playing, etc.

D. Evaluation:
1. Parents retain self-esteem.
2. Parents understand the disorder and its management.
3. Parents able to choose a course of action that fits within their family's values and goals.

STATISTICS

1. Fertility rate—number of births per 1000 women between the ages of 14 and 44 years in a given population.

2. Birth rate
A. Number of live births per 1000 population.
B. Factors influencing birth rate, for example:
   1. Socioeconomic depression.
   2. Accessibility of contraception and abortion.
   3. Trend toward smaller families (one to three children).

3. Maternal death
A. *Definition:* deaths from *any* cause during pregnancy or within 42 days after termination of pregnancy.
B. Maternal mortality: number of deaths per 100,000 live births.
   1. 1967—28/100,000; 1977—9.4/100,000.
   2. Nonwhite—three times higher rate than for Whites.
   3. Obstetric death—not used often; deaths related directly to pregnancy and its complications.
   4. Causes of maternal mortality:
      a. Hemorrhage—22%.
      b. Infection—20%.
      c. Hypertensive disorders—15%.
      d. Other—43%.

4. Infant mortality
A. Deaths per 1000 live births; deaths before one year per live births during that year.
B. Has been a traditional indicator of environmental factors such as nutrition, prenatal care.
C. United States ranked fifteenth among nations in 1970.
D. Causes of infant deaths:
   1. Congenital anomalies.
   2. Immaturity and related causes.
   3. Asphyxia.
   4. Influenza/pneumonia.
   5. Birth injury.
   6. Gastrointestinal diseases.

5. Fetal death—deaths in utero, 20 weeks' gestation or more.

6. Neonatal mortality—number of deaths of neonates 28 days of age or less per 1000 live births.

7. Perinatal mortality—combined fetal and neonatal deaths per 1000 live births.

8. Use of statistics—*caution*, it is easy to misinterpret statistical data.

A. To project health care needs of childbearing families in a particular community.
B. To evaluate adequacy of maternal health care services and resources in a community.
C. To plan for hospital services such as number of units, need for ICN, postpartum beds, staffing.
D. To determine health priorities.
E. To plan services such as preparation-for-childbirth classes, screening programs, adolescent services.

LEGAL ASPECTS

All nurses have a clear responsibility to keep current in all areas of their changing, expanding specialty, including the legal ramifications of their actions. Some general legal concepts, their definitions, and examples from maternity/gynecologic situations are given below. (For more information, see Unit 6.)

1. *Accountability*—As nurses become more independent in their role as health care providers, they are considered more accountable for their actions. Boundaries between medicine and nursing are indistinct; nurses must know the boundaries of nursing in their area of specialization.

2. *Statutory law*—legislated definitions of nursing practice; vary from state to state.

3. *Reasonably prudent nurse*—nurse must react as a reasonably prudent nurse trained in that specialty area would react. For example, if a nurse works with fetal monitors, she must know how to use the monitors, know how to read the strips, and know what actions to take based on the findings.

4. *Malpractice*—negligent act performed by a professional person, such as instilling wrong-strength silver nitrate into neonate's eyes.

5. *Charting*—written documentation of the nurse's actions. The statute of limitations does not begin to run its course until the client reaches "legal age," usually 21 years after birth.

6. *Informed consent*—implies that significant benefits and risks of any procedure, as well as alternate methods of treatment, have been explained; person has had time to ask questions and have these answered; and person has agreed to the treatment voluntarily, is legally competent to give consent; and communication is in a language known to the client.

TRENDS AND OPTIONS

1. Consumerism

A. Consumer push for humanization of health care during the childbearing cycle.

B. Increase in options available for conduct of birth experience and setting for birth: birthing homes, alternative birth center (ABC) in hospitals; birthing chairs; side-lying position for birth; family-centered cesarean delivery; and more.

C. Increased consumer awareness of legal issues.

2. Social trends

A. Alternative life styles of families—single parenthood, communal living, surrogate motherhood, marriages without children.

B. Earlier sexual experimentation—availability of assistance to emancipated minors.

C. Increase in number of older (over 38) primiparas.

D. Legalization of abortion; availability to emancipated minors.

E. Smaller families.

F. Rising divorce rates.

3. Technologies

A. Development of genetic and bioengineering techniques.

B. Development of prenatal diagnostic techniques, with options for management of each pregnancy.

C. In-vitro fertilization and embryo transplantation.

FAMILY PLANNING: DECISION-MAKING REGARDING REPRODUCTION

If a woman chooses to be sexually active, and if she is capable of becoming pregnant, she has several choices available. She (or her partner) can prevent conception temporarily or permanently. If she conceives, she can confirm the diagnosis with a pregnancy test, along with a history and physical examination. Several methods are available to estimate the length of gestation. The woman (or couple) then has the option to interrupt the pregnancy, utilizing a method appropriate to the age of gestation, or to continue the pregnancy.

1. Factors influencing implementation of family planning

A. Attitudes toward use of contraceptive methods:
  1. Deterrents to implementation—
    a. Religious objections.
    b. Social objections—many teens state that "being prepared" negates spontaneity.
    c. Magical thinking—"It (pregnancy) can't happen to me."
    d. Psychologic need to confirm virility or fertility.
    e. Ignorance of methods available.
    f. Lack of available information and/or supplies.
  2. Factors supporting implementation—
    a. Social recognition of need for responsible parenthood, leading to regulation of the number and spacing of children to provide optimal maternal readiness (nutritional stores); delay of pregnancy until she (or the couple) is "ready"; concern for world population and changing environment.
    b. Increasing acceptance of alternative life styles.

B. Factors affecting choice of method of contraception:
  1. Safety of method.
  2. Degree of effectiveness.
  3. Amount of involvement each (man or woman) is willing to have.
  4. Cost.
  5. Influence of culture or life style.
  6. Attitude toward voluntary abortion as a back-up to contraceptive failure.

2. Several methods of contraception

are presented in Table 3–4. In addition, the mode of action; the advantages, disadvantages and/or side effects; and the effectiveness are also presented. Before the client chooses a method, the nurse/physician must first assess the following: the woman's desire to use a contraceptive method, her physical condition, and her plans for a family. The client makes a decision based on information contained in this table. If the woman chooses to use the symptothermal method, for example, the nurse determines what the woman needs to know and proceeds to teach her. The nurse evaluates her effectiveness in teaching the woman when the latter is able to use the contraceptive method successfully and is satisfied with the results.

3. Sterilization procedures

—discussed in Table 3–5—are available to those who wish a permanent form of contraception. The client needs to give an "informed consent" prior to the procedure (see p. 170).

4. Conception confirmed by pregnancy test

A. Enough human chorionic gonadotropin (HCG) is produced to give a positive test (Gravindex and

TABLE 3–4.   *Contraception**

Method	Action	Advantages	Disadvantages and side effects	Effectiveness
ORAL MEDICATION Combination of estrogen and progesterone or sequential—estrogen during first half of cycle; progesterone during second half of cycle, for example. (Sequentials have been removed from the US market.)	Suppresses ovulation by suppressing production of FSH and LH; needs to be taken for full month initially before woman is "safe"; a second form of contraceptive should be used during first month of use. Pill must be taken at same time each day to maintain pituitary suppressive action. If dosage is inadequate, ovulation and conception may occur.	Easy to take for those motivated to remember to take pill as directed. Disassociated from sex act. Helps regulate cycle for woman who wishes to conceive later. Menstrual cycles are predictable. No egg matures, so conception is not possible. May decrease menstrual cramps.	*Discomforts* simulating those of pregnancy include breast tenderness, water retention, nausea, chloasma—may persist even after discontinuing the pill—and fatigue. *Hazards* include thrombus formation, thrombophlebitis, pulmonary embolus, and hypertension. *Contraindicated* in obesity; hypertension, sickle cell disease, heavy smokers, diabetes, migraine headaches, and women over 35 years. Possible closure of epiphyses of the long bones in early adolescence. Must discontinue for at least 6 weeks before elective surgery.	Most efficient form of contraception (99.7%) if used consistently. *If one pill is missed*, it should be taken when woman remembers; next pill should be taken as scheduled. *If two pills are missed*, follow directions above; in addition, a second form of contraceptive should be used for the rest of that month. *If more than two pills are missed*, pills should be discontinued for rest of month and another form of contraceptive used; pill-taking schedule should be resumed on fifth day of menstrual cycle.
Minipill—progesterone (norethindrone 0.35 mg daily).	Antifertility effect. Makes cervical mucus impervious to sperm and alters endometrium. Ovulation does occur most of the time.	Supposedly reduces side effects found with other oral preparations.	Menstrual irregularity. Lumps in breast.	Undetermined. Can reach 98% reliability if used exactly as prescribed.
Morning-after pill—estrogen in very high levels (25 mg) (DES).	Suppresses anterior pituitary or alters endometrium. Menstruation within 5 days.	Can be taken within 24 hours after coitus; two tablets should be taken each day for 5 days.	Nausea and vomiting. Dilatation and curettage (D & C) if no menstruation ensues. Predispose female fetus to reproductive-tract cancer in adolescence and adulthood.	100% effective only when followed by D & C.

INTRAUTERINE DEVICES (IUDs) The following are made of soft plastic and/or nickel-chromium alloy, a nonreactive metal: Lippes Loop, Saf-T-Coil; the Cu-7 is wound in copper wire. One IUD releases progesterone for a 2-year period.	Interferes with fertilization. Alters rate of egg's passage through fallopian tube. Or, discourages implantation by altering endometrium, preventing sperm from entry into fallopian tube.	No interference with hormonal regulation of menstrual cycle. No need to remember to take a pill each day or engage in other manipulation prior to or between coitus. May be removed by physician when pregnancy is desired.	*Hazards*—unnoticed expulsion, must check for presence of IUD after each menses; uterine perforation with intraabdominal trauma and/or intrauterine or fallopian infection. *Side effects*—heavy flow, spotting between periods, and cramping, especially during early months of use. May increase the incidence of tubal pregnancy and infections of the reproductive structures. Some are allergic to copper and develop a rash.	Not as effective as the pill. Failure rate—during first year, about 2% to 3%; later, under 2%.
MECHANICAL BARRIERS Diaphragm—shallow rubber device that fits over cervix.	Barrier preventing sperm from entering cervix if it is correct size and correctly placed; refitted for size after each baby, every 2 years, and/or when woman has gained or lost 10 pounds.	Safety—no side effects. May be inserted several hours before (however, 1 hour prior is recommended) intercourse and is left in place for 6 hours afterward; for additional intercourse before 6 hours are over, foam is used prior to each time.	Some women find insertion and removal objectionable. Device requires washing with warm water and soap, careful drying, storage away from heat, and checking for tears. Spermicides may be allergenic.	Failure rate—10 to 15 pregnancies per 100 users per year. Effectiveness is improved somewhat if a spermicidal foam, jelly, or cream is also used.

(Continued)

TABLE 3-4. *(Continued)*

Method	Action	Advantages	Disadvantages and side effects	Effectiveness
Condom—thin, stretchable rubber sheath to cover penis.	Barrier preventing sperm from entering vagina. Is applied over erect penis.	Safety—no side effects. Protective measure against spread of sexually transmitted infections, to some extent.	Some couples object to taking time to apply sheath on erect penis. Preejaculatory drops also contain sperm; conception possible even when drops fall around *external* vaginal opening. Sheath may tear during intercourse.	Failure rate—3% if spermicidal foam, jelly, or cream is also used and sheath is held in place as penis is withdrawn to prevent emptying of sperm in or near vagina.
CHEMICAL BARRIERS				
Spermicide, tartaric acid, and bicarbonate—foam, jelly, cream, or vaginal suppository.	Kills sperm. Decreases sperm motility. Sperm cannot pass through chemical barrier.	Increases effectiveness of mechanical barriers. Ease of application. Aids lubrication of vagina. Does not harm delicate vaginal tissue. Does not require previous medical examination or prescription.	Described as "messy" by some. If it is only method being used, each intercourse should be preceded (by 30 minutes) by a fresh application. Felt to decrease tactile sensation by some users. May be allergenic.	High failure rate, especially when used without diaphragm or condom.
OTHER METHODS				
Rhythm—rectal temperature each morning before any physical activity (BBT).†	Conception is avoided by sexual abstinence during woman's fertile period: no sperm may be present while egg is present. The "fertile" period includes 3 days before ovulation plus 1 day after; sperm may live up to 3 days; the egg from 24 to 36 hours.	Physically safe to use—no drugs or appliances are used. Meets requirements of most religions.	Effectiveness depends on the following: high level of motivation and diligence, daily temperature-taking and record-keeping for duration of childbearing years, and willingness to abstain. Requires fairly predictable menstrual cycle. Ovulation almost invariably occurs 14 days *before* the next menstrual flow. Ovulation may occur at atypical times.	Very low rate of effectiveness. Temperature varies with tension, infection, staying up late the night before, or any prior activity. Irregular cycles require long periods of abstinence. Effectiveness may be increased by using litmus paper and/or checking changes in cervical mucus. Failure rate—14% to 40%.

Litmus paper—when oral mucus turns paper blue (basic), couple must abstain for five days.	Identifies fertile period so that the couple knows when to prevent conception or to get pregnant.	Physically safe. Acceptable to most religions.	Effectiveness unknown. Requires daily check of oral mucus.	Unknown at present.
Observe for change in cervical mucus—ovulation method (Billings).	Identifies fertile period: cervical mucus is clear, stretchable (Spinnbarkeit) like raw egg white; lubricative, ferns when dried. Nonfertile ("safe") period: cervical mucus is opaque, nonstretchable; feels sticky.	Physically safe. Acceptable to most religions.	Requires couple to learn cervical mucus changes during 1 month of total abstinence and engage in the internal vaginal manipulation necessary to assess mucus. Vaginal discharge from infection and presence of semen may confuse couple.	Unknown at present.
NOT RECOMMENDED				
Coitus interruptus	Avoids ejaculation of sperm into vagina.	None.	Requires discipline. Psychologically unsound—strains sexual relationship. Preejaculatory drops contain sperm. Sperm deposited anywhere near vagina may lead to conception.	Low rate of effectiveness.
Douching	Washes out vagina.	None.	Sperm enter cervix as it dips into ejaculatory pool in vagina during orgasm. Douching may force more sperm into cervix.	Ineffective.

*From Jensen, Margaret Duncan, and Bobak, Irene M.: Handbook of maternity care: a guide for nursing practice, St. Louis, 1980, The C. V. Mosby Co; modified from Section IV, Maternity Nursing, Bobak, I. M., in Addison-Wesley's nursing examination review, edited by Sally L. Lagerquist, Addison-Wesley Publishing Co., Medical/Nursing Division, Menlo Park, Calif, 1977.
†The combination of the BBT and the ovulation method is also known as the symptothermal method, or "natural family planning."

TABLE 3–5. Sterilization*

Method	Action	Advantages	Disadvantages and side effects	Effectiveness
MEN				
Vasectomy	Vas deferens is ligated and severed, interrupting passage of sperm.	Relatively simple surgical procedure. Does not affect endocrine function, production of testosterone. Does not alter volume of ejaculate.	Some men become impotent due to psychologic response to procedure. Reversible in 20% to 40% of cases.	100% effective after ejaculate is free of sperm that was in vas deferens (about 3 months or ten ejaculations).
WOMEN				
Tubal ligation	Both fallopian tubes are ligated and severed, preventing passage of eggs; fulguration of the tubes at the cornu is most effective.	Abdominal surgery utilizing 1-inch incisions and laparoscopy.	Major surgery (if done by laparotomy) with possible complications of anesthesia, infection, hemorrhage, and trauma to other organs. Trauma to surrounding vasculature may alter ovary's production of estrogen/progesterone and therefore alter the menstrual cycle. If woman wishes to have tuboplasty in hopes of reestablishing fertility, the altered cycle may still render her infertile. Psychologic trauma in some.	100% effective if ligatures do not slip, recanalization does not occur, or fistula does not form.
Hysterectomy with salpingooophorectomy	No egg is produced.	No possibility of pregnancy. No further menstruation.	Abrupt loss of ovarian hormones, simulating menopause. Major surgery complications. Psychologic trauma in some—loss of femininity and sexuality.	100% effective.

*From Jensen, Margaret Duncan, and Bobak, Irene M.: Handbook of maternity care: a guide for nursing practice, St. Louis, 1980, the C. V. Mosby Co.; modified from Section IV, Maternity nursing, Bobak, I. M., in Addison-Wesley's nursing examination review, edited by Sally L. Lagerquist. Addison-Wesley Publishing Co., Medical/Nursing Division, Menlo Park, Calif, 1977.

UCG) within two weeks of implantation or by the end of the fifth week since LMP (if the cycle would have been 28 days in length).

B. Over-the-counter pregnancy test kits may present a problem with false negatives since they lack the physical assessment and counseling by an objective examiner found in a clinical setting.

C. The Friedman and A-Z (Aschheim-Zondek) tests are no longer done (take longer, cost more, and require the sacrifice of animals).

5. Estimation of length of gestation

A. Nägele's rule—the estimated date of confinement (EDC) is calculated by noting the first day of the last normal menstrual cycle (LMP), counting back three months, and adding seven days; length of gestation—280 days, ten lunar months (four weeks each), or nine calendar months plus one week. For example:

1. LMP January 15 (1/15)

   12 months + 1 month = 13 months
   $$\underline{-\quad 3 \text{ months}}$$
   10th month and 15 days
   $$\underline{+\qquad\qquad 7 \text{ days}}$$
   10th month and 22 days
   EDC = October 22

2. LMP June 17 (6/17)

   6th month − 3 months = 3rd month and 17 days
   $$\underline{\qquad\qquad\qquad\qquad + 7 \text{ days}}$$
   3rd month and 24 days
   EDC = March 24

B. Haase's rule—fetal length by lunar months; this is frequently used to determine age of abortus:

   Month No. $1 \times 1 = 1$ cm (0.4 in.), 4 weeks
   $2 \times 2 = 4$ cm (1.5 in.), 8 weeks
   $3 \times 3 = 9$ cm (3.5 in.), 12 weeks
   $4 \times 4 = 16$ cm (6 in.), 16 weeks
   $5 \times 5 = 25$ cm (10 in.), 20 weeks
   $6 \times 5 = 30$ cm (12 in.), 24 weeks
   $7 \times 5 = 35$ cm (14 in.), 28 weeks
   $8 \times 5 = 40$ cm (16 in.), 32 weeks
   $9 \times 5 = 45$ cm (18 in.), 36 weeks
   $10 \times 5 = 50$ cm (20 in.), term

C. Fundal height: above the symphysis pubis (SP) and in relation to umbilicus (U) or ensiform cartilage (EC).*

   12 weeks—at SP.

16 weeks—halfway between SP and U.
20 weeks—just below U.
22 weeks—about at level of U.
24 weeks—just above U.
28 weeks—⅔ of way between U and EC.
32 weeks—just below EC.
36 weeks—at EC.
38–40 weeks—below EC after lightening.

D. Quickening—"feeling life," usually first noted about 18 to 20 weeks' gestation by the nullipara, but noted earlier by the multipara.

E. Sonography (ultrasound)—"A" scan is used to measure the biparietal diameter, starting with week 16.

6. Interruption of Pregnancy—also known as elective, voluntary, or therapeutic abortion. Once the diagnosis of pregnancy and the length of gestation are established, the woman faces the decision to interrupt or to maintain the pregnancy. An "informed consent" (see p. 170) is mandatory.

A. Legal status of abortion:

1. 1973 Supreme Court decision legalized abortion with the following stipulations:
   a. First trimester—woman and physician make decision.
   b. Second trimester—woman and physician make decision; individual state may stipulate where and how abortion may be performed.
   c. Third trimester—increased state regulation, abortion may be prohibited except when health of mother is jeopardized.

2. 1978 Congressional passage of the Hyde Amendment severely restricts the use of federal funds for abortions. Medicaid funds may be used for abortions if:
   a. The woman's life is endangered by the pregnancy.
   b. The pregnancy would cause severe and long-lasting physical health damage to the woman.
   c. The pregnancy is a result of rape or incest.*

B. Nursing and medical management:

1. Assessment—
   a. Psychologic status: perception of the event; feelings about abortions; age and maturity level; if decision was already made before she came to clinic, how was decision made?; does she have a support system?

---

*Ensiform cartilage is also known as xiphoid process.

*Federal funds may not be available for this reason either.

b. Laboratory tests: Type, Rh, hemoglobin, hematocrit, urinalysis, pregnancy test, other tests dependent on her health status.
c. Health history and physical examination.
d. Information needs.
2. Plan and implementation—
a. Verbally prepare her for the procedure (Table 3–6).
b. Prior to procedure, reassess her as detailed above; refer any questions to physician (such as ambivalence).
c. Assist with procedure* and talk the woman through it, explaining what is happening, what sensations she may feel, etc.
d. Monitor blood loss, woman's affect, vital signs; administer medications, prn.
e. Provide and explain postprocedure care: monitor vital signs, blood loss, IVs (if any); administer Rho (D antigen) immune globulin (RhoGAM) if gestation is eight weeks or more, if indicated; administer oxytocin as ordered.
f. Predischarge anticipatory guidance (also provide in written form):
    (1) Immediately report any cramping, excessive bleeding, signs of infection.
    (2) Provide name and phone number of person to call if she has questions.
    (3) Schedule a postabortal check-up.
    (4) Discuss contraception, if woman indicates interest; or give her place and name to call for information later.
3. Evaluation—the nurse knows interventions were successful if:
a. Woman returns for postabortal appointment.
b. Woman suffers no adverse physical sequelæ to the procedure.
c. Woman suffers no adverse psychologic sequelae to the procedure.
d. Woman is successful in achieving her goal of either contraception or conception at the time she desires.
4. Postabortion psychologic impact:
a. Majority—relieved and happy.
b. Small number (5% to 10%)—negative feelings, such as guilt or low self-esteem.

---

*"Conscience" clauses allow nurses to refuse to assist with procedures that go against their moral, religious, or medical judgment.

Part B / NORMAL PREGNANCY

CONCEPTION AND PLACENTATION

1. General comments
A. *Egg*—the life span of the egg (ovum) is about 24 hours after ovulation.
B. *Sperm*—the life span of the sperm is about 72 hours after ejaculation into the female reproductive tract.
C. *Conception* (fertilization) usually occurs 12 to 24 hours after ovulation, within the distal two-thirds of the fallopian tube.
D. *Implantation* (nidation) occurs within 7 days (6 to 9 days) of conception, or about day 21 of a 28-day cycle.

2. Placenta
A. Development of placenta (afterbirth):
    1. Primitive placenta—24 hours after implantation, syncytiotrophoblast begins to invade the endometrium; HCG production begins; exchange between mother and embryo begins.
    2. Developed from the decidua basalis and chorion of the embryo.
    3. Formed by the end of the third month of gestation.
    4. Cotyledon—subdivision of placenta on maternal surface.
    5. At term—one-sixth the weight of the neonate; rounded, flat, approximately 1 to 1½ lb, 1 inch thick in center, and 7 to 8 inches in diameter.
    6. Fetal surface—glistening grayish (Schultz).
    7. Maternal surface—beefy red and rough; cotyledons evident (Duncan).
B. *Decidua*—hypertrophied endometrium of pregnancy; sloughed off in lochia following delivery.
    1. *Decidua basalis*—lies between embryo and decidua.
    2. *Decidua capsularis*—covers developing embryo.
C. *Chorion*—outermost fetal membrane continuous with placenta.
D. *Amnion*—innermost fetal membrane, containing amniotic fluid and fetus.
E. Function of placenta:
    1. Effective lung, kidney, stomach, intestine, and endocrine gland for the fetus. Also has anabolic and catabolic functions.

TABLE 3–6.   *Interruption of pregnancy**

Methods	Advantages	Disadvantages and side effects	Effectiveness
FIRST-TRIMESTER PROCEDURES†			
Menstrual extraction—forced endometrial extraction through undilated cervix.	Performed 14 days after missed period.	Cervical trauma may occur, may lead to incompetence. Hemorrhage.	100% if implantation site is not missed.
Prostaglandin—IV or injection into cul-de-sac of Douglas or by vaginal suppository or pessary.	Stimulates contraction of smooth muscle. Causes degeneration of corpus luteum.	About 24 hours to work. May cause vomiting, diarrhea, chills, local tissue reaction (retained placenta necessitates D & C).	100%.
Vacuum (suction) curettage—cannula suction following cervical dilatation with woman under local anesthesia.	Effective with relatively few complications—minimal bleeding, minimal discomfort. 5- to 15-minute duration. Done on come-and-go basis.	Pregnancy 12 weeks or less. Cervical trauma may occur (decreased if dilatation accomplished by laminaria inserted 4 to 24 hours prior to procedure); endometrial trauma possible.	100%.
D & C—cervix dilated with metal sounds; endometrium is scraped with a spoonlike instrument.	15-minute duration. Usually complications are few.	Pregnancy 12 weeks or less. Hazards—uterine perforation, infection (25%), effects of general anesthesia, cervical trauma.	100%.
SECOND-TRIMESTER PROCEDURES			
Intraamniotic infusion between weeks 14 and 16 (uterus in abdominal cavity and sufficient amniotic fluid present). Transabdominal extraction of amniotic fluid and replacement with equal amount of saline (20%) (or 30% urea in 5% D/W).	Does not require laparotomy. Woman may ambulate until labor starts (within 24 hours) and during early labor.	Complications increase proportionately with weeks of gestation. Hazards—requires hospitalization; 6% readmitted. Reaction to saline (hypernatremia)—tinnitus, tachycardia, and headache. Water intoxication symptoms—edema, oliguria (< 200 ml/8 hr), dyspnea, thirst, and restlessness. Hemorrhage and possible disseminated intravascular coagulation (DIC); may require postabortal D & C or vacuum extraction as well; fever with sepsis. Experiences labor.	Fetal death within 1 hour of injection, abortion completed within 36 to 40 hours. Two-thirds of fetuses are aborted in 24 hours.
Instillation of 40 to 45 mg prostaglandin F_2, E_2.	Labor is usually shorter than with saline. Avoids complications of water intoxication and hypernatremia.	May cause vomiting, diarrhea, nausea. Fetus may be born alive. D & C may be required to remove placental fragments.	100%.

(Continued)

TABLE 3–6. *(Continued)*

Methods	Advantages	Disadvantages and side effects	Effectiveness
D & E (dilatation and evacuation).	Does not experience labor. Hospitalization is shortened. With a skilled operator, complication rate is lower than with intraamniotic injection methods.	Few skilled operators are available at present. Fetus may be born alive. 24 hours before procedure, 2 to 3 laminaria are inserted to dilate the cervix to the required 2 cm.	100%.
SECOND- AND THIRD-TRIMESTER PROCEDURES			
Hysterotomy—cesarean delivery.	Preferred method if woman wishes a tubal ligation or hysterectomy to follow.	Post–major surgery complications—hemorrhage and infection. Fetus may be born alive, opening ethical, moral, religious, and legal problems. Mortality risk—combination hysterotomy-hysterectomy carries 40% greater risk than D & C. As above.	100%.
Hysterectomy—at or before 24 weeks without first emptying uterus.	As above.	As above.	100%.

*From Jensen, M. D., and Bobak, I. M. 1980. Handbook of maternity care: a guide for nursing practice. St. Louis: The C. V. Mosby Company; modified from Section IV, Maternity Nursing, Bobak, I. M., in Addison-Wesley's Nursing Examination Review; edited by Sally L. Lagerquist, Addison-Wesley Publishing Co., Medical/Nursing Division, Menlo Park, Calif., 1977.

2. Transfer of gases, nutrients, wastes, antibodies, drugs, and microorganisms between mother and fetus across the placenta is by diffusion and osmosis, pinocytosis, and active selective transport.
3. Maternal and fetal blood do not generally mix. Leakage through small defects in trophoblastic surface permits slight mixing.
4. Most versatile endocrine organ in the body. Produces steroid hormones (except ACTH) plus analogues of all the pituitary hormones.
   a. Steroid hormones—progesterone (pregnanediol) and estrogen (estrone, estradiol, estriol) produced by the fetal-placental unit.
   b. Protein hormones—human chorionic gonadotropin (HCG) and human chorionic somatomammotropin (HCS). HCS has an immunochemical action similar to growth hormone; also referred to as human placental lactogen (HPL).

3. *Amniotic fluid*—for more information, see p. 210.
A. Amount: about 1000 ml at term.
B. Composition: changes throughout pregnancy.
   1. Chemicals: Albumin, urea, uric acid, phospholipids (lecithin [surfactant], phosphotidylglycerol), sphingomyelin, enzymes, fat, fructose, inorganic salts.
   2. Epithelial cells.
   3. Leukocytes.
   4. Lanugo.
C. Origin: multiple sources; not fully understood.
D. Functions:
   1. Protection from direct trauma—shock absorber.
   2. Allows fetus freedom of movement.

3. Protects against rapid temperature changes.
4. Source of oral fluids.
5. Medium for excretion collection.

4. Fetal circulation

A. Fetal structures—four intrauterine structures differ from extrauterine structures:
   1. *Umbilical vein* carries oxygen- and nutrient-enriched blood from the placenta to the ductus venosus and liver. Ductus venosus connects to inferior (ascending) vena cava and allows most of the blood to bypass the liver.
   2. *Foramen ovale* allows fetal blood to bypass fetal lungs by shunting it from the right atrium into the left atrium.
   3. *Ductus arteriosus* allows fetal blood to bypass fetal lungs by shunting it from the pulmonary artery into the aorta.
   4. *Umbilical arteries* (two) allow return of deoxygenated blood to the placenta.
B. Umbilical cord (funis)—extends from the fetus to the center (usually) of the placenta; it is usually 50 cm (20 to 21 inches) long and 1 to 2 cm (½ to 1 inch) in diameter. This protective structure contains:
   1. Wharton's jelly.
   2. One vein—carrying oxygen and nutrients from placenta to fetus.
   3. Two arteries—carrying deoxygenated blood and fetal wastes from fetus to placenta; absence of one artery signals need to examine newborn to rule out intraabdominal anomalies.
C. Fetal hemoglobin (Hb_F) and RBCs.
   1. Produced in yolk sac until week six; then produced in fetal liver until the fifth month; from the fifth month on, produced in bone marrow.
   2. Hb_F has a higher oxygen saturation level than adult hemoglobin (Hb_A) at any given tension, and it releases oxygen to fetal tissues easily. Fetal hemoglobin and a cardiac output that is twice that of the adult, assure adequate oxygenation of fetal tissues.
   3. Hb_A replaces Hb_F by three to six months after birth.
   4. Values at term are shown in Table 3–7.
D. Total blood volume: 85 ml/kg body weight (higher in the preterm neonate).

5. Fetal development

A. Fetal development normally progresses in an orderly and predictable pattern.
   1. Trimester one: period of organogenesis, in which the developing tissues and organs are most susceptible to teratogenic insult.

TABLE 3–7. *Values at term*

	Mean	Range
Hb	16.6 g/dl	12 g to 22 g/dl
RBC	4.9 million/mm^3	3.3 to 6 or 7 million/mm^3
Hct	52%	38% to 62%

   2. Trimester two: period of continued growth and development of tissues and organs.
   3. Trimester three: period of storage. Fetus stores subcutaneous fat and tissue mass, minerals and vitamins, and immune bodies from the mother.
B. See Table 3–9 (p. 184) for a summary of the normal development of the placenta and embryo/fetus, and of maternal adaptations to pregnancy.

MATERNAL ADAPTATIONS

1. Physiologic-anatomic adjustments

A. Bases of functional alteration:
   1. Hormonal—Table 3–8, hormones of pregnancy, provides the knowledge base for anticipatory guidance regarding such maternal adaptations as vascular spiders, palmar erythema, breast changes, joint relaxation, edema of the lower extremities, and lactation, and for early identification of deviations from the norm.
   2. Mechanical—enlarging uterus causes displacement and pressure; increased weight of uterus and breasts causes changes in posture and pressure (Table 3–9).
B. Reproductive organs (Table 3–9):
   1. Uterus—
      a. Growth is due to hypertrophy of existing muscle cells and connective tissue and some hyperplasia of existing muscle cells and connective tissue.
      b. Increased vascularity adds to increase in size and to softening of the isthmus (lower uterine segment) (Hegar's sign).
      c. Amenorrhea. Occasional spotting is common, especially at time of first missed period.
   2. Cervix—
      a. Increase in vascularity results in softening (Goodell sign) and in deepened blue-purple coloration (Chadwick's sign).
      b. Edema, hyperplasia, thickening of mucous lining, and increased mucous gland

TABLE 3–8. *Hormones of pregnancy*

Primary effects	*Clinical implications for nursing actions*
ESTROGEN	
Level rises in serum and urine.	Basis of test for maternal/placental/fetal well-being.
Uterine development.	Probable sign of pregnancy.
Breast development.	Probable sign of pregnancy; increased tingling, tenderness.
Genital enlargement: increased vascularization, hyperplasia.	Vaginal growth facilitates vaginal birth.
Softens connective tissue.	Results in back- and legache; relaxes joints to increase size of birth canal and rib cage.
Altered nutrient metabolism: Decreases HCl and pepsin. Antagonist to insulin—to make glucose available to fetus—therefore β-cells of pancreas normally undergo hyperplasia and hypertrophy to meet increased demand for insulin during the second half of gestation.	GI and metabolic changes: Digestive upsets. Antiinsulin effect challenges maternal β-cells in pancreas to produce more insulin; sluggish response or failure of β-cells to respond leads to "gestational" diabetes. For the insulin-dependent woman, insulin requirements increase by an average of 67% during the second half of pregnancy.
Supports fat deposition.	Protect source of energy for fetus.
Sodium and water retention; edema of lower extremities (nonpitting).	Meet increased plasma volume needs and maintain fluid reserve.
Hematologic changes: Increased coagulability.	Increased tendency to thrombosis.
Increased sedimentation rate (SR).	SR loses diagnostic value for heart disease.
Vasodilation: spider nevi; palmar erythema.	Resolve spontaneously after delivery.
Increased production of melanin-stimulating hormone.	Resolves spontaneously after delivery.
PROGESTERONE	
Development of decidua.	High levels result in tiredness, listlessness, and sleepiness.
Reduces uterine excitability.	Protection against early delivery.
Development of mammary glands.	Prepares breasts for lactation.
Alters nutrient metabolism:	Nutritional significance:
Antagonist to insulin.	Diabetogenic.
Favors fat deposition.	Energy reserve.
Decreases gastric motility and relaxes sphincters.	Favors heartburn and constipation.
Increased sensitivity of respiratory center to CO_2.	Increased depth, some dyspnea, increased sighing as mother "breathes for two."
Decreased smooth muscle tone:	Decreased tone can lead to:
Colon.	Constipation.

TABLE 3–8. *(Continued)*

Primary effects	*Clinical implications for nursing actions*
Bladder, ureters.	Stasis or urine with infection.
Veins.	Dependent edema; varicosities.
Gallbladder.	Gallbladder disease.
Increased basal body temperature (BBT) by 0.5 C.	Discomfort from hot flashes and perspiration.
HCG Maintains corpus luteum during early pregnancy.	Placenta must be ready to "take over" after a few weeks.
Stimulates male testes.	Increased testosterone in male fetuses.
May suppress immune response.	May inhibit response to foreign protein, for example, fetal portion of placenta.
	Diagnostic value: 　Hydatidiform mole. 　Basis for pregnancy test. 　Decreased level with threatened abortion. 　Increased level with multiple pregnancy.
HCS Antagonizes insulin.	Diabetogenic.
Mobilizes free fatty acids in maternal organism.	
PROLACTIN Suppressed by estrogen and progesterone.	No milk produced before delivery.
Increased level after placenta is born.	Milk production 2 to 3 days after birth.
FSH Production depressed during pregnancy; level returns to prepregnant levels in 3 weeks after birth.	No ovulation during pregnancy. Ovulation usually returns 　within 6 weeks for 15%, 　within 12 weeks for 30%.
OXYTOCIN Causes uterus to contract when the oxytocin levels exceed those of estrogen and progesterone.	Labor induction or augmentation. Treatment for postpartum uterine atony.

　production; formation of mucous plug by end of month two.
　c. Becomes shorter, thicker, and more elastic.
3. Vagina—
　a. Increased vascularity deepens the color (Chadwick's sign).
　b. Hypertrophy and thickening of walls.
　c. Relaxation of connective tissue.

　d. pH—acidic (4.0 to 6.0).
　e. Leukorrhea—nonirritating.
　f. Storage of glucose.
4. Perineum—
　a. Increase in size—hypertrophy of muscle cells, edema, and relaxation of elastic tissue.
　b. Deepened color—increased vascularization.
　c. Varices.

TABLE 3–9. *Summary of development by week and trimester in calendar months**

Menstrual or gestational age†	Embryo-fetus development	Uterine changes	Possible maternal signs and physiologic changes in pregnancy
MONTH ONE			
Week 1		*Menstruation* Weight—57 gm (2 oz); length—6.5 cm (2½ inches); and capacity—30 ml (1 oz).	
Week 2		Phase—estrogenic, preovulatory, or proliferative.	Cervical mucus becoming clear, slippery, stretchable, with a lubricative sensation; dried mucus shows fern arborization at midcycle; receptive to sperm.
Week 3		*Fertilization-conception* Phase—progestational, secretory, or luteal.	Basal body temperature remains elevated, decreased appetite due to decreased gastric motility; cervical mucus cloudy, thick, impenetrable by sperm.
Week 4	Digestive system forming, germ layers differentiated, primitive blood cells present.	*Implantation* Mucosa invaded by trophoblasts, endometrium becomes *Decidua*.	Nausea, fatigue, and breasts tense and tingling.
MONTH TWO			
Week 5	Embryonic stages begin 3 weeks after ovulation. Brain, nervous system, and reproductive system forming; heart developing and beginning to beat. Susceptible to teratogenic effect. Length: ⅛ inch.	*Amenorrhea* Human chorionic gonadotropin (HCG) secreted in quantity by chorionic villi.	Basal temperature elevated and constant, blood sugar low, and endocrine test (for HCG) positive. Some painless bleeding (spotting) experienced by 25% of women—cause unknown.
Week 6	Length: 3/16 inch; facial features forming, circulation starts; embryo may be seen by ultrasonography.	Mild contractions start; cervix and vagina blue—Chadwick's sign; lower uterine segment soft—Hegar's sign. Cervix soft—Goodell sign.	Pressure on bladder from enlarging uterus and turgescence of bladder and urethral walls from estrogen and progesterone stimulation cause urinary frequency and urgency.
Week 7	½ inch (1¼ cm) long, arm and leg buds appear, and umbilical cord forming.	Mucus plug forming in cervical canal.	Profuse vaginal secretions, thick and acid; nausea subsiding; epulis may occur. Salivation (ptyalism), breasts larger and nodular, and Montgomery's follicles appear.
Week 8	Hands, feet, fingers, and toes forming (with thalidomide, phocomelia); 1 inch long; thin skin covers body; becoming a fetus—ossification of skeleton begins.		

TABLE 3–9. *(Continued)*

Menstrual or gestational age†	Embryo-fetus development	Uterine changes	Possible maternal signs and physiologic changes in pregnancy
MONTH THREE			
Week 9	Eyelids forming, and genital ridge visible but sexless in character as yet. Length: 1¼ inch.	*Placenta* is now secreting progesterone (corpus luteum is decreasing function).	
Week 10	Human appearance, respiratory activity evident, can swallow. Begins to secrete insulin now. Becomes a fetus.	Placenta covers one-third of uterine wall.	
Week 11	Eyelids fused, *sex is distinguishable,* 20 tooth buds forming; kidney begins to secrete urine; bile now present in intestines. FHTs may be heard by Doppler method by 11 to 12 weeks.		A precolostrum fluid may be expressed from nipples.
Week 12	External genitals now show definite signs of male or female sex; fingernails and toenails forming. Length: 3½ inches.	Size of orange, fundus at level of symphysis pubis (SP).	Nausea and vomiting rare now.
Week 13	Muscles contract occasionally, weakly.	Rising from pelvic cavity.	Bladder pressure less and blood sugar up.

END OF FIRST TRIMESTER—period of organogenesis (organ differentiation) and hyperplasia ends; fetus is less susceptible to teratogenic effect from now on; and growth continues primarily by hypertrophy (increase in cell size).

MONTH FOUR			
Week 14	Nearly 10 cm (4 inches) long, sex easily distinguishable; thyroid and liver functional; blood forming in bone marrow. Skeleton visible on X ray, a positive sign of pregnancy.	Becoming an abdominal organ.	Blood volume starts to increase, cardiac output is 24% to 50% greater, and heart size increases.
Week 15	*Lanugo* appearing, head hair forming.	Enough amniotic fluid (200 ml) to permit amniocentesis.	Physiologic anemia; free HCl in gastric juices declines, making it harder to absorb iron; and blood pressure lower.
Week 16	Weight—114 g (4 oz); length—16 cm (6½ inches); and muscles contract more vigorously. Skin transparent.	Uterine contractions, but not yet palpable; fundal height‡ halfway between SP and U; 3–4 fingerbreadths (FB) above SP.	Increased fibrinogen, plasma volume, and RBC; decreased hemoglobin concentration; and a few mothers may experience quickening; colostrum may be expressed.
Week 17		Uterine souffle or bruit can be heard.	Pigmentation changes may occur after the sixteenth week: chloasma, nipples, areolae.

TABLE 3–9.   *(Continued)*

Menstrual or gestational age†	Embryo-fetus development	Uterine changes	Possible maternal signs and physiologic changes in pregnancy
MONTH FIVE			
Week 18	*Vernix* caseosa forming on skin and *meconium* collecting. FHR heard by fetoscope. Length: 7 inches.	Walls thin; fetal movements may be palpated by the examiner in most instances.	Decisive increase in blood volume (30%) starts; nitrogen storage increasing due to increased metabolic demands for new tissue formation and increased steroids causing retention of Na and water; increase in vascular system.
Week 19	Onset of rapid growth; iron starts to be stored; enamel-dentin deposited.	Ballottement may be elicited by examiner (mo. 4 to 5).	Most women have experienced quickening by now.
Week 20	FHTs may be heard more easily with a stethoscope—a positive sign of pregnancy; downy lanugo covers almost entire body; some scalp hair. Length: 25 cm (10 in.); weight: 300 g (10 oz).	Fundal height: just below U.	Secondary areolae appear and internal ballottement may be felt.
Week 21	Eyebrows and eyelashes visible; head hair forming.		Umbilicus flush with skin and relaxation of smooth muscle, veins, bladder, etc.
MONTH SIX			
Week 22	Body and head more proportionate.	Fundal height at about the umbilicus.	
Week 23	25 mg of iron stored. Skin less transparent and wrinkled; vernix accumulating.		Ureteral dilatation marked and *linea nigra* and *chloasma* (mask of pregnancy) may appear.
Week 24	Length—30 cm (12 inches); weight—680 g (1½ lb); may be viable; if born, will attempt to breathe.	Fundal height: just above umbilicus.	Period of greatest weight gain starts (4 to 5 lb/month); abdomen slightly distended.
Week 25	Skin red and shiny and face wrinkled.		*Striae gravidarum* may appear.
Week 26	Outline may be felt abdominally, positive sign of pregnancy.	Amniotic fluid—1000 to 1500 ml.	Period of lowest hemoglobin starts—iron therapy may be started now, if not started earlier.

END SECOND TRIMESTER

MONTH SEVEN			
Week 27	Much iron stored, storage of subcutaneous fat starts, and testes descend.	Wall soft and yielding and start of placental senility.	Weight gain continues— 4 lb/month.
Week 28	Length—35 cm (14 inches); weight—1134 g (2½ lb); eyelids open; fingerprints set;	Fundus—22 cm above SP and elastic tissue wall thickening.	Period of lowest hemoglobin continues.

TABLE 3–9.   *(Continued)*

Menstrual or gestational age[†]	Embryo-fetus development	Uterine changes	Possible maternal signs and physiologic changes in pregnancy
	in female—all eggs are present and have completed first stage of development; viable now (although many at 22–24 weeks are surviving with expert care).		
Weeks 29 to 30	Weak cry, more rapid growth starts, much calcium deposit/ storage.	Braxton-Hicks contractions palpable.	Marked protein storage; blood volume highest—30% to 50% over nonpregnant amounts.
MONTH EIGHT Week 31	15.5 mg nitrogen is stored, lanugo begins to be shed, and fingernails grow rapidly.	Fundus—25 cm above SP, halfway between umbilicus and ensiform cartilage.	Large amount of calcium lost to fetus; BMR: + 2.
Week 32	Length—40 cm (16 inches); weight—1800 g (4 lb); presentation—usually vertex, 3% breech; chance of extrauterine survival greater now; testicles may descend into scrotal sac.	Fundal height—3 FB below xiphoid; McDonald—28 cm; Spiegelberg—30 cm; other— 32 cm.‡	3 to 4 lb gained this month; striae gravidarum more marked; pelvic joints more relaxed—mother may feel her pelvis is loose; duck-waddle walk common.
Weeks 33 to 35	227.6 mg iron and 31.6 mg nitrogen stored; largest deposit of calcium starts; body covered with vernix.	Braxton-Hicks contractions stronger.	Large amount of iron lost, stomach flaccid and on top of uterus, heartburn common.
MONTH NINE Week 36	Length—45 cm (18 inches); weight—2268 g (5 + lb); increased amount of subcutaneous fat, storage of minerals and vitamins; and acquisition of immune bodies from mother.	Fundus—at ensiform cartilage or 1–2 FB below; McDonald and Spiegelberg—32 cm; other—36 cm.	Umbilicus protrudes, shortness of breath, Hgb starts to rise, BP rises a bit, BMR: + 4.
Weeks 37 to 38	58.5 mg nitrogen stored, high Hgb, low O_2 tension (cyanotic), and body well formed.	Engaged (nullipara): fundus— slightly below ensiform cartilage.	*Lightening* (nullipara), breathing easier, varicosities, ankle edema, and urinary frequency.
Weeks 39 to 40	246.2 mg iron stored; length— 50 cm (20 inches); weight— 3175 to 3400 g (7 to 7½ lb). Lanugo shed except for shoulders, generally; body contours plump; decreased amount of vernix; scalp hair 2 to 3 cm long; cartilage in nose, ears is well developed. Male: testes within well-wrinkled scrotum. Female: labia well developed and covering vestibule.	Weight—1000 g (2 lb); capacity—4000 ml; length— 32 cm; amniotic fluid—500 to 1200 ml. Fundal height— McDonald: 35 cm. Spiegelberg: 37.7 cm.	Lightening with start of labor in multigravida; cervix generally soft, slightly patulous, and partially (nullipara) or totally (multipara) effaced.

TABLE 3–9.   *(Continued)*

Menstrual or gestational age†	Embryo-fetus development	Uterine changes	Possible maternal signs and physiologic changes in pregnancy
END THIRD TRIMESTER	Survival at term—optimal.	Placenta—1/6 of fetal weight.	BMR + 7.
POSTTERM Over 42 weeks	Vernix, lanugo absent; breast tissue—7 mm; skin dry, thick, desquamating, with superficial or deep cracks—parchmentlike. Length, bone growth continue; weight—fetus may need to mobilize own subcutaneous fat to meet metabolic needs. If postmature—subcutaneous fat and glycogen reserves decrease; hypoxia with passage of meconium; skin dry and wrinkled; nails long; survival jeopardized.	Placental degeneration continues; metabolic exchange diminishing.	Impatient for delivery: concern heightened by physician's request for tests to determine fetal well-being; cesarean delivery may be indicated. Increased fatigue and danger of dystocia.

*Study this chart primarily by *trimester,* not week by week.

†Menstrual or gestational age is considered to be 2 weeks' more than conceptional age.

‡Fundal height scales for the various weeks gestation differ from author to author. Two or more values are given to emphasize differences.

5. Ovaries—
   a. No maturing follicles.
   b. Only corpus luteum is active; its activity is limited to the first trimester.
C. Breasts (Tables 3–8 and 3–9).
D. Metabolism:
   1. Weight gain 20 to 30 lb (average gain 24 lb); pattern of weight gain: 1 lb/mo for first trimester; 0.9 to 1 lb/week during rest of gestation.
   2. Basal metabolic rate (BMR) increases as pregnancy progresses, due to increased oxygen consumption.
   3. Protein—increased need for fetal and uterine growth and maternal blood (500 g needed for hemoglobin and plasma protein).
   4. Increased water retention.
   5. Carbohydrates—
      a. Need increased amount to spare protein stores and intake.
   b. During first half of pregnancy, glucose is rapidly and continuously siphoned across placenta to meet growth needs of conceptus. May lead to hypoglycemia and feeling of faintness.
   c. During second half of pregnancy, antiinsulin hormones, normal maternal hyperglycemia to meet fetal needs, challenge the β-cells of pancreas to maintain high levels of insulin.
      (1) Pregnancy aggravates existing diabetes mellitus.
      (2) Gestational diabetes may occur.
   6. Fat—levels of plasma lipids rise.
   7. Iron—supplementation recommended to meet increased need for RBC by maternal/placental/fetal unit.
E. Cardiovascular system:
   1. Heart displaced upward and to the left; systolic murmurs common.

2. Circulation—
    a. Cardiac volume increases by 30% to 50% during the last two trimesters.
    b. Cardiac output increases by 35% during last two trimesters.
    c. Heart rate increases five to ten beats/minute.
    d. Labor—with each contraction, cardiac output increases by 15% to 20%, regardless of regional anesthesia.
3. Hematocrit and hemoglobin values diminish approximately 10% in the last two trimesters (physiologic anemia).
4. Vena caval syndrome or supine hypotensive syndrome—bradycardia, reduced cardiac output, and a drop in systolic blood pressure from uterine compression of inferior vena cava when the mother is supine; additional maternal symptoms include faintness, sweating, and nausea; fetal symptoms include marked bradycardia (deceleration).

F. Urinary tract:
1. Relaxation of smooth muscle (see K below, *Musculoskeletal system*) leads to dilatation of ureters (especially on right side) and decreased bladder tone, increasing possibility of urinary stasis and infection; persists for four to six weeks after delivery.
2. Glucosuria evident and normal; later, lactosuria as well (urine glucose level is not a reliable index of diabetic status).
3. Frequency during early and late pregnancy due to hormone-induced turgescence and weight of gravid uterus.
4. Glomerular filtration rate increases by 50% during last two trimesters without a similar rise in renal plasma flow; that is, increases efficiency without raising blood pressure.

G. Gastrointestinal tract:
1. Gingivae soften and enlarge (epulis) and have a greater tendency to bleed due to increased vascularity.
2. Ptyalism—increased salivation.
3. General decrease in smooth-muscle tone and motility.
    a. Movement of food slows, increasing reabsorption of water from bowel, predisposing to constipation, hemorrhoids.
    b. Stomach—emptying time is delayed.
    c. Cardiac sphincter relaxes—may result in indigestion, heartburn, and reflex esophagitis.

    d. Increasing size of uterus and displacement of intraabdominal organs results in constipation, heartburn, and flatulence.
4. Increased acidity leads to heartburn and requires special consideration of aspiration during labor.

H. Respiratory tract:
1. Increased ventilation with increased oxygen consumption; increased sensitivity to CO_2 levels; may be short of breath with normal exertion at times.
2. Respiratory rate—relatively unchanged, 16/minute (woman breathes deeper, not faster).
3. Diaphragm is elevated and anterior-posterior diameter of rib cage is increased.
4. Vital capacity—unchanged.

I. Endocrine system:
1. Progressive increase in BMR (up 25%).
2. Increase in size and activity of some glands—pituitary, parathyroid, and adrenals, for example.
3. Twenty percent increase in thyroid function may result in palpitations, tachycardia, emotional lability, heat intolerance, fatigue, perspiration.
4. Pancreas, during second half of pregnancy, must be able to increase production of insulin. By term, maternal insulin needs to increase by an average of 67%.

J. Integument:
1. Increased pigmentation from second trimester of pregnancy—linea nigra, darkened genitalia, chloasma, and areolae due to melanin-stimulating hormone from the pituitary gland.
2. Striae gravidarum (stretch marks).
3. Increased sebaceous and sweat gland activity.
4. Estrogen-induced vascular changes—palmar erythema, vascular "spiders."

K. Musculoskeletal system:
1. Progesterone-, estrogen-, and relaxin-induced relaxation of joints, cartilage, and ligaments.
    a. Subjective symptoms—
        (1) Feeling of pelvic looseness.
        (2) Duck-waddle walk.
        (3) Tenderness of symphysis pubis.
    b. Function in childbirth—increase in anteroposterior diameter of rib cage and enlargement of birth canal.
2. Posture—increasing weight of uterus tilts the pelvis forward; the woman throws her head and shoulders backward to compensate, exaggerating the lumbar spinal curvature (lordosis).
    a. Results in leg and back strain and fatigue.

b. Treatment:

(1) Good body alignment—tuck pelvis under baby; tighten abdominal muscles.

(2) Pelvic rock exercise.

(3) Squat, bend at the knees, not with the back.

(4) Wear low-heeled, sturdy shoes.

(5) Wear maternity girdle.

2. *Emotional changes*—affected by age, maturity, support system, number of concurrent stresses, coping repertoire, physical and mental health status.

A. Tasks of pregnancy (Reva Rubin and others):

1. Accept the pregnancy, from the symbiotic relationship with the fetus to the emergence of the child as a separate individual.

2. Seek and ensure acceptance of child by others.

3. Seek safe passage for self and infant through pregnancy and labor.

4. Prepare realistically for the coming child and be ready to separate from it physically; "I am going to be a parent."

5. Adopt maternal role.

B. Physical bases of changes:

1. Increased metabolic demands may lead to fatigue and anemia.

2. Increased levels of hormones—steroids, estrogen, and progesterone—affect mood as well as physiology.

C. First trimester:

1. Mood swings; emotional lability may be disturbing to self and significant others.

2. Nursing actions—

a. Validate normalcy of mood swings, ambivalence, displeasure with subjective symptoms of early pregnancy.

b. Provide information regarding pregnancy, its management, and her resources.

D. Second trimester—ambivalence toward pregnancy *now*—usually gives way to acceptance when fetal movements are felt; introversion and passivity usually begin.

1. Old, unresolved conflicts emerge—feelings toward mother, sexual intimacy, and masturbation; movement toward resolution is possible now.

2. Reevaluates herself, her life style, and her marriage (if applicable).

3. Daydreams, fantasizes herself as "mother"; may acquire pet, babysit, or seek out other pregnant women or new mothers with whom to interact.

4. Nursing actions—validate normalcy of libidinal

and other mood swings, and feelings of dependency and introversion. Fill in informational gaps. Discuss preparation for childbirth classes.

E. Third-trimester fears:

1. Loss of body image.

2. Bodily mutilation—growth and stretching of body tissues, especially birth canal; episiotomy; cesarean delivery.

3. Loss of control of body function—ptyalism; leaking of colostrum, leukorrhea, urinary frequency, constipation, and stress incontinence.

4. For baby—deformity or death.

5. Pain.

6. Exposing fears and thoughts to others.

7. Nursing actions—validate feelings regarding discomfiture of late pregnancy and anticipation of labor; help meet dependency needs; help her prepare for labor and for the baby's, the family's, and her personal needs in early puerperium.

F. Spouse:

1. Frequently shares her fears and period of introspection, but often each is unaware of this fact.

2. Requires same nursing interventions as she does—

a. Reassurance that these fears and feelings are expected and acceptable.

b. Assistance in opening or keeping open lines of communication.

c. Opportunity to ventilate feelings and concerns.

d. Validation that it is normal for the father to experience some discomforts of pregnancy too.

e. Information regarding childbearing and expectant and new parenthood.

G. Reaction of other family members, including siblings and grandparents:

1. Siblings—

a. Encourage sibling-neonate relationship by taking pictures of neonate in hospital and arranging visits and time for sibling to discuss fears.

b. Alert parents to sibling's increased needs for demonstrations of love, especially the preverbal toddler; if child is older, he or she needs honest verbal explanations.

c. Alert parents to sibling's possible use of misbehavior to get attention or to vent feelings.

2. Grandparents—

a. Alert parents to possible negative reactions of grandparents such as criticism of one or

both parents or in-laws, decreased self-esteem.
   b. Encourage ventilation of feelings.

3. Sexuality and sexual expression during pregnancy and postpartum

A. Sexual appetite may increase or decrease during pregnancy; because of the perineal vasocongestion, some women are orgasmic for the first time during pregnancy.

B. First trimester:
1. Decline in interest, usually—nausea, fatigue, breast tenderness.
2. If woman is an habitual aborter, it may be wise to avoid intercourse and/or orgasm during the times when she would normally be having her menstrual period.

C. Second trimester:
1. A relative increase in orgasmic activity and sexual interest.
2. Women may feel a responsibility to show interest to keep their men at home.
3. Some men are repulsed by the increased vaginal show (leukorrhea).

D. Third trimester:
1. In the absence of pathology, bleeding, or ruptured membranes, there is no proven reason why sexual activity cannot continue until labor begins or membranes rupture.
2. Positions need to be varied to accommodate enlarging abdomen; may prefer mutual masturbation at this time.
3. Men may experience an attraction or aversion to viewing a pregnant body or to feeling fetal movement, or may express concern regarding fetal welfare and therefore prefer nonintercourse sexual expression.
4. Avoid oral-genital manipulation—for example, man blowing into vagina, as this may cause an air embolus and possible maternal death.

E. Postpartum:
1. May resume intercourse after lochia stops, about the third week.
2. May have some dyspareunia with first intercourse after delivery due to "dry" vaginal mucosa from hormone deprivation between birth of placenta and resumption of menstrual cyclic activity; episiotomy and other trauma to the birth canal should be healed by now.
3. To check vaginal readiness, partner should coat one finger with coconut oil and insert into vagina gently, then two fingers; if no discomfort, intercourse should not be painful.
4. Use some form of contraception.

F. Sexual arousal during breastfeeding (see sections below on infant-feeding, breastfeeding, and lactation).

NURSING CARE AND OBSTETRIC SUPPORT DURING ANTEPARTAL PERIOD

1. Discomforts from maternal adaptations to pregnancy

A. Maternal adaptations to pregnancy may lead to discomfort. The woman and her family need reassurance when this discomfort is a normal expression of adaptation. She also benefits from learning ways to prevent or to cope with the discomfort (Table 3–10).

B. To assist women in active participation in their own health care, and to identify potential serious complications during the antepartal period, women need a printed list of danger signs and symptoms that require immediate attention. A summary follows. (The specific disease processes involved are discussed below under *Complications*.)
1. Visual disturbances—blurring, double vision, and spots.
2. Swelling of face or fingers.
3. Severe, frequent, or continuous headaches.
4. Muscular irritability or convulsions.
5. Persistent vomiting beyond first trimester or severe vomiting any time.
6. Epigastric pain.
7. Fluid discharge from vagina—bleeding or amniotic fluid (anything other than leukorrhea).
8. Chills or fever.
9. Severe or unusual pain in the abdomen.
10. Absence of fetal movements after quickening.
11. Burning on urination.

2. Nutrition for childbearing

A. Recommended daily allowances (RDA) for nonpregnant, pregnant, and lactating women of differing ages are discussed in Appendix A.

B. Weight gain—average, about 24 lb (Table 3–11).
1. If underweight at conception, gravida should gain more than 24 lb.
2. If obese at conception, gravida *should not diet* now; she should gain at least 24 lb.

TABLE 3–10.   *Discomforts during pregnancy*

Discomfort and cause	Prevention	Treatment
Morning sickness—first three months; nausea and vomiting; may occur anytime, day or night; *cause:* hormonal, psychologic, and empty stomach.	Eat five to six times daily, small amounts; avoid empty stomach, offending odors, and food difficult to digest (food high in fat, for example).	Alternate dry carbohydrate one hour, fluids (hot tea, milk, or clear coffee) next hour; take dry carbohydrate before rising, stay in bed 15 more minutes.
Fatigue (sleep hunger)—first three months; *cause:* hormones? Often returns late pregnancy when physical load is great.	Not preventable—may be modified with rest and diet (prevent anemia).	Iron supplement if anemic—foods high in iron, folic acid, and protein of high biologic value.
Fainting (syncope)—early pregnancy, due to slightly decreased arterial blood pressure; late pregnancy, due to venous stasis in lower extremities.	When standing, do not lock knees; avoid prolonged standing; may come with prolonged fasting.	Elevate feet; sit down when necessary.
Urinary frequency—enlarging uterus presses on bladder, turgescence of structures from hormone stimulation; relieved somewhat as uterus rises from pelvis; recurs with lightening.	Unpreventable—modified by Kegal's exercises.	Kegal's exercises; limit fluids just before bedtime to ensure rest. Rule out urinary-tract infection.
Vaginal discharge—months two to nine; mucusy, acid, and increases in amount.	Not preventable; cleanliness important.	Treatable only if infection sets in; douche only with prescription.
Hot flashes—heat intolerance, increased metabolism, increased sweating.	None.	No treatment or prevention is necessary—alter clothing, bathing, and environmental temperature as necessary.
Headache—cause unknown; blood pressure change? nutritional? tension? (unless associated with preeclampsia).	Be aware of sources of tension; practice relaxing; eat adequate diet.	If pain relief needed, consult physician (avoid aspirin without prescription).
Nasal stuffiness—due to increased vascularization; allergic rhinitis of pregnancy.	Not avoidable if woman has this tendency; will return to normal postpartum.	Antihistamines and nasal sprays by prescription only.
Heartburn—not related to heart; enlarging uterus and hormones slow digestion; progesterone causes reverse peristaltic waves resulting in reflux of stomach contents into esophagus.	Instead of leaning over, bend at the knees, keeping torso straight; sit on firm chairs; limit fatty and fried foods in diet; small, frequent meals.	Sips of milk may provide temporary relief; physician may prescribe an antacid; "flying exercise"; avoid use of baking soda or seltzers.
Flatulence—altered digestion from enlarging uterus and hormones.	Not preventable—maintain regular bowel habits, avoid foods that are gas formers.	Same as prevention; antiflatulent may be prescribed.
Insomnia—fetal movements, fears or concerns, and general body discomfort from heavy uterus.	Exercise; side-lying positions of comfort with pillow supports; change position often; backrubs from spouse; time to ventilate feelings.	Same as prevention; medication by prescription only.
Shortness of breath—enlarging uterus limits expansion of diaphragm.	Not preventable—relieved with delivery.	Good posture; cut down on smoking, position—supine and upright.

TABLE 3–10.   *(Continued)*

Discomfort and cause	Prevention	Treatment
Backache—increased elasticity of connective tissue, increased weight of uterus, and increased lumbar curvature.	Avoid fatigue; eat good diet; posture; low-heeled, wide-base shoes; pelvic rock; good body mechanics.	Correct posture, shoes, and diet; do pelvic rock often, on hands and knees; tuck pelvis under the baby.
Pelvic joint pain—hormones relax connective tissue and joints and allow movement within joints.	Not preventable—needed to increase the birth passage.	Rest; good posture; will go away after delivery, in six to eight weeks.
Leg cramps—pressure of enlarging uterus on nerve supplying legs; lack of calcium? Fatigue, chilling, and tension?	Avoid pointing toes, especially when arising; rest legs; keep warm; maintain recommended daily intake of calcium.	Stretch affected muscle and hold until it subsides; *do not rub* (may release a blood clot, if present).
Constipation—decreased motility (hormones, enlarging uterus) and increased reabsorption of water; iron therapy (oral).	Diet—prunes, fruits, vegetables, roughage, and fluids; regular habits; exercise; sit on toilet with knees up.	Same as prevention—avoid enemas (damages mucosa, hemorrhoids); never use mineral oil, inhibits vitamin absorption.
Hemorrhoids—varicosities around anus; aggravated by pushing with stool and by uterus pressing on blood vessels supplying lower body.	Avoid constipation; do not strain at stool, sit on toilet with feet on foot stool.	Pure Vaseline or Desitin are mild and sometimes soothing; use any other preparation with prescription only.
Ankle edema—normal and nonpitting; gravity.	Rest legs often during day with legs and hips raised.	Same as prevention.
Varicose veins—lower legs, vulva, pelvis; pressure of heavy uterus; relaxation of connective tissue in vein walls; hereditary.	Progressively worse with subsequent pregnancies and obesity; elevate legs on pillows above level of heart; support hose may help.	Same as prevention; avoid restrictive clothing (knee-high hose); avoid long periods of standing.
Cramp in side or groin—round ligament pain; stretching of round ligament with cramping.	To get out of bed, turn to side, use arm and upper body and push up to sitting position.	Same as prevention.

3. Appropriate weight gain pattern:
   a. First trimester—2 to 4 lb.
   b. Second and third trimesters—0.9 to 1.0 lb/week.
4. Consequent to this weight increase and pattern of weight gain is the lowest incidence of pre-eclampsia/eclampsia, small-for-gestational-age infants, and perinatal mortality.
C. "Basic four" food groups:
   1. See Appendix C for RDA.
   2. Nutrient needs change during pregnancy (Table 3–12).
   3. Fluids—at least four glasses per day (about 1 liter).
D. Assessment for nutritional status:
   1. Physical findings suggestive of poor nutritional status—skin rough, dry, scaly; lesions on lips in corners of mouth; dull, brittle hair; caries; pale mucous membranes.
   2. Height, weight, age.
   3. Assessment tools—three-day diet history; variety of different check-list, history-taking forms.
   4. Laboratory values—hemoglobin, hematocrit, others.
E. Counseling:
   1. Example of nutritional assessment, plan, and implementation is found in Table 3–13. The woman is of adequate weight for height and age; no anemia or other risk factors; woman is at 20 weeks' gestation.
   2. Counseling in selected situations:
      a. *Pica*—the regular and excessive ingestion of

TABLE 3–11. *Average weight gain during pregnancy (40 weeks' gestation)*

	Grams	Pounds, ounces
Fetus	3150	7
Placenta	675	1, 15
Amniotic fluid	900	2
Subtotal	4725	10, 15
Uterus	900	2
Mammary gland	450	1
Maternal blood volume	1350	3
Tissue fluids	1350	3
Fat	4050	9
Subtotal	8100	18
Total	12825	28 lb, 15 oz

nonfood items (Argo starch, red clay from Kentucky, plaster) or of foods with limited nutritional value, often related to cultural and geographic factors. Nurse needs to stress the importance of adequate nutrition. The woman's appetite may be dulled with the nonfood.

b. *Smoking, drug addiction, and alcoholism*—psychological problems may affect compliance with sound nutrition. Person may not consume sufficient quantities; alcohol affects B vitamin absorption and utilization. May need additional supplementation with vitamins, minerals; referral to USDA Food Stamp Program and Supplemental Food Program for Women, Infants, and Children (WIC).

c. *Adolescence* (especially women under 15 years of age)—metabolic needs of pregnancy are superimposed on those of adolescent growth spurt; peer pressure to follow dietary habits is great; may need to rebel against eating a "good" diet (a reminder of dependent childhood days). See page 200.

d. *Culture/ethnicity, religion*—assess individual's diet for the types and amounts of nutrients versus foods commonly eaten by the major culture. Help woman explore types of foods she would or could consider adding to or deleting from her current diet if inadequacies exist (Table 3–14).

e. *Vegetarian*—lacto-ovovegetarian and lacto-vegetarian diets contain complete proteins; eaten in adequate quantity, no problems are inherent. Pure vegetarian diets must be carefully planned to achieve complete proteins; vitamin B_{12} deficiency is most common problem. Fruitarian diet is most likely to be inadequate. Refer families to F.M. Lappé, *Diet for a Small Planet*.

F. Evaluation:
1. Weight gain—pattern is gradual and steady; minimum weight gain of 24 lb.
2. Laboratory results are within normal; e.g., Hgb, Hct, other.
3. Fetal maturity and size is appropriate to gestational age.
4. Improvement in family's nutritional knowledge and status is demonstrated.

G. Sodium-restricted diets:
1. Degrees of restriction per 24 hours—
   a. Mild—2 to 4 g (2000 to 4000 mg).
   b. Moderate—1000 mg (1 g).
   c. Strict—500 mg.
2. Care must be taken with these diets, since sodium needs normally increase during pregnancy; protein foods of high biologic value contain large amounts of sodium; therefore, two needed nutrients are compromised; these diets in preeclampsia are falling out of favor for women, since for the most part preeclampsia may be a disease of malnutrition (diets low in good protein).
3. Many studies show prevention and cure of preeclampsia by increasing protein (and therefore salt) in diets and by preventing hypovolemia.
4. It is wise to limit foods with excess sodium, such as canned foods, potato chips, cokes, etc., because caloric value of these is high, the nutritional value low, and salt intake excessive.

3. Prenatal management

A. Goals for initial assessment:
1. To establish baseline for health supervision, teaching, emotional support, and/or referrals (for genetic counseling, voluntary abortion, family planning, and social services).
2. To determine gravidity and parity.

TABLE 3–12. *Nutrient needs during pregnancy*

Nutrient	Maternal need	Fetal need	Food source
Protein	Maternal tissue growth: uterus, breasts, blood volume, storage.	Rapid growth—see Table 3–9.	Milk and milk products. Animal meats: muscle, organs. Grains, legumes. Eggs.
Calories	Increased BMR.	Primary energy source for growth of fetus.	Carbohydrates 4 Kcal/g; Proteins 4 Kcal/g; Fats 9 Kcal/g
Minerals: Calcium (and phosphorus).	Increase in maternal Ca^{++} metabolism.	Skeleton and tooth formation.	Milk and milk products, especially Swiss cheese.*
Iron.	Increase in RBC mass.	Liver storage (especially in third trimester).	Organ meats: liver, animal meat; egg yolk, whole or enriched grains; green leafy vegetables; nuts.
Vitamins A	Tissue growth.	Cell development—tissue and bone growth and tooth bud formation.	Butter, cream, fortified margarine; green and yellow vegetables.
Bs	Coenzyme in many metabolic processes.	Coenzyme in many metabolic processes.	Animal meats, organ meats; milk and cheese; beans, peas, nuts; enriched grains.
Folic acid	Meet increased metabolic demands in pregnancy. Production of blood products.	Meet increased metabolic demands, including production of cell nucleus material.	Liver; deep-green, leafy vegetables.
C	Tissue formation and integrity. Increase iron absorption.	Tissue formation and integrity.	Citrus fruit, berries, melons; peppers; green, leafy vegetables; broccoli; potatoes.
D	Absorption Ca^{++}, phosphorus.	Mineralization of bone tissue and tooth buds.	Fortified milk and margarine.
E	Tissue growth; cell wall integrity; RBC integrity.	Tissue growth; cell integrity; RBC integrity.	Widely distributed: meat, milk, eggs, grains, leafy vegetables.

*Swiss cheese contains twice the amount of calcium as 8 oz of whole milk, but only 0.09 as much lactose. Therefore, a good source for those with lactose intolerance. Tofu (soybean cake) is high in calcium and contains no lactose.

TABLE 3–13. *Example of nutritional counseling*

Present diet	Comments	Revised diet
Breakfast: 7 A.M. with husband—1 slice toast with butter, coffee.	Feels "worn out" by 11 A.M. Lactose intolerance. Lacks: Vitamin C, protein, calories.	6 oz fresh strawberries, 1 soft-cooked egg on 1 slice toast with butter, coffee.
		Morning snack: 2 slices swiss cheese, 1 medium apple.
Lunch: picks at whatever is available—does not like to eat alone.	Suggest she thinks of preparing and sitting down to lunch with her unborn child; or have lunch with a friend. May need to supplement with calcium gluconate or lactate.	1 tuna fish sandwich made of: 2 slices whole wheat, ½ C tuna (packed in water); diced celery, green pepper, onion, optional; mayonnaise, lettuce, tomato, optional; fresh fruit; coffee or tea.

a. *Gravida*—a pregnant woman.
  (1) *Nulligravida*—woman who has never been pregnant.
  (2) *Primigravida*—woman with a first pregnancy.
  (3) *Multigravida*—woman with a second or later pregnancy.

b. *Para*—refers to *past pregnancies* (not number of babies) that reached viability, whether or not the infant or infants were born alive.
  (1) *Nullipara*—woman who has not carried a pregnancy to viability, e.g., may have had one or more abortions.
  (2) *Primipara*—woman who has carried one pregnancy to viability.
  (3) *Multipara*—woman delivered of two or more pregnancies that had reached viability (24 weeks' gestation or more).
  (4) *Grandmultipara*—woman delivered of six or more pregnancies that had reached viability.

c. Examples of recordings of women's gravidity/parity:
  (1) A woman who is pregnant now for the fifth time and whose previous pregnancies yielded two full-term neonates, no premature infants, and two abortions (spontaneous or therapeutic), and who now has two living children, may be designated as: 5–2–0–2–2.
  (2) A woman who is pregnant for the first time and is yet undelivered is designated as: 1–0–0–0–0. After she delivers a full-term living neonate, she becomes 1–1–0–0–1.
  (3) If a woman's second pregnancy results in an abortion and she has a living child from her first pregnancy that had been delivered at term, she is designated as: 2–1–0–1–1.
  (4) Others record as follows: number gravida/number para. Using the examples given in a, b, c, above, those women would be designated as follows: (1)—5/2; (2)—1/0; (3)—2/1.

3. To validate diagnosis of pregnancy. Diagnosis must be accurate. A false diagnosis can lead to personal, marital, and relationship problems and can have legal repercussions for the physician/ nurse as well. The physician makes the differential diagnosis between the presumptive/probable signs/symptoms commonly seen in early pregnancy and other disorders that may underlie the signs/symptoms.

a. Presumptive symptoms—woman's subjective experiences:
  (1) Amenorrhea—more than ten days past missed period.
  (2) Breast changes.
  (3) Nausea and vomiting.
  (4) Striae gravidarum, linea nigra, chloasma, and quickening (after week 16).
  (5) Urinary frequency.
  (6) Fatigue.

TABLE 3–14.   *Cultural food patterns*

Ethnic group	Cultural food patterns	Possible dietary excesses or omissions
Mexican (native)	Basic source of protein—dry beans; flan; cheese; many meats, fish, eggs. Chili peppers and many deep-green and yellow vegetables; fruits include zapote, guava, papaya, mango, citrus. Tortillas (corn, flour); sweet bread; fideo.	Limited meats, milk, and milk products. Some are using flour tortillas more than the more nutritious corn. Excessive use of lard (manteca), sugar. Tendency to boil vegetables for long periods of time.
Filipino (Spanish-Chinese influence)	Utilize most meats, eggs, nuts, legumes. Use many different kinds of vegetables. Large amounts of rice and cereals.	May limit meat, milk, and milk products (the latter may be due to lactose intolerance). Tend to prewash rice. Tend to fry many foods.
Chinese (mostly Cantonese)	Use cheese, tofu, many meats, chicken and pigeon eggs; nuts; legumes; soybean curd (tofu). Many different vegetables, leaves, bamboo sprouts. Rice and rice-flour products; wheat, corn, millet seed.	Tendency among some immigrants to use excess grease in cooking. May be low in protein, milk, and milk products (the latter may be due to lactose intolerance). Often wash rice before cooking. Use large amounts of soy and oyster sauces, both of which are high in salt.
Puerto Rican	Milk with coffee. Pork, poultry, eggs, dried fish; beans (habichuelas). Viandas (starchy vegetables; starchy ripe fruits). Avocados, okra, eggplant, sweet yams. Rice, cornmeal.	Utilize large amounts of lard for cooking. Limited use of milk and milk products. Limited amounts of pork and poultry.
Black American	Milk and milk products (if no lactose intolerance). Variety of meats, eggs, nuts, legumes, fish. Deep leafy vegetables, other vegetables; variety of fruits. Variety of breads and cereals (including grits, hominy, hot breads). Molasses (dark molasses is especially good source of calcium, iron, vitamins B_1 and B_2, and niacin).	Limited use of milk group (lactose intolerance). Extensive use of frying, "smothering," simmering for cooking. Large amounts of fat: salt pork, bacon drippings, lard, gravies. May have limited use of citrus and enriched breads.
Middle Eastern (Greek, Syrian, Armenian)	Yogurt. Predominantly lamb, nuts, dried peas, beans, lentils. Deep-green leaves and vegetables; dried fruits. Dark breads and cracked wheat.	Tend to use excessive sweeteners, lamb fat, olive oil. Tend to fry meats and vegetables. Insufficient milk and milk products (almost no butter—use olive oil, which has no nutritive value except for calories). Deficiency of fresh fruits.
Middle European (Polish)	Many milk products. Pork, chicken. Root vegetables (potatoes); cabbage; fruits. Wheat products.	Tend to use excessive sweets and to overcook vegetables. Limited amounts of fruits (citrus), raw vegetables, and meats.
Native American (American Indian—much variation)	If "Americanized," use milk and milk products. Variety of meats: game, fowl, fish; nuts, seeds, legumes. Variety of vegetables, some wild; variety of fruits, some wild, rose hips; roots. Variety of breads, including tortillas, cornmeal, rice.	Nutrition-related problems: obesity, diabetes, dental problems, iron-deficiency anemia; alcoholism. Limited quantities of high-protein foods depending on availability (flocks) and economic situation. Excessive use of sugar.

(7) Deeper vulvar color.
(8) Braxton Hicks contractions.
(9) Weight gain.
(10) Finger- and toenail changes.
(11) BBT elevation.
(12) Abdominal enlargement.
b. Probable signs—examiner's objective findings:

(1) Positive pregnancy test.
(2) Enlargement of abdomen (after third month) along with uterine enlargement.
(3) Reproductive-organ changes (after sixth week).
  (a) Hegar's sign—softening of lower uterine segment.
  (b) Goodell sign—cervical softening.

        (c) Chadwick's sign—bluish vagina.

    (4) Ballottement (after fourth or fifth month).

    (5) Outline of fetus palpated through abdominal wall (after fourth or fifth month).

    (6) Braxton Hicks contractions.

    (7) Uterine souffle—after week 16.

  c. Positive signs of pregnancy:

    (1) Fetal heart tones—

      (a) Doptone—12 weeks.

      (b) Fetoscope—20 weeks.

    (2) Examiner feels fetal movements, usually after 24 weeks.

    (3) X ray of fetal skeleton (3 months).

    (4) Sonographic examination (after week 14, when fetal head is sufficiently developed to assure accurate diagnosis).

    (5) Fetal EKG by week 12.

    (6) Radioimmunoassay (RIA) test for the β-subunit of HCG (not available everywhere) almost 100% accurate as early as 24 hours after implantation.

B. Physical aspects—assessment:

  1. Weight.

  2. Vital signs.

  3. Blood work—hematocrit and hemoglobin for anemia; type and Rh; tests for sickle cell trait, syphilis, and rubella antibody titer.

  4. Urinalysis—glucose, protein, acetone, signs of infection, and pregnancy test (HCG).

  5. History—

    a. Familial—inheritable diseases and reproductive problems.

    b. Personal, medical, and past obstetrical.

    c. Present pregnancy—LMP and calculation of EDC, symptoms, drugs taken, and exposure to X ray or infectious diseases.

  6. Pelvic examination—

    a. Signs of pregnancy.

    b. Adequacy of pelvis and pelvic structures.

    c. Size and position of uterus.

    d. Papanicolaou smear (see p. 271).

    e. Smears for monilial and trichomonal infections (see p. 268).

    f. Signs of pelvic inflammatory disease (see p. 269).

C. Psychosocial aspects:

  1. *Assessment*—various tools (such as checklists) are available.

    a. Note whether pregnancy was planned or not, whether wanted or not; ascertain the plans for this pregnancy (voluntary abortion, desire for pregnancy, or relinquishment for adoption); cultural or ethnic influences, if pertinent.

    b. Explore development of parenting role during pregnancy:

      (1) Are parents actively and appropriately seeking medical care, information regarding pregnancy, childbirth, parenthood?

      (2) Do they show involvement and growth by practicing: babysitting, getting a new pet, changing patterns in friendship groups?

      (3) Are they mobilizing support groups for themselves?

      (4) Are they role-playing with potential names, the possibility of having a boy or a girl, choice of feeding?

    c. Assess family readiness for childbearing: example—Duvall's framework; what provisions have they made for the following:

      (1) Physical maintenance.

      (2) Allocation of resources.

      (3) Division of labor.

      (4) Socialization of family members.

      (5) Reproduction, recruitment, launching of family members.

      (6) Maintenance of order (relationships within family).

      (7) Maintenance of motivation and morale.

      (8) Placement of members in larger society (relationships outside of family).

  2. Plan and implementation—

    a. Provide anticipatory guidance and support for ambivalent feelings, negative feelings, and mood swings and changes.

    b. Support both partners.

      (1) Encourages mutuality between them.

      (2) Increases the tendency for the mother to turn to the father as the most significant person (as opposed to turning toward the obstetrician).

      (3) Decreases the probability of postpartal psychologic problems.

    c. If the couple is unwed, encourage both to participate in the decision regarding this pregnancy.

    d. Refer to or provide education for childbirth

and parenting classes. Although these classes are a source of information to assist expectant parents through the antepartal period, a major component relates to the process of giving birth. See *Education for Childbirth*, p. 210.

3. Evaluation—
   a. Parents express satisfaction with their decision regarding this pregnancy.
   b. Parents demonstrate development in the parenting role.
   c. Parents are prepared for the birth and for early parenthood.

D. Prenatal management *following the initial visit:*
1. Schedule—
   a. Once per month until week 32.
   b. Every 2 weeks until week 36.
   c. Every week until she goes into labor.
2. Assessments—
   a. General well-being, concerns, questions.
   b. Weight.
   c. Urinalysis for protein and sugar.
   d. Blood pressure (right arm, sitting).
   e. Abdominal palpation.
      (1) Fundal height (Table 3–9); tenderness, masses, hernias.
      (2) Fetal heart rate: start at 10–12 weeks with Doppler; start at 18–20 weeks with a fetoscope.
      (3) Fetal presentation—after week 24.
      (4) Leopold's (abdominal) palpation—after week 32.
   f. Vaginal or rectal examination, prn (if not bleeding).
   g. Laboratory tests: venous blood.
      (1) Repeat Hct, Hgb, anti-Rh titer, VDRL.
      (2) Cultures, prn (vaginal discharge; cervical scraping for chlamydia trachomatis, for example).
   h. Follow-up on medications (vitamins, iron) and nutrition.

PARENTS WITH SPECIAL CONSIDERATIONS

1. The pregnant adolescent
A. High-risk factors:
1. Obstetric/perinatal—only one problem is directly related to physiologic age. The female who becomes pregnant within three years of menarche delivers a neonate who is small for gestational age (SGA). Cause is unknown.
2. Psychosocial, emotional, nutritional, and physical demands of adolescence are compounded by those of pregnancy.
   a. Nutrition-related risk factors—
      (1) Inappropriate weight gain—under 10 lb or over 35 lb.
      (2) Increased incidence of pregnancy wastage—spontaneous abortion, premature labor, premature rupture of membranes, stillbirth, neonatal deaths.
      (3) Increased incidence of preeclampsia/eclampsia.
      (4) Increased incidence of anemia, which predisposes to hemorrhage and infection at any time during the childbearing cycle.
   b. Concurrent infections—
      (1) Communicable diseases such as Rubella, scarlet fever, pneumonia.
      (2) Sexually transmitted diseases such as gonorrhea, herpes II, syphilis.
      (3) Urinary-tract infections.
   c. Delay in initiating, and inconsistent compliance with, prenatal care.
      (1) Magical thinking—"It can't happen to me," "If I ignore it, it will go away"; concept of invulnerability.
      (2) Distrustful of medical personnel and other adults.
      (3) Ashamed.
   d. Increased incidence of suicidal attempts prior to and during pregnancy.
   e. Conflict between developmental tasks of adolescence and those of pregnancy (Table 3–15).
   f. Concurrent social problems.
      (1) Previous out-of-wedlock pregnancy.
      (2) Other family members had an out-of-wedlock pregnancy.
      (3) Presence of parents who are physically abusive to children.
      (4) Mental illness in family.
      (5) Alcoholism in family.
      (6) Disorganized family.
      (7) Single-parent family.
      (8) History of involvement in courts of law (as law breakers).
B. Etiology of adolescent pregnancy:
1. Experimentation with changing body and feelings.

TABLE 3–15. *Developmental tasks*

Adolescence	*Pregnancy*
1. *Piaget*—intellectual development: Early adolescence—concrete operations, for example, must have an experience to know what it is like. Late adolescence—formal operations, for example, capable of abstract thinking, of projecting a result from a certain set of circumstances.	1. *Tasks of pregnancy:* Need to accept the reality of pregnancy and to accept one's initial reaction (anger/guilt) to it. Need to incorporate growing fetus into own body image (accept it, attach to it). Need to separate self from the growing fetus (toward the end of pregnancy). Need to separate self physically from the fetus during labor/delivery.
2. *Erikson*—developmental tasks: Early adolescence—identity versus role diffusion; peers and leadership models are influential. Late adolescence—intimacy, solidarity versus isolation; chosen partners of same and opposite sex are influential.	2. *If marriage occurs*, the tasks that couples face in marriage are superimposed: financial support system, mutually satisfying sexual relationship, and satisfying relationship with friends and others in the community. Adolescent couple may be forced to live with parents.
3. *Need to accept* and live comfortably with body that is changing physically and developing sexual feelings to ensure a positive self-image.	3. *In addition* to adolescent changes, pregnancy imposes further changes in shape and functioning; adolescence and pregnancy require additional nutrients; society favors the slim figure.
4. *Thought reorganization*—needs to become less egocentric.	4. *Thought reorganization*—pregnancy imposes introspection, egocentricity, dependence (emotional).
5. *Increased independence* from parents and growth toward interdependence; responsible for own actions.	5. *Financial, physical supportive dependence* needed; occasionally, alienation between parents and daughter occurs.
6. *Identity*—first with peers of the same sex and then with those of opposite sex.	6. *Difference* (of being pregnant) isolates one from peers of own sex and often from those of opposite sex as well.
7. Most do not have a wide repertoire of social skills, for example, often cannot ask for help or express appreciation verbally or nonverbally; nurses and others may misinterpret their behavior.	7. *Need for additional support*—see Psychosocial aspects, p. 198.

2. Need for someone to love them—being held and caressed by partner during love-making and/or being loved by the new baby.
3. Cultural expectation.
4. "It can't happen to me."
5. Group pressure not to remain a virgin.
6. May repeat a pregnancy to obtain a supportive, caring relationship with a social worker or nurse.

7. "Getting even with" a parent; giving a present to a parent.
8. Confirmation of fertility and adequate biologic functioning.

C. Nursing management:
  1. Avoid blaming, scolding, and moralizing.
  2. Nutritional counseling—start where woman is; she may equate "milk and square meal" approach

as reverting back to childhood; peer pressure in food preferences; stress value of nutrition for character of skin, hair, return to prepregnant figure; pizza, hamburgers, milkshakes all can be incorporated into diet plan.

3. Provide atmosphere in which woman may ventilate feelings and fears (during entire childbearing cycle).
4. Involve woman in problem-solving and planning for her future.
5. Do not criticize the father of the child, as this reflects on the woman as well.
6. Observe for complications.
7. Ask her if or what she wishes to know about any contraceptives; inform her where she can get information when she wants it.
8. Provide continuity of care throughout, through one primary nurse in charge of her "case" or through an effective communication system such as POR (problem-oriented record) to help adolescent develop trust (there is a natural distrust of adults and need to test their limits) and to prevent isolation/abandonment during any part of the cycle.

2. Older parents

A. The multipara who gets pregnant during *menopause*.
  1. Assessment:
    a. Response may vary from extreme pleasure (to find oneself "still young enough") to despair, especially if she faces decision whether or not to abort.
    b. Associated physical complications—hypertension, preeclampsia/eclampsia, other medical problems (such as diabetes), hemorrhage, chromosomal aberrations, physical stamina.
    c. Economic, social conditions.
    d. Other family members, their ages, and their responses to this pregnancy.
  2. Plan, implementation:
    a. Refer to appropriate resource, for example, for abortion, for prenatal care, for preparation-for-childbirth classes.
    b. Involve family in preparation for the birth and the newborn.
  3. Evaluation:
    a. Woman and family are satisfied with decision regarding this pregnancy.
    b. If woman chooses to carry pregnancy, the experience is satisfying and both mother and neonate are healthy.

B. The nullipara who chooses to delay parenthood until her *late 20s and 30s*.
  1. Assessment:
    a. During pregnancy, same as for other women.
    b. Reaction to reality of pregnancy *now*.
  2. Plan and implementation:
    a. Anticipatory guidance regarding new parenthood—change from career environment to home environment.
    b. Management—same as for other women.
  3. Evaluation:
    a. Woman (couple) is able to adopt parent role and find satisfaction in it.
C. The nullipara with a long history of *infertility*.
  1. Assessment:
    a. Reaction to reality of pregnancy *now*.
      (1) Pleased.
      (2) Angry that it happened now after she had altered her life's plans and/or life style.
      (3) Feeling regarding management: abortion, carry and keep, or carry and relinquish.
    b. Physical status—what was cause of her infertility? Was it a hormonal problem that may compromise this pregnancy or its outcome?
  2. Plan and implementation:
    a. Support for her feelings, even if she is very angry and hostile.
    b. Refer to appropriate resource for abortion, antepartal care, etc.
    c. Physical and psychosocial management same as for other women.
  3. Evaluation:
    a. Woman (couple) is satisfied regarding management (and decision) regarding this pregnancy.
    b. If parenthood is chosen, woman (couple) adopts parent role.

INTRAPARTAL PERIOD

1. Components of labor process

A. Uterus—see *Reproductive system in women,* p. 160.
  1. Contractions—involuntary, intermittent contractile activity of the uterine musculature.
    a. Purpose:
      (1) Move presenting part forward.
      (2) Effacement of the cervix—process of thinning out, pulling up, or shortening the cervix.

A. Nullipara   B. Multipara

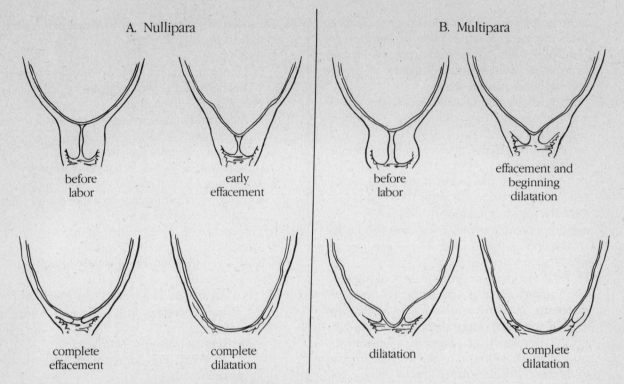

FIGURE 3–1. *Cervical effacement and dilatation*
(a) Nullipara.   **(b)** Multipara. (Courtesy Ross Laboratories, Columbus, Ohio. Redrawn from Clinical Education Aid No. 13.)

(3) Dilatation of the cervix—process of being opened, as the cervix enlarges from 0 to 10 cm (Figure 3–1).
  b. Effect of contractions:
    (1) Raises maternal blood pressure due to increased peripheral arteriole pressure.
    (2) Decreases blood flow to uterus.
    (3) Dilates the cervix during the first stage of labor.
    (4) With bearing-down efforts, expels the fetus (second stage of labor) and the placenta (third stage of labor).
  2. Uterine changes during labor—the beginning of involution.
    a. Upper uterine segment becomes thicker and shorter.
    b. Lower uterine segment becomes thinner and longer.
B. Maternal pelvis:
  1. *Engagement*—widest diameter of presenting part has passed through the pelvic inlet (or brim), for example, biparietal diameter of fetal head.
  2. *Station*—relationship of presenting part to the level of the ischial spines (IS).

  a. *Floating*—presenting part is still in false pelvis, above the inlet.
  b. *Dipping*—presenting part is still in false pelvis, above the inlet.
  c. Station − 5 cm to − 1 cm—presenting part above IS.
  d. Station 0—presenting part at the IS.
  e. Station + 1 cm to + 5 cm—presenting part has descended to level of ischial tuberosities.
3. *False pelvis*—lying above the linea terminalis (the line travels across top of symphysis pubis around to the sacral promontory); it supports the gravid uterus during gestation.
4. *True pelvis* (Figure 3–2)—lies below linea terminalis; divided into:
  a. Inlet—"brim," demarcated by linea terminalis; transverse diameter is widest at 13.5 cm; anterior-posterior (or true conjugate from the top of symphysis to sacral promontory) diameter is 11 cm.
  b. Pelvic cavity.
  c. Outlet—anterior-posterior diameter is widest measurement, thereby facilitating delivery in occiput anterior (OA) position.

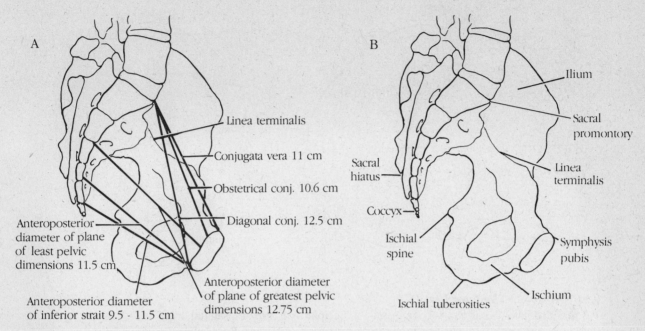

FIGURE 3–2. *Maternal pelvis*
(a) Diameters of pelvic planes. **(b)** True and false pelvis. (Courtesy Ross Laboratories, Columbus, Ohio. Redrawn from Clinical Education Aid No. 18.)

5. Classifications—structure and configuration of inlet:
   a. Gynecoid—true female pelvis; circular.
   b. Android—triangular or wedge-shaped.
   c. Anthropoid—oval.
   d. Platypelloid—flattened, transverse oval.
C. Fetus:
   1. *Fetal head* (Figure 3–3)—
      a. Bones—one occiput, one frontal, two parietals, and two temporals.
      b. Suture—line of junction or closure between bones: sagittal (longitudinal), coronal (anterior), and lambdoidal (posterior).
      c. Fontanels—membranous space between cranial bones during fetal life and infancy.
         (1) Anterior "soft spot"—diamond-shaped; 2.5 cm × 2.5 cm; forms junction with coronal and sagittal sutures; ossifies (closes) in 12 to 18 months.
         (2) Posterior—triangular shape; 1 cm; junction of the sagittal and lambdoidal sutures; ossifies in approximately two months.
         (3) Sphenoid—at termination of coronal suture at junction of frontal, parietal, and temporal bones.
         (4) Mastoid—at termination of lambdoidal

suture between occipital, parietal, and mastoid bones. Mastoid and sphenoid fontanels are palpated and assessed for widening when hydrocephalus is suspected or diagnosed.
   2. Fetal lie—relationship of fetal axis to maternal axis (spine).
      a. Transverse—shoulder presents.
      b. Longitudinal—vertex or breech presents.
   3. Presentation—that fetal part which enters the inlet first.
      a. Cephalic—vertex (most common), face, or brow.
      b. Breech:
         (1) Complete—feet and legs are flexed on thighs; buttocks and feet presenting.
         (2) Frank—legs extended so feet are up by shoulder; buttocks present.
         (3) Footling—single foot; double or two feet; or both knees.
      c. Shoulder.
   4. Attitude—flexion or extension of fetal parts on itself.
   5. Position (Figure 3–4)—the quadrant of the pelvis in which the presenting occiput, mentum, or sacrum is located; could be located on maternal left, anterior or posterior, or on her right side,

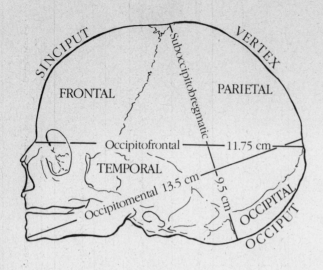 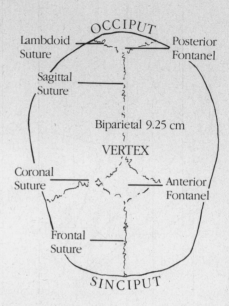

FIGURE 3–3. The fetal head
Bones: frontal—2, parietal—2, temporal—2, occipital—1. *Sutures:* sagittal, frontal, coronal, lambdoid. *Fontanels:* anterior, posterior. (Courtesy Ross Laboratories, Columbus, Ohio. Redrawn from Clin. Ed. Aid No. 13.)

anterior or posterior; examples: LOA, most frequent; LMA; LSA; determined by Leopold's maneuvers and rectal or vaginal examination.

6. Denominator (fetal reference point)—occiput, mentum, or sacrum.

2. Overview of labor process

A. *Lightening*—process of "dropping" or sinking of the fetus into the pelvic inlet, with the accompanying descent of the uterus (see *Engagement*).
   1. Effects—pressure of diaphragm alleviated and breathing is easier; pressure in pelvis increases with return of urinary frequency, a worsening of varices (legs, vulva, and perianal) and increasing pressure in the thighs.
   2. Usually occurs two to three weeks before term in the nullipara and during labor in multiparas. If lightening does not occur, the cause must be determined.

B. Initiation of labor—exact mechanism unknown; theories include:
   1. Overdistention of uterus.
   2. Altered levels of estrogen and progesterone.
   3. High levels of prostaglandins.
   4. Fetal hormone secretion.
   5. Combination of two or more of these mechanisms.

C. False and true labor—differentiation:
   1. False—
      a. Uterine contractions or abdominal sensations.
         (1) Braxton Hicks contractions intensify (or seem to) at night.
         (2) Short and irregular.
         (3) Stop with a change in position or activity.
         (4) Abdominal discomfort may be due to GI upset or bladder spasms.
      b. Cervical assessment.
         (1) No cervical dilatation or effacement.
         (2) No progress in dilatation or effacement if some change had been noted on first examination.
   2. True—
      a. Uterine contractions.
         (1) Fairly regular; may be 20 to 30 minutes apart at first, with frequency, duration, and intensity increasing.
         (2) Not stopped by moderate analgesia, change of position, or activity.
         (3) Felt in lower back, radiating to abdomen.
      b. Cervical dilatation and effacement—progressive.

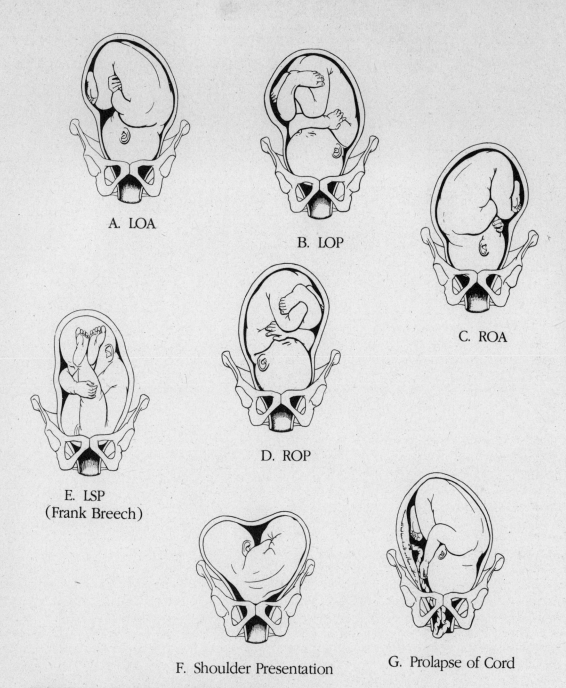

A. LOA

B. LOP

C. ROA

D. ROP

E. LSP
(Frank Breech)

F. Shoulder Presentation

G. Prolapse of Cord

FIGURE 3–4. *Categories of presentation*
(a) LOA: fetal occiput is in left anterior quadrant of maternal pelvis. **(b)** LOP: fetal occiput is in left posterior quadrant of maternal pelvis. **(c)** ROA: fetal occiput is in right anterior quadrant of maternal pelvis. **(d)** ROP: fetal occiput is in right posterior quadrant of maternal pelvis. **(e)** LSP: fetal sacrum is in left posterior quadrant of maternal pelvis. **(f)** Shoulder presentation with fetus in transverse lie. **(g)** Prolapse of umbilical cord with fetus in LOA position. (Courtesy Ross Laboratories, Columbus, Ohio. Redrawn from Clinical Education Aid No. 18.)

TABLE 3–16. *First stage of labor*

Phases of first stage	Expected maternal behaviors	Nursing actions
0 to 4 cm—latent phase and early active phase. 1. Time—nullipara 8–10 hours, average.	1. Usually comfortable, euphoric, excited, talkative, and energetic, but may be fearful and withdrawn.	1. Provides encouragement, feedback for relaxation, companionship.
2. Contractions—regular, mild 5–10 minutes apart, 20–30 seconds' duration.	2. Relieved or apprehensive that labor has begun.	2. Coaches during contractions: signals beginning of contraction, marks the seconds, signals end of contraction; "follow my breathing," "watch my lips," etc.
3. Low back pain and abdominal discomfort with contractions. 4. Cervix thins; some bloody show. 5. Station— Multipara: −2 to +1. Nullipara: 0.	3. Alert, usually receptive to teaching, coaching, diversion, and anticipatory guidance.	3. Provides comfort measures: position for comfort; praise; keep aware of progress.
4 to 8 cm—midactive phase, phase of most rapid dilatation. 1. Average time—nullipara 1–2 hours.	1. Tired, less talkative, and less energetic.	1. Continues to coach during contractions; husband (coach) may need some relief too.
2. Contractions—2 to 5 minutes apart, 30–40 seconds' duration, intensity increasing.	2. More serious, malar flush between 5 and 6 cm, tendency to hyperventilate, may need analgesia, needs constant coaching.	2. Provides comfort measures (to husband too—as needed): positions for comfort while preventing hypotensive syndrome; encourages relaxation, focusing her on areas of tension; provides counterpressure to sacrococcygeal area, prn; praises; keeps aware of progress; minimizes distractions from surrounding environment (loud talking, other noises): offers analgesics and anesthetics, as appropriate; provides hygiene: mouth care, ice chips, clean perineum; provides warmth as needed.
3. Membranes may rupture now. 4. Increased bloody show.		3. Continues to monitor progress of labor and maternal/fetal response. 4. If monitors are in use, focuses attention on mother; periodically checks accuracy of monitor read-outs.
5. Station: −1 to 0.		
8 to 10 cm—transition, deceleration period of active phase. 1. Average time: Nullipara—40 minutes to 1 hour. Multipara—20 minutes.	1. If not under regional anesthesia, more introverted; may be amnesic between contractions.	1. Stays with woman (couple) and provides constant support.

2. Contractions—1½–2 minutes 60–90 seconds, strong intensity:	2. Feeling she cannot make it; increased irritability, crying, nausea, vomiting, and belching; increased perspiration over upper lip and between breasts; leg tremors; and shaking.	2. Continues to coach with contractions; may need to remind, reassure, and encourage her to reestablish breathing techniques and concentration with each contraction; coaches panting or "he-he" respirations to prevent pushing.
3. Increased vaginal show; rectal pressure with beginning urge to bear down.	3. May have uncontrollable urge to push at this time.	3. Provides comfort measures: reminds her and husband that her behavior is normal and "OK"; coaches breathing to quell nausea.
4. Station: + 3 to + 4.		4. Assists with countertension techniques woman requested: effleurage. Continues to monitor contractions, FHR (after each contraction), vaginal discharge, perineal bulging, maternal vital signs; records every 15 minutes. Assesses for bladder filling. Keeps mother (couple) aware of progress. Prepares husband for birth (scrub gown, etc.).

D. Stages of labor:
1. *First* (stage of the uterus/cervix)—from beginning to complete dilatation and effacement, from 0 cm to 10 cm. It is divided into three phases (Table 3–16):
   a. Latent and early active.
   b. Mid-active.
   c. Transitional.
2. *Second* (stage of the neonate)—from 10 cm cervical dilatation through birth of infant.
3. *Third* (stage of the placenta)—from birth of infant through birth of placenta.
4. *Fourth* (arbitrary stage of stabilization of maternal system)—from birth of placenta until maternal condition is stabilized, about one to four hours.

E. Normal time limits for phases of first stage:
1. Nullipara—
   a. Latent—8½ hours, normal; 20 hours, upper limit.
   b. Active—5 hours, normal; 13 hours, upper limit.
2. Multipara—
   a. Latent—5 to 6 hours, normal; 12 hours, upper limit.
   b. Active—2½ hours, normal; 10 hours, upper limit.
3. Normal—S-curve on Friedman chart.
4. Dystocia—exaggeration or prolongation of normal S-curve.

F. Mechanisms of labor—vertex presentation (Figure 3–5):
1. Descent—head engages and proceeds down birth canal.
2. Flexion—head flexes on chest, allowing smallest diameter of vertex to present.
3. Internal rotation—during second stage of labor, transverse diameter of fetal head enters pelvis; occiput rotates 90° to bring back of neck under symphysis pubis, for example, LOT to LOA to OA for delivery.
4. Extension—back of neck pivots under symphysis pubis to allow head to be born by extension.
5. Restitution—*head* turns 45° back to normal position with shoulders; with LOA, after restitution, infant faces mother's right thigh.
6. External rotation—*shoulders* rotate 45° so that upper shoulder delivers under symphysis pubis.
7. Expulsion—delivery of neonate is completed.

3. Assessment techniques
A. Leopold's maneuvers or abdominal palpation:
1. First—place fingers just above symphysis pubis

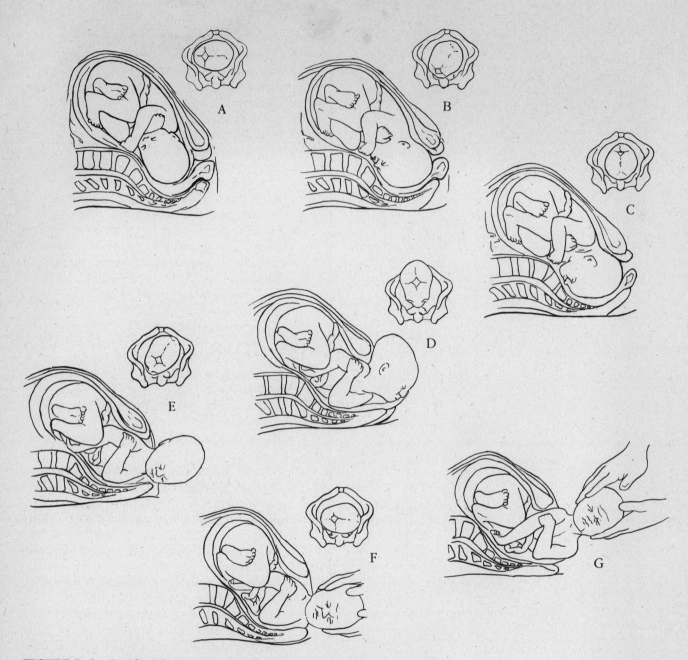

FIGURE 3–5. Cardinal movements in the mechanism of labor with the fetus in vertex presentation
(a) Engagement, descent, flexion. (b) Internal rotation. (c) Extension beginning (rotation complete). (d) Extension complete. (e) External rotation (restitution). (f) External rotation (shoulder rotation). (g) Expulsion. (Courtesy Ross Laboratories, Columbus, Ohio. Redrawn from Clinical Education Aid No. 13.)

to feel presenting part (head presents in 90% of cases).

2. Second—locate fetal back and small parts by running hands up sides of abdomen.

3. Third—bring hands over fundus to feel fetal breech; breech in fundus feels softer, not as round or mobile as the head would be.

4. Fourth—while facing gravida's feet, run hands down sides of abdomen to symphysis to check for cephalic prominence (usually on gravida's right side) and to check whether head is floating or engaged.

B. Vaginal examination:
1. Condition of cervix—soft ("ripe") or rigid.
2. Dilatation and effacement.
3. Station and position of presenting part.
4. Palpable fontanels, and sutures, and caput succedaneum, if vertex; degree of molding.
5. Membranes—
   a. Intact.
   b. Ruptured—fluid should be opaque (milky) with white flecks and have no offensive odor; test with litmus (Nitrazine) paper: amniotic fluid is alkaline (blue on litmus).
6. *Ferguson reflex.* Increase in myometrial contractility that follows mechanical stretching of the cervix. Reflex is blocked by spinal or epidural anesthesia.

C. Locate and monitor fetal heart rate (FHR).
1. Location of most audible FHR and fetal position.
   a. Breech presentation—usually *above* the umbilicus.
   b. Vertex presentation—usually *below* the umbilicus.
   c. Shift in the point where most audible FHR is heard is a useful indicator of fetal descent.
2. Rate—between 120 and 160 beats per minute; bradycardia $\leq$ 100/minute, or 30/minute lower than baseline reading; tachycardia $\geq$ 160/minute, or $\geq$ 30/minute above baseline reading.
3. Factors affecting audibility:
   a. FHR heard best through fetal back or chest; harder if arms and legs intervene.
   b. Polyhydramnios.
   c. Obesity.
   d. Faulty equipment.
   e. Noise in room.
   f. Maternal position.
   g. Maternal gastrointestinal sounds.
   h. Loud uterine bruit—maternal origin, blood moving through uterine vessels, synchronous with maternal pulse.
   i. Loud funic souffle—fetal origin, hissing of blood through umbilical arteries, synchronous with FHR.

D. Contractions:
1. Assessing contractions—
   a. Place finger tips over fundus, use gentle pressure.
   b. Contraction is felt as a tensing or hardening (acrement), reaching a peak intensity (acme), then diminishing slowly (decrement).
   c. Report if contraction begins other than in fundus.
2. Assessing intensity—
   a. Weak—fingers easily indent into fundus.
   b. Moderate—fingers indent slightly; some tension felt.
   c. Strong—fingers cannot indent fundus.
3. Timing contractions—
   a. Frequency—time from beginning of one contraction to beginning of the next, normally not less than two minutes.
   b. Duration—time from beginning to end of a contraction, normally 90 seconds or less.

4. *Nursing actions during first stage of labor*

A. Assessment:
1. Careful evaluation of antepartal history—genetic and familial problems; concurrent medical condition; infectious diseases, past and present; blood type, Rh, serology; EDC; obstetric history; pelvic measurements and present size of fetus; urinalysis, vital signs, weight gain; reassess for allergies.
2. Perform assessment techniques (see above).
3. Monitor labor—ongoing assessment of:
   a. Contractions—check at least every 30 minutes.
   b. Fetal response to labor—check and record every 15 to 20 minutes for FHR, fetal activity level, and amniotic fluid.
   c. Maternal response to labor (Table 3–16).
   d. Maternal vital signs.
      (1) Obtain between contractions.
      (2) Response to pain or use of special breathing technique alters the pulse and respiration.
      (3) BP if normotensive, take on admission, then every four hours and prn; after regional anesthesia, every 30 minutes.
      (4) TPR on admission, then every four hours and prn if within normal range.

(5) Prior to and after analgesia-anesthesia.

(6) After rupture of membranes (see *Amniotic fluid embolism,* p. 245).

e. Observe character and amount of show.

f. Monitor output and observe for bladder-filling (palpate abdomen just above symphysis. A full bladder may impede progress, or result in trauma to bladder.

4. Obtain admission urine (if membranes are intact).

a. Send to laboratory for routine urinalysis.

b. Check for protein and glucose.

5. Observe for signs of second stage.

a. Increased bloody-mucous vaginal drainage.

b. The mother saying, "It's coming!"

c. Bulging perineum.

6. Rupture of membranes—note, record, and report.

a. Time—danger of infection if ruptured more than 24 hours.

b. FHRs stat and ten minutes later (to check for prolapsed cord).

c. Amount—*polyhydramnios* (excessive fluid ≥ 2000 ml) is associated with anomalous development, high gastrointestinal-tract obstruction, for example; *oligoamnios* is associated with anomalous development of urinary tract.

d. Character—thick consistency and/or odor suggests infection.

e. Color:

(1) *Yellow* fluid may represent fetal distress about 36 hours previous, or Rh or ABO incompatibility.

(2) *Green* fluid and fetus in vertex position may indicate recent or current hypoxia.

(3) *Port-wine*-colored fluid may indicate abruptio placentae.

f. Check perineum for prolapsed cord and signs of imminent birth (crowning or bulging perineum).

g. Vaginal exam—effacement, dilatation, and check for cord.

B. Plan and implementation:

1. Psychosocial management—general comments. (See also Table 3–16, and *Education for childbirth*).

a. Respect gravida's desires concerning management of labor—degree of participation by self and significant other (husband or friend), and breathing and relaxation techniques.

b. Nurse the woman rather than the equipment.

c. Women in labor fear and dread being left alone, and can sue for "abandonment" if left alone.

d. Keep woman and family informed of progress.

e. Foster rest—keep noise level down and eliminate unnecessary talking and bright lights.

f. Coach throughout labor.

2. Physical management.

a. Perineal prep—shaving the perineum is still done in some hospitals for cleanliness.

b. Enema—soapsuds enema should never be given, as it is potentially dangerous; if needed, a Fleet's enema or equivalent is physiologically compatible; enema is *never* given if:

(1) There is vaginal bleeding.

(2) In presence of premature labor.

(3) Fetus is in abnormal presentation or position.

c. Encourage frequent emptying of bladder.

d. Encourage gravida to lie on side when she must be in bed.

(1) Allows gravity to help in anterior rotation of fetal head.

(2) Promotes relaxation.

(3) Prevents supine hypotension syndrome.

(4) Prevents aortoiliac compression by the contracting uterus (Poseiro effect).

e. Food and fluids per hospital and physician preference.

(1) Natural childbirth—may have clear fluids throughout.

(2) Ice chips or sips of water until delivery.

(3) NPO with IV.

(4) IV if regional anesthesia is started.

C. Continue ongoing evaluation for continual updating of plan and its implementation.

5. Management of discomfort during first stage of labor

A. Education for childbirth:

1. Grantly Dick-Read.

a. Basic premises—childbirth is a natural event; *tension* plus *fear* equals increased *pain* and increased pain perception.

b. Tension and fear are often reduced in prepared couples if the gravida comprehends contractions and the work and physiology of labor.

   c. Breathing techniques help the work of uterine contractions and relax the perineum for the birth process.

2. Psychoprophylactic childbirth—*Lamaze method.*

   a. Basic premises—a conditioned response to stimuli occupies nerve pathways thus dulling pain perception; education for the birth process replaces misconceptions and superstitions.

   b. Conditioned responses:

    (1) Concentration on a focal point.

    (2) Breathing techniques to cope with and to assist contractions, to prevent bearing down too soon by panting or use of pant-blow and to bear down when appropriate; the first and last two breaths should be cleansing breaths.

   c. The woman and her coach (husband or other) are also taught physiology and anatomy, psychology (of man and woman), and what to expect in the hospital setting.

   d. The woman requires active coaching to enable her to use breathing techniques appropriate for the phase of labor and to prevent hyperventilation (Figure 3–6).

    (1) First stage of labor—early: slow, deep chest-breathing pattern.

    (2) First stage of labor—"transition": rapid, shallow breathing pattern with panting, pant-blow technique, or "he-he" pattern to prevent pushing.

    (3) Second stage of labor: pushing or bearing down to aid fetal descent through birth canal; panting aids in relaxation between contractions and prevents head from "popping out" during delivery (see *When the nurse must assist the mother giving birth,* p. 217).

3. Other types of preparation-for-childbirth classes include classes for siblings, multiparas, and those who are planning a cesarean birth.

B. General nursing actions, irrespective of method used.*

   1. When necessary, remind the partner/coach of the appropriate breathing pattern or assist with effleurage.

2. Provide supplies for comfort measures: cool, wet washcloth, ice chips, or other fluid (approved by the physician or midwife).

3. Apply lip balm (Chapstick, petroleum jelly).

4. Offer moral support, encouragement, and praise as appropriate.

5. Exert firm counterpressure over the sacrococcygeal area or to the groin if the woman finds these offer relief.

6. Keep the woman and her partner/coach updated regarding her progress and any procedures she experiences.

7. Relieve the partner/coach for breaks as necessary.

8. Insist that the partner/coach get nourishment and fluids; offer these when possible.

9. If the woman and/or her partner/coach hyperventilates, suggest one of the following actions to increase $Paco_2$ and relieve symptoms (e.g., carpopedal spasms, faintness, dizziness):

   a. Breathe into a paper bag.

   b. Breathe into one's own cupped hands.

   c. Hold one's breath.

10. Then demonstrate the appropriate breathing pattern for a few contractions to help them reestablish the rate and rhythm.

11. Reassure the woman and her partner/coach that her irritability is all right.

12. Provide scrub clothes for the partner/coach early enough in labor to avoid a last-minute rush.

13. Direct the parturient to push out through the *vagina* (the directive to push as though one is having a bowel movement activates the wrong set of muscles).

14. Provide a mirror so the woman can see the efforts of her bearing-down and thus be motivated further.

15. Insist that only one person give her directions from the acceleration phase through delivery to avoid confusing her. Permit no extraneous chatter at this time, when she is most egocentric and vulnerable.

16. Support the woman and her partner/coach in decision-making regarding medication for relaxation or pain relief. Childbirth should not be an endurance test, nor should the woman be made to feel that she "failed" if she requests medicated relief.

---

*From Jensen, M. D., Benson, R. C., and Bobak, I. M.: Maternity care: the nurse and the family, ed. 2, St. Louis, Missouri, 1981, The C. V. Mosby Co.

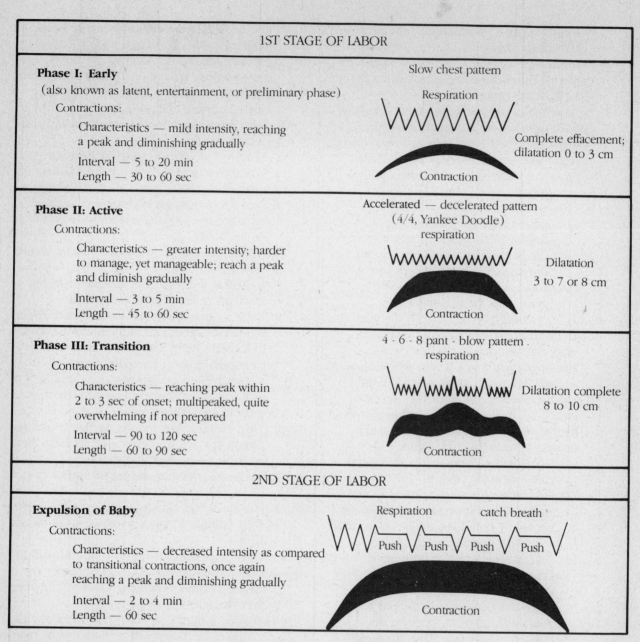

1ST STAGE OF LABOR

Phase I: Early

(also known as latent, entertainment, or preliminary phase)

Contractions:

    Characteristics — mild intensity, reaching a peak and diminishing gradually

    Interval — 5 to 20 min

    Length — 30 to 60 sec

Slow chest pattern

Respiration

Contraction

Complete effacement; dilatation 0 to 3 cm

Phase II: Active

Contractions:

    Characteristics — greater intensity; harder to manage, yet manageable; reach a peak and diminish gradually

    Interval — 3 to 5 min

    Length — 45 to 60 sec

Accelerated — decelerated pattern (4/4, Yankee Doodle) respiration

Contraction

Dilatation 3 to 7 or 8 cm

Phase III: Transition

Contractions:

    Characteristics — reaching peak within 2 to 3 sec of onset; multipeaked, quite overwhelming if not prepared

    Interval — 90 to 120 sec

    Length — 60 to 90 sec

4 - 6 - 8 pant - blow pattern respiration

Contraction

Dilatation complete 8 to 10 cm

2ND STAGE OF LABOR

Expulsion of Baby

Contractions:

    Characteristics — decreased intensity as compared to transitional contractions, once again reaching a peak and diminishing gradually

    Interval — 2 to 4 min

    Length — 60 sec

Respiration   catch breath

Push   Push   Push   Push

Contraction

FIGURE 3–6. Stages of labor, their characteristics, and Lamaze breathing techniques

Breathing techniques are used according to need. Phase does not dictate which technique should be used. (From Huprich, P.A. 1977. Assisting the couple through a Lamaze labor and delivery. *MCN: The American Journal of Maternal Child Nursing*, July/August. New York: American Journal of Nursing Company.

17. Some authorities are questioning the rigid adherence to breathing patterns advocated by proponents of prepared childbirth practices. The nurse must remember that these patterns need to be individualized to the woman and the situation. Relaxation, diversion, and disassociation may be achieved through the use of various techniques.

18. Share in the couple's joy (or in their grief).

C. Analgesia-anesthesia may be required or desirable (Table 3–17).

6. Nursing management during second stage of labor

A. Characteristics:
1. Average time—two minutes to one hour.
2. Vaginal discharge increases.
3. If regional anesthesia has not been given, reflex bearing down occurs with grunting sounds; may experience nausea, vomiting, shaking, and amnesia between contractions.
4. Perineum bulges with contractions—fetal head crowns, then head is born by extension.
5. Episiotomy may be performed now (medial or mediolateral) and head may be delivered by low forceps.
6. After restitution and external rotation of head, first shoulders, then rest of baby slips out with a gush of amniotic fluid.
7. Expulsion is accomplished by abdominal muscles (bearing down) and uterine contractions every 1½ to 3 minutes, lasting 60 to 90 seconds.

B. Assessment:
1. Assess mother's (or parents') response to labor and to the neonate.
2. Monitor FHR continuously by electronic monitor or by fetoscope after each contraction.
3. Time contractions and check BP every five minutes if mother has received regional anesthesia, to check for slowing of labor and hypotension.
4. Watch perineum for increased vaginal mucus, bulging, or crowning.
5. Assess environment for noise and unnecessary light.

C. Plan and implementation.
1. Never leave mother and father alone now, whether she is in labor or delivery room.
2. Keep mother and father informed; see that father is comfortable; reassure regarding mother's behavior if she is unanesthetized.
3. Coach breathing, bearing down with each con-

traction; encourage; adjust mirror so she can see bulging or crowning.
4. Ensure safety.
   a. Precautions when putting legs in stirrups:
      (1) Never put legs in stirrups if there are extensive varicosities.
      (2) Avoid pressure points to popliteal veins; pad stirrups.
      (3) Assure proper alignment by adjusting stirrups.
      (4) Move legs simultaneously when putting them into and taking them out of stirrups to avoid nerve, ligament, and muscle strain.
   b. Support woman in whatever position she will be giving birth.
   c. Cleanse perineum, thighs, and lower abdomen, using sterile technique.
5. Facilitate parent-child attachment.
   a. While protecting neonate from cold stress, facilitate and encourage parent(s) to see, hold, massage the neonate.
   b. Comment about neonate's individuality, characteristics, and behaviors.
   c. Mother breastfeeds newborn, if she wishes, after the neonate is assessed for congenital anomalies, such as esophageal atresia.
6. Maintain a comfortable environment, free of unnecessary noise and light, warm.

7. Third stage of labor—time between the delivery of the neonate and the complete delivery of the placenta.

A. Average time—five minutes.
B. Signs of placental separation:
1. Increase in bleeding.
2. Cord lengthens.
3. Uterus changes from a discoid to a globular shape.
4. Woman feels a contraction (if she is not anesthetized).
C. If placenta is retained, an "hourglass" shape to the uterus is noted.
D. Types of delivery:
1. Schultz—"shiny"; shiny fetal surface presents; most common.
2. Duncan—"dirty"; maternal surface presents.
E. Check for intactness and number of vessels in the cord.
F. If mother is to bottle feed, a drug to suppress lactation may be given as the placenta is delivered;

TABLE 3–17.   *Analgesia-anesthesia during childbirth**

Types	Characteristics	Nursing care
PSYCHOPROPHYLACTIC CHILDBIRTH Read Lamaze		Know method so as to be able to assist woman and her family.
ANALGESIA	Relieves pain or its perception.	Explain expected action of drug; *safety measures*—siderails and call bell; *record*—amount, route given, time, and woman's response; *monitor labor*—vital signs, contractions, bladder filling, and FHR; augment effect with comfort measures.
Barbiturates Secobarbital (Seconal) sodium Pentobarbital sodium (Nembutal) Amobarbital (Amytal)	Sedation; may depress neonate; produces excitement if given alone in presence of pain.	Best given in early latent phase of first stage of labor; must *not* be given with existing maternal or renal disorders.
Ataractics Promethazine HCl (Phenergan) Propiomazine (Largon) Hydroxyzine pamoate (Vistaril) Promazine HCl (Sparine)	Tranquility and sedation; potentiate narcotic; antiemetic.	Same as for Analgesia.
Narcotics Meperidine (Demerol) HCl	Slows labor, or accelerates labor as mother relaxes; may depress neonate; sedation.	Given in active phase, first stage, but *not* when delivery is expected in two hours; maternal vital signs and FHR before and every 15 to 30 minutes after administering.
Amnesics Scopolamine (belladonna alkaloid)	Dulls memory and parasympathetic nervous system.	Not recommended in Lamaze; given with narcotic to decrease possibility of excitation and hallucinations; stay with her.
Trichlorethylene (Trilene)	Given by inhalation, self-administered (usually) from a capsule and mask strapped to wrist; may cause cardiac arrhythmias.	Stay with woman; note pulse every 30 minutes and FHR every 15 minutes.
ANESTHESIA	Produces local or general loss of sensibility to touch, pain, or other stimulation.	Explain to woman; note history of allergy.
General Nitrous oxide (N_2O)—40%	Mother is not awake; *danger*—aspiration and respiratory depression; safer than regional anesthesia for hypovolemic clients; does not depress neonate unless mother is anesthetized deeply.	NPO with IVs.
Halothane (Flouthane)	Relaxes uterus quickly—facilitates intrauterine manipulation: version and extraction.	Observe for postpartum hemorrhage (from uterine atony); recovery room care.
Thiopental (Pentothal) sodium	Produces rapid induction of anesthesia; depresses neonate.	Recovery room care.

TABLE 3-17.   *(Continued)*

Types	Characteristics	Nursing care
REGIONAL ANALGESIA-ANESTHESIA		
Common agents in 0.5–1.0% solution Procaine HCl (Novocaine) Lidocaine (Xylocaine) Bupivacaine (Marcaine) HCl Tetracaine (Pontocaine) HCl Mepivacaine HCl (Carbocaine)	Used with epinephrine (or other vasoconstrictor drug) to (a) delay absorption, (b) prolong anesthetic effect, and (c) decrease chance of hypotension.	Note any history of allergy; note woman's response: (a) allergic reaction, (b) hypotension, and (c) lack of or wearing off of anesthetic effect.
Peripheral nerve block Pudendal (5–10 ml each side) anesthetizes lower two-thirds of vagina and perineum.	Perineal anesthesia of short duration (30 minutes) given for delivery and repair; local anesthesia; may be done by physician; simple and safe; does not depress neonate; may inhibit bearing-down reflex.	Explain to woman to get her cooperation during procedure.
Paracervical block (5–10 ml given into each side) anesthetizes cervix and upper two-thirds of vagina.	May be given between 3 and 8 cm by physician when woman is having at least three contractions in ten minutes; lasts 45–90 minutes, during which time woman may rest; can be repeated in 90 minutes; can be followed by local, epidural, or other; may cause temporary fetal bradycardia, which does not respond to treatment.	Explain to woman, especially length and type of needle; take maternal vital signs and FHR; have her void; help position her; monitor FHR continuously; monitor contractions; and watch for return of pain.
Local infiltration	Useful for perineal repairs.	No special nursing care.
Nerve root block	(a) Need trained anesthesiologist, (b) with proper administration, relieves pain completely, (c) may prolong labor if given too early, (d) hypotension from vasodilation (below anesthesia level) is likely, (e) fetal bradycardia from maternal hypotension, (f) bearing-down reflex is partially or completely eliminated, necessitating outlet forceps at delivery, (g) postanesthesia headache if medication mixes with cerebrospinal fluid, (h) fosters postpartum uterine and bladder atony, (i) woman is awake, and (j) can be used for women with metabolic, lung, and heart diseases.	Note history of allergy, skin infection over back, previous neural or spinal injury or disease, and attitude toward anesthesia; explain to her: (a) expected feeling as anesthesia begins, warm toes and as it wears off, tingling, (b) positioning—help position her, offering reassurance and support; take maternal vital signs and FHR; have her void; monitor labor; siderails; record; observe for return of pain.
Caudal	Useful during first and second stages; can be given "one-shot" or continuously; given in peridural space through sacral hiatus.	Treatment of hypotension (with resultant fetal bradycardia): (a) turn from supine to lateral, or elevate legs, (b) administer humidified oxygen by mask at 8–10 liters/minute, (c) increase rate of IV fluids (use infusate *without* Pitocin).

(Continued)

TABLE 3–17. *(Continued)*

Types	Characteristics	Nursing care
REGIONAL ANALGESIA-ANESTHESIA		
Epidural	Useful during first and second stages; can be given "one-shot" or continuously; given on top of (or over) dura through 3rd, 4th, or 5th lumbar interspace; risk of dura puncture.	Same as for Caudal.
Saddle (low spinal or subarachnoid)	Usually given "one-shot" when head is on perineum; medication is mixed with cerebrospinal fluid in subarachnoid space; injected through 3rd, 4th, or 5th lumbar interspace.	Postdelivery: encourage oral fluids; lying flat in bed for 8 to 12 hours; observe for headache and bladder and uterine atony.

*The medications presented are representative of those used for labor and birth.

otherwise, birth of placenta triggers the production of lactogenic hormone by the posterior pituitary.*

G. Oxytocin preparation to prevent uterine atony may be given after expulsion of placenta.

H. Continue to facilitate parent-child attachment (see above).

8. **Fourth stage of labor**—first hour postpartum (see p. 222).

9. **Newborn management during and immediately after birth**

A. As neonate's head is being born, or soon after neonate's birth, its oropharynx and nasopharynx are aspirated or drained.

B. Infant is usually held on same level as placenta until pulsation stops before cord is clamped and cut—to prevent fetal blood loss or overloading fetal cardiovascular system.

C. Dry infant quickly, and note Apgar score. Note and record at one minute and at five minutes of age (Table 3–18).
   1. Score of 7–10—infant is in good condition.
   2. Score of 4–6—infant is in fair condition; clear airway, give O_2 as needed; assess for CNS depression.
   3. Score of 0–3—infant is in poor condition; requires resuscitative measures immediately.
   4. Asphyxia neonatorum is defined as the absence of spontaneous breathing within the first 30 to 60 seconds after birth: hypercapnia (increase in CO_2) and hypoxia (decrease in O_2) result.

D. Maintain body temperature—quickly dry and warm infant.
   1. Conserves energy and preserves store of brown fat.
   2. Decreases need for oxygen and prevents acidosis.
   3. Assists respiratory efforts or resuscitative measures.

E. Ensure patent airway.
   1. Suction mouth first, then nose; sensitive receptors around entrance to nares, when stimulated, initiate a gasp, therefore mouth should be free of mucus first.
   2. Suction with bulb syringe.
   3. If deeper suctioning is needed, use a DeLee mucus trap; long and vigorous suctioning should be avoided because:
      a. Laryngospasm may result.
      b. Oxygen and air may be removed.
      c. Tissue trauma may result, with edema and bleeding.
      d. Cardiac arrhythmia may occur.
   4. Trendelenburg's and side-lying position—assist gravity drainage of fluids.

F. Identify infant by identiband or beads and footprints.

G. Prevent eye infection—silver nitrate, 1% (two drops in each eye) or penicillin ophthalmic ointment to prevent gonorrheal ophthalmia neonatorum; given within two hours of birth.

*Because antilactogenic drugs containing estrogens may be implicated in endometrial carcinoma, women are asked to sign an "informed consent" prior to receiving this medication.

TABLE 3–18. *Apgar score*

Sign	0	1	2
Heart rate	Absent	Below 100	Over 100
Respiratory effort	Absent	Slow and irregular	Good and crying
Muscle tone	Flaccid	Some flexion of extremities	Active motions, general flexion
Reflex irritability	No response	Weak cry or grimace	Cry
Color	Blue, pale	Body pink, extremities blue	Completely pink

H. Assess neonate's condition—gross, incomplete assessment at this time; record and report findings.
  1. Check cord for one vein and two arteries.
  2. Collect and send cord blood for appropriate test: Rh, Coombs', etc.
  3. Note any malformations and birth trauma (dislocated shoulder, lacerations, or scalp edema).
  4. Identify the preterm or postterm neonate; identify the dysmature neonate.
  5. Note skin color (cyanosis, jaundice) and condition (maceration, lesions).
  6. Note meconium staining—umbilical cord, skin, and nails.
  7. Note neonate's cry—presence, pitch, and quality.
  8. Note respirations and respiratory effort (nasal flaring, retractions, and expiratory grunt).
  9. Neurologic status.
I. Record significant data from mother's chart, diabetes, hypertension, course of labor, and fetal distress, for example; record delivery events.

10. When the nurse assists the mother giving birth

A. Nursing function when *mother* is giving birth:
  1. Reassure her.
  2. Assist infant with respirations—mucus, warmth, and resuscitative measures.
  3. Protect mother from injury, infection, and hemorrhage.
B. Follow these steps until physician arrives or you can get the mother and newborn to a medical facility; use aseptic technique if possible or be as clean as possible; do not touch birth canal without aseptic conditions prevailing.
  1. Delivery of the head—with clean or sterile towel, if available.
    a. Place gentle pressure with the palm of your hand on the head as it emerges from the introitus and ask mother to pant-breathe to prevent rapid perineal stretching and perhaps lacerations and to prevent injury to fetal head.
    b. As head emerges, feel with finger down nape of neck for cord; slip it over the head if possible, or down over the shoulders; if it is tight and you have sterile ties and scissors, tie the cord in two places, cut between the ties, unwrap cord, and proceed with delivery of shoulders.
    c. If membranes are not yet ruptured, as head is emerging, tear the membranes (caul) at the neck quickly so that the infant's first breath is in air; note color and character of fluid.
  2. Delivery of shoulders—hold head in both hands; after restitution, apply gentle pressure downward to deliver the anterior shoulder under the symphysis pubis, and then raise head gently to deliver the posterior shoulder.
  3. Support infant as rest of body slips out with a gush of amniotic fluid.
  4. Hold infant with head down—*do not hold by ankles or feet* as this may cause injury to cerebral capillaries by gravity and to the spine by overextension; do Apgar score.
    a. Infant can be cradled in arms while being held head down to allow drainage of fluids to prevent aspiration; hold infant at same level as placenta until cord stops pulsating; cradling also provides warmth.
    b. Suction mouth and nose with bulb syringe, if available.
    c. Cover infant with what is available; lay infant on its side, over mother's abdomen,

...es for
... as stimulating
... ate placenta.

... separation (see
... o deliver.
... ...in one to two
... by the expansion
... rd and by the
... piration; therefore, it
nee... ...en tied. May be cut
safely after on... even without sterile
equipment.

6. For added warmth, wrap infant and placenta together and give to mother.
7. To prevent maternal hemorrhage:
   a. Put infant to breast.
   b. Gently massage fundus; express clots gently when uterus is contracted.
   c. If mother's bladder is full, have her void.
8. Record the events of delivery.
9. Stay with mother and child until assistance arrives; give appropriate praise to mother for her efforts, encourage her to talk about the experience with you if she wishes.
10. If placenta does not separate *do not pull* on cord.
    a. If no sterile supplies are available, *do not cut cord;* take mother to medical facility.
    b. Place baby in mother's arms and at breast to feed if cord is long enough—may stimulate placental separation.
    c. Place baby on mother's abdomen or between legs if cord is short.
    d. Rationale:
       (1) Pulling on cord before placenta separates may invert uterus and result in infection and massive hemorrhage.
       (2) Abnormal implantation of placenta—
          (a) Placenta accreta has partially grown into myometrium; treatment—hysterectomy.
          (b) Placenta increta has completely grown into myometrium (no decidua present); treatment—hysterectomy.
11. If neonate *does not breathe spontaneously:*
    a. Maintain body temperature—dry and cover.
    b. Clear airway—turn head to side, lower head, and clear mouth with finger.
    c. Stimulate gently—rub back and flick soles of feet.

   d. Slightly extend neck to "sniffing position," place mouth over neonate's nose and mouth and exhale air in cheeks, saying "ho" (prevents excessive pressure).
   e. If in hospital, use other techniques (see p. 216).
   f. Cardiopulmonary resuscitation (CPR)— with two fingers over middle third of sternum, compress ½ to ¾ inches, 100–120 times per minute. Breathe neonate (with your mouth over the neonate's nose and mouth) on the upstroke of each fifth sternal compression. The ratio is 1:5.

11. **Operative obstetrics**—surgical procedures during labor or delivery.
A. Episiotomy—incision of perineum to facilitate the birth of the infant.
   1. Types:
      a. Midline—greater chance of extension into anal sphincter than mediolateral.
      b. Mediolateral—healing is more painful than midline.
   2. Rationale:
      a. Substitutes a surgical incision for a possible laceration.
      b. Easier to heal than a laceration.
      c. Protects infant's head from being forced against a resistant perineum (as in premature delivery).
      d. Shortens second stage.
      e. Prevents overstretching of maternal perineum.
   3. Nursing assessment:
      a. Observe and assess for hematoma and infection.
      b. Evaluate pain in area—if excessive and episiotomy is not the source, report immediately; a vulvar, paravaginal, or ischiorectal abscess or hematoma may be the underlying cause of the pain.
   4. Nursing plan/implementation:
      a. Cleanliness.
      b. Ice bag during first hour postpartum to decrease edema formation and discomfort.
      c. Analgesics, topical sprays, Tucks, heat lamps, and sitz baths for comfort and to promote healing. Teach her proper way to sit; avoid sitting on one hip.
B. Forceps delivery—delivery of the head with the aid of forceps.
   1. Types:
      a. Low—outlet forceps.

b. Mid—applied after head is engaged.

c. High—applied before engagement has taken place; rarely done; very hazardous.

d. Piper—applied on the after-coming head in breech deliveries.

2. Conditions for applying forceps:
   a. Engaged fetal head.
   b. Ruptured membranes.
   c. Full dilatation.
   d. Absence of cephalopelvic disproportion.
   e. Some anesthesia has been given and an episiotomy has usually been performed.
   f. Empty bladder and rectum.

3. Indications for forceps delivery:
   a. Fetal distress.
   b. Maternal need.
      (1) Exhaustion.
      (2) Concurrent disease condition such as cardiac disorder.
      (3) Poorly progressing second stage, secondary inertia, for example.
      (4) Persistent transverse or posterior fetal position.

4. Possible complications:
   a. Maternal—lacerations of birth canal, rectum-bladder injury, or uterine rupture.
   b. Birth injury—cephalhematoma, skull fracture, brain damage, intracranial hemorrhage, facial paralysis, cord compression, and direct tissue trauma (abrasions and ecchymoses).

5. Nursing assessment:
   a. Listen to FHR after forceps application—forceps blade may compress cord.
   b. Observation of mother-newborn for complications or injury.

6. Nursing plan/implementation:
   a. Support mother, who may feel that baby was taken from her—that she did not give birth to baby.
   b. Support for the parents if bruising or complications occur.

C. Cesarean birth—incision through abdominal wall and uterus to deliver the products of conception.
   1. Types:
      a. Low segment—preferred method, transverse incision into lower uterine segment, and skin incision is longitudinal or transverse.
         (1) Fewer immediate complications—less blood loss, more comfortable convalescence, and less intestinal obstruction.
         (2) Fewer future complications—less chance of uterine rupture and less adhesion formation.
      b. Classical—longitudinal incision through skin and into body of uterus.
         (1) More bleeding, scar tissue, and adhesion formation.
         (2) Necessary for anterior placenta previa and transverse lie.
      c. Extraperitoneal—transverse incision through skin and into lower uterine segment without entering peritoneal cavity; used less now with availability of blood replacement and antibiotic therapy.
      d. Porro's—hysterotomy followed by hysterectomy—necessary in presence of hemorrhage from atony, placenta previa, abruptio placentae, placenta accreta, ruptured uterus, fibromyomata, or cancer of cervix or ovary.

   2. Indications:
      a. Cephalopelvic disproportion (CPD).
      b. Previous surgery on uterus.
      c. Uterine dysfunction.
      d. Placental condition—placenta previa and abruptio placentae with Couvelaire uterus.
      e. Maternal disease—diabetes, preeclampsia/eclampsia, genital herpes (active).
      f. Malposition or malpresentation of fetus—some favor a cesarean delivery for all nulliparas with a breech presentation.
      g. Fetal distress.
      h. Postterm pregnancy.
      i. Neoplasms of the birth canal or uterus.
      j. Fetal jeopardy—Rh incompatibility and diabetic or preeclamptic/eclamptic mother.
      k. Prolapsed cord.

   3. Nursing care—same as for other preoperative and postoperative patients except for:
      a. Monitoring FHR prior to surgery.
      b. Alerting pediatrician for delivery.
      c. Postpartum check (see p. 222).

D. *Induction of labor*—initiation or augmentation of labor.
   1. Indications for induction:
      a. Maternal—
         (1) Woman with history of fast or silent labors or who lives far from the hospital.
         (2) Premature separation of low-lying placenta with uncontrolled bleeding; after artificial rupture of membranes, presenting part moves down and acts as a tamponade during labor.

(3) Uncontrolled progressive preeclampsia or diabetes.

(4) Active herpes, intact membranes.

(5) Premature rupture of membranes (PROM) that increases the possibility of intrauterine infection and prolapsed cord.

b. Fetal—

(1) Maternal diabetes.

(2) Rh or ABO incompatibility.

(3) Postterm date.

(4) Congenital anomaly, anencephaly, for example.

2. Conditions for successful induction:

a. Absence of CPD, malposition, or malpresentation.

b. Engaged vertex of single gestation.

c. Close to, or at, term.

d. Fetal lung maturity—better survival rate if 32 weeks or more with an L/S ratio greater than 2:1, or, if the mother is diabetic, if phosphotidylglycerol is found in amniotic fluid.

e. "Ripe" cervix—softening, partially effaced, or ready for effacement or dilatation if it has not yet begun (intravaginal or paracervical application of prostaglandin gel or laminaria may be used to prepare the cervix for labor).

3. Amniotomy:

a. Definition—artificial rupture of membranes to:

(1) Induce labor.

(2) Increase efficiency of contractions.

(3) Shorten labor.

(4) Apply (pressure of) presenting part to low-lying placenta to minimize separation.

b. Nursing assessment—same as for spontaneous rupture of membranes.

(1) Monitor FHR and assess for fetal distress (p. 245).

(2) Observe for prolapsed cord.

(3) Observe fluid (p. 210).

(4) Assess fetal activity.

(a) Excessive activity may indicate fetal distress.

(b) Absence of activity may indicate fetal demise.

4. Intravenous infusion of oxytocin (Pitocin or Syntocinon):

a. With physician on the unit and with a double set-up running (one bottle of fluid with oxytocin and one without) connected to a three-way stopcock at the point where the needle enters the vein.

(1) Monitor drop rate continuously (best to use a controlled-infusion pump).

(2) Monitor each contraction—must not be closer together than two minutes, nor last longer than 90 seconds (a fetal monitor with a continuous read-out of FHR and uterine activity is appropriate).

(3) Monitor maternal vital signs, especially blood pressure.

(4) Monitor output because of Pitocin's slight antidiuretic effect.

b. Danger to fetus—

(1) Decreased oxygen concentration in cord blood with hypoxia; followed by asphyxia neonatorum.

(2) Anoxia with tetanic contractions; death.

(3) Arrhythmias.

c. Danger to mother—

(1) Uterine rupture.

(2) Postpartum hemorrhage.

(3) Oxytocin toxicity.

(4) Water intoxication following infusion over long periods.

(5) Allergic reaction.

(6) Abruptio placentae.

(7) Hypertensive crisis with possible cerebral hemorrhage.

5. Buccal oxytocin (Pitocin):

a. 200-unit tablet placed between gums and cheek.

b. Rate of absorption unpredictable.

c. Monitor FHR, maternal blood pressure, and contractions.

d. To deactivate tablet, ask woman to spit it out or swallow it; rinse mouth.

e. Toxicity—allergy or hypertension.

PUERPERIUM

Puerperium is the period of time spanning the first six weeks after the birth of the placenta. It is characterized by anabolic activity of lactation and catabolic activity in the uterus known as involution. During the puerperium, body tissues, especially reproductive organs, return to near prepregnant state; rate of involution or retrogression increases if the woman breastfeeds.

1. *Theoretic basis*

A. Uterus:
1. Reduction in size and weight.
   a. Autolysis—breakdown of muscle protein (decrease in myometrial cell size) and connective tissue collagen and elastin; excreted in the urine.
   b. Lochia—sloughing of the decidua and blood.
   c. Size—after delivery 1000 g (2.2 lb); one week 500 g (1.1 lb); and two weeks 350 g (11 oz).
2. Formation of new endometrium.
   a. Twenty-one days—newly formed except for placental site.
   b. Six weeks—placental site healed without scarring by process of exfoliation.
3. Height of fundus.
   a. After delivery—at umbilicus, size of grapefruit and firm.
   b. Day one—one finger above umbilicus.
   c. Involutes by one finger's breadth each day, until day ten.
   d. Day ten—behind symphysis pubis.
4. "After pains"—discomfort of uterine contractions; intensity, frequency, and regularity decrease after first postpartum day.
   a. Primipara—uterus remains contracted, often does not feel "after pains."
   b. Multipara—uterus relaxes and contracts, felt as "after pain."
   c. Increased by *breastfeeding,* after delivering a large baby, and in presence of retained placental fragments.
5. Lochia—blood from placental site, decidua, and mucus.
   a. Amount lost in six weeks—225 g.
   b. Days *one to three*—rubra (bright red).
   c. Days *three to seven*—serosa (pink to brown).
   d. By day ten—alba (creamy white), contains many microorganisms and leukocytes.
   e. Investigate—
      (1) If bright red after day three—possible retention of placental fragments.
      (2) Clots—hemorrhage.
      (3) Putrid odor—infection.
      (4) Lochia beyond three weeks—subinvolution (see page 253).

B. Cervix:
1. After delivery—bruised, small tears, and admits a hand.
2. Eighteen hours—becomes shorter, firmer, and regains its shape.
3. One week—admits two fingers.
4. Never fully returns to prepregnant state.
   a. Os is wider and not perfectly round, as it is in nullipara.
   b. Lacerations heal as scars radiating from os.

C. Vagina and pelvic floor:
1. Vagina—never fully returns to prepregnant state.
   a. After delivery—thin-walled from hormone (estrogen) deprivation; few rugae.
   b. Week three—rugae reappear.
   c. Hymen, if torn, may heal as fibrosed mucosal nodules, called curunculae myrtiformes.
2. Pelvic floor—
   a. After delivery—infiltrated with blood, stretched, and torn.
   b. Month six—considerable tone regained.

D. Perineum:
1. After delivery—edematous, may have episiotomy (or repaired lacerations) or hemorrhoids.
2. Hematoma—blood in connective tissue beneath skin; mass is painful, tense, and fluctuant.

E. Abdominal wall:
1. Overdistention during pregnancy may cause rupture of elastic fibers, persistent striae, and diastasis of the rectus muscles.
2. Usually takes six to eight weeks to retrogress.
3. Strenuous exercises are discouraged until after eight weeks postpartum.

F. Cardiovascular system:
1. After delivery—increased cardiac load as uterine blood flow is redirected to general circulation.
2. Blood volume returns to prepregnant state (5 to 6 liters down to 4 liters) in about three weeks (two-thirds of this reduction occurs by the end of the first week through diuresis and diaphoresis).
3. Blood values (Table 3–19)—
   a. High white-cell count during labor (25,000/ml) returns to normal level within the first few days.
   b. Week one—hemoglobin, RBC, hematocrit, and elevated fibrinogen return to normal.
4. Blood coagulation—
   a. During pregnancy, there is an increased concentration of clotting factors, with a large deposition of fibrin in the placental bed.
   b. During labor, there is a rapid consumption of clotting factors that formed during pregnancy.

TABLE 3–19. *Blood values*

Component	Pregnant	Prepregnant
WBC	9–16,000 (25,000–labor)	4–11,000
RBC volume	1900 ml	1600 ml
Plasma volume	3700 ml	2400 ml
Hct (PCV)	32–42%	37–47%
Hgb (at sea level)	10–14 g/dl	12–16 g/dl
Fibrinogen	400 mg/dl	250 mg/dl

    c. During puerperium, although consumption of clotting factors increases, extensive activation of clotting factors (platelets, fibrinogen, factor VIII) keeps levels above prepregnant levels during the first week postpartum.

    d. The secondary increase in clotting factors during the puerperium, together with immobility, sepsis, or trauma during delivery, predisposes to thromboembolic complications (pulmonary emboli).

  5. Vital signs—

    a. Temperature—normal, except if dehydrated or fatigued; puerperal infection, 38 C (100.4 F) on two consecutive postpartal days, starting with day two.

    b. Pulse—bradycardia (50 to 70) common on days one and two, but may persist seven to ten days; cause unknown.

    c. Blood pressure—generally unchanged.

G. Urinary tract:

  1. Twelve hours to five days—diuresis (daily output may reach 3000 ml).

  2. Urine constituents—

    a. Sugar—primarily lactose.

    b. Acetonuria—following prolonged labor.

    c. Proteinuria for first three days.

  3. Edema, trauma, and anesthesia may result in retention with overflow.

  4. Dilatation of ureters subsides in a few weeks.

H. Integument—skin:

  1. Striae—persist as silvery lines.

  2. Diastasis recti abdominis—some midline separation may persist (see Abdominal wall, p. 221).

  3. Diaphoresis—excessive perspiration for first few days (approximately five).

I. Legs:

  1. Should have no redness, tenderness, local areas of increased skin temperature, or edema.

  2. Homan's sign should be negative (no calf pain when knee is extended and gentle pressure is applied to dorsiflex the foot).

  3. May have soreness from delivery position.

J. Weight:

  1. After delivery—

    a. Loss—fetus, placenta, amniotic fluid, tissue fluid.

    b. Abdomen protrudes.

    c. Mother weighs more than in prepregnant state.

  2. Week six—weight reduction is individual.

K. Menstruation and ovarian function: first menstrual cycle may be anovulatory.

  1. Nonnursing—ovulation four to six weeks and menstruation six to eight weeks.

  2. Nursing—anovulatory period varies (39 days to six months or more); some for duration of lactation; some for 8 to 14 months; contraceptive value, very unreliable.

L. Breasts:

  1. Nonlactating—lactosuppressant, testosterone enanthate and estradiol valerate (Deladumone OB) IM given as placenta starts to separate. The FDA (1977) specifies that women must sign an informed consent prior to receiving estrogens for any reason.

  2. Lactating (see p. 229).

M. Postpartal checkup—six weeks:

  1. Weight, vital signs, urine for protein, and complete blood count (CBC).

  2. Breast exam—lactating or not.

  3. Pelvic exam—involution and position of uterus, perineal healing, and tone of pelvic floor.

  4. Contraception implemented.

2. Nursing management: first hour postpartum (fourth stage of labor)

A. Assessment—every 15 minutes four times (then every 30 minutes two times or until stable).

  1. Height and firmness of fundus.

  2. Blood pressure.

  3. Pulse.

  4. Lochia—amount, color, number of clots, character, and odor.

  5. Perineum—healing and drainage.

  6. Bladder fullness.

  7. Rate of IV if present; note any added medication.

8. Recovery from analgesia-anesthesia.
9. Interaction between woman and husband (or other): verbal, nonverbal (posture, expressions).
10. Interaction between parent(s) and newborn infant.

B. Interventions and rationale—every 15 minutes for one hour or until stable. Most frequent complication is hemorrhage (leading cause of maternal death; see p. 170).

1. Boggy fundus—gentle massage to avoid uterine fatigue; express clots after fundus is firm.
2. Note and report hypotension (see p. 252) that may be caused by hemorrhage, reaction to anesthesia, or other.
3. Report increase in blood pressure—postpartum preeclampsia/eclampsia is possible, especially during the first 48 hours.
4. Rapid pulse—assess blood pressure, pulse, and bleeding; report.
5. Lochia—more than one soaked pad (100 ml) in one hour and clots, report to and save for physician; order blood; add oxytocin to IV as ordered; or give oxytocin orally.
6. Perineum—apply covered ice pack over episiotomy during the first hour after delivery to discourage edema and numb the area; assess for hematoma formation and pain: report to physician and/or medicate prn. Apply clean pad and give peri-care after each voiding and/or every three hours—teach good handwashing.
7. Bladder—check frequently for full bladder because as it fills, the bladder causes the uterus to rise and relax and bleed. Record voiding or catheterization; character of urine, time, and amount.
8. IV—discontinue when finished or add new bottle if bleeding is excessive or if not fully recovered from anesthesia.
9. Caution woman not to get out of bed (after caudal and epidural); keep her flat in bed after saddle block for the time specified by the physician. Even if woman delivered without any medication, caution her to have assistance the first time she ambulates.
10. Mate and newborn may visit continuously (some units have double beds for the new family); newborn may nurse.

C. Parent-child attachment.*

---

* "Attachment" is used instead of "bonding."

1. Mother and father should see, touch, hold, and fondle infant immediately following birth if physically possible, to begin attachment.
2. Early sustained contact with child facilitates the process of grieving for the loss of the fantasy baby and the identification and acceptance of the real baby.
3. Nursing at the breast stimulates uterine contractions and hastens involution.

3. Nursing management: subsequent postpartal care

A. Assessment—minimum two times per day—
1. Vital signs.
2. Fundus, lochia, and perineum.
3. Voiding and bowel function.
4. Breasts.
5. Legs.
6. Emotional status and response to baby.

B. Interventions and rationale—
1. Follow prescribed treatment for excessive bleeding, fever, urine retention, and constipation.
2. Medicate as ordered.
   a. Stool softeners.
   b. Analgesics; sedatives for sleep.
   c. Uterine contraction—ergot products (Methergine, Ergotrate, and Ergonovine); give if woman is normotensive, usually 0.2 mg (1/300 or 1/320 gr) q4h × 6 doses. Oxytocins may be substituted for ergot products if she is hypertensive.
3. Perineal care—teach regarding:
   a. Shower for cleanliness.
   b. Wash hands, wipe from front to back once per tissue, apply clean pad from front to back, and wash hands.
   c. Comfort—Tucks, anesthetic sprays, heat lamp, and sitz baths; keep buttocks together and tightened when in process of standing up, sitting down, and getting out of bed.
4. Breasts—lactating mothers (see p. 229). Teach regarding breast self-examination (SEB).
5. Meet nutritional needs.
6. Meet need for rest.
7. Anticipatory guidance:
   a. Process of involution (see p. 221).
   b. Resumption of intercourse (see p. 191).
   c. Contraception—pills are resumed *after* first menstrual period (if not breastfeeding); use of IUDs or diaphragms is generally determined at six-week check-up (if she is

using diaphragm, size and fit must be readjusted after birth of baby).

d. Exercises—

   (1) Many organizations and agencies sponsor exercise programs for new mothers, such as YWCA, parent education groups, community colleges, private agencies.

   (2) Purposes: regain muscle tone and relieve tension and backache.

   (3) Some exercises suggested for weeks one through eight:

      (a) Deep abdominal breathing.
      (b) Head raising.
      (c) Stretching from head to toe.
      (d) Lower back exercise.
      (e) Kegal (to strengthen pubococcygeal muscles, regain perineal tone).

   (4) More strenuous exercises that are not suitable until much later in the puerperium, such as those used to strengthen and firm the abdominal muscles. If these are done, the woman starts by lying recumbent with knees slightly bent: leg-raising; sit-ups (only as far as lifting head and shoulders off floor).

8. Assist with psychologic tasks—maternal role- taking.

   a. See *Attachment,* p. 223.

   b. Need to *integrate* labor and delivery experience by talking about it; need to express disappointment, if any; and need for compliments for what she (and spouse) did well.

   c. Early phase (days one to three)—labeled by R. Rubin as *"taking-in,"* is characterized by passivity; dependency; talkativeness; concern for self needs, such as eating, sleeping, and eliminating; and desire to be taken care of.

   d. "Taking-hold" phase (third day to two weeks)—mother is impatient to have control over own body functions, to learn how to care for own baby ("mothering tasks") with assurance that she is doing a good job now; builds foundation for future success in mother-child relationship.

   e. "Letting-go" phase—begins during pregnancy and continues in the puerperium; mother must give up or "let go" of her former role and self-concept and integrate her new role and self-concept as a mother; may have concerns about ability or willingness to incorporate several roles.

   f. "Postpartum blues" (often experienced by the father as well).

      (1) Thought to be the result of a combination of hormonal changes, the realization of the need to change to take on the new role and let go of the old, and the extent of maternal responsibilities and fatigue (sleep deprivation).

      (2) This can be frightening, if unprepared; she and spouse should be assured that crying helps (if she chooses to cry).

      (3) May appear by fourth or fifth day as hormone levels drop.

   g. Lag in experiencing "maternal feelings"— first described by Gerald Caplan; each must be prepared that this experience is possible, especially for the primipara; "maternal lag," with resultant guilt feelings, may contribute to "blues"; lag is possible to extend over six months, but usually is resolved by four to six weeks; maternal lag may be greatly diminished or avoided if the mother is able to see and hold her newborn immediately after giving birth.

   h. Parents' groups are now being offered in many cities to help people deal with these postpartal feelings.

THE NEWBORN INFANT

1. Admission to the nursery

A. Delivery nurse reports significant events from mother's history, labor, and delivery and newborn's condition.

B. Place newborn in warm environment, take rectal temperature, weigh, and measure—length, and head and chest circumferences; check respirations q1h × 5; take apical pulse q1h × 3; and give IM vitamin K (if ordered) into anterior or lateral thigh muscle.

C. Assess for gestational age. (For detailed discussion, see *Classification of infants by weight and gestational age,* p. 255, and Tables 3–25 and 3–26.)

D. Do *physical assessment* of term neonates (Table 3–20).

E. Neonate may be bathed when temperature is stable.

TABLE 3–20. *Physical assessment of the term neonate*

Criterion	Average values and normal variations	Deviations from normal
VITAL SIGNS		
Heart rate	120–140/minute, irregular, especially when crying, and functional murmur.	Faint sound—pneumomediastinum; and heart rate under 100 or over 180/minute.
Respiratory rate	30–60/minute with short periods of apnea, irregular; cry—vigorous and loud.	Distress—chin tug, flaring of nares, retractions, tachypnea, grunting, excessive mucus, under 30 or over 60 per minute and weak, high-pitched cry.
Temperature	Stabilizes about 8 to 10 hours after birth; 36.5–37 C (97.7–98.6 F) axillary.	Unreliable indicator of infection.
Blood pressure	80/46; varies with change in activity level.	Hypotension: with RDS. Hypertension: coarctation of aorta.
MEASUREMENTS		
Weight	3400 g (7½ lb)	See Table 3–9.
Length	50 cm (20 inches)	
Chest circumference	2 cm (¾ inch) less than head circumference	If relationship varies, check for reason.
Head circumference	33–35 cm (13–14 inches)	Check for microcephalus and macrocephalus (4 cm or more larger than chest circumference).
GENERAL ASSESSMENT		
Muscle tone	Good tone and generalized flexion; full range of motion; spontaneous movement.	Flaccid, and persistent tremor or twitching; limited movement; asymmetric movement.
Skin color	Mottling, Harlequin's syndrome, acrocyanosis, and physiologic jaundice. Petechiae (over presenting part), ecchymoses (from forceps), milia, mongolian spotting, telangiectases, lanugo, and vernix caseosa.	Pallor, plethora, cyanosis, and jaundice within 24 hours of birth. Petechiae or ecchymoses elsewhere; all rashes, except newborn rash (erythema toxicum); pigmented nevi; hemangioma; and yellow vernix.
Skin character	Thick with superficial or deep cracking, pinch test negative.	Thin texture; parchmentlike texture; pinch test positive.
Head	Molding of fontanels and suture spaces; comprises 1/4th of body length.	Cephalhematoma, caput succedaneum, sunken or bulging fontanels, and closed sutures; wide fontanels and wide space between sutures.
Hair	Silky, single strands; lies flat; grows toward face and neck.	Fine, wooly; unusual swirls, patterns, hair line; coarse.
Eyes	Edematous eyelids, conjunctival hemorrhage; grayish-blue to grayish-brown in color; blink reflex; usually no tears; uncoordinated movements, although may focus for a few seconds; good placement on face; white discharge from silver nitrate; cornea is bright and shiny; pupillary reflex equal and reactive to light; red reflex; eyebrows distinct.	Epicanthal folds (in non-Orientals); discharges; agenesis; small eyeballs; opaque lenses; lesions (coloboma); strabismus; "doll's eyes" beyond 10 days; absence of reflexes: red, pupillary, corneal, blink.
Nose	Appears to have no bridge; should have no discharge; obligate nose breathers; sneezes to clear nose.	Discharge and choanal atresia; malformed; flaring of nares beyond first few moments of life.

(Continued)

TABLE 3–20.   *(Continued)*

Criterion	Average values and normal variations	Deviations from normal
GENERAL ASSESSMENT		
Mouth	Epstein's pearls on gum ridges; symmetrical lip movement; tongue does not protrude and moves freely, symmetrically; uvula in midline; reflexes present: sucking, rooting, gag, extrusion.	Cleft lip or palate; teeth; cyanosis; circumoral pallor; asymmetric lip movement; macroglossia; excessive saliva; micrognathia; thrush; incomplete or absent reflexes.
Ears	Well formed, firm; notch of ear should be on straight line with outer canthus.	Low placement, clefts; and tags; malformed; lack of cartilage.
Face	Symmetrical movements and contours.	Facial palsy (7th cranial nerve); looks "odd" or "funny."
Neck	Short, freely movable, and sternocliedomastoid muscles are even; thyroid not palpable; some head control.	Wry neck, webbed neck; restricted movement; masses; distended veins; absence of head control.
Chest	Enlarged breasts, "witch's milk," barrel-shaped, especially when asleep; both sides move synchronously; well-formed nipples, symmetrically placed.	Misshapen, flattened, funnel-chested, and asynchronous movement; lack of breast tissue; fracture of clavicle(s); supernumerary or widely spaced nipples; bowel sounds (see diaphragmatic hernia).
Abdomen	Dome-shaped, abdominal respirations, soft, and may have small umbilical hernia; umbilical cord well formed, containing 2 arteries and 1 vein; dry around base; linea nigra; bowel sounds within 2 hours of birth; no bladder distention and is voiding; passage of meconium.	Scaphoid-shaped, omphalocele, diastasis of recti abdominis muscles (in midline), and distention; umbilical cord containing 1 artery; redness or drainage around base of cord with or without offensive odor.
Genitalia 1. Female	Large labia, may have some bloody discharge per vagina, smegma, and tags; vaginal orifice open; increased pigmentation; ecchymosis and edema following breech birth; vaginal tags; pink-stained urine (uric acid crystals).	Agenesis and imperforate hymen; ambiguous; labia widely separated, fecal discharge per vagina; epispadias or hypospadias.
2. Male	Pendulous scrotum covered with rugae and testes usually descended; voids with adequate stream; increased pigmentation; edema and ecchymosis following breech birth.	Phimosis and epispadias or hypospadias; ambiguous; scrotum smooth and testes undescended.
Extremities	Synchronized movements, freely movable through full range of motion, legs appear bowed, and feet appear flat; attitude of general flexion; arms longer than legs; grasp reflex; normal palmar and sole creases; normal contour.	Fractures (clavicle and femur), brachial nerve palsy, clubbed foot, phocomelia or amelia, unusual number or webbing of digits, and abnormal palmar creases; poor muscle tone; asymmetric movement; increased muscle tone; unusual hip contour with "shortened" leg and click sign (hip dysplasia); hypermobility of joints.
Back	Spine straight, easily movable, and flexible; may have small pilonidal dimple at base of spine; may raise head when prone; reflexes present; trunk incurvation, magnet reflex, crossed extension.	Fusion of vertebrae; pilonidal dimple with tuft of hair, spina bifida, and agenesis of part of vertebral bodies; limitation of movement; weak or absent reflexes.

TABLE 3–20. *(Continued)*

Criterion	Average values and normal variations	Deviations from normal
GENERAL ASSESSMENT		
Anus	Patent, well placed, and "wink" reflex.	Imperforate, and absence of "wink" (absence of sphincter muscle); fistula.
Stools	Meconium within first 24 hours; transitional—days 2 to 5; breastfed: loose, golden yellow; bottle-fed: formed, light yellow.	Light-colored meconium, inspissated (dry, hard), or absent with distended abdomen (cystic fibrosis or Hirschsprung's disease); diarrhetic.
REFLEXES	Well-developed and complete Moro reflex; tonic neck; grasp—palmar and plantar; rooting; suck; swallow; gag; cough; sneeze; stepping; pupillary; Babinski's; tongue extrusion.	Incomplete, absent, or asynchronous responses need to be evaluated for neurologic development and musculoskeletal intactness.
LABORATORY VALUES		
Hemoglobin (cord)	13.6–19.6 g/dl	Evaluate for anemia and persistent polycythemia.
Serum bilirubin	2–6 mg/dl	Identify and treat hyperbilirubinemia (term: 12 mg or more; preterm: 15 mg or more) to prevent kernicterus.
Blood glucose	Over 30–40 mg/dl for term, and over 20 mg/dl for preterm.	Identify hypoglycemia prior to overt or asymptomatic hypoglycemia—do Dextrostix on all suspects (large- or small-for-gestational-age neonates, or neonates of diabetic mothers).
NEUROLOGIC EXAMINATION*	Specific to gestational age and state of wakefulness.	
1. Behavioral patterns	Cortical control and responsiveness.	
a. Feeding	Variations in interest, hunger. Usually feeds well within 48 hours.	Lethargic. Tires easily or may perspire while attempting to feed. Poor suck, poor coordination with swallow. Cyanosis, choking.
b. Social	Crying is lusty, strong, and soon indicative of hunger, pain, attention-seeking. Smiling, vocalizing evident within first week. Responds by quietness and increased alertness to cuddling, voice.	Absent; no focusing on person holding him/her; unconsolable.
c. Sleep-wakefulness	Transitional period with 2 periods of reactivity: at birth, and 6–8 hours later. Stabilization with wakeful periods about every 3–4 hours.	Lethargy, drowsiness. Disorganized pattern.
d. Elimination	Develops own pattern within first 2 weeks. Stooling: see Stools. Urination: first few days: 3–4 qd. end of first week: 5–6 qd. later: 6–10 qd, with adequate hydration.	See Stools. Diminished number: dehydration.

(Continued)

TABLE 3–20. *(Continued)*

Criterion	Average values and normal variations	Deviations from normal
NEUROLOGIC EXAMINATION*		
2. Reflex response	Brain stem development and musculoskeletal intactness.	Present in anencephalic infants also.
	Well-developed and intact response: startle, Moro, tonic neck, palmar and plantar grasp, rooting, suck and swallow present and coordinated, gag, cough, stepping, pupillary, Babinski, cremasteric.	Absent, hyperactive, incomplete, asynchronous.
3. Sensory capabilities		
a. Vision	Limited accommodation with clearest vision within 7–8 inches.	Absence of these responses may be due to absence of or diminished acuity or to sensory deprivation.
	Detects color by 2 months but attracted by black-white pattern by 5 days. Focuses and follows by 15 minutes of age. Prefers patterns to plain. Prefers changes in patterns by 2 months. At birth, can gaze intently (comes well equipped for early attachment process).	
b. Hearing	By 2 minutes of age, can move in direction of sound. Responds to high pitch by "freezing," followed by agitation; to low pitch (crooning) by relaxing. Ability to hear begins in last trimester of fetal life.	Absence of response: deafness.
c. Touch	Sensitivity to pain may be diminished (?). Soothed by massaging, warmth, weightlessness (as in water bath).	Unable to be comforted: possible drug dependence.
d. Smell	By 5th day can distinguish between mother's breasts and those of another woman.	
e. Taste	Under 3 days, can distinguish between sucrose and glucose and grimace in response to drop of lemon juice on tongue.	
f. Motor	Coordinates body movement to parent's voice and body movement; imitates parent's actions by 2 weeks.	Absence.

*Based on Brazelton's method.

2. Routine nursing care
A. Assess neonate's responses and appearance continuously: general assessment, Dubowitz gestational age assessment; Brazelton assessment (Table 3–20).
B. First feeding:
1. Selected infants may breastfeed stat after birth.
2. Nurse or parent, with supervision, does first feeding otherwise—sterile water (preferable to glucose, which irritates respiratory tree if aspirated); observe infant's suck-swallow reflex, color, respirations, regurgitation, and fatigability.
3. Check infants susceptible to hypoglycemia with Dextrostix at 30 minutes and one, two, and four hours of age; feed if hypoglycemic.
4. Start feedings at four to eight hours of age to prevent dehydration, prevent hypoglycemia, keep bilirubin levels lower, and stimulate GI tract.
5. May regurgitate mucus and amniotic fluid.
C. Weigh daily if bottle fed, or before and after breastfeeding. (However, some are no longer weighing babies before and after feeding; some start weighing baby only after mother's milk supply is established.)
1. May lose 5% to 10% of birth weight in first few days.

2. Regain birth weight in 7 to 14 days.
D. Note and record all voidings.
E. Note and record stools:
   1. Meconium—deep green-black, sticky, odorless, unformed stools; first day, sterile.
   2. Transition—greenish yellow and loose (days two to five).
   3. Bottle fed (after five days)—firmer, passed less frequently, yellow, pH neutral to alkaline, foul odor; can be normal to have occasional liquid stool.
   4. Breastfed (after five days)—unformed but not watery, one or two each day or one after each feeding, bright golden yellow, occasionally light green, some odor, pH is acidic.
   5. Diarrhea—yellowish-green; increased amount of mucus; water ring on diaper around stool; forcefully expelled; causes—overfeeding, infection (usually *Escherichia coli*), or wrong formula.
   6. Constipation—can be a feature of organic disease, such as obstruction, pyloric stenosis (although usually not until after first month), starvation, megacolon, or rectovaginal fistula.
F. Cord care:
   1. Observe for abnormalities—bleeding, redness, drainage, or odor.
   2. Keep clean and dry; apply alcohol or thimerosal (Merthiolate) to cord.
   3. Normal—separates and drops off in seven to ten days.
G. Observe for jaundice—sclera, mucosa, and skin.
H. Circumcision care—check for bleeding, replace petrolatum gauze prn (if ordered), and keep clean and dry.
I. Order PKU, galactosemia, and T₄ tests for third day.*
J. Teach parents characteristics and care of newborn.

3. Nutrient needs
A. Calories—42–50 calories/lb/day.
B. Protein: 1.5–2 g/lb/day or 3.5 g/kg/day (1 g protein = 1 oz milk).
C. Fluids—2–3 oz/lb/day.
D. Vitamin D—400 IU daily for bottle-fed babies after week two.

4. Infant feeding
A. Suppression of lactation:
   1. Antilactogenic drugs.

---

*Parents may refuse to sign permit for infant to have these tests. The parents are asked to sign a release for the hospital and physician for any damage that can occur if any one of these diseases does develop.

a. Testosterone enanthate and estradiol valerate injection (Deladumone OB)—engorgement, rare.
   b. Chlorotrianisene (Tace)—less effective, given in several doses.
   2. Other methods—tight binder, avoid emptying breasts; restricting fluids is unwarranted.
   3. Engorgement (see following discussion).
   4. Teach regarding bottle feeding—holding and burping.
B. Breastfeeding and lactation:
   1. Colostrum (yellowish fluid)—continues for the first two to three days; may have some antibiotic and nutritive value; infant suckles to give mother and self chance to learn, to meet infant's sucking needs, and to stimulate milk production and "let-down" reflex.
   2. Milk (bluish white, thin-looking)—comes on about the third day; "let-down" reflex, a function of the posterior pituitary, stimulates the ejection or release of milk from the alveoli into the nipple ducts.
   3. Procedure—takes patience for mother and nurse.
      a. Teach regarding rooting reflex and putting infant on breast, burping, what to do if infant chokes, and removing infant from breast.
      b. Infant must grasp nipple and areola over the location of milk sinuses.
   4. Factors influencing successful breastfeeding—emptying both breasts at each feeding, rest, fluids, relaxation (adrenalin suppresses lactation), and additional calories and fluids.
   5. Infant should nurse at both breasts at each feeding—emptying breasts is best stimulus for milk production and prevents mastitis; it takes three weeks for supply to meet demand; alternate the "beginning breast."
   6. Engorgement—stasis of venous and lymphatic circulation immediately preceding lactation.
      a. A painful condition, lasts about 24 hours.
      b. Relieved by warm packs, analgesics, emptying breasts, and good supporting bra.
      c. Should not be accompanied by fever.
      d. Collecting ducts around areola may have to be emptied manually before infant can take hold to suck.
   7. A restful environment free of emotional and physical discomfort is necessary for adequate milk production.
   8. One thousand additional calories are needed daily for milk production: 500 calories need to

come from diet; 500 calories from maternal energy (fat) stores (120 calories needed to produce 100 ml milk; eventually 1000 ml or more produced per day), protein, minerals, vitamins, and fluids (3000 ml/day); may need to divide this large quantity of food into five or six feedings to manage it.

9. Nipple care—
   a. Prevention. Good handwashing; infant should grasp areolar tissue into mouth; infant nurses on each breast for short lengths of time at first until nipple toughens; infant is removed from breast after mother breaks suction; nipple is dried after each feeding; no soap is used in cleansing breasts.
   b. Cracked or fissured nipples. Encourage and support mother; use heat lamp to dry nipples after each feeding (40–watt, 18 inches from breast); limit sucking time to five minutes at each breast; use pacifier if baby's sucking needs have not been met; use a nipple shield; discontinue nursing for 48 hours while maintaining milk supply by expression of milk; change position for holding infant during feeding (from usual position to football hold).

10. Drugs—avoid use except under medical supervision, as drugs and their metabolites appear in breast milk and may affect baby; some drugs (oral contraceptives) may also suppress milk production and predispose to thrombus formation.

11. Sexual sensation—some women feel sexual pleasure or are sexually aroused by the nursing process; this natural, pleasurable feeling may upset some women and be a cause to terminate breastfeeding.

12. During orgasm, milk may squirt out of nipples.

13. Contraceptive value of nursing is a *myth*. Lactation can prevent ovulation for up to eight months or more in some women. For other women, ovulation occurs about 40 days after delivery even with lactation. Women can be taught to assess their cervical mucus to help determine time of ovulation.

Part C / COMPLICATIONS OF CHILDBEARING AND THE HIGH-RISK NEONATE

ANTEPARTAL PERIOD

1. Reproductive hemorrhagic problems
A. Spontaneous abortion:
   1. Etiology—defective germ plasm, insufficient progesterone production, acute infections, abnormalities of reproductive system, and injuries (physical or emotional).
   2. Types and assessment—
      a. Threatened—mild bleeding, spotting, cramping, and cervix closed; no loss of fetal parts.
      b. Inevitable—moderate bleeding, painful cramping, and cervix dilated; membranes ruptured.
      c. Imminent—profuse bleeding, severe cramping, and urge to bear down.
      d. Recurrent (habitual)—three or more successive pregnancies lost through spontaneous abortion.
      e. Incomplete—fetal parts or fetus expelled and placenta and membranes retained.
      f. Complete—all products of conception expelled.
      g. Missed—fetal death with no abortion within four weeks; may exhibit symptoms of anorexia, malaise, and headache; clotting time may be increased due to hypofibrinogenemia (disseminated intravascular coagulation is a potential problem); saline injection via amniocentesis is preferred method to stimulate expulsion of products of conception.
      h. Septic abortion—usually following introduction of instruments or chemical; may accompany a "criminal" abortion. Death may result from septicemia, endotoxic shock (*E. coli* is most common; pseudomonas is often fatal), and DIC. Symptoms include fever, chills, constant lower abdominal pain with distention and diminished bowel sounds and rebound tenderness. Severe symptoms include oliguria, dark urine, jaundice. Vaginal examination reveals

malodorous discharge, pain when cervix is moved, and a soft, tender uterus. Laboratory values: increase in WBC (a decrease in WBC carries a poor prognosis).

3. Treatment—threatened abortion—
   a. Notify physician stat; bring all perineal pads, all clots or other matter passed from the vagina, to the hospital or doctor's office.
   b. Bedrest and sedation; reduce physical and emotional stress.
   c. Avoid coitus and orgasm.
4. Treatment—inevitable, imminent, or incomplete abortion—
   a. Pain medication.
   b. IVs; type and crossmatch; replace blood loss; assess platelets, serum fibrinogen, clotting time.
   c. Prevent (sterile technique) or treat infection.
   d. Dilatation and curettage or dilatation and evacuation.
   e. IV oxytocin or intrauterine saline induction if abortus is 14 weeks' gestation or more.
   f. Observe for blood loss, shock, and infection.
   g. Administer RhoGAM if woman is Rh negative and gestation is eight weeks or more.
   h. Supportive counseling to the woman for the loss.
5. Treatment—habitual or recurrent abortion—
   a. Treat as for inevitable, imminent, or incomplete abortion.
   b. Diagnose etiology—endocrine, genetic, anomaly or disorder of reproductive tract (uterine fibroma or incompetent cervical os, for example), blood incompatibility, or psychologic.
6. Voluntary or "therapeutic" abortion (see p. 177).

B. Incompetent cervix:
1. Defective cervix (internal os) allowing dilatation and effacement in the middle of the second or early in the third trimester when the fetus weighs about 1¼–1½ lb.
2. Etiologies—
   a. Unknown.
   b. Injury to cervix during previous birth or repeated cervical dilatation, as in abortion (spontaneous or therapeutic).
3. Succeeding pregnancies may be retained following cerclage procedures, such as McDonald or Shirodkar, after the first trimester, may be delivered vaginally (after purse-string suture is cut at onset of labor) or by cesarean delivery.
   a. Supportive care prior to and after surgery.

   b. Following procedure—observe for signs of labor and bleeding; generally, no complications are expected.

C. Hydatidiform mole:
1. Pathology—anomalous development of placenta in which chorionic villi develop into a grape-cluster-like mass of vesicles; may be antecedent to choriocarcinoma, a rapidly spreading, highly malignant tumor of the trophoblast.
2. Etiology—incidence 1 out of 2000 pregnancies; seen more frequently in women over 45 years of age.
3. Assessment—
   a. Rapid enlargement of uterus not congruous with age of gestation.
   b. Brownish discharge, beginning about week 12 of gestation; discharge may contain vesicles.
   c. Symptoms of preeclampsia that appear early in pregnancy (before third trimester).
   d. No fetal parts palpable or seen on X ray, sonography, or amniography.
   e. High HCG levels.
4. Medical treatment—
   a. Empty the uterus—hysterectomy may be necessary.
   b. Chemotherapy (methotrexate) and/or radiation, if malignant cells are seen.
   c. Follow-up for one year for HCG levels; persistent HCG level is consistent with choriocarcinoma.
   d. Strict contraception for a minimum of one year to permit accurate assessment.
5. Nursing management—
   a. Observe for hemorrhage, passage of retained vesicles, and abdominal pain or infection (perforation of uterine wall highly probable).
   b. Assist woman (or couple) in selecting contraceptive method best suited to her (them).
   c. Supportive care for woman after evacuation or hysterectomy and during follow-up care.

D. Ectopic pregnancy—one of the most serious emergencies (6% maternal mortality) 6–12 weeks after LMP.
1. Pathology—implantation outside of uterine cavity.
2. Types—tubal (95% of cases), cervical, abdominal, and ovarian.
3. Etiologies—

a. Inflammatory disease (PID)—pelvic, salpingitis, and endometriosis.
b. Anomalous tubes or uterus, tubal spasm, and tumors in or pressing on the reproductive organs; following tuboplasty.
c. Adhesions from pelvic inflammatory disease (PID) or past surgeries.
d. IUD in place.
4. Assessment—
a. Dependent on site of implantation.
b. Early signs—abnormal menstrual period usually following a missed period, spotting, and some symptoms of pregnancy; possible dull pain on affected side.
c. Following tubal rupture—pain, usually sudden, in lower abdomen; nausea and vomiting; symptoms of shock, referred pain in shoulder (Kehr's sign) or neck from blood in peritoneal cavity; blood in cul-de-sac of Douglas may be experienced as rectal pressure.
d. Sharp, localized pain when cervix is touched during pelvic examination; shock and collapse occurs in 10%, usually after vaginal examination.
e. Pregnancy test is positive in 50% of women.
5. Treatment—surgery.
6. Nursing management—
a. Usual preoperative and postoperative care (IV, O$_2$, blood—see Unit 5).
b. Supportive care for grief reaction (see p. 251).
(1) Loss of a pregnancy.
(2) Loss of a part of the reproductive tract.
(3) Threat to self-image as a woman and as a childbearer.
E. Placenta previa:
1. Pathology—abnormal implantation of placenta near or over the internal os.
2. Types—
a. Low-lying or marginal placenta previa.
b. Partial placenta previa—partially covers the internal os.
c. Complete placenta previa—covers the internal os of the cervix; may be accompanied by unusual fetal presentations.
3. Etiology—
a. Unknown.
b. Occurs more frequently with multiparity and advanced maternal age.
c. Fibroid tumors or old scars (from cesarean delivery) or endometriosis may be factors.

4. Assessment—
a. Bleeding that usually appears in the eighth month, when there is some cervical effacement and dilatation.
b. Bleeding is usually painless (unless accompanied by abruptio placentae as well) and is not accompanied by uterine contractions; bleeding may be intermittent.
c. Possibility of low implantation may be suspected prior to eighth month by palpating a boggy lower-uterine segment during vaginal examination.
d. If in labor, contractions are usually normal.
5. Treatment—dependent on location of placenta and amount of bleeding.
a. Vaginal delivery is possible with low-lying placenta and minimal bleeding, active labor with good progress, and if presenting part is acting as a tamponade.
b. Vaginal examination under double set-up:
(1) Woman is prepared for cesarean birth (abdominoperineal preparation).
(2) In an operating room set up for emergency cesarean delivery.
6. Nursing management—
a. Do not permit vaginal or rectal exams or enemas.
b. Place on bedrest in high-Fowler's position if placenta is marginal.
c. Monitor FHRs continuously.
d. Monitor maternal vital signs and bleeding.
e. General preoperative and postoperative care (see Unit 5).
f. Postpartum—observe for hemorrhage; placental site is located in a less contractile part of uterus.
g. Postpartum—observe for infection; ascending infection can reach placental site more easily.
F. Abruptio placentae:
1. Pathology—premature separation of the placenta; placenta is usually normally implanted.
a. Incidence—1/500 pregnancies.
b. Types—
(1) Partial abruptio placentae—small portion of placenta separates.
(2) Complete abruptio placentae—total placenta separates.
(3) Abruptio placentae with *concealed* bleeding—blood remains within uterus.
(4) Abruptio placentae with *external* bleeding—blood escapes into vagina.

c. Complications possible—
   (1) Afibrinogenemia and disseminated intravascular coagulation (DIC)—result of clot formation behind placenta.
   (2) Couvelaire uterus—bleeding into myometrium, necessitating hysterectomy.
   (3) Amniotic-fluid embolus (see p. 245).
   (4) Hypovolemic shock.
2. Etiologies:
   a. Preeclampsia/eclampsia.
   b. Preceding the delivery of second twin.
   c. Traction on placenta (short cord or impatient accoucheur).
   d. Rupture of membranes.
   e. Injudicious use of oxytocin in induction or augmentation of labor.
   f. High parity.
   g. Chronic vascular renal disease with hypertension.
3. Assessment—
   a. Bleeding, concealed or external.
      (1) Concealed—central separation; prior to onset of labor.
      (2) External—marginal separation with or without central separation, allowing passage of blood through cervix; usually during labor.
      (3) Amniotic fluid may be port-wine colored.
   b. Shock is usually more profound than amount of observed bleeding would support.
   c. Pain—often sudden and severe (may contribute to shock).
   d. Increased uterine muscle tonus—uterus may contract unevenly; does not relax completely between contractions.
   e. Fetal hyperactivity that may indicate fetal distress; bradycardia; or loss of fetal heart tones with fetal demise.
4. Treatment—medical and nursing management—
   a. Control hemorrhage.
   b. Control neurogenic and hypovolemic shock; maintain in side-lying position to avoid pressure on vena cava.
   c. Determine clotting ability; give fibrinogen if necessary; fibrinogen injection is avoided if possible since there is a high incidence of hepatitis with this treatment.
   d. Deliver infant:
      (1) Cesarean delivery.

   (2) If vaginal delivery is imminent, membranes are ruptured to speed up delivery.
   e. Postpartum:
      (1) Be alert for uterine atony, hemorrhage, and puerperal infection.
      (2) Monitor urinary output (anuria, oliguria) or hematuria from renal failure.
      (3) Observe for pulmonary emboli (see p. 222).
      (4) Give heparin if necessary.
      (5) Support the parents.

2. Preeclampsia/eclampsia—toxemias of pregnancy.
A. Pathophysiology:
   1. Generalized arteriospasm—results in hypertension and decreased perfusion of tissues.
   2. Renal lesion—glomerular capillary endotheliosis.
   3. As intravascular protein is lost in the urine, fluid moves out of vascular bed and into tissues.
B. Incidence:
   1. 7% to 10% of all pregnancies.
   2. Develops after week 24 of gestation.
   3. Fourth leading cause of maternal mortality in the United States today.
C. Assessment—results from decreased blood flow to the kidney, brain, and uterus.
   1. Kidney:
      a. Water and sodium retention—edema.
      b. Proteinuria.
      c. Hypertension (from kidney release of angiotensin).
      d. Oliguria.
   2. Brain:
      a. Cerebral and visual disturbances—due to arteriospasm and edema.
      b. Convulsions and coma—due to increased irritability of central nervous system (CNS).
   3. Uterus:
      a. Small-for-gestational-age baby.
      b. Abruptio placentae.
D. Types:
   1. Preeclampsia—*mild:*
      a. Hypertension—systolic increase of 30 mm Hg or more over baseline and diastolic rise of 15 mm Hg or more over baseline.
      b. Proteinuria $\geq$ 1 g/day.
      c. Edema—especially digital and periorbital; weight gain over 0.45 kg (1 lb) per week.
   2. Preeclampsia—*severe:*
      a. Increased hypertension—systolic pressure at

or above 160 mm Hg or 50 mm Hg above baseline and diastolic, 110 mm Hg or more.

b. Proteinuria—5 g or more in 24 hours.

c. Oliguria—400 ml or less in 24 hours.

d. Cerebral or visual disturbances, such as disorientation and somnolence; severe frontal headache; increased irritability; and blurring, halo vision, dimness, and blind spots.

e. Persistent vomiting.

f. Epigastric pain—edema of liver capsule.

g. Hemoconcentration.

3. Eclampsia—*convulsions* (clonic and tonic); a more severe form of toxemia; symptomatology same as severe preeclampsia, but usually accompanied by convulsions, coma, and renal shutdown.

E. Etiologies:

1. Pregnancy—to initiate and continue this condition, a functioning trophoblast must be present.

2. Age—under 17 and over 35 years; multiple gestation, diabetes, or first pregnancy.

3. Diet—low in protein.

4. Polyhydramnios.

5. Unknown.

F. Prognosis—

1. Good—symptoms mild and respond to treatment.

2. Poor—convulsions (number and duration); persistent coma; hyperthermia; tachycardia, 120 bpm or more; and cyanosis.

3. Terminal—pulmonary edema, congestive cardiac failure, acute renal failure, and cerebral hemorrhage.

G. Medical-*nursing management*—moderate to severe condition:

1. Dietary—improve protein intake to replace low serum protein; low serum protein leads to movement of fluid out of vascular and into interstitial fluid compartments.

2. Drugs (Table 3–21—also see Appendix D)—

a. Anticonvulsants.

b. Antihypertensives.

c. Diuretics.

d. Blood volume expanders.

3. Monitor progress of preeclampsia—

a. Blood pressure.

b. Weight—evaluation of edema.

c. Intake and output—Foley catheter.

d. Reflex responses.

e. Laboratory values—blood (hematocrit, serum protein) and electrolytes.

4. Monitor fetal status (see *Fetus in jeopardy*, p. 245).

5. Monitor for signs and symptoms of labor.

6. Observe for abruptio placentae (a high blood pressure or a rapid drop may initiate abruptio).

7. Observe for DIC (unusual bleeding).

8. Convulsion care—

a. Maintain patent airway; administer O_2 prn.

b. Observe for signs and symptoms of impending convulsion—sharp cry; frontal headache; epigastric pain, and facial twitching.

c. Safety—keep padded tongue blade or plastic airway on hand; pad siderails; reduce environmental stimulus, for example, keep lights dim, maintain quiet.

d. Observe, report, and record onset and progression of convulsion and whether it was followed by bladder and bowel evacuation and/or coma.

e. *Remain alert* for *48 hours postpartum* for convulsions, even if no convulsions occurred prior to delivery.

3. Cardiac disorders

A. *Normal* alterations during normal pregnancy that mimic cardiac disorder:

1. Systolic murmurs, palpitations, tachycardia, and hyperventilation with some dyspnea with normal moderate exertion.

2. Edema of lower extremities.

3. Red blood cell sedimentation rate tends to rise near term.

4. Cardiac enlargement.

B. Anticipatory guidance and *nursing care* of the gravida with cardiac involvement.

1. Signs and symptoms of cardiac decompensation and congestive failure—if any of these appear, the woman should notify physician (hospitalization is mandatory)—

a. Pedal edema.

b. Moist cough.

c. Dyspnea with minimal physical activity.

d. Rapid weak pulse.

e. Cyanosis of lips and nail beds.

2. Methods of decreasing work of heart—

a. Rest—sleep at least ten hours per night and rest for half an hour after each meal.

b. Avoid heavy work (including housework), excessive weight gain, and emotional stress.

c. Prevent and/or treat anemia.

TABLE 3–21. *Pharmacologic control of hypertension and its sequelae in pregnancy and labor**

Medication	Target tissue	Effects of medication		Nursing actions
		Maternal	*Fetal/neonatal*	

ANTICONVULSANTS

Medication	Target tissue	Maternal	Fetal/neonatal	Nursing actions
Magnesium sulfate IV or IM. Dosage: Pritchard—first dose: 4 g 20% IV at 1 g/min and 10 g 50% IM, subsequently; 5 g 50% IM q 4 hr; Zuspan—first dose: 6 g 20% IV, subsequently: 10–24 g/L of 5% D/W at 1 g/hr.	*Myoneural junction:* decreases acetylcholine, thereby depressing neuromuscular transmission. *Thyroid:* decreases parathormone secretion, resulting in increased urinary excretion of calcium. Placental perfusion dynamics not altered.	Minimum hypotensive effect. Minimum, if any, direct effect on CNS because of blood-brain barrier to magnesium. Hypocalcemia. CAUTION: Do not give excessive dosages that tend to decrease urinary output and to depress DTRs. DANGER: Muscular paralysis (cardiopulmonary). Antidotes: calcium gluconate, neostigmine, pentylenetetrazol (Metrazol).	Mild depression in small number (6%). Neonatal hypermagnesemia easily treated: calcium; exchange transfusion with citrated blood.	Notify perinatal staff. Decrease CNS irritability. Arrange environment to promote rest. Provide continuous nursing care. Encourage kidney perfusion with left side-lying position and insert indwelling urinary catheter; monitor urinary output every hour. Under 30 ml/hr—do not repeat dose. Diuresis—good prognostic sign. Repeat dose per order if: DTRs present. Respirations 12/min or more. Urinary output over dl/4 hr. Assess maternal condition: Hydration. Affect. Other signs or symptoms of preeclampsia. Keep 20 ml of 10% calcium gluconate at bedside, with linen/equipment for delivery, eclamptic tray, oxygen, and suction equipment.
Diazepam (Valium)	*Thalamus* and *hypothalamus:* direct depressant effect.	Effective in initial management of eclamptic convulsions.	Flattens fetal heart rate (FHR) baseline (loss of beat-to-beat variability), an important criterion in assessing fetal oxygenation. High levels in newborn: Depressed sucking ability. Hypotonia. Temperature instability (decrease). Decreased respiratory rate.	Notify perinatal staff. Assess DTRs, respirations, signs of labor. Monitor labor: see Normal labor.

(Continued)

TABLE 3–21.   *(Continued)*

| | | Effects of medication | | |
Medication	Target tissue	Maternal	Fetal/neonatal	Nursing actions
ANTICONVULSANTS				
Barbiturates (rapid-acting) Sodium phenobarbital 0.2–0.3 mg IV. Sodium amobarbital 0.25–0.5 g IV.	CNS: depressant effect.	Controls seizures.	Depressant effect on fetus. May minimize hyperbilirubinemia.	See Diazepam.
ANTIHYPERTENSIVES**				
Hydralazine (Apresoline, Neopresol)	Peripheral arterioles: decreases muscle tone, thereby decreasing peripheral resistance. Hypothalamus and medullary vasomotor center: minor decrease in sympathetic tone.	Headache. Flushing. Palpitation. Tachycardia. Some decrease in uteroplacental blood flow.	Minimum effects: some decrease in PO_2	Assess for effects of medications. Alert mother (family) to expected effects of medications. Assess BP (precipitous drop can lead to shock and perhaps to abruptio placentae) and urinary output. Maintain bedrest with siderails.
Methyldopa (Aldomet) (used if maintenance therapy is needed): 250–500 mg orally q 8 hr.	Postganglionic nerve endings: interferes with chemical neurotransmission to reduce peripheral vascular resistance.	Sleepiness. Postural hypotension. Constipation. Rare: drug-induced fever in 1% of women and positive Coombs' test in 20%.	After 4 mo of maternal therapy, positive Coombs' test in infant.	See Hydralazine.
DIURETICS†				
Thiazides	Arteriolar smooth muscles: reduces responsiveness to catecholamines.	Ineffective in preventing preeclampsia. Further reduces already present decreased plasma volume of preeclampsia. Complications: Fluid and electrolyte imbalance. Pancreatitis. Decrease in CHO intolerance. Hyperuricemia.	Hyponatremia. Thrombocytopenia.	Arrange to have blood drawn to measure levels of Na, Cl, CO_2, K, and H^+, to prevent hyponatremia, hypokalemia, hypochloremia, metabolic acidosis.
Furosemide (Lasix): 40 mg IV.	Loop of Henle.	Relieves pulmonary edema. Excessive use results in hypokalemia and hyponatremia.	No abnormalities noted.	See Thiazides.
Ethacrynic acid (Edecrin)	Similar to furosemide.	Similar to furosemide.	Deafness.	See Thiazides.
Mannitol (for impending renal failure, oliguria, DIC): 12.5–25 mg IV.	Osmotic diuretic: pulls fluid into vascular bed (therefore not recommended for persons with congestive heart failure).	Increases renal plasma flow and urinary output. Flushes out kidneys. Reduces swelling in ischemic cells in kidney and myocardium.	No known effect.	See Thiazides.

TABLE 3–21.   *(Continued)*

| Medication | Target tissue | Effects of medication | | Nursing actions |
		Maternal	Fetal/neonatal	
BLOOD VOLUME EXPANDERS				
(Salt-poor, serum albumin‡)	Intravascular volume.	Increases blood volume.		

*From: Jensen, M.D., Benson, R.C., and Bobak, I.M. 1981. Maternity care: the nurse and the family. St. Louis: The C. V. Mosby Company, ed. 2.

**By midpregnancy, diastolic and systolic blood pressure normally fall by 10–15 mm Hg. If diastolic blood pressure is 75 mm Hg or more in second trimester and 85 mm Hg or more in third trimester, there is statistical increase in fetal mortality.
NOTE: For the obese woman, use a thigh cuff to obtain accurate readings (or use ultrasound).

†For control of chronic hypertension, pulmonary edema, renal oliguria, acute renal failure, chronic nephrotic syndrome. If used, physician must be ready to justify action.

‡May not be appropriate for the woman with severe preeclampsia/eclampsia.

d. Avoid infection—avoid crowds, fatigue, anemia, and cold drafts; eat well-balanced diet.
e. Avoid situations of reduced ambient O_2, such as high altitudes, flight in unpressurized plane, smoking, and prolonged exposure to a smoke-filled or *highly polluted* environment.
f. Avoid excessive salt intake.
3. Management of labor—
   a. NPO for foods and fluids.
   b. Frequent vital signs, especially pulse (over 110), which is the most sensitive and reliable indicator of impending congestive heart failure, and respirations over 24.
   c. Semirecumbent position, with arms and legs supported.
   d. No bearing down efforts; low-outlet forceps and episiotomy are used to shorten second stage.
   e. Regional (conduction) anesthesia such as epidural, caudal, or saddle block (inhalation anesthesia is contraindicated)—
      (1) To relieve stress of pain.
      (2) To eliminate bearing-down reflex.
   f. Digitalis prn; diuretics with KCl supplementation, prn; antibiotics, prn.
4. Referral to social services if gravida needs help in home.
C. Medical management:
   1. Determination of cardiac involvement.
      a. Class I—least affected; no dyspnea with ordinary activity for example; best pregnancy risk.
      b. Class II—activity somewhat limited.
      c. Class III—activity markedly limited.
      d. Class IV—most affected; symptoms apparent at rest; should not get pregnant.
   2. Drug therapy (see Appendix D).
      a. Diuretics with supplementation for lost electrolytes.
      b. Digitalis.
      c. Antibiotics—prophylaxis against recurrence of rheumatic fever.
      d. Oxygen.
   3. Hospitalize gravida for several days or weeks prior to EDC and after delivery.
   4. Special evaluation and supervision stat after delivery.
      a. Delivery results in rapid decrease in intraabdominal pressure, with resultant vasocongestion and rapid increase in cardiac output.
      b. Blood loss—prevent hypovolemic shock.
      c. Pain relief—prevent neurogenic shock.
      d. Rapid alterations in water metabolism that occur after delivery present an added stress to the new mother with heart involvement—observe for tachycardia and/or respiratory distress.
   5. Operative procedures, therapeutic abortion and cesarean delivery, for example, are avoided if at all possible.

4. Diabetes and prediabetes
A. Pathology—inability of the beta cells of the islets of Langerhans in the pancreas to produce sufficient insulin to metabolize glucose properly.

B. White's classification considers age at onset, duration, and vascular or renal changes, if any.
   1. Class A—abnormal glucose tolerance test (GTT), dietary regulation, no insulin needed.
   2. Class B—onset after 20 years of age, duration less than ten years, no associated vascular involvement.
   3. Class C—onset between 10 and 19 years of age, duration of 10 to 19 years, no associated vascular involvement.
   4. Class D—onset under 10 years of age, duration of more than 20 years, early vascular disease (legs, retina).
   5. Class E—X ray verification of pelvic arteriosclerosis.
   6. Class F—vascular nephropathy.
   7. Class G—duration over 20 years, vascular disease and nephropathy, history of many obstetric failures.
C. Etiology:
   1. Heredity—recessive trait.
      a. Age—incidence increases with age.
      b. Rapid hormone change—necessity to make rapid metabolic changes compromises the genetic diabetic; rapid changes occur during menarche, pregnancy, menopause.
   2. Environment—affects the expression of the trait.
      a. Obesity—imposes excessive demands on beta cells.
      b. Stress—added demands on beta cells with infection, surgery, and other emotional and physical trauma.
   3. Tumor or infection of the pancreas may damage the beta cells so that diabetes occurs secondary to the trauma.
D. Normal metabolic alterations (during normal pregnancy) that aggravate the diabetic condition:
   1. Hormone production (see p. 182).
      a. HCS (HPL).
      b. Cortisol.
      c. Estrogen.
      d. Progesterone.
   2. Effects of hormones—
      a. Decreased glucose tolerance—changes in metabolic rate; increased production of adrenocortical and pituitary hormones; glucosuria is common.
      b. Decreased effectiveness of insulin (increased resistance to insulin by peripheral tissues) is a glucose-sparing mechanism that assures an abundant supply of glucose to the fetus because glucose is the primary substrate to meet the fetal energy needs; increased gluconeogenesis.
      c. Increased size and number of islets of Langerhans to meet increased maternal needs.
      d. Increased mobilization of free fatty acids.
      e. Decreased CO_2- combining power of blood; an increase in BMR increases the tendency to acidosis.
E. Effect of diabetes *on pregnancy*—increased incidence of:
   1. Preeclampsia/eclampsia (occurs in one-third to one-half of cases).
   2. Polyhydramnios.
   3. Spontaneous abortion.
   4. Stillbirths.
   5. Infertility.
   6. Congenital anomalies (Three times more prevalent—see p. 241).
   7. Premature labor and delivery.
   8. Urinary-tract infection (UTI).
   9. Vaginal infections.
F. Effect of pregnancy *on diabetes:*
   1. Nausea and vomiting—predisposes to ketosis and acidosis.
   2. Insulin requirements—relatively stable during the first trimester; increase rapidly during the second and third trimesters.
   3. Pathophysiologic sequelae of diabetes—nephropathy, retinopathy, and arteriosclerotic changes, for example, may appear now, or existing pathology may be aggravated.
G. Assessment of diabetes:
   1. History—
      a. Familial history.
      b. Previous infant weighing 4000 g or more.
      c. Unexplained fetal wastage—abortion, stillbirth.
      d. Obesity with a very rapid weight gain.
      e. Hydramnios (polyhydramnios).
      f. Previous infant with congenital anomalies.
      g. Increased incidence and intensity of vaginal infections, especially with *C. albicans*.
   2. Laboratory tests—GTT abnormal if two or more of the following are abnormal. Normal values follow—
      a. FBS—under 100 mg/dl (90 mg/dl may be normal during first trimester).
      b. One hour—under 200 mg/dl.
      c. Two hours—under 150 mg/dl.
      d. Three hours—under 120 mg/dl.
   3. Abdominal assessment—

a. Excessive fundal height.
b. Polyhydramnios.
c. Large fetus for gestational age or, if woman has vascular pathology, small fetus for gestational age.
4. Symptoms—
a. Polydipsia.
b. Polyphagia.
c. Weight loss.
H. Medical management—*antepartum:*
1. Early identification of diabetes (gestational) to minimize incidence of congenital anomalies, decrease perinatal mortality, and minimize excessive fetal growth (macromia).
2. Control diabetes to minimize—
a. Incidence of maternal complications (such as preeclampsia/eclampsia or macrovascular problems from deposit of lipoproteins within vessels).
b. Cardiovascular damage (such as nephropathy, retinitis).
c. Incidence of infections.
3. Schedule of visits—every 2 weeks until 30 weeks, then every week until delivery.
4. Diet—
a. Optimal weight gain about 24 lb.
b. Needs 35 calories/kg of ideal body weight.
c. Protein—1/5–2 g/kg, or about 70 g.
d. CHO—30% to 45%; bulk should be in complex form (bread, milk). If woman is larger, she may need more CHO to prevent ketoacidosis.
e. Fats—unsaturated.
5. Exercise—
a. Needed for feeling of well-being, to regulate weight gain, and to control level of blood sugar.
6. Insulin: regular, NPH.
a. Urine-testing—double-voided specs.
b. No oral medication, such as tolbutamide, that crosses the placenta and does not prevent ketoacidosis.
c. Requirements:
(1) First trimester—may decrease with periods of hypoglycemia because of fetal drain; HCS and other hormone levels are still low.
(2) Second trimester—insulin needs begin to increase.
(3) Third trimester—insulin needs may increase to as much as three to four times prepregnant dose.

d. Diabetic acidosis more common late in pregnancy—precipitated by increase in stress (emotional, concurrent illness).
7. Identification and treatment of infection—
a. Urinary-tract infection (UTI).
b. Mycotic vaginitis is more common and harder to control (see p. 268).
8. Hospitalization frequently required for—
a. Regulation of insulin; change from tolbutamide to regular insulin during pregnancy.
b. Control of infection.
c. Determination of fetal jeopardy—basis for possible early termination of pregnancy (see p. 245).
I. Medical management—*intrapartum* (labor):
1. Timing—see *Determination of fetal jeopardy,* p. 245.
2. Day of delivery—management varies widely.
a. Insulin is added to intravenous infusion of 5% to 10% D/W that may be titrated to keep the plasma glucose level between 100–150 mg/dl, but definitely under 200 mg/dl; D/W is needed to prevent hyperglycemia (that can lead to neonatal hypoglycemia) or hypoglycemia (that can lead to maternal ketoacidosis).
b. Side-lying position is imperative because polyhydramnios or a large infant can cause severe supine hypotension and because hypotension increases the incidence of RDS or aggravates it in the neonate.
c. Electronic fetal monitoring and ultrasound or X-ray pelvimetry may be indicated to identify possible fetal jeopardy and CPD.
J. Medical management—postpartum:
1. Insulin requirements may be one-half to two-thirds of prepregnant dose on first postpartum day if she is eating a full diet because of rapid fall of HCS when placenta is delivered and serum glucose is being converted to lactose.
2. Preeclampsia/eclampsia precautions—
a. Incidence—in one-fourth of all diabetic new mothers in classes A and B, and in one-third of all diabetic new mothers in classes C and D.
3. Hemorrhage, especially after—
a. Polyhydramnios.
b. Large fetus.
c. Induction of labor.
4. Infections—

a. Do not catheterize if at all possible and do make sure she is voiding.

b. Good nipple care to prevent fissures and mastitis.

c. Good hygiene to prevent vaginitis with *C. albicans.*

5. Breastfeeding—

a. Advantages—besides satisfaction and pleasure, it has an antidiabetogenic action which results in decreased insulin need and lowered serum glucose and helps to prevent weight gain (maternal).

b. Women requiring large doses of insulin may need to triple caloric intake and decrease insulin by one-half.

c. If acetonuria occurs, mother must stop breastfeeding (baby's liver enlarges) while physician supervises readjustment of insulin/diet balance (mother may pump breasts until nursing can be restarted).

d. If mother becomes hypoglycemic, her adrenalin level increases and this decreases the milk supply and the let-down reflex response.

6. Counseling (with the couple)—

a. Risk of infant inheriting gene for diabetes is 4% if diabetes is of maturity onset and 22% if diabetes is of juvenile onset.

b. Increased risk of congenital anomalies.

c. Cannot use oral contraceptives because they decrease CHO tolerance. Barrier contraceptives are recommended, such as diaphragms and condoms; IUDs are used with caution because of possible infection.

d. If she has renal disease or proliferative retinopathy, there is an increased risk for mother and fetus with another pregnancy.

K. Nursing management:

1. Ongoing care—ambulatory:

a. Assess woman's knowledge and acceptance of the disease and its management to facilitate her compliance with management.

b. The nurse's caring actions assist her acceptance of the disease, herself and her new self-image, attachment to the neonate, and appropriate grieving if fetus/neonate succumbs.

c. Coordinate teaching—using POR and checklists, and assigning the gravida to a primary-care-giver.

d. Refer her to group of other high-risk women to help maintain motivation, follow diet,

cope with being "high risk" as well as with approaching parenthood.

e. Teach hygiene even though her disease may be mild.

f. Reinforce physician's explanations, advice, directions for diet and exercise.

g. Record pattern of weight gain; blood pressure; and urine test for glucose, acetone, and protein.

h. Encourage woman to report problems such as vomiting and infection.

i. Check FHR and height of fundus.

2. Antepartal hospitalization—

a. Assist with fractional urine, insulin regulation, and diet.

b. Check FHR, height of fundus, amount of amniotic fluid, and signs of labor.

c. Vital signs, I & O, and daily weight.

d. Assist with tests for fetal status.

e. Encourage bedrest (if prescribed), provide diversions (side-lying position).

f. Provide atmosphere conducive to expression of feelings and concerns; keep her (and family) informed. Support reduces anxiety and tension, which contributes to insulin/glucose balance.

g. Prepare for possibility of cesarean delivery.

h. In event of fetal demise, provide emotional support.

3. Labor and delivery—

a. Fractional urines, q2–3h; regular insulin.

b. IVs (Ringer's); I & O.

c. Monitor FHR continuously; monitor maternal vital signs frequently.

d. Order blood sugar to be done q1–3h.

e. Support to reduce anxiety and tension.

4. Postpartum—

a. Observe for hypoglycemia or insulin reaction; assist with regulation of insulin.

b. Fractional urines.

c. Observe for and avoid exposure to infection.

d. Observe for signs and symptoms of preeclampsia/eclampsia.

e. Reinforce counseling by physician and/or genetic counselor, family-planning counselor, or other.

f. Discuss with her how she plans to cope with the care of her other children (if there are any), this child, and her diabetes.

g. Discuss with her the importance of eating on time, even if the infant has to wait to eat.

h. Discuss with her her need to rest and have

exercise so as to maintain an insulin/glucose balance.

L. Infant of the diabetic mother (IDM)— *assessment:*

1. Macrosomia—excessive weight for gestational age due to excessive tissue growth, deposit of subcutaneous fat, and retention of interstitial fluids.

   a. Caution—excessive size may mask premature status; evaluate each infant for maturity since function is related to gestational age and not fetal size.

   b. Possible etiologies of macrosomia—

      (1) Maternal production of large amounts of pituitary growth hormone and adrenocortical hormones.

      (2) Fetal production of large amounts of insulin.

      (3) Fetal hyperglycemia reflecting maternal hyperglycemia.

2. Cardiac enlargement; hepatomegaly and splenomegaly.

3. Subject to hypocalcemic tetany, acidosis, hypoglycemia, and hyperbilirubinemia.

4. Increased incidence of respiratory distress syndrome (RDS), which is related in part to elective premature delivery and control of the diabetic condition. (Maternal hypotension may contribute to RDS or aggravate it.)

5. Increased incidence of congenital anomalies or defects (five times the average incidence) that include cardiac, pelvic, and spinal anomalies.

M. Nursing management of infant of diabetic mother (IDM):

1. Assess for characteristics of IDM (described previously).

2. Assess blood sugar (or order lab work) at 30 minutes and 1, 2, 4, 6, 9, 12, and 24 hours of age; feed per order, prn (term: under 30–40 mg/dl; preterm: under 20 mg/dl).

3. Observe for behavioral indications of hypoglycemia (see p. 261).

4. Assess for gestational age; institute premature care prn (incubator care).

5. Observe for jaundice.

6. If baby is large, assess for birth injuries—fractures (clavicle, humerus), brachial palsy, intracranial hemorrhage (symptoms of increased intracranial pressure), and cephalhematoma.

7. Assess for hypocalcemia that occurs in 20% of infants of women with gestational diabetes (usually within 24 hours) and in 30% of IDMs.

   a. Symptoms: similar to hypoglycemia, such as irritability, coarse tremors, twitching, convulsions.

   b. Treatment: calcium gluconate, po or IV.

N. Prognosis—overall prognosis is now less than 10% morbidity.

1. Worsens with increasing severity of the disease and with intrapartum asphyxia or maternal bleeding, and the incidence of RDS increases accordingly.

2. Gestational diabetes and classes A through C that are diagnosed later in pregnancy predispose to macrosomia, increased risk of perinatal death, hypoglycemia, and congenital anomaly, all of which may be related to the period of time before diagnosis when the disease was uncontrolled.

3. Stillbirths, 4% to 12%.

4. Neonatal mortality (if premature), 4% to 10%.

   a. Class A, 8%.

   b. Classes B, C, D with polyhydramnios, 17% to 18%.

O. Perinatal mortality by gestational age:

1. Age 32 to 34 weeks: 19% (prematurity).

2. Age 36 weeks: 11%.

3. Age 37 to 40 weeks: 26% (intrauterine death, usually).

5. *Polyhydramnios*—amniotic fluid in excess of 2000 ml (normal—500 to 1200 ml).

A. Incidence—associated with:

1. Maternal diabetes (in 25% of gravidas).

2. Multiple pregnancies.

3. Erythroblastosis fetalis.

4. Preeclampsia/eclampsia.

5. Congenital anomalies—anencephaly and upper GI anomalies, such as esophageal atresia.

B. Assessment:

1. Height of fundus higher than appropriate for gestational age.

2. Fetal parts difficult to feel and small in proportion to size of uterus.

3. Increased discomfort due to large, heavy uterus—increased edema in vulva and legs, shortness of breath, and GI discomfort.

4. Supine hypotension.

C. Complications:

1. Maternal respiratory embarrassment.

2. Premature rupture of membranes (PROM) with prolapsed cord and/or amnionitis.

3. Premature labor.

4. Postpartum hemorrhage.

D. Medical management:
1. Amniocentesis—to diagnose anomalies, erythroblastosis.
2. Sonogram—diagnose multiple pregnancy; gross fetal anomaly.
3. Voluntary abortion or hysterotomy.

E. Nursing management:
1. Support of mother for diagnostic or therapeutic procedures, loss of pregnancy, or treatment plan if pregnancy is to be continued.
2. Observe for signs of preeclampsia and premature labor.

6. Hyperemesis gravidarum

A. Pathology—intractable vomiting during the first 14 to 16 weeks' gestation with a peak incidence at 10 weeks; excessive vomiting any time during pregnancy; potential hazards are:
1. Dehydration with fluid and electrolyte imbalance.
2. Starvation, with loss of 5% or more of body weight.

B. Incidence—1 out of 300 pregnancies.

C. Etiology:
1. Psychologic—thought to be related to rejection of pregnancy and/or sexual relations.
2. Physiologic—secretion of HCG, decrease in free gastric HCl, reduced gastrointestinal motility, and displacement of stomach.
   a. Incidence increases in presence of hydatidiform mole.
   b. Incidence increases with twin or multiple gestation because the production of HCG is increased.

D. Assessment:
1. Abdominal pain.
2. Hiccups.
3. Weight loss—dehydration, starvation with metabolic acidosis, and increased BUN.

E. Treatment and nursing management:
1. Rule out other diseases, infection and tumors, for example.
2. Mild cases—give emotional support, dry crackers on awakening, frequent small feedings every two hours, prochlorperazine dimaleate (Compazine) or other medication.
3. Severe cases—hospitalization:
   a. NPO with intravenous fluids containing calories, vitamins, and minerals for 24 hours, careful I & O records.
   b. Antiemetics—promazine HCl (Sparine) IV

and prochlorperazine dimaleate (Compazine) IM.
   c. Bedrest.
   d. Restrict visitors, including mate.
   e. Observe for acetone breath.
   f. Therapeutic abortion is considered if any of the following conditions appear—
      (1) Jaundice.
      (2) Neurologic disturbances, somnolence.
      (3) Pulse 130 or more per minute.
      (4) Fever, after woman is adequately hydrated.
      (5) Retinal hemorrhage.
4. Discharge home when gravida demonstrates weight gain.

INTRAPARTAL PERIOD

1. Mechanical dystocia

A. Definition—prolonged (over 24 hours), difficult labor.

B. Uterine dysfunction:
1. Definition—significant prolongation of descent of fetus, effacement, and dilatation.
2. Types:
   a. Inertia—deficient forces of expulsion; hypotonic contractions.
      (1) Primary—prolongation of latent phase.
         (a) Nullipara—over 20 hours.
         (b) Multipara—over 14 hours.
      (2) Secondary—prolongation or abnormality of active phase.
         (a) Nullipara—less than 1.2 cm/hour.
         (b) Multipara—less than 1.5 cm/hour.
   b. Excessive contractions—hypertonic.
      (1) Precipitate labor-delivery—under three hours; possible trauma to mother and fetus.
      (2) Clonic contractions.
      (3) Tetanic contractions—last more than 90 seconds; danger of fetal asphyxia or uterine rupture.
   c. Failure of uterine contractions—missed abortion or labor.
3. Inertia:
   a. Primary inertia—poor uterine muscle tone; contractions are inefficient from the start.
      (1) Cause—"unripe" cervix; early or heavy sedation, especially during latent phase; false labor; cause may be unknown.

(2) Diagnosis—vaginal examination, X-ray pelvimetry; Leopold's maneuvers for fetal position and station.

(3) Nursing care—stimulate labor through walking, monitor oxytocin (Pitocin) induction, give enema, and assist with artificial rupture of membranes.

b. Secondary inertia—previously normal contractions become ineffectual or stop.

(1) Causes—related to maternal exhaustion, injudicious use of analgesia-anesthesia, minor pelvic contractures, CPD, fetal position, overdistended uterus, overdistended bladder, or cervical rigidity.

(2) Nursing care—careful observation to assist physician diagnosis, morphine rest, reassurance, prepare for cesarean delivery if labor prolonged beyond 24 hours.

4. Excessive contractions—hypertonic dysfunction.

a. Symptoms—incomplete relaxation between contractions and frequent prolonged contractions.

b. Hazards:

(1) Decreased oxygen concentration in cord blood.

(2) Rapid molding of fetal skull may result in intracranial hemorrhage.

(3) Possibility of uterine rupture or lacerations of cervix, vagina, or perineum.

c. Treatment and *nursing care:*

(1) Supportive care to assist mother to cope with fear, pain, and discouragement.

(2) Careful monitoring of maternal and fetal vital signs.

(3) Oxygen by mask, as necessary.

(4) Morphine to promote rest.

(5) Regional anesthesia to slow down contractions.

5. Failure of uterine contractions—hypotonic dysfunction.

a. Cause—etiology unclear.

b. Nursing care:

(1) Assist with X-ray pelvimetry.

(2) Supportive care—explain procedures and remain at bedside.

(3) Monitor contractions during oxytocin infusion induction or augmentation.

(4) Monitor maternal and fetal vital signs.

(5) Prepare for cesarean delivery.

c. Dangers to mother:

(1) Maternal fatigue, exhaustion, and dehydration evidenced by an increased pulse rate and temperature.

(2) Infection—preventive treatment includes fluids and antibiotics, especially if membranes are ruptured for prolonged period or if mother has a fever.

d. Dangers to fetus—injury and death.

6. Some conditions of the uterus make conception, pregnancy, or labor difficult if not impossible:

a. Anomalous uterus or fallopian tube.

b. Myomata of wall of uterine body or cervix.

c. Pathologic or Bandl's contraction ring.

C. Fetal abnormalities or conditions—fetopelvic disproportion and cephalopelvic disproportion (CPD).

1. Excessively *large* fetus:

a. Macrosomia—large newborn of a diabetic mother.

b. Large newborn—4500 g (10 + lb).

c. Enlarged fetal body—erythroblastosis fetalis (edema).

2. Fetal malformations—hydrocephalus (1 out of 2000 pregnancies).

3. Abnormal presentations of fetus:

a. Breech—3% of term deliveries; labor prolonged, soft buttocks do not dilate cervix as efficiently as hard vertex.

b. Occiput posterior (OP)—labor prolonged and woman experiences severe backache; may result in deep transverse arrest.

c. Face or brow—presenting diameter may be too large to negotiate through bony pelvis.

d. Transverse lie–shoulder (scapula) presenting—delivery usually by cesarean, although spontaneous version may occur.

e. Compound presentation—hand alongside head, for example.

4. Multiple births—*twinning.*

a. Comparison—identical and fraternal (Table 3–22).

b. Associated problems—increased risk of:

(1) Preeclampsia/eclampsia.

(2) Premature delivery.

(3) Hyperemesis gravidarum.

(4) Dystocia.

(5) Danger of asphyxia of second fetus (placenta may begin separating or cervix may close after birth of first twin).

TABLE 3–22. *Comparison of identical and fraternal twins*

Identical (monozygotic)	Fraternal (dizygotic)
Union of one egg and one sperm.	Union of two eggs and two sperm.
One or two placentas (fused, double).	Two placentas (fused, double).
One or two chorions.	Two chorions.
Always same sex.	Same or different sexes.
Usually hereditary.	Incidence increases with maternal age.
Greater chance of twin-to-twin transfusion (one polycythemic and one anemic).	Fare better than single-ovum twins.

  (6) Postpartum hemorrhage.
 c. Indications of multiple pregnancy:
  (1) Height of fundus—too high for dates.
  (2) Sonography.
  (3) High urine estriol.
 5. Nursing care—depends on type of dystocia.
  a. Observe mother for contour of uterus, presentation (vaginal examination or Leopold's maneuvers), contractions, and location of discomfort to help identify possible CPD early.
  b. Relieve back pain with sacral pressure, change of position, and pelvic rock if trial labor is indicated.
  c. Discuss with gravida her perceptions and knowledge of old wives' tales, "dry births," for example, which may increase her discomfort.
  d. Provide anticipatory guidance, for example, newborn's face will be swollen and discolored in face or occiput posterior delivery.
D. Birth canal dystocias:
 1. Soft tissue obstacles—
  a. Full bladder.
  b. Full rectum.
  c. Myomata of wall of cervix.
 2. Pelvis—
  a. Congenital deformities.
  b. Diseases of pelvic bone—rickets, tuberculosis, or osteomalacia.

  c. Abnormalities of spine—lordosis, scoliosis, or kyphosis.
  d. Old fractures.
 3. Nursing care:
  a. Support woman through a trial labor.
  b. Keep bladder and rectum empty.
  c. Prepare for cesarean delivery.
  d. Monitor maternal and fetal condition continuously.
E. Common problems associated with dystocia:
 1. Prolapse of cord.
 2. Prolonged labor.
 3. Fetal distress.
 4. Postpartum—increased incidence of hemorrhage and infection.

2. Uterine rupture
A. Pathology and etiology—uterus ruptures when the strain on muscle exceeds its strength; potential stresses include:
 1. Excessive distention—large baby or multiple gestation.
 2. Old scars—previous cesarean deliveries.
 3. Contractions against fetus who does not progress through birth canal because of malpresentation or CPD, for example.
 4. Injudicious obstetrics—malapplication of forceps or application without full dilatation and effacement.
 5. Folk medicines—some herbs cause uterine rupture.
B. Assessment:
 1. Complete rupture—
  a. Sudden sharp abdominal pain followed by cessation of contractions; abdominal tenderness.
  b. Shock, fetal heart tones cease, and vaginal bleeding.
  c. Presenting part not palpable during vaginal examination.
 2. Incomplete rupture—progresses over several hours:
  a. Contractions continue but are accompanied by abdominal pain and failure to dilate.
  b. Symptoms of maternal shock—pallor, tachycardia, air hunger, and exhaustion.
  c. May have some vaginal bleeding.
  d. Cessation of fetal heart tones.
C. Treatment—laparotomy, hysterectomy, transfusions, and antibiotics.
D. Nursing care:
 1. Prevention of uterine rupture—

a. Identify predisposing factors early (see previous discussion).

b. Judicious initiation and monitoring of oxytocin induction.

2. Be alert for predisposing conditions and developing signs of uterine rupture—report stat and initiate shock treatment (positioning, O_2, and IVs).

E. Prognosis:

1. Fetus—grave.
2. Mother—guarded.

3. *Amniotic fluid embolus*—amniotic fluid (with any meconium, lanugo, or vernix) enters maternal circulation through open venous sinuses at placental site and travels to pulmonary arterioles.

A. Etiology—rare complication, usually following rupture of membranes with some abruptio placentae and difficult labor.

B. Prognosis—poor; often fatal to mother.

C. Assessment:

1. Sudden dyspnea and cyanosis.
2. Pulmonary shock due to anaphylactic vascular collapse.
3. Evidence of blood coagulapathy (DIC).

D. Treatment:

1. Assist ventilation—position in semi-Fowler's, suction, oxygen, and mechanical ventilatory assistance.
2. Give whole-blood transfusion and injections of heparin. Platelets may be given.
3. Deliver stat—preferably with forceps, vaginally.
4. Digitalize.

4. *Prolapsed umbilical cord*—descent of cord in advance of presenting part.

A. Etiologies:

1. Spontaneous or artificial rupture of membranes before engagement of presenting part.
2. Excessive force of fluid escaping, as with hydramnios.
3. Malposition—breech, compound presentation, and transverse lie.
4. Premature or small fetus, allowing space for descent of cord.

B. Assessment:

1. Visualization of cord outside or inside vagina.
2. Fetal distress—variable deceleration and persistent bradycardia.

C. Treatment:

1. Place mother on absolute bedrest in exaggerated Trendelenburg's position, knee-chest, or Sims's position with pillows to elevate hips.

2. Push presenting part off cord with sterile gloved hand in vagina.

3. Cover exposed cord with sterile dressing, preferably wet with warm saline.

4. Oxygen by mask (8–10 liters/minute).

5. Deliver stat:

a. Vaginally with forceps.

b. Cesarean delivery, if vaginal delivery is not imminent.

6. Monitor FHR continuously or every two minutes.

5. *Inverted uterus*

A. Pathology and etiology—uterus is turned inside out, usually during birth of placenta when:

1. Cord is excessively short.
2. Cord is pulled before placental separation.
3. Fundal pressure is exerted when uterus is relaxed.

B. Assessment—shock, hemorrhage, and severe pain.

C. Treatment—replace uterus, hysterectomy, fluid and blood replacement, antibiotic therapy, and treatment for shock.

6. *Fetus in jeopardy*

A. Pathology—a compromised fetus suffering from hypoxia, anemia, or ketoacidotic environment.

B. Etiologies:

1. Maternal preeclampsia/eclampsia, heart disease, or diabetes.
2. Insufficient uteroplacental circulation due to—
   a. Maternal hypotension or hypertension.
   b. Cord compression.
   c. Hemorrhage.
   d. Malformation of the placenta/cord.
   e. Postterm gestation (placental senility).
   f. Maternal infection.
   g. Hydramnios.
   h. Hypertonic contractions.
   i. Placental infarcts.
3. Rh or ABO incompatibility.
4. Chorioamnionitis.
5. Dystocia (from CPD, for example).

C. Assessment:

1. Fetal heart rate (FHR) (Figure 3–7).
   a. Persistent irregularity.
   b. Persistent tachycardia of 160 or more per minute.
   c. Persistent bradycardia of 100 or less per minute.
   d. Early deceleration—head compression.

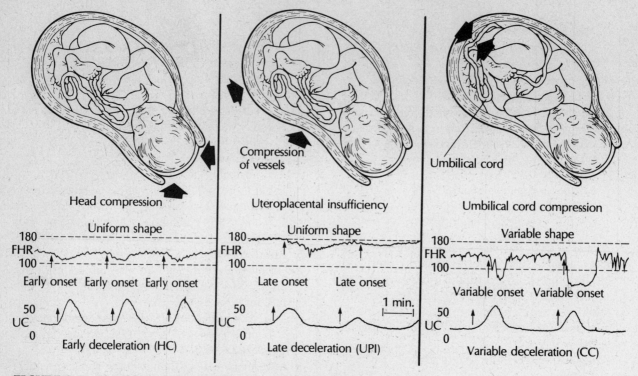

FIGURE 3-7. *Fetal heart rate (FHR) deceleration patterns*
(a) Early deceleration—head compression. **(b)** Late deceleration—uteropla-cental insufficiency. **(c)** Variable deceleration—umbilical cord compression. (From Olds, S. B., et al. *Obstetric nursing.* 1980. Menlo Park, California, Addison-Wesley Publishing Co. Adapted from Hon, E., 1976. An introduction to fetal heart rate monitoring (2 ed.). Los Angeles: University of Southern California School of Medicine.)

e. Late deceleration—uteroplacental insufficiency.
f. Variable deceleration—umbilical-cord compression.
g. Flatness of variability in FHR pattern.
2. Passage of meconium in vertex position; relaxation of anal sphincter, and gasping are consequences of cerebral anoxia.
3. Fetal activity:
   a. Hyperactivity—symptom of CO_2 retention.
   b. Cessation—possible fetal demise.
D. Fetal heart rate monitors:
1. Stethoscope or fetoscope.
2. Phonocardiography with microphone amplification.
3. Internal fetal electrode attached directly to fetus through the dilated cervix after membranes are ruptured.
4. Doppler probe using ultrasound flow.
5. Cardiotocograph—picks up sound through transducers placed on abdomen.
E. Evaluative tests:
1. Amniocentesis—

a. Definition—transabdominal placement of a needle into the amniotic cavity for the purposes of aspirating or injecting fluid; after 14th week of gestation.
b. Purposes:
   (1) Assessment of fetal maturity.
   (2) Diagnosis of fetal jeopardy.
   (3) Treatment of fetal hemolytic anemia after week 24.
   (4) Assessment of placental function (sufficiency).
   (5) Induction of abortion.
   (6) Identification of chromosomal aberrations.
c. Preparation:
   (1) Explain to woman.
   (2) Assist with sonography (to locate placenta).
   (3) Ask her to empty bladder.
   (4) Do surgical prep of skin.
   (5) FHR.
d. Studies—the aspirant is centrifuged to separate the cellular components from the

supernatant fluid for the purpose of:

(1) Cytogenetic study—genetic disorders, such as trisomy 21 (Down's syndrome), fetal sex determination (for sex-linked disorders), and fetal ABO incompatibility.

(2) Amniotic fluid study—

   (a) Spectrophotometric analysis for breakdown products of bilirubin (in presence of ABO or Rh incompatibility); in absence of hemolytic disease, bilirubin disappears after 38 weeks.

   (b) Lecithin/sphingomyelin ratio ("shake test" or "foam test") for fetal lung maturity—lecithin to sphingomyelin ratio of 2 to 1 (after week 35) usually indicates lung maturity (sufficient surfactant [lecithin] to initiate and maintain respirations).

   (c) Detection of inborn errors of metabolism—enzyme deficiency disease such as Tay-Sachs disease.

   (d) Creatinine level—2 mg/dl at week 36.

   (e) Level of alpha-1-feto protein (AFP) to identify neurotube defects.

e. Injection procedures:

(1) Saline solution to induce abortion (see Table 3–6).

(2) Radiopaque dye for fetus to swallow prior to transfusion of packed red blood cells, type O, Rh negative into the peritoneal cavity of a fetus compromised by maternal isoimmunization, after week 24, to relieve fetal anemia (see p. 265).

f. Hazards—under 1% for combined total for mother and fetus.

(1) Stimulation of labor when not desired.

(2) Puncture of fetus—monitor FHR.

(3) Puncture of placenta or placental vessels.

(4) Infection—request woman to notify physician if fever or malaise develop.

2. Evaluation of amniotic fluid after rupture of membranes (see p. 210).

3. Estriol assays:

a. Definition—index of placental functioning or sufficiency and fetal well-being; estriol is produced by fetal adrenals, processed by placenta, and excreted by maternal kidney; 24-hour levels increase as pregnancy progresses:

(1) Serial studies are begun about week 34, but may be done as early as week 28.

(2) Adequate functioning—12 mg or more per 24 hours.

b. Specimens—

(1) Urine—if maternal renal function is normal.

(2) Blood—not dependent on renal function.

4. Oxytocin challenge test (OCT)—determination of FHR response to uterine contractions.

a. Gravida is hospitalized; the FHR baseline is recorded; oxytocin induction is started; IV drip is regulated until three contractions occur in every ten minutes, then it is discontinued; contractions and FHR are monitored by cardiotocograph or fetal monitor.

b. If placental function is normal, fetal oxygenation is unimpaired by contractions.

c. If late or variable deceleration patterns are noted, or FHR falls below 100, fetal lung maturity tests are done and the gravida may be prepared for cesarean delivery, since fetus is most likely unable to withstand the process of labor.

d. This test is most frequently done on the diabetic or prediabetic gravida.

e. Complication—sustained or continuing uterine contractions.

f. No deaths (intrauterine) have been reported within one week of a negative test.

5. Nonstress test:

a. Test may be conducted on an out-patient basis.

b. Test is performed in same manner as OCT except that the woman's contractions are spontaneous and not induced by exogenous oxytocin.

6. Fetal activity acceleration determination (FAD).

a. Gestation of 28 weeks or more.

b. Externally monitored: FHR recorded in relation to fetal movement.

c. Difficult to determine if lack of fetal response reflects a problem or a sleeping fetus.

7. Fetal blood sampling:

a. Conditions—ruptured membranes, engaged vertex, and some cervical dilatation.

b. Signs of fetal distress—
   (1) pH below 7.20 (normal range is 7.3 to 7.4).
   (2) Increased arterial Pco_2.
   (3) Decreased arterial Po_2.

8. Summary of tests for estimating fetal maturity.
   a. Ultrasound—"A" scan may be done weekly for biparietal diameter after week 16.
   b. X ray—distal femoral epiphyses usually formed by week 36.
   c. Hormone levels—estriol and human placental lactogen (HPL) rise with normal pregnancy.
   d. Analysis of amniotic fluid (discussed previously).

F. Prevention and treatment of fetal jeopardy:
   1. Prenatal care to identify and treat concurrent medical conditions.
   2. Positioning gravida on her side for labor to prevent hypotensive syndrome.
   3. Judicious initiation and monitoring of induction.
   4. Intravenous fluids and oxygen prn.
   5. Astute frequent monitoring of fetal-maternal vital signs, labor, and response to labor.
   6. Prevention of maternal exhaustion, infection, dehydration, and hemorrhage.

7. Summary of danger signs during labor

A. Tonic contractions—every two minutes, lasting more than 90 seconds, with poor relaxation in between.

B. Sudden sharp abdominal pain followed by board-like abdomen and shock—abruptio placentae or ruptured uterus.

C. Bleeding from vagina.

D. FHR deceleration—late; variable; bradycardia, below 100; and tachycardia, 160 or more.

E. Amniotic fluid—excessive or diminished amount; presence of odor; meconium-stained, port-wine-colored, or yellow-colored; 24 hours or more since rupture of membranes.

F. Wide fluctuation in blood pressure—hypotension or hypertension.

G. Increased temperature, pulse, and blood pressure.

H. Fetal hyperactivity or cessation of activity.

I. Prolapsed cord.

J. Dyspnea and cyanosis following rupture of membranes.

8. Premature labor

A. Etiology:

1. Unknown. Labor may be stimulated by factors from the fetus when the placental function begins to diminish.

2. Medical conditions—
   a. Incompetent cervix.
   b. Multiple gestation.
   c. Polyhydramnios.
   d. Hypertension.
   e. Infections that may cause premature rupture of membranes (PROM).
   f. PROM of unknown etiology.
   g. Third-trimester bleeding.
   h. Iatrogenic:
      (1) Miscalculate EDC for repeat cesarean delivery.
      (2) Diabetes.
      (3) Other maternal conditions.

B. Prevention:
   1. Primary—maternal nutrition, decrease maternal stress (good mental and physical health).
   2. Secondary—cerclage for incompetent cervix.
   3. Tertiary—suppression of premature labor.
      a. Rest: bedrest in side-lying position.
      b. Pharmacologic: follow hospital protocol (Table 3–23).
         (1) Beta-adrenergic agents that make uterine myometrial cells less reactive to oxytocic and prostaglandin stimulation while increasing blood flow to uterus. Examples: isoxsuprine (Vasodilan) and ritodrine.
         (2) Alcohol (decreasing in popularity).
         (3) Terbutaline.
         (4) Magnesium sulfate.

C. Suppression of premature labor. Obtain a signed "informed consent."
   1. Maternal/fetal contraindications for suppression:
      a. Placenta previa or abruptio placentae.
      b. Chorioamnionitis.
      c. Erythroblastosis fetalis.
      d. Severe preeclampsia.
      e. Severe diabetes.
      f. Increasing placental insufficiency from any etiology.
      g. Cervical dilatation of 4 cm or more.
      h. Ruptured membranes.
   2. Nursing actions:
      a. Help mother maintain positive self-concept as a whole biologic woman (she has not finished tasks of pregnancy and is still not ready to let go of pregnancy).
         (1) Acknowledge her feelings of fear, guilt;

TABLE 3–23. *Pharmacologic inhibition of premature labor**

Pharmacologic substance	Side effects/precautions	Nursing actions
Ethyl alcohol 9.5% solution, IV (blocks secretion of oxytocin by the maternal pituitary).	Requires hospitalization. Fetotoxicity? Personal injury. Aspiration of emesis. Hypotension from excessive urinary output. Oral treatment for follow-up; outpatient treatment has no definitive guidelines or guaranteed results.	Monitor rate of IV infusion; rate determined by hospital protocol. Observe intoxicated woman closely: Keep siderails up. Assign someone to sit with her during treatment. Prevent aspiration if emesis occurs. Maintain careful record of urinary output. Monitor uterine activity, FHR, maternal vital signs. Provide emotional support to mother and family.
Isoxsuprine† (Vasodilan) (β_2-receptor stimulant; sympathomimetic).	Requires hospitalization. Bedrest with physician or nurse in constant attendance during intravenous infusion. Continuous cardiac monitoring (maternal); pulse irregularity. Arteriosonde monitoring: blood pressure fall. May require sedation or tranquilization to counter the effects of β-stimulation. If labor is suppressed, woman requires close supervision (on a weekly basis) for the duration of the pregnancy. No effect on fetus. It increases blood flow to fetus by maternal vasodilation. *Antidote:* Propranolol, 0.25 mg IV; may be repeated q 5 min, times 3 doses.	Initially administer IV infusion by calibrated pump. Increase rate of flow q 10 min until contractions diminish or cardiovascular effects indicate need to slow or stop infusion. After good control of uterine activity is achieved, continue infusion at maintenance dose for 12–24 hr longer. Position her as per physician order: Trendelenburg's or side-lying position. After therapy by IV infusion is discontinued, administer IM dose as ordered; then give orally, as ordered. Monitor uterine activity, FHR, maternal vital signs. Monitor emotional response because agitation and fear states may accompany β-stimulation; administer sedative or tranquilizer as ordered.
Ritodrine† (Premar) (an improved analogue of isoxsuprine).	Requires hospitalization. IV infusion with 1000 ml normal saline needed to hydrate woman prior to infusion with ritodrine; many hours of intravenous infusion are required. Constant monitoring of mother and fetus necessary. If labor is suppressed, requires close supervision (on weekly basis) for duration of pregnancy.	Baseline period: Assist with history and physical and admission procedures. Order laboratory tests before and at 48 hr and 6 wk after delivery: CBC, urinary analysis, CSB-I and -II for electrolytes, direct bilirubin. Initiation of therapy: Monitor FHR and uterine activity continuously. Monitor q 15 min; report BP < 90/60 or pulse > 140 beats/min. Maintenance dose period (oral medications)—outpatient status. Advise woman (couple) of doses per day, daily intake never exceeds 120 mg or 12 tablets per 24 hr.

(Continued)

TABLE 3–23.   *(Continued)*

Pharmacologic substance	Side effects/precautions	Nursing actions
		Order repeat of laboratory tests. Schedule weekly visits and assess FHR, maternal pulse, BP, uterine contractions, side effects.
Terbutaline sulfate† (Brethine, Bricanyl) (β_2-receptor stimulant; sympathomimetic).	Requires hospitalization. Side effects: Tachycardia, palpitations, sweating. Headache, nervousness, tremors, restlessness, anxiety, lethargy, drowsiness, tinnitus, dizziness. Nausea, vomiting.	Assist with history and physical and admission procedure. Order laboratory tests: CSB-II (electrolytes); urinary analysis; CBC: creatinine; serum ε_3 (before and 24 hr after treatment is started). Administer medication per hospital protocol. Monitor FHR and uterine activity. Monitor maternal BP q 15 min × 4 after each dose; if < 90/60 or pulse > 140 beats/min, hold next dose and call physician. Assess all urine for protein and glucose. If she is to be an outpatient on maintenance doses (5 mg tid for 4 wk), caution her (couple) regarding side effects. Phone physician. Home care for dizziness: increase fluid intake and lie down in lateral decubitus position (side-lying).
Magnesium sulfate	Cannot be given to woman who is digitalized. Requires hospitalization. Depresses CNS. Depresses muscles (cardiac, skeletal, smooth). Side effects: flushing and sweating, hypotension. Magnesium sulfate toxicity: severe CNS toxicity: Initial symptoms and signs: feeling "hot all over" and thirsty; diminished or absent patellar reflex. Flaccid paralysis, hypothermia, circulatory collapse, depressed cardiac function. Serum levels of magnesium > 10–12 mg/dl. IV injection of magnesium sulfate may cause neuromuscular or respiratory depression in neonate if administered to mother within 2 hr of delivery. *Antidote:* For magnesium toxicity in mother, calcium gluconate, 10% solution, 10–20 ml.	Assist with history and physical examination and admission procedure; check history to rule out digitalization. Have antidote readily available. Never leave woman alone. Before repeating doses per physician order, check patellar and other reflexes, respiratory rate, and urinary output. Monitor FHR and uterine activity; monitor maternal vital signs, intake and output, presence of side effects.

*From Jensen, M. D., Benson, R. C., and Bobak, I. M. 1981. *Maternity care: the nurse and the family.* St. Louis: The C. V. Mosby Company, ed 2. (Protocols vary because treatment is not yet fully tested or standardized.)

†Effects resemble the response to stimulation of β-adrenergic nerves: contractility and rate of heart muscle are increased, arterioles to skeletal muscle are dilated, bronchi relax, uterine muscle relaxes. These drugs may result in extreme agitation and fear states.

provide factual information.
(2) Explain proposed management.
(3) Familiarize her (family) with environment.
(4) Facilitate, support her feelings about fetal/neonatal prognosis.
(5) Provide comfort measures.
  b. Maximize oxygenation of fetus during labor.
(1) Side-lying position.
(2) Coach her breathing to prevent hyperventilation.
  c. Monitor—
(1) Response to suppression protocol: FHR and uterine activity.
(2) Maternal vital signs: BP, P, R; I & O; temp.
(3) For signs of continuing dilatation and of descent (change in point of maximal FHT impulse).
(4) Affect: maternal emotional response (may be denying reality or trying to cover up an intense guilt reaction); evaluate family's reaction to event.
(5) Maternal hydration: increased temperature and pulse; intake and output; assess urine.
(6) Temperature: if increased, assess for dehydration, anxiety, infection, exhaustion.
(7) Urine values.
  d. Stimulation of fetal lung maturity with beta-methasone (if premature delivery is deemed inevitable).
D. Labor (also see *Nursing actions, suppression of labor,* above):
1. Notify perinatal team.
2. Provide emotional support to parent(s): do not leave alone; keep them informed; provide comfort measures to mother (family).
3. Monitor labor: uterine activity, descent of fetus, bladder, etc.
4. Fetal monitoring: FHR (electronically, if possible); biochemical (blood gases, pH).
5. Coach: breathing and relaxation, positioning.
6. Preparation for delivery: May deliver before complete dilatation has occurred.
  a. May be delivered in side-lying (Sims) position.
  b. May have an extensive episiotomy.
  c. May be delivered with low forceps.
  d. Oxygen by mask.
  e. Continued monitoring of FHR.
7. Avoid using other medications during labor.

E. Postpartum care:
1. Facilitate attachment between infant and parents: emotional support during entire experience facilitates attachment by preventing drain of energy to fear and other negative feelings; foster couple's sense of mutual experience and closeness; help her (them) maintain a positive self-concept; encourage touching of infant before it is transported to nursery or premature center; father may accompany infant and report back to mother; encourage early contact; facilitate maternal need to ventilate feelings.
2. Routine postpartum care.
3. Assist parent(s) with grief and grieving process, if necessary.

9. *Grief and the childbearing experience*—the loss of a pregnancy or a newborn, or the birth of a child with a disorder, is a crisis situation (Table 3–24). The unexpected outcome (a small, sickly baby rather than a healthy, cute, full-term baby) can cause the parent(s) to lose self-esteem. In addition, the woman who does not conceive and/or complete a pregnancy, including labor and delivery, in the manner she expected, also suffers a sense of loss, for example, of self-esteem, self-concept, positive body image, feelings of worthiness.

POSTPARTAL PERIOD

1. *Hypofibrinogenemia*
A. Pathology—decrease of the clotting factor, fibrinogen in the blood; may be accompanied by disseminated intravascular clotting.
B. Etiologies:
1. Missed abortion or missed labor following intrauterine fetal death.
2. Clot formation following abruptio placentae.
C. Nursing management:
1. Order blood work.
2. Observe woman for bleeding and clot formation.

2. *Postpartal hemorrhage*—see also *Nursing management, fourth stage of labor,* p. 222).
A. Definition—loss of 500 ml blood or more during first 24 hours.
B. Etiology (in order of frequency):
1. Uterine atony—uterine relaxation secondary to:
  a. Overdistended pregnant uterus—multiple gestation, large baby, or hydramnios, for example.

TABLE 3-24.   *Loss of pregnancy*

Stage of grief	Possible maternal response	Nursing intervention
Shock, disbelief	Pulls back, withdraws: not interested in events around her; may stay in bed, staring at wall with shades drawn.	Since mother cannot communicate effectively now, nurse demonstrates caring behaviors by staying with her, touching or massaging her; providing physical care; giving her opportunity to talk if she wants to. Do not make light of her situation.
Anger, fear	Verbal fault-finding and possible physical aggression, irritability, insomnia.	State that it is normal to be angry; help her identify her questions and concerns (guilt); be available to her (and her family).
Helplessness, despair	Dependent behaviors—may become demanding, may cry, may exhibit regressive behaviors; may see no purpose to anything; may feel very guilty, worthless.	Help her verbalize her feelings: "It is hard to understand," "you probably feel you are to blame. . . .'"; "The way you feel may seem strange or even 'crazy' to you." Do provide physical care, give massage, keep her physically comfortable.
Reorganization (after discharge)	Begins to be interested in events around her, to have increased amounts of energy. Inquires again about events leading to the situation, the etiology, the medical and nursing management, as she tries to integrate the experience. Older siblings may show regressive behavior; fear of the dark, fear of school, or behavioral difficulties.	Community health or clinic nurse listens, clarifies, fills in gaps. Reexplain the grieving process—that her (their) behaviors were normal; that acute grief lasts 6 weeks, while the entire process lasts about 1 year. Talk about what older siblings or other family members may be feeling—a young child's return to bed-wetting may be a response to the parents' tension, etc.

b. Multiparity.
c. Prolonged labor or precipitous labor.
d. Anesthesia—deep inhalation or regional anesthesia, especially saddle block.
e. Myomata.
f. Oxytocin induction of labor.
g. Postpartum overmassage of uterus.
h. Distended bladder.
2. Lacerations—cervical, vaginal, or perineal.
3. Retained placental fragments.
4. Hematoma—deep pelvic, vaginal, or episiotomy site.
C. Assessment of shock—air hunger, restlessness, anxious facial expression, weak rapid pulse, cool and clammy skin, dropping blood pressure, and tachypnea.
D. Nursing care:
1. Note—
a. Lab values on prenatal chart—check for clotting time, hematocrit, and hemoglobin.

b. Estimated blood loss during labor-delivery.
c. Estimated blood loss postpartum.
2. Observe for and report—
a. Lacerations—bright red bleeding; bleeding continues when fundus is firm.
b. Atony—constant dark seepage, large clots expressed after firming fundus, and boggy uterus, a sign of relaxation of the "living ligature."
c. Hematoma—pain, discoloration, and swelling; can lose 500 ml or more into hematoma.
d. Retained placental tissue—boggy uterus and dark bleeding.
E. Treatment:
1. Uterine atony—primarily nursing responsibility (see *Postpartal care,* p. 222).
2. Lacerations—repair; replace fluid and blood prn.
3. Retained placental fragments—hemorrhage often occurs after woman is discharged; instruct concerning observation for bleeding, fever, and who

and when to call; return to hospital for D & C to remove tissue.

4. Hematoma—evacuation and fluid and blood replacement prn.

5. Prevent infection.

6. Remain with woman—check fundus, bleeding, and vital signs every 15 minutes until stable, then every two to four hours for one day.

7. Keep warm.

3. *Subinvolution*—failure of complete closure of the vessels in the placental site.

A. Assessment: persistent lochia; brisk hemorrhagic episodes.

B. Treatment: curettage.

C. Nursing care: explain condition and treatment; provide support to assist her with fatigue, irritability, delay in return to "normal."

4. *Postpartal infections*

A. "Childbed fever," *puerperal fever*—a genital-tract infection usually localized in the endometrium.

1. Predisposing conditions:
    a. Anemia.
    b. Premature rupture of membranes (PROM).
    c. Long labor.
    d. Intrauterine manipulation—manual extraction of placenta; version.
    e. Retained placental fragments.
    f. Postpartum hemorrhage.
    g. Numerous vaginal exams during labor.

2. Assessment:
    a. Fever 38 C (100.4 F) or more, chills, and malaise.
    b. Increased pulse rate.
    c. Pain—pelvic or abdominal.
    d. Vaginal discharge is foul smelling and profuse.
    e. Abscess formation elsewhere in body.
    f. Thrombophlebitis.
    g. Dysuria.

3. Prevention:
    a. Prevent anemia.
    b. Aseptic technique during labor and delivery.
    c. Labor—avoid prolonged labor, treat long labor or PROM with IVs containing calories and electrolytes, antibiotics, or deliver by cesarean.
    d. Avoid lacerations and retained fragments (allow spontaneous separation of placenta if possible) or diagnose early and treat.

    e. Perineal cleanliness.

4. Nursing care, see *Endometritis,* p. 254.

B. Urinary-tract infection:

1. Predisposing factors—
    a. Birth trauma to bladder, urethra, or meatus.
    b. Bladder hypotonia with retention (from anesthesia or birth trauma).
    c. Catheterization.

2. Symptoms may not appear for several days—dysuria, frequency, pus, and fever.

3. Nursing care—prevention:
    a. Ice pack to perineum during first hour postpartum to discourage edema and facilitate voiding.
    b. Encourage fluids and voiding.
    c. Aseptic catheterization technique and complete emptying of bladder.

4. Nursing care—treatment:
    a. Obtain urine for culture and sensitivity.
    b. Instruct woman concerning fluids, medications, general hygiene, and diet.

C. Mastitis—inflammation of breast tissue:

1. Cause—commonly caused by *Staphylococcus aureus* from infant's nasopharynx and oropharynx, clogged milk duct, bruised tissue, unclean hands, cracked or fissured nipples.

2. Assessment—
    a. Fever, chills, increased pulse, malaise, flu-like symptoms.
    b. Breast may be engorged, reddened, very hard and hot to palpation, tender or painful; a hard "moth ball" lump may be felt.

3. Nursing care—prevention:
    a. Nurse should be free of infection and use good handwashing technique.
    b. Instruct mother about cleanliness—handwashing, washing breasts and nipples with warm water *only* (so as not to dry out tissues and remove protective oils), and clean baby and linens.
    c. Assist mother with good breastfeeding technique to prevent fissures.
        (1) Proper support of infant at breast.
        (2) Gradual increase in infant's nursing time as nipples toughen.
        (3) Proper removal of nipple from infant's mouth.

4. Nursing care—treatment:
    a. Medications and ice packs, as ordered.
    b. Encourage wearing of bra or good support.
    c. Assist mother to stop nursing, if ordered—

encourage ventilation of feelings and treat for engorgement (see p. 229).

    d. If mother is to continue nursing, teach her how to "milk" breasts to stimulate continued production of milk until nursing from that breast is resumed.

D. Breast abscess: a localized complication of a more generalized infection (mastitis) in which pus accumulates in a local area in the breast.

  1. Nursing care—prevention (see *Mastitis* above).

  2. Nursing care—treatment:

    a. Discontinue nursing on the affected side.

    b. Express milk from affected side and discard it until abscess heals.

    c. Continue to nurse on the unaffected side.

E. Thrombophlebitis—inflammation of a vein.

  1. Causes:

    a. Extension of infection from uterine cavity (placental site) into pelvic and femoral veins.

    b. Clot formation in pelvic veins following cesarean delivery, or in calf of leg, due to poor circulation.

  2. Assessment:

    a. Pelvic—abdominal or pelvic discomfort and tenderness.

    b. Calf—positive Homan's sign, pain as foot is flexed while knee is extended.

    c. Femoral—leg swelling and pain, fever, chills, or "milk leg."

  3. Nursing care:

    a. Support bandage or stocking and elevate hip and/or leg.

    b. Medications—antibiotics and anticoagulants.

    c. Heat therapy, as ordered.

    d. Bedrest with bed cradle to support bedding.

    e. Caution mother not to massage "cramp" in leg.

F. Endometritis—infection of lining of uterus:

  1. Mild, local—no symptoms, or slight fever.

  2. Severe—

    a. Symptoms of infection—fever, chills, malaise, anorexia, headache, and backache.

    b. Uterus—large, boggy, and tender; dark brown lochia having a foul odor.

    c. If it remains localized, lasts ten days.

    d. Treatment:

      (1) Isolate.

      (2) Discontinue breastfeeding—depletes mother's energy.

      (3) Medications—antibiotics and ergot products.

      (4) Semi-Fowler's to promote lochial drainage.

      (5) High-calorie nourishment, fluids up to 4000 ml/day (oral or IV), and I & O.

      (6) Emotional support.

5. Postpartal psychiatric problems—sometimes seen in both the new mother and the new father. In women, psychiatric intervention is required in 4–5% of cases. Usually occurs within two weeks of delivery.

A. Etiology not fully understood. Probable etiology includes:

  1. Reaction to newborn and responsibilities for care.

  2. Surfacing of deep-seated feelings about femaleness and self-concept.

  3. Increased incidence among single parents (unwed, separated).

  4. Lack of adequate support system (familial, medical, nursing) in the early puerperium.

  5. Ambivalence regarding dependency/independency.

B. Most common symptomatology: affective disorders.

C. Assessment:

  1. Withdrawal.

  2. Paranoia.

  3. Refusal to eat.

  4. Depression may alternate with manic behaviors.

  5. May injure self and/or infant.

D. Management:

  1. Maintain her contact with infant.

  2. Pharmacologic—

    a. Schizophrenia—use phenothiazines.

    b. Depression—use mood-elevating medications.

    c. Mania—use sedatives.

  3. Maintain support systems.

E. Prognosis:

  1. Good.

  2. Recurrence risk after subsequent pregnancies is 10–20%.

NEONATE AT RISK

1. Neonatal disorders—effects of environmental events on embryonic/fetal development are detailed above in Table 3–9.

A. Assessment of environmental influences:

  1. Teratogens—"monster formers," environmental agents that interfere with normal cell differentiation during the period of organogenesis (the first

trimester); proven teratogens are X ray, rubella (German or three-day measles), and thalidomide.

   a. *Rubella*—congenital cataracts, microcephalus with mental retardation, congenital deafness of the Cranial VIII nerve, and cardiac malformations.

   b. *Thalidomide*—abnormalities in formation of extremities and craniofacial anomalies.

   c. *X ray*—specific malformations are not known; however, damage to the chromosomes within the sperm/ova is probable.

2. Harmful drugs—drugs primarily affect physiologic response when the fetus is exposed during the second and third trimesters.

   a. *Anticoagulants* (except for heparin)—hemorrhage and death of fetus.

   b. *Aspirin* (salicylates)—even one dose during week prior to birth—hypoprothrombinemia resulting in increased tendency to hemorrhage.

   c. *Corticosteroids*—possible cleft palate and anencephaly.

   d. *Diethylstilbestrol* (DES)—vaginal adenocarcinoma in childhood and adolescence; uterine, oviduct, and vaginal anomalies; higher percentage of abnormal sperm.

   e. *Dilantin*—cleft lip and palate, congenital heart disease, neonatal hemorrhage.

   f. *Amphetamines*—neonatal withdrawal, possible congenital heart disease, biliary atresia.

   g. *Oral progestins, androgens, estrogens*—masculinization of fetus, advanced bone age with growth failure occurring later.

   h. *Tolbutamide* (Orinase)—thrombocytopenia, multiple-birth anomalies, ketoacidosis.

   i. *Sedatives*—excessive amounts result in hemorrhage and death.

   j. *Sulfonamides*—kernicterus.

   k. *Tetracyclines*—teeth discoloration, hypoplasia of enamel, inhibition of bone growth; "grey syndrome."

   l. *Smoking* (20 cigarettes or more per day)—small-for-gestational-age (SGA) neonates, possible increased tendencies toward respiratory-tract illnesses during childhood.

   m. *Alcohol* (excessive, chronic use)—"fetal alcohol syndrome," intrauterine growth retardation (IUGR), respiratory depression at birth, withdrawal, craniofacial anomalies; later physical, cognitive, social-growth retardation.

   n. *Narcotic dependence* (morphine, heroin, methadone, meperidine)—increased fetal activity when drug level goes down; withdrawal syndrome in neonatal period; possible sudden infant death (SID) in later months.

3. Infections—many infections are hazardous to the fetus during the second and third trimesters.

   a. *Rubella*—SGA, bleeding tendency, enlarged liver and spleen, hepatitis (often with jaundice), bone lesions, encephalitis, pneumonia, abnormal EKGs, and abnormal fingerprints and palm creases.

   b. *Herpes simplex II* (genital herpes)—may be lethal to fetus, skin eruptions on newborn, and septicemia with respiratory and circulatory failure.

   c. *Syphilis*—snuffles (rhinitis), rhagades (scars around mouth), hydrocephaly, and corneal opacity; later: saddle nose, saber shin, Hutchinson's teeth (notched, tapered canines), and diabetes; no residual fetal-newborn effects if mother is treated adequately before fifth month.

   d. *Gonorrhea*—ophthalmia neonatorum acquired during passage through birth canal and neonatal sepsis with temperature instability, hypotonia, poor feeding, and jaundice; may be cause of premature labor, premature rupture of membranes, maternal fever, and chorioamnionitis.

   e. *Chlamydial disease*—conjunctivitis appears after three to four days; pneumonia (the adult male harbors this bacterium in his urethra and transmits it to his partner).

   f. *Cytomegalic inclusion disease* (virus in parotid glands) and toxoplasmosis (protozoan disease frequently acquired from household cats)—both produce similar symptoms: microcephaly, chorioretinitis, and cerebral calcification with seizures, progressive anemia, and hepatomegaly.

   g. *Mumps*—abortion, premature labor, fetal death, and congenital anomalies.

2. Classification of infants by weight and gestational age

A. Terminology:

1. Preterm or premature—37 weeks' gestation or under (usually 2500 g—5½ lb—or less).

2. Term—38 to 42 weeks' gestation.

TABLE 3–25.   *Estimation of gestational age—some common clinical parameters*

Physical characteristics	Preterm	Term
Head	Oval—narrow biparietal diameter ($\leq$ 35 cm, $\leq$ 13 inches); head large in proportion to body size; face looks like an "old man."	Square-shaped; biparietal prominences; head one-fourth body length.
Ears: form, cartilage	Soft, flat, and shapeless.	Pinna firm; erect from head.
Hair: texture, distribution	Fine, fuzzy, or wooly; clumped; appears at 20 weeks.	Silky; single strands apparent.
Sole creases	Starting at ball of foot, one-third covered with creases by 36 weeks; two-thirds by 38 weeks.	Entire sole heavily creased.
Breast nodules	0 mm at 36 weeks; 4 mm, 37 weeks	10 mm or more
Nipples	No areolae.	Formed; raised above skin level.
Genitalia		
Female	Clitoris large and labia gaping.	Labia larger, meet in midline.
Male	Small scrotum, rugae on inferior surface only, and testes undescended.	Scrotum pendulous and covered with rugae; testes usually descended.
Skin: texture, opacity	Visible abdominal veins; thin, shiny.	Only some larger veins may be seen indistinctly; thick, cracked, dry, peeling.
Vernix	Covers body between 31 to 33 weeks.	Small amount at term; absent and skin appears dry and wrinkled postterm.
Lanugo	Apparent at 20 weeks; between 33 to 36 weeks, covers shoulders.	No lanugo, or minimal amount.
Musculoskeletal signs		
Muscle tone	Hypotonia; extension of arms and legs.	Hypertonia; well flexed.
Posture	Froglike.	Attitude of general flexion.

3. Postterm—over 42 weeks.
4. Postmature—see characteristics in Table 3–9.
5. Appropriate for gestational age (AGA)—for each week of gestation, there is a normally expected range of weight:
   a. Small for gestational age (SGA) or dysmature—weight falls below normal range for age.
      (1) Cause—toxemia, malnutrition, smoking, placental insufficiency, alcohol syndrome, rubella, syphilis, twins, or genetic.
      (2) A term infant weighing 2500 g is usually mature in physiologic functioning and frequently may be discharged with the mother.
      (3) If respiratory distress occurs, it is usually due to aspiration syndrome.
   b. Large for gestational age (LGA)—above expected weight for age.
      (1) Cause—diabetic or prediabetic mother,

maternal weight gain over 35 lb, maternal obesity, or genetic.
      (2) A preterm infant weighing 7½ lb should be treated as a premature infant; if respiratory distress occurs, it is usually due to respiratory distress syndrome (RDS).
      (3) Associated problems—hypoglycemia, hypocalcemia, hyperbilirubinemia, and birth injury.
B. Estimation of gestational age—to plan for adequate care, it is essential to differentiate between the premature and the term infant. For a guide to clinical assessment, see Tables 3–25 and 3–26.

3. *Premature infant*—neonate of 37 weeks' gestation or less.

A. Etiology (see *Premature labor,* p. 248):
   1. Iatrogenic—EDC is miscalculated for repeat cesarean deliveries.

TABLE 3–25.   *(Continued)*

Physical characteristics	Preterm	Term
Traction response (head lag)	Head lags and arms have little or no flexion.	Head follows trunk and strong arm flexion.
Owl sign	Head capable of being rotated past point of shoulder.	Head can only be rotated to point of shoulder.
Scarf sign	Elbow is capable of being moved beyond midline to opposite axilla.	Elbow can only be brought close to midline, infant resists.
Square window	90°.	0°.
Ankle dorsiflexion	90°.	0°.
Popliteal angle	180°.	Under 90°.
Heel-to-ear maneuver	Touches ear easily.	90°.
Ventral suspension	Hypotonia; "rag doll."	Quite good caudal and cephalic tone.
Neurologic responses		
Moro reflex	Apparent at 28 weeks; good but no adduction.	Complete reflex with adduction, disappears four months postterm.
Grasp reflex	Fair at 28 weeks; arm is involved at 32 weeks.	Grasp response, strong enough to sustain weight for few seconds when infant is pulled up; hands, arm, and shoulders are involved.
Cry	24 weeks, weak; 28 weeks, high-pitched; 32 weeks, cry is good.	Good cry; lusty and can persist for some time.
Length	Under 47 cm (18½ inches), generally.	See Table 3–9.
Weight	Under 2500 g (5 lb 5 oz), generally.	

2. Placental factors—abruptio placentae, placenta previa, and insufficiency.
3. Uterine factors—multiple gestation, incompetent cervix, and uterine anomalies (including fibroids).
4. Fetal factors—malformations, infections (rubella, toxoplasmosis, and cytomegalic inclusion disease), and erythroblastosis.
5. Maternal factors—malnutrition, overwork, severe physical or emotional trauma, preeclampsia, hypertension, diabetes, heart disease, and infections (syphilis, leukemia, pyelonephritis, pneumonia, and influenza).
6. Miscellaneous—close frequency of pregnancy, advanced age of parents, heavy smoking, and high altitudes.

B. Cause of mortality (in relative order):
1. Abnormal pulmonary ventilation.
2. Infection—pneumonia, septicemia, diarrhea, and meningitis.
3. Intracranial hemorrhage.
4. Congenital defects.

C. Physiologic disadvantages—infant born before term is anatomically and physiologically disadvantaged; environment and care must be planned to meet special needs.
1. Respiratory system—insufficient surfactant and number and maturity of alveoli; immature musculature and rib cage; *problems:* respiratory distress syndrome, atelectasis, apnea, and poor gag and cough reflex.
2. Digestive system—poorly developed suck, swallow, and gag reflexes; small stomach capacity; immature enzyme system; *problems:* aspiration, malabsorption, diarrhea, abdominal distention, and fat intolerance; intake of tocopherol (vitamin E) is adequate in the breastfed neonate, but must be supplemented in the formula-fed; edema and anemia are attributed to a deficiency.
   a. Vitamin E (alpha-tocopherol): fat-soluble vitamin, and antioxidant. Functions: maintains structure and function of smooth,

TABLE 3-26. Clinical estimation of gestational age*

Examination First Hours

WEEKS GESTATION

PHYSICAL FINDINGS		Findings across weeks 20–48
Vernix		Appears (20) · Covers body, thick layer (24–37) · On back, scalp, in creases (38–39) · Scant, in creases (40–41) · No vernix (42+)
Breast tissue and areola		Areola and nipple barely visible, no palpable breast tissue (20–33) · Areola raised (34) · 1–2 mm nodule (36–37) · 3–5 mm (38–39) · 5–6 mm (40) · 7–10 mm (41) · ?12 mm (44)
Ear	Form	Flat, shapeless (20–32) · Beginning incurving superior (33–34) · Incurving upper 2/3 pinnae (36–37) · Well-defined incurving to lobe (39+)
	Cartilage	Pinna soft, stays folded (20–32) · Cartilage scant, returns slowly from folding (33) · Thin cartilage, springs back from folding (36–37) · Pinna firm, remains erect from head (39+)
Sole creases		Smooth soles without creases (20–32) · 1–2 anterior creases (33) · 2–3 anterior creases (35) · Creases anterior 2/3 sole (37) · Creases involving heel (39) · Deeper creases over entire sole (42+)
Skin	Thickness & appearance	Thin, translucent skin, plethoric, venules over abdomen, edema (20–31) · Smooth, thicker, no edema (33) · Pink (36–37) · Few vessels (38) · Some desquamation, pale pink (40) · Thick, pale, desquamation over entire body (42+)
	Nail plates	Appear (20) · Nails to finger tips (34) · Nails extend well beyond finger tips (44)
Hair		Appears on head (20) · Eye brows and lashes (23) · Fine, woolly, bunches out from head (28) · Silky, single strands, lays flat (37) · ?Receding hairline or loss of baby hair, short, fine underneath (42)
Lanugo		Appears (20) · Covers entire body (22–24) · Vanishes from face (34) · Present on shoulders (38) · No lanugo (42)
Genitalia	Testes	Testes palpable in inguinal canal (28) · In upper scrotum (37) · In lower scrotum (41)
	Scrotum	Few rugae (29) · Rugae, anterior portion (36) · Rugae cover (40) · Pendulous (42)
	Labia & clitoris	Prominent clitoris, labia majora small, widely separated (30–32) · Labia majora larger, nearly cover clitoris (36) · Labia minora and clitoris covered (42)
Skull firmness		Bones are soft (20) · Soft to 1" from anterior fontanelle (29) · Spongy at edges of fontanelle, center firm (35) · Bones hard, sutures easily displaced (38) · Bones hard, cannot be displaced (42+)
Posture	Resting	Hypotonic, lateral decubitus (20–24) · Hypotonic (26) · Beginning flexion, thigh (30) · Stronger hip flexion (32) · Frog-like (34) · Flexion, all limbs (36) · Hypertonic (38) · Very hypertonic (42)
	Recoil – leg	No recoil (20) · Partial recoil (33) · Prompt recoil (39)
	Arm	No recoil (20) · Begin flexion, no recoil (34) · Prompt recoil, may be inhibited (38) · Prompt recoil after 30" inhibition (42)

Week scale: 20 21 22 23 24 25 26 27 28 29 30 31 32 33 34 35 36 37 38 39 40 41 42 43 44 45 46 47 48

Confirmatory Neurologic Examination To Be Done After 24 Hours

Weeks Gestation

Category	Physical Findings	Findings across weeks (20–48)
Tone	Heel to ear	No resistance → Some resistance (≈31) → Impossible (≈36+)
	Scarf sign	No resistance (20–) → Elbow passes midline (≈33) → Elbow at midline (≈37) → Elbow does not reach midline (≈43)
	Neck flexors (head lag)	Absent (20–) → Holds head (≈43)
	Neck extensors	Head begins to right itself from flexed position (≈34) → Good righting cannot hold it (≈36) → Holds head few seconds (≈39) → Keeps head in line with trunk > 40 (≈41) → Turns head from side to side (≈45)
	Body extensors	Straightening of legs (≈33) → Straightening of trunk (≈37) → Straightening of head and trunk together (≈43)
	Vertical positions	When held under arms, body slips through hands (≈28) → Arms hold baby, legs extended? (≈34) → Legs flexed, good support with arms (≈39)
	Horizontal positions	Hypotonic, arms and legs straight (≈27) → Arms and legs flexed (≈37) → Head and back even, flexed extremities (≈40) → Head above back (≈44)
Flexion angles	Popliteal	No resistance (20); 150° (29); 110° (33); 100° (35); 90° (39); 80° (41)
	Ankle	45° (33); 20° (37); 0° (41); A pre-term who has reached 40 weeks still has a 40° angle (43)
	Wrist (square window)	90° (29); 60° (33); 45° (37); 30° (39); 0° (41)
Reflexes	Sucking	Weak, not synchronized with swallowing (26); Stronger, synchronized (33); Perfect (35); Perfect, hand to mouth (38); Perfect (43)
	Rooting	Long latency period slow, imperfect (26); Hand to mouth (31); Brisk, complete, durable (35); Complete (44)
	Grasp	Finger grasp is good, strength is poor (26); Stronger (33); Can lift baby off bed, involves arms (39); Hands open (46)
	Moro	Barely apparent (22); Weak, not elicited every time (26); Stronger (33); Complete with arm extension, open fingers, cry (35); Arm adduction added (39); ?Begins to lose Moro (47)
	Crossed extension	Flexion and extension in a random, purposeless pattern (26); Extension, no adduction (33); Still incomplete (36); Extension, adduction, fanning of toes (39); Complete (43)
	Automatic walk	Minimal (31); Begins tiptoeing, good support on sole (32); Fast tiptoeing (36); Heel-toe progression, whole sole of foot (39); A pre-term who has reached 40 weeks walks on toes (43); ?Begins to lose automatic walk (47)
	Pupillary reflex	Absent (20); Appears (30)
	Glabellar tap	Absent (20); Appears (33)
	Tonic neck reflex	Absent (20); Appears (32)
	Neck-righting	Absent (20); Appears (35); Present after 37 weeks (38)

Weeks: 20 21 22 23 24 25 26 27 28 29 30 31 32 33 34 35 36 37 38 39 40 41 42 43 44 45 46 47 48

skeletal, and cardiac muscles and vascular tissue; maintains liver integrity; maintains red blood cell integrity; functions as a coenzyme in tissue respiration; is the treatment for malnourished infants with macrocytic anemia. If the neonate is receiving a formula rich in polyunsaturated fats and fortified with iron, the need for vitamin E increases. Often a significant part in meeting the nutritional needs of the preterm neonate.

b. Necrotizing enterocolitis (NEC) is an inflammatory disease of the GI mucosa. Perinatal asphyxia is the most probable cause—if asphyxia persists beyond 30 minutes, blood is distributed to the heart and brain and away from GI mucosa. Other probable causes: immaturity, high-solute feedings, or excessive numbers of feedings. Septicemia may follow initial intestinal events. Abdominal distention is most frequent sign, but there may also be gastric residuals of 2 ml or more and/or occult blood in stool. Diagnosis is by X ray. Treatment is supportive: GI tract is rested and neonate is fed intravenously; antibiotics; surgery, prn. Complications (adhesions, etc.) may prolong recovery.

3. Heat regulation—unstable:
   a. Lack of subcutaneous fat.
   b. Large body surface area in proportion to body weight.
   c. Small muscle mass.
   d. Absent sweat or shiver responses.
   e. Poor capillary response to change in environmental temperature.

4. Resistance to *infection* is low—lack of immune bodies from mother (these cross placenta from mother late in pregnancy); inability to produce own immune bodies (immature liver); poor WBC response to infection; thin skin.

5. Central nervous system immature—weak or absent reflexes and fluctuating primitive control of vital functions.

6. Immature *liver*—susceptible to hyperbilirubinemia and hypoglycemia; immature production of clotting factors and immune globulins; anemia.

7. Retrolental fibroplasia—increased susceptibility of immature retina to high levels of arterial oxygen.

8. Immature *renal* function—cannot concentrate urine; precarious fluid and electrolyte balance.

9. Capillary fragility—increased susceptibility to hemorrhage in all tissues, including brain.

D. Factors influencing survival of premature newborn:
   1. Lung maturity.
   2. Anomalies.
   3. Size.
   4. Gestational age.

E. Assessment:
   1. Symptoms of respiratory distress.
   2. Feeding behaviors—color changes, abdominal distention, fatigue, and respiratory distress.
   3. Jaundice—susceptible to kernicterus at lower bilirubin levels.
   4. Voiding and stooling.
   5. Congenital anomalies.
   6. Skin—color, petechiae, ecchymoses, turgor, and edema.

F. Respiratory distress syndrome (RDS):
   1. Pathophysiology—lack of surfactant (lecithin) and immature alveoli predispose to atelectasis; ventilation is compromised; alveolar ducts and terminal bronchioli become lined with a fibrous glossy membrane.
      a. Primarily a function of prematurity.
      b. Other predisposing factors—
         (1) Fetal hypoxia—from maternal bleeding or hypotension, for example.
         (2) Birth asphyxia.
         (3) Postnatal hypothermia, metabolic acidosis, or hypotension.
      c. Factors protecting neonate from RDS—
         (1) Chronic fetal stress, from maternal hypertension, toxemia, and heroin addiction, for example.
         (2) Premature rupture of membranes (PROM).
         (3) Maternal ingestion of steroids, such as beta-methasone.
         (4) Low-grade chorioamnionitis.
   2. Assessment:
      a. Usually appear during first or second day of life.
      b. Signs of respiratory distress—
         (1) Retractions.
         (2) Tachypnea—60/minute or more.
         (3) Cyanosis.
         (4) Expiratory grunt.
         (5) Chin tug.
         (6) Increase in number and length of apneic episodes.

(7) Flaring of nares.

(8) Increasing exhaustion.

c. Hypercapnia with increased CO_2 level (respiratory acidosis).

d. Metabolic acidosis due to increased lactic acid.

3. Nursing care—supportive:

a. Ensure warmth (isolette at 97.6 F).

b. Provide O_2—amount sufficient to relieve cyanosis.

(1) Warmed, humidified, and at lowest concentration.

(2) Via hood, nasal prongs, endotracheal tube, bag, or mask.

c. Monitor continuous positive airway pressure (CPAP)—oxygen-air mixture is given under pressure during inhalation *and* exhalation; functions to keep alveoli open on exhalation.

d. Position to support respiratory efforts—side-lying, or supine with arms at sides, and neck slightly extended in "sniffing" attitude.

e. Keep airway clear—

(1) Postural drainage and percussion, as ordered.

(2) Suction.

f. Suction the neonate with an endotracheal tube.

(1) Disconnect tubing at the adaptor.

(2) Inject up to 0.5 ml sterile normal saline.

(3) Insert sterile suction tube, start suction, rotate tube between fingers and withdraw.

(4) Suction up to five seconds.

(5) Ventilate neonate with bag and mask during procedure.

(6) Reconnect tubing to adaptor securely.

(7) Take apical pulse and listen to chest for breath sounds.

g. Fluids, electrolytes, calories, vitamins, and minerals; intake and output records.

h. Protect against infections.

i. Meet neonate's psychologic needs—touch without pain; hear soft voices; see faces; and experience pleasurable motion, such as rocking.

j. Parents need support, information on condition and progress, and early sight and touch contact to foster attachment.

G. Oxygen toxicity:

1. Retrolental fibroplasia—primarily a disease of immaturity and high levels of arterial oxygen concentration; arterial oxygen concentrations should be kept between 50 and 60 mm Hg, if possible and should be measured by blood gas determinations; sequelae include various degrees of poor vision to blindness.

2. Bronchopulmonary dysplasia—primarily a disease of immaturity of the pulmonary system and high levels of arterial oxygen concentrations administered under pressure (CPAP and PEEP).

4. *Hypoglycemia*—low blood glucose level.

A. Assessment:

1. Lethargy and hypotonia or jitteriness; convulsions.

2. Sweating; unstable temperature.

3. Tachypnea or apneic episodes.

4. Cyanosis.

5. Shrill cry.

6. Feeding difficulty.

B. Predisposing conditions:

1. Birth asphyxia.

2. Gestational malnutrition (placental dysfunction; postmaturity).

3. Stress—infection, respiratory distress, abrupt discontinuation of parenteral fluids, and chilling.

4. Erythroblastosis.

5. Maternal disease—renal, cardiac, preeclampsia, and diabetes.

C. Nursing care:

1. Diagnose by noting preceding symptoms and predisposing conditions.

2. Diagnose by ordering lab work or doing a heel Dextrostix.

3. Normal lab values:

a. Term neonate—30–40 mg/dl blood.

b. Preterm neonate—20 mg/dl blood.

4. If hypoglycemic:

a. Feed glucose orally or parenterally, as ordered.

b. Record and report to physician.

5. *Drug-dependent neonate*—maternal addiction to heroin, morphine, methadone (see also p. 255).

A. Most drug-dependent neonates (50–90%) show withdrawal.

B. Assessment—degree depends on type and duration of addiction and level of drug in maternal blood at delivery.

1. Hyperactivity, hypertonicity; exaggerated reflexes, tremors, twitching, irritability, and difficulty sleeping; high-pitched cry. Note when assessing for hypertonicity:

a. Reddened nose, chin, knees from rubbing on linens.

b. When checking for the "step" or "pacing" reflex, the nurse notes that the addicted neonate places both feet onto surface and assumes a rigid, upright stance instead of stepping.

c. When checking for the "head-righting" reflex, the nurse notes that the neonate's head does not lag, but is held rigidly.

2. Feeding problems—regurgitation, vomiting, poor feeding, diarrhea, and increased mucus production.

3. Hunger—sucks on fists.

4. Nasal stuffiness and sneezing.

5. Respiratory distress, cyanosis and/or apnea, and pallor; yawning; tachypnea; exaggerated acrocyanosis and/or mottling in the warm infant.

6. Sweating.

7. Convulsions with abnormal eye-rolling and chewing motions.

C. Acute nursing care:

1. Monitor apical pulse and respirations.

2. Keep airway open—position on side and suction.

3. Collect all urine during first 24 hours for toxicologic studies.

4. Food/fluids—oral or parenteral, I & O, and weigh daily.

5. Decrease stimuli—keep noise down, handle infrequently, and offer pacifier.

6. Keep warm and swaddle for comfort.

7. Skin care—clean; dry; zinc oxide ointment and karaya powder q2–4h to excoriated buttocks, expose excoriated skin to air; and mitts over hands.

8. Medications, as ordered:

a. Paregoric gtt po, to wean neonate from drug.

b. Phenobarbital.

c. Chlorpromazine (Thorazine).

d. Diazepam (Valium)—do not give it to jaundiced neonate, as it predisposes to hyperbilirubinemia.

9. Emotional support to mother; encourage visits and participation in care; refer to social service or public-health nurse prn.

6. Postterm—over 42 weeks' gestation.

A. Labor may be hazardous for mother and fetus.

1. Large size may contribute to dystocia; diagnosis by ultrasound, "A" scan, and/or X ray.

2. Placental insufficiency may exist, exposing infant to intrauterine hypoxia; diagnosis by oxytocin challenge test, nonstress test, maternal urine estriol levels.

B. If also postmature, neonate may exhibit the following characteristics:

1. Wrinkled, dry skin—fetus may have needed to metabolize reserves of fat and glycogen to meet energy needs.

2. Long finger- and toenails.

3. No vernix and no lanugo.

4. Wide-eyed, alert expression, probably due to chronic hypoxia (oxygen hunger).

C. Prognosis—higher incidence of infant morbidity and mortality, especially during labor.

D. Nursing care:

1. Emotional support of mother during labor—may require cesarean delivery for CPD or because fetus cannot tolerate stress of labor contractions.

2. Monitor FHR continuously—report late or variable deceleration stat.

3. Diagnose and treat neonatal hypoglycemia.

4. If delivered vaginally, observe neonate for birth injuries.

7. Congenital disorders

A. Early recognition and treatment of structural or metabolic problems is a priority.

1. Early repair or treatment.

2. Emotional support of parents who must go through a grieving process soon after birth (see pp. 251).

3. Genetic counseling or family planning when appropriate; nutritional counseling, prn.

B. Types frequently seen:

1. Gastrointestinal tract—

a. Cleft lip and/or palate.

b. Tracheoesophageal fistula and/or esophageal atresia.

c. Imperforate anus.

d. Intestinal obstruction.

e. Omphalocele—protrusion of abdominal contents into base of umbilical cord.

f. Gastroschisis.

2. Orthopedic problems—

a. Clubbed foot (talipes equinovarus).

b. Congenital hip dysplasia.

c. Phocomelia—absence of all or part of a limb.

d. Supernumerary digits or polydactyly.

3. Central nervous system—

a. Anencephalus—absence of the cerebrum, its overlying bones, skin, and hair.

b. Microcephalus or hydrocephalus.

c. Spina bifida.

d. Intracranial bleeding or lesion—signs of increased intracranial pressure: tremors, eye-rolling, convulsion, respiratory distress with cyanosis or apnea, poor feeding and/or sucking, bulging fontanel, high-pitched cry, and incomplete or absent Moro reflex.

e. Dysfunction—evident by absent or abnormal reflexes; respiratory distress with cyanosis or apnea; weak and/or high-pitched, whining cry; poor feeding with regurgitation or vomiting; hypotonia or hypertonia; bradycardia; and hypothermia.

4. Urinary system:

   a. Hypospadias or epispadias—urinary meatus on the undersurface or the oversurface of the penis.

   b. Exstrophy of the bladder—absence of anterior of bladder wall exposing bladder wall; urine seeps onto abdominal skin.

   c. Agenesis—absence of development.

   d. Ambiguous genitalia.

5. Respiratory system:

   a. Diaphragmatic hernia with scaphoid abdomen—hernia of abdominal contents into thoracic cavity.

   b. Choanal atresia—partial or complete blockage of posterior nares.

6. Chromosomal aberrations:

   a. Down's syndrome (mongolism).

   b. Cri-du-chat syndrome—cry sounds like meowing of a cat.

   c. Turner's or Klinefelter's syndromes.

7. Cardiovascular system—congenital heart defects:

   a. Examples—tetralogy of Fallot, valvular atresias, and transposition of major vessels.

   b. Symptoms—cyanosis that may not respond to O_2; X ray shows an abnormal heart; respiratory distress; lethargy; hypotonia; easy fatigability; weak cry; poor feeding; sweating with exertion, such as crying or feeding; and edema.

8. Metabolic—inborn errors of metabolism:

   a. Phenylketonuria (PKU)—missing enzyme (phenylalanine hydroxylase) prevents conversion of phenylalanine (essential amino acid present in all animal protein) to tyrosine.

      (1) Inherited as a recessive gene.

      (2) Incidence—1 in 10,000 live births.

      (3) Build-up of phenylalanine results in mental retardation.

      (4) Treatment to minimize or prevent mental retardation—phenylalanine-poor diet, Lofenalac infant formula, for example.

   b. Galactosemia—inborn error of sugar metabolism, leads to mental retardation.

C. Nursing care:

   1. Preoperative and postoperative care—prevent infections, ensure adequate nutrition, and assist with laboratory work and other diagnostic tests.

   2. Parental support—assist parents to express feelings and ask questions; simplify and clarify physician's explanations; prepare them for sight of neonate and equipment needed for the neonate's care; allow for parents to see, hold, and touch neonate and to assist with nursing care as soon as possible; involve parents in decision-making process; make referrals to community resources as necessary.

   3. Emotional support of the neonate at risk (see p. 266).

8. Hemolytic disease of the neonate

A. Rh incompatibility (Figure 3–8):

   1. The Rh factor is an antigen that appears on the red blood cells of some people; these people are then Rh-positive; the Rh factor is dominant; a person may be (a) homozygous for Rh factor or (b) heterozygous for Rh factor.

   2. An Rh-negative person is homozygous for this recessive trait; does not carry the antigen.

   3. Isoimmunization is the process by which the Rh-negative person develops antibodies against the Rh factor.

   4. Pregnancy and the Rh factor:

      a. An Rh-positive mother may carry either an Rh-negative infant or Rh-positive infant with no consequence to the infant.

      b. An Rh-negative mother may carry an Rh-negative infant with no consequence to the infant.

      c. An Rh-negative mother carrying her first Rh-positive child usually does not develop antibodies to a level harmful to the fetus unless she was previously sensitized by an inadvertent transfusion with Rh-positive blood. Fetal cells usually do not enter the maternal blood stream until the time the placenta separates from the uterus, at abortion, abruptio placentae, and at delivery.

      d. After the delivery of an Rh-positive child, some of the child's Rh-positive cells enter

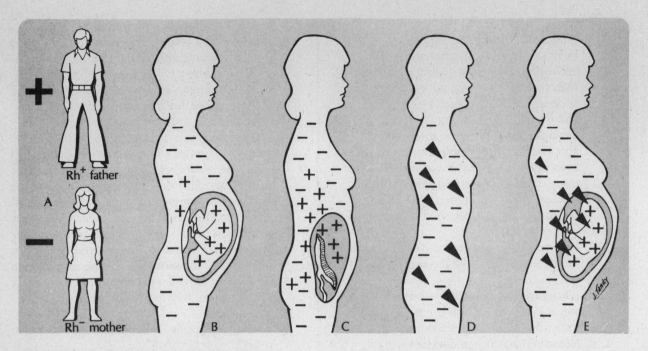

FIGURE 3–8. Erythroblastosis fetalis
Rh isoimmunization sequence. **(a)** Rh positive father and Rh negative mother.
(b) Pregnancy with Rh positive fetus. Some Rh positive blood enters the mother's
blood. **(c)** As placenta separates, further inoculation of mother by Rh positive
blood. **(d)** Mother sensitized to Rh positive blood; anti-Rh positive antibodies
are formed. **(e)** With subsequent pregnancies with Rh positive fetus, Rh positive
red blood cells are attacked. (From Olds, S.B., et al. Obstetric nursing. 1980.
Menlo Park, California: Addison-Wesley Publishing Co.)

the maternal blood stream and the mother
begins to develop antibodies against the red
blood cells carrying the Rh factor.

e. The anti-Rh-positive antibodies remain in
her blood stream with no consequence to
her; but at the time of the next pregnancy
with an Rh-positive fetus, these antibodies
will cross the placenta and enter the fetal
blood stream; hemolysis of fetal red blood
cells begins; degree of hemolysis is
dependent on amount of maternal
antibodies.

5. Assessment of isoimmunization—presence of
antibodies against Rh-positive red blood cells; Rh
sensitization or isoimmunization.
   a. Amniocentesis during pregnancy, beginning
   as early as 26 weeks (see p. 246, and 247).
   b. Indirect Coombs' test—to determine titer
   (amount) of antibodies mother has
   produced.

(1) Specimen—mother's blood.
(2) Test—mix mother's blood with Rh-
positive red blood cells.
(3) Positive test result—Rh-positive red
blood cells agglutinate (clump).
c. Direct Coombs' test:
(1) Specimen—neonate's blood (from
umbilical cord).
(2) Test—fetal red blood cells are "washed"
and mixed with Coombs' serum.
(3) Positive test result—neonate's Rh-
positive red blood cells agglutinate.

6. Summary of factors predisposing Rh incompatibility:
   a. Rh-negative woman.
   b. Pregnancies with Rh-positive fetuses.
   c. Accidental transfusion with Rh-positive
   blood.
   d. Small, concealed abruptio placentae where
   pregnancy continues for several days.

7. Rho(D) immune globulin:
   a. This drug is given to Rh-negative mothers of Rh-positive infants within 72 hours of delivery; the mothers should have *no* titer.
   b. This drug (Rh antibodies) removes fetal Rh-positive red blood cells that have entered the maternal blood stream; therefore, the mother does not develop antibodies.
   c. This drug *does not* remove anti-Rh antibodies from the maternal blood stream; that is, it cannot reverse any sensitization that has already occurred.
   d. This drug is given after every abortion and after every birth of an Rh-positive baby.
   e. If the fetus requires transfusion, Rh-negative blood is used.

B. ABO incompatibility—less severe hemolytic disease, usually.
   1. The person with type O blood carries anti-A and anti-B antibodies.
   2. The type O mother carrying a fetus who is type AB passes the anti-A and anti-B antibodies across the placenta to the fetus and hemolysis of fetal red blood cells commences.
   3. Because these antibodies are already present, even the first pregnancy with a type AB fetus is jeopardized; this incompatibility usually does not result in the severe hemolytic conditions possible with Rh incompatibility.
   4. If the fetus needs a transfusion, type O Rh-negative blood is used.

C. Assessment of hemolytic disease:
   1. Spectrophotometric analysis of amniotic fluid (between 26 and 31 weeks' gestation) identifies amount of hemolytic activity as seen by the amount of breakdown products of bilirubin present; this analysis is done after the mother has demonstrated a rising titer by indirect Coombs' test for anti-Rh antibodies or has a history of ABO incompatibility.
   2. Birth of a child with hydrops fetalis—the most severe form of hemolytic erythroblastosis; infant is grossly *edematous* from severe *anemia* and cardiopulmonary failure; infant is usually stillborn.
   3. Birth of an icteric infant, most common type.
   4. Development of *jaundice* within 48 hours of birth, mildest type.
   5. High bilirubin levels lead to the deposit of the yellow pigment in the basal ganglia of the brain, causing kernicterus; kernicterus may result in

death or varying degrees of neuromuscular dysfunction.
   a. Early signs—poor feeding, depressed reflexes, and increased muscle tone.
   b. Treatment—see following discussion of hyperbilirubinemia; if severe, postnatal blood exchange or intrauterine transfusion is performed.

D. Hyperbilirubinemia:
   1. Pathology—bilirubin, a breakdown product of hemolyzed red blood cells, appears at increased levels in the blood, more than 13–15 mg/dl blood; *warning:* there is no set serum bilirubin level that is safe; kernicterus is a function of the bilirubin level and the age and condition of the infant; poor fluid and caloric balance subjects the infant (especially the premature) to kernicterus at low serum levels of bilirubin, for example.
   2. Etiologies—
      a. Rh or ABO incompatibility, during first one or two days.
      b. During resolution of an enclosed hemorrhage, such as cephalhematoma.
      c. Infection-induced.
      d. Drug-induced—injection of vitamin K, maternal ingestion of sulfisoxazole (Gantrisin), and "breastfeeding jaundice" (pregnanediol in milk), for example.
      e. Immature liver.
   3. Assessment—
      a. Jaundice noted after blanching skin to suppress hemoglobin color; or noted in sclera or mucosa of dark-skinned neonates.
      b. Blood-level determination—hemoglobin or indirect bilirubin.
      c. Pallor.
      d. Concentrated, dark urine.
      e. Kernicterus—clinical manifestations are similar to those of intracranial hemorrhage.
         (1) Poor feeding and/or sucking and regurgitation and vomiting.
         (2) High-pitched cry.
         (3) Temperature instability.
         (4) Hypertonicity or hypotonicity.
         (5) Progressive lethargy; diminished Moro reflex response.
         (6) Respiratory distress.
         (7) Cerebral palsy, mental retardation, or death.
   4. Treatment—
      a. Prenatal treatment—transabdominal injection of packed Rh-negative, type O, red

blood cells into fetal peritoneal cavity to relieve fetal anemia.

b. Phototherapy—fluorescent light breakdown of bilirubin into water-soluble products.

c. Nursing care of infant receiving phototherapy:

(1) Cover closed eyelids while neonate is under light; with light off, remove eye pads for short periods during feeding or cuddling sessions or when parent visits.

(2) Expose as much skin as possible.

(3) Change position q1h.

(4) Note any loose green stools, provide good skin care, and offer fluids (about 25% more) between feedings.

d. Exchange transfusion—Rh incompatibility:

(1) Purpose—

(a) Remove anti-Rh antibodies and fetal Rh-positive red blood cells coated with antibodies; remove bilirubin when 20 mg/dl blood in term neonates and 16 mg/dl blood in preterm neonates.

(b) Correct anemia with red blood cells that will not be destroyed by maternal antibodies, Rh-negative, type O, for example; maximum amount exchanged is 500 ml; duration of exchange is 45 to 60 minutes.

(2) Hazards—

(a) If blood is not at room temperature, cardiac arrest may occur.

(b) If blood is not fresh, there is an increased possibility of hypocalcemia, tetany, and convulsions; to counteract this, have on hand calcium gluconate; 1 ml of calcium gluconate is given after every 100 ml of donor blood transfused.

(3) Nursing care during transfusion—

(a) Have equipment ready—monitors, resuscitation, radiant heater, and light.

(b) Monitor and record vital signs—baseline and continuous every 15 to 30 minutes.

(c) Record time and amount of blood withdrawn, donor blood injected, and medications given.

(d) Observe for dyspnea, listlessness, bleeding from transfusion site, cyanosis, cyanosis and coolness of lower extremities, and cardiovascular irregularity or arrest.

(4) Nursing care posttransfusion—

(a) In addition to preceding symptoms, observe for jaundice; continued observation for cardiac arrest or irregularities, hypoglycemia, and sepsis.

(b) Keep warm.

(c) Take frequent vital signs.

(d) Give oxygen to relieve cyanosis.

(e) Keep cord moist (in case of repeat transfusion).

(f) Feed per schedule.

9. Neonatal sepsis

A. Etiology:

1. Prolonged rupture of membranes.

2. Long, difficult labor.

3. Resuscitation procedures.

4. Maternal infection.

5. Aspiration—amniotic fluid, formula, or mucus.

6. Iatrogenic (nosocomial)—caused by infected personnel or equipment.

B. Assessment—generalized, usually nonspecific:

1. Respirations—irregular, periods of apnea.

2. Irritability or lethargy.

3. Jaundice or pallor.

4. Poor feeding (and/or sucking), vomiting, diarrhea, weight loss, and dehydration.

5. Hypothermia or hyperthermia.

C. Diagnosis:

1. Cultures—skin (before bath), throat, blood, urine, spinal fluid, and umbilicus.

2. Stomach contents—examined for polymorphonuclear cells.

D. Nursing care:

1. Isolate.

2. Keep warm.

3. Medications, as ordered.

4. Vital signs.

5. Oxygen to relieve respiratory distress, prn.

6. Food/fluids, as ordered; I & O; weigh daily; observe for dehydration (soft eyeballs, sunken fontanels, and poor skin turgor on thighs or abdomen).

7. Emotional support for neonate and parents.

10. Emotional support of the high-risk neonate

A. The neonate at risk has the same developmental needs as the healthy neonate—social and tactile stimulation that interest and comfort, and removal

of discomforts (hunger and soiling) by a consistent, parenting person.
B. It is more difficult to meet these needs, as the neonate:
  1. Listens to the sound of motors, hiss of oxygen, and sounds of human voices distorted by the incubator.
  2. Views the outside world distorted through the incubator and oxygen hood.
  3. Feels needle sticks and application and removal of monitors.
C. *Some* suggestions to modify effects:
  1. Assign the same nurses whenever possible.
  2. Arrange times to stroke skin, hold hand, hum or sing to neonate in enface position (nurse looking into neonate's eyes), comfort when crying, and hold during feeding if possible.
  3. Avoid loud, discordant radio music and loud voices.
  4. Arrange for parents to do above as often as possible for them to form attachment and to prevent later child abuse (much higher incidence of child abuse against child who had been a high-risk neonate).
D. Signs of emotional ill health of neonate:
  1. Does not look at person performing care tasks.
  2. Does not cry or protest.
  3. Shows poor weight gain and fails to thrive.

11. Neonatal infections
A. General infections (see pp. 255 and 268).
B. Oral thrush—mycotic stomatitis.
  1. Etiology:
    a. Organism—*Candida albicans,* a fungus.
    b. Vulnerable newborns—sick, debilitated newborns; those receiving antibiotic therapy; newborns with cleft lip or palate, neoplasms, or hyperparathyroidism.
  2. Spread of infections by direct contact with:
    a. Maternal birth canal, hands, and linens.
    b. Contaminated feeding equipment.
    c. Contaminated hands.
  3. Assessment:
    a. Appearance of white patches on oral mucosa, gums, and tongue that bleed when touched.
    b. Occasionally, some neonates may have difficulty swallowing.
  4. Treatment and *nursing management:*
    a. Cleanliness and good handwashing technique.
    b. Chemotherapy:
      (1) Aqueous gentian violet 1% to 2%

applied with a swab to infected areas.
      (2) Nystatin (Mycostatin) instilled into mouth with a medicine dropper or applied with a swab to lesions, after feedings; prior to medicating, feed sterile water to wash out milk.

Part D | REPRODUCTIVE-SYSTEM DISORDERS IN WOMEN AND MEN

REPRODUCTIVE-SYSTEM DISORDERS IN WOMEN*

1. Menstrual conditions
A. Amenorrhea—absence of menstruation.
B. Dysmenorrhea—painful menstruation.
C. Menorrhagia—excessive menstrual bleeding.
D. Metrorrhagia—bleeding between menstrual periods and after menopause.
E. Menopause—cessation of ovulation and menstruation, occurring at approximately 40 to 50 years of age.

2. Abnormal uterine bleeding in nonpregnant women
A. Menstrual disorders: may be treated with oral-contraceptive medications.
B. Trauma—from attempted self-abortion, IUD, rape—may be treated with surgery as needed, removal of IUD, counseling.
C. Infection: may be treated with antibiotic or other chemotherapy.
D. Neoplasms: may be treated with surgery, radiation, chemotherapy.
E. Contraceptive medications: alter the brand and dosage.
F. Drugs such as anticoagulants, salicylic acid (aspirin), sulfa drugs, thiazide diuretics, quinine: medication is discontinued and alternative is prescribed as necessary.
G. Endometriosis: heat coagulation by laparoscopy, hormonal therapy, surgery may be used in treatment.

---

*For anatomy and physiology, see pp. 160–166.

H. Iron deficiency anemia: may treat with iron supplement and diet.
I. Congenital or acquired blood coagulation disorders: may be treated with infusion of platelets, cryoprecipitate, whole blood, or packed red blood cells.

3. Gynecologic procedures
A. Abortion (detailed above in Table 3–6).
B. Cold-knife conization of cervix—rotary coring or excision of the endocervix for removal of diseased or abnormal tissue.
C. Colporrhaphy—anterior (repair of cystocele) and posterior (repair of rectocele).
D. Culdoscopy—visualization of the cul-de-sac for evidence of PID, bleeding, ectopic pregnancy, and ovarian cysts.
E. Dilatation and curettage (D & C) (Table 3–6).
F. Hysterectomy—types:
  1. Subtotal—fundus excised; cervical stump remains.
  2. Total—entire uterus excised; tubes and ovaries remain.
  3. Pan—entire uterus, tubes, and ovaries excised.
G. Laparoscopy—visualization of intraabdominal cavity with a scope inserted through small incision in abdomen.
H. Culposcopy—magnified visualization of cervix that permits visualization of cellular dysplasia and vascular or tissue abnormalities. Useful in monitoring abnormal Pap smears and DES daughters.
I. Culdocentesis—passage of a needle (culdotomy) into the cul-de-sac through the posterior fornix of the vaginal vault. Can obtain fluid from peritoneal cavity and perform tubal ligation.
J. Oophorectomy—removal of the ovaries.
K. Salpingectomy—removal of the fallopian tubes.
L. Biopsy—removal of a small amount of tissue for microscopic examination.
M. Endometrial smear—removal of cells for microscopic examination.
N. Pap smear—removal of cells for microscopic examination.
O. Vulvectomy—removal of the vulva.

4. Infections
A. Vaginal infections—types and care.
  1. *Candida albicans* (moniliasis):
    a. Fungus—likes dark, wet environment.
    b. Assessment—pruritus, redness, and thick cheesy discharge.
    c. Medications—local, 5% gentian violet; insertion propionate compound (Propion gel), ointment or suppository; nystatin (Mycostatin); and antibiotics.
    d. Those more prone—diabetics, those taking oral contraceptives, pregnant women, and those on medications (antibiotics and steroids).
    e. Causes *thrush* in newborn.
  2. *Trichomonas vaginalis:*
    a. Protozoa—thrives in alkaline environment.
    b. Assessment—increased thin, frothy vaginal discharge, pruritus, burning, redness, and punctate (strawberry) cervix.
    c. Medication—change pH to acid with vinegar douche; oral medication (for both partners), metronidazole (Flagyl).
  3. Nursing care:
    a. Instruct woman about medications and general hygiene.
    b. Instruct about douching.
    c. Instruct about avoiding intercourse until cured.
  4. Douching—douche only when prescribed during pregnancy; do not douche until after six-week postdelivery check-up.
    a. Fill can or bag with prescribed fluid.
      (1) Acidic douche—Massengill or white vinegar, 15 ml to 1000 ml water (1 tbsp to 1 qt water).
      (2) 1000 to 2000 ml of the prescribed solution is warmed to 40 to 43 C (105 to 110 F).
    b. Connect via tubing to vaginal *nozzle* (do not use bulb as this may force fluid into uterus and cause embolus).
    c. Hang bag two feet or less above the hips.
    d. Sit in clean tub or on toilet.
    e. Void prior to procedure.
    f. Insert nozzle 1½ to 2 inches downward and backward; rotate to wash all surfaces.
    g. If sitting on toilet, hold labia together, fill vagina, release labia; fluid and debris will be washed out.
    h. Continue until required solution is used up.
B. *Gonorrhea* is the most common contagious bacterial disease in North America (see E below).
  1. Bacterium—*Neisseria gonorrhea,* gram-negative diplococcus.
  2. May be mildly symptomatic or asymptomatic and persist undetected.
  3. If symptoms occur, they appear within days of contact and include: vaginitis, cervicitis with

infection, then ascending up the reproductive tract into the peritoneum.

4. May result in adhesions and infertility.

5. Fetal effects: premature rupture of membranes, amnionitis, low birth weight, premature labor, ophthalmia neonatorum (see p. 255).

6. In postpartum period, woman may exhibit signs of acute salpingitis, dermatitis, arthritis.

7. Treatment: woman and sexual partner(s) are treated to prevent reinfection. Penicillin is drug of choice, but erythromycin or cephalosporins may be used. In acute stage of salpingitis, bedrest may be prescribed.

C. *Syphilis* remains a major cause of late abortion throughout the world. Congenital syphilis still occurs. The chancre (which appears three to four weeks after contact) is the primary infection and is transient. Therefore the chancre may be overlooked; the woman may become infected after her initial obstetric examination and VDRL.

1. Spirochete—*Treponema pallidum.*

2. Diagnosis by various serologic tests:
   a. Nontreponemal serologies: screening, less expensive.
      (1) VDRL—venereal disease research laboratory.
      (2) RPR—rapid plasma reagin.
      (3) False positives are possible if client has a collagen disease or infectious mononucleosis.
   b. Treponemal-specific serologies: specific for treponemal organism and more expensive.
      (1) TPI—treponema pallidum immobilization test.
      (2) FTA-ABS—fluorescent treponemal antibody absorption test.

3. Treatment: preferably with penicillin, but drugs such as erythromycin may also be used.

4. If woman is treated by the eighteenth week of gestation, both the infection and the stigmas of congenital syphilis (see p. 255) are prevented; if treated after that time, the infection will be controlled but the destruction of tissue that has occurred is irreversible.

D. *Herpes virus, type II,* is increasing in incidence.

1. This viral infection may involve the external genitals, vagina, and cervix. It is characterized by painful papulovesicles that develop, drain, and then remain as superficial ulcerations until healed.

2. May result in stillbirths, abortions; leukorrhea, vaginal bleeding, and genital pain.

3. The woman in labor with genital herpes:
   a. If genital lesions are present and the membranes have not ruptured, delivery is by cesarean surgery to prevent contamination of the fetus during birth.
   b. If genital lesions are present and the membranes are ruptured for longer than four hours, vaginal delivery is allowed. Ascending infection has already infected the fetus.

4. The newborn with congenital herpes is severely compromised. There is no treatment; many of these newborns succumb (see p. 255).

5. Repeated infections with herpes are implicated in cervical carcinoma, especially if the woman has been very sexually active prior to age 17 and has had repeated infections from that time.

6. Treatment is for comfort. As yet there is no cure. Local anesthetic applications may bring comfort. Nystatin (Mycostatin) suppositories may be given to prevent candidiasis.

E. Pelvic inflammatory disease (PID)—inflammation of pelvic contents, which may include fallopian tubes (salpingitis), ovaries (oophoritis), pelvic-vascular system, and peritoneum.

1. Etiology:
   a. Pathogens are usually introduced through cervical canal and spread by direct extension and by the lymphatic and vascular systems.
   b. Pathogens—*Streptococcus; Staphylococcus;* sexually transmitted (venereal) herpes virus II, syphilis, gonorrhea, and *Trichomonas;* and tubercle bacillus (from lungs via blood stream).

2. Assessment—fever and malaise.
   a. Abdominal and low-back pain.
   b. Nausea, vomiting, and diarrhea.
   c. Leukocytosis.
   d. Foul-smelling vaginal discharge with pruritus.
   e. Urinary-tract infection.

3. Complications—
   a. Chronic discomfort and disease.
   b. Sterility—from scar tissue in fallopian tubes.
   c. Ectopic pregnancy—passage to uterus blocked by scar tissue.
   d. Adhesions—pelvic organs.

4. Nursing care and treatment—acute care:
   a. Semi-Fowler's to facilitate drainage.
   b. Heat—external to abdomen; internal via douching.
   c. Shower preferable to tub bathing.

5. Nursing care and treatment (ongoing)—
   a. Administer medications.
   b. Prevent spread.
      (1) Good handwashing by woman and personnel.
      (2) Isolation technique for care or disposal of equipment, supplies, linen, and perineal pads.
      (3) To handle equipment and supplies, wear gloves and use instruments (forceps).
      (4) Avoid catheterization.
   c. Provide emotional support.
   d. Nutrition—fluids to 3000 ml/day.

5. Pelvic-support relaxation

A. Cystocele—descent of part of posterior bladder wall into vagina.
   1. Etiology: delivery of large baby, numerous deliveries, prolonged labors.
   2. Assessment: sensation of vaginal fullness, "falling out," incomplete bladder-emptying or stress incontinence; bulge seen in vagina with Valsalva maneuver.
   3. Complications: urinary retention with recurring UTIs.
   4. Prevention: Kegal exercises; prevent obesity, chronic cough, straining, traumatic deliveries.
   5. Treatment: pessary, exercises (Kegals), surgery (colporrhaphy).
B. Rectocele—rectovaginal hernia:
   1. Etiology—delivery of large infant or breech delivery, numerous deliveries; poor bowel habits (chronic constipation with straining).
   2. Assessment—difficulty evacuating stool, sensation of vaginal fullness; soft, reducible mass bulging into posterior wall of vagina.
   3. Complications—fecal impaction.
   4. Prevention—episiotomy for prolonged second stage or large infant; good bowel habits, for example, avoid prolonged use of laxatives or enemas, avoid constipation with straining.
   5. Treatment—correct faulty diet and bowel habits, pessory, surgery.
C. Other conditions:
   1. Enterocele—intestinal hernia.
   2. Urethrocele—prolapse of the female urethra through the urinary meatus.
   3. Prolapsed uterus—protrusion of uterus into vagina, partially or completely through the vaginal orifice.

6. Endometriosis—abnormal growth of endometrial tissue outside of the uterus.

A. Etiology—unclear.
   1. Embryonic tissue remnants.
   2. Transport of endometrial tissue to ectopic sites during surgery, with menstrual flow, or via vascular system.
B. Assessment:
   1. Infertility or sterility.
   2. Abnormal uterine bleeding.
   3. Pain—backache, rectal pain, and dyspareunia (painful intercourse), and dysmenorrhea.
C. Diagnosis:
   1. Vaginal-rectal pelvic examination—fixed nodes, ovaries, and uterus; pain.
   2. Barium enema—adhesions and constrictions.
   3. Presence of a bluish spot on cervix.
D. Nursing management and treatment:
   1. Emotional support.
   2. Ovulation suppressants to relieve dysmenorrhea.
   3. Surgeries—relieve adhesions, resection of tissue, and total hysterectomy.

7. Neoplasms

A. Tumors of the breast:
   1. Types—
      a. Fibroadenoma—benign, firm, round, movable, and painless.
      b. Cancer, malignant—leading cause of mortality in women; survival rate, approximately 50%.
   2. Incidence—increases in women who are childless, have not breastfed, have a family history of breast cancer, or have a late menopause.
   3. Injuries are not a cause.
   4. Assessment—elevation and asymmetry of breast, bleeding from nipple, orange-peel skin, nipple retraction, and painless lump (especially in upper, outer quadrant).
   5. Diagnosis—breast self-examination (95%), physician examination, mammography, thermography, xerography, and biopsy.
   6. Stages and treatment (the following reflects traditional thinking; today lumpectomy is the preferred treatment in many cases)—
      a. Stage I (localized nodes negative)— mastectomy with or without radiation.
      b. Stage II (localized, axillary nodes positive)— mastectomy with or without radiation.
      c. Stage III (local extension, area nodes positive)—masectomy and excision of large axillary nodes; radiation alone if mass is fixed.
      d. Stage IV (distant metastasis)—variable surgery, radiation, hormone treatment, and chemotherapy.

7. Treatment and nursing care—
   a. Emotional support.
   b. Preoperative and postoperative care.
   c. For women receiving localized radioisotope therapy:
      (1) Follow directions on precaution sheet accompanying therapy.
      (2) Wear film badge when near woman.
      (3) Limit time near her, provide only essential care, for example.
      (4) Limit time spent within 1 m (3 ft) of woman.
      (5) Encourage her to remain in own room.
      (6) Watch for loosened or lost implants in bedding, clothing, bedpan, dressings, etc.; *do not pick it up;* call the radiology laboratory.
      (7) Follow precautions when handling the following:
         (a) Iodine—excreted in urine and sweat; present in blood and vomitus.
         (b) Colloidal gold—present in wound seepage; excreted in urine.
         (c) Phosphorus—excreted in urine and feces; present in vomitus.
   d. Predischarge teaching regarding exercises, follow-up care.

B. Stages—Papanicolaou test (cytology test for cancer):
   1. Class I—normal.
   2. Class II—atypical cells, nonmalignant; follow-up with repeat pap smears.
   3. Class III—suspicious cells; cytology evaluated by biopsy, D & C.
   4. Class IV—abnormal cells; suspicious of malignancy; cytology evaluated by biopsy, D & C.
   5. Class V—malignant cells present.
   6. Herpesvirus, type II—may be a major etiologic factor in cervical dysplasia, cancer (also may cause fetal death).
C. Cervical carcinoma (Table 3–27)—general nursing actions (see also Unit 5):
   1. Assessment:
      a. Woman's (family's) perception and knowledge of the condition and its treatment.
      b. General health history.
      c. Situational supports, coping skills.
      d. Wound-healing; infection.
      e. Colostomy stoma and drainage, and/or ileal conduit and urine.
      f. Fluid/electrolyte status; I & O; IVs.
      g. Readiness for oral intake: fluids, progressive diet.
      h. Amount of time spent at her bedside if she

TABLE 3–27. *International system of staging for cervical carcinoma*

Stage	Location	Prognosis	Treatment
0	In situ.	Highly curable.	Conization.
I	Cervix.	Cure rate decreases as stage progresses.	Radiation.
II	Cervix to upper vagina.		Radiation.
III	Cervix to pelvic wall or lower ⅓ of vagina.		Surgeries: 1. Panhysterectomy with wide vaginal excision with removal of lymph nodes; ileal conduit. 2. Pelvic exenteration: a. Anterior: removal of vagina and bladder; ileal conduit. b. Posterior: removal of rectum and vagina; colostomy. c. Total: both anterior and posterior. 3. Chemotherapy.
IV	Cervix to true pelvis, bladder, or rectum.		

has a radioactive implant; wear a dosimeter; limit time to 15 min/day.

   i. Later: assess adjustment to changes: elimination, sexual life; activity of daily living, etc.

2. Interventions—plan and implementation:
   a. Explain and reexplain.
   b. Nasogastric tube to decompress the GI tract.
   c. Progress diet based on individual's preferences.
   d. Teach regarding colostomy care, ileal conduit functioning, infection, exercises (legs, deep breathing).
   e. Listen actively, facilitate ventilation and decision-making, etc.: grief, loss, mutilation, possible death; changed relationships with others; changes in life styles; sexual counseling; loss of fertility; cultural meaning to woman and her family.
   f. Link up with self-help groups (stoma groups); Meals-on-Wheels.
   g. If receiving radiation—side effects, such as change in appetite, fatigue, nausea: counsel regarding diet modification, rest.
   h. If receiving chemotherapy: side effects as above and also loss of hair.
   i. Do not allow pregnant women or children to visit at bedside—help woman maintain contact with family, friends, through phone calls, notes, pictures.

D. Uterus—*endometrium:*
   1. High-risk population: perimenopausal women.
   2. Pap smear: may be negative in 20% to 30% of cases.
   3. Conditions—
      a. Benign fibroid tumors (myomata)—20% to 40% of women, aged 25 to 40 years, causes menorrhagia, low-back pain, urinary and bowel problems, and infertility or sterility.
      b. Malignant tumors—women, aged 30 to 50 years; second highest cause of mortality; metrorrhagia; leukorrhea; surgery may be followed by radiation.
   4. Stages of invasiveness:
      a. 0, in situ; atypical adenomatous hyperplasia; treated by hysterectomy.
      b. I, uterus is of normal size; treated by hysterectomy with no radiation.
      c. II, uterus is slightly enlarged, but tumor is undifferentiated; treated by radiation: implant, X ray; four to six weeks after radiation, hysterectomy is performed.
      d. IV, advanced, metastatic; progestin may

diminish pulmonary lesions; radiation, chemotherapy, surgery are choices of treatment depending on condition of client.

E. Ovarian neoplasms:
   1. Benign ovarian cysts—more common than malignant neoplasms.
   2. Malignant changes—less frequent than carcinoma of the endometrium or cervix.

REPRODUCTIVE-SYSTEM DISORDERS IN MEN*

1. Conditions affecting the reproductive tract in men
A. Venereal disease:
   1. Syphilis—chancre begins as a dull, red, hard, and insensitive papule on or near glans about three to four weeks after infection; treatment by penicillin or tetracycline.
   2. Gonorrhea—causes urethritis, purulent discharge about four to ten days after infection; inflammation of meatus with burning on urination developing; treatment by penicillin or tetracycline.
B. Prostate:
   1. Prostatitis—inflammation caused by bacteria, prostatic stones and urethral stenosis, alcohol, and irregular sexual activity.
   2. Benign hypertrophy—enlargement due to hyperplasia of normal glandular and muscular tissue (interferes with normal urination).
   3. Malignant neoplasm—cancer of the prostate (incidence of this rather rare neoplasm may be increased in men whose mothers were treated with DES during that pregnancy).
C. Scrotum:
   1. Hydrocele—abnormal accumulation of fluid in scrotum following local trauma, infection (epididymitis or orchitis), tumor, or in conjunction with congestive heart failure or hepatic cirrhosis.
D. Testes:
   1. Tumor—usually malignant.
   2. Epididymitis—inflammation due to infection (prostatic, urinary tract, or septicemia).
   3. Orchitis—inflammation of testes most often due to mumps; mumps orchitis may lead to sterility.
   4. Cryptorchidism (cryptorchism)—undescended testes; if one or both testes remain in abdominal cavity, testosterone will be produced, but spermatogenesis will not occur; orchiopexy is best performed at five to seven years of age.

---

*For anatomy and physiology, see pp. 166–168.

5. Vasectomy—ligation-transection of a section of the vas usually done to sterilize the man.
   a. Prevents the transport (but not the production) of sperm.
   b. No physical effect on production of testosterone or sexual performance (potency, erection, and ejaculation); seminal fluid continues to be produced by the seminal vesicles and prostate glands; psychologic response may alter sexual performance, however.
   c. Reanastamosis possible in 20% to 40% or more of cases. However, autoimmunity (antibodies against his own sperm) may result in permanent sterility.
E. Penis:
   1. Glans—ulceration may be caused by cancer; syphilis; herpes virus, type II (genital); psoriasis; and others.
   2. Cancer—rare, usually of prepuce or glans.
   3. Balanitis—inflammation of glans penis.
   4. Phimosis—constricted prepuce that cannot be retracted over glans; treated by circumcision.
   5. Circumcision—excision of prepuce or foreskin.
   6. Paraphimosis—following retraction, prepuce cannot be brought forward over the glans again; this is a surgical emergency (circumcision) to prevent gangrene of glans.

INFERTILITY IN WOMEN AND MEN

1. **Infertility**—or the inability to conceive with unprotected intercourse of a year's duration—occurs in about 12% to 15% of couples. The emotional impact of infertility requires judicious and sensitive counseling and physical evaluation. A complete history and physical examination are necessary. Factors in women are responsible in 40% of cases; factors in men, 50%; couple factors, 10%; no medical factors identified, 5% to 10%.

2. **General factors implicated in infertility for both women and men**
A. Hormonal.
B. Mechanical:
   1. Adhesions.
   2. Tumors.
C. Infection/inflammation.
D. Congenital anomalies.
E. Lack of sexual knowledge.
F. Immune response.

3. **Infertility in women**
A. Irregular menstrual cycles or anovulatory cycles may be causative factors; usually during a hospitalization of one or two days, several endocrine tests may be done; one is a urine test for FSH, estrogen, and 17-ketosteroids.
B. Hysterosalpingography is done during the woman's follicular phase (first half of cycle) to evaluate the uterine cavity and tubal patency (often, this test alone clears any minor obstruction and pregnancy may be possible); tubal patency is assessed by transuterine insufflation with carbon dioxide gas (Rubin test).
C. The Sims/Huhner test for motility of sperm in vaginal/cervical secretions is performed within 24 hours of intercourse; this postcoital test determines the receptivity of the cervical-vaginal mucus to the sperm.
D. Culdoscopy may reveal any structural anomalies present in the intraabdominal cavity and reproductive organs.
E. Occasionally a female develops antisperm antibodies to her mate's sperm, thus altering their ability to fertilize.

4. **Infertility in men**
A. A low sperm count (40 million/ml or less) is a primary factor in 20% of cases and a contributing factor in another 20%.
B. Occasionally, a man develops autoimmunity to his own sperm; the sperm is altered in such a way that fertilization is not possible.

Questions / NURSING CARE DURING THE REPRODUCTIVE YEARS

Select the one answer that is best. (Answer blanks are provided at the back of this book.)

The nurse who teaches young men and women of childbearing age in a family-planning clinic must have a sound foundation of knowledge of the menstrual cycle. Questions 1 through 6 refer to this situation.

1. Factors that influence whether or not contraceptives are used and the type of contraceptive method chosen include all of the following, *except:*
   1. Religious teachings.
   2. Cultural influences.

3. Legalization of abortion.
4. Consumer push for return to naturalness.

2. The rhythm method of birth control depends on basal body temperature (BBT) during the menstrual cycle. The hormone responsible for the elevation in BBT is:
1. FSH.
2. HCS.
3. Estrogen.
4. Progesterone.

3. At the time of ovulation, the BBT:
1. Falls slightly, then increases by about 0.5 C.
2. Rises slightly, then falls by about 0.2 C.
3. Is affected by a surge of FSH.
4. Is affected by a surge of progesterone.

4. The reliability of the BBT in determining the time of ovulation depends on all of the following *except:*
1. Level of motivation of the woman.
2. Level of tension.
3. Regularity of the menstrual cycle.
4. Level of formal education completed.

5. At the time of ovulation, the cervical mucus has all of the following characteristics, *except:*
1. Clear.
2. Good spinnbarkeit.
3. Sticky.
4. Fern pattern appears when dried.

6. Under the influence of progesterone, the cervical mucus has all of the following characteristics, *except:*
1. Opaque.
2. Stretchable.
3. Sticky.
4. Does not dry into a fern pattern.

7. In which of the following contraceptive methods is the production of an egg suppressed?
1. Intrauterine device.
2. Spermicidal foam or jelly.
3. Oral-contraceptive pills.
4. Tubal ligation.

8. One form of contraception is to take the "morning after" pill, which contains 25 mg of estrogen. If menstruation does not occur within five days after treatment is completed:
1. Nothing further is needed. Pregnancy has not occurred.
2. D & C needs to be performed.
3. The treatment is repeated.
4. The treatment is 100% effective.

9. In a 30-day cycle, ovulation probably occurred on which day of the menstrual period?
1. Day 5 or 6.
2. Day 13 or 14.
3. Day 16 or 17.
4. Day 28 or 29.

10. Which of the following is *not* a normal side effect of oral contraceptives?
1. Nausea and weight gain.
2. Chloasma.
3. Leg cramps and headaches.
4. Breast tenderness.

11. The Hyde Amendment (1978) severely restricts the use of federal funds for:
1. Family-planning clinics.
2. Abortions.
3. In-vitro fertilization and embryo transplantation.
4. Bioengineering such as cloning.

12. Signs and symptoms of water intoxication do *not* include:
1. Headache.
2. Oliguria (under 200 ml/8 hr).
3. Dyspnea.
4. Restlessness.

13. Signs of hypernatremia, a condition that can occur during saline abortion, do *not* include:
1. Thirst.
2. Tinnitus.
3. Tachycardia.
4. Headache.

Joan states that her last menstrual period (LMP) was six weeks ago (April 10) and that she spotted two weeks ago (May 8). Questions 14 through 19 refer to this situation.

14. Joan's expected date of confinement (EDC) is:
1. January 17.
2. January 3.
3. February 15.
4. February 1.

15. Joan is anxious to hear when a pregnancy test can be done. Counting from the last menstrual cycle, sufficient HCG is present in the urine to give a positive test by the end of the:
1. Fourth week.
2. Fifth week.
3. Sixth week.
4. Seventh week.

16. Joan is undergoing a pelvic examination. You can assist her by all of the following nursing actions, *except:*
1. Explain what to expect and why the examination is being done.
2. Offer your hand for her to squeeze.
3. Suggest breathing techniques to help her to relax.
4. Ask her to empty her bladder before the examination.

17. Joan's vaginal discharge is thick, white, cheese-like, and pruritic. The nurse's therapeutic and educational actions are based on the following theory:
1. No action needed. This is the normal leukorrhea of pregnancy.

2. Metronidazole (Flagyl) is the best drug for this condition.
3. Even if untreated, this condition presents no hazard for the neonate.
4. This is more likely to occur in women who are pregnant, taking oral contraceptives or antibiotics, or who are diabetic.

18. You know that Joan understands how to decrease her discomfort from "morning sickness" when she tells you she feels good after doing any one of the following, *except:*
1. Avoids an empty stomach.
2. Takes an antacid between meals.
3. Snacks on dry (unsalted) carbohydrates before arising in the morning.
4. Eats small servings of bland foods.

19. The person who examines Joan will probably find:
1. The FHT is detected with an ultrasound device, over the symphysis pubis.
2. The urine test for pregnancy is positive.
3. The uterine fundus is at the level of the symphysis.
4. Joan's pregnancy is not advanced enough for any of the above findings.

20. During the first eight weeks of gestation, progesterone and estrogen are produced principally by the:
1. Trophoblasts.
2. Placenta.
3. Anterior pituitary.
4. Corpus luteum.

21. Inadequate nutrition during pregnancy may contribute to fetal-newborn problems such as:
1. Premature delivery and small-for-gestational-age infants.
2. Oversized fat babies with immature functional responses.
3. Hyperbilirubinemia.
4. Acrocyanosis.

22. In addition to one liter of water, an adequate daily minimum intake for women who are within normal weight for age and height when they conceive includes all of the following (or the equivalents), *except:*
1. 1500 ml milk (6 cups).
2. Meat—three servings.
3. Vegetables and fruits—four servings, including at least one of citrus.
4. Breads and cereals—two slices bread, 1 oz cereal, and one serving of food like grits, spaghetti, or rice.

23. Ms. M tells you she cannot tolerate citrus fruits in any form. Which of the following foods are rich in vitamin C (ascorbic acid) and can be taken to meet the daily requirement?
1. Broccoli, papaya, and cantaloupe.
2. Dried beans (cooked) and peanut butter.
3. Yellow cheeses, spinach, and prunes.
4. Egg yolk, winter squash, and enriched bread.

24. Ms. M should be advised that the following foods are rich in iron:
1. Citrus fruits, sweet potatoes, and bananas.
2. Dry beans (cooked), chicken, prunes, and broccoli.
3. Enriched bread or cereal, cheddar cheese, and egg.
4. Peanut butter, carrots, and cornmeal or corn oil.

25. To relieve heartburn, a common discomfort during pregnancy, Ms. M may be advised to:
1. Eat dry bread products before rising in the morning.
2. Bend at the knees, not at the waist, when reaching down.
3. Eat fewer, larger meals per day and avoid nibbling.
4. Do pelvic rock exercise in standing position.

26. Although there is considerable diversity in individual life experiences that affect the adaptive process, there are certain psychic trends common to each trimester of pregnancy. During the second trimester, the woman generally:
1. Is ambivalent about the pregnancy.
2. Is ready to begin learning breathing exercises.
3. Fantasizes about the child and may withdraw from other relationships.
4. Becomes more outgoing.

27. During normal pregnancy, islets of Langerhans increase in size and increase insulin production due to:
1. Antiinsulin effect of human chorionic somatomammotropin (HCS).
2. Proinsulin effect of HCS.
3. Increased maternal tissue sensitivity to insulin.
4. None of the above. Islets of Langerhans do not change in size or production.

28. All of the following are within normal limits during pregnancy, *except:*
1. Elongation of urethra by 1½ to 3 inches.
2. Hydroureter, especially on the right side.
3. Esophageal regurgitation.
4. Loss of teeth due to drain on calcium/phosphorus stores.

For questions 29 through 31, indicate those groupings of physical-emotional changes that are most characteristic of a particular trimester of pregnancy.

29. Umbilicus flush with skin; chloasma and secondary areolae appear; external ballottement is felt; and iron therapy is started:
1. First trimester.
2. Second trimester.
3. Third trimester.
4. Fourth trimester.

30. Weight gain about 1 lb per week; pelvic joints relax; varicosities increase; and woman is anxious to be done with pregnancy:

    1. First trimester.
    2. Second trimester.
    3. Third trimester.
    4. Fourth trimester.

31. Test for HCG positive; lower uterine segment softens; urinary frequency common; and colostrum appears:
    1. First trimester.
    2. Second trimester.
    3. Third trimester.
    4. Fourth trimester.

32. Anticipatory guidance during the prenatal period includes instructing the mother to recognize abnormal symptoms that require immediate notification of the physician; these include:
    1. Excessive saliva, "bumps" around her areolae, and increased vaginal mucus.
    2. Fatigue, nausea, and urinary frequency.
    3. Ankle edema, enlarging varices, and heartburn.
    4. Severe pain in abdomen, fluid discharge from vagina, and fingers swelling.

33. Placental functions include all of the following, *except:*
    1. Secrete HCG, HCS (HPL), estrogen, and progesterone.
    2. Act as the organ of respiration for the fetus.
    3. Screen out viruses, large bacteria, and toxins.
    4. Provide for the passage of nutrients to the fetus and for removal of fetal wastes.

34. Antibodies produced by the mother are transmitted to the fetus because:
    1. Fetal and maternal blood mix in the intervillous spaces.
    2. Osmotic exchange occurs through capillaries between pooled maternal blood and fetal circulation.
    3. There is active secretion of the antibodies by the placenta.
    4. Antibodies cannot cross the placental barrier.

Melissa is in her 34th week of pregnancy. She states that her legs become swollen by late afternoon, she is uncomfortable with hemorrhoids and constipation, and she can feel her womb tighten and relax "a lot." Questions 35 through 37 refer to this situation.

35. During Melissa's routine prenatal visit, the nurse can expect the following normal findings:
    1. Braxton Hicks contractions, hypermobility of joints, backache.
    2. Dysuria, constipation, hemorrhoids, lightening.
    3. Feeling of tranquility and a heightened introspection.
    4. Morning sickness, breast tenderness.

36. The nurse reviews with Melissa those symptoms that require immediate medical intervention; these include all of the following, *except:*
    1. Epigastric pain.

    2. Periorbital edema.
    3. Brownish spotting occurring within 48 hours after vaginal examination.
    4. Seeing double.

37. Melissa also complains of groin pain, which is noticeably worse on her left side. This is most likely due to:
    1. Bladder infection.
    2. Constipation.
    3. Tension on the round ligaments.
    4. Beginning of labor.

In questions 38 to 41, indicate in which period you would expect to find the following groupings of characteristics of fetal-neonatal development.

38. Lanugo and vernix caseosa appear, quickening is first noted, FHR is first heard (with a stethoscope), and enamel and dentin are deposited:
    1. First trimester.
    2. Second trimester.
    3. Third trimester.
    4. In the postterm neonate.

39. Fetus assumes a human appearance and is vulnerable to teratogenic effects, period of organogenesis, and placenta begins to secrete progesterone:
    1. First trimester.
    2. Second trimester.
    3. Third trimester.
    4. In the postterm neonate.

40. Fingernails extend well beyond fingertips, skin is wrinkled and dry, eyes are wide open and appear alert, and vernix and lanugo are absent:
    1. First trimester.
    2. Second trimester.
    3. Third trimester.
    4. In the postterm neonate.

41. Length 20 inches (50 cm), eyes are open, cry is good, testes are descended, lanugo is shed, and storage of fat and nutrients occurs:
    1. First trimester.
    2. Second trimester.
    3. Third trimester.
    4. In the postterm neonate.

42. All of the following may decrease a gravida's anxiety of labor and delivery, *except:*
    1. An introduction to some breathing techniques to practice at home.
    2. A tour of maternity unit and meeting the personnel.
    3. Preparation-for-parenthood classes.
    4. A description in detail of the events of labor and some common complications and how these are managed.

43. In fetal circulation, the presence of the foramen ovale allows for the flow of blood:
    1. From the right atrium into the left atrium.

2. From the left atrium into the right atrium.

3. From the right ventricle into the left ventricle.

4. From the pulmonary artery into the aorta.

44. In fetal circulation, the presence of the ductus arteriosus allows for the flow of blood:

1. From the pulmonary artery into the pulmonary vein.

2. From the right atrium into the left atrium.

3. From the left ventricle into the pulmonary artery.

4. From the pulmonary artery into the aorta.

45. Rubella infection during the second or third trimesters is hazardous to the unborn fetus. The fetus/neonate may exhibit all of the following, *except:*

1. Hepatitis (often with jaundice).

2. Abnormal fingerprints and palm creases.

3. Snuffles.

4. Encephalitis.

46. The woman who contracts rubella during the first trimester may have a child with all of the following disorders, *except:*

1. Congenital cataracts.

2. Cranial VIII nerve injury.

3. Cardiac malformations.

4. Hydrocephaly.

47. If a woman smokes 2½ packs of cigarettes per day during her pregnancy, the nurse:

1. Tells her that if she keeps that up, the baby will be small in size and have a greater chance for respiratory-tract infections during childhood.

2. Tells her how to substitute snacking on cheese or raisins or dried apricots to curb her desire for smoking.

3. Asks her to think of ways she may be able to cut down.

4. Asks her how she plans to cut her smoking down to ten cigarettes per day.

48. Which of the following groups of findings is most indicative of a 20-week gestation?

1. Lightening, FHR audible with Doptone, and height of fundus at one fingerbreadth below umbilicus.

2. Braxton Hicks contractions, ballottement, and height of fundus at umbilicus.

3. Quickening noted, FHR audible by fetoscope, and height of fundus just below the umbilicus.

4. Goodell, Hegar, and Chadwick signs appear; fundus halfway between symphysis and umbilicus.

49. Douching during pregnancy:

1. Is unnecessary.

2. Should never be done, as it may induce abortion.

3. Becomes a necessity because of the copious vaginal secretions.

4. Depends on the woman's routine of personal hygiene.

50. Gravidas should know that labor has progressed sufficiently to go to the hospital when:

1. Contractions are three to five minutes apart, lasting 50 seconds, and a malar flush appears.

2. Contractions are three to five minutes apart and low-back pain and urinary frequency is experienced with contractions.

3. Contractions are regular, lasting 30 to 45 seconds or more, with some bloody show.

4. Contractions are two to three minutes apart, lasting 60 to 90 seconds.

51. Which of the following symptoms should the gravida report to the physician immediately?

1. Edema of lower extremities, vulval varices, and copious clear vaginal discharge.

2. Heartburn, shortness of breath, change in appetite.

3. Leg cramps, back pain, and increased pigmentation over bridge of nose and cheeks and in vulval area.

4. Headache, feeling of fullness in face and hands, and a few spots of brown discharge from vagina.

52. The mechanism that initiates labor is unknown. Which one of the following is definitely *not* a factor?

1. Decrease in progesterone as placenta matures.

2. Maternal pituitary production of oxytocin and fetal hormone production.

3. Reflex uterine response to overdistention.

4. Increasing fetal activity.

53. During her last month of pregnancy, Ms. L tells you she is "sick and tired of this whole thing. I can hardly wait to get this out of me." The nurse's most appropriate response at this time would be:

1. Refer her to the psychiatric social worker, since she should be experiencing a positive response to her infant now.

2. Tell her you know exactly how she feels and that you've been through it all yourself.

3. "Well, it sounds like you are ready for labor. Do you have any questions about your coming labor?"

4. "Your pregnancy is getting a bit wearisome and the time is dragging?"

54. Ms. L tells you that she is planning to breastfeed because "you don't have to take contraceptives until you wean the baby." The nurse's response should be:

1. Lactation does suppress ovulation so you are pretty safe.

2. You are safe just as long as you do not menstruate.

3. When a woman is breastfeeding, she may not menstruate, although she may ovulate; it is best to use some type of birth control.

4. You will find that you won't be interested in resuming intercourse until you wean the baby.

55. During her pregnancy, Ms. L developed moniliasis. All of the following are true about moniliasis, *except:*

1. Caused by *Candida albicans,* a fungus.

2. Causes ophthalmia neonatorum in the newborn.

3. Treated by drugs such as nystatin (Mycostatin) and gentian violet.

4. Most prevalent in women who are taking oral contraceptives or who are diabetic.

56. When assessing the frequency, duration, and intensity of contractions, the nurse:
    1. Spreads the fingers of one hand lightly over the fundus.
    2. Moves the fingers of one hand over the uterus, pressing into the muscle.
    3. Holds her hand (fingers and palm) over the area just below the umbilicus.
    4. Indents the uterus in several places during and between contractions to check for uniform uterine response.

57. Vaginal examinations during labor are done to ascertain all of the following, *except:*
    1. Station.
    2. Dilatation and effacement.
    3. Beginning separation of low-lying placenta.
    4. Presenting part and fetal position.

58. Mr. S is staying with his wife throughout labor. As Mrs. S progresses in labor, she becomes increasingly irritable with her husband, complaining of lower back pain and fatigue. The nurse appropriately responds by:
    1. Having Mrs. S turn on her side and giving her a back rub.
    2. Asking Mrs. S if she would like the doctor to give her something for the discomfort.
    3. Reassuring Mr. S that irritability is normal now and teaching him to apply pressure to her lower back.
    4. Encouraging Mrs. S to try and get some rest and asking Mr. S if he would like to take a break for some coffee.

59. When the physician checks Mrs. S, she reports that the cervix is dilated to 7 cm. To provide pain relief, the physician gives Mrs. S an epidural block. Which nursing action is vitally important during regional anesthesia?
    1. Monitoring blood pressure for possible hypertension.
    2. Giving oxytocin to counteract the effect of the epidural (or caudal) in slowing contractions.
    3. Having the gravida lie flat in bed to avoid postanesthesia headache.
    4. Monitoring blood pressure for possible hypotension.

60. Mrs. M is unmedicated. As she approaches the second stage of labor, her expected behavior may include all of the following, *except:*
    1. Becoming more talkative and alert.
    2. Shaking legs, nausea, and vomiting.
    3. Amnesia between contractions.
    4. Increase in bloody show and urge to push.

61. During the process of labor, the uterine muscle:
    1. Undergoes no change in thickness or size.

2. Becomes longer and thinner in both the upper and lower segments.
3. Thins in the lower uterine segment but remains the same in the upper.
4. Thins in the lower uterine segment and becomes shorter and thicker in the upper.

62. On vaginal examination, the fetus is found to be LOA. This means that:
    1. A bony prominence can be felt in the left front abdomen just above the symphysis; a hard, round, movable mass is felt in the fundal area.
    2. After the birth of the head, the infant will restitute and face the mother's left thigh; the infant may have to be turned with forceps, because it is posterior.
    3. The fetus is breech; a hard, round, movable prominence is felt in the fundal area; labor will probably be prolonged.
    4. A bony prominence can be felt in the left front abdomen just above the symphysis; after the birth of the head, the infant will restitute and face the mother's right thigh; the posterior fontanel can be palpated vaginally.

The first stage of labor is divided into three phases. Identify the phase described in questions 63 through 65.

63. In this phase, the mother becomes more introspective and irritable; she feels she cannot make it; and increased perspiration is noted on her upper lip and between her breasts.
    1. Latent phase.
    2. Active phase.
    3. Phase of transition.
    4. Pushing phase.

64. In this phase, the mother is apt to be excited, euphoric, and eager to learn; she likes to walk around.
    1. Latent phase.
    2. Active phase.
    3. Phase of transition.
    4. Pushing phase.

65. In this phase, the mother becomes increasingly more serious; a malar flush is noted; and she has a tendency to hyperventilate.
    1. Latent phase.
    2. Active phase.
    3. Phase of transition.
    4. Pushing phase.

66. When the midwife finally says that she can push, Mrs. T feels tremendous relief. Her husband assists her in delivery by supporting her shoulders while she pushes the baby out. When the baby is delivered, the midwife announces that the baby is a boy. Mrs. T asks if he is OK and does he have all his fingers and toes? The nurse would reply most appropriately:
    1. "Yes, he looks just fine. I can see that from here."

2. "Yes, he looks fine. As soon as the cord is cut, you can see for yourself."
3. "Yes, he looks fine. You can rest assured that the pediatrician will check him over thoroughly."
4. "Yes, he is fine. There is nothing for you to worry about."

67. During oxytocin induction, discontinue the infusion containing the drug if you observe:
    1. Increased amount of bloody show from the vagina.
    2. Increased pain over sacral area.
    3. Increased fetal heart rate from 145 to 160 bpm between contractions.
    4. Decrease in fetal heart rate below 100 with contractions.

The nurse who monitors the woman in labor is held legally responsible for knowledgeable assessment and appropriate intervention. Questions 68 through 75 pertain to assessment and intervention during labor.

68. Abdominal palpation (Leopold's maneuvers) reveals: soft, rounded mass in the fundus; irregular nodules on mother's right side; hard prominence on mother's right just above the symphysis. This means that the fetus is:
    1. RSP.
    2. LSA.
    3. ROP.
    4. LOA.

69. In the example in question 68 above, the nurse can expect to find the FHT:
    1. Below umbilicus, on mother's left side.
    2. Below umbilicus, on mother's right side.
    3. Above umbilicus, on mother's left side.
    4. Above umbilicus, on mother's right side.

70. The term that refers to that portion of the fetus that enters the pelvis first and covers the internal cervical os is:
    1. Lie.
    2. Presentation.
    3. Attitude.
    4. Station.

71. In an ROA presentation, during vaginal examination, the nurse can expect to feel the fetal:
    1. Anterior fontanel.
    2. Posterior fontanel.
    3. Buttocks.
    4. Shoulder.

72. The vaginal examination provides data regarding all of the following, *except:*
    1. Descent, flexion.
    2. Position of the placenta.
    3. Dilatation, effacement.
    4. Condition of the membranes.

73. Ms. M is 4 to 5 cm dilated, 100% effaced, − 3 station, with bulging membranes. She wants to get up and walk around awhile. The nurse's best response is:
    1. "Yes, but lie down if your water bag breaks."
    2. "No. The baby is not down far enough yet. If your membranes ruptured now, the cord could slip down ahead of the baby."
    3. "Only to go to the bathroom."
    4. "Let's ask the doctor if it is alright."

74. Mrs. L is lying flat, supine, in bed during labor. She insists on remaining supine. The nurse's best response would be:
    1. "It is best for the baby for you to lie on your side."
    2. "These two pillows under your knees will be good for the baby and more comfortable for you."
    3. "You will get nauseated and light-headed if you stay that way."
    4. "This rolled towel placed under your one hip will do the job just as well."

75. Under which of the following conditions is passage of meconium *before* birth "normal"?
    1. Prolonged first stage of labor.
    2. Transverse lie.
    3. Breech presentation, during second stage.
    4. Under no condition is passage of meconium normal prior to birth.

The following statements refer to effects of anesthesias used in obstetrics. Questions 76, 77, and 78 refer to this situation.
1. *Loss of bearing-down reflex.*
2. *Depression of contractions.*
3. *Maternal hypotension.*
4. *Fetal bradycardia.*
5. *Low forceps delivery.*
6. *Postnatal bladder atony.*
7. *Postnatal uterine atony.*
8. *Need to remain flat in bed for some hours after delivery.*

76. When a parturient is given a paracervical block, the nurse can expect:
    1. Low forceps delivery.
    2. Depression of contractions, maternal hypotension, fetal bradycardia, postnatal uterine atony.
    3. Depression of contractions and fetal bradycardia.
    4. Loss of bearing-down reflex, low forceps delivery.

77. When a parturient is given an epidural (or caudal) anesthesia, the nurse can expect:
    1. Maternal hypotension, low forceps delivery, need to remain flat in bed for some hours after delivery.
    2. Loss of bearing-down reflex, depression of contractions, maternal hypotension, fetal bradycardia, low forceps delivery.
    3. Loss of bearing-down reflex, depression of contractions, maternal hypotension, fetal bradycardia, low forceps delivery, postnatal bladder atony, postnatal uterine atony.
    4. Depression of contractions, maternal hypotension.

78. When a parturient is given a saddle block (low spinal) anesthesia, the nurse can expect:
1. Loss of bearing-down reflex, maternal hypotension, low forceps delivery, need to remain flat in bed for some hours after delivery.
2. Fetal bradycardia, low forceps delivery, postnatal uterine atony, need to remain flat in bed for some hours after delivery.
3. Loss of bearing-down reflex, low forceps delivery, postnatal bladder atony, postnatal uterine atony.
4. Loss of bearing-down reflex, maternal hypotension, low forceps delivery, need to remain flat in bed for some hours after delivery, fetal bradycardia, postnatal uterine atony, postnatal bladder atony.

79. All of the following are thought to assist in initiating respirations in the neonate at the moment of birth, *except:*
1. An increase in oxygen and a decrease in carbon dioxide.
2. A drop in oxygen and an increase in carbon dioxide.
3. The change in skin temperature and tactile stimulation to the body.
4. Change from weightlessness to gravity environment.

80. After the physician cuts the cord and before the infant is given to the mother to hold, the nurse does all of the following. Which of the following would the nurse do *first?*
1. Confirm identification of infant and apply bracelets to mother and infant.
2. Examine the infant for any observable abnormalities.
3. Dry the infant in prewarmed blankets and place in warm environment.
4. Instill silver nitrate drops in each eye.

81. All of the following factors contribute to rapid heat loss in the normal newborn immediately after birth, *except:*
1. Large body surface compared to body weight.
2. Room temperature of 72 F.
3. Neonate's inability to shiver.
4. Wrapping and placing neonate on mother's abdomen.

82. All of the following are normal characteristics of the newborn, *except:*
1. The circumference of the newborn's chest is normally equal to or slightly less than that of the head.
2. Abdomen is dome shaped.
3. The newborn's hemoglobin and hematocrit are equal to or less than that of an adult.
4. Irregular patterns of respiratory activity, including occasional short periods of apnea.

83. Following a precipitous delivery, the neonate appeared in good condition. The physician's orders: "Observe for subdural hematoma." You would be on the alert for all of the following, *except:*

1. Telangiectases and subconjunctival hemorrhage.
2. Separation of cranial sutures.
3. Repeated vomiting.
4. Bulging fontanel.

84. Ms. K is concerned that her two-day-old infant is losing too much weight. She tells you her baby weighed 7 lb at birth and now weighs only 6 lb 8 oz. What is the maximum number of ounces you could expect this baby to lose and still be within normal limits?
1. 6 oz (170 g).
2. 8 oz (227 g).
3. 11 oz (312 g).
4. 16 oz (454 g).

85. The first feeding for a formula-fed baby usually is sterile water rather than glucose water or formula. This is done because:
1. If aspiration occurs, it causes less harm.
2. It is less irritating to the gastric mucosa.
3. It is assimilated more easily.
4. It stimulates gastric secretions and initiates peristalsis.

86. The Moro reflex is a reflex response to all of the following, *except:*
1. Sudden or loud noises.
2. The sensation of falling.
3. A jolt to the crib.
4. Hypoglycemia and hypocalcemia.

87. Physiologic jaundice in the newborn is consequent to:
1. Liver immaturity and fetal polycythemia.
2. Oliguria and kidney immaturity.
3. Infection.
4. Dehydration.

88. Observations during the "fourth" stage of labor (first hour postpartum) include all of the following, *except:*
1. Checking every 30 minutes.
2. Assessing the condition and height of fundus.
3. Assessing for bladder distention.
4. Observing the episiotomy, the perineal pad, and the linens under the buttocks.

89. During the first postpartum day or two, the new mother may be expected to display which of the following behaviors:
1. Talkativeness, dependency, and passivity.
2. Autonomy and independence.
3. Disinterest in her own body functions.
4. Interest in learning to bathe the baby.

90. Mrs. P has been looking at her two-day-old infant; she has a frown on her face. She turns to you and asks if her baby's looks and actions are normal. You know that the following are normal variations of the newborn, *except:*
1. Enlarged breasts and a spot of pink drainage from her baby's vagina.

2. The light line between the baby's umbilicus and symphysis.
3. The little "black heads" covering the nose and chin.
4. The dark discoloration over her shoulders and upper back.

91. Phyllis calls you over to ask you about the "lump" on the side of her baby's head. You note that the tense lump does not cross suture lines. You know that this is caused by:
1. Bleeding between the periosteum and the parietal bone from pressure against the bony pelvis during delivery.
2. Edema of the scalp from pressure of the vertex against the cervix during dilatation.
3. Intracranial hemorrhage from either the pressure against the bony pelvis or the obstetric forceps.
4. A hemangioma.

92. "Afterpains" can be very disturbing, especially in the multipara who is also breastfeeding. Which of the following would you do *first?*
1. Give her a pain medication as per order.
2. Have her lie on her abdomen with a rolled towel at the level of the fundus.
3. Ask her to walk around for a while.
4. Ask her to empty her bladder.

93. For the mother who is breastfeeding, good nipple care includes:
1. Washing nipples and breasts every day with soap and water.
2. Keeping nipples clean with warm water and then drying.
3. Applying a diluted alcohol solution on them after each feeding to toughen the nipples.
4. Covering the nipples with a plastic-lined shield to protect clothing.

94. During her hospital stay, Mrs. C asks you what she should expect as far as physiologic changes now. She wonders if she is all right. Normal changes that occur during the first three to four postpartum days include all of the following, *except:*
1. Headaches and muscular pains in legs, until hormone and metabolic reversals are accomplished.
2. Diaphoresis and diuresis.
3. Strong uterine contractions.
4. Pulse between 50 and 70/minute.

95. Jane wishes to breastfeed. On the third day, there is no indication that her milk is coming in. To initiate lactation, the physician orders:
1. Testosterone enanthate and estradiol valerate injection (Deladumone OB).
2. Methylergonovine (Methergine) tartrate or ergonovine (Ergotrate) maleate.
3. Stilbestrol.
4. Oxytocin (Syntocinon, Pitocin).

96. Mrs. Q delivered in the car on the way to the hospital. In the emergency room, the physician examined the mother while the nurse's priority intervention was to:
1. Gently tug on the cord and massage the uterus to see if the placenta could be delivered now.
2. Clamp and cut the cord with sterile scissors.
3. Note and record the Apgar score.
4. Clear the mucus from the neonate's mouth and nose.

97. Jennie tells you that she is breastfeeding her son because she can't stand the thought of her newborn having to get vaccinations. You respond:
1. "That's great. Vaccinations are not necessary when you're breastfeeding."
2. "Oh, you still need to have him vaccinated against DPT, measles, and polio before he is six months old."
3. "You can only protect him temporarily against those diseases that you have had yourself."
4. "The most protection comes from the colostrum right after birth, and you didn't start feeding him until the second day."

98. The infant mortality rate is:
1. The number of deaths during the first four weeks per 1000 live births.
2. The number of deaths before 1 year of age per 1000 live births.
3. Lowest in the United States and Canada.
4. The number of illnesses before age 1 year per 1000 live births.

99. Perinatal mortality is:
1. The number of maternal and fetal-newborn deaths within four weeks after term.
2. Deaths between 28 weeks' gestation (1000 g or more) and 4 weeks of age.
3. The number of stillborns between 28 weeks' (1000 g or more) and 40 weeks' gestation.
4. The number of deaths occurring in the first four weeks of life per 1000 live births.

100. Birthrate refers to the number of births per:
1. 1000 population.
2. 1000 women aged 14 to 44.
3. 100,000 population.
4. 1000 women and men aged 14 to 44.

101. In some hospitals, new mothers are being asked to read and sign informed-consent forms prior to receiving antilactogenic drugs containing estrogens (Deladumone OB). To have a legally effective consent, it must provide all of the following elements, *except:*
1. It must be given voluntarily, without coercion.
2. The person must be given information about the procedure, its consequences and any alternate procedures and their consequences.

3. The person giving consent must be capable of comprehending the information.

4. Oral consent is sufficient if the person giving the consent is not medicated and can understand the information.

102. A woman who is giving birth at home wonders if her baby will need silver nitrate drops in the eyes because she knows that neither she nor her husband have gonorrhea. Your best answer to her is that:

1. It is all right then not to have the drops.

2. The baby must have the drops and must receive them within a few minutes after birth.

3. The baby needs the drops, but does not have to receive them for up to two hours after birth.

4. The drops are needed to prevent the eye condition known as retrolental fibroplasia.

103. It is safe to delay instillation of silver nitrate or erythromycin into the neonate's eyes for two hours after delivery. This delay:

1. Facilitates the process of attachment to the mother (father).

2. Facilitates neonatal transition to extrauterine life.

3. Permits extra time for assessing the neonate's condition.

4. Decreases the amount of time the neonate is exposed to cool temperatures.

104. Mrs. T is three months' pregnant. Her first pregnancy ended in abortion at 10 weeks. She delivered a live-born female at 36 weeks' gestation, who is now alive and well. Her gravidity/parity is:

1. Gravida III, Para I.

2. Gravida II, Para II.

3. 2-0-1-1-1.

4. 3/2.

105. Ms. H has just delivered twin boys at 38 weeks. Her first pregnancy was aborted electively. She is now:

1. Gravida II, Para II.

2. Gravida II, Para I.

3. Gravida I, Para I.

4. Gravida III, Para II.

106. "Natural childbirth" has come to mean different things to different people. Some erroneous concepts have sprung up as well. One of the myths that has developed is:

1. Medications may be used to reduce tension and pain.

2. Labor and delivery are rendered almost painless.

3. Labor is easier for women who are self-assured, relaxed, and cooperative with the labor process.

4. Preparation for childbirth may include body-building exercises, breathing techniques, and comfort aids.

107. Breathing techniques for women using the Lamaze method of childbirth include all of the following, *except:*

1. Slow, deep chest-breathing during first stage.

2. Woman involves intercostal muscles but keeps diaphragm relaxed during the first stage of labor.

3. Slow, shallow breathing alternating with panting is recommended just before full dilatation.

4. Woman begins and ends each contraction and breathing pattern with two cleansing breaths.

108. Many women (couples) are opting for early discharge from the hospital. Some leave at the end of six hours. The nurse must be very careful that this woman (couple) has received sufficient instruction regarding the care of the mother and the infant and that they are not discharged if any complication or suspicion of a possible complication is present because the nurse (physician and hospital) may be legally charged with:

1. Malpractice.

2. Negligence.

3. Abandonment.

4. Assault and battery.

109. If a circumcision is performed on a newborn without parental permission (with a signed informed consent), but the parents decide not to press charges, the infant may, *when he reaches the age of majority* (21 in most states), hold the physician, hospital, and nursery nurses legally responsible and charge them with:

1. Malpractice.

2. Negligence.

3. Abandonment.

4. Assault and battery.

110. Ms. J is an unwed pregnant 14-year-old who is giving her baby up for adoption. Nurses and social workers can help her best if they:

1. Provide a safe environment to facilitate ventilation of her feelings but do not give answers or direction so that she makes her own decisions.

2. Help her understand the existing situation, place it in perspective in terms of her life goals, and begin to plan for the future.

3. Assure her that her decision to place the baby up for adoption is the best suited for her needs.

4. Help her see ways of not making the same mistake again so that she can grow in self-esteem and self-respect.

111. Adoption agencies such as the Children's Home Society and Family Service Association carefully screen prospective adoptive parents by evaluating all of the following, except:

1. Ages of spouses, duration of marriage, and financial stability.

2. Physical and mental health of spouses and motivation underlying desire to adopt.

3. Other children, if any, in the home.

4. The parents' professions.

112. Medical and nursing management of moderate to

severe hyperemesis gravidarum consists of all of the following, *except:*

1. NPO for 24 hours and parenteral therapy with B complex and C vitamins added.
2. Restriction of visitors, including family.
3. Immediate therapeutic abortion.
4. Observation for jaundice, delirium, and tachycardia.

113. Hydatidiform mole may be diagnosed by all of the following clinical features, *except:*
1. Preeclampsia.
2. Continuous or intermittent brownish discharge, starting about the end of the first trimester.
3. Uterus excessively large for gestational age and high serum levels of HCG.
4. Tenderness and rigidity of abdomen and uterus.

114. Mrs. T missed two menstrual periods. One day she experienced a sharp, stabbing pain in her lower abdomen. Entering the emergency room, she began spotting and became dizzy and pale. These clinical manifestations are most probably indicative of:
1. Incompetent cervix.
2. Placenta previa.
3. Abruptio placentae.
4. Ectopic pregnancy.

115. The gravida carrying twins must be carefully observed for all of the following frequently associated conditions, *except:*
1. Hyperemesis gravidarum.
2. Premature labor and/or preeclampsia.
3. Dystocia and/or postpartum hemorrhage.
4. Placenta previa.

116. Identical twins differ from fraternal twins in that for identical twins:
1. Advanced maternal age is an accepted predisposing factor.
2. They result from the union of two eggs and two sperm.
3. Tissue transplants are readily accepted from one another.
4. They frequently are of the same sex.

117. Abnormal symptoms during pregnancy that require immediate notification of the physician include:
1. Ptyalism, enlarged Montgomery follicles, and leukorrhea.
2. Fatigue, nausea, and urinary frequency.
3. Ankle edema, enlarging varices, and heartburn.
4. Severe pain in abdomen, fluid discharge from vagina, and fingers swelling.

118. A gravida is admitted to the maternity unit directly from the clinic with a blood pressure of 146/98. Without waiting for a physician's order, the nurse would do all of the following, *except:*
1. Evaluate amount and distribution of edema, if present.

2. Place her on bedrest in a room with three new postpartum women so that they could call the nurse for her if needed.
3. Take her weight on admission and daily thereafter.
4. Test her urine for protein; start an I & O sheet.

119. When preparing a room for a woman who is about to be admitted for preeclampsia, the nurse adds all of the following to the ordinary room equipment in readiness for an eclamptic emergency, *except:*
1. Urinary catheter tray.
2. Intravenous solutions and infusion equipment.
3. Suction apparatus.
4. Restraints.

120. Any woman being treated for preeclampsia must be carefully assessed for intake of fluids and output of urine, because:
1. Oliguria is a grave sign.
2. Intake per day should never exceed 2000 ml.
3. Sudden diuresis can precipitate a convulsion.
4. When urinary output is less than 100 ml/4 hours, a repeat dose of magnesium sulphate is indicated.

121. The hospitalized gravida being treated for severe preeclampsia is closely observed for all of the following, *except:*
1. Hyperemesis gravidarum.
2. Urinary output, reflex response, and respiratory rate.
3. Severe frontal headache and/or epigastric pain.
4. Tone of uterus and sensitivity of abdomen and uterus to touch.

122. The nurse should be alert to possible sequelae of abruptio placentae, which include all of the following, *except:*
1. Fetal hyperactivity or fetal demise.
2. Hypertension.
3. Disseminated intravascular coagulation.
4. Amniotic-fluid embolism.

123. Postpartum nursing care of a woman who had preeclampsia is influenced by the following knowledge:
1. This mother may convulse any time during the first 48 hours after delivery, even if she did not convulse before.
2. Once the baby is delivered, the nurse can be assured of an immediate cure of the preeclampsia.
3. The woman should be advised that she will undoubtedly be left with chronic renal damage.
4. The woman should be advised regarding contraceptives, since a subsequent pregnancy is hazardous.

124. Gravida-nurse-physician relationship is especially important when the gravida is diabetic because her motivation and cooperation are essential for all of the following, *except:*
1. Early identification and treatment of infection.
2. Conversion to use of regular insulin during the pregnancy.

3. Restriction of daily activity or exercise.

4. Frequent urine tests daily in the home.

125. Obstetric complications encountered more frequently with the diabetic gravida include all of the following, *except:*
    1. Spontaneous abortion.
    2. Preeclampsia.
    3. Dystocia.
    4. Erythroblastosis fetalis.

126. The diabetic gravida may be hospitalized during pregnancy for all of the following, *except:*
    1. Regulation of insulin dosage.
    2. Determination of placental functioning.
    3. Control of morning sickness.
    4. Amniocentesis to determine if fetus carries gene for diabetes.

127. Anticipatory guidance for the new mother who is diabetic includes all of the following, *except:*
    1. Breastfeeding is contraindicated.
    2. Nipple and/or vaginal monilial infection is a possible problem.
    3. She must eat on time herself, even if baby must wait to be fed.
    4. She must prevent hypoglycemia because that would inhibit the let-down reflex and decrease her milk supply.

128. During the postpartum period, the mother who is diabetic is counseled about all of the following, *except:*
    1. With mature-onset diabetes (before age 40), 4% of offspring will inherit the disorder; with juvenile onset, 22% will inherit the disorder.
    2. Oral contraception, IUDs, foams, and gels are all acceptable methods of birth control.
    3. The woman's ability to cope with both small children in the home and her disease (especially if the diagnosis has been made recently).
    4. If she has renal disease or proliferative retinopathy, there is an increased risk with another pregnancy.

129. On the first postpartum day, the diabetic mother's insulin dose is one-half to one-third of her prepregnant dose (if she is eating a full diet) because of the rapid fall of HCS when the placenta is delivered. You are making rounds on the postpartum unit at night and want to assess the sleeping woman for insulin reactions. Any of the following are signs of insulin reaction, *except:*
    1. A flash of light in the woman's face does not result in a squint or turn of the head.
    2. The woman seems restless, her face is flushed, pulse rapid, and respiration deep.
    3. The woman perspires while sleeping.
    4. The woman wakes up with a headache.

130. Congestive heart failure in the gravida with rheumatic valvular damage may be precipitated by all of the following, *except:*
    1. Insufficient physical exercise.
    2. Loss of a loved one.
    3. Urinary-tract infection.
    4. Eating peanut butter, canned meats and vegetables, and cheeses.

131. A gravida with cardiac failure is admitted to your unit with symptoms of dyspnea following ordinary physical activity, moist cough, and a rapid pulse. "Complete bedrest" for her consists of all of the following, *except:*
    1. Assisting her with grooming and changing.
    2. Preparing her food on her tray and feeding her.
    3. Bathroom privileges.
    4. Assisting her with position changes in bed.

132. Nursing care of a gravida with class I cardiac involvement during labor and delivery would include all of the following, *except:*
    1. Helping her maintain a semirecumbent position.
    2. Monitoring her pulse more frequently than other vital signs.
    3. Preparing her for regional anesthesia (epidural or caudal).
    4. After complete dilatation, coaching her to bear down only once per contraction.

133. The early postpartum period for the new mother with cardiac involvement is a critical one. All of the following are essential components of her care, *except:*
    1. Administer fluids (oral or parenteral) slowly for first day or two.
    2. Force fluids so her water metabolism returns to normal more quickly.
    3. Minimize blood loss.
    4. Stay with her and monitor vital signs and condition continuously through the first hour postpartum.

Mrs. O is a 37-year-old primigravida whose labor is being induced. The physician is on the unit. She has a double infusion set-up with 1000 ml lactated Ringer's in 5% dextrose, and 500 ml 5% D/W containing Pitocin 5 units. There is a three-way stopcock attached to the needle entering her vein. At this time, the stopcock is set so that the 5% D/W with Pitocin is infusing. Mrs. O's contractions and FHR are being monitored electronically. Questions 134 through 140 refer to this situation.

134. Medical indications for induction of labor include all of the following, *except:*
    1. Uterine inertia.
    2. Gravida who is 35 years old or older.
    3. Preterm delivery of infant with severe isoimmunization.
    4. Prolonged rupture of membranes.

135. The "shake" test is used to determine the presence, in the amniotic fluid, of:
    1. Creatinine.

2. Bilirubin.

3. Lecithin.

4. Estriol.

136. The labor and delivery unit has become very busy so that you, a float nurse, have been assigned to help out. You have never worked with Pitocin induction or fetal monitors. If any abnormal tracing appears and you do not recognize fetal distress:
    1. You will not be held accountable because you were floated to help out in an understaffed situation.
    2. The physician is held accountable for the care given to his/her patients.
    3. You are held accountable because you accepted a responsibility for which you were not trained.
    4. The head nurse is held accountable because he/she did not assess your capability before assigning you to the care of this parturient.

137. During the Pitocin induction, the physician leaves the unit to attend a case in another hospital. The nurse:
    1. Continues the Pitocin induction.
    2. Readjusts the stopcock so that the 1000 ml lactated Ringer's without Pitocin infuses during the physician's absence.
    3. Reduces the flow from the Pitocin bottle to "keep open" only.
    4. Asks another physician to be "on hand" until the first physician returns.

138. During Pitocin induction, in addition to monitoring uterine contractions and FHR, the nurse monitors another Pitocin-related factor:
    1. Urinary output.
    2. Blood pressure.
    3. Deep-tendon reflexes.
    4. Level of consciousness.

139. Which of the following FHR deceleration patterns *does not* have to be reported stat:
    1. Uniform in shape, onset coincides with contraction, returns to baseline at end of contraction.
    2. Uniform in shape, onset after contraction is established, returns to baseline seconds after end of contraction.
    3. No uniformity in shape, onset any time before, during, or after a contraction.
    4. FHR persisting at, or less than, 20 bpm below baseline, following a contraction, or persisting through several contractions.

140. You notice an abnormal FHR tracing. The nurse's first action is to:
    1. Notify the physician.
    2. Prepare the woman for cesarean delivery.
    3. Turn stopcock so that the lactated Ringer's is infusing.
    4. Give the woman oxygen by mask at 8 to 10 l/min.

141. Which one of the following women is *least* likely to experience uterine atony during the fourth stage of labor at term:
    1. Mrs. W, who had spinal anesthesia to deliver a 7½-pound female, after a 10-hour labor.
    2. Mrs. X, who used LaMaze method to deliver a 6¾-pound male, after a 14-hour labor.
    3. Mrs. Y, who, with Pitocin induction (due to premature rupture of membranes), delivered after a 12-hour labor.
    4. Mrs. Z, who delivered twins under pudendal anesthesia after a 10-hour labor.

142. When a woman is experiencing a dystotic labor, therapeutic nursing actions include all of the following, *except:*
    1. Clear and repeated descriptions of progress and explanations for delay.
    2. Careful assessment for maternal exhaustion.
    3. Acceptance of her hostility.
    4. Reassurance that her physician is "the best there is."

143. Mrs. J had an emergency cesarean delivery after 18 hours of a dystotic labor. Nursing actions in the postnatal period which facilitate recovery include all of the following, *except:*
    1. Tell her that a birth is a birth whether it is cesarean or vaginal.
    2. Discuss events preceding the cesarean birth.
    3. Position her in bed with pillows.
    4. Teach her how to splint the incision.

144. The nurse scans the prenatal record to identify factors that may adversely affect the newborn's immediate adaptation to extrauterine life. All of the following conditions affect the vascular supply to the placenta, *except:*
    1. Syphilis.
    2. Hypertension.
    3. Anemia.
    4. Posture.

145. Which of the following events would alert the nurse to the possibility of postpartum hemorrhage?
    1. Labor of nine hours, baby weighing 6 lb 10 oz, no anesthesia, and primipara.
    2. Second baby, weighing 7 lb 2 oz, and paracervical block with local anesthesia for episiotomy repair.
    3. Labor prolonged in latent phase and nitrous oxide for delivery of an 8-lb girl, first baby.
    4. Labor of two hours, fourth pregnancy, twins weighing 4 lb 8 oz and 5 lb, and spinal anesthesia.

146. If there is a possibility that Mrs. T has retained some placental fragments, which of the following drugs *would not* be given?
    1. Testosterone enanthate and estradiol valerate injection (Deladumone OB).
    2. Methylergonovine (Methergine) or tartrate ergonovine (Ergotrate) maleate.

3. Stilbestrol.
4. Oxytocin (Syntocinon, Pitocin).

147. Judicious management of the third stage of labor is vital in the prevention of hemorrhage and its complications. Which one of the following is the preferred method for the delivery of the placenta:
1. Ritgen maneuver.
2. Brandt-Andrews maneuver.
3. Schultze mechanism.
4. Manual separation and removal.

Mrs. M arrives at the hospital with the following signs and symptoms: painless bleeding that is continuous and sufficient in amount to trickle down her leg; blood pressure 102/68, pulse 92; some uterine cramping with complete relaxation between contractions. Questions 148 to 151 refer to this situation.

148. Mrs. M presents the classic symptoms of:
1. Placenta accreta.
2. Beginning second stage of labor.
3. Abruptio placentae.
4. Placenta previa.

149. While awaiting the physician, the nurse:
1. Does a vaginal examination to assess fetal presentation, descent, cervical dilatation, and effacement.
2. Positions her on her side, with a small pillow under her head.
3. Adjusts the bed in semi-Fowler's position.
4. Prepares her for cesarean delivery.

150. Mrs. M's vaginal bleeding is increasing, her contractions indicate she is in good labor, and this is her third child. Assuming that a proper assessment has been completed (by the physician and radiologist), the physician decides to rupture the membranes. The woman had expressed her desire to have as natural a labor as possible and is very concerned about artificial rupture of membranes. The nurse's response is based on the principle underlying artificial ROM in this case:
1. Uterine contractions, and therefore labor, will be enhanced.
2. The hard fetal head (that is presenting) will increase pressure on the placenta.
3. Umbilical-cord compression, a possible complication in this case, will be prevented.
4. Artificial rupture of membranes is an individual physician's preference.

151. In the immediate postpartum period, this woman is more likely to experience a hemorrhage for the following reason:
1. The placenta was located in the lower uterine segment where there are fewer muscle fibers to contract the placental site.
2. The area under the abrupted placenta never contracts as strongly as if there were no placenta abruption.

3. Since the placenta was surgically removed, the uterine muscle under the site does not contract as efficiently.
4. There is no greater possibility of hemorrhage in this case.

Mrs. K arrives at the hospital with the following signs and symptoms: severe pain in the abdomen, "my womb is so hard"; no vaginal bleeding; complains of feeling light-headed and sweaty. Questions 152 to 157 refer to this situation.

152. Mrs. K presents the classic symptoms of:
1. Placenta accreta.
2. Rupture of ectopic pregnancy.
3. Abruptio placentae.
4. Abdominal pregnancy.

153. While awaiting the physician, the nurse:
1. Does a vaginal examination to assess fetal presentation, descent, cervical dilatation, and effacement.
2. Positions her on her side, with a small pillow under her head.
3. Adjusts her bed in the semi-Fowler's position.
4. Prepares her for surgical intervention.

154. The nurse completes the assessment of Mrs. K's condition. The nurse is likely to evaluate all of the following, *except:*
1. State of contraction of the uterus and the degree of relaxation between contractions.
2. Rate and rhythm of fetal heart tones.
3. Deep-tendon reflexes.
4. Blood pressure and pulse.

155. If hemorrhage is concealed in this condition, which one of the following can occur?
1. Placenta accreta.
2. Couvelaire uterus.
3. Hyperfibrinogenemia.
4. Uterine rupture.

156. Nursing care is planned based on knowledge of the priority of medical management, which consists of:
1. Artificial rupture of membranes to enhance labor.
2. Eradication of the coagulation problem.
3. Immediate cesarean delivery.
4. Augmentation of labor with intravenous oxytocin.

157. Mrs. K's condition is most likely to develop in women with a history of all of the following, *except:*
1. Multiparity or multiple pregnancy.
2. Tumultuous labor or labor induced with Pitocin.
3. Severe preeclampsia.
4. Previous uterine surgery, such as cesarean delivery.

158. Two hours after delivery, Mrs. Evan's perineal pad is saturated; bleeding occurs in gushes; uterus contracts spasmodically. The nurse suspects:
1. Atonic bleeding.
2. Traumatic bleeding.

3. Retained placental fragments.
4. Inverted uterus.

159. After firming and expressing Mrs. Evan's uterus, the nurse's next action is to:
1. Call the physician, because she needs surgery.
2. Call the physician, because the site of bleeding must be located.
3. Administer oxytocin according to prn order.
4. Reapply perineal pad and ask her to keep her thighs together.

160. One hour after delivery, Mrs. Faris's perineal pad is saturated; bleeding occurs in a trickle; uterus is firm and smooth. The nurse suspects:
1. Atonic bleeding.
2. Traumatic bleeding.
3. Retained placental fragments.
4. Inverted uterus.

161. The nurse's next action for Mrs. Faris is to:
1. Call the physician, because she needs surgery.
2. Call the physician, because the site of bleeding must be located.
3. Administer oxytocin according to prn order.
4. Reapply perineal pad and ask her to keep her thighs together.

162. Postpartum hemorrhage is a leading cause of maternal death. The definition of postpartum hemorrhage is:
1. Blood loss greater than 1% of body weight (for a 50 kg woman, that would mean a 500 ml blood loss).
2. Blood loss greater than 300 ml at delivery.
3. Blood loss greater than 200 ml during the first hour postpartum.
4. Blood loss of 1000 ml during the entire puerperium.

163. All of the following complications predispose to disseminated intravascular coagulation, *except:*
1. Retained placental fragments.
2. Severe eclampsia.
3. Amnionitis.
4. Amniotic-fluid embolus.

164. The mother's well-being following hemorrhage in the postpartum period is further jeopardized by all of the following possible sequelae, *except:*
1. Severe eclamptogenic toxemia.
2. Puerperal infection.
3. Anemia.
4. Embolism.

165. Amniotic-fluid embolism is a rare complication of childbirth. During which of the following times is the nurse on the alert for the appearance of amniotic-fluid embolism:
1. Any time after the membranes rupture.
2. During the second stage of labor.
3. During the postpartum period if she has been on bedrest for several days.
4. Until the presenting part is at least at 0 station.

166. Symptoms of amniotic-fluid embolism are identical to any embolism. These symptoms include all of the following, *except:*
1. Sudden dyspnea.
2. Profound shock.
3. Rise in blood pressure and hypertonia.
4. Cyanosis and pulmonary edema.

167. The test designed to identify the fetus at risk from placental insufficiency is:
1. Amniocentesis for L/S ratio.
2. Nonstress test.
3. Sonography.
4. Coombs' determination.

168. If the expectant mother's membranes rupture more than 24 hours prior to delivery, the neonate's immediate adaptation may be adversely influenced by the possibility of:
1. Amnionitis.
2. A "dry" birth.
3. Hypofibrinogenemia.
4. Couvelaire uterus.

169. In addition to FHR, the nurse is constantly alert to two other signs of fetal distress:
1. Crowning and increased fetal activity.
2. Crowning and secondary uterine inertia.
3. Increased fetal activity and meconium-stained amniotic fluid.
4. Secondary uterine inertia and meconium-stained amniotic fluid.

170. All of the following factors contribute to fetal anoxia, *except:*
1. Contractions of the uterine muscle.
2. Maternal supine position.
3. High or low blood pressure of the mother.
4. Umbilical cord that is 50 cm long.

171. In the presence of fetal hypoxia, the amniotic fluid appears:
1. Opaque with white flecks, if hypoxia is recent.
2. Opaque with white flecks and some streaks of pink, if hypoxia is more than 36 hours past.
3. Greenish-black if hypoxia is recent.
4. Port-wine colored.

172. Should fetal distress be noted, the nurse can often relieve the distress by taking appropriate actions. These actions include all of the following, *except:*
1. Turn gravida from back to side-lying position.
2. Turn gravida from side to back-lying position.
3. Administer oxygen.
4. Stop oxytocin induction, if in progress, and increase rate of intravenous fluid (without oxytocin) if running (or start an IV).

173. The nurse knows that the actions taken have improved fetal well-being when:

1. Contractions decrease in frequency, duration, and intensity.
2. Maternal blood pressure remains stable.
3. FHR pattern indicates early deceleration.
4. FHR pattern indicates late deceleration.

174. Yellowish vernix on a newborn may indicate:
1. Rh or ABO incompatibility or maternal ingestion of sulfisoxazole (Gantrisin).
2. A gonorrheal infection.
3. Maternal diabetes mellitus.
4. Fetal postmaturity.

175. What is the Apgar score of an infant who at one minute after birth has the following characteristics: heart rate over 100, respiratory effort—slow and irregular, muscle tone—flaccid, response to slap on soles of feet—weak cry, color—body, pink, and extremities, blue?
1. 5.
2. 6.
3. 7.
4. 8.

176. Asphyxia neonatorum is a condition that exists when the infant, following birth, gives no indication of breathing within:
1. 30 to 60 seconds.
2. 60 to 90 seconds.
3. Two minutes.
4. Five minutes.

177. Hyaline membrane disease or respiratory distress syndrome is most likely to occur in the infant who is:
1. 38 weeks' gestation and over and who weighs under 2500 g (5 lb 8 oz).
2. 38 weeks' gestation and over and who weighs over 2500 g.
3. 37 weeks' gestation and under and who weighs under 1500 g (3 lb 5 oz).
4. 44 weeks' gestation or more and who weighs 2500 g.

178. The nurse recognizes respiratory distress when the infant exhibits all of the following, *except:*
1. Respiratory rate over 60 per minute.
2. Much activity of the intercostal muscles.
3. Expiratory grunting.
4. Absence of flaring of nasal alae.

179. An infant begins to show signs of respiratory distress. The nursing actions listed below are all appropriate responses in this situation.
A. Notify the physician.
B. Give oxygen if cyanosis occurs.
C. Record—time, symptoms, degree of symptoms, and whether oxygen relieved symptoms.
D. Apply electrodes from apnea monitor.
E. Maintain an open airway.
Which answer best ranks the first and second nursing actions:
1. Give oxygen if cyanosis occurs (B), then notify the physician (A).

2. Notify the physician (A), then maintain an open airway (E).
3. Apply electrodes from apnea monitor (D), then give oxygen if cyanosis occurs (B).
4. Maintain an open airway (E), then give oxygen if cyanosis occurs (D).

180. Signs and symptoms of RDS include all of the following, *except:*
1. Abdominal or see-saw respirations.
2. Acrocyanosis in room air.
3. Flaring of the nares.
4. Expiratory grunt.

181. Prolonged and deep suctioning of the throat with a catheter:
1. Is necessary when the infant has aspirated meconium and amniotic fluid.
2. Can cause pulse irregularities and laryngospasm.
3. Minimizes the development of the respiratory distress syndrome.
4. Is done prior to each feeding of an infant with severe respiratory distress.

182. During the first 24 hours after birth, an infant whose gestational age is 37 weeks or less begins to show signs of respiratory distress. His symptoms are most likely indicative of:
1. Aspiration syndrome.
2. Respiratory distress syndrome (hyaline membrane disease).
3. Oxygen toxicity.
4. Bronchopulmonary dysplasia.

183. During the first 24 hours after birth, a term infant (38 to 41 weeks) begins to show signs of respiratory distress. Her symptomatology is most likely indicative of:
1. Aspiration syndrome.
2. Respiratory distress syndrome (hyaline membrane disease).
3. Oxygen toxicity.
4. Bronchopulmonary dysplasia.

184. During the first 24 hours after birth, a postterm infant (over 42 weeks) begins to show signs of respiratory distress. His symptomatology is most likely indicative of:
1. Aspiration syndrome.
2. Respiratory distress syndrome (hyaline membrane disease).
3. Oxygen toxicity.
4. Bronchopulmonary dysplasia.

You are working in a newborn nursery. The delivery room nurse brings you an infant weighing 6 lb 1 oz. Prenatal history regarding EDC is unclear. You note that the infant's ears are pliable, plantar sole creases cover the top half of the foot, he has no breast nodules, and his elbow can cross over his midline. Questions 185 through 189 refer to this situation.

185. You know that this infant is:

1. Preterm, and large for gestational age (LGA).
2. Term, and adequate for gestational age (AGA).
3. Postterm, and small for gestational age (SGA).
4. Postmature.

186. Your first nursing action is to:
1. Feed him dextrose and water to prevent hypoglycemia.
2. Place him in an incubator and maintain temperature.
3. Make no alterations from normal newborn care.
4. Do a complete assessment for gestational age.

187. Preterm infants are more susceptible to anemia. Nursing management to minimize anemia and its effects includes all of the following, *except:*
1. Handle the infant gently.
2. Accurately record blood drawn for laboratory tests.
3. Detect early signs of hyperbilirubinemia.
4. Utilize good technique for phototherapy.

188. Gavage feedings are often indicated for preterm infants because of all of the following, *except:*
1. Feeding can be accomplished rapidly and handling of neonates is minimized.
2. Gag and cough reflexes are weak or absent.
3. Neonates' energy must be conserved.
4. Neonates' suck and swallow reflexes are weak and uncoordinated.

189. Premature labor and delivery has many causes; many of these are preventable. As a nurse giving anticipatory guidance to young people before they get pregnant, which of the following would you discuss with them in the hopes of preventing premature labor and delivery:
1. Ages of male and female; number and spacing of pregnancies; obesity; smoking; frequency of intercourse during pregnancy.
2. Ages of male and female; number of pregnancies; smoking; frequency of intercourse during pregnancy.
3. Ages of male and female; obesity; smoking.
4. Age of female; number of pregnancies; spacing of pregnancies.

190. Scanning a prenatal record of a gravida, you are alert to factors associated with small-for-gestational-age infants. These factors include:
1. Second pregnancy, other child is 2½ years old.
2. Single fetus.
3. Hypertension.
4. Obesity.

191. Which of the following infants would you monitor for hypoglycemia:
1. 8-pound infant at 40 weeks' gestation.
2. 7½-pound infant at 43 weeks' gestation.
3. 7½-pound infant at 40 weeks' gestation.
4. 6½-pound infant at 38 weeks' gestation.

192. Early feedings are initiated for term infants who are small for gestational age for all of the following reasons, *except:*
1. Decrease the risk of hypoglycemia.
2. Minimize respiratory distress.
3. Begin rehydration of dehydrated state.
4. Facilitate immediate and continuous weight gain.

193. Hypoglycemia may be asymptomatic yet contribute to cerebral impairment, infant morbidity, and mortality. All of the following predispose the neonate to hypoglycemia, *except:*
1. Respiratory distress syndrome.
2. Hyperbilirubinemia.
3. Septicemia.
4. Cooling.

194. An infant at risk frequently receives parenteral therapy. The nurse assists the physician in the evaluation of an infant's needs for intravenous fluids by all of the following, *except:*
1. Measuring the width of the cranial sutures.
2. Careful weighing once or twice per day.
3. Measuring amount of specific gravity of urine.
4. Checking skin turgor q 4 hours.

195. Mrs. G is admitted to the labor suite for induction of labor. By menstrual dates and sonography, fetal gestational age is more than 42 weeks. Your nursing management in the labor room would include all of the following, *except:*
1. Constant electronic monitoring of the fetus.
2. An oxygen supply and oxygen equipment readily available.
3. "Eclamptic tray" in labor room.
4. Notification of pediatrician and nursery staff.

196. The labor of a woman whose pregnancy is past 42 weeks' gestation may be hazardous because the:
1. Placental function diminishes, causing fetal problems.
2. Placenta may separate prematurely.
3. Mother is overly tired and worn out after such a long pregnancy.
4. Fetus continues to gain weight and may cause fetopelvic disproportion.

197. Mrs. V is in her eighth month of gestation (between 34 and 36 weeks). She asks you what the baby would be like if she were to be born now. After determining what prompted her question, your most appropriate response would be:
1. She is still not fully developed and is not viable if born now.
2. In general, she looks and acts just about like a full-term baby and has a good chance for survival.
3. Physiologically and anatomically she is just like a full-term baby and has the same chances for survival.
4. She looks like a term baby, but weighs much less and this makes her chances for survival very slim.

198. Accurate monitoring of the neonate's temperature in an incubator involves all of the following, *except:*
1. Checking and recording the temperature of the infant and incubator frequently.
2. Placing incubator away from air-conditioning vents.
3. Touching the infant's body and extremities to check for coolness.
4. Positioning a gooseneck lamp directly over incubator for better visualization of distress indicative of hypothermia or hyperthermia.

199. All of the following may be early signs of kernicterus, *except:*
1. A depressed or absent Moro reflex.
2. Passage of yellowish-brown stool.
3. Weak or whiny, high-pitched cry.
4. Refusal or regurgitation of feedings.

200. The purposes of an exchange transfusion for Rh incompatibility include all of the following, *except:*
1. Combat anemia.
2. Remove and dilute maternal antibodies.
3. Decrease serum bilirubin levels.
4. Inactivate the maternal antibodies.

201. Rho (D) immune globulin is given to mothers who are:
1. Rh-negative, have just given birth to an Rh-negative baby, and have some titer.
2. Rh-negative, have just given birth to an Rh-positive baby, and have no titer.
3. Rh-positive, have just given birth to an Rh-positive baby, and have no titer.
4. Rh-positive, have just given birth to an Rh-negative baby, and have some titer.

202. Phenylketonuria is:
1. Inherited as a recessive trait and necessitates that the infant drink Lofenalac.
2. A congenital defect and necessitates infant feedings with human breast milk.
3. Due to a viral disease of the mother during the first trimester and necessitates infant feedings with nonallergenic formulas.
4. A congenital defect and necessitates infant feedings with nonallergenic formulas.

203. When caring for a premature infant, which of the following precautions should be taken to guard against retrolental fibroplasia?
1. Maintain the oxygen content in the incubator at less than 40%.
2. When the infant is under the fluorescent light, the eyes should be kept well covered.
3. Regulate the amount of ambient oxygen on the basis of arterial blood levels of oxygen.
4. Order daily serum bilirubin levels; levels above 10 mg/dl blood predispose to this disorder.

204. Katey gave birth to a little girl with a cleft lip and palate last night. This morning she tells you that she doesn't want to see her physician. She just knows that the antihistamine she took for her allergy three months ago was wrong. The most appropriate response by the nurse would be:
1. "This kind of problem is very easily repaired. Just wait until you see her after surgery!"
2. "The antihistamines you took had nothing to do with this. Drugs during the last trimester don't affect babies like this."
3. "The baby is really quite cute otherwise, and it would be wise to get used to feeding the baby now, while you are still in the hospital with someone to help you."
4. "It must be very difficult for you to have a baby like this."

205. Baby Kelly is with his mother, who is a diabetic. He appeared pink and alert, and his temperature was stable when he left the nursery 15 minutes before. His mother calls you over and brings your attention to his legs. You observe spontaneous jerky movements. Your *first* response is to:
1. Tell his mother this is normal behavior for a newborn.
2. Tell her to feed him his glucose water now.
3. Take him back to the nursery to do a Dextrostix.
4. Take him back to the nursery and observe him for other behaviors and neurologic symptoms.

206. The absence of one umbilical artery is of concern because it is frequently associated with:
1. Respiratory distress syndrome.
2. Renal agenesis.
3. Patent ductus arteriosus.
4. Premature ossification of cranial bones.

207. Syphilis in the newborn is recognized by all of the following characteristics, *except:*
1. Conjunctival hemorrhages and/or telangiectases over the bridge of the nose and at the nape of the neck.
2. Superficial ulcerations or cracks surrounding the anus and/or mouth.
3. Snuffles.
4. A skin rash of rose spots and plantar and palmar lesions or blebs.

208. In addition to ophthalmia neonatorum, gonorrhea may be responsible for any or all of the following, *except:*
1. Premature rupture of membranes and chorioamnionitis.
2. Neonatal temperature instability.
3. Congenital anomalies.
4. Neonatal hypotonia and poor feeding.

209. Statistics pertaining to maternal death in the United States show that the causes of death in order of frequency are:
1. Preeclampsia/eclampsia, hemorrhage, cardiac disease.
2. Hemorrhage, infection, preeclampsia/eclampsia.

3. Cardiac disease, diabetes, preeclampsia/eclampsia.
4. Infection, hemorrhage, cardiac disease.

210. During which of the following pregnancies is perinatal mortality the lowest:
1. First pregnancy.
2. Second pregnancy.
3. Third pregnancy.
4. There is no difference in perinatal mortality among the first, second, or third pregnancies.

211. If a female experiences childhood undernutrition, the effects on her subsequent pregnancy and the developing fetus:
1. Are negligible if nutrition during her pregnancy is adequate.
2. Cannot be completely removed by improved nutrition during this pregnancy.
3. Have no influence on the woman's pregnancy or developing fetus.
4. Can be prevented if she ingests a high-protein diet and vitamin and mineral supplements.

212. Giving birth to a neonate with a defect is a crisis situation and anxiety is a dominant response. Sources of this anxiety in the parents include all of the following, *except:*
1. Feeling a loss of self-esteem.
2. Concern about social status.
3. Threat to their sense of adequacy as a male/female.
4. People do not take solace from religion anymore.

213. The woman who experiences a stillbirth is in crisis. Therapeutic (emotionally supportive) nursing actions include:
1. Reassuring the mother that she can have another child.
2. Listening to her and encouraging her to talk it out.
3. Telling her it is God's will and we must accept what has happened.
4. Reassuring her that the stillbirth was not due to anything that she had done.

214. Baby Earl's mother becomes concerned about the growth and development of her baby, who was born at 34 weeks' gestation. She asks the nurse, "Will my baby be retarded?" Which of the following would be the most appropriate response by the nurse:
1. "I'm sure that your physician will be talking to you soon about your concerns."
2. "It is too soon to give an answer to that question. Any evaluation of his motor and intellectual ability will have to wait until he has begun to walk and talk."
3. "You have no cause for concern. Your baby has survived the critical period of this life. Just offer extra inducement to stimulate him to higher achievements."
4. "Your baby's rate of development may be slower than that of a full-term baby, but most premature infants eventually catch up with their age group."

215. All of the following features are characteristic of the premature infant and distinguish him from the full-term infant, except:
1. The body temperature is unstable and thus he responds readily to temperature changes in the environment.
2. The infant is usually puny and weighs less than 2000 g.
3. The infant's head is proportionately large, his skull is round or ovoid in shape, and his facial features are small and angular.
4. The skin is soft and transparent, and may be covered by lanugo.

216. Maternal vaginal infection that may cause thrush in the newborn is:
1. Leukorrhea.
2. Gonorrhea.
3. Moniliasis.
4. *Trichomonas vaginalis.*

217. Cytology report on a Papanicolaou smear reveals cell dysplasia, class III. Your anticipatory guidance includes:
1. Preparation of woman for biopsy and D & C.
2. Preparation of woman for cold-knife conization of cervix.
3. Scheduling woman for a repeat pap smear.
4. No further diagnostic tests or treatment are needed, since the cells are normal.

218. In performing nursing care for a woman with a cobalt implant in the cervical canal, the nurse does all of the following, *except:*
1. Wear an X ray film badge.
2. Maximize the time spent with the woman, since she is in isolation and suffers from lack of social stimulation.
3. Limit the time spent within 1 m (3 ft) of woman.
4. Check linen, clothes, and bathroom floor for any pencil-shaped object.

219. Functions of the seminal vesicles include all of the following, *except:*
1. Produce prostaglandin.
2. Store sperm until mature and capable of motility.
3. Add fluid to semen.
4. Add nutrients and favorable pH to semen.

220. All of the following statements about vasectomy are true, *except:*
1. Each vas deferens is ligated and a small segment is excised.
2. Testosterone production ceases.
3. Sexual potency is maintained.
4. Ejaculation and volume of seminal fluid production are unaffected.

221. The male climacteric occurs:
1. At no specified age.
2. Between the ages of 10 and 16.

3. Between 55 and 65 years of age.
4. In conjunction with benign hypertrophy of the prostate.

222. Which reproductive structure in man is analogous to the fallopian tube:
1. Vas deferens.
2. Epididymis.
3. Seminal vesicle.
4. Seminiferous tubules.

223. Conditions that may lead to infertility or sterility include all of the following, *except:*
1. Endometriosis.
2. Pelvic inflammatory disease.
3. Phimosis.
4. Mumps orchitis.

224. Diagnostic tests for infertility-sterility include all of the following, *except:*
1. Immune reactions.
2. Sims/Huhner.
3. Rubin test.
4. Bioassay for HCG.

225. A complete history is taken to identify possible factors implicated in infertility. These factors include all of the following, *except:*
1. A menstrual cycle varying from 26 to 28 days.
2. Age of each of the couple.
3. Length of unprotected exposure to conception.
4. Frequency and pattern of intercourse during the month.

226. A complete assessment for suspected sterility includes all of the following, *except:*
1. Testicular biopsy.
2. Cervical smear for cytology.
3. Genetic evaluation.
4. Cervical smear for antisperm antibodies.

227. All of the following are useful in treating infertility, *except:*
1. Record of basal body temperature (BBT) over a period of several months.
2. Use of condom and diaphragm until cervical mucosal antibody titer drops.
3. Use of an oral contraceptive over a period of time.
4. Engaging in intercourse every day and twice per day at the time of ovulation.

228. In March 1979, an Ethics Advisory Board made a recommendation to the Secretary of the Department of Health and Welfare concerning in-vitro fertilization and embryo transplantation. This recommendation stated that:
1. The procedure is not ethically acceptable.
2. The procedure is ethically acceptable.
3. Other methods are available to treat infertility.
4. Further experimentation along these lines is not ethical.

229. The next diagnostic step after mass screening utilizes a method of direct magnified visualization of the cervix. This method is known as:
1. Culdoscopy.
2. Laparoscopy.
3. Culposcopy.
4. Culdocentesis.

230. Which technique is used for inspection of the pelvic structures through an incision in the posterior cul-de-sac?
1. Culdoscopy.
2. Laparoscopy.
3. Culposcopy.
4. Culdocentesis.

231. Which of the following is a transperitoneal endoscopic technique that allows excellent visualization of the internal pelvic structures and limited surgery:
1. Culdoscopy.
2. Laparoscopy.
3. Culposcopy.
4. Culdocentesis.

232. Which of the following refers to the technique of passing a needle into the cul-de-sac of Douglas through the posterior fornix:
1. Culdoscopy.
2. Laparoscopy.
3. Culposcopy.
4. Culdocentesis.

Answers— Rationale / NURSING CARE DURING THE REPRODUCTIVE YEARS

1. (3) Legalization of abortion is the least likely factor to influence choice or use of contraceptive method. No. 1 is incorrect because religious teachings do influence a person's choice or use of contraceptive method, for example, the Catholic Church accepts only the rhythm and cervical mucus (Billings) methods for family planning. No. 2 is incorrect because culture influences one's attitudes toward childbearing, family size, touching one's genitalia, and the like. No. 4 is incorrect because the consumer push for naturalness and concern for possible complications following the use of some contraceptive methods has indeed influenced choice of methods used for family planning.

2. (4) Progesterone is responsible for the rise in BBT.

Nos. 1, 2, and 3 are incorrect because FSH is responsible for the maturation of a graafian follicle, HCS is produced by the placenta and has a growth hormone-like action, and estrogen is produced in the first half of the menstrual cycle and is responsible for the proliferative phase of the endometrium.

3. (1) The BBT falls slightly, then increases by about 0.5 C and remains elevated until about the 25th day (in a 28-day cycle) or until the woman conceives. No. 2 is incorrect because the BBT does not rise slightly, then fall by about 0.2 C. No. 3 is incorrect because the BBT is affected by a surge of LH, luteinizing hormone (not FSH), that is responsible for ovulation and the development of the corpus luteum of the second half of the menstrual cycle. No. 4 is incorrect because the BBT is maintained by progesterone that is produced during the second half of the menstrual cycle, but the original change in BBT is more related to the surge of LH at the time of ovulation.

4. Answer 4 is correct because level of formal education has the least impact on the reliability of BBT method. 1, 2, 3 are incorrect. Motivation and diligence are required to remember to take one's temperature at the same time each day; tension, infection, staying up late the night before and other factors result in temperature changes; fairly predictable menstrual cycles increase reliability by helping the woman evaluate the slight fall, then rise in BBT at time of ovulation. Nos. 1, 2, and 3 are incorrect because they are incomplete.

5. (3) At the time of ovulation, the cervical mucus is lubricative, not sticky. No. 1 is incorrect because the cervical mucus is clear, like egg white. No. 2 is incorrect because spinnbarkeit is greatest at time of ovulation. No. 4 is incorrect because the fern pattern does appear when dried.

6. (2) Under the influence of progesterone, the cervical mucus is nonstretchable (virtually no spinnbarkeit). No. 1 is incorrect because, under the influence of progesterone, the cervical mucus is opaque. No. 3 is incorrect because the mucus is sticky. No. 4 is incorrect because the cervical mucus dries in a variable (not fern-like) pattern that serves to block the passage of sperm.

7. (3) Oral contraceptive pills contain combinations of estrogen and progesterone, which suppress anterior pituitary activity so that no egg matures in the graafian follicle. No. 1 is incorrect because the IUD has no effect on egg production; eggs may be fertilized but generally do not implant. No. 2 is incorrect because spermicidal jelly works locally to kill sperm outside the external cervical os. No. 4 is incorrect because tubal ligation only interrupts the passage of the egg from the ovary into the fallopian tubes and uterus.

8. (2) D & C needs to be performed to avoid the risk of reproductive-tract adenocarcinoma if pregnancy (with a female fetus) has occurred. No. 1 is incorrect because pregnancy may have occurred and a D & C is advocated. No. 3 is incorrect because a D & C, not a repeat treatment, is indicated. No. 4 is incorrect because the "morning after" pill can only be considered 100% effective if it is followed by a D & C.

9. (3) Ovulation occurs most frequently 14 days *prior to* the first day of the next menstrual cycle. Nos. 1, 2, and 4 are incorrect because the second half of the cycle (after ovulation) is almost always 14 days.

10. (3) Headache and leg cramps may be signs of thromboembolism caused by the change in clotting factors that occurs under estrogen-progesterone stimulation. Nos. 1, 2, and 4 are incorrect because nausea, weight gain, chloasma, and breast tenderness, although annoying side effects, are not clinically significant.

11. (2) The Hyde Amendment severely restricts the use of federal funds for abortion. Nos. 1, 3, and 4 are incorrect because the Hyde Amendment does not pertain to operation of family-planning clinics, to in vitro fertilization and embryo transplantation, or to bioengineering projects.

12. (1) Headache is a sign of hypernatremia, not of water intoxication. Nos. 2, 3, and 4 are incorrect because oliguria, dyspnea, and restlessness, along with edema and thirst, are all signs and symptoms of water intoxication.

13. (1) Thirst is a symptom of water intoxication, not hypernatremia. Nos. 2, 3, and 4 are incorrect because tinnitus, tachycardia, and headache are all signs and symptoms of hypernatremia.

14. (1) Nägele's rule states: from the LMP subtract 3 months and add 7 days. You get the same result by counting forward 9 months and adding 7 days to the LMP. Do not count the "spotting"; about 25% of women spot during their first missed periods when pregnant. No. 2 is incorrect because 7 days has been subtracted rather than added. Nos. 3 and 4 are incorrect because the EDC was calculated from the date of spotting.

15. (2) HCG can be detected by the usual slide and test tube tests 20 days after fertilization (fifth week of cycle). Test results are more accurate after the sixth week, however. No. 1 is incorrect because a sophisticated radioassay test is necessary to detect HCG this early. Nos. 3 and 4 are incorrect because Joan wants to know the earliest date the test could be done.

16. (2) Offering her your hand to squeeze encourages her to tense her muscles, including the pubococcygeus muscle of the pelvic floor. No. 1 (explain what to expect and why the examination is being done), No. 3 (suggest breathing techniques to help her relax), and No. 4 (ask her to empty her bladder before the examination) are all nursing actions that tend to reduce the stress of undergoing a pelvic examination.

17. (4) This condition (moniliasis or candidiasis caused by *Candida albicans*—a fungus) is more likely to occur in women whose vaginal pH is changed due to pregnancy, ingestion of oral contraceptives, or diabetes, or if the normal flora are altered (as when one is taking antibiotics). No. 1 is incorrect because normal leukorrhea of pregnancy is not pruritic or cheese-like. No. 2 is incorrect because Flagyl is used to treat trichomonas vaginalis vaginitis, a protozoan infection. No. 3 is incorrect because candidiasis is readily transmitted to the neonate as a local lesion in the mouth (thrush) or as a disseminated septicemia.

18. (2) Take an antacid between meals. Drugs of any kind are best used only sparingly, if at all, during pregnancy. No. 1 is incorrect because avoiding an empty stomach by keeping small quantities in it at all times seems to decrease morning sickness. No. 3 is incorrect because dry carbohydrates ingested prior to getting out of bed (at least 15 minutes) seem to decrease morning sickness. No. 4 is incorrect because eating small servings of foods seems to decrease morning sickness.

19. (2) The urine test for pregnancy is positive. Sufficient HCG is present in the urine at this time to give a positive response, if pregnant. No. 1 is incorrect because the FHTs cannot be heard at this time, even with an ultrasound device. No. 3 is incorrect because, in normal pregnancy, the fundus does not reach the top of the symphysis pubis until about the 12th week. No. 4 is incorrect because it contradicts No. 2.

20. (4) Some spontaneous abortions occur at this time (8 to 12 weeks), when hormonal production by corpus luteum decreases, and this function should be taken up by the developing placenta. Nos. 1, 2, and 3 are incorrect because trophoblasts and corpus luteum do not produce progesterone and estrogen and the placenta is not mature enough in this time period.

21. (1) Inadequate nutrition depletes maternal stores and subjects her to preeclampsia, anemia, and infection. It is responsible for a higher incidence of congenital disorders or anomalies. No. 2 is incorrect because incidences of oversized babies with immature functional responses are not directly related to inadequate nutrition. No. 3 is incorrect because hyperbilirubinemia is a result of hemolytic disease. No. 4 is incorrect because acrocyanosis is a neonatal condition related to an immature vascular system and body temperature.

22. (1) Only 1000 ml of milk are recommended per day for the pregnant woman. Too much milk can result in leg cramps from an imbalance in calcium and phosphates. No. 2 is incorrect because three (to four) servings of meat are recommended to ensure the proper amount of protein, iron, and B vitamins, among other nutrients. No. 3 is incorrect because four (to five) servings of vegetables and fruits are recommended, including one serving of a citrus fruit and green and yellow vegetables to provide many vitamins, minerals, and roughage. No. 4 is incorrect because four (to five) servings of bread and cereal foods are recommended.

23. (1) Vitamin C is found in many foods. When working with people of different cultures, the nurse evaluates nutrient content of the foods preferred by the individual and family. No. 2 is incorrect because dried beans and peanut butter, although rich in protein, are not rich in vitamin C. Nos. 3 and 4 are incorrect because the listed foods do not provide vitamin C in large enough quantities.

24. (2) Dry beans, chicken, prunes, and broccoli are all rich in iron. Nos. 1, 3, and 4 are incorrect because none of these groups contains as much iron as the foods in No. 2.

25. (2) Bending at the waist facilitates movement of food out of stomach through relaxed cardiac sphincter; good posture and stooping by bending at the knees is better. No. 1 is incorrect because it is the treatment for morning sickness. No. 3 is incorrect because this would aggravate heartburn. Pressure from enlarging uterus compresses stomach and facilitates reflux of food into esophagus. No. 4 is incorrect. Pelvic rock relieves lower back pain, not heartburn.

26. (3) The mother does fantasize about the child and may withdraw from other relationships (period of introspection and introversion). No. 1 is incorrect because ambivalence about the pregnancy is usually an early response. No. 2 is incorrect because the woman is ready to begin learning breathing exercises during her third trimester when she is approaching labor. No. 4 is incorrect because it contradicts No. 3.

27. (1) During normal pregnancy, the islets of Langerhans in the pancreas do increase in size and increase insulin production in response to antiinsulin effect of HCS and reduced maternal tissue sensitivity to insulin. This maternal adaptation ensures an adequate supply of glucose, the main substrate to meet fetal energy needs. No. 2 is incorrect because HCS (others refer to this hormone as growth hormone or HPL) has an antiinsulin, not a proinsulin, effect. No. 3 is incorrect because there is reduced, not an increased, sensitivity to insulin in maternal tissues. No. 4 is incorrect because islets of Langerhans do increase in size and do increase the production of insulin in normal women during pregnancy.

28. (4) Loss of teeth due to drain on calcium/phosphorus stores is not within normal limits of pregnancy because, if calcium intake is inadequate, maternal stores other than the teeth are tapped to meet the tremendous fetal need. No. 1 is incorrect because the urethra does elongate by 1½ to 3 inches because perineal structures are enlarged due to increase in vasculature, hypertrophy of perineal body, and deposition of fat. No. 2 is incorrect because hydroureter does occur, primarily on the right side, due to general dilatation and loss of tone from estrogen and progesterone effect and compression of the ureters against the pelvic brim by the enlarged uterus. The right ureter is more involved because the uterus is shifted to that position by the large intestine. No. 3 is incorrect because esophageal regurgitation is common during pregnancy. It is caused by progesterone-influenced decreased tone in the entire GI tract, delayed emptying time of the stomach, and upper pressure from the enlarging uterus. The condition is known as "heartburn."

29. (2) The physical and emotional changes described are seen during the second trimester.

30. (3) The physical and emotional changes described are seen during the third trimester. Fetus is gaining weight rapidly while the maternal system is preparing for physical and emotional separation from the fetus.

31. (1) The physical and emotional changes described are seen during the first trimester, and are known as presumptive signs and symptoms of pregnancy.

32. (4) Severe pain in the abdomen may be due to abruption or other abdominal emergency; fluid discharge from vagina may indicate premature rupture of membranes; finger swelling may indicate developing preeclampsia. Nos. 1, 2, and 3 are incorrect because they all represent normal maternal adaptations to pregnancy. Anticipatory guidance may relieve anxiety caused by normal changes.

33. (3) The placenta inhibits the passage of large molecules only; viruses and many toxins cross the placenta. Nos. 1, 2, and 4 are incorrect because all of these are functions of the placenta.

34. (2) Antibodies produced by the mother are transmitted by osmotic exchange. No. 1 is incorrect because maternal and fetal blood do not mix. No. 3 is incorrect because the placenta does not secrete antibodies. No. 4 is incorrect because maternal antibodies do cross the placenta.

35. (1) Braxton Hicks contractions, hypermobility of joints, and backache are all normal findings during this time of pregnancy. No. 2 is incorrect because dysuria must be investigated further. If a UTI exists and goes untreated, the well-being of both mother and fetus is compromised. Lightening should not occur now. Constipation and hemorrhoids are common discomforts resulting from decreased GI muscle tone, increased water absorption, pressure from the enlarging uterus, and oral iron supplementation. No. 3 is incorrect because a feeling of tranquillity and a heightened introspection are common to the second trimester. No.

4 is incorrect because these findings are seen early in pregnancy.

36. (3) Brownish spotting is a normal finding within 48 hours after vaginal examination (or coitus) because of the increased friability and vascularity of the cervix during pregnancy. No. 1 is incorrect because "epigastric pain" is the subjective feeling that results from edema of the liver capsule in severe preeclampsia/eclampsia. No. 2 is incorrect because periorbital edema is a sign of preeclampsia. No. 4 is incorrect because seeing double and other visual disturbances are signs of preeclampsia, resulting from retinal edema and arteriolar changes.

37. (3) Tension on the round ligaments occurs because of the human's upright posture; the enlarging uterus and poor body mechanics all contribute to this discomfort. No. 1 is incorrect because bladder infection is accompanied by other symptoms as well. The nurse does assess for signs of bladder infection, however. No. 2 is incorrect because discomfort from constipation is accompanied by other symptoms, and the location of the discomfort differs. No. 4 is incorrect because left-sided groin pain is not descriptive of beginning of labor.

38. (2) These findings are consistent with the second trimester. Data are helpful in anticipatory guidance regarding nutrition and estimation of gestational age (e.g., FHR first heard with stethoscope at about 20 weeks).

39. (1) These data are consistent with the first trimester. Data are helpful in anticipatory guidance regarding effects of drugs, X rays, and diseases on fetal development.

40. (4) These data are consistent with postterm gestation. The nurse needs to be aware that the mortality rate is four times that of term infants.

41. (3) These data are consistent with the third trimester. Data are helpful in assessing the gestational age of the neonate; the term infant generally is the least likely to be at risk.

42. (4) A detailed description is overloading—may inspire fears parent(s) had not thought of before. Nos. 1, 2, and 3 are incorrect because all of these activities tend to *decrease* a gravida's anxiety of labor and delivery.

43. (1) The fetal blood is shunted from the right atrium into the left atrium; the mechanism allows blood to bypass pulmonary circulation. Hence, Nos. 2, 3, and 4 are incorrect.

44. (4) The ductus arteriosus allows blood to be shunted from the pulmonary artery to the aorta, a mechanism that allows blood to bypass pulmonary circulation. Nos. 1, 2, and 3 are therefore incorrect.

45. (3) Snuffles are symptomatic of the rhinitis of congenital syphilis. Nos. 1, 2, and 4 are all incorrect because hepatitis, abnormal fingerprints and palm creases, and encephalitis are often seen along with bleeding tendency, enlarged liver and spleen, bone lesions, and abnormal EKG. The child may have the rubella virus present in mucous secretions for up to two years after birth.

46. (4) Hydrocephaly does not occur with rubella infection during the first trimester. Microcephaly with mental retardation occurs instead. Nos. 1, 2, and 3 are incorrect because cranial VIII nerve injury (congenital deafness), cardiac malformations, and congenital cataracts occur in 50% of fetuses exposed to rubella during the first trimester.

47. (3) Asking her to think of ways she may be able to cut down implies your respect for her ability to think for herself; and she will be more apt to comply with her self-made rules. No. 1 is incorrect because telling her that she is injuring the baby if she doesn't decrease her smoking is a threat and does not show respect for her needs. No. 2 is incorrect because telling her to substitute snacking, even with "good" foods, is your choice and not hers. No. 4 is incorrect because asking her how she plans to cut down her smoking to 10 cigarettes per day implies that you are not giving her a choice but an ultimatum; goals for the client are best determined mutually.

48. (3) These findings are indicative of a 20-week gestation. No. 1 is incorrect because lightening usually occurs about the 36th to 38th week and the FHR is first heard with a Doptone by the 11th to 12th week. No. 2 is incorrect because Braxton Hicks contractions are usually palpable around the 30th week; the fundus is at the umbilicus at about the 22nd week. No. 4 is incorrect because Goodell, Hegar, and Chadwick signs are usually first noted about the 6th week; the fundus is halfway between the umbilicus and the symphysis at about the 16th week.

49. (1) Injudicious douching may alter the normal vaginal environment. No. 2 is incorrect because there may be an instance with vaginal infection when a medicated douche may be ordered; however, the douche given with a bulb syringe is potentially dangerous—it may result in embolus. No. 3 is incorrect because douching does nothing to prevent the copious secretions. No. 4 is incorrect because of answer No. 1.

50. (3) These instructions vary with the gravida—distance from the hospital, mode of transportation, previous labor history, and other factors may modify the individual's directions. No. 1 is incorrect because she really should have gone sooner—the malar flush usually appears about 5 cm. No. 2 is incorrect because these findings may be due to urinary-tract infection. No. 4 is incorrect because these contractions indicate that delivery may not be too far off and she should already be at the hospital.

51. (4) Headache and feeling of fullness in face and hands may indicate preeclampsia, and brown discharge from vagina (along with other symptoms) may indicate hydatidiform mole. Nos. 1, 2, and 3 are incorrect because these are normal changes during pregnancy.

52. (4) Fetal activity level does not initiate labor. Nos. 1, 2, and 3 are incorrect because any or all of these may have a role in initiating labor.

53. (4) The gravida needs support for her feelings and needs to know that this reaction is natural and understandable. Nos. 1, 2, and 3 are incorrect because they do not validate the naturalness of her feelings and do not allow for further ventilation.

54. (3) The bottle-feeding mother's ovulation and menstrual cycle has been noted to occur as early as 36 days; the breastfeeding mother's, as early as 39 days. In both cases, ovulation usually does not occur until later, however. Hence, Nos. 1 and 2 are incorrect. No. 4 is incorrect because the couple may wish to resume intercourse when the lochia stops at three weeks.

55. (2) Moniliasis does not cause ophthalmia neonatorum. Nos. 1, 3, and 4 are incorrect because all of these are related to moniliasis.

56. (1) This describes the correct way to assess contractions. Nos. 2, 3, and 4 are likely to cause uterine dysfunction because of excessive manipulation.

57. (3) No vaginal examination is done if one suspects an abnormal implantation of the placenta—hemorrhage is likely to result. Nos. 1, 2, and 4 are incorrect because all of these assessments are possible with vaginal examinations.

58. (3) This usually helps assuage the mate's feelings of guilt, impotence, and helplessness and fosters the couple's sense of mutual experience. Nos. 1, 2, and 4 are incorrect because none of these meets the goals achieved by No. 3 above.

59. (4) Hypotension is a frequent side effect. Maternal hypotension causes fetal bradycardia and hypoxia. No. 1 is incorrect because epidural anesthesia causes hypotension, not hypertension. No. 2 is incorrect because, although the nurse may be monitoring oxytocin augmentation of labor after contractions slow due to epidural block, hypotension is the most important side effect of this form of anesthesia, and must be avoided. No. 3 is incorrect because the gravida must lie flat after spinal (saddle block) anesthesia, not after epidural anesthesia.

60. (1) These behaviors are more indicative of the early first stage of labor. Nos. 2, 3, and 4 are incorrect because they are indicative of approaching the second stage of labor.

61. (4) This process is necessary to expel the fetus from the uterus and to propel it through the birth canal. Hence, Nos. 1, 2, and 3 are incorrect.

62. (4) These findings are consistent with LOA presentation and position. No. 1 is incorrect because the fetus is not breech—the "hard, round mass" refers to the fetal head. No. 2 is incorrect because the fetus is not posterior, but anterior. No. 3 is incorrect because the fetus is not breech, nor is labor going to be prolonged. Left occiput anterior position is considered optimal for delivery.

63. (3) These behaviors are indicative of the phase of transition; the woman needs constant supportive care as she approaches 10 cm, or complete dilatation.

64. (1) These behaviors are indicative of the latent phase of the first stage of labor.

65. (2) These behaviors are indicative of the active phase of the first stage of labor; she is about 5 cm. These behaviors are not noted in women who have received regional anesthesia.

66. (2) The mother must see her infant for herself for reassurance and for beginning the process of attachment (bonding). Nos. 1, 3, and 4 are incorrect because they do not achieve the goals mentioned above.

67. (4) A decrease in fetal heart rate below 100 with contractions connotes fetal distress. No. 1 is incorrect because there is normally an increased amount of bloody show from the vagina as the presenting part descends down the birth canal. No. 2 is incorrect because the pain is most probably due to persistent posterior. No. 3 is incorrect because minimal acceleration in FHR, without loss of variability or significant changes in periodic patterns, is usually benign. Close observation is maintained, however.

68. (4) LOA (left occiput anterior)—with the breech in the fundus, the occiput is the only possible presentation from among the choices. Since the irregular nodules (elbows, fist, knees, feet) are on the mother's right, the fetal back must be on her left. Therefore the occiput and the back are on the left. Nos. 1 and 2 are incorrect because the denominator—the S or sacrum—is not presenting, vertex is. No. 3 is incorrect because the fetal back is to the mother's left side. Since the fetal back is on the same side as the occiput, the occiput is also to the maternal left.

69. (1) Below umbilicus, on mother's left side. In vertex presentations, the FHTs are generally heard clearest below the umbilicus. In LOA the fetal back is to the maternal left; the FHTs are generally easiest to hear through the fetal back. No. 2 is incorrect because in an LOA position, the fetal back is toward the maternal left side. Nos. 3 and 4 are incorrect because, with a vertex presentation (occiput presenting), FHTs are loudest below the umbilicus.

70. (2) Presentation refers to that portion of the fetus that enters the pelvis first and covers the internal cervical os. No. 1 is incorrect because lie refers to the relationship of the fetal spine to the maternal spine. For example, in vertical lie (vertex, breech) the fetal spine parallels the maternal spine and in transverse lie (shoulder) the fetal spine is horizontal. No. 3 is incorrect because attitude refers to the relationship of one fetal part to another, for example, general flexion, general flexion with extension of neck. No. 4 is incorrect because station refers to the relationship of the fetal biparietal diameter (in vertex presentation) to the ischial spines of the mother.

71. (2) In most cases, the fetus assumes an attitude of general flexion to allow the smallest diameter of the fetal head to present; this positions the posterior fontanel over the cervical os. No. 1 is incorrect because the fetal neck would have to be extended to present the anterior fontanel over the cervical os. No. 3 is incorrect because the vertex, not the breech, is presenting. No. 4 is incorrect because the fetus is in the vertex presentation and in vertical lie, therefore the shoulder cannot be the presenting part.

72. (2) Position of the placenta is determined by sonography. No vaginal examinations are performed if the placenta is abnormally implanted. No. 1 is incorrect because the descent (station) and flexion can be determined by vaginal examination. No. 3 is incorrect because dilatation and effacement of the cervix can be determined by vaginal examination. No. 4 is incorrect because the condition of the membranes (ruptured, intact, bulging) can be determined by vaginal examination.

73. (2) The danger of prolapse of the cord is exceptionally great when there are bulging membranes and the presenting part is at − 3 station. When the membranes rupture, the cord could be washed down ahead or to the side of the presenting part. Nos. 1 and 3 are incorrect because of the danger of prolapsed cord when the membranes rupture. No. 4 is incorrect because this is common knowledge expected of the labor room nurse.

74. (4) Tilting the hip moves the heavy uterus off the vena cava, thus preventing supine hypotension and fetal bradycardia. No. 1 is incorrect since the statement denies her need for comfort now. No. 2 is incorrect since the statement is only half correct. The pillows may increase her comfort but will not prevent supine hypotension. No. 3 is incorrect since the statement sounds more like a threat and does not acknowledge her present need to remain supine and flat.

75. (3) Breech presentation—pressure exerted on the presenting breech is sufficient to force emptying of the rectum. Nos. 1 and 2 are incorrect because relaxation of the anal sphincter and release of meconium are the direct result of fetal hypoxia or anoxia. No. 4 is incorrect because it contradicts No. 3.

76. (3) Depression of contractions and fetal bradycardia are expected effects of paracervical block. No. 1 is incorrect because the bearing-down reflex is not affected by this anesthesia. No. 2 is incorrect because maternal blood pressure and postnatal uterine contractility are not affected by paracervical block. No. 4 is incorrect because the bearing-down reflex is not affected and therefore forceps delivery is usually not needed.

77. (3) The medication never mixes with cerebral spinal fluid and therefore there is no need for the woman to lie flat for several hours after receiving this form of anesthesia. Nos. 1, 2, and 4 are incorrect because their lists are incomplete.

78. (4) All of the listed effects are to be expected following spinal anesthesia: loss of bearing-down reflex, depression of contractions, maternal hypotension, fetal bradycardia, low forceps delivery, postnatal bladder atony, need to remain flat in bed for some hours after delivery, and postnatal uterine atony. Nos. 1, 2, and 3 are incorrect because their lists are incomplete.

79. (1) A drop, not an increase, in oxygen is thought to stimulate respirations (if the hypoxia is neither excessive nor of long duration). No. 2 is incorrect because hypoxia, if not too prolonged, seems to be the most powerful stimulant to initiate respiration. No. 3 is incorrect because changes in skin temperature and tactile stimulation aid in initiating respirations. No. 4 is incorrect because changes from weightlessness to gravity environment aid in initiating respirations.

80. (3) The first priority is to maintain the neonate's temperature; the second, to note any abnormalities; the third, to identify the neonate; the fourth, to instill silver nitrate drops (which may be delayed for two hours while neonate attaches to mother/father). Hence, Nos. 1, 2, and 4 are incorrect.

81. (4) The temperature of the wrapped (normal, full-term) infant in the mother's arms does not differ significantly from that of the infant in a warmed incubator. Nos. 1, 2, and 3 are incorrect because all of these factors do contribute to rapid heat loss.

82. (3) Hgb and Hct are very high at birth. The excess red blood cells (needed for the relative hypoxic intrauterine environment) are hemolyzed soon after birth, resulting in "physiologic" jaundice by about the third day. Nos. 1, 2, and 4 are all normal characteristics of the newborn.

83. (1) Telangiectases and subconjunctival hemorrhage (from capillaries ruptured from increased pressures experienced passing through the birth canal) are normal newborn characteristics. Nos. 2, 3, and 4 are incor-

rect because they are all signs of increased intracranial pressure.

84. (3) Term infants may lose 5% to 10% of body weight. Arithmetic: 7×16 oz = 112 oz and 10% of 112 oz = 11.2 oz (3175 g $\times$ 10% = 317.5 g).

85. (1) If aspirated, sterile plain water is less irritating to the respiratory tract. Hence, Nos. 2, 3, and 4 are incorrect.

86. (4) The Moro reflex is not stimulated by hypoglycemia or hypocalcemia. Nos. 1, 2, and 3 are incorrect because all of these stimulate the Moro reflex in the neonate with an intact neuromuscular system from the brain stem down.

87. (1) Physiologic jaundice in the newborn infant is related to liver immaturity and fetal polycythemia. Nos. 2, 3, and 4 are incorrect because, although they may cause jaundice, it would not be "physiologic."

88. (1) The newly delivered woman should be checked every 15 minutes because the tendency to hemorrhage is greater during the first hour after delivery. Nos. 2, 3, and 4 are incorrect because all of these assessments are appropriate during the fourth stage of labor (the first hour after delivery or until the woman's condition stabilizes).

89. (1) Talkativeness, dependency, passivity, and interest in her own body functions are all characteristic of the "taking-in" phase of this period of the puerperium. No. 2 is incorrect because she is interested instead in being cared for; needs food, fluids, rest, and praise for a job well done; and needs someone with whom to discuss her delivery experience. No. 3 is incorrect because she is very interested in her body functions, e.g., her ability to void and defecate, to walk and sit. No. 4 is incorrect because she is not ready to "take hold," to learn mothering tasks, until she is rested, has integrated the delivery experience, and has regained control over her body functions.

90. (3) Milia, unopened sebaceous glands, look like "whiteheads," not blackheads. No. 1 is incorrect because both enlarged breasts and pink spotting (pseudomenstruation) are effects of the high levels of maternal hormones to which she had been exposed in utero. No. 2 is incorrect because the linea nigra (dark line) is present due to maternal hormones. No. 4 is incorrect because the dark discoloration ("mongolian spotting") is found over the lower back and sacrum in darker skinned peoples—darker Whites, Orientals, and Blacks.

91. (1) The "lump" is a cephalhematoma that requires no treatment because it resolves spontaneously in a few weeks; the mother needs to be on the alert for increased jaundice as the clot resolves, however. No. 2 is incorrect because this is a description of caput succedaneum. No. 3 is incorrect because this birth injury

is outside of the fetal skull, between the bone and its periosteum. No. 4 is incorrect because a hemangioma is a benign tumor made up of newly formed blood vessels, clustered together.

92. (4) A full bladder may be the direct cause of discomfort. No. 1 is incorrect because the nurse gives a pain medication only after trying other comfort measures. No. 2 is incorrect because the nurse would use this therapeutic measure after the bladder is empty—a warmed, rolled towel is very soothing. No. 3 is incorrect for this problem, because walking does not relieve afterpains.

93. (2) Nipples cleaned with warm water and dried carefully are less likely to fissure. No. 1 is incorrect because soap is very drying and washes off natural and protective oils. No. 3 is incorrect because alcohol would be too drying and would thus facilitate fissure formation. No. 4 is incorrect because the plastic shields would keep moisture close to the skin and possibly cause maceration.

94. (1) Headaches and leg pains must be evaluated to rule out thromboembolytic disease, a condition more common during and just after pregnancy because of the change in clotting factors from progesterone influence. Headache may also herald postpartum preeclampsia/eclampsia. Nos. 2, 3, and 4 are all normal findings in the postpartum period.

95. (4) Oxytocin stimulates the "let-down" reflex but is not always successful. Nos. 1 and 3 are incorrect because these drugs have an antilactogenic effect. No. 2 is incorrect because it is used to contract the uterus.

96. (4) A clear airway is the first priority. No. 1 is incorrect—never tug on the cord until after the placenta has separated. Nos. 2 and 3 are incorrect because these actions are taken only after a clear airway is assured.

97. (3) The mother can only pass on those antibodies she herself produced to counteract a disease. No. 1 is incorrect because any antibodies present in breastmilk do not protect against DPT, measles, or polio. No. 2 is incorrect because the measles vaccination is ineffectual if given before the first birthday. No. 4 is incorrect because antibodies in mother's milk do not protect against the above-named diseases.

98. (2) "Infant" refers to the first year of life. No. 1 is incorrect because the first four weeks of life are known as the neonatal period. No. 3 is incorrect because the United States and Canada rank around 15th to 17th when compared to the mortality rates of other countries of the world. Hence, No. 4 is incorrect because mortality refers to deaths while illnesses are referred to by morbidity.

99. (2) "Perinatal" refers to the period of time between 28 weeks' gestation and the 28th day after birth. No. 1 is incorrect because perinatal refers only to the fetus/neonate and to the period of time between the 28th week of gestation and the 28th day after birth. No. 3 is incorrect because perinatal period includes the 28 days after birth as well. No. 4 is incorrect because perinatal period includes the time from the 28th week of gestation as well as the 28 days after birth.

100. (2) The birth rate is figured per 1000 women of childbearing age. Hence Nos. 1, 3, and 4 are incorrect.

101. (4) Oral consent is only sufficient if the person giving the consent is not medicated and can understand the information, *and* the oral consent is witnessed by a reliable individual. No. 1 is incorrect because an informed consent must be given voluntarily, without coercion. No. 2 is incorrect because the person must be given information about the procedure, its consequences and any alternate procedures and their consequences. No. 3 is incorrect because the person giving consent must be capable of comprehending the information. Interpreters are to be used when necessary.

102. (3) Silver nitrate drops still have to be instilled into the neonate's conjunctival sacs to prevent infection, not just from gonorrhea but also from such pathogens in the birth canal as pneumococcus and streptococcus. No. 1 is incorrect because of the presence in the birth canal of pathogens other than gonorrhea. No. 2 is incorrect because it is safe to wait up to two hours to instill the drops. This allows time for maternal-child eye contact and interaction, which facilitates attachment. No. 4 is incorrect because retrolental fibroplasia results from too high an oxygen concentration in immature retinal vessels during oxygen therapy for the compromised neonate.

103. (1) The delay does facilitate the process of attachment to the mother (father). Nos. 2, 3, and 4 are incorrect because none of these options relates to delaying the instillation of silver nitrate into the neonate's conjunctival sacs.

104. (1) This is her third pregnancy: one pregnancy ended in abortion, one pregnancy was preterm, and the child was born alive and is now living and well. Gravida = number of times the uterus was pregnant. Para = number of pregnancies carried to viability. No. 2 is incorrect because this is her third pregnancy and she has carried only one pregnancy to viability. No. 3 is incorrect because this is the third time her uterus is gravid. No. 4 is incorrect because she has carried only one pregnancy to viability.

105. (2) She has just been delivered of her second pregnancy. The first ended in abortion; the second was carried to viability and resulted in twins. Para refers to the number of pregnancies carried to viability regardless of the number of fetuses delivered from one preg-

nancy. She is 2-1-0-1-2. Hence, Nos. 1, 3, and 4 are incorrect.

106. (2) Preparation for natural childbirth does not guarantee freedom from discomfort during labor. No. 1 is incorrect because medications may be used. However, women prepared for childbirth tend to require much less medication when it is needed. Nos. 3 and 4 are incorrect because both these statements are true about natural childbirth and preparation for childbirth.

107. (3) The breathing technique for "transition" is *rapid* and shallow, not slow and shallow. Nos. 1, 2, and 4 are incorrect because all of these breathing techniques are correct as stated.

108. (3) "Abandonment" is the term used when a client is discharged before it is safe. Nos. 1, 2, and 4 are incorrect because they describe other legal charges.

109. (4) Even after 21 years, the nurse, physician, and hospital are legally responsible for what happened to the person as a newborn infant. In this case, assault and battery is used when something is done to a person without his (or his guardian's) consent.

110. (2) Only No. 2 meets the adolescent's needs, which include (a) respect and concern for her welfare and involvement in her care and feelings about her future, including her sexual behavior, and (b) assistance with problem-solving techniques and alternatives for action.

111. (4) All of the other factors listed are considered by adoption agencies in choosing parents for children. "Hard-to-place" infants are usually adopted out to older couples; younger couples get the infants. Adoptions from agencies or in private contracts are not finalized for six months.

112. (3) Therapeutic abortion is considered only if gravida develops jaundice and fever while adequately hydrated, tachycardia of greater than or equal to 130, retinal hemorrhage, and delirium. Nos. 1, 2, and 4 are incorrect because these include the major nursing actions for women suffering from hyperemesis gravidarum.

113. (4) Tenderness and rigidity of abdomen and uterus are indicative of severe abruptio placentae. Nos. 1, 2, and 3 are incorrect because all of these are associated with hydatidiform mole.

114. (4) Rupture of ectopic pregnancy is often experienced as a sharp, stabbing pain in the lower abdomen and is usually seen after two missed menstrual periods. Nos. 1, 2, and 3 are incorrect because her symptoms appear too early for incompetent cervix (12 weeks), placenta previa (near term and usually painless) and abruptio placentae (near term).

115. (4) Placenta previa is not associated with a multiple gestation. Nos. 1, 2, and 3 are incorrect because all of the conditions listed are associated with multiple gestation.

116. (3) Tissue transplants are readily accepted from one another because identical twins share the same chromosomes. No. 1 is incorrect because chance and heredity, not advanced maternal age, are implicated in identical twins. No. 2 is incorrect because identical twins arise from the union of one egg and one sperm. No. 4 is incorrect because identical twins are *always* of the same sex.

117. (4) Severe pain in abdomen may be due to abruptio placentae or an abdominal emergency; fluid discharge from the vagina may be due to premature rupture of the membranes; and swelling of the fingers may indicate developing preeclampsia. Nos. 1, 2, and 3 are incorrect because all of these are normal maternal adaptations to pregnancy.

118. (2) She should be housed in a quiet room. Nos. 1, 3, and 4 are incorrect because all are important nursing actions when caring for a gravida with preeclampsia.

119. (4) Restraints are inappropriate for someone who is apt to have, or who is having, a convulsion—restraints could cause severe injury. Nos. 1, 2, and 3 are all incorrect because a urinary catheter tray, IV solutions and insertion equipment, and suction apparatus are all needed for severe preeclampsia and eclampsia. In addition, the nurse adds the eclamptic tray (drugs) and oxygen.

120. (1) Oliguria is indeed a grave sign when the woman has severe preeclampsia or eclampsia. No. 2 is incorrect because daily intake is calculated on individual needs. No. 3 is incorrect because sudden diuresis is a good prognostic sign. No. 4 is incorrect because urinary output must *exceed* 100 ml in four hours before magnesium sulphate, if needed, can be given again.

121. (1) Hyperemesis is not a sign of preeclampsia, eclampsia, or its sequelae. Hyperemesis occurs primarily during the first trimester and is thought to have a strong psychologic overlay. No. 2 is incorrect because the nurse monitors urinary output, reflex response, and respiratory rate to assess drug therapy and disease status. No. 3 is incorrect because the nurse is alert to symptoms of frontal headache and/or epigastric pain (due to liver capsule edema) that herald imminent convulsions. No. 4 is incorrect because increased uterine tone accompanied by increased sensitivity of the abdominal wall are indicative of abruptio, a sequela to hypertension of any etiology.

122. (2) Hypertension is a cause of abruptio, not a sequela. Nos. 1, 3, and 4 are all sequelae of abruptio placentae.

123. (1) The possibility of postpartum eclampsia, while high, is often overlooked. Nos. 2, 3, and 4 are incorrect because none of these statements is true.

124. (3) Normal, moderate (not "restricted") activity is necessary for good insulin control and mental well-being. No. 1 is incorrect because early treatment is imperative to maintain adequate metabolism and prevent ketoacidosis, a condition that is fetotoxic. No. 2 is incorrect because the gravida who is not on regular insulin needs to convert to regular for the duration of pregnancy, especially if she had been taking tolbutaline. Tolbutaline does not protect the fetus from ketoacidosis. No. 4 is incorrect because the woman will need to be meticulous in checking her urine (or blood sugar) because her insulin requirements change during pregnancy.

125. (4) Erythroblastosis fetalis usually results from Rh incompatibility. Nos. 1, 2, and 3 are incorrect because among diabetic gravidas there is an increased incidence of spontaneous abortion, preeclampsia, and dystocia.

126. (4) Amniocentesis cannot determine whether the fetus carries the gene for diabetes. No. 1 is incorrect because the diabetic woman may be hospitalized for regulation of insulin. No. 2 is incorrect because tests for placental functioning (sufficiency) are utilized to determine safety of intrauterine environment for the fetus. No. 3 is incorrect because uncontrolled morning sickness may lead to acidosis.

127. (1) Breastfeeding is actually encouraged because it has an antidiabetogenic effect (it decreases blood glucose and therefore insulin requirement). No. 2 is incorrect because nipple and/or vaginal monilial infection is one of the minor problems which can affect the diabetic woman. No. 3 is incorrect because she must eat on time, even if her baby must wait to be fed, to maintain an adequate blood glucose level for the amount of insulin she takes. No. 4 is incorrect because she must prevent hypoglycemia (which stimulates adrenalin production) because that would inhibit the let-down reflex and decrease her milk supply.

128. (2) Oral contraception is contraindicated because the hormones decrease carbohydrate tolerance, necessitate readjustment of insulin dosage, and may increase her chances for coronary heart disease and myocardial infarction, especially in the older woman. IUDs may predispose to infection in the reproductive tract. No. 1 is incorrect because, with mature onset of diabetes, 4% of offspring can inherit the disease; juvenile onset, 22% of offspring can inherit the disease. No. 3 is incorrect because the woman's ability to cope with both small children and the disease may be too stressed, making it difficult to adjust the insulin dosage properly. No. 4 is incorrect because, with renal disease or proliferative retinopathy, she faces increased risk with another pregnancy and must be informed of these risks as well as of sterilization procedures.

129. (2) The woman who seems restless, with flushed face, rapid pulse, and deep respirations, is exhibiting signs of hyperglycemia, not insulin reaction. No. 1 is incorrect because a flash of light in the sleeping person's face does not result in a squint and turn of the head if she is having an insulin reaction. No. 3 is incorrect because the woman does perspire while sleeping during an insulin reaction. No. 4 is incorrect because the woman does wake up with a headache if she is having an insulin reaction.

130. (1) This woman's need for rest is paramount. Nos. 2, 3, and 4 are incorrect because any or all of these may precipitate congestive heart failure in the gravida with rheumatic valvular damage. No. 4 lists high-salt foods contraindicated for this woman.

131. (3) Bathroom privileges may be too stressful physically. She should be assisted on and off bedpan or bedside commode. Nos. 1, 2, and 4 are incorrect because all of these are therapeutic nursing actions for a gravida with cardiac failure.

132. (4) Bearing-down is too strenuous for a woman with cardiac disease. No. 1 is incorrect because propping her into a semirecumbent position facilitates cardiac function. No. 2 is incorrect because an increase in pulse rate is an early sign of cardiac decompensation. No. 3 is incorrect because regional anesthesia eliminates pain and anxiety and thus helps prevent cardiac decompensation. Regional anesthesia also helps pool blood in the legs.

133. (2) Fluids should not be forced or cardiac overload may occur. Nos. 1, 3, and 4 are incorrect because all of these actions are therapeutic and/or diagnostic. The immediate postpartal period is critical because the sudden release of intraabdominal pressure (from the emptying of the uterus) may cause collapse.

134. (2) Maternal age alone is not an indicator for induction. No. 1 is incorrect because induction is appropriate for stimulating labor when there is uterine inertia. No. 3 is incorrect because the fetus with severe isoimmunization is delivered before term to prevent serious sequelae to hemolytic disease. No. 4 is incorrect because the gravida with prolonged rupture of membranes is delivered within 24 hours to prevent chorioamnionitis.

135. (3) Lecithin, a phospholipid, rises abruptly at about the 35th week and, if present in a ratio to sphingomyelin of 2:1 or more, fetal lung maturity is assumed. Other names include foam test or test for surfactant activity. No. 1 is incorrect because, although creatinine indicates fetal maturity, the test for it is not known as the shake test. No. 2 is incorrect because bilirubin (assessed by spectrophotometric analysis) should have disappeared from amniotic fluid by 37 weeks unless the fetus is suffering from hemolytic disease. No. 4 is incorrect because estriol levels are used to assess maternal-placental-fetal well-being, especially if the mother is diabetic or suffers from hypertension of any etiology. The test specimen is usually urine.

136. (3) If you accept the assignment, you are expected to perform as a trained and reasonably prudent nurse would perform in that area. No. 1 is incorrect because you are responsible for your actions and are expected to refuse an assignment for which you are unprepared. Nos. 2 and 4 are incorrect because you hold the primary responsibility for your behavior; the physician or head nurse may share in a legal action, but you are primarily accountable under the law.

137. (2) Pitocin is a potentially dangerous drug that may result in tetanic contractions leading to maternal injury (uterine rupture, lacerations of the lower uterine segment and birth canal) and fetal asphyxia and death. Pitocin induction must be closely monitored by a physician who is either at the bedside or close by. Hence, Nos. 1, 3, and 4 are incorrect.

138. (1) Pitocin has an antidiuretic effect, so woman may retain fluids. Urinary output is assessed to check for adequacy. Nos. 2, 3, and 4 are incorrect because changes in blood pressure, deep-tendon reflexes, and level of consciousness are not directly related to Pitocin induction.

139. (1) Early deceleration is thought to be related to head compression and is of no clinical significance. No. 2 is incorrect because late deceleration is caused by uteroplacental insufficiency, requiring interventions such as (a) placing woman on her left side, increasing rate of IV fluids (Pitocin-free), and administering oxygen; (b) cesarean delivery. No. 3 is incorrect because lack of uniformity in shape (may be "U," "V," "W" in shape), with onset anytime before, during, or after a contraction (variable deceleration), is caused by umbilical-cord compression and requires immediate intervention, such as stated under No. 2 above. No. 4 is incorrect because this pattern of bradycardia may indicate cord compression or separation of the placenta, requiring immediate intervention as stated under No. 2 above.

140. (3) The highest priority in care is to stop artificial stimulation of the uterus to facilitate adequate perfusion of the uterine-placental-fetal unit. No. 1 is incorrect because, unless this could be done concurrently by a second person, the nurse would waste valuable time that should first be spent improving the FHR. No. 2 is incorrect because this action is taken after the physician evaluates the maternal-fetal condition, and a cesarean delivery is deemed necessary. No. 4 is incorrect because this action is second in priority after steps are taken to improve perfusion—a necessary condition before any oxygen can reach the fetus.

141. (2) Uterine muscle tone is generally good when no analgesia/anesthesia affects innervation, when fetal size does not overstretch uterine muscle, and when labor is not overlong. No. 1 is incorrect because the factor in this case is the spinal anesthesia that interrupts innervation to the uterine muscle and other abdominal organs, such as the bladder, thereby predisposing to atony. No. 3 is incorrect because Pitocin overstimulates the uterine muscle, thereby predisposing to muscle fatigue and later to atony. No. 4 is incorrect because the uterus is generally overly stretched to accommodate twin gestation. Overstretching predisposes to atony.

142. (4) This is a defensive statement that does not recognize the mother's concern. No. 1 is incorrect because clear and repeated descriptions of progress and explanations for delay help her cope with the long labor. The "unknown" is ego-weakening. No. 2 is incorrect because preventing or identifying and treating maternal exhaustion is necessary for good maternal and fetal outcome. No. 3 is incorrect because the expression of hostility caused by the frustration of a difficult labor is therapeutic for the woman.

143. (1) Telling her that a birth is a birth, whether by cesarean or vaginal route, is the nurse's opinion and denies the mother's need to work out her feelings about the change from her expectations. No. 2 is incorrect because discussing events preceding the cesarean birth does assist her in sifting out, clarifying, and filling in details of the experience so that she is better equipped to integrate the event into her self-concept and self-image in a positive manner. No. 3 is incorrect because positioning her in bed with pillows eases her discomfort directly and indirectly indicates to her the respect the nurse has for her as an individual—all of which assist her to "rest." No. 4 is incorrect because knowing how to splint the incision and decrease pain does help her "rest."

144. (1) Syphilis does not impair uterine perfusion, although the spirochete is very harmful to the fetal tissues. No. 2 is incorrect because hypertension does diminish perfusion of the uterus. No. 3 is incorrect because anemia does diminish perfusion of the uterus. No. 4 is incorrect because poor posture can diminish perfusion of the uterus, e.g., supine hypotension syndrome.

145. (4) Precipitate labor (under three hours), multiparity, overdistention of uterus (twins), and relaxation of uterus by spinal anesthesia predispose this woman to postpartum hemorrhage. Hence, Nos. 1, 2, and 3 are incorrect.

146. (2) Methergine or Ergotrate contract the cervix as well, which would interfere with the expulsion of the fragments. No. 1 is incorrect because this is an antilactogenic hormone, with no effect on uterine activity. No. 3 is incorrect because stilbestrol (Diethylstilbestrol), when given in the postpartum period, acts as an antilactogenic. No. 4 is incorrect because oxytocin is given to increase uterine tone, which would increase uterine effectiveness in passing the fragments or in helping keep the uterus firm after a D & C.

147. (2) The Brandt-Andrews maneuver involves gentle removal of the detached placenta while safely supporting the uterus. No. 1 is incorrect because the Ritgen maneuver refers to a method of assisting the delivery of the fetal head while controlling the speed of delivery and supporting the fetal head. No. 3 is incorrect because the Schultze mechanism refers to the fetal membrane side of the placenta that delivers first. Designating this mechanism in regard to delivery of the placenta is now considered archaic and insignificant. No. 4 is incorrect because this mechanism favors excessive manipulation of the intrauterine cavity and artificial detachment of the placenta, predisposing the woman to uterine atony, retained placental fragments, and puerperal infection. In some instances, it is an appropriate method to remove the placenta.

148. (4) The signs and symptoms are classic for placenta previa. Hence, Nos. 1, 2, and 3 are incorrect.

149. (3) Semi-Fowler's position allows the presenting part to apply pressure to the previa. No. 1 is incorrect because a vaginal (or rectal) examination is likely to increase the separation and cause massive hemorrhage. No. 2 is incorrect because this position does not allow the presenting part to apply direct pressure to the separating placenta. No. 4 is incorrect because some women with placenta previa can deliver vaginally.

150. (2) The hard fetal head pressing on the low-lying placenta can effectively stop bleeding and further separation and can permit her to delivery vaginally. Hence, Nos. 1, 3, and 4 are incorrect.

151. (1) This woman had a placenta previa. Nos. 2, 3, and 4 are incorrect because the problem was implantation of the placenta in the lower uterine segment.

152. (3) These signs and symptoms are classic for abruptio placentae. No. 1 is incorrect because placenta accreta refers to placenta in which the chorionic villi have grown into the myometrium. No. 2 is incorrect because the woman would not be able to feel a "hard" womb—the womb is not enlarged, and ectopic pregnancy generally ruptures during the first trimester. No. 4 is incorrect because the woman would not feel a "hard" womb; in addition, this condition should have been diagnosed and a delivery date and method determined by now!

153. (2) The side-lying position will prevent hypotension, will increase perfusion of the uterus, and will not cause a rapid change in her blood pressure. No. 1 is incorrect because the nurse's time would be better spent continuingnuing assessment of FHR, etc., checking her chart to see that all data needed for surgery (should that be required) have been collected. No. 3 is incorrect because it contradicts No. 2. No. 4 is incorrect because the physician must order this first. However, the nurse can have all equipment, etc., ready.

154. (3) Deep-tendon reflexes are not directly related to abruption. This assessment may be warranted if abruption was the result of maternal hypertension, however. Nos. 1 and 2 are incorrect because uterine activity and FHR are priority assessments. The majority of fetal deaths is attributed to anoxia due to abruption. No. 4 is incorrect because hypertension may be the underlying cause of the abruption, or hypotension may be indicative of maternal blood loss.

155. (2) Couvelaire uterus results from bleeding into the myometrium, especially when bleeding is concealed. No. 1 is incorrect because placenta accreta cannot separate—chorionic villi have grown into the myometrium and no cleavage line exists between the placenta and uterus. No. 3 is incorrect because *hypo-* rather than *hyper*fibrinogenemia occurs frequently. No. 4 is incorrect because uterine rupture is not associated with this condition.

156. (3) Immediate cesarean delivery is needed to try to save the fetus and also to stop the consumption of clotting factors in the blood that can lead to hypofibrinogenemia and DIC (disseminated intravascular coagulation). Nos. 1 and 4 are incorrect because vaginal delivery (unless the head is on the perineum at the time) is rarely indicated with moderate to severe abruption. No. 2 is incorrect because there is insufficient time for laboratory testing and treatment before delivery must be effected.

157. (4) Previous uterine surgery is not one of the predisposing factors for abruption. Nos. 1, 2, and 3 are incorrect because multiparity, tumultuous labor, and severe preeclampsia are associated with abruptio placentae. In addition, maternal age, diabetes, and an abnormally short cord are all factors.

158. (1) Bleeding occurs in gushes when the uterus contracts spasmodically but not firmly. Uterus is somewhat boggy; clots must be expressed by massaging fundus with right hand while left hand supports the uterus with pressure superior to the symphysis pubis. No. 2 is incorrect because traumatic bleeding occurs in trickles if flow is not impeded by clots and the uterus is firm, smooth, and free of clots. No. 3 is incorrect because uterus can feel firm, although lochia rubra may persist beyond the usual three days. No. 4 is incorrect because the bleeding from inverted uterus is excessive and life-threatening. This condition is diagnosed prior to leaving the delivery area.

159. (3) Atonic bleeding can be controlled with oxytocic stimulation. No. 1 is incorrect because it refers to inverted uterus. No. 2 is incorrect because the bleeding does not seem to be from lacerations. No. 4 is incorrect because this treatment is inappropriate for treating any but the most superficial tears, and then only if stitches cannot be taken to close them.

160. (2) Traumatic bleeding is characterized by a firm,

smooth uterus and a continuous trickle. Nos. 1, 3, and 4 are incorrect (see question 158 above).

161. (2) The tear or laceration must be located and treated before the bleeding will stop. Nos. 1, 3, and 4 are incorrect (see question 159 above).

162. (1) The correct way to evaluate whether postpartum hemorrhage has occurred is to relate the amount of blood lost to her body weight in kilograms. However, most clinicians arbitrarily regard a 500-ml blood loss as a postpartum hemorrhage. Nos. 2, 3, and 4 are incorrect because none constitutes a postpartum hemorrhage. The blood lost at delivery is added to that lost during the puerperium to evaluate blood loss.

163. (1) Retained placental fragments are not thought to predispose the woman to DIC. Nos. 2, 3, and 4 are incorrect because severe eclampsia, amnionitis, and amniotic-fluid embolism do predispose her to DIC. Other obstetric causes include placenta abruptio and dead fetus (missed abortion) retained longer than four weeks before delivery.

164. (1) Hemorrhage does not predispose the woman to eclampsia during the early puerperium. Nos. 2, 3, and 4 are incorrect because hemorrhage does predispose the woman to puerperal ("childbed") fever, anemia (and therefore tiredness and irritability during early parenthood), and embolism.

165. (1) Amniotic-fluid embolism is possible any time after rupture of membranes. It occurs if fluid is able to get behind a partially separated portion of the placenta. The fluid enters the maternal blood stream via the placental lakes. Hence, Nos. 2, 3, and 4 are incorrect.

166. (3) Blood pressure and deep-tendon reflexes are unrelated to amniotic-fluid embolism. Nos. 1, 2, and 4 are incorrect because sudden dyspnea, profound shock, and cyanosis and pulmonary edema are all symptoms/signs of embolism.

167. (2) The nonstress test identifies the fetus whose heart rate pattern undergoes late deceleration. No. 1 is incorrect because the L/S ratio is used to determine the lung maturity of the fetus. No. 3 is incorrect because sonography is used to assess placental location, fetal biparietal diameter, and the like. No. 4 is incorrect because the Coombs' test is used to determine the level of maternal anti-Rh-positive antibodies.

168. (1) Intrauterine infection of the membranes and fluid may occur from ascending contamination from the birth canal. The upper limits of safety are 48 hours. Neonatal pneumonia may follow. No. 2 is incorrect because there is no such thing as a "dry birth"; amniotic fluid is produced continuously and replaced entirely six times per day. No. 3 is incorrect because hypofibrinogenemia and disseminated intravascular disorder are not related to ruptured membranes. No. 4 is incor-

rect because Couvelaire uterus is a complication that can follow abruptio placentae.

169. (3) Significantly increased fetal activity and meconium-stained amniotic fluid are signs of fetal distress. Nos. 1 and 2 are incorrect because crowning is followed quickly by birth and should fetal distress occur now, the physician can deliver the baby quickly with forceps after an episiotomy. No. 4 is incorrect because of the two signs given, only one—meconium-stained fluid—is correct.

170. (4) The umbilical cord's length is normal for a term pregnancy and, unless compressed, presents no problems. No. 1 is incorrect because long, strong contractions can diminish the oxygen supply to the fetus. These tetanic contractions (over 90 seconds long and two minutes apart) can result from precipitous labor or vigorous Pitocin induction. No. 2 is incorrect because, in the supine position, the heavy uterus compresses the ascending vena cava, resulting in supine hypotension and fetal bradycardia. No. 3 is incorrect because blood flow to tissues is diminished in the presence of hypo- or hypertension.

171. (3) The greenish-black coloration comes from meconium released from the rectum during hypoxia. (Anal sphincter relaxes with hypoxia.) No. 1 is incorrect because amniotic fluid can normally appear opaque with white flecks (of vernix caseosa). No. 2 is incorrect because amniotic fluid can normally appear opaque with white flecks and some pink streaking (from "bloody show"). No. 4 is incorrect because this color is indicative of abruptio placentae.

172. (2) Side-lying, not supine, position increases uterine perfusion by moving the uterus off the ascending vena cava, thus relieving hypotension. No. 1 is incorrect because the side-lying position prevents supine hypotension. No. 3 is incorrect because administering oxygen does increase uterine perfusion. No. 4 is incorrect because decreasing uterine contractility does increase uterine perfusion.

173. (3) FHR pattern indicates early deceleration—a benign sign of head compression. No. 1 is incorrect because, although contractions that decrease in frequency, duration, and intensity can result in better perfusion of the fetus, a good FHR pattern is reassuring. No. 2 is incorrect because in this case maternal blood pressure was not relevant. No. 4 is incorrect because late deceleration pattern is a sign of fetal distress.

174. (1) Yellowish vernix results from the breakdown of hemoglobin and/or bile pigments in meconium. Both maternal anti-Rh antigen antibodies and ingestion of Gantrisin are implicated in breakdown of fetal RBCs. No. 2 is incorrect because gonorrheal infection renders the amniotic fluid opaque, thick, and odorous, without discoloring the vernix. No. 3 is incorrect because diabetes mellitus does not affect the color of vernix. No. 4 is incorrect because the postmature fetus does not have vernix.

175. (1) Heart rate, 2; respiratory effort, 1; muscle tone, 0; reflex response, 1; and color, 1. Total Apgar score is 5. Hence, Nos. 2, 3, and 4 are incorrect.

176. (1) Definitions of asphyxia vary from 30 to 60 seconds, depending on the author. Hence, Nos. 2, 3, and 4 are incorrect.

177. (3) These infants have a greater tendency to be deficient in surfactant (lecithin) necessary to maintain alveolar stability on exhalation. Hence, Nos. 1, 2, and 4 are incorrect.

178. (4) Flaring of nasal alae is a sign of respiratory distress. Nos. 1, 2, and 3 are incorrect because all are signs of respiratory distress.

179. (4) Adequate ventilation is the top priority, and one never administers oxygen unless the airway is clear first. Nos. 1, 2, and 3 are incorrect because the airway should be opened first.

180. (2) Acrocyanosis in room air is a common finding, especially when the neonate is chilly. Deepening acrocyanosis when the neonate is warm is a sign of respiratory or cardiac disorder. Nos. 1, 3, and 4 are incorrect because all are signs and symptoms of RDS.

181. (2) Injudicious suctioning can cause pulse irregularities and laryngospasm. It may also decrease the amount of oxygen available to the neonate and cause tissue trauma, resulting in bleeding and/or edema. Hence, Nos. 1, 3, and 4 are incorrect.

182. (2) Preterm neonates are more prone than more mature neonates to RDS due to the former's insufficient amount of surfactant. No. 1 is incorrect because RDS is suspected first when respiratory distress is noted in the preterm neonate. No. 3 is incorrect because the neonate is only 24 hours old and oxygen toxicity takes time to develop. No. 4 is incorrect because bronchopulmonary dysplasia is a complication of oxygen therapy that takes a period of time to develop.

183. (1) Respiratory distress in the term infant would be due most likely to aspiration rather than to RDS because the term infant has sufficient surfactant to support ventilation. No. 2 is incorrect because RDS is most closely related to prematurity and insufficient surfactant, that is, an L/S ratio of 2:1 or more. (L refers to lecithin—or surfactant.) Nos. 3 and 4 are incorrect because, even if the neonate were receiving oxygen therapy, 24 hours is insufficient time for oxygen toxicity and bronchopulmonary dysplasia to develop.

184. (1) Aspiration syndrome occurs commonly among postterm neonates, especially if they are postmature. Hypoxia accompanies the progressing placental insuf-

ficiency with advancing gestational age. Physiologic response to hypoxia is relaxation of the anal sphincter, release of meconium into the amniotic fluid, and a gasp reflex. The result is aspiration of amniotic fluid and its particulate matter. No. 2 is incorrect because RDS is closely related to prematurity and insufficient amounts of surfactant (lecithin) in the fetal lung to sustain extrauterine ventilation. Nos. 3 and 4 are incorrect because, even if the neonate were receiving oxygen therapy, 24 hours is not enough time for oxygen toxicity or bronchopulmonary dysplasia to develop.

185. (1) Six lb 1 oz is too large for a normal preterm neonate (pliable ear cartilage, top half of sole covered with creases, no breast tissue, and positive scarf sign). No. 2 is incorrect because the term neonate's ear cartilage is firm, sole creases cover foot, breast nodules are present, and elbow does not cross the midline. Nos. 3 and 4 are incorrect because findings are consistent with prematurity.

186. (2) The preterm infant is prone to temperature instability. Cold stress compromises any neonate, but especially the preterm. No. 1 is incorrect because feeding is ordered after the neonate is assessed. No. 3 is incorrect because signs indicate prematurity, and special precautions for maintaining temperature are taken until the neonate is assessed. No. 4 is incorrect because maintaining the neonate's temperature takes priority over any of the other options given here.

187. (4) Phototherapy, to remove excess breakdown products of bilirubin from the neonate's blood, is not a cause of anemia. No. 1 is incorrect because rough handling of the preterm neonate can lead to rupture of the friable surface or of deeper capillaries. No. 2 is incorrect because it is vital to monitor the amount of blood removed so that it can be replaced to prevent anemia. No. 3 is incorrect because detection of early signs of hyperbilirubinemia opens the way to prevent continued breakdown of RBCs or to perform an exchange transfusion to correct anemia.

188. (1) The neonate's feeding should *not* be accomplished quickly so as to prevent abdominal distention and regurgitation, with possible respiratory distress and aspiration. No. 2 is incorrect because preterm neonates do have weak gag and cough reflexes, which predispose them to regurgitation and aspiration. No. 3 is incorrect because preterm neonates need all of their energy for metabolism and growth. No. 4 is incorrect because preterm neonates' suck and swallow reflexes are weak and uncoordinated, so they are in danger of aspiration and use of excessive energy.

189. (4) Female's age, spacing of pregnancies (repeated pregnancies less than two years apart), and number of pregnancies (four or more) are all related to premature labor. These factors are closely related to nutrition and the maternal stores available. Nos. 1, 2, and 3 are incorrect because the male's age, obesity, smoking, and frequency of intercourse during pregnancy are not associated with premature labor.

190. (3) Hypertension decreases perfusion to tissues. No. 1 is incorrect because, if nutrition were adequate, her stores of nutrients would have been replenished or would not have depleted excessively, based on the age of her first child and the fact that this is just her second pregnancy. No. 2 is incorrect because a single fetus is not competing with others in the womb. No. 4 is incorrect because, in most cases, obese women have larger babies than do smaller women.

191. (2) The postmature neonate has had to utilize its glycogen stores to meet metabolic and growth needs that could no longer be met by the progressively insufficient placenta. Nos. 1, 3, and 4 are incorrect because these weights are appropriate for gestational age and in themselves do not predispose the neonate to hypoglycemia in the early neonatal period.

192. (3) The small-for-gestational-age infant is not dehydrated. No. 1 is incorrect because early feeding does decrease the risk of hypoglycemia. No. 2 is incorrect because hypoglycemia is evidenced by respiratory distress. No. 4 is incorrect because early feeding does facilitate early weight gain.

193. (2) Hyperbilirubinemia does not use up available glucose. Nos. 1, 3, and 4 are incorrect because all of these conditions use up available glucose.

194. (2) Weight is the definitive assessment tool for evaluating amount of fluid therapy necessary. Hence, Nos. 1, 3, and 4 are incorrect.

195. (3) Eclampsia is not a complication associated with postterm gestation. Nos. 1, 2, and 4 are incorrect because all of these are related to a postterm labor.

196. (1) The placenta does become progressively less efficient, and fetal problems (hypoxia, anoxia) do occur. Nos. 2, 3, and 4 are incorrect because they do not relate to postterm labor. The placenta does not separate prematurely just because of postterm age; the mother may be tired but this does not cause a hazard to her; the fetus grows in length, and this may cause fetus-pelvic disproportion, but it may decrease in weight (needs to burn own stores to meet metabolic needs because of placental insufficiency).

197. (2) The 34- to 36-week fetus looks and acts just about like a full-term baby and has a good chance for survival. Hence, Nos. 1, 3, and 4 are incorrect.

198. (4) Heat from the lamp may increase the neonate's temperature. Nos. 1, 2, and 3 are incorrect because these nursing actions are part of accurate monitoring of the neonate's temperature.

199. (2) This describes a normal transitional stool. Nos. 1, 3, and 4 are all neurological signs consistent with kernicterus.

200. (4) There is *no* treatment that can inactivate maternal antibodies. Nos. 1, 2, and 3 are incorrect because exchange transfusion does help combat anemia, remove and dilute maternal antibodies, and decrease serum bilirubin levels.

201. (2) Rho (D) immune globulin destroys Rh-positive RBCs, therefore the recipient must be Rh-negative. The mother must be in the position to receive an inoculation of Rh-positive RBCs, so the fetus must be Rh-positive. Rho (D) immune globulin does not deactivate antibodies already formed against the Rh antigen, so the mother must be Coombs' negative. Given to the mother, it destroys fetal Rh-positive RBCs before the mother can form antibodies against them. No. 1 is incorrect because the mother is not exposed to Rh-positive RBCs if the neonate is Rh-negative. Nos. 3 and 4 are incorrect because the mother is Rh-positive, and Rho (D) immune globulin, if given to her, would destroy her own Rh-positive RBCs.

202. (1) PKU is inherited as a recessive trait. The neonate's inability to metabolize phenylalanine necessitates feeding with Lofenalac, a special protein preparation that does not contain the amino acid. Hence, Nos. 2, 3, and 4 are incorrect.

203. (3) Retrolental fibroplasia is a disease of immaturity and high arterial oxygen levels. No. 1 is incorrect because ambient oxygen does not reflect arterial oxygen concentration. No. 2 is incorrect because the effect of fluorescent light on the neonate's eyes is unknown as yet, but there is no indication that it is in any way related to retrolental fibroplasia. No. 4 is incorrect because serum bilirubin levels do not provide data regarding oxygen levels.

204. (4) The mother needs assistance to express her feelings now. Nos. 1, 2, and 3 are incorrect because they either ignore her feelings or are defensive.

205. (3) The nurse needs more data on which to make an assessment prior to intervening. Dextrostix is a test for blood sugar. If this term infant's blood sugar is 35 mg/dl or less, the infant is fed with glucose water, the data recorded, and the physician notified. (This procedure will vary with the protocol of the institution.) No. 1 is incorrect because persistent, spontaneous jerky movements of the extremities are generally not within normal limits. No. 2 is incorrect because the nurse would be intervening before assessing all the necessary data. No. 4 is incorrect because it is not the priority action, although the nurse would do this following the assessment and primary intervention.

206. (2) The infant with one umbilical artery requires a comprehensive physical examination. The prenatal history must be reviewed. The presence of oligoamnios as well is suspicious of renal anomalies. Nos. 1, 3, and 4 are incorrect because these conditions are not associated with the occurrence of one umbilical artery.

207. (1) Conjunctival hemorrhage and/or telangiectases over the bridge of the nose and at the nape of the neck are normal occurrences following vaginal delivery. Nos. 2, 3, and 4 are all signs of congenital syphilis. Wear gloves when handling this infant for about 12 hours after antibiotic therapy is started.

208. (3) Congenital anomalies have not been attributed to gonorrhea. Nos. 1, 2, and 4 are incorrect because premature rupture of membranes, chorioamnionitis, neonatal temperature instability, neonatal hypotonia, and poor feeding are all sequelae of maternal gonorrhea infection.

209. (2) The causes of maternal mortality, in order of occurrence, are hemorrhage, infection, preeclampsia/eclampsia. Hence, Nos. 1, 3, and 4 are incorrect.

210. (2) The "safest" pregnancy is the second one. This may be due to the fact that maternal problems (small pelvis, medical problems, etc.) were identified during the first pregnancy, while the woman's nutritional stores are probably not depleted yet. No. 1 is incorrect because the woman has not proven herself yet during childbearing. No. 3 is incorrect because the care of the other children and repeated demands on her nutritional stores may put added stress on this pregnancy. No. 4 is incorrect because it contradicts No. 2.

211. (2) It takes two generations to eradicate the effects of poor nutrition in a female's childhood. If she has good nutrition during this pregnancy (first generation), and if her baby is female and has good nutrition during her pregnancy (second generation), then *her* children (third generation) will reap the benefits of good nutrition. Hence, Nos. 1, 3, and 4 are incorrect.

212. (4) Although many people take solace from their religion, there are predictable responses to loss. Nos. 1, 2, and 3 are incorrect because the birth of a child with a defect does result in feelings of lost self-esteem (the child is seen as an extension of the self and the child is defective), concern about social status (society expects the couple to produce children who will contribute to, rather than drain, its resources), and inadequacy (what did I produce; what kind of parent can I be to this child, etc.).

213. (2) This mother needs to talk, to review events, and to put them into perspective. Nos. 1 and 3 are incorrect because they do not acknowledge her right to feel the way she does. No. 4 is incorrect because it serves only to reassure the nurse.

214. (4) If the premature infant did not suffer severe RDS or the like, its rate of development will be slower in the early months. No. 1 is incorrect because the nurse is refusing to take any responsibility for assisting this woman with her concerns. Nos. 2 and 3 are incorrect because they are not supported by the data given.

215. (2) The primary criterion identifying the premature infant is gestational age. The infant may weigh more than 2500 g (5 lb 8 oz) but must be 37 weeks' gestation or less. Nos. 1, 3, and 4 are incorrect because these statements are all true regarding premature characteristics.

216. (3) *Candida albicans* is the causative agent of thrush and moniliasis. Hence, Nos. 1, 2, and 4 are incorrect.

217. (1) Class III results refer to the presence of suspicious cells. Cytology results are confirmed by biopsy and D & C. Hence, Nos. 2, 3, and 4 are incorrect.

218. (2) The nurse should minimize, not maximize, time spent with the woman. Nos. 1, 3, and 4 are all incorrect because the nurse would do all of these when performing nursing care for a woman with a cobalt implant.

219. (2) Sperm are stored in the epididymis until they are mature and capable of motility. Nos. 1, 3, and 4 are incorrect because all of these are functions of the seminal vesicles.

220. (2) Testosterone production continues in the Leydig cells. Nos. 1, 3, and 4 are incorrect because all of these statements are true about vasectomy.

221. (1) There is no "usual" age for the appearance of the male climacteric. Hence, Nos. 2, 3, and 4 are incorrect.

222. (1) The vas deferens is the transport duct for the sperm, as the fallopian tube is the transport duct for the egg. Hence, Nos. 2, 3, and 4 are incorrect.

223. (3) Phimosis, stricture of the prepuce, is not related to infertility. Nos. 1, 2, and 4 are incorrect because all of these conditions may lead to infertility.

224. (4) The bioassay for HCG is the test for pregnancy, not for infertility-sterility. Nos. 1, 2, and 3 are incorrect because they are all tests for infertility-sterility.

225. (1) A normal menstrual cycle (26 to 28 days) is usually not implicated in infertility. Nos. 2, 3, and 4 are incorrect because these factors may be implicated in infertility.

226. (2) The cervical smear for cytology (Pap smear) is a screening test for cervical cellular dysplasia. Nos. 1, 3, and 4 are incorrect because a work-up for suspected sterility does include all of these assessments.

227. (4) Engaging in intercourse this frequently does not allow the man to store up sperm, a necessity for the man with a low sperm count. A period of abstinence prior to the expected day of ovulation is recommended for men who have a low sperm count. No. 1 is incorrect because this activity helps in determining the date of ovulation. No. 2 is incorrect because this technique helps to decrease the number of antibodies that the woman develops to the male's sperm. No. 3 is incorrect because oral-contraceptive therapy has been used successfully to "readjust" the woman's menstrual cycle so that she is able to conceive after she completes the course of treatment.

228. (2) In March 1979, an Ethics Advisory Board recommended that in vitro fertilization and embryo transplantation be ethically acceptable. Hence, Nos. 1, 3, and 4 are incorrect.

229. (3) After mass screening, if a suspicious pap smear is found, the health care provider may view the cervix under magnification. This procedure is known as culposcopy. Hence, Nos. 1, 2, and 4 are incorrect.

230. (1) Culdoscopy is used for inspection of the pelvic structures through an incision in the posterior cul-de-sac. Hence, Nos. 2, 3, and 4 are incorrect.

231. (2) Laparoscopy refers to the transperitoneal endoscopic technique that allows for excellent visualization of the internal pelvic structures and for limited surgery. Hence, Nos. 1, 3, and 4 are incorrect.

232. (4) Culdocentesis refers to the technique of passing a needle into the cul-de-sac of Douglas through the posterior vaginal fornix. Hence, Nos. 1, 2, and 3 are incorrect.

ANNOTATED BIBLIOGRAPHY

Jensen, M., Benson, R., and Bobak, I. Maternity care: the nurse and the family (2 ed.). 1981: St. Louis, The C. V. Mosby Company. A comprehensive nursing text. Psychosocial and biophysical content is presented in depth providing the basis for nursing management. Nursing care plans are organized for ease of application. Content is easily retrieved and well indexed. Unique features—chapters on nutrition, genetics and genetics counseling, fathers, grief and grieving incorporated throughout, identification and management of the high-risk neonate, legal aspects, and human sexuality and sexual expression.

Jensen, M. D., and Bobak, I. M. Handbook of maternity care: a guide for nursing practice. 1980: St. Louis, The C. V. Mosby Company. A handbook to assist the nurse clinician or nurse practitioner in the clinic, hospital, or home setting. It provides guidelines for nursing actions: diagnostic, therapeutic, and educational. Written to expand basic knowledge.

Clark, A. L., and Affonso, D. Childbearing: a nursing perspective. 1976: Philadelphia, F. A. Davis Company. A comprehensive obstetric nursing textbook. Several notable physicians and nurses contributed to the content of this book, adding considerable depth and breadth to the physical and behavioral bases of nursing on most topics pertinent to the subject.

Olds, S. B., et al. Obstetric nursing. 1980: Menlo Park, Addison-Wesley Publishing Company. Clearly presented obstetric textbook for the beginning practitioner. Several contributors were involved in writing this text thereby presenting a wide scope of experience in applying relevant nursing knowledge to the care of the childbearing family.

Reeder, S. R., et al. Maternity nursing, ed. 14. 1980: Philadelphia, J. B. Lippincott Company. This edition has been updated to include recent advances in fetology and neonatology, alternative lifestyle family living, family planning, and abortion. It retains features such as posttests and numerous illustrations.

Ziegel, E. E. and Cranley, M. S. Obstetric nursing, ed. 7. 1978: New York, Macmillan Publishing Company. Well organized, comprehensive nursing text for obstetrics. Readable, easily understood, well illustrated.

GLOSSARY

acini cells   milk-producing cells in the breast

acrocyanosis   cyanosis of hands and feet, common in the neonate up to 7–10 days

adnexa   accessory organs of the uterus (tubes, ovaries)

asphyxia   hypoxemia (lowering of Po_2) and hypercapnia (increase in Pco_2)

attitude   in utero, the relationship of fetal parts to each other (flexed, extended)

ballottement   probable sign of pregnancy; the examiner feels the fetus "bounce" in response to pressure on the cervix

breast milk jaundice   yellowing of skin resulting from interference with conjugation of bilirubin caused by pregnanediol in mother's milk

bregma   anterior fontanel; junction of sagittal and coronal sutures

brown fat   exceptional source of energy found only in neonates

bruit, uterine   sound of movement of blood through uterine vessels, synchronous with maternal pulse (see souffle, uterine)

caul   unruptured fetal membranes covering fetal head during delivery

climacteric   "change of life"; period of time during which gonads respond less and less to gonadotropic hormones and many physiologic and psychologic changes occur

consanguinity   blood relationship between people

diastasis recti abdominis midline separation of abdominal muscles

dysmaturity intrauterine growth retardation

dystocia difficult labor and delivery

effleurage light fingertip massage of the abdomen

erythema toxicum "newborn rash" of unknown etiology that resolves spontaneously

ferning under estrogen influence, cervical mucus dries in a fernlike pattern

funis cord, umbilical

gravidity number of time the uterus of a woman has been pregnant

hydramnios polyhydramnios; amount of amniotic fluid in excess of 2,000 ml

iatrogenic a disorder or condition caused by treatment (e.g., retrolental fibroplasia resulting from high arterial levels of oxygen)

inertia lack of activity

intrathecal within the subarachnoid space

isoimmunization autoimmunization or sensitization, such as an Rh-negative woman developing antibodies to Rh-positive, or a man developing immunity to his own sperm

karyotype systematic arrangement of photographed chromosomes to assess numbers and morphology

Kegal exercises exercises of perineal muscles around the anus, vagina, urinary meatus

let-down reflex oxytocin-induced release of milk from alveoli of the breasts into the milk ducts

lie maternal and fetal spines are parallel (longitudinal: vertex or breech), or fetal spine is perpendicular to maternal spine (transverse lie: shoulder)

macrosomatia, macrosomia large body size

parity the number of pregnancies that have been carried to viability (24–28 weeks)

position relationship between an anatomic landmark of the presenting part of the fetus (occiput, sacrum, shoulder) to the front, back, and sides of the maternal pelvis

presentation the part of the fetus that enters the pelvis first (head, breech)

pseudocyesis false pregnancy

restitution external rotation of the newly born head to the right or left

souffle, funic sound of the rush of blood through umbilical cord; rate is synchronous with FHR

subinvolution failure of the uterus to return to prepregnant state during puerperium

surfactant lecithin; present in alveoli in mature neonates and serves to keep alveoli open on expiration

toco, toko pertaining to childbirth or labor

TORCH pertaining to the following infections: toxoplasmosis, other (syphilis), rubella, cytomegalovirus, herpes simplex

version act of "turning" a fetus from one lie to another to facilitate delivery (usually no longer done because cesarean delivery is safer)

viable "capable of living," e.g., a fetus of 28 weeks' gestation or more

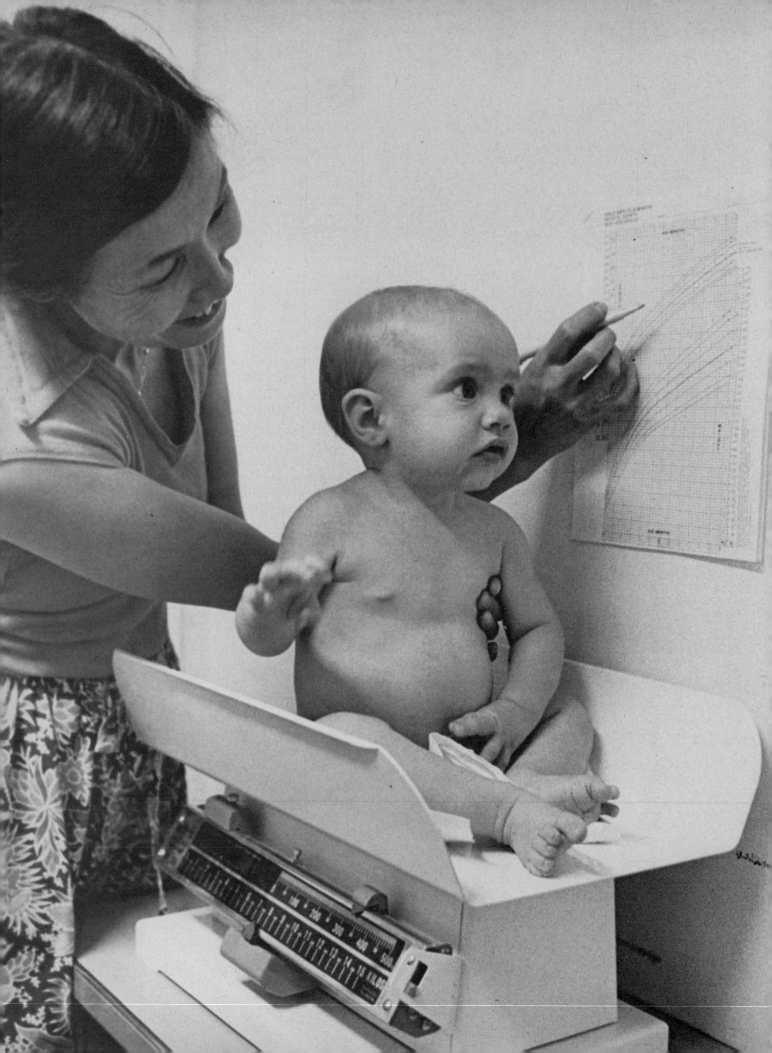

Unit 4 / NURSING CARE OF CHILDREN AND FAMILIES

Introduction

This unit presents a review of basic pediatric concepts and entities with which the nurse should be familiar. Each section contains a discussion of growth and development followed by an outline of the most common conditions encountered by children in a specific age group.

Presented in outline form, the material includes information on assessment and nursing management, following the nursing process, which will form the basis of the nursing licensure examination. When nurses are not specifically mentioned, their involvement is assumed because they are the people to whom this book is addressed.

The unit's scope has been extended to include more preventive health concepts and well-child topics that the nurse must know to counsel family, parents, and children effectively. Among the disease entities that have been added or expanded in the second edition are congenital heart disease, Down's syndrome, osteomyelitis, oncology, scoliosis, and herpes simplex. The special concerns for each age group have been expanded to encompass issues of sex education and psychosocial behavior problems. Additional information is also offered in tables on Piaget's theories of cognitive development, major developmental milestones, and management of pediatric emergencies.

A new part of this unit addresses the special issues of administering medications to pediatric patients, and of death and dying.

For more detailed coverage of any subject, please refer to the annotated bibliography at the end of the unit. There you will also find questions to test application of your knowledge and ability to reason, followed by detailed answer/rationales.

Sandra Forrest Fritz

Part A | INFANCY AND TODDLERS— BIRTH TO 2 YEARS

NORMAL GROWTH AND DEVELOPMENT

In caring for children, the nurse must be familiar with theories of normal growth and development. To provide a basis for this chapter, two of the most prevalent theories utilized in pediatrics today are presented (Tables 4–1, 4–2, and 4–3; *see also* Table 1–2).

1. Birth to 6 months

A. Assessment of physical development (birth to 6 months):
1. Height—gains approximately 2.5 cm (1 inch) per month.
2. Weight—gains 150 to 210 g (5 to 7 oz) per week.
3. Posterior fontanel closes at 2 months.
4. Begins to drool saliva at 4 months.

B. Assessment of behavior patterns (birth to 6 months):
1. Motor development (see Table 4–4)—
   a. Age 2 months—visually follows objects horizontally and vertically.
   b. Age 3 months—discovers hands and reaches for objects.
   c. Age 4 months—recognizes familiar objects and increases body movements at their sight.
   d. Age 5 to 6 months—turns over completely; bangs with object held in hand.
2. Socialization and vocalization—
   a. Newborn—cries when hungry or uncomfortable.
   b. Age 2 months—crying becomes differentiated; smiles in response to another's smile.
   c. Age 3 months—babbles and coos.
   d. Age 4 months—laughs aloud; recognizes maternal figure and shows interest in other members of family.
   e. Age 5 to 6 months—vocalizes displeasure

TABLE 4–1. *Erikson's stages of personality development**

Stage	Approximate age (years)	Central problem	Influencing persons
Infancy	0–1	Trust versus mistrust†	Maternal figure
Toddler	2–3	Autonomy versus shame, doubt	Parental figures, with focus on independence
Preschool	4–5	Initiative versus guilt	Basic family unit, with focus on establishment of values
School	6–12	Industry versus inferiority	School and neighborhood figures
Puberty and early adolescence	12–18	Identity versus role-diffusion	Peers, leadership and sexual models
Late adolescence Young adult	18–30	Intimacy, solidarity versus isolation	Chosen partners of same and opposite sex; work relationships
Middle-age adult	30–60	Generativity versus self-absorption, stagnation	Shared household, with focus on mate and children
Elderly adult	60–end of life	Ego integrity versus despair	"Mankind," with focus on acceptance of physical change and living arrangements

*Reprinted from *Childhood and society,* 2nd Edition, by Erik H. Erikson. By permission of W. W. Norton & Company, Inc. Copyright 1950. © 1963 by W. W. Norton & Company, Inc.

†The central problem of each stage must be successfully solved to provide a basis for the solution of the next problem. It should be noted that each problem is not completely solved for each stage but that habits of both continuums remain with most people throughout life.

TABLE 4–2. *Piaget's theories of cognitive development**

Stage/substage	Approximate age	Characteristics
SENSORIMOTOR	0–2 years	
Reflexes	Birth–1 month	Reliance upon reflexes to interact with environment; e.g., sucking, shivering, sneezing.
Primary circular reactions or habits	1–4 months	Anticipatory behavior such as sucking when placed in nursing position. Purposeful behavior such as hand to mouth. Imitative behavior—laugh or vocalize in response to others.
Secondary circular reactions	4–10 months	Behavior and interest extend to external environment. Discovery of cause and effect, although initially this is by accident; e.g., kicking in crib causes mobile to move.
Coordination of secondary schemes	10–12 months	Behavior is systematic and goal-directed. Concept of object permanence is shown by actively searching for an object, such as moving a pillow to find toy *beneath* the pillow. Imitate and initiate activities that symbolize an event; wave "bye-bye" when someone leaves.
Tertiary circular reactions	12–18 months	Experiment with new ways of attaining a goal. Walk and actively explore environment, show signs of using memory; e.g., retrieve toy from toy box.
Beginning of thought	18 months–2 years	Transition to symbolic thought. Do not need to see object to know what it is; e.g., follow directions to get doll from another room. Use language to refer to absent objects. Imitate behaviors that have occurred in the past, suggesting internalization of these behaviors.
PREOPERA-TIONAL	3–7 years	
Preconceptual thought	3–4 years	Increased use of language for symbolization, unable to put self in another's place; i.e., imagine how someone else feels. Do not understand relationships of size, weight, volume; e.g., believe nickel is more than a dime because it is bigger.
Intuitive thinking	5–7 years	Magical thinking—trees have feelings, sun goes to bed.
CONCRETE OPERATIONS	8–12 years	Reasoning is inductive and children can classify and organize facts to solve concrete problems. Cannot deal with abstract situations. Are able to understand reversibility of states, e.g., if shown two clay balls of equal size, when one is flattened they will know that volume is the same although shape has changed.

(Continued)

TABLE 4–2. (Continued)

Stage/substage	Approximate age	Characteristics
FORMAL OPERATIONS	13–16 years	Thought is qualitative. Capable of introspection and able to solve complicated problems based upon theories, regardless of experience. Able to formulate and test hypotheses.

*Development is progressive through each stage.

TABLE 4–3. Developmental milestones in children and suggested activities

Approximate age	Major developmental milestones	Suggested activities
INFANTS		
1–6 months	Smile in response to other persons, discover hands, begin vocalization.	Most often posture is supine or prone in horizontal plane; do need to develop measures to enhance developing senses: music, use of voice, mobiles, touching.
6–12 months	Sit alone, creep or crawl, cruise around furniture.	Peek-a-boo, pat-a-cake, container or nesting toys, fabric books; allow to hold spoon during feedings.
12–18 months	Walk, throw objects, feed selves.	Pull and push toys; read to child, name objects, encourage vocabulary development.
TODDLERS		
18 months–2 years	Jump, climb up and down, fear separation from family; becoming toilet trained; say "no" and "mine" constantly.	Provide security toy/object, wagons/buggy, small toys for manipulation, consistency in setting limits; use suggestion rather than choice, diversion rather than force.
PRESCHOOLERS		
3–5 years	Dress selves, know name, identify colors, curious.	Puzzles, crayons and paper; ride on toys (tricycle); trips outside home (zoo, store); contact with other children.
SCHOOL-AGE		
6–8 years	Lose teeth, tell time; fine hand movements.	Table games, kits, erector sets, tinkertoys, bicycle.
9–11 years	Eye-hand coordination well developed; enjoy secrets, privacy important; begin secondary sex characteristics.	Books, musical instruments, handicrafts; give factual information to any queries.
ADOLESCENTS		
12–18 years	Peer group of major importance; completing sexual development; independent actions.	Games involving abstract thought: chess, dungeons and dragons; classic literature, sports involvement; discussions involving goals, aspirations, attitudes; allow choices in action/care.

TABLE 4–4. *Reflexes of the newborn*

Reflex	Description	Present and/or disappears
Babinski	Extension of great toe on stroking sole of foot.	Disappears at 12 to 18 months.
Blinking	Aroused by bright light; protective reflex.	Present at birth.
Coughing and sneezing	Clear respiratory tract, rid respiratory system of amniotic fluid, and protect newborn from inhaling foreign substances.	Present at birth.
Crying	Protective or defensive; to indicate a need.	Present at birth.
Dancing	When held in upright position with feet touching a solid surface, infant responds with prancing movements.	Present at birth, but disappears very soon.
Gagging and vomiting	Provide for rejection of irritating or toxic substances from GI tract; gag reflex activated when infant has more in mouth than can successfully be swallowed.	Present throughout life.
Moro or "startle"	Response to sudden loud noise or jarring, causing body to stiffen; legs will draw up with soles of feet turned toward each other, and arms will go up and out, then forward in embracing position; movements are symmetrical.	May be *absent first 24 hours* after birth, appear second day, be *strongest* during first *8 weeks* of life, and disappear about *5 months* of age.
Neck-righting	When head is turned to one side, the shoulder and trunk will turn to that side, followed by the pelvis.	Disappears at 9 to 12 months.
Palmar grasp	Pressure on palm of hand will elicit grasp.	Reflex at birth, later develops into purposeful grasping; reflex disappears at 6 to 7 months.
Parachute	Infant in horizontal position who is suddenly thrust downward will extend hands forward as if protecting self from falling.	Appears at 7 to 9 months, persists indefinitely; absent in blind infants.
Plantar grasp	Pressure on sole of foot behind toes will cause flexion of toes.	Disappears at 9 to 12 months.
Pupillary	Ipsilateral constriction to light.	Present at birth.
Rooting	When corner of mouth is touched and object is moved toward cheek, infant will turn head toward object and open mouth; way of reaching for food.	Disappears at 4 months.
Shivering	Protective reflex when cold.	Present at birth.
Sucking	Sucking movements when anything touches lips; necessary for feeding.	Present *before* birth.
Swallowing	Follows sucking; necessary for ingestion of food subtances.	Present before birth.

(Continued)

TABLE 4-4.   (Continued)

Reflex	Description	Present and/or disappears
Tonic neck reflex—"fencing position"	*Postural* reflex of infant lying on back; turns head to one side and extends arm and leg on that side; arm and leg on opposite side are flexed.	Present until 18 to 20 weeks of age; disappears at 5 to 6 months.
Yawn	Draws in added supply of oxygen when rate of respiratory exchange is insufficient to meet needs; protective reflex.	Present at birth.

when objects are taken away; vocalizes syllables.

C. Nursing goals and implementation (birth to six months):

1. Goals: provide appropriate play activities based on developmental level—child develops cephalocaudally (from head progressing downward and from trunk outward to extremities); each sensory mode must be stimulated to develop perception of that sense organ; deprivation of any sensory mode obstructs development of that modality, partially or completely.

   a. Age 1 to 3 months—
      (1) Smile, talk, and sing to infant for visual and hearing senses.
      (2) Provide tactile stimulation—hold, pat, caress, cuddle, and touch infant.
      (3) Crinkle different kinds of paper, tissue, newsprint, and cellophane near infant's ear for differentiation of hearing sense.
      (4) Use mobiles, wind chimes, and bright dangling objects for visual, hearing, and attention modalities.
      (5) Utilize cradle gym and infant seat for posture changes.

   b. Age 4 to 6 months—
      (1) Use mirror play for increased visual awareness.
      (2) Supply soft squeeze toys in vivid colors with varying textures for visual and tactile stimulation.
      (3) Collect a box of textures—sandpaper, velvet, fur, silk, wood, screening, corrugated cardboard, cotton, and items with smooth, highly polished surfaces—to increase tactile awareness.
      (4) Give the infant a very small, soft balloon with a jingle bell in it to stimulate tactile and auditory senses.

2. Goals: provide guidance—
   a. Hold infant during feeding.
   b. Support head and back when lifting infant.
   c. Allow infant sufficient sleep for development, 16–20 hours per day.
   d. Hold toys in front of infant to encourage reaching.
   e. Be aware of safety concerns for teaching:
      (1) Place infant seat where it will not tip over.
      (2) Strap infant into high chair or infant seat.
      (3) Use toys without buttons, wires, or removable parts.
      (4) Bath—avoid scalding infant by checking water with elbow; keep one hand on baby under 4 months; do not leave 6-month-old infant alone in bath because of danger of drowning.
      (5) Do *not* leave infant alone where it could wriggle and roll off of surface, bed, counter, etc.
      (6) Keep filmy plastics, harnesses, zippered bags, and pillows away from infant to prevent smothering and suffocation.
      (7) Use a good car bed that can be strapped or securely fastened onto the car seat for safety.
      (8) Keep pins and other sharp objects out of reach.

2. *Age 6 to 12 months*
A. Assessment of physical development (6 to 12 months):
   1. Height—66 to 74 cm (26 to 29 inches).
   2. Weight—6 months: twice the birth weight; 12 months: three times the birth weight.
   3. Age 12 months—has six teeth (Table 4–5).

TABLE 4–5. *Dentition*

Primary teeth—20 in number

	Eruption		Shedding	
	Lower	Upper	Lower	Upper
	(age in months)		(age in years)	
Central incisors	6	7½	6	7½
Lateral incisors	7	9	7	8
Cuspids	16	18	9½	11½
First molars	12	14	10	10½
Second molars	20	24	11	10½

Permanent-teeth eruption—32 in number

	Lower	Upper
	(age in years)	(age in years)
Central incisors	6–7	7–8
Lateral incisors	7–8	8–9
Cuspids	9–10	11–12
First bicuspids	10–12	10–11
Second bicuspids	11–12	10–12
First molars	6–7	6–7
Second molars	11–13	12–13
Third molars	17–21	17–21

B. Assessment of behavior patterns (6 to 12 months):
  1. Motor development—
     a. Age 6 to 8 months—begins to show good coordination and sits alone.
     b. Age 7 to 9 months—plays with feet.
     c. Age 6 to 9 months—transfers toys from one hand to the other.
     d. Age 7 to 9 months—begins to crawl and creep.
     e. Age 10 to 12 months—pulls self to feet, walks with help and cruises.
  2. Socialization and vocalization—
     a. Age 6 to 8 months—shy, shows fear of strangers other than self and family members by crying when approached, hiding face.
     b. Age 7 to 9 months—cries when scolded.
     c. Age 10 to 12 months:
        (1) Claps hands on request.
        (2) Responds to own name.
        (3) Imitates.
        (4) Smiles at image in mirror.
        (5) Recognizes meaning of no.
        (6) Says three words other than Ma-Ma and Da-Da.
C. Nursing goals and implementation (6 to 12 months):
  1. Goals: provide appropriate play activities based on developmental level—the child is now acquiring the capacity to differentiate self from environment; there is active exploratory behavior plus a beginning perception of space and depth.
     a. Give large, round nesting toys to encourage space and size differentiation.
     b. Use squeeze toys in bath to stimulate curiosity in changes of objects.
     c. Play peek-a-boo, bye-bye, and pat-a-cake to reinforce concept of reappearance after separation.
     d. Give toys to stimulate curiosity (milk carton, fabric book, and containers to fill and spill).
     e. Blow bubbles for infant and encourage infant to catch them to stimulate hand-eye coordination.
     f. Play whistles and horns of different sounds for auditory differentiation.
     g. Play table-slapping game to encourage imitation.
     h. Place several cereal bowls on the table with a different consistency in each one, such as sand, flour, cornflakes, water, cotton balls, sugar, wet coffee grounds, marbles, and beans; help the infant dig into each bowl with both hands to feel and learn the differences of each material. Aids in tactile stimulation and differentiation.
  2. Goal: provide guidance—
     a. Allow infant to play with an extra spoon during feeding to prepare for self-feeding.
     b. Begin to set limits on areas infant can play in and on expected behavior; for example, "no-no" for forbidden behavior.
     c. Reward positive or desired behavior by smiling, gentle pats, verbal reinforcement.
     d. Alleviate teething pain, which often causes irritability.
        (1) Aids for teething pain—topical ointments, although they may be short-acting and cause sensitivity reactions.
        (2) Teething rings.
        (3) Aspirin.
     e. Be aware of safety concerns:
        (1) Fence stairways.

(2) Pick up loose objects from floor, including buttons, peanuts.

(3) Keep hot liquids, hot foods, and electrical cords on small appliances out of reach.

(4) Keep tablecloth from hanging within infant's reach.

(5) Keep medicines and poisons in a locked cabinet.

(6) Place guards in front of open heaters and around registers and floor furnaces.

(7) Use safety plugs for wall sockets.

(8) Keep scissors, knives, and breakable objects out of reach of infant.

(9) Keep easily overturned floor lamps and sharp-edged furniture away.

3. Age 12 to 18 months

A. Assessment of physical development (12 to 18 months):

1. Height—76 to 81 cm (30 to 32 inches).
2. Weight—9.5 to 11 kg (21 to 24 lb).
3. Anterior fontanel closed.
4. Abdomen protrudes.

B. Assessment of behavior patterns (12 to 18 months):

1. Motor development—
   a. Age 12 to 14 months—starts to walk.
   b. Age 14 to 18 months—throws a ball.
   c. Age 15 to 18 months:
      (1) Pulls a toy while walking.
      (2) Climbs up stairs and onto furniture.
      (3) Builds a tower with up to three blocks.
   d. Age 16 to 18 months:
      (1) Walks and runs with a stiff gait and wide stance.
      (2) Stoops to pick up toys.
   e. Age 18 months:
      (1) Seats self in child's chair by backing into it.
      (2) Holds cup with two hands.
      (3) Scribbles; differentiates between circular and straight lines.

2. Socialization and vocalization—
   a. Age 12 to 14 months:
      (1) Develops new awareness of strangers.
      (2) Wants to explore everything in reach.
      (3) Imitates simple things.
      (4) Hugs a favorite doll or stuffed toy.
   b. Age 16 to 18 months:
      (1) Finds security in some object.
      (2) Knows ten words.

c. Age 18 months:
   (1) Uses phrases.
   (2) May begin to have temper tantrums.
   (3) Enjoys solitary play or watching others.
   (4) May control bowel movements.

C. Nursing goals and implementation (12 to 18 months):

1. Goal: provide appropriate play activities based on developmental level—this is a period of increased locomotion as well as one of improving eye-hand coordination. Small-muscle coordination is steadily becoming differentiated. Verbal communication with the child encourages language development and a meaningful vocabulary. Security from favorite object begins.
   a. Give pull toys and push toys.
   b. Bring teddy bears, dolls, pots and pans, telephone, and fabric picture books.
   c. Collect bells of different tones and have child shake them.
   d. Give child a pan of warm soapy water in which to splash hands and feet.
   e. When you pick up the child, say "up" and when you put the child down, say "down."
   f. Hold the child around the trunk in front of a mirror and tilt forward, backward, and sideways, telling child the direction of each tilt.
   g. Put the child in a box and tilt it gently in all directions.
   h. Age 18 months—collect empty spice bottles to introduce smells to the child by putting various odors on a cotton ball and putting one in each jar.

2. Goal: provide guidance.
   a. Begin teaching infant to brush teeth and wash hands.
   b. Read nursery rhymes.
   c. Assess readiness factors in toilet-training (18 months):
      (1) Nervous system growth makes standing possible and child demonstrates need to defecate.
      (2) Child makes grunting sounds or strains.
      (3) Tugs at diaper.
      (4) Tells parents of bowel movement or brings diaper to them.
      (5) Bowel movements come at regular times.
      (6) Child knows what toilet seat or potty chair is for.

(7) Child is willing to sit on seat and defecate.

d. Toilet-training guidelines:
   (1) Do not force child to sit on toilet.
   (2) Small seat or potty chair should be acquired and child allowed to explore it.
   (3) Supports or height should be adjusted so child's knees are even or above level of anus to allow easy passage of feces and to avoid straining and impediment of circulation to lower extremities.
   (4) Do not shame child for accidents; praise child for success. (This is Erikson's stage of autonomy versus shame and doubt.)

e. Be aware of safety concerns:
   (1) Safely fasten doors that lead to stairways, driveways, and storage areas.
   (2) Lock or nail screens on windows.
   (3) Fence play yard.
   (4) Turn pot handles on the stove to the wall.
   (5) Lock up matches, furniture polish, and cleaning agents, especially lye and detergents.
   (6) Store medicines and home products in child-safe containers.
   (7) Never leave child alone in tub or wading pool or around open or frozen bodies of water.
   (8) Make sure toys have no removable parts and are unbreakable.
   (9) In autos, use seat restraints or "approved" car seats, properly attached.

4. Age 2 years

A. Assessment of physical development (2 years):
   1. Height—gains 7.5 to 10.5 cm (3 to 4 inches).
   2. Weight—12 to 13 kg (26 to 28 lb).
   3. Approximately 16 temporary teeth.

B. Assessment of behavior patterns (2 years):
   1. Motor development—
      a. Walks up and down stairs.
      b. Jumps crudely.
      c. Opens doors and turns knobs.
      d. Drinks from cup held in one hand.
      e. Assists with dressing.
      f. Imitates vertical stroke when scribbling.
      g. Uses spoon without spilling.
      h. Builds a tower of five or more blocks.
      i. Kicks a ball with one foot without falling.
   2. Socialization and vocalization—
      a. Uses word "mine" constantly.
      b. Has vocabulary of 300 words and makes short sentences or phrases.
      c. Fears separation from parents; has *no* concept of time, length of separation, or of object permanence when out of sight.
      d. Treats other children as objects.
      e. Is toilet-trained in daytime.
      f. Helps to undress self; can put on some clothing.
      g. Obeys simple commands.
      h. Does not know right from wrong.
      i. Begins to have temper tantrums when frustrated.

C. Nursing goals and implementation (2 years):
   1. Goal: provide appropriate play activities based on developmental level—the curiousness and the newness of situations are sources of never-ending excitement to this child. The 2-year-old is aware of self as distinct from other beings and is now striving to gain a sense of autonomy without loss of control. As the child becomes less "babyish" and more demanding of self-rights, behavior problems may arise and maternal figures may become upset about losing a baby and be alarmed by the child's signs of autonomy. Manual dexterity is quite refined. The concept of object permanence is acquired during this year.
      a. Give small toys to investigate.
      b. Use large toys such as wagon or buggy.
      c. Provide mud and sand (pounding and patting).
      d. Read aloud, as child enjoys hearing stories.
      e. Keep in mind child's short attention span.
   2. Goal: provide guidance—
      a. Recognize that child needs peer companionship, although will not share.
      b. Have child eat meals with family.
      c. Be aware that child says "no" even if he or she does not mean it.
      d. Be consistent in discipline—parents need to agree and be consistent concerning when and how to discipline.
         (1) Excessively strict measures will deflate child's self-image and child may become antagonistic and rebellious or passive with little self-assertion or initiative.

    (2) Provide parental example and praise in lieu of excessive discipline.

    (3) With children under 2 years of age, chief use of discipline is to enforce rules for safety, such as removing child from situation.

  e. Allow doll or toy in bed.

  f. Be aware that child will try to delay sleeping by calling for drink of water or asking to go to the bathroom.

  g. Provide diversion to achieve cooperation, as child is impatient with restraints.

  h. Be aware of safety concerns:

    (1) Keep child away from the street and driveway with fence and firm discipline.

    (2) Supervise play when playmates are present, as they may injure one another with rough play.

    (3) Use large sturdy toys without sharp edges or small removable parts for safety.

    (4) Keep matches and cigarette lighters from child.

    (5) Store dangerous tools and garden equipment in safe place.

3. Goal: prevent frequent temper tantrums—

  a. Normal at 2 to 5 years (most frequent during second year).

  b. Provoked by sudden feeling of frustration.

  c. Nursing goals and implementation—health-teaching of parents.

    (1) Avoid abrupt withdrawal from play activities, or other precipitating factor.

    (2) Avoid excessive demands on child, especially if child is hungry, tired, or ill.

    (3) During tantrum, ignore behavior but stay close so child will not feel abandoned, use distraction.

    (4) Encourage consistency in parental reactions to temper tantrums and not allow temper tantrums to modify their behavior or their view of the child.

SPECIAL CONCERNS FROM BIRTH TO 2 YEARS

1. **Response to illness and hospitalization**—birth to 2 years.

A. Assessment of discomfort or pain (Tables 4–6 and 4–7):

1. Crying frequently.
2. Excessive irritability.
3. Elevated temperature.
4. Lethargy.
5. Prostration.
6. Decreased appetite.

B. Assessment of reaction to stage of illness:

1. Initial illness or hospitalization—

  a. Expected coping or adaptive behaviors:

    (1) Rejects everyone except mother figure.

    (2) Cries loudly—*phase one* of separation anxiety.

  b. Undesirable or maladaptive behaviors:

    (1) Monotonous crying and sad moans—*phase two* of separation anxiety.

    (2) Thumb-sucking, nose-picking, and body-rocking.

2. Prolonged hospitalization and convalescence—

  a. Expected coping or adaptive behaviors:

    (1) Demands attention.

    (2) May be difficult to handle.

    (3) Some regression (toilet-trained toddler begins to wet pants).

  b. Undesirable or maladaptive behaviors:

    (1) Indifferent to mother or maternal figure—*phase three* of separation anxiety.

    (2) Clings to nurse instead of mother figure.

    (3) Preoccupied with material things.

    (4) Behaviors do not return to normal after returning home.

    (5) No protest when mother leaves.

3. Assessment of phases of separation anxiety in toddlers (Table 4–8).

2. **Nutrition and feeding**—birth to 2 years.

A. Caloric requirements:

1. Birth to 2 months—115–120 cal/kg/24 hours.
2. Age 2 to 6 months—110 cal/kg/24 hours.
3. Age 6 to 12 months—100 cal/kg/24 hours.
4. Age 1 to 2 years—1000/24 hours.
5. Age 2 to 3 years—1250/24 hours.

B. Normal diets:

1. Infant—

  a. Fluid requirement—70 to 130 ml/kg (2 to 3 oz per pound of body weight) per 24 hours.

  b. Solid food and supplements—add one new food at a time to observe toleration and sensitivity, rash or diarrhea, for example.*

---

*Please note: This is a general outline. Current trend is to begin solid food when infant requires milk q 2 h p̄ previously q 4 h.

TABLE 4–6.   *Vital signs and laboratory values (newborn to 18 years)*

Age	Heart rate (beats/minute)	Average heart rate	Respirations/ minute	Blood pressure (systolic/ diastolic)*
Newborn	120–180		30–50	80/46
1–6 months	80–160		30–60	80–90/60
1 year	100–140	120	20–40	90/60
2 years	80–130	110	20–35	95/65
4 years	80–120	100	18–26	90/65
6 years	75–115	100	18–26	95/60
10 years	70–110	90	20–26	100/65
12–14 years	80–90	85–90	15–24	115/60
14–18 years	70–80	70–75	10–22	120/60

Temperature
Oral—36.4–37.2 C (97.6–99 F)
Rectal—37–37.8 C (98.6–100 F)
Axillary—35.9–36.7 C (96.6–97.8 F)

Urine
pH 5–7
Specific gravity
   Infant 1.002–1.006
   Child 1.005–1.018

*Wide variations are normal in children, so serial readings should be taken to provide a baseline reading from which upward or downward trends can be determined.

TABLE 4–7.   *Blood values (newborn to 18 years)*

Age	Hemoglobin (Hgb) (g/100 ml)	Hematocrit (% volume of cells)
Birth	16–22	45–65
1 month	11–22	53
3 months	16	35–40
6 months	12	33–42
1 year	11–12.5	35–40
2–8 years	13	34–43
8–10 years	13–14	46
12–14 years	14–16	34–46
14–18 years	14–16	42–47

c. 0–3 months:
   (1) Nonformula-fed infants—vitamin supplement of A, D, C once daily.
   (2) Iron supplement 1–2 mg/kg daily, particularly *nonbreastfed* infants. If not receiving iron, hemoglobin check should be made 6–9 months of age.
d. 3–4 months:
   (1) Iron-fortified dry cereal—2–4 tbsp/day mixed with equal amount formula.
   (2) Because of possible allergic response, begin with rice cereal and progress to oats; barley, wheat after 6 months of age.
   (3) Coincides with appearance of drooling and pancreatic enzymes necessary for digestion and with absence of tongue protrusion reflex.
e. 4–5 months:
   (1) Add vegetable—4 tbsp/day.

TABLE 4–8. *Phases of separation anxiety in toddlers**

Phase	*Assessment/Description*	*Nursing goals and actions*
Phase one—protest	Lasts a few hours to several days, expressed by violent crying and intense aggression; child may feel punished; newly gained sense of control and autonomy is threatened.	Goal: important for nurse to be close, even though behavior is difficult to tolerate; nurse only needs to remain in visual field, not necessarily attempting to touch or hold child; use of primary nurse would be most beneficial in preventing progression of stages.
Phase two—despair	Increased hopelessness characterized by sad moans; a perpetually sad countenance; declining activity; thumb-sucking, nose-picking, and body-rocking are seen; few or no demands; and accepts care passively.	Goal: encourage social interaction with other children, nurse, and staff.
Phase three—denial	Often erroneously interpreted as recovery, cheerful, actively interested in ward, indifferent to mother or maternal figure, and preoccupied with material things.	Goal: continuity of care is extremely important; help mother understand situation and encourage her to visit; *try to prevent this stage,* as it is difficult to cure and may cause long-lasting problems in the child's life.

*Based on studies and findings of Bowlby, J.: *Maternal care and mental health,* Geneva, World Health Organization, 1952.

(2) Add fruit—4–8 tbsp/day.

(3) Encourage pureed, unseasoned table food as opposed to commercial, more expensive preparation.

(4) Add one fruit *or* vegetable every three days to allow observation of effect of specific food.

(5) Because of possibility of nitrate intolerance (and/or poisoning), postpone use of carrots, beets, spinach.

(6) May add egg *yolk*—once daily; white may be source of allergic response.

f. 5–6 months:

  (1) Add meat, may mix with vegetable to total 4 tbsp/day.

  (2) Give fortified juice as source of vitamin C—begin with apple, reserving orange juice until after age 6 months.

g. 6–8 months:

  (1) Encourage self-feeding by giving finger foods such as pieces of fruit, frankfurter, cheese.

  (2) Self-feeding decreases opportunity for overfeeding as infant will eat only until satisfied.

h. 8–12 months:

  (1) Begin transition to all table foods by cutting up meat, offering nonpureed foods; withhold seasonings, including sugar and spices.

  (2) Encourage self-feeding using spoon, fork, and hands.

  (3) Encourage to eat with family.

i. Since stomach-emptying varies, a rigid feeding schedule is not advisable.

j. If infant cries often, reasons other than hunger should be investigated:

  (1) Wet diapers.

  (2) Fever.

  (3) Pain.

  (4) Boredom.

  (5) Immobilization.

k. Do not force child to eat.

l. Breastfeeding:

  (1) Usually mother's preference.

  (2) Advantages—

    (a) Readily available and at proper temperature.

    (b) Feeding difficulties are less common; less allergy-prone.

    (c) Antibodies from mother (polio and mumps, for example) transferred to infant, thus providing temporary immunity.

    (d) Less expensive.

    (e) Promotes good maternal-infant relationship.

    (f) Less contamination.

  (3) Disadvantages:

    (a) Often inconvenient for parents;

lactation diet is necessary for mother; and causes greater fatigue.

  (b) May produce jaundice in neonates.

  (c) May interfere with mother's returning to work.

 (4) Contraindications:

  (a) Active tuberculosis in mother.

  (b) Severe chronic disease in mother or infant.

  (c) Severe maternal malnutrition.

2. Toddler—

 a. Daily requirements include foods from basic four groups.

 b. Spacing of meals coincides with three meals plus snack (crackers, cheese, and pieces of fruit).

 c. Give small portions.

 d. Allow child to eat with rest of family.

 e. Usual to have decreased appetite due to decreased rate of growth.

C. Special concerns of infant-feeding:

1. Burping—

 a. Infant may swallow air during feeding.

 b. Infant should be burped or bubbled at least once during feeding and at end of feeding.

 c. Support infant with head elevated (over shoulder or sitting slightly forward on adult's lap) and gently pat or stroke back until infant burps.

2. Colic—

 a. Recurrent sharp abdominal pain occurring in infants under 3 months of age.

 b. Assessment:

  (1) Crying suddenly and loudly.

  (2) Face flushed.

  (3) Abdominal distension and tenseness.

  (4) Legs drawn up to abdomen.

 c. Analysis of etiology:

  (1) Undetermined, with some infants more susceptible than others; may be immaturity of GI tract.

  (2) Usually associated with hunger, air-swallowing, overfeeding, and maternal insecurity.

  (3) Certain foods may be responsible, but change in diet usually has no effect.

 d. Nursing implementation:

  (1) Reassure parents that attacks usually do not occur after 3 months of age.

  (2) Hold infant upright over shoulder.

  (3) Feed 1 to 2 oz of warm water or weak tea.

  (4) Learn feeding and burping techniques.

  (5) Establish stable emotional environment.

  (6) Sedation *may* be recommended by physician for severe, prolonged attacks.

3. Spitting up—

 a. Because of immature swallowing mechanism, regurgitation of small amounts (spitting up) is common for infants for first 6 months.

 b. Differentiate from vomiting (emptying of stomach contents).

 c. Unless other symptoms are present and if baby is gaining weight, spitting up should be ignored.

4. Vomiting—

 a. Most common cause is overfeeding.

 b. If accompanied by other symptoms such as fever, decreased urine output, blood in stool, or severe abdominal pain, seek medical attention.

5. Diarrhea (as differentiated from disease entity)—

 a. Overfeeding of formula may be cause—decrease feeding, give clear fluids (water or apple juice), and offer no solids at next meal or feeding.

 b. Frequent watery stools should be referred to physician for possible infectious etiology.

 c. Diarrhea that is not stopped within 24 hours should be investigated and treated.

6. Constipation—

 a. *Hard* stools that are difficult to pass.

 b. Recommend increased intake of fluids, such as water or juice.

 c. If diet is adequate and problem persists, pathology must be ruled out.

7. Weaning—

 a. About 6 months, offer sips of milk from a cup before and after regular feedings; weaning needs to be gradual process.

 b. Most infants are weaned to a cup at about 12 to 14 months of age.

 c. Discourage bottle in bed because of the likelihood of causing dental caries; also, older infant does not need the extra calories obtained from the bottle.

 d. Since sucking needs differ, infants are weaned at different ages.

8. Nutritional anemia (iron deficiency)—
   a. Often seen in infants 6 months to 2 years of age.
      (1) Infants have iron store from mother to age 6 months.
      (2) Most of food intake comes from milk, which is a poor source of iron.
      (3) Symptoms—chubby, pale, irritable, poor muscle tone, prone to infection.
   b. Analysis of cause:
      (1) Failure to assimilate.
      (2) Intake (diet).
      (3) Hemorrhage.
   c. Goal: replenish iron supply.
      (1) Sources include iron supplement (1–2 mg/kg/day), iron-fortified cereal, meat (frankfurters and hamburger are easy for toddlers to eat), egg yolks, peanut butter, and green vegetables.
      (2) Administering iron:
         (a) Best given between meals accompanied by fruit or juice (vitamin C is necessary for iron utilization) for greatest absorption. If not tolerated (vomiting and diarrhea) may administer with meals.
         (b) Give with medicine dropper or straw to decrease likelihood of stained teeth.
         (c) Prepare parents for appearance of tarry, greenish-black stools.
9. Overfeeding—
   a. Leads to obesity in infancy and later child- and adulthood, with possible consequent psychological problems and hypertension.
   b. May contribute to gastrointestinal symptoms such as vomiting and diarrhea.
10. Overuse of carbohydrates—
   a. Increases development of dental caries.
   b. Contributes to obesity and possible malnutrition.

3. Thumb-sucking
A. If prior to mealtime, may signify hunger.
B. Between meals—indicates need for more sucking.
   1. Breastfed infants—allow more time at breast.
   2. Bottle-fed infants—fewer and smaller holes in nipple.
   3. Nipple comforter or pacifier may be used between meals to satisfy sucking instincts.
C. Do not bind arms to side, or cover hands with mitts to prevent thumb-sucking.
D. Usually disappears by 2 years of age.

CONDITIONS AND DISEASE ENTITIES FROM BIRTH TO 2 YEARS

1. Immunizations—for an immunization schedule and outline of side effects and contraindications, see Tables 4–9 and 4–10.

2. Tuberculin skin test
A. Keep area dry for two to four hours after test.
B. Positive reading—2 mm or more diameter of *raised* reaction; redness itself is not necessarily indicative of positive reaction.
C. False negative reading may result from:
   1. Recent vaccination with live vaccine (measles, mumps, or smallpox).

TABLE 4–9.   Immunization schedule

Age	Immunizations*
2 months	DPT, TOPV
4 months	DPT, TOPV
6 months	DPT, TOPV
12 months	Tuberculin test
14 months	MMR
18 months	DPT, TOPV
4–6 years	DPT, TOPV
14–16 years, and every 10 years thereafter	TD

*Descriptions:
   DPT—diphtheria and tetanus toxoids combined with pertussis vaccine.
   TOPV—trivalent oral polio vaccine.
   Tuberculin test—given at least six weeks prior to MMR, as measles vaccine may give a false negative reading or may activate latent tuberculosis.
   MMR—combined measles, mumps, rubella vaccine.
   TD—tetanus and diphtheria toxoids (adult type); differs from DT, which contains a larger amount of diphtheria antigen. Pertussis is contraindicated over age 6 years due to possibility of severe complications and decreased risk of contracting pertussis.
Adapted from recommendations by the American Academy of Pediatrics.

TABLE 4–10.   *Side effects and contraindications*

Immunization	Assessment of side effects	Contraindications
DT: diphtheria toxoids	Local tenderness and pain, fever, and swelling.	Infectious process or history of febrile convulsions in child.
PV: pertussis vaccine (whooping cough)	Local redness, swelling and tenderness, fever, convulsions, and thrombocytopenia.	Not given to child over age 6 years because risk of complications from pertussis decreases and risk of febrile and vaccine-induced convulsions increases; child with brain damage or history of convulsive disorders— these children may receive a minute test dose, and if no reaction occurs, normal schedule is followed.
Tetanus toxoid	Rare in childhood; itching; painful, swollen injection site; and fever.	Child sensitive to horse serum and history of antitoxin formation.
Polio vaccine	Virtually no side effects.	Acute illness or gastroenteritis.
Measles vaccine	Occur 7–10 days after administration—anorexia, rash, and fever.	Not recommended for infants under 1 year unless epidemic present, then reimmunize after 1 year of age; acute infection and skin rash.
Rubella vaccine	Joint pain and arthritis, more common in older children.	Child with egg allergy, child whose mother is pregnant, and child under one year of age.
Mumps vaccine	Virtually no side effects.	Child with egg allergy, with immune deficiency, with pregnant mother, on steroid therapy, or undergoing radiation therapy.

2. Acute fever.
3. Child on steroid therapy.
D. Contraindications:
1. Previous history of positive reaction.
2. Previous vaccination with BCG.

3. Congenital diseases

A. Ophthalmia neonatorum (gonorrheal conjunctivitis):
1. Analysis of cause-pathophysiology—
   a. Gram negative organism, *Neisseria gonorrhoeae.*
   b. Acquired by infant during birth process by direct contact with infected vagina.
2. Assessment—
   a. Redness and swelling of eyelids.
   b. Profuse purulent discharge.
3. Nursing goals and implementation—
   a. Be absolutely certain to instill eyedrops (1% silver nitrate in the conjunctival sac) that are required by law in newborn within 72 hours of birth. Explain action to parents.
   b. Note any of the signs and report them so a smear or culture can be taken.
   c. Isolate infected infant.
   d. Utilize sterile technique when irrigating infected eye or eyes and move from inner to outer canthus to prevent self-infection.
B. Congenital syphilis (lues):
1. Analysis of cause-pathophysiology—
   a. Organism—spirochete, *Treponema pallidum.*
   b. Transmitted to fetus by direct inoculation into blood stream through placenta during latter half of pregnancy.
2. Assessment—
   a. Prior to age 6 weeks—corresponds to secondary stage in adults.
      (1) Persistent rhinitis "snuffles."
      (2) Generalized rash, including soles and palms.
      (3) Signs of anemia (confirmed by lab)— low hemoglobin count and prolonged bleeding time (see Table 4–7).
      (4) Bleeding ulcerations of mucous membranes.
      (5) Pseudoparalysis or pathologic fractures.
      (6) Jaundice.
   b. After age 2 years, corresponds to tertiary stage in adults.

(1) Saddle nose—destruction of nose bones.

(2) Saber shins—sharp forward curve of tibia.

(3) Hutchinson's teeth—permanent central incisors are peg shaped with a notch.

(4) Neurosyphilis—characterized by hemiplegia, spastic paralysis, and mental retardation.

3. Nursing goals and implementation—

a. Prevention of transmission of disease to other infants and staff by strict isolation of infant and use of gown and glove technique; not contagious after 48 hours of treatment.

b. Clean infant's nose before feeding because of rhinitis so infant can breathe while eating.

c. Handle infant carefully—pain on movement caused by bone lesions.

d. Take axillary temperature every 3–4 hours.

e. Administer medication, usually penicillin. If mother treated prior to seventh month of gestation, infant will be cured.

4. Congenital anomalies

A. Congenital heart disease (CHD)—each type will be discussed separately, but generally the signs and symptoms can be explained by understanding the effects of increased pulmonary artery pressure; this results in right-to-left shunting in the lungs, causing a decrease in the oxygen–carbon dioxide exchange; the infant's rate of respiration increases, which leads to easy fatigability with resultant feeding and weight-gain problems.

1. Analysis of etiology and incidence:

a. 8–10/1000 live births.

b. Prenatal factors which may contribute to increased incidence:

(1) Rubella or virus infection in mother.

(2) Poor maternal nutrition.

(3) Mother over age 40 years.

(4) Maternal alcoholism.

c. Genetic factors:

(1) Chromosomal defect such as Down's syndrome.

(2) Siblings or parents with CHD.

2. Assessment—classification of cardiac defects:

a. Cyanotic type—there is a communication between pulmonary and systemic circulations where the blood is continually flowing from venous to arterial side; the blood going to the periphery of the body is never fully saturated, so tissues have a blue tint.

(1) Tetralogy of Fallot.

(2) Tricuspid atresia.

(3) Transposition of great vessels.

(4) Truncus arteriosus.

b. Acyanotic type—there is no abnormal communication between pulmonary and systemic circulations.

(1) Coarctation of the aorta.

(2) Aortic stenosis.

c. Potentially cyanotic—an abnormal communication exists between the pulmonary and systemic circulations, but the pressure is such that blood flows through the shunt from arterial to venous side so that no cyanosis is present; however, it is possible that the flow could reverse direction (unusual stress or myocardial failure) and produce cyanosis by mixing venous blood with arterial blood.

(1) Patent ductus arteriosus.

(2) Atrial septal defects.

(3) Ventricular septal defects.

3. Types:

a. Patent ductus arteriosus (PDA)—a vascular connection that directs blood from the pulmonary artery to the aorta during fetal life, normally closes soon after birth; if this connection remains open after birth, the direction of the blood flow in the ductus is reversed by the higher pressure in the aorta; commonly seen in premature infants and usually closes spontaneously within first three months of life in these infants.

(1) Assessment—

(a) Slow weight gain.

(b) Machinery-like murmur heard over pulmonary artery in upper left sternal border.

(c) Feeding difficulties.

(d) Pale, scrawny appearance.

(e) Usually acyanotic because of mingling of blood between pulmonary and systemic circulations.

(f) Low diastolic blood pressure.

(2) Treatment—

(a) Surgical ligation and division of the patent ductus arteriosus.

(b) Usually elective at 2 to 3 years of age, as patency involves increased risk of bacterial endocarditis.

(c) After treatment, the diastolic blood pressure rises but stabilizes four to five days postoperatively.

b. Atrial septal defect (ASD)—an abnormal opening between right and left atria, causing left-to-right shunting of blood; this means that oxygenated blood that flows from the left to the right atrium is recirculated through the lungs, causing an increased total blood flow through the lungs with resultant enlargement of the right heart and distension of the pulmonary vessels.

(1) Assessment:
   (a) Systolic murmur over pulmonary artery heard over second interspace of left sternal border.
   (b) Dyspnea with exertion.
   (c) Tires easily.
   (d) Slow weight gain.
   (e) Enlargement of the heart.
   (f) Frequent respiratory infections.
   (g) Usually acyanotic due to mingling of pulmonary and systemic circulations, but may become cyanotic if flow reverses through shunt or defect.

(2) Diagnosis:
   (a) Murmur.
   (b) Cardiac catheterization.

(3) Treatment, usually done prior to entering school:
   (a) Surgical closure by suture or patch.
   (b) May utilize open-heart or closed technique.

c. Ventricular septal defect (VSD)—this is an abnormal opening between right and left ventricles; during systole, there is shunting of blood from left to right, causing an increase in pulmonary arterial pressures.

(1) Assessment:
   (a) Usually acyanotic, but pulmonary hypertension may occur, causing right-to-left shunting in lungs and cyanosis.
   (b) Small defects may be asymptomatic, but large defects develop symptoms at 1 to 2 months.

(c) Loud systolic murmur heard over left lower sternum.
(d) Left ventricular hypertrophy evidenced on ECG (electrocardiogram); may have right ventricular hypertrophy.
(e) Dyspnea, tires easily.
(f) Repeated respiratory infections.
(g) Feeding difficulties with slow weight gain.
(h) Congestive heart failure may develop with cardiac enlargement and pulmonary engorgement.

(2) Diagnosis:
   (a) Cardiac catheterization.
   (b) EKG (electrocardiogram).

(3) Treatment:
   (a) In low septal defects with murmur as only symptom, no treatment is indicated; 50% close spontaneously by age 3 years; *risk*—bacterial endocarditis.
   (b) Larger defects require open-heart surgery by direct closure or by suturing a patch into the opening at 3–4 years of age.
   (c) Success of treatment depends on the amount of resistance that has developed in the pulmonary vascular bed; if resistance is high, child will not do well with or without surgery.

(4) Complication—congestive heart failure.

d. Coarctation of aorta—a narrowed aortic lumen producing obstruction to flow of blood through aorta, causing increased left ventricular pressure and work load; the severity of symptoms depends on the degree of constriction.

(1) Assessment:
   (a) Murmur may or may not be heard.
   (b) Elevation of blood pressure in arms and low pressure in legs, with leg pains; systolic and diastolic hypertension.
   (c) During later childhood, may have slow growth and complain of fatigue and weakness in legs.
   (d) Headache and nose bleeds due to increased upper-body blood pressure.

(e) In severe coarctation, the infant develops congestive heart failure (see p. 330).

(2) Diagnosis:
   (a) Electrocardiogram.
   (b) Chest X ray.

(3) Treatment:
   (a) In infancy—treat congestive heart failure; surgery only as emergency procedure.
   (b) Surgery in middle childhood consists of excision of constricted area and anastomosis of excised ends.

e. Complete transposition of great vessels—the aorta originates from the right ventricle and the pulmonary artery originates from the left ventricle, thus there are two separate circulations; an abnormal opening between the two circulations must be present to sustain life.

(1) Assessment:
   (a) Severe cyanosis.
   (b) Shallow, rapid respirations.
   (c) Clubbing of fingers and toes.
   (d) Development of congestive heart failure (see p. 330).
   (e) Thrombosis.
   (f) Severe hypoxia.
   (g) Polycythemia and increased hemoglobin and hematocrit verified by lab tests.

(2) Treatment:
   (a) Create opening so two circulatory systems can mingle; life-saving.
      i. Rashkind—use of balloon catheter to create atrial septal defect via cardiac catheterization.
      ii. Blalock-Hanlon—create atrial septal defect via surgery.
   (b) Permanent correction with Mustard's procedure—use of cardiopulmonary bypass, atrial septum is removed and a graft is sutured into the atrium to direct pulmonary venous blood to right ventricle and systemic venous blood to left ventricle; usually done during preschool years.

f. Tetralogy of Fallot—this is characterized by pulmonary stenosis, ventricular septal defect, overriding aorta, and hypertrophy of the right ventricle; there is an obstruction of the blood from the right ventricle into the pulmonary artery; the ventricular septal defect allows unoxygenated blood into the aorta; high right ventricular pressure causes right ventricular hypertrophy.

(1) Assessment:
   (a) Variable signs and symptoms—dependent on the obstruction.
   (b) Cyanosis—usually becomes more severe as child gets older and stenosis becomes more severe.
   (c) Paroxysmal dyspnea—occurs during first two years of life, air hunger, hypoxia, deep cyanosis, and loss of consciousness, with or without convulsions.
   (d) Dyspnea on exertion.
   (e) Squatting to relieve chronic hypoxia when child reaches walking stage; self-limiting of activities due to fatigue and dyspnea.
   (f) Clubbing of fingers and toes.
   (g) Slow weight gain, delayed growth and development.
   (h) Fainting or mental slowness due to hypoxia.
   (i) Usually systolic murmur heard on lower left sternal border.
   (j) Tachycardia.

(2) Diagnosis:
   (a) Cardiac catheterization.
   (b) Angiocardiography.

(3) Treatment:
   (a) Relieve paroxysmal dyspnea by placing child in knee-chest position to increase cardiac efficiency and by administering oxygen to increase oxygen saturation of blood.
   (b) Surgery usually between 3 and 14 years, delaying as long as possible to ensure successful outcome.
   (c) The following procedures increase pulmonary blood flow by creating a patent ductus arteriosus:
      i. Waterston's shunt—anastomosis of ascending aorta and right pulmonary artery.
      ii. Blalock-Taussig shunt—anastomosis of branch of aorta

(in infants) or subclavian artery (in older child) to the right pulmonary artery.
iii. Potts-Smith-Gibson— anastomosis of aorta and left pulmonary artery.
(d) Total correction is achieved by removal of the shunt (one of the preceding procedures), repair of ventricular septal defect, and relief of right ventricular obstruction.
g. Truncus arteriosus—the aorta and pulmonary artery are fused into a single tube that receives blood from right and left ventricles simultaneously; a VSD is always present.
(1) Assessment:
(a) Loud murmur heard over truncus point of origin.
(b) Degrees of cyanosis, dyspnea, and retarded growth.
(c) Pulmonary vascular congestion develops after a few weeks, resulting in: marked cyanosis, dyspnea, activity intolerance, left ventricular hypertrophy.
(d) Signs/symptoms of CHF (see *Congestive heart failure,* p. 330).
(2) Treatment:
(a) Palliative—banding both pulmonary arteries to decrease amount of blood flow through lungs.
(b) Surgical correction—Rastelli's procedure, which involves closing VSD, allowing truncus arteriosus to arise from left ventricle, excising pulmonary arteries from aorta and utilizing a prosthetic, valved conduit to attach them to right ventricle. Best results obtained in children 5–12 years of age.
h. Tricuspid atresia—there is no opening between right atrium and right ventricle; that is, no tricuspid valve. Characterized by a small right ventricle and a large left ventricle and diminished pulmonary circulation; unless a ventricular septal defect or patent ductus arteriosus is present, there is no way for the blood to circulate through the lungs.
(1) Assessment:

(a) Severely cyanotic infant who does not improve with oxygen.
(b) Dyspnea, lack of energy.
(c) Polycythemia.
(d) Prone to infections.
(e) Failure to thrive.
(2) Treatment:
(a) Palliative: create a ventricular septal defect or patent ductus arteriosus surgically or via shunt (see *Tetralogy of Fallot,* p. 328).
(b) Total correction: placement of valved conduit between pulmonary artery and right atrium, and closing ASD.
4. Nursing goals and implementation:
a. Know signs and symptoms of heart defects.
b. Assess child's behavior and physical appearance with accurate recording as a basis for observing and reporting changes.
(1) Palpate and record femoral (inguinal area) and brachial pulse.
(2) Chest—appearance of one-sided prominence.
(3) Skin and mucous membrane coloring—cyanotic or pink.
(4) Note effect of feeding on cyanosis.
(5) Clubbing of phalanges.
(6) Listen and record type and location of murmur heard or absence of murmur.
(7) Motor coordination.
(8) Muscle development.
(9) Slow weight gain.
(10) Poor feeding habits.
(11) Frequent respiratory infections.
c. Relieve respiratory distress associated with increased pulmonary blood flow or decreased oxygen available to child.
(1) Position child at 45° angle to relieve pressure of organs on the diaphragm and to allow expansion of lung volume and better venous return to lungs and heart.
(2) Pin diapers loosely to decrease likelihood of pressure on infant's diaphragm.
(3) Feed slowly to decrease chance of aspiration due to rapid respirations.
(4) Suction mouth and nose if child cannot cough up secretions.
d. Provide environment conducive to rest so

that less oxygen will be required, thus reducing workload of heart.
(1) Organize nursing care to provide periods of undisturbed rest.
(2) Avoid excessive crying and expenditure of energy by feeding baby when hungry, using a pacifier, and holding child.
(3) Provide diversional activities to avoid fatigue—
  (a) Sing to infant.
  (b) Read to young child.
  (c) Offer books, crayons, or quiet activity appropriate to developmental level.
e. Protect child from exposure to infections.
f. Explain condition to child and family.
(1) Help parents understand true limits of child's activities, if any, so they can avoid overprotection and indulgence, as this is common among parents of children with congenital heart disease.
(2) Encourage parents to be truthful with child.
(3) Explain condition to child as soon as old enough to understand so child will be more likely to follow restrictions and understand symptoms.
g. Assess for signs and symptoms of congestive heart failure (CHF): inability to meet body's metabolic demands—
(1) Tachycardia.
(2) Tachypnea.
(3) Dyspnea.
(4) Nasal flaring.
(5) Retractions.
(6) Cyanosis or pale color.
(7) Periorbital edema in infants; swelling of hands and feet in older children.
(8) Murmurs.
(9) Decreased urine output.
(10) Weak cry.
(11) Irritability.
(12) Poor feeding.
(13) Perspiration, especially with activity, feeding, for example.
h. Implement medical treatment of CHF— goals and methods:
(1) Improve myocardial efficiency— digitalization.
(2) Decrease energy requirements— bedrest.

(3) Remove accumulated fluid and sodium—diuretics and low-sodium diet.
(4) Improve tissue oxygenation—administer oxygen.
i. Assess for signs and symptoms of infectious endocarditis: infection of valves and inner lining of heart.
(1) Spiking fever.
(2) Petechiae.
(3) Anorexia.
(4) Fatigue.
(5) Pallor.
j. Prepare family and child for diagnostic procedures:
(1) Chest X ray.
(2) Electrocardiography.
(3) Laboratory tests.
(4) Cardiac catheterization.
(5) Angiocardiography.
k. Prepare family and child for surgical repair.
(1) Preoperative nursing goals and implementation:
  (a) Determine from physician what type of repair is planned.
  (b) Appropriately explain procedure to family and child by drawing a picture, for example.
  (c) Tour ICU or CCU facilities.
  (d) Allow child to observe and touch equipment as appropriate; for example, oxygen mask, blood-pressure cuff, suction machine and tubing, IV equipment. Demonstrate use.
  (e) Prepare for pain and how child will look and feel on recovering from anesthesia.
  (f) Record all vital signs, activity level, and exercise tolerance, intake and output, and preparation done.
(2) Postoperative nursing goals and implementation:
  (a) Plan nursing care to provide optimal rest.
  (b) Monitor and record all vital signs, noting respiratory status and reporting promptly any deviations or unexpected alterations in any of the vital signs.
  (c) Record all intake and output, noting type, color, specific gravity of urine;

record daily weight as measure for fluid calculations.
  (d) Observe for symptoms indicative of complications, such as hemorrhage, congestive heart failure, pulmonary edema, elevated temperature.
  (e) Provide emotional support to patient and parents by explaining phenomena, answering queries, and allowing them to participate in care as appropriate.
  (f) Explain that regressive behaviors are normal postoperatively, soiling pants, return to bottle, for example.
  (3) Convalescent nursing goals and implementation:
  (a) Encourage child to continue progressive activity.
  (b) Explain any medications that the child may receive, their intended action, side effects.
  (c) Assist family in accepting feelings of change in physical status of child and relinquishing sick role.
  (d) Refer to public health nurse for home follow-up and encourage family to keep appointments for follow-up care.
5. Medical management of congenital heart disease:
  a. Prescribe medication to improve myocardial efficiency and observe for side effects and actions.
  b. Prescribe diuretics to assist in removal of accumulated fluid and sodium. Low-salt diets are rarely prescribed in infants and young children due to normally limited range of child's diet.
  c. Prescribe rest to lessen work load on heart; semi-Fowler's position for easier breathing.
  d. Prescribe oxygen to further enhance tissue oxygenation.
B. Congenital dislocation of hip:
  1. Analysis of cause-pathophysiology—
  a. Etiology unknown but predisposing factors may include intrauterine posture, maternal hormone secretion, newborn posture (swaddling, for example).
  b. Malposition or head of femur not in acetabulum.

  c. Incidence—1:700 births, more often found in females than males.
2. Assessment—
  a. Asymmetry of major gluteal folds.
  b. Limited ability to abduct leg on affected side to no more than 45° while on back with knees and hips flexed; audible click may be heard, Ortolani's click.
  c. Trendelenburg sign—pelvis drops on normal side if child stands on affected leg.
  d. Affected leg shorter.
  e. Delayed walking.
  f. Child limps; ducklike waddle when walking.
3. Treatment—
  a. In infant, double or triple diapering or splint to hold hip in full abduction may be only treatment.
  b. Surgery followed by hip spica cast may be required for older infant or toddler.
4. Nursing goals and implementation—
  a. Report positive assessment findings.
  b. Maintain abduction utilizing method prescribed and teach parents proper care of device such as splint.
  c. Special measures while in hip spica cast:
  (1) Circulation checks for cyanosis of toes.
  (2) Prevention of cast soiling from urine and feces by using plastic between child and cast and by elevating upper trunk so excrement will not flow into cast.
  (3) Petal cast edges and cover with adhesive tape to protect skin.
  (4) Maintain in position with upper body elevated to avoid urine and feces contamination.
  (5) Space between cast and abdomen should not be constrictive.
  d. Provide diversified environment through use of visual and auditory stimulation; no wet toys or toys small enough to fall into cast.
  e. Teach parents care of cast and offer suggestions for activities, such as use of wagon to move child.
C. Cleft lip:
  1. Analysis of cause-pathophysiology—
  a. Hereditary factor involved.
  b. Failure of the embryonic development

when fusion of the first brachial arch does not occur during sixth week of gestation.

  c. Incidence—1:600 births; males affected more.

2. Assessment—

  a. Obvious appearance of incompletely formed lip.

  b. May be bilateral or unilateral, involve only lip, or extend to nostril(s) or upper gum.

  c. Treatment involves lip surgery, either immediately or within two to three months, or when child weighs 10 lb.

3. Nursing goals and implementation—

  a. Preoperatively:

    (1) Show acceptance of infant by maintaining composure and not showing shock or disgust when handling.

    (2) Anticipate parental grief for perfect infant they did not have.

    (3) Feeding—

      (a) May feed well with a regular nipple with enlarged holes, or use special nipple now available.

      (b) Bubble frequently as infant swallows much air.

      (c) Feed in upright position to decrease possibility of aspiration.

    (4) Prepare parents for newborn's surgery, which may occur several hours after birth rather than later in infancy.

  b. Postoperatively:

    (1) Prevent injury to suture line of lip.

      (a) Use elbow restraints.

      (b) Logan bow—wire placed cheek to cheek across top of suture line to prevent lateral tension, gauze covers suture line. Keep moist with saline.

      (c) Place infant on side or back, *never* on stomach.

    (2) Prevent child from crying, this increases tension.

    (3) Maintain nutritional needs with rubber tip dropper or syringe for about three weeks; encourage frequent burping.

    (4) Cleanse suture line frequently with half-strength hydrogen peroxide applied with cotton tip applicator; prevent crusting to decrease scarring from tissue infection.

    (5) Gently dry mouth by patting.

    (6) Observe for respiratory distress—edema of tongue, nostrils, and mouth.

    (7) Give water after feeding to rid mouth of milk to decrease bacteria growth and infection.

    (8) Teach parents proper suctioning, cleansing, restraining, and feeding.

D. Cleft palate:

1. Analysis of cause-pathophysiology—

  a. Hereditary factor involved.

  b. Failure of embryonic development when fusion of the secondary palate does not occur during week 7–12 of gestation.

2. Analysis of etiology and incidence—

  a. 1:2500 births.

  b. Occurs more often in females.

3. Assessment—

  a. Opening in roof of mouth.

  b. Usually associated with cleft lip.

  c. May involve soft palate or soft and hard palate.

  d. Sucking difficulties.

4. Nursing goals and implementation—

  a. Preoperatively:

    (1) Support parents when they see child for the first time; show acceptance of child.

    (2) Treatment is done in stages, repair may begin between 18 and 36 months.

    (3) Feeding techniques and equipment—

      (a) Hold infant in upright position to decrease chance of aspiration.

      (b) Do not allow infant to suck, as this will not be allowed postoperatively.

      (c) Equipment—Lamb's nipple, Brecht feeder, and Duckey nipple prior to repair in infant; toddler should drink from cup. Give water after feeding to cleanse mouth.

    (4) Prevent infection by keeping child away from others with any infections and by keeping cleft clean.

    (5) Teach parents what to expect postoperatively.

  b. Postoperatively:

    (1) Observe for airway obstruction, shock, and hemorrhage.

    (2) Prevent injury to suture line by use of elbow restraints.

(3) Irrigate child's mouth with ear syringe frequently and following meals; child should be sitting and leaning forward or placed on abdomen.

(4) Do not allow child to suck—feed with rubber tip syringe.

(5) Administer antibiotics, as prescribed.

(6) Provide diversion and play activities to maintain normal growth and development; provide tactile stimulation.

(7) Child should be placed on side and back until sutures are removed, following immediate postoperative period.

(8) Otitis media is a common complication—any signs of an earache, such as crying and pulling on ear, should be reported immediately.

(9) Be sure parents are aware that follow-up care and repair will be on a *long-term basis*, usually involving plastic surgeon, orthodontist, speech therapist, and possibly others.

E. Gastrointestinal disorders:

1. Tracheoesophageal atresia—an abnormal connection between esophagus and trachea; the cause for the failure of this embryonic closure is unknown. Most affected infants are of low birth weight.

   a. Assessment—
      (1) Excessive amount of secretions exhibited by continual drooling from mouth and nose.
      (2) Intermittent cyanosis relieved by suctioning.
      (3) Abdominal distension.
      (4) Coughing, choking, cyanosis, and return of liquid through nose when feeding attempted.

   b. Treatment—
      (1) Primary repair—surgical esophageal anastomosis and fistula division.
      (2) Palliative surgery—gastrostomy and cervical esophagostomy until infant gains weight; usually choice for premature infants.

   c. Nursing goals and implementation—
      (1) Preoperatively:
         (a) Maintain body position in semi- to high-Fowler's to prevent aspiration of gastric juices.
         (b) Suction secretions frequently to prevent accumulation in blind pouch and to maintain patent airway.
         (c) Administer parenteral feedings to maintain hydration and electrolyte balance.
      (2) Postoperatively:
         (a) Maintain patent airway to prevent oxygen starvation, apnea, and aspiration of secretions.
         (b) Mark suction catheter so it can be inserted to desired depth for suctioning.
         (c) Assist in progression of feedings—
            i. Parenteral or gastrostomy feedings first week.
            ii. Oral feeding 7 to 14 days postoperatively or as prescribed; feed slowly, watch for vomiting and difficulty in swallowing, which may indicate stricture of anastomosis site.
         (d) Give emotional and physical support to infant and family—
            i. Hold infant upright to feed.
            ii. Assist mother in feeding her infant.
            iii. Offer pacifier to infant who is not eating by mouth, so sucking needs will be met.

2. Imperforate anus—failure of embryonic development resulting in an intact anal membrane or internal blind pouch of lower bowel. Occurs 1:5000 births.

   a. Assessment:
      (1) No anal opening and inability to insert thermometer or small probe.
      (2) Absence of meconium stool.
      (3) Gradual increase of abdominal distension.

   b. Treatment choices:
      (1) Anoplasty.
      (2) Abdominoperineal pull-through.
      (3) Colostomy with abdominoperineal pull-through when child is older.

   c. Nursing goals and implementation:
      (1) Report any of the preceding signs immediately.
      (2) Observe infant for stool-tinged urine or feces coming from a fistula.

(3) Pass nasogastric tube to prevent abdominal distension.

(4) Explain defect and planned surgical technique to parents.

(5) Postoperatively—
   (a) Position child so perineum is exposed for cleaning with minimal irritation, on abdomen or on back with legs suspended at 90° angle to trunk, for example.
   (b) Observe for abdominal distension, bleeding from perineum, and respiratory difficulties.
   (c) Oral feedings should begin when peristalsis returns.
   (d) Perform anal dilatation to prevent stricture at site of anastomosis.

3. Pyloric stenosis—congenital hypertrophy of the muscle of the pylorus; the constriction of the lumen of the pyloric canal causes the stomach to become dilated, resulting in delayed gastric emptying, which causes vomiting after feeding.
   a. Analysis of etiology and incidence:
      (1) Five times more common in males.
      (2) Majority are full-term, Caucasian infants.
   b. Assessment:
      (1) Nonprojectile progressing to projectile vomiting.
      (2) Non-bile-stained vomitus—narrowing located above common bile duct.
      (3) Constipation.
      (4) Visible left-to-right peristaltic waves during or after eating.
      (5) Palpable olive-shaped mass in upper-right quadrant.
      (6) Excessive hunger.
      (7) Dehydration leading to alkalosis.
      (8) Weight loss.
      (9) Decreased urinary output and number of stools.
   c. Treatment:
      (1) Medical treatment—refeeding, use of thickened formula, gastric lavage, and medication to relax pyloric muscle spasm.
      (2) Surgical—Fredet-Ramstedt; longitudinal incision in pyloric muscle permitting it to gape.
   d. Nursing goals and implementation:
      (1) Preoperatively—

         (a) Administer IV fluids to restore hydration and electrolyte balance.
         (b) Record output accurately, including specific gravity of urine.
         (c) Preventive measures to decrease vomiting, that is, NPO or use of thickened formula.
         (d) Prepare parents for surgery by explaining procedure and use of gastric tube.
      (2) Postoperatively—
         (a) Assist in resuming oral feedings—two to eight hours postoperatively, begin with glucose water and progress from half-strength to regular formula.
         (b) Elevate head and shoulders after feeding and position on right side to aid in gastric emptying.
         (c) Encourage parents to care for and feed infant.

4. Chalasia—abnormal continual relaxation of lower end of esophagus, cardiac sphincter, causing vomiting; self-limiting; treatment consists of measures to decrease vomiting.
   a. Assessment:
      (1) Regurgitation immediately after feeding.
      (2) Weight loss.
      (3) Dehydration.
   b. Nursing goals and implementation:
      (1) Administer IV fluids to restore hydration and electrolyte balance.
      (2) Measures to decrease vomiting—
         (a) Thickening formula.
         (b) Place infant upright after feeding.
         (c) Minimal handling during feeding.
      (3) Teach parents to play with infant *before* feeding.
      (4) Explain that problem is self-limiting—usually disappears by three months.

5. Hirschsprung's disease—the congenital absence or decreased number of ganglion cells in muscle wall of intestinal tract, usually at distal end; no peristalsis in this area.
   a. Analysis of etiology and incidence:
      (1) A familial pattern is demonstrated; four times more common in males.
      (2) Often associated with Down's syndrome.
   b. Assessment:
      (1) Early infancy—

(a) No meconium.
(b) Bile-stained vomitus.
(c) Constipation with overflow diarrhea.
(d) Anorexia.
(e) Abdominal distension.
(2) Later childhood—
(a) Progressive distension of abdomen.
(b) Peristalsis observable.
(c) Constipation with malodorous, ribbonlike stool.
(d) Failure to grow.
(e) Palpable fecal mass.
(f) Anemia due to malabsorption.
c. Treatment:
(1) Relieve fecal impaction with enema and digital removal.
(2) Medical management—stool softeners and low-residue diet to decrease bulk of stool.
(3) Surgical intervention by removal of aganglionic area and anastomosis of two ends of colon, utilizing Duhamel pull-through or Soave procedure; sometimes a temporary colostomy is performed to allow bowel to rest, with anastomosis performed later.

(4) May be placed on parenteral hyperalimentation preoperatively.
d. Nursing goals and implementation:
(1) Preoperatively—
(a) Utilize proper measures to empty bowel—enema, digital removal, and liquid diet.
(b) Take axillary temperature.
(c) Note any abdominal distension.
(d) Prepare for colostomy if necessary (pictures, doll play).
(2) Postoperatively—
(a) Observe for any complications—respiratory difficulties, abdominal distension, and hemorrhage.
(b) Keep child NPO until bowel sounds return.
(c) Monitor IV fluids to maintain hydration and electrolyte balance.
(d) Prevent infections of operative site by careful cleansing.
(e) If colostomy is present, keep clean to prevent skin breakdown.

(f) Have nasogastric tube available to prevent abdominal distension.
(g) Continue axillary temperatures to avoid injury.
(h) Observe stools for return to normal pattern.
(i) Provide emotional support to child and parents by encouraging them to talk about fears and anxieties and answering their questions.
(j) If colostomy is temporary measure, explain this to parents in order to decrease their anxiety.
6. Intussusception—the telescoping of a portion of intestine into adjacent distal section; possibly due to increased mobility of intestine and rapid peristalsis; it can lead to gangrene of the bowel.
a. Analysis of etiology and incidence:
(1) Occurs three times more often in males.
(2) Usually seen 3–12 months of age.
(3) Increased incidence in cystic fibrosis and celiac diseases.
b. Assessment:
(1) Sudden onset in latter half of first year of life.
(2) Intermittent, severe abdominal pain and distension accompanied by screaming and knees drawn to chest.
(3) Currant-jelly-like stools—stools with pus and mucus.
(4) Vomiting.
(5) Sausage mass palpable in upper right quadrant accompanied by nothing palpable in lower right quadrant due to less involvement of bowel distal to obstruction.
(6) Dehydration and fever.
c. Treatment:
(1) May reduce spontaneously or be reduced by exerting slight retrograde pressure to barium instilled by enema to confirm diagnosis.
(2) May require emergency surgical intervention to reduce or, if gangrene has set in, to resect portion of colon.
d. Nursing goals and implementation:
(1) Maintain IV to restore hydration and electrolyte balance.
(2) Insert nasogastric tube to prevent abdominal distension and vomiting.

(3) Take axillary temperatures to avoid injury and stimulation.

(4) Offer support to family and child to allay fears and anxieties.

(5) Postoperatively—observe for signs of shock and hemorrhage; check for return of bowel sounds; report passage of normal stool.

7. Diarrhea—as a disease entity, diarrhea is an excessive loss of water and electrolytes through repeated passing of unformed stools; it is indicative of some type of condition or disease; it may indicate an infectious process (bacterial or viral infection), noninfectious process (allergic

response or metabolic disorder), or a mechanical or congenital disorder (intussusception or Hirschsprung's disease).

a. Assessment:
   (1) Diarrhea of gradual or sudden onset.
   (2) Anorexia.
   (3) Low-grade fever (below 105 F).
   (4) Rapid respirations.
   (5) Signs of dehydration.
   (6) Irritability, restlessness, stupor, and/or convulsions.
   (7) Signs of metabolic acidosis (Table 4–11).

b. Treatment goals:

TABLE 4–11. *Comparison of metabolic and respiratory acidosis-alkalosis*

	Metabolic	Respiratory
ALKALOSIS		
Definition	Deficit of acid (H^+, hydrogen ions) and excess of base (HCO_3, bicarbonate, more than 25 mEq/liter).	Deficit of acid (H_2CO_3, carbonic acid, less than 25 mEq/liter).
Causes	Vomiting, lavage, and diuretics.	Hyperventilation.
Assessment	Nausea, vomiting, diarrhea, tremors, convulsion, and altered degree of alertness.	Tachypnea, numbness, tingling of hands and face, and altered degree of alertness.
Treatment	Replace fluid loss, especially potassium and chloride.	Sedation and have patient hold breath.
Nursing management	Record intake and output, take seizure precautions, and administer prescribed medications.	Give prescribed medications, have child breathe into paper bag, and stay with child to make child feel secure.
ACIDOSIS		
Definition	Excess of acid (H^+, hydrogen ions) and deficit of base (HCO_3, bicarbonate, less than 25 mEq/liter).	Excess of acid (H_2CO_3, carbonic acid, more than 25 mEq/liter) and elevated PCO_2 (above 38 mm Hg, arterial).
Causes	Diabetes, renal failure, and diarrhea.	Hypoventilation and muscular weakness.
Assessment	Headache, nausea, vomiting, diarrhea, tremors, convulsions, and altered degree of alertness.	Decreased respirations, drowsiness, semicomatose, tachycardia, arrhythmia, and altered degree of alertness.
Treatment plan	Treat underlying cause (give glucose, insulin to diabetic); rid body of protein and excess H^- by resins or dialysis; administer oxygen (encourages carbohydrate metabolism); and give bicarbonate IV.	Treat cause and take measures to improve ventilation—intermittent positive pressure breathing (IPPB), antibiotics, postural drainage, suction, endotracheal tube, tracheostomy, and ventilator.
Nursing implementation	Administer bicarbonate, take seizure precautions (padded siderails, tongue blade at bedside; remove toys that could cause injury) and record intake and output; fluid therapy may be forced or restricted.	Improve ventilation—semi-Fowler's position, low-flow oxygen, chest physiotherapy (postural drainage), change positions frequently, and encourage coughing.

(1) Restore electrolyte balance and hydration.

(2) Laboratory studies to diagnose cause—

    (a) Serum studies.

    (b) Urinalysis.

    (c) Stool cultures.

(3) Isolation of infant to protect infant and others from possible pathogens.

c. Nursing goals and implementation:

(1) Monitor IV amount and rate to avoid circulatory overload and to restore electrolyte balance and hydration. Keep strict recording of I and O.

(2) Weigh infant daily to determine fluid needs.

(3) Keep child NPO to allow bowel to rest; offer pacifier for sucking needs and observe for abdominal distension (bubbling infant or passage of nasogastric tube may be necessary).

(4) Talk to and hold child during diagnostic procedures to reassure.

(5) Explain procedures and treatment to parents.

(6) Practice meticulous skin care to lessen excoriation caused by alkaline stool.

(7) Explain follow-up care and teach parents regarding diet, hygiene measures.

F. Neurologic disorders:

1. Meningomyelocele—a congenital condition in which both spinal cord and cord membranes protrude through defect in spinal canal; it occurs during the fourth to sixth week of embryonic development, but exact cause is unknown.

a. Incidence—1:1000 births. Possible genetic predisposition.

b. Assessment—

(1) Round bulging sac on infant's back.

(2) No response to sensation below level of sac due to neurologic dysfunction.

(3) Constant dripping of urine or urinary retention.

(4) Incontinence or retention of stool.

(5) Spontaneous movements below defect are absent or minimal.

(6) May develop hydrocephalus.

c. Treatment—

(1) Surgical correction:

    (a) Closure of sac to prevent infection and rupture.

    (b) Laminectomy to prevent deterioration of neural functioning.

(2) Orthopedic measures to prevent deformities and ulcerations of lower extremities:

    (a) Support ankles with foam or roll to keep toes off bed when infant is placed on abdomen; place foam between knees when infant is placed on side.

    (b) Range of motion exercises.

    (c) Casting of clubbed feet—so child can learn to walk with braces when older.

d. Nursing goals and implementation—

(1) Preoperatively:

    (a) Prevent leakage or rupture of sac by positioning infant on side or abdomen.

    (b) Prevent infection of sac by avoiding contamination.

    (c) Prevent urinary infection by using—

        i. Credé's method to expel urine (apply gentle rolling pressures with hand, beginning at umbilicus and continue downward under symphysis pubis).

        ii. High vitamin C diet.

        iii. Force fluids.

    (d) Provide normal handling and sensory stimulation, for example, hold while feeding, hang a mobile over crib, or place a music box near crib.

    (e) May use a Bradford frame to ensure good body positions, facilitate gravity flow of urine and feces without contamination, and avoid injury to sac. (Bedpan is placed in center opening of frame and child can be positioned so sac is in opening of frame, thus alleviating any pressure.)

(2) Postoperatively:

    (a) Prevent postoperative complications.

        i. Infection—keep surgical site clean.

        ii. Pneumonia—keep airway clear, suction infant, and change position often.

    (b) Observe for signs/symptoms of increased intracranial pressure.

(c) Contribute to interdisciplinary approach for planning of infant's future, which will include physical therapy, neurology, orthopedics, and urology.

(d) Provide support for family by referrals to other disciplines and assistance in accepting long-term care of child.

2. Hydrocephalus—the inability to absorb cerebrospinal fluid, causing an increase of fluid under pressure, or an obstruction between source of cerebrospinal fluid and area of reabsorption; it may be a sequela to developmental defects, inflammatory reactions (such as meningitis), neoplasm, and hemorrhage (following trauma).

   a. Assessment—
   (1) Rate of increase of more than 1 inch/month in head size.
   (2) Tense, bulging, widened fontanel.
   (3) Signs/symptoms of increased intracranial pressure (ICP).
   (4) Eventual development of "sunset" eyes and shiny scalp, with noticeable scalp veins.
   (5) Developmental lag and failure to thrive.
   (6) High-pitched cry in infants.
   (7) Hyperactive reflexes.

   b. Treatment—involves surgical procedure to insert a tube (shunt) that carries fluid from brain to the bloodstream or some body cavity such as inferior vena cava, peritoneal cavity, or ureter.

   c. Nursing goals and implementation—
   (1) Preoperatively:
      (a) Measure head circumference each day and record.
      (b) Provide adequate nutrition by planning meal times and rest periods as child is anorexic and lethargic; feed after treatment and bath, for example.
      (c) Perform range-of-motion (ROM) exercises to prevent development of contractures.
      (d) Prevent skin breakdown of head by frequent turning of infant, as infant may be unable to turn self.
   (2) Postoperatively:
      (a) Observe infant for respiratory difficulties, increased ICP, sodium imbalance, abdominal distension, and dehydration.
      (b) Position flat to prevent subdural hematoma; too rapid drainage of fluid evidenced by sunken fontanel.
      (c) Monitor fontanels.
      (d) Observe shunt site for obstruction and early signs of infection—
         i. Redness.
         ii. Swelling.
         iii. Tender to touch.
         iv. Elevated temperature.
         v. Exudate at suture site.
      (e) Explain procedure and anticipated outcomes to parents.

3. Cerebral palsy—a nonprogressive disorder of the motor centers and pathways of the brain, causing difficulty in control of voluntary muscles; it is caused by prenatal, natal, and postnatal factors such as maternal anoxia and infections, anoxia or cerebral trauma at birth, and infections or trauma after birth. Exact incidence not known. Most are low birth weight.

   a. Assessment—
   (1) Spastic type—fixed postures due to loss of smooth movement of voluntary muscles; scissoring (legs crossed and toes pointed) due to increased deep-tendon reflexes; attempts to move a joint cause muscles to contract.
   (2) Athetosis—involuntary, uncoordinated, uncontrollable movements of muscle groups due to lesions of basal ganglia.
   (3) Dystonia—rigid attitudes; posturing; slow moving; muscles remain semicontracted and resist movement.
   (4) Ataxia—loss of balance due to cerebellar involvement; visual disturbance.
   (5) Early signs:
      (a) Asymmetry in motion.
      (b) Twitching.
      (c) Stiffness.
      (d) Difficulty with sucking and swallowing.
      (e) Deviation from normal growth and development—no weight gain and persistence of abnormal reflexes or lack of normal reflexes; inertia.
      (f) Delayed or defective speech

(often diagnosed as mentally retarded).
- (g) Convulsions.
- (h) Hyperactive gag reflex.

b. Treatment goals—
- (1) Establish optimal locomotion, communication and self-help.
- (2) Correct associated defects.

c. Nursing goals and implementation—
- (1) Anticipate possible respiratory problems by having suction machine available.
- (2) Diet:
  - (a) High-calorie diet as child is likely to eat less than usual for age because of difficulty eating and to have increased energy requirements due to motion.
  - (b) Foods that can be easily chewed and swallowed.
  - (c) Relaxed mealtime with little emphasis placed on cleanliness or perfect manners.
- (3) Provide measures to ensure periods of relaxation, such as quiet activities (reading or listening to music) and organize nursing care to minimize interruptions.
- (4) Prevent contractures through use of physical therapy, splints, braces, and active motions when playing.
- (5) Assist child to develop maximum potential by being alert to visual disturbances and hearing and speech problems; often child has normal intelligence.
- (6) Help child play—use puppets, tell stories, or any activities to develop eye-hand coordination.
- (7) Explain the necessity of long-term-care planning with parents—involves physical therapists, occupational therapists, physicians, speech therapists, and other professionals as needed.
- (8) Preparation for discharge is extremely important and is accomplished over time.

G. Mental retardation—term applied to persons with *impaired intelligence* and inadequate development in childhood that affects their ability to adapt to environment (Table 4–12).

1. Analysis of causes and frequency (1% of general population):
   a. Before birth (50% to 60% of the 1% total)—
      - (1) Genetic (Down's syndrome).
      - (2) Toxic conditions (Rh or ABO incompatibility).
      - (3) Endocrine imbalance (PKU; galactosemia, hypothyroidism, cretinism—early treatment needed to prevent retardation).
      - (4) Trauma.
      - (5) Nutrition.
      - (6) Anoxemia.
      - (7) Infections (German measles in first trimester of pregnancy, or syphilis).
   b. At birth (8% of 1% total)—
      - (1) Hemorrhage.
      - (2) Prolonged and difficult birth.
      - (3) Forceps delivery (trauma).
      - (4) Anoxemia.
   c. Following birth (32% to 42% of 1% total)—
      - (1) Encephalitis or meningitis.
      - (2) Toxemia.
      - (3) Malnutrition.
      - (4) Vitamin deficiency.
      - (5) Lead poisoning.
      - (6) Trauma—head injury.
2. Assessment:
   a. Neuromuscular development does not progress consistently.
      - (1) Infant does not suck; toddler does not learn to feed self.
      - (2) Slow to sit, stand, and walk.
   b. Unable to learn or profit from experience.
   c. May have other sensory defects—
      - (1) Language disorders.
      - (2) Speech and language disorders.
      - (3) Visual and/or hearing defects.
   d. Unable to respond in accepted manner in social situations (culturally determined).
   e. Labile emotional reactions—often placid.
3. Nursing goals and implementation:
   a. If child is hospitalized, obtain a nursing history of child's routine at home so a care plan can be developed to help child feel secure and to minimize regression.
      - (1) Feeding habits—how, when, and what to feed infant.
      - (2) Sleeping—times and any "security" toy.
      - (3) Toilet habits—words used.

TABLE 4–12. *Mental deficiency**

Level (IQ)	Preschool (0–5 years)— maturation and development	School-age (6–21 years)— training and education	Adult (21 years and over)— social and vocational adequacy
Profound: 0–19	Gross retardation; minimal capacity for functioning in sensorimotor areas; need nursing care.	Obvious delays in all areas of development; show basic emotional responses; may respond to skillful training in use of legs, hands, and jaws; need close supervision.	May walk, need nursing care, have primitive speech; usually benefit from regular physical activity; incapable of self-maintenance.
Severe: 20–35	Marked delay in motor development; little or no communication skills; may respond to training in elementary self-help, for example, self-feeding.	Usually walk, barring specific disability; have some understanding of speech and some response; can profit from systematic habit training.	Can conform to daily routines and repetitive activities; need continuing direction and supervision in protective environment.
Moderate: 36–51	Noticeable delays in motor development, especially in speech; respond to training in various self-help activities.	Can learn simple communication, elementary health and safety habits, and simple manual skills; do not progress in functional reading or arithmetic.	Can perform simple tasks under sheltered conditions; participate in simple recreation; travel alone in familiar places; usually incapable of self-maintenance.
Mild: 52–67	Often not noticed as retarded by casual observer but are slower to walk, feed self, and talk than most children.	Can acquire practical skills and useful reading and arithmetic to a third- to sixth-grade level with special education; can be guided toward social conformity.	Can usually achieve social and vocational skills adequate to self-maintenance; may need occasional guidance and support when under unusual social or economic stress.

*Classification developed by the American Association of Mental Deficiency.

(4) Play—what activities are usual.

b. Plan nursing interventions on child's *developmental level,* not chronologic age.

c. Use of three Rs in helping child learn new activities:

  (1) Relaxation—provide calm, nonthreatening environment for activity to be learned.

  (2) Repetition—the retarded child learns by demonstration and repeated attempts at an activity or behavior.

  (3) Reinforcement—positive reinforcement is needed as a reward for behaviors or tasks accomplished or desired.

d. Explain to parents necessity of teaching child acceptable standards of behavior—

  (1) Establish daily routine so child will know what is expected.

  (2) In discipline, use language child can understand to explain misdeed.

  (3) If punishment is necessary, it should *immediately* follow the misdeed, as child cannot recall past misdeed.

  (4) Give child responsibilities that can be mastered (dependent on level of retardation).

e. Summary: general goals in management—stimulation needs, motor control, sensory training, sociability, safety, self-care, and independence to maximum developmental, not chronologic, ability.

f. See *Behavior modification* in Unit 2.

H. Down's syndrome—an abnormality resulting from an extra chromosome causing mental retardation; the extra chromosome may be evident as three number 21 chromosomes (trisomy 21) for a total of 47 chromosomes, or the parent may have an abnormal attachment of chromosome 21 to number 15, thus transmitting an extra chromosome 21 plus a normal chromosome 21 (resulting in 46 chromosomes); the latter is therefore inherited but the former is not; chromosomal analysis shows which type of chromosome 21 attachment is present.

1. Analysis of etiology and incidence:
   a. Incidence of trisomy 21 increases with maternal age; 1:1000 under age 30 years, 15:1000 over age 35 years. Amniocentesis is recommended for pregnant women over age 35.
   b. Normal fetal growth is affected, causing complications—
      (1) Congenital heart defects (atrial septal defect is most common).
      (2) Intestinal obstruction.
2. Assessment:
   a. Hypotonia.
   b. Hyperextension of extremity joints.
   c. Inner epicanthic folds of eyes (oriental appearance).
   d. Flat nasal bridge.
   e. Excess skin on back of neck.
   f. Small, low-set ears.
   g. Simian crease—transverse line on palm.
   h. Shortened fourth finger and flat, square hands.
   i. Plantar furrow—line runs vertically down sole of foot.
   j. Brachycephaly with flat occiput.
   k. Mouth open, with thick, protruding tongue.
   l. Slow development.
3. Nursing goals and implementation:
   a. Look at physical appearance to help decide appropriate intervention.
   b. Provide nipple that allows minimal sucking effort because of protruding tongue and difficulty swallowing.
   c. Be aware of abdominal distension as sign of intestinal obstruction.
   d. Note apical pulse, cyanosis, and respiratory distress as signs of cardiac defects.
   e. Encourage self-help and activities to promote development.
   f. Utilize previous discussion of mental retardation for further nursing approaches.
4. Counseling goals:
   a. If amniocentesis is performed, support parents' decision to abort or to have child.
   b. Explain prolonged need for sensorimotor play and need for observation of URI, GI, and cardiac problems.
   c. Verbal skills are delayed due to mental retardation and lack of control of tongue and facial muscles.
   d. Emphasize *consistency* and *immediacy* in discipline and limit-setting on behavior.
   e. Provide anticipatory guidance for socialization and sexual development, emphasizing need for simple, repetitive explanations to reduce frustration of failure.
   f. Encourage involvement in clubs, hobbies, and sports to reduce isolation.
   g. Discuss concerns of older child such as birth control, marriage, employment capabilities.
   h. Explore parental concerns: other children's and relatives' reaction to the child, decisions about present and future life of child, possible rejection of child, strain on marital relations.
   i. Assist parents to express fears, confusion, guilt, disappointments concerning their child by listening and answering questions.
5. Placement, other than family home:
   a. Usually dependent upon degree of retardation, age of parents, home environment, family situation.
   b. Infant and young children—
      (1) Foster home.
      (2) Institution for those requiring special care, treatment.
   c. Adolescent/young adult—
      (1) Foster home.
      (2) Boarding home with other retarded adults who have high degree of self-care.
   d. Older adult—
      (1) Boarding home.
      (2) Minimal-care residential facility.
I. Metabolic disturbances:
1. Hypothyroidism (cretinism)—a congenital or acquired endocrine disease; deficient production of thyroid hormone; it is noted at 2 to 3 months of age.
   a. Assessment—
      (1) Jaundice.
      (2) Nasal stuffiness and obstructions.
      (3) Episodes of apnea.
      (4) Hoarse cry.
      (5) Constipation.
      (6) Subnormal temperature.
      (7) Poor muscle tone and short, stubby extremities.
      (8) Thick, coarse, dry hair.

(9) Thick protruding tongue causing feeding difficulties, that is, infant has difficulty swallowing and takes a long time to eat.

(10) Slow motor and mental development and lack of interest in environment.

(11) Umbilical hernia.

b. Diagnosis—
(1) Clinical manifestations.
(2) Thyroid function tests.

c. Treatment—
(1) Oral administration of desiccated thyroid as replacement for deficient thyroid hormone.
(2) Untreated child becomes a mentally deficient dwarf; treatment results in normal growth and development if instituted early, although child may still be slightly retarded.

d. Nursing goals and implementation—
(1) Administer thyroid as ordered and observe for toxic effects.
   (a) Tachycardia.
   (b) Cramps.
   (c) Diarrhea and vomiting.
   (d) Elevated temperature.
   (e) Excitability, hyperactivity.
(2) Provide well-balanced diet with special attention to intake of iron, vitamin D, and roughage (see Appendix A).

2. Cystic fibrosis—believed to be hereditary as recessive trait, more often occurring in white males; the secretions of exocrine glands are viscous and tenacious, affecting mainly pulmonary, gastrointestinal, and sweat gland functioning; thick mucus plugs in the bronchi and bronchioles cause overinflation of lungs and atelectasis, leading to infections and fibrotic changes in the lungs; thick mucus also plugs the pancreatic ducts, preventing pancreatic enzymes from entering the small intestines and causing impairment of digestion—of fats, in particular.

a. Diagnostic test—
(1) Sweat test.
(2) Stool test for trypsin.

b. Assessment—
(1) Infant's skin tastes salty when kissed because secretions contain excessive amount of salt.
(2) Coughing and wheezing.
(3) Recurrent pulmonary infection.

(4) Failure to gain weight despite voracious appetite caused by impaired digestion.
(5) Stools bulky and foul smelling due to lack of digestive enzymes in small intestine.
(6) Protruding abdomen (caused by meconium ileus, a plug of meconium blocking lumen of small intestine) and thin extremities.

c. Treatment goals—
(1) Administration of pancreatic enzymes with meals, pancreatin (Viokase) or pancrelipase capsules (Cotazym), for example.
(2) Broad-spectrum antibiotics for prophylaxis.
(3) Expectorants to thin bronchial mucus secretions.
(4) Bronchodilators to increase width of bronchial tubes to allow greater passage of air into lungs.

d. Nursing goals and implementation—
(1) Administer pancreatic enzymes immediately prior to or with feedings to replace absent pancreatic enzymes—amount of enzyme given is determined by amount of fat in diet.
(2) Diet:
   (a) High-calorie, high-protein, low-fat diet, as absorption of food is incomplete.
   (b) Water-soluble vitamins (fat absorption is affected).
   (c) Increased salt intake during hot weather to prevent salt depletion because of sweat gland problems.
(3) Assist in IPPB therapy and postural drainage to aid in clearing secretions from respiratory tract.
(4) Teach breathing exercises to assist in prevention of lung disease and to increase capacity.
(5) Assist in parental teaching:
   (a) Genetic counseling (1 in 4 chance of inheriting disease with each pregnancy).
   (b) Care and use of IPPB equipment and postural drainage technique.
   (c) How to cope with insecure, frightened child.

3. Celiac disease—an inborn error of metabolism of wheat and rye products, characterized by chronic intestinal malabsorption causing malnutrition; commonly diagnosed about 6 months of age or after child begins ingesting grains.
   a. Assessment—
      (1) Progressive malnutrition symptoms; similar to cystic fibrosis.
      (2) Foul, bulky, greasy stools because of malabsorption of food.
      (3) Anorexia, general malnutrition.
      (4) Chronic diarrhea and abdominal distension.
      (5) Celiac crisis, which is an emergency, life-threatening complication.
          (a) Causes—upper respiratory infection, ingestion of gluten, prolonged fasting, infection.
          (b) Signs/symptoms—vomiting, large watery stools, drowsy, restless, increased sweating, extremely cold, signs of metabolic acidosis.
   b. Diagnosis—
      (1) Stool test for fat excretion.
      (2) Blood studies.
      (3) Peroral jejunal biopsy is definitive test.
   c. Treatment is by dietary means—
      (1) No wheat, oats, barley, or rye products or foodstuffs, gluten-free diet.
      (2) Add foods slowly and one at a time to observe effect.
      (3) High-protein, high-calorie, low-fat, low-residue, and starch-free foods.
   d. Nursing goals and implementation—
      (1) Follow prescribed diet calculations, as suggested in treatment section, precisely and record accurately any reaction to diet.
      (2) Use preventive measures to avoid infections and prevent celiac crisis.
          (a) Avoid exposure.
          (b) Keep child warm and dry.
      (3) Note any changes in behavior and intervene appropriately:
          (a) Whining or crying.
          (b) Irritability or restlessness.
      (4) Involve parents in care and teach diet and signs/symptoms of celiac crises.
4. PKU (phenylketonuria)—a recessively transmitted, inborn error of metabolism of phenylalanine caused by lack of an enzyme (phenylalanine hydroxylase); phenylalanine is one of the amino acids in protein; the substance collects in the blood of affected infants after one or two days of milk feedings.
   a. Diagnosis—definitive test is blood phenylalanine.
   b. Assessment—
      (1) High level of blood phenylalanine (correlated later with level of mental retardation).
      (2) Urine contains products of unmetabolized phenylalanine substance verified by a Phenistex test (impregnated paper).
      (3) Signs of mental retardation by age 2 years.
      (4) Child is usually blond and blue-eyed because of interference with normal development of pigment.
      (5) Eczema.
      (6) Convulsions.
   c. Treatment—
      (1) Diet—free of lactose (low-protein and no milk), not very palatable and quite expensive.
      (2) Irreparable damage occurs if child is not treated by *6 months* of age; diet therapy useless after *2 years* of age.
   d. Nursing goals and implementation—
      (1) Explain genetic inheritance to parents (1 out of 4) (see *Cystic fibrosis*).
      (2) Be certain blood and urine tests are done on infants.
      (3) Refer to dietitian and assist in selection of diet.

5. **Respiratory conditions**
   A. Croup:
      1. Analysis of cause-pathophysiology—
         a. Epiglottitis—inflammatory disease of the epiglottis; life-threatening.
         b. Laryngotracheitis—inflammatory disease of vocal cords and trachea.
      2. Assessment—
         a. Epiglottis:
            (1) Mucous membranes of glottis and epiglottis appear red and swollen.
            (2) Airway partially or totally obstructed by inflammation and edema.
            (3) Severe inspiratory stridor.
            (4) Hoarseness.

(5) Elevated temperature (104 F).

(6) Cyanosis.

b. Laryngotracheitis:

(1) Early characteristic symptom—inspiratory stridor.

(2) Slightly elevated temperature (below 102 F).

(3) Cyanosis.

(4) Child restless and frightened.

B. Bronchiolitis—an infection of bronchioles and involves a generalized inflammation of respiratory mucosa, with tenacious exudate in brochiol lumens.

1. Analysis of cause-pathophysiology—

a. Infection or virus.

b. Occurs under age 1 year with peak age of 6 months, mostly in winter and early spring.

c. Air enters alveoli during inspiration; orifice closes, trapping air during expiration, causing atelectasis and expiratory wheezing.

2. Assessment—

a. Expiratory wheezing and sternal retractions.

b. Nonproductive cough.

c. Dyspnea.

d. Cyanosis.

e. Lethargy with fever and restlessness due to oxygen hunger.

C. Bronchopneumonia—

1. Analysis of cause-pathophysiology:

a. Caused by bacteria or virus.

b. Inflammation of the bronchi with exudate formation.

2. Assessment:

a. Anorexia.

b. Vomiting and diarrhea.

c. Cyanosis.

d. Increased pulse and respirations with retractions.

e. Progressive respiratory distress (dyspnea).

f. Sudden high fever and productive cough.

3. Nursing goals and implementation in respiratory conditions:

a. Note respiratory rate and pattern to detect impending airway obstruction.

b. Note and record presence of cyanosis. Monitor temperature.

c. Place child in croupette—to provide cool, humidified environment with oxygen, if ordered, to alleviate anoxia, liquefy secretions and ease respirations.

d. Maintain adequate hydration via IV if in respiratory distress or small sips of *clear liquid* if in no acute distress (use cup or straw).

e. Record amount and specific gravity of urine to determine hydration.

f. Keep emergency equipment available for intubation and tracheostomy.

g. Reposition frequently and provide postural drainage as necessary—head down, on side.

h. Sit up in semi-Fowler's position for comfort and ease of breathing.

i. Allow child to conserve energy by resting and by adjusting environment.

j. Keep constant vigilance on child and promote feelings of security—talk to child and give child comforting toy as appropriate.

k. Instruct parent to take child in bathroom, if croup (laryngotracheitis) occurs at home, turn on hot-water faucets, and close door to provide wet, steamy environment to relieve edema.

l. Place in croupette—avoid fatigue; no sharp toys.

6. Skin conditions

A. Infantile eczema:

1. Analysis of cause-pathophysiology—

a. Usually a common early sign of allergy (onset—2 to 6 months of age); 50% develop hayfever and asthma later.

b. Inflammatory dermatosis.

c. Most common cause in infancy is cow's milk, eggs.

d. Spontaneous remission usually occurs at 3 years of age.

2. Assessment—

a. Erythematous, papular, weeping lesions involving epidermis due to dilatation of capillaries.

b. Oozing and crusting of lesions.

c. Pruritus, often accompanied by secondary infection.

d. Irritable child.

e. Unaffected area dry and rough.

3. Nursing goals and implementation—

a. Utilize measures to keep child from scratching lesions—prevent irritation and further infection.

(1) Protective devices—elbow or jacket restraints and cotton mitts.

(2) Trimmed nails.

(3) Soft toys.

(4) Medication, as prescribed, usually chloral hydrate, benadryl, or Periacton.

(5) Avoid woolen clothing or blankets.

b. Bathe using prescribed method—*do not use soap* because of allergic response. Tepid water with cornstarch to decrease itching.

c. Use soaks, paste, and coal tar, as prescribed.

d. Loosen crusts with prescribed mineral oil.

e. Help child adhere to dietary regimen, which is usually an elimination diet (all foods stopped, one new food every two or three days; observe for reaction—hives, further eczema, or itching, for example); usually no milk, wheat, or eggs.

f. Protect child from sources of infection; place child in protective isolation if necessary.

g. Provide play activities—reading stories or using puppets.

h. Avoid immunizations of live vaccines to child or siblings because of likelihood of overwhelming reaction.

B. Oral thrush:

1. Analysis of cause-pathophysiology—

   a. Caused by *Candida albicans.*

   b. Fungus infection of mouth or throat.

   c. Often contracted during birth via infected vagina.

2. Assessment—

   a. Small white patches on tongue, gums, or oral mucous membranes.

   b. Dry mouth.

   c. Fever may be present.

   d. No pain noted.

   e. Most important differentiation—patches rinse away if they are milk particles but will bleed when scraped if fungus.

3. Nursing goals and implementation—

   a. Look for signs/symptoms in high-risk patients.

      (1) Infants who are ill.

      (2) Infants receiving antibiotics.

      (3) Infants with cleft lip and palate.

   b. Prevent spread of disease.

      (1) Careful handwashing.

      (2) Proper cleansing of nipples.

      (3) Apply medication, as ordered.

      (4) Prevent infant from putting fingers or toys in mouth.

7. *Nephrotic syndrome*

A. Analysis of pathophysiology and etiology:

1. Etiology unknown; occurs more often in males.

2. A complex renal disorder with multiple and varied pathological manifestations and causes.

3. Increased glomerular permeability to plasma protein, which results in massive urinary protein loss.

B. Assessment:

1. Generalized edema—child retains sodium as homeostatic adjustment to hypoproteinemia.

2. Marked proteinemia.

3. Hematuria.

4. Hypertension.

5. Average age 1½–3 years at onset.

C. Treatment goals:

1. Reduce excretion of urinary protein.

2. Prevent infection.

3. Administer steroids to reduce edema and proteinuria.

   a. Exact mode of action is unknown.

   b. Prednisone is choice due to toleration and less sodium retention and potassium loss.

   c. Tapered dosage.

4. Symptomatic care.

D. Nursing goals and implementation:

1. Acute phase—bedrest.

2. Edema—

   a. Skin care.

   b. Daily weights.

   c. Strict reporting of intake and output.

   d. Administration of prescribed diuretics.

3. Decrease chances of infection, especially upper respiratory.

   a. Turn frequently when on bedrest.

   b. Protect from others with URI.

   c. Monitor vital signs.

   d. Provide warm, dry environment.

4. Administer prescribed steroids.

   a. Be alert to diuresis 10–12 days after administration.

   b. Prepare for Cushing's syndrome (weight gain, acne, hirsutism, hypertension, infection) by explaining to child and family; reassure of reversibility of symptoms.

5. Diet:

   a. High protein because of nitrogen balance and tissue-wasting due to heavy proteinuria.

   b. High potassium because of loss in potassium and ammonia (cations) in urine.

   c. Low sodium, because all sodium is

retained as edema fluid; but needs some sodium since edema is an attempt at homeostasis.

6. Counsel family that treatment and syndrome are very long term, reoccurring; no short-term cure.

8. **Child abuse**—the nonaccidental abuse of a child, usually by person caring for child; may be physical or emotional abuse.

A. Analysis of causes:
  1. May be result of disciplinary action.
  2. Child may not fulfill need of caretaker.
  3. Abuser may be under much stress and use child to vent feeling of frustration.
  4. Abusive parents—any socioeconomic group; they have often been abused themselves as children; loners, no affiliations with groups; immature emotional responses.

B. Assessment:
  1. Incidence—
     a. History is incompatible with extent of injury.
     b. Victim—child is most likely under 3 years of age, possibly under 6 months.
  2. How diagnosed—
     a. General characteristics of physical neglect.
     b. History of previous emergency-room visits, usually at more than one hospital.
     c. Type of lesions:
        (1) Welts.
        (2) Bruises (may appear from specific causes, but usually are not consistent with history given or type of accident reported).
        (3) Wringer fractures caused by twisting or "wringing" extremity.
        (4) Burns, especially with characteristic quality, such as those caused by cigarettes.
     d. Fractures in different stages of healing (X-ray examination).
     e. Child appears withdrawn; monotonous crying; no or little emotional response.
     f. Child becomes happier and no new lesions are present upon hospitalization.

C. Nursing goals and implementation:
  1. Nurses are bound by law to report suspected cases of child abuse to law enforcement authorities.
  2. Be alert to possible abuse in high-risk families—
     a. Unwanted pregnancy.
     b. Lack of knowledge of child development.

     c. Deficient child-rearing models.
     d. Lack of attachment.
        (1) Prematurity of infant or child with defect, especially.
        (2) Immature or retarded parent.
     e. Many stresses on family.
  3. Take a thorough history from person bringing child to hospital.
  4. Avoid direct confrontation or accusation of caretaker.
  5. Inspect child carefully upon admission and note any lesions (as listed previously, usually bruises) and state of healing.
  6. Observe and record caretaker-child relationship—eye contact, comforting measures, manner of talking (gentle or gruff), and body contact, for example.
  7. Assign one nurse per shift to care for child in hospital to establish relationship of trust.
  8. Foster relationship with caretaker so guidance and help may be provided.
  9. Teach caretaker principles of normal growth and development; many caretakers attribute attitudes, thoughts, and behaviors to the child that are beyond the child's developmental capabilities.
  10. Refer caretakers for help as appropriate—Parents Anonymous, public health nurse, or counseling.

9. **Sudden infant death syndrome (SIDS), or crib death**

A. Analysis of cause-pathophysiology:
  1. Exact cause unknown—most common cause of death in first year of life (excluding first week); 1 out of 300.
  2. Various theories include suffocation caused by large thymus, cardiac arrhythmia resulting from inappropriate diving reflex (apneic spells), or abnormal respiratory center, which does not respond appropriately.
  3. Death is caused by occluded airway while child is sleeping; death is silent.
  4. Occurs more often in premature infants.

B. Assessment:
  1. An apparently normal infant is found dead in crib.
  2. Usually between 2 and 3 months of age, but within first year: rare before 3 weeks or after 8 months.
  3. Often have history of prior viral infection and low birth weight, and often from lower socioeconomic group.
  4. Most often occurs in late fall or winter.

C. Nursing goals and implementation:
1. Be aware of nature of SIDS—sudden, unpredictable, unpreventable.
2. Anticipate parental feelings of guilt and provide factual information to parents.
3. Counsel family that SIDS is not contagious and has no known hereditary causes.
4. Consider referral to community nurse or parents' group.

10. Failure to thrive (maternal deprivation)

A. Definition: Children who, without apparent organic cause, are below the third percentile in physical growth; this is secondary to the lack of emotional and sensory stimulation from the primary parent.
B. Analysis of data:
1. Possible etiology—congenital heart defects, UTI, neurologic disorders, renal insufficiency, malabsorption syndrome, and endocrine problem; severe malnutrition (e.g., kwashiorkor, marasmus).
2. Parental deprivation may be the cause in 10% of the situations.
3. Characteristics of families—
   a. Emotionally detached primary parent who is unable to fulfill nurturing role due to:
      (1) Own deprived background.
      (2) Child who is difficult to relate to.
      (3) Inability to pick up cues from child seeking attention.
      (4) Perceived need to turn away to other activities.
      (5) Inability to tell cry of hunger from cry of pain, etc.
   b. Multiple-problem families: emotional, social, economic, and marital.
   c. Lack of knowledge of age-appropriate toys or expected behavior at a given developmental age.
   d. Mothers who do not have support from mate or baby's father and who lead solitary lives with little outside relief from child care.
4. Psychologic damage is severe if emotional starvation occurs before age 3.
C. Assessment:
1. Signs of malnutrition and delayed development.
2. History of sleep and feeding disturbances and irritability.
3. Body language—
   a. Rigid, unresponsive to cuddling and holding; or floppy like a rag doll.
   b. No eye-to-eye contact; slow to smile or respond to another person.
   c. No signs of comfort or pleasure when given attention.
D. Nursing goals and implementation:
1. Attend to physical needs while hospitalized for diagnostic tests to rule out organic causes; protect from exposure to other children with infections, as child is vulnerable while debilitated and/or malnourished.
2. Help parents learn new ways of relating to and caring for the child; meet their needs for emotional nurturance.
   a. Teach parents about child's physical care, developmental skills, and emotional needs via example and demonstration; allow time to learn.
   b. Give opportunity to talk about own lives and feelings about child.
   c. Promote self-respect and instill confidence by positive reinforcement.
3. Provide appropriate *developmental* stimulation, after administering the Denver Developmental Screening Test (DDST), which gives approximate age for present achievement in gross and fine motor skills, social adaptiveness, and language.
4. Reverse cycle of frustration-dissatisfaction—
   a. Provide consistent, patient, and understanding primary nurse for all three shifts (with relief for time off).
   b. Provide additional time for bathing, feeding, rocking, and cuddling; encourage eye-to-eye contact, tactile stimulation, and vocalization.
E. Evaluation of outcome:
1. Weight gain after a period of adequate nurturing/parenting.
2. Negative lab results, ruling out systemic or congenital problems that may cause growth failure.
3. Improvement in level of developmental retardation after a period of time of appropriate stimulation.
4. Diminishing clinical signs of deprivation when placed in a more nurturing environment.

11. Hernia

A. Inguinal:
1. Protrusion of abdominal structures into inguinal or scrotal area.
2. More common in boys; noticeable 3 to 4 months of age when increased activity causes protrusion on crying or straining.

3. Danger—strangulation when protrusion does not retract into abdominal cavity.
4. Treatment—
   a. Direct pressure and ice pack.
   b. Surgical intervention.
5. Explain procedure to parents and teach them how to keep dressing clean until wound heals.

B. Umbilical or navel:
1. Imperfect closure or weakness of umbilical ring.
2. Appears at 6 months of age and disappears spontaneously by 5 years of age.
3. If large hernia or strangulation occurs, surgical intervention may be indicated.
4. Parents should be instructed that taping and use of binder or coin is not necessary and may cause infection or irritation of skin.

Part B / PRESCHOOLER—AGE 3 TO 5 YEARS

NORMAL GROWTH AND DEVELOPMENT OF THE PRESCHOOLER

1. The 3-year-old

A. Assessment of physical development:
1. Height—grows 5 to 7 cm (2 to 2½ inches) per year; 91 cm (36 inches).
2. Weight—gains less than 2 kg (5 lb); 15 kg (32 lb).
3. Vision—gross testing is 20/30.

B. Assessment of behavior patterns:
1. Motor development—
   a. Can brush teeth.
   b. Can wash hands.
   c. Can eat with fork.
   d. Can button.
   e. Dresses self with supervision.
   f. Tries to draw a picture.
   g. Copies a circle or cross.
   h. Imitates a three-block bridge.
   i. Pours fluid from a pitcher.
   j. Helps dry dishes and dusts.
   k. Climbs and jumps well.
   l. Can hit large pegs in a pegboard with a hammer.
   m. Can go to the toilet.
2. Socialization, vocalization, and mental development—
   a. Can tolerate short separation without undue anxiety.
   b. Exaggerates, boasts, and tattles on others.
   c. Talks with imaginary companion.
   d. Uses language fluently and confidently.
   e. Knows first and last name.
   f. Refers to self as I.
   g. Can identify longer of two lines.
   h. Can name figures in a picture.
   i. Understands simple explanations of cause and effect.
   j. Cautious about common dangers.

C. Nursing goals and implementation:
1. Goals: provide appropriate play activities—
   a. Peer-group play.
   b. Toys and games—record player, nursery rhymes, housekeeping toys, tricycles, cars, wagons, blocks, blackboard and chalk, easel and brushes, clay, fingerpaints, outside toys (sandbox or swing), books, and drum.
2. Goals: provide guidance—
   a. Give child small errands to do around house, such as dusting or drying silverware.
   b. Expand world with trips to zoo or market or take child out to lunch.
   c. Aid toileting by dressing child in simple clothing so child can go to the toilet with little trouble; remind child to go occasionally to prevent accidents.
   d. Set realistic limits, as child may delay bedtime by ritualistic behaviors; use night light and/or security toy or doll.

2. The 4-year-old

A. Assessment of physical development:
1. Weight—16 to 18 kg (34 to 40 lb), average.
2. Height—approximately 102 cm (42 inches).
3. Vision—gross testing is 20/20.

B. Assessment of behavior patterns:
1. Motor development—
   a. Hops two or more times.
   b. Walks upstairs without grasping handrail.
   c. Walks backwards.
   d. Uses scissors to cut out picture.
   e. Throws a ball overhand.
   f. Copies a square and a triangle.
   g. Can lace shoes.
   h. Dresses and undresses with little assistance.

2. Socialization, vocalization, and mental development—
   a. May have imaginary companion.
   b. Can go on errands outside of home.
   c. Is obedient and reliable.
   d. Has a sense of order.
   e. Is developing conscience, which influences behavior.
   f. Has increased self-confidence.
   g. Is cooperative in playing games.
   h. Can name three objects in succession.
   i. Knows primary colors.
   j. May run away from home.
   k. Asks many questions.
   l. Has vocabulary of 1500 words.
   m. Knows own age.
   n. Has poor space perception.
C. Nursing goals and implementation:
   1. Goal: provide appropriate play activities—
      a. Use costumes.
      b. Give rope to jump and skip.
      c. Plan group play and cooperative projects.
      d. Offer simple puzzles.
   2. Goal: provide guidance—
      a. Provide quiet time after lunch in lieu of afternoon nap.
      b. Prepare for kindergarten by exposing child to other children and allowing child to go on errands outside of home.
      c. Provide opportunities for group play—invite friends over or send child to preschool for half day several days a week.
      d. Make up stories.
      e. Allow child to select own food at table and serve self; food jags are common but harmless—will soon pass if attention is not drawn to them.

3. **The 5-year-old**
A. Assessment of physical development:
   1. Height—gains more in inches than pounds so appears taller and slimmer, 104 to 114 cm (43 to 45 inches).
   2. Weight—approximately 19 to 21 kg (42 to 44 lb).
   3. Posture—lordosis has disappeared.
B. Assessment of behavior patterns:
   1. Motor development—
      a. Begins to attempt riding two-wheel bike.
      b. Runs and plays games at same time.
      c. Can use hammer to hit nail on head.
      d. Can wash self without wetting clothes.
      e. Can rollerskate.
      f. Puts toys away neatly in box.
      g. Can fold paper diagonally.
      h. Can form some letters correctly.
      i. Prints first name and possibly some other words.
      j. Draws recognizable man or woman.
   2. Socialization, vocalization, and mental development—
      a. Likely to do what is expected.
      b. Takes some responsibility for actions.
      c. Interested in meaning of relatives (uncle and cousin, for example).
      d. Vocabulary of 2100 words.
      e. Talks constantly.
      f. Repeats syllables of 10 or more in sentence.
      g. Can name at least four colors.
      h. Can identify penny, nickel, and dime.
      i. Knows names of days of week, and week as unit of time.
      j. Views death as reversible process.
C. Nursing goals and implementation:
   1. Goals: provide appropriate play activities—
      a. Encourage play with other children.
      b. Play house; may begin to imitate firefighters and teachers.
      c. Give bicycle to ride.
      d. Play games involving large muscles.
      e. Have child tell you stories.
   2. Provide guidance—
      a. Start kindergarten.
      b. Allow opportunity for self-expression through talking or play activities.
      c. Adult supervision, as is interested in conforming to rules and regulations.
      d. Avoid giving responsibility to care for younger children. While children of this age are protective of younger children, they are *not* capable of caring for them and should not be given that responsibility.

SPECIAL CONCERNS OF THE PRESCHOOLER

1. **Response to illness and hospitalization**—3 to 5 years.
A. Assessment of discomfort or pain:
   1. Crying.
   2. Irritable.
   3. Elevated temperature.
   4. Decreased appetite.

5. Lethargy.
6. Prostration.
7. Holding affected area.
8. Verbalizations, such as "my tummy hurts."
9. Regressive behaviors.

B. Assessment of reaction to stage of illness:
1. Initial illness or hospitalization—
   a. Expected coping or adaptive behaviors—rejects everyone except maternal figure, cries loudly, physically aggressive, occasionally withdrawn (not wanting to play), and has fantasies about illness and procedures.
   b. Maladaptive behaviors stem from feeling of abandonment—withdrawal from everyone, monotonous moaning, completely passive or excessively aggressive, and regressive.
2. Prolonged hospitalization and convalescence—
   a. Expected coping or adaptive behaviors—some regression to earlier behaviors, that is, bed-wetting and baby talk; demands attention; wants needs met immediately; and may be difficult to handle.
   b. Maladaptive behaviors arising from lack of trust of anyone meaningful to child—complete rejection of parents, behaviors that do not return to normal, and superficial relations with everyone.
   c. Nursing goals and implementation:
      (1) Since child views illness as punishment for some wrong, real or imagined, nurse must explain illness or hospitalization to child, emphasizing that child is *not* bad.
      (2) Involve child in peer-group activity.
      (3) Meet needs or demands as soon as possible, since child is insecure in new or different surroundings, but help child set limits on behavior, for example, "You can go to the playroom after I put on your new dressing."
      (4) Establish rapport and trust by providing continuity of caretakers; if this is done on admission, most positive behaviors will be maximized and negative behaviors avoided.

2. Nutrition and feeding—3 to 5 years.
A. Calorie requirements:
   1. Age 3 to 4 years—1400 cal/24 hours.
   2. Age 4 to 6 years—1600 cal/24 hours.
B. Normal diet:

1. Transition from baby food to regular diet—
   a. Keep variety of nutritious finger foods on hand for snacks, such as cheese, fruit, raw vegetables, crackers, pieces of frankfurter. (Include raw vegetables and fruits to aid muscle development via chewing.)
   b. Allow child to be messy as normal part of learning to eat by self.
   c. Since calorie intake needs are lower and growth is slower, allow child to eat less.
   d. Handle normal food jags by ignoring.
2. Call child to meal at least 15 minutes before meal is served to allow time for toilet, handwashing, and settling down from active play.
3. Keep mealtimes pleasant and free from discipline and arguments.
4. Avoid using desserts as rewards.
5. Serve small portions to entice the child to eat more; large portions may appear overwhelming.
6. Accept the fact that child has preferences and offer acceptable substitutes.
7. Do not force a child to eat, as it usually results in rebellious behavior.

3. Immunizations—3 to 5 years.
A. Age 4 to 6 years—DPT and TOPV.
B. Tuberculin test every one to two years.

4. Safety measures—3 to 5 years.
A. Keep medicines, gasoline, kerosene, paint products, and *matches* locked up.
B. Store tools and equipment in a safe place.
C. Check play area for attractive hazards, such as old refrigerators, deep holes, construction, trash heaps, and rickety buildings.
D. Check on child's activities frequently.
E. Teach child safe ways to handle tools and kitchen equipment.
F. Teach child danger of water and start swimming instructions.
G. Have child learn rules and dangers of traffic.
H. Teach child danger of open flames.
I. Teach child not to go with strangers.

5. Fears—3 to 5 years.
A. Most often between 2 and 6 years of age.
B. Child's fear is real to the child—avoid laughing, strict punishment, or leaving child alone to "get over it."
C. Remain with child until acute fright has subsided, then divert child's attention with toy or talk of something pleasant.

D. Common fears:
1. Animals—
   a. In time, child will see that the animal is harmless.
   b. Hold the animal and allow child to touch, but *not* during child's acute fright.
2. Dark—
   a. Part of normal separation anxiety—offer favorite toy or blanket as comfort during bedtime.
   b. Use night light or leave door open and talk loudly in another room to assure child of another's presence in the house.

6. Thumb-sucking
A. Many children suck their thumb prior to going to sleep and should be considered normal.
1. Way of comforting self.
2. Lonely just after being put to bed.
B. Child may suck thumb when nervous or frustrated, which is not a serious problem unless persists into school age and occurs day and night.
C. Need to assess child's behavior patterns:
1. If there is a new sibling, may need reassurance of love and self-confidence.
2. May need companionship such as preschool or kindergarten.
3. May feel need for more attention if change in household. (Mother returns to work, house guests occupy mother's time, etc.)
4. May be bored and need more play outlets (out of doors, with others, new skills to learn such as feeding, dressing self).
D. Parents need to be counseled as to reasons why child may be thumb-sucking; suggest alternate activities.
E. Parents need to ignore actual thumb-sucking and recognize their own anxieties.
F. Harsh measures such as spanking, chemical on hands, mitts, bandaging thumbs may work but often lead to other symptoms of nervousness such as nail-biting, enuresis, stuttering, school failure.
G. Malocclusion: a problem if continuous thumb-sucking after 7–9 years of age.

7. Sibling rivalry
A. Most common when sibling is same sex and between 2 and 4 years old.
B. Behaviors seen: *regressive,* such as wetting pants when already toilet-trained, wanting to suck bottle when already weaned; *aggressive,* such as hitting new baby.

C. Interventions:
1. Allow older child to help in baby's care.
2. Grant special privileges to increase status.
3. Set limits; do not allow physical attacks on baby.

8. Masturbation
A. Normal exploration and source of pleasure in infants and young children. Not a manifestation of immature sexuality.
B. Masturbation is not physically harmful, but cultural values will often dictate acceptance or nonacceptance of masturbation as regular practice.
C. If child masturbates frequently and regularly, may be handled similarly to thumb-sucking or nail-biting, as may be reaction to frustration or anxiety. Ignore or distract older child who masturbates in public.

9. Telling lies
A. Between 2 and 6 years of age, reality and fantasy are not clearly delineated, so child incorporates fantasies into stories.
1. Do not view it as deliberate lying.
2. Use humor and let child know that adult appreciates and recognizes child's game of pretending.
B. Older child may consciously lie to cover shame and guilt over misdeed, to compensate for feelings of weakness or inferiority, or because of parental example.
1. Let child know you are aware of lie and help child clarify problem and find better solutions.
2. Praise child for capabilities and encourage to build self-confidence and feeling of self-worth.
3. Avoid telling child white lies or having child tell lies for you; do not make promises that cannot be or are not intended to be fulfilled.

10. Swearing
A. Assessment of stages:
1. Age 2–3 years—lavatory words are expression of interest in playing with dirt.
2. Age 3–5 years—learns words from other children and adults and uses them when angry or as means of upsetting parents.
3. Later childhood and adolescence—uses swearing as means of pretending to be more grown up or of compensating for feelings of ignorance of secrets of adulthood.
B. Nursing goals and implementation:
1. *Avoid* overreacting, emotional appeals, moral lectures, or strict discipline.

2. Attempt to devalue the emotional meaning of words—
   a. Change subject to divert attention if small child.
   b. Repeat word with indifference and lack of emotion.
   c. Give substitute word for child to master, such as delicious or atrocious.

11. Stuttering
A. Common 2–4 years old; more often among boys.
B. Child has not mastered thought transference to speech.
C. Nursing goals and implementation:
   1. Do not draw attention to stuttering; child may not notice; attention accentuates stuttering and problem persists as speech pattern.
   2. Reassure parents that there is no correlation between stuttering and intellect.
   3. Do not interrupt or finish sentence for child, as leads to insecurity and stuttering persists.

CONDITIONS AND DISEASE ENTITIES OF THE PRESCHOOLER

1. Sickle cell disease—severe chronic hemolytic anemia.
A. Analysis of pathophysiology/etiology/incidence:
   1. Genetically determined, inherited as recessive disorder, and more prevalent in Black and Mediterranean races (Figure 4–1).
   2. Red blood cells sickle (shape of crescent) under low oxygen concentration.
   3. Pathologic changes result from increased blood viscosity and increased red blood cell destruction.
   4. Present in 1:400 Black Americans.
B. Assessment:
   1. Sporadic and variable severity of symptoms, depending on severity of disease.
   2. Anorexia.
   3. Paleness.
   4. Weakness.
   5. Pain in abdomen, legs, and arms due to occlusion of small vessels by sickled red cells.
   6. Swelling of joints.
   7. Jaundice caused by increased red blood cell destruction.
   8. Growth retardation.
   9. Delayed sexual maturation.
   10. Thrombocytic crisis—

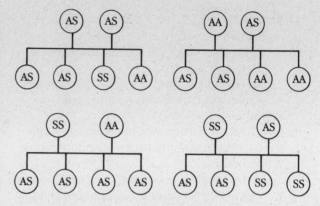

AA = person with normal hemoglobin.
AS = person with sickle cell trait; asymptomatic.
SS = person with sickle cell disease/anemia.

FIGURE 4–1.
These charts show the chances in four of *each pregnancy* for children to inherit A and S hemoglobin from their parents. Nurses may use this type of chart in counseling.

   a. Distal ischemia resulting from occluded small vessels.
   b. Splenomegaly and abdominal pain.
   c. Cerebral occlusion, causing blindness, strokes, and hemiplegia.
   11. Sequestration crisis—
   a. Blood pools in liver and spleen.
   b. Circulatory collapse and death.
C. Nursing goals and implementation:
   1. Prevent sickling—
   a. Promote tissue oxygenation—avoid strenuous exercise and prevent infection.
   b. Promote hydration—encourage adequate fluid intake, avoid overheating and resultant fluid loss.
   2. Encourage quiet activities such as reading, puzzles, and table games.
   3. Provide emotional support to child and parents and factual information based on child's level of development and parent's knowledge of physiology and prognosis (no known cure).
   4. Offer preventive education: screening programs, genetic counseling.

2. Hemophilia—a congenital blood dyscrasia characterized by absence or malfunction of blood-clotting factor.
A. Analysis of cause-pathophysiology:
   1. Hereditary, sex-linked, recessive disease that appears in men but is transmitted by women.

2. Types and clotting factor involved—
   a. Type A (classic)—VIII (antihemophilic factor).
   b. Type B (Christmas disease)—IX.
   c. Type C—XI.
3. Type A and Type B comprise 75% of all hemophilia.

B. Assessment:
1. Child bruises easily.
2. Prolonged bleeding from lacerations or mucous membranes.
3. Intramuscular hematomas from minor trauma.
4. Hemarthrosis causing pain, swelling, and limited movement of affected joint.
5. Repeated hemorrhages produce degenerative changes—osteoporosis and muscle atrophy.

C. Treatment:
1. Immediate or prophylactic (presurgical procedures)—whole blood or plasma (freshly drawn or frozen), contains clotting factor, especially Type VIII, which is not stable for long at regular room or refrigerated temperatures.
2. Administration of cryoprecipitate is often treatment of choice.
3. Splinting—decrease excessive motion and further acute bleeding; long-term use causes ankylosis and atrophy.

D. Nursing goals and implementation:
1. Provide emergency treatment for bleeding wound—cleansing, applying pressure and ice, and immobilization.
2. Alleviate pain—
   a. Administer prescribed medication, avoid aspirin.
   b. Avoid manipulation.
   c. Use bed cradle.
3. Prevent further bleeding—oral medications, no sharp toys or rough play.
4. Prevent permanent deformities and crippling—passive exercise and gentle massage.
5. Focus on main concern of parents—avoid overprotection of child.
6. Be aware of slow development due to curtailed activities; encourage independence.
7. Offer genetic counseling; identify carrier offspring.

3. **Skin conditions—burns** (refer also to Unit 5, Nursing Care of the Acutely or Chronically Ill Adult).
A. Analysis of cause-pathophysiology:
1. Causes vary and include the following—
   a. Hot water.
   b. Open flames.
   c. Electrical burns.
   d. Caustic acid or alkali, as in household cleaners.
   e. Chemicals.
   f. Child abuse.
   g. Smoke inhalation.
2. Types—
   a. First degree—superficial epidermis (slight edema, red, and painful).
   b. Second degree—epidermis, intradermal (very edematous, red, blistered, moist, painful, and regenerates without grafting).
   c. Third degree—dermis, subdermal, fat, muscle, and bone (marked edema; white, dry, or charred; may or may not be painful; and will not regenerate without graft).
3. Physiologic effects—
   a. Dilatation of capillaries, increased permeability.
   b. Plasma to interstitial fluid shift, resulting in edema around burn area.
   c. *Fluid and electrolyte* imbalance—decreased potassium and increased water loss due to damage of evaporative water barrier.
   d. Decreased efficiency of temperature control due to water loss.
   e. Skin is first line of defense against infections; burn is a medium for bacterial, fungal, and viral invasions.
   f. *Circulatory changes*—RBC hemolysis, decreased cardiac output, and decreased blood volume.
   g. Increased cell volume—increased hematocrit.
   h. *Renal changes*—hypotension leads to renal perfusion and renal shutdown → decreased urinary output → increased urinary tract infections.
   i. Gastrointestinal changes—congested capillaries, acute gastric dilatation, paralytic ileus, and hemorrhagic gastritis ("coffee grounds" aspirant).

B. Assessment:
1. Immediate due to fluid shift.
   a. Appearance of burned area.
   b. Increased pulse rate.
   c. Decreased or subnormal temperature.
   d. Pallor.
   e. Low blood pressure.
2. Toxemia development after one to two days due

to reduction in blood volume and blocked capillaries.
   a. Fever.
   b. Rapid pulse.
   c. Cyanosis.
   d. Vomiting.
   e. Edema.
3. Respiratory-tract signs/symptoms—due to fluid shifts, when neck and face are burned.
   a. Dyspnea.
   b. Stridor.
   c. Rapid respirations.
4. Smoke inhalation after 6 to 48 hours—
   a. Pulmonary edema.
   b. Signs/symptoms of airway obstruction.
   c. Bronchiolitis.
C. Treatment:
1. First aid—*do not use ointments or salve.*
   a. Apply cold to burn.
   b. Cover burn with sterile dressing, clean cloth to prevent contamination and decrease pain by blocking air flow.
   c. Irrigate chemical burns.
   d. Cover child to prevent body heat loss.
   e. Transport to treatment facility for all burns except minor first-degree burns.
2. Open method—burn area exposed to maintain dry surface, form eschar, and decrease infection.
3. Closed method—burn area covered with dressings; dressings can be soaked in solution or applied dry after topical medication is applied to skin.
4. Topical agents—
   a. Silver nitrate—0.5% solution as a continuous wet soak in combination with large, bulky dressings.
   b. Mafenide (Sulfamylon)—"burn butter," applied in even coating to partial- and full-thickness burns following initial débridement.
   c. Gentamicin cream—specific effect against *Pseudomonas*, applied in even coating.
   d. 1% silver sulfadiazine—used in open, semiopen, and closed method; soothing; softens eschar, making débridement less painful.
D. Nursing goals and implementation:
1. Recognize signs/symptoms of shock and hypovolemia—thirst, vomiting, increased pulse, decreased blood pressure, and decreased urine output.

2. Administer oxygen via mask, tent, or catheter to combat anoxia.
3. Note urine output, which is most important sign of fluid balance.
4. Keep accurate intake and output record—circulatory overload is common complication three to five days after burn.
5. Prevent respiratory distress—suction secretions, provide humidified oxygen, cough, deep breathe, and position and turn child frequently.
6. Provide source of heat to maintain body temperature.
7. Observe vital signs for increased pulse and temperature, which are signs of infection.
8. Maintain sterility, "super-clean" environment, or reverse isolation to reduce or prevent infection.
9. Provide adequate nutrition via high-protein (usually three to four times normal), high-calorie diet (usually two times normal), as metabolic demands are greatly increased.
10. Use ingenuity to provide diversion and play for child—use puppets or act out stories.
11. Prevent contractures—keep in body alignment, active-passive ROM, use whirlpool, and splint extremities in position of function during sleep.

4. *Meningitis*—an inflammation of the meninges caused by a bacterial or viral organism.
A. Bacterial:
1. Preceded by febrile upper respiratory infection or otitis media.
2. Causative agents—*Hemophilus influenzae*, meningococcus, pneumococcus, *Streptococcus, Staphylococcus,* or *Escherichia coli.*
3. Assessment—chills, fever, vomiting, headache, stupor, convulsions, and opisthotonos (head and feet touch bed with body arched, caused by tetanic spasm).
B. Viral:
1. Causative agents include coxsackie virus B, echovirus, rubella, mumps, or herpes virus.
2. Assessment—fever, headache, vomiting, lethargy, stupor, and stiff neck.
3. Herpes virus type—rapid onset, severe rapid deterioration, brain damage, and death usually results.
C. Diagnosis—symptoms, culture of spinal fluid and nasopharyngeal material, lumbar puncture (increased CSF pressure and cloudy in bacterial).

D. Sequelae—subdural effusion, hydrocephalus, seizure disorders, impaired intelligence, and visual and hearing defects.

E. Treatment—IV medications; antibiotics if bacterial, symptomatic if viral.

F. Nursing goals and implementation:
1. Observe for convulsions and monitor vital signs for signs and symptoms of increased intracranial pressure.
2. Position flat in bed; on side if opisthotonos is present.
3. Provide quiet, restful environment.
4. Prevent spread of infection—isolation may not be utilized, but excretory precautions should be taken in viral type.
5. Ensure adequate hydration—offer fluids in ways not requiring sitting (straw, gelatin dessert, and popsicle).
6. Observe site for inflammation and infiltration—medications are toxic and irritating to vein.

5. **Tuberculosis**—in children, tuberculosis is considered a single disease entity with initial infection of tubercle bacillus, *Mycobacterium tuberculosis,* in the lungs and complications seen in all parts of the body.

A. Analysis of pathophysiology:
1. Bacillus inhaled through droplets, ingested, and enters through abrasion or mucous membranes.
2. Inflammatory area created by bacilli, primary focus.
3. Bacilli migrate through lymphatics.
4. Incubation two to ten weeks.

B. Assessment—diagnostic procedures:
1. Positive skin test indicating that child has been infected with tuberculosis bacillus.
   a. Mantoux test—0.1 ml; old tuberculin (OT), purified protein derivative (PPD), or tuberculin intradermally, results in 48 to 72 hours, 10 mm induration indicates positive reaction.
   b. Heaf test—PPD injected with gun (six punctures), three to seven days for results; appearance of four or more papules indicates positive reaction.
   c. Tine test—predipped OT pressed into skin, four tines, 48 to 72 hours, one to two papules 2 mm or larger indicates positive reaction.
2. Gastric lavage done after positive skin test—produces bacillus.

C. Treatment goal: arrest condition and prevent complications.
1. Isoniazid (INH)—penetrates cell membrane, moves freely into CSF, oral (usual) or intramuscular; neurotoxic.
2. Para-aminosalicylic acid (PAS)—bacteriostatic, oral; causes gastrointestinal disturbances.
3. Streptomycin SO_4—inhibits growth of tubercle bacillus, intramuscular, toxicity involves eighth cranial nerve.
4. INH and PAS frequently used in combination; streptomycin is used in severe forms, for example, miliary tuberculosis and tubercular meningitis.
5. Bacille Calmette-Guérin (BCG) vaccine—lasts ten years, given to child who lives with persons with tuberculosis, given only to child with negative skin test and negative chest X ray within previous two weeks; more effective than other tested vaccines.

D. Nursing goals and implementation:
1. Encourage bedrest as necessary for short period—play activities such as puppets, puzzles, and stories.
2. Do not isolate; child on medication and afebrile is not contagious.
3. Counteract anorexia by choosing favorite, high-nutrition foods (high-calorie, protein, calcium, and phosphorus).
4. *Important on discharge*—stress chemotherapy maintenance.
5. Instruct family of patient to have regular skin tests.
6. Discuss routine skin-testing of all children every year if negative.

E. Serious types:
1. Acute miliary tuberculosis—multiple tubercles develop due to bacilli lodging in capillaries; seen within two weeks on X ray; 100% mortality if untreated, lower with triple therapy.
2. Tubercular meningitis—bacilli in subarachnoid space; convulsion is first sign; 100% mortality unless treated with triple therapy; may still have residual neurologic damage (see *Meningitis*).

6. **Legg-Calvé-Perthes disease**—an aseptic necrosis of capital femoral epiphysis caused by disturbance of circulation to that area.

A. Analysis of cause-pathophysiology:

1. Unknown etiology, mostly boys 4 to 10 years old, white population.
2. Disease is self-limiting.
3. Stages—each lasts 9 to 12 months.
   a. Stage I, aseptic necrosis—femoral head necrotic, swelling of soft tissues, and widening of joint space.
   b. Stage II, revascularization—epiphysis fragmented and femoral head density increases.
   c. Stage III, reossification—femoral head reforms, new bone develops, and dead bone is removed and replaced with new bone.
   d. Stage IV, post recovery period—with treatment, complete recovery; without treatment, femoral head flattens; incongruity between femoral head and acetabulum remains; and degenerative changes occur later in life.
B. Assessment:
   1. Limping with pain in hip caused by synovitis.
   2. Referred pain to knee, front of thigh, and groin.
   3. Limited abduction and rotation of hip.
   4. Mild to moderate muscle spasm.
C. Treatment goals:
   1. Avoid weight-bearing on affected extremity, accomplished by braces, casting.
   2. Keep head of femur in acetabulum.
D. Nursing goals and implementation:
   1. Provide carts, wagons, and stretchers for mobility during long-term convalescence (two to five years) and restriction of movement by surgery, cast, or braces.
   2. Suggest activity as appropriate to maintain continued development of child while immobilized; encourage collections, crafts, art work.
   3. Teach techniques of skin care and provide opportunity for use and exercise of unaffected limb and upper extremities.
   4. Provide adequate nutrition, such as high-residue diet, since activity level decreased.
   5. Teach exercises for lungs—use blow bottles or blow up balloons.

7. Oncology
A. Wilms' tumor (nephroblastoma):
   1. Analysis of cause-pathophysiology—
      a. Unknown etiology; classified as embryoma.
      b. Malignant renal tumor.
      c. Metastasis is a complication through ve-
nous extension or lymphatic channels to any organ; most common is to lungs.
   2. Etiology and incidence—
      a. Occurs 1:10,000 children.
      b. Peak age 3 years old.
      c. Kidney most commonly affected.
   3. Assessment—
      a. Firm abdominal mass.
      b. Abdominal pain occurs as tumor grows and causes pressure, which in turn causes constipation, vomiting, weight loss, hematuria, and interference with kidney function (pressure causes dislocation of pelvis of kidney).
      c. Fever.
      d. Hypertension due to kidney ischemia.
   4. Diagnosis—IVP demonstrates how mass distorts, rather than displaces, collecting system.
   5. Treatment—usually consists of nephrectomy, radiation therapy, and chemotherapy—usually actinomycin D and Vincristine (see Appendix D).
   6. Nursing goals and implementation—
      a. Most important nursing measure—avoid manipulation of the abdomen to prevent metastasis.
      b. Give emotional support to parents on diagnosis.
      c. Be aware that tumor is often encapsulated so prognosis is good; highest survival rate of all childhood cancers.
      d. Prepare parents and child for diagnostic tests and surgical procedure (blood-drawing and IVP); especially important since surgery is frequently done within 24–48 hours after diagnosis.
      e. Postoperatively, observe for decreased blood pressure, urinary output or oliguria, signs of infection.
      f. Prepare parents and family for side effects of radiation, if used—nausea, vomiting, diarrhea, skin irritation, lethargy, and anorexia; or of chemotherapy.
      g. Support child and family if tumor metastasizes and child is dying—stay with child, cope with fear of being alone, maintain comfort measures (skin and mouth), and do not leave parents alone at time of death.
B. Acute lymphocytic *leukemia*—most common type of leukemia in children.
   1. Analysis of cause-pathophysiology:

a. Exact etiology unknown.
b. Rapid and abnormal proliferation of leukocytes in blood-forming organs and presence of immature leukocytes in peripheral circulation.
c. Peak incidence at 3 to 4 years of age.
d. Types—acute and chronic lymphatic and chronic myelocytic.

2. Assessment:
   a. Early—onset usually rapid, two to three months.
      (1) Abdominal and bone pain.
      (2) Persistent fever.
      (3) Enlarged lymph nodes.
      (4) Petechiae.
      (5) Easily tired and general malaise.
      (6) Anemia and pallor.
   b. Later—
      (1) Oral and rectal ulcers.
      (2) Hemorrhage.
      (3) Infection.

3. Diagnosis:
   a. Stained smear of peripheral blood.
   b. Bone marrow aspirate.

4. Treatment goals:
   a. Initial phase is to induce remission by administration of corticosteroids, Vincristine, L-asparaginase.
   b. Second phase is designed to destroy leukemic cells or prevent them from invading parts of body protected from action of drugs used in initial phase; accomplished by cranial irradiation and/or intrathecal administration of methotrexate as prophylactic treatment of CNS.
   c. Third phase is maintenance treatment to preserve remission accomplished by administration of drugs, such as 6-mercaptopurine and methotrexate, p.o. This phase is continued for approximately three years.

5. Nursing goals and implementation:
   a. Be supportive of parents and child on learning diagnosis; do not discuss time limits or offer false hope that child will be okay; remissions are occurring more frequently than in past and are of longer duration.
   b. Maintain adequate nutrition by making meal a pleasant time—offer food preferences, soft foods because of gum-bleeding, and high-protein and high-calorie diet; leu-

kemic cells require increased metabolic needs, thereby depriving body of necessary nutrients.
   c. Record intake and output.
   d. Utilize measures to prevent infections.
   e. Be alert to signs of hemorrhage.
   f. Plan nursing care to give child periods of rest.
   g. Prepare child and parents for return visits to hospital; activity as tolerated during remission.
   h. Prepare child for tests, transfusions, and IV.
   i. Prepare child for, and be alert to, symptoms of effects of treatment—
      (1) Nausea and vomiting.
      (2) Anorexia.
      (3) Alopecia.
      (4) Headache.
      (5) Hyperpigmentation.
   j. If death is imminent, be supportive of child and family.

8. **Ingestion of poisons and drugs**
   A. Analysis of cause-pathophysiology:
      1. Caused by immaturity of child, availability of substance, or accidental rendering by another person.
      2. Ingestion of some substance may harm tissues and disturb body functioning; two most frequent are aspirin and bleach.
   B. Assessment:
      1. Gastrointestinal—
         a. Abdominal pain and/or distension.
         b. Nausea.
         c. Vomiting.
         d. Diarrhea.
         e. Difficulty swallowing.
         f. Anorexia.
         g. Odor of breath.
      2. Central nervous system—
         a. Lethargy.
         b. Restlessness.
         c. Delirium.
         d. Dilated pupils or pinpoint pupils.
         e. Coma.
         f. Convulsions.
      3. Respiratory—
         a. Obstruction.
         b. Respiratory depression.
         c. Difficulty breathing.
      4. Cardiovascular—

a. Increased or decreased heart rate.
b. Irregular heart rate.
c. Cardiac failure.
5. Skin symptoms—
a. Burns around mouth.
b. Cyanosis.
C. Nursing goals and implementation:
1. Determine, if possible, what was ingested and how much.
2. Contact poison control center as necessary to determine treatment; administer antidote as described on product; universal antidote—2 parts burned toast (powdered charcoal), 1 part milk of magnesia, and 1 part strong tea (tannic acid).
3. Remove poison from body.
a. Induce vomiting by sticking finger down throat unless child is convulsing, comatose, or has ingested acid, alkali, kerosene, or gasoline.
b. Gastric lavage—use tap water and follow with cathartic to hasten removal of material from gastrointestinal tract.
4. Be aware of signs and symptoms of systems involvement and treat symptomatically.
5. Remain calm and encourage parents to do so also, even though they may feel guilty.
6. Instruct about measures to prevent poisoning.
a. Keep medicines and poisons out of reach.
b. Lock up highly toxic substances such as Drāno.
c. *Do not* store foods, drugs, and poisons in same area.
d. Leave medicines, drugs, and chemicals in original container.
e. *Do not* store dish detergent and cleaning agents under sink.
f. Dispose of poisonous substances where child cannot get to them.
g. Use medicine only for person intended; discard unused portions (for example, flush down toilet).
h. Do not hide medicine in food for child or tell child that medication is candy.
i. Teach child not to taste or eat unfamiliar foods or substances.

9. Lead poisoning

A. Occurs most often at 1 to 5 years of age.
B. Ingestion of lead-base paint in repainted furniture such as cribs, banisters, and windowsills; certain lead toys, plaster, putty, and face powder; water from lead pipes, fruit covered with insecticides; lead-glazed earthenware pottery; and industrial crayons and oil paints.
C. Lead accumulates in body—assessment:
1. Early—anorexia, crying without reason, listlessness, constipation, vomiting, weight loss, anemia, headache, and insomnia.
2. Later—difficulty in coordination, ataxia, loss of recently acquired developmental skills (walking and buttoning clothes, for example), joint pains, bradycardia, and encephalopathy.
D. Diagnosis: blood level concentrations.
E. Anemia develops due to interference of lead with metabolism of iron and synthesis of hemoglobin.
F. X rays show lead lines and increased density at end of long bones and along margins of flat bones, indicating temporary cessation of growth.
G. Treatment goals:
1. Excrete lead via kidneys by medication that assists urinary excretions.
2. Remove source of lead ingestion.
H. Nursing goals and implementation:
1. Know early symptoms of lead poisoning.
2. Observe child for neurologic involvement.
3. Assist in ascertaining source of lead and ways of removing that source.
4. Offer emotional support to family, which often experiences guilt concerning child's condition.
5. Refer to public health nurse or community resources as appropriate.

10. Otitis media

10. *Otitis media*—Common infection of middle ear, usually a complication of upper respiratory infection in infants and young children because eustachian tube is short and crooked; horizontal position of tube hinders drainage due to usual prone or supine position of infant.
A. Assessment:
1. Fever—may be 104 F.
2. Pain indicated by pulling at ear and crying.
3. Irritability.
4. Rhinorrhea, vomiting, and diarrhea may be present.
B. Treatment:
1. Antibiotic, usually ampicillin or penicillin, even after symptoms disappear.
2. Aspirin or acetaminophen may be given to reduce fever.
3. Occasionally, decongestants are also ordered.
C. Nursing goals and implementation:
1. Assist parent in establishing schedule for antibiotics to maintain adequate blood level.

2. Encourage administration of medication even after symptoms disappear in order to prevent chronic otitis media.
3. Educate parents in proper feeding position to prevent bacteria from milk from entering eustachian tubes.
   a. Elevate head when feeding child.
   b. Do not prop bottle or allow child to fall asleep with bottle in mouth.

11. *Tonsillitis (pharyngitis)*
A. Inflammation of structures in pharynx.
B. Viral—assessment:
   1. Gradual onset of fever, malaise, anorexia.
   2. White exudate on tonsils.
   3. Treatment is symptomatic—aspirin to control fever and soothing throat lozenges or gargling with warm salt water.
C. Bacterial (group A, β-hemolytic streptococci)—assessment:
   1. Abrupt onset of high fever; sore throat; headache; localized, tender, firm cervical nodes; and petechiae on soft palate.
   2. Treatment—penicillin (or other antibiotic in case of allergy) for ten days.
D. Treatment of bacterial tonsillitis essential to prevent serious complications such as rheumatic fever, scarlet fever, and acute glomerulonephritis.
E. Tonsillectomy—surgical removal performed if child has repeated infections; tonsils hypertrophy, causing obstruction (difficulty breathing and swallowing and blockage of eustachian tubes).
   1. Nursing goals and implementation:
      a. Preoperatively—
         (1) Tell child what a hospital is for and why it is necessary to be there—use books and preadmission hospital visit.
         (2) Tell child what will be felt after surgery—sore throat.
         (3) Take vital signs, check signs of infection (increased temperature), and check for loose teeth to avoid aspiration.
         (4) Bleeding is most common serious complication—lab tests for clotting time, prothrombin time, and platelets.
      b. Postoperatively—
         (1) Place child in semiprone or prone position to allow patent airway, draining of secretions, and prevent aspiration.
         (2) When child is alert, offer cool liquids—soothe sore throat and prevent dehydration.
         (3) Since milk products are mucus-producing, *do not* offer immediately postoperatively.
         (4) Ice collar to reduce swelling and promote comfort.
         (5) Signs/symptoms of hemorrhage—frequent swallowing, vomiting bright red blood, *rapid pulse,* restlessness, and pallor.

Part C / SCHOOL-AGE CHILDREN—AGE 6 TO 12 YEARS

NORMAL GROWTH AND DEVELOPMENT OF SCHOOL-AGE CHILDREN

1. *Age 6 to 8 years*
A. Assessment of physical development:
   1. Growth spurt begins.
   2. Gains 2 to 4 kg (4 to 7 lb) per year.
   3. Begins to lose baby teeth; has 10 to 11 permanent teeth by 8 years of age.
   4. Eyes fully developed.
   5. At age 8 years, the arms grow longer in proportion to body; some girls may begin to develop secondary sex characteristics.
B. Assessment of behavior patterns:
   1. Motor development—
      a. The 6-year-old child is very impulsive and active.
      b. Balance and rhythm good.
      c. Capable of fine hand movements.
      d. Can throw and catch a ball.
      e. Prefers to bathe self.
      f. Nervous habits are common.
      g. Descriptive gestures accompany speech.
   2. Social, vocal, and mental development—
      a. Plays well alone.
      b. Enjoys group play with small groups.
      c. Prefers to play with same sex.
      d. Uses telephone.
      e. Knows comparative value of coins.
      f. Knows right and left.
      g. Learns to read.

h. The 7-year-old child counts by 1s, 2s, 5s, and 10s.

i. Aware of differences between own home and that of friends.

j. Begins to tell time; oriented to time and space (day of week and month).

k. Enjoys holiday celebrations; counts days until anticipated event takes place.

l. Has sense of humor.

m. Recognizes property rights.

C. Nursing goals and implementation:

1. Goal: provide appropriate play activities—

   a. Painting, coloring, pasting, and drawing.

   b. Imaginary dramatic play with "real" costumes.

   c. Table games—tiddlywinks, marbles, and dominoes.

   d. Handicrafts.

   e. Collections.

   f. Radio, TV, records.

   g. Magic tricks.

   h. Papier-mâché.

   i. Cooking sets, erector sets, and tinker toys.

   j. Books the child can read.

2. Goal: provide guidance—

   a. Give some responsibility for household duties.

   b. Teach safety in crossing streets.

   c. Accept aggressiveness as normal.

   d. Accept quiet days and periods of shyness as part of growing up.

   e. Reassure about nightmares and various fears.

   f. Treat with consideration; give small responsibilities.

   g. Give simple, honest answers to questions related to sexuality.

   h. Work through common problems—teasing, quarreling, nail-biting, enuresis, whining, poor manners, and swearing; causes for these behaviors should be investigated and dealt with constructively (for example, trying to find why, substituting other activities, and removing cause), not by negative handling (that is, do not use harsh punishment or belittling).

2. Age 9 to 12 years

A. Assessment of physical development:

1. Height increases at 9 years.

2. Weight gain may intensify at 10 years.

3. Eye-hand coordination is well developed.

4. Dentition—

   a. Shed cuspids and first and second molars.

   b. Have approximately 26 permanent teeth by 12 years.

5. Sexual maturation—

   a. Girls—breast enlargement, appearance of pubic and axillary hair, and menarche may begin by age 11 years.

   b. Boys—growth spurt, growth of external genitalia, appearance of pubic and axillary hair, change of voice, and transient enlargement of nipples may begin to appear by age 11 years.

B. Assessment of behavior patterns:

1. Motor development—

   a. Plays and works hard.

   b. Cares for own physical needs completely.

   c. Uses tools fairly well.

   d. Uses both hands independently.

   e. A marked difference in motor skills according to sex at 10 years.

   f. Constant activity.

   g. Very active—finger-drumming and foot-tapping, for example.

2. Social and mental development—

   a. Play is varied and companionship becomes more important than play.

   b. Likes to have secrets.

   c. Can do multiplication and division.

   d. Sex differences in play; antagonism between the sexes.

   e. Interested in family life.

   f. Interested in how things are made.

   g. Growing capacity for thought and conceptual organization.

   h. Courteous and well-mannered behavior with adults.

   i. Seeks others' ideas and opinions.

   j. Thinks about social problems and prejudices.

   k. Occasional privacy is important.

   l. Sees physical qualities as constant despite changes in size, shape, weight, and volume.

   m. Has ability to plan ahead.

   n. Can be quite critical of own work.

   o. An 11-year-old child has hero worship; characters in book become real for child.

   p. Operating in Erikson's *sense of industry or accomplishment* versus *feelings of inferiority* stage.

C. Nursing goals and implementation:

1. Goal: provide appropriate play activities based on developmental level—
   a. Books.
   b. Musical instruments.
   c. Clubs and organizations.
   d. Experiments.
   e. Jewelry.
   f. Ceramics.
   g. Handicrafts—sewing; copper, leather, and metal work; knitting; and crocheting.
2. Goal: provide guidance —
   a. Investigate causes if lying and stealing become problems (give recognition or remedy inadequacies).
   b. Accept child as is—active or quiet.
   c. Encourage participation in organized clubs and youth groups.
   d. Give information concerning sex changes.
   e. Use "power of suggestion" rather than dictums.
   f. Avoid harsh and severe punishment.
   g. Support and give democratic guidance as child works through dependence and independence; set realistic limits.
   h. Help channel energy into purposeful endeavors.
   i. Recognize that 11-year-old child may withdraw rather than verbalize.
   j. Recognize need to rebel and deprecate others.
   k. Do not reinforce child's feeling of being "picked on" when not in control of situation.

SPECIAL CONCERNS OF SCHOOL-AGE CHILDREN

1. *Response to illness and hospitalization*—age 6 to 12 years.
A. Assessment of discomfort or pain:
   1. Expresses that something is wrong, such as, "I feel sick."
   2. Cries.
   3. Tells adult of illness so adult can do something about it.
B. Assessment of reaction to stage of illness:
   1. Initial illness or hospitalization—
      a. Expected coping or adaptive behaviors:
         (1) Anger.
         (2) Guilt.
         (3) Fantasies and fears of mutilation; body image threatened.
         (4) Increased activity as response to anxiety.
         (5) Reaction to immobility (depression, anger, and crying).
         (6) Increased imagination about surgery or treatments.
         (7) Cries or aggressively resists treatment.
         (8) Needs parents and authority.
      b. Maladaptive behaviors—stemming from loss of control, insecurity, and feelings of inferiority:
         (1) Excessive guilt and anger and inability to express it.
         (2) Night terrors.
         (3) Excessive hyperactivity.
         (4) Not talking about experience.
         (5) Regression and complete withdrawal.
         (6) Excessive dependency.
         (7) Insomnia.
   2. Prolonged hospitalization and convalescence—
      a. Expected coping or adaptive behaviors:
         (1) Shows desire to get well.
         (2) Wants to do things for self.
         (3) Talks about going home.
         (4) Shows interest in play, peers, and school.
      b. Maladaptive behaviors:
         (1) Gives up hope.
         (2) Shows no inclination to get well.
         (3) Not interested in happenings outside hospital.
C. Nursing goals and implementation:
   1. Explain procedures, treatments, and condition to child to allay fears and misconceptions.
   2. Encourage child to verbalize feelings in order to discover conceptions, fears, and expectations.
   3. If maladaptive behaviors appear, help child explain fears; give punching bag or clay to allow outlet for aggressive feelings.
   4. Have same group of nurses care for child to provide security and predictability.
   5. Set limits—child expects to be disciplined for misbehavior (take away a privilege, TV, for example).
   6. Encourage visits from peers, friends; letters, telephone calls, pictures.
   7. Maintain school work, if appropriate.

2. *Nutrition*—age 6 to 12 years.
A. Age 6 to 8 years: 2000–2100 cal/24 hours.
B. Age 8 to 10 years: 2100–2200 cal/24 hours.

C. Age 10 to 12 years: boy, 2500 cal/24 hours; girl, 2250 cal/24 hours.
D. Tends to choose own foods; needs nutritional education.
E. Displays good table manners and enjoys having guests to dinner.
F. Nutritional snack foods should be kept on hand for extra food during growth spurts.

3. Safety concerns—age 6 to 12 years.
A. Be role model as safe driver.
B. Use safety belts while riding in auto.
C. Teach rules of pedestrians.
D. Do not allow play in streets or alleys.
E. Teach bicycle "rules of the road."
F. Firearms:
  1. Store safely.
  2. Handle carefully.
  3. Teach proper use.
G. Provide supervision during sports activities.
H. Provide adult supervision and teaching for swimming and boating.
I. Teach respect for fire and its dangers.
J. Recognize that as part of group, child may try anything once; set good examples for child to follow.

4. Nail-biting
A. Rare in preschoolers.
B. Usually a sign of nervousness, tension, or stress; often unconscious.
C. Nursing goals and implementation:
  1. Attempt to remove chronic sources of tension in child's environment, such as high expectations of child's capabilities in home or school.
  2. Instill sense of pride in nails.
  3. Suggest toys or activities which require manipulation of fingers.
  4. Constructive activity: opportunity for destructive play to vent aggressive feelings, such as tearing newspapers for papier mâché.

5. Bed-wetting (enuresis)
A. Under age 4–5 years: occasional accidents not uncommon.
B. Seven- and eight-year-olds: may occur during stress, change in family structure or environment, or undue excitement.
C. Chronic bed-wetters should be evaluated by physician for physiologic problems.
D. If no physiologic basis, emotional factors should be evaluated.
E. Training program:
  1. Accurate record of fluid intake and output for a few days to determine how frequently child urinates in relation to how much he or she drinks.
  2. Encourage child to drink many fluids and hold urine as long as possible; usual pattern may be several, small-quantity urinations; accidents are expected.
  3. May require three to six months for child to develop bladder capacity to sleep through night without wetting bed.

6. Sex education
A. Parents need to acknowledge own understanding and feelings regarding sex education.
B. Answer in simple terms, responding only to the child's queries, as he or she is unable to equate moral lectures with information.
C. Answer honestly and immediately or child may seek information elsewhere that may be erroneous.
D. Help the child understand that this interest is expected but that he or she need not ask questions outside of family circle, as most people consider sex questions a private affair.
E. If a child has not asked questions about sex or body changes by ten years of age, offer this information and prepare preadolescents for normal changes of adolescence.

CONDITIONS AND DISEASE ENTITIES OF SCHOOL-AGE CHILDREN

1. Childhood communicable diseases—most common in this age group (Table 4–13).

2. Acute rheumatic fever
A. Analysis of cause-pathophysiology:
  1. Most cases preceded by Group A β-hemolytic streptococcal infection.
  2. Systemic disease with changes caused by inflammatory lesions of connective tissue and endothelial tissue, specifically of the heart, joints, blood vessels, and subcutaneous tissues.
  3. Presence of Aschoff's bodies—cellular response of inflammation to the perivascular connective tissue; nodules; and myocardial lesion.
B. Analysis of incidence and etiology:
  1. Peak age 6–8 years.
  2. Predisposition to streptococcal infection.
  3. Possible autoimmune process causing streptococci to initiate tissue damage.

TABLE 4–13. *Childhood communicable diseases*

Disease	Analysis of data			Assessment	
	Incubation period	Isolation of child	Observation of contact	Clinical manifestations	Nursing actions
Varicella (chickenpox)	11–21 days.	Until pustules and most of scabs have disappeared.	11–17 days from first exposure.	General malaise, slight fever, anorexia, headache; successive crops of maculae, papules, vesicles, and crust; pruritus.	Prevent child from scratching; use lotions.
Parotitis (mumps)	14–24 days.	Duration of swelling.	3 weeks from first exposure.	Swelling and pain may occur in salivary, parotid, sublingual, and submaxillary glands; unilaterally or bilaterally, difficulty swallowing, headache, fever, and malaise.	Liquid or soft foods; bedrest for duration of swelling; and heat or cold application to reduce discomfort.
Roseola	10–15 days.	Duration of rash.	2 weeks from first exposure.	Elevated temperature, drowsy, irritable, and anorexic; after temperature falls (2–4 days), macular or maculopapular rash appears on trunk and neck.	Symptomatic—cool clothing, tepid baths; offer liquids frequently.
Rubella (German measles)	14–21 days.	Duration of rash.	12–21 days from first exposure.	Slight fever; mild coryza; rash of small pink or light red maculae, which fade in three days; *no* Koplik's spots.	Bedrest until fever subsides; otherwise, symptomatic.
Rubeola (measles)	10–14 days.	5 days after appearance of rash.	2 weeks from last exposure.	Coryza, conjunctivitis, photophobia, Koplik's spots in mouth; hacking cough, high fever, rash, and enlarged lymph nodes; rash goes from maculae to papules, which fade with pressure, last 5 days.	Bedrest until fever and cough subside; dim lights in room; use tepid baths and lotion for itching; encourage fluids.
Scarlet fever	2–4 days.	About 1 week.	1 week from last exposure.	Headache, fever, rapid pulse, rash, thirst, vomiting, and red-strawberry tongue; often seen poststreptococcal sore throat.	Penicillin usually administered; encourage fluid intake, bedrest, and mouth care.

(Continued)

TABLE 4–13. *(Continued)*

| Disease | Analysis of data | | | Assessment | |
	Incubation period	Isolation of child	Observation of contact	Clinical manifestations	Nursing actions
Pertussis (whooping cough)	7–14 days.	1 week from last paroxysm.	2 weeks from last exposure.	Coryza, dry cough becomes worse at night; cough is distinctive—paroxysms of sharp coughs in single expiration followed by deep inspiration with "whoop" sound; dyspnea, fever, and occasional vomiting.	Bedrest with emotional support, warm humid air; offer frequent small feedings; child may require small amounts of sedative to ensure adequate rest and relaxation to decrease coughing.

C. Assessment—modified Jones criteria for diagnosis: two major criteria or one major and two minor criteria present in child.
  1. Major criteria:
     a. Carditis.
     b. Erythema marginatum (pink rash).
     c. Polyarthritis.
     d. Chorea.
     e. Subcutaneous nodules.
  2. Minor criteria:
     a. Pain in one or more joints, with no inflammation, tenderness, or limited motion.
     b. Fever.
     c. Abdominal pain.
     d. Rapid pulse during sleep.
     e. Anemia.
     f. Epistaxis.
     g. Malaise.
     h. Previous streptococcal infection.
     i. Leukocytosis.
     j. Elevated erythrocyte sedimentation rate.
     k. Prolonged P-R interval on ECG.
     l. Positive reactive protein.
D. Treatment:
  1. *Major aim*—prevent permanent *heart damage;* bedrest during febrile stage (mitral valve most affected).
  2. Eradication of streptococcal *infection*—penicillin or, if allergic, erythromycin; long-term, *chemoprophylaxis.*
  3. *Corticosteroids*—used only when congestive heart failure is present.
  4. *Aspirin*—helps comfort child when febrile and when joint pain is present.

E. Nursing goals and implementation:
  1. Be alert to signs/symptoms of carditis—
     a. Listen to heart to identify changes in murmur or onset of murmur.
     b. Tachycardia, especially during sleep.
     c. Precordial pain.
  2. Provide quiet diversional activity (stories, handicrafts, or TV) while on *bedrest* during febrile stage to prevent cardiac damage.
  3. When joints are painful, move child carefully, supporting joints; in acute phase—goal is to prevent deformity.
  4. If febrile, take frequent temperatures.
  5. Low-sodium diet—to prevent fluid retention, should be as palatable as possible so child will eat; offer several small portions rather than three large meals; *avoid excessive fluids,* which augment congestive heart failure.
  6. Be aware that two to six months following infection, girls may develop *chorea* (St. Vitus' dance)—muscular twitching, purposeless movements, facial grimacing, and weakness; subsides after period of time; relieved by rest/sleep; pad bedrails to prevent injury; rectal temperature, as child may bite thermometer if taken orally.
  7. Explain that prognosis depends on amount of cardiac damage.
  8. Prevent recurrence—long-term antibiotic therapy, avoid exposure to infections and seek treatment in acute stage of disease. Recurrence depends on further streptococcal infections; if there is no treatment in acute phase, extensive cardiac damage may occur.

9. Discuss physical activity allowed when discharged.
10. Encourage continuing school work as appropriate.

3. Acute glomerulonephritis
A. Analysis of cause-pathophysiology:
1. Antigen-antibody reaction secondary to initial infection, usually Group A β-hemolytic streptococcal infection.
2. Causative organism contains antigens similar to basement membrane of renal glomeruli, so antibodies attack organism *and* the glomerular tissue, causing an inflammatory reaction in kidney-glomerulus and resulting in destruction of basement membrane with loss of blood protein due to general vascular disturbances (loss of capillary integrity and spasm of arterioles).
3. Kidneys enlarged, glomerular capillaries are obstructed, causing decreased glomerular filtrate and decreased amount of sodium and water passed to tubules for reabsorption.
4. Incidence—peak age is 6 years; 2:1 males to females.
5. Usually five- to ten-day course.
B. Assessment:
1. Hematuria—first sign, oliguria and proteinemia (characteristic symptoms).
2. History of streptococcal infection approximately 10–14 days prior to onset of symptoms.
3. Headache.
4. Malaise.
5. Fever—initially over 104 F; stays at approximately 100 F for duration of illness.
6. Edema—extremities and cerebrum, present in most patients (characteristic symptom).
7. Hypertension—present in 50% of patients after four or five days.
8. Anorexia and vomiting (characteristic symptom).
9. Bradycardia.
10. Congestive heart failure (CHF).
C. Treatment—generally supportive and symptomatic.
1. Bedrest.
2. Limited sodium in diet.
3. Antibiotics, if evidence of infection.
4. Strict monitoring of intake and output.
5. Daily weights to monitor fluid balance for edematous child.
6. Antihypertensive therapy if indicated.
D. Nursing goals and implementation:
1. Maintain bedrest to prevent complications—hypertensive encephalopathy and cardiac involvement by increased glomerular filtration.
2. Protect child from infection—avoid exposure to contagious diseases and upper-respiratory infection.
3. Use hygiene measures; good skin care especially if edematous.
4. Follow dietary regimen and explain modifications to child (low-salt or salt-free diet because of renal failure or decreased potassium or protein, for example).
5. Record exact intake and output to identify fluid retention and prevent fluid overload.
6. Weigh child daily—check for fluid retention.
7. Limit fluid intake to reduce hypertension.
8. Toys—avoid games and articles that require fine eye work.
9. Observe for signs of complication indicating decreased kidney function and increased metabolic end products in blood—
   a. Restlessness.
   b. Stupor.
   c. Convulsions.
   d. Severe headache.
   e. Visual disturbances.
   f. Vomiting.
   g. Tachycardia.
   h. Dyspnea.
   i. Muscular twitching.

4. Asthma
A. Analysis of cause-pathophysiology:
1. Varied etiology.
   a. Antigen-antibody response.
   b. Infection.
   c. Hereditary tendency—75% have other family members afflicted.
   d. Irritants.
   e. Exercise.
   f. Emotional factors.
2. Spasm of bronchial muscle, causing reversible obstruction of air passage by accumulation of thick mucus.
3. Status asthmaticus—severe attack not alleviated by treatment.
4. Incidence: onset rare in first year of life; prior to puberty more often seen in males but as reach adolescence and young adulthood more common in females.
B. Assessment:

1. Gradual increase of nasal congestion and sneezing.
2. Wheezing on expiration, nasal flaring, and rales.
3. Diaphoresis.
4. Coughing and expectoration of viscous mucus secretions.
5. Anxiety.
6. Paroxysmal dyspnea.
7. Cyanosis.
8. Increased pulse and respiration.
9. Distended neck veins.

C. Treatment goals:
1. Acute attack—relief of bronchospasm by dilating of bronchi, decreasing mucosal edema, removing excess bronchial secretions, and using bronchodilators, corticosteroids, and expectorants.
2. Antibiotic treatment for an infectious process, as this may precipitate an attack.
3. Sedation to relieve anxiety.

D. Nursing goals and implementation:
1. Acute phase—
   a. Observe breathing pattern—shallow, rapid respiration, chest retractions, and wheezing.
   b. Vital signs—observe for nasal flaring; use stethoscope to hear if all areas of chest are aerated.
   c. Place in high-Fowler's position or slightly leaning forward to allow maximum lung expansion.
   d. Administer oxygen cautiously; low PO_2 may be necessary for spontaneous breathing.
   e. Remain with child during acute attack.
   f. Provide calm, quiet environment.
   g. Provide adequate hydration to liquefy bronchial secretions and maintain electrolyte balance.
   h. Know effects and side effects of drugs (bronchodilators) administered.
2. Convalescent phase—
   a. Teach child and family breathing exercises to increase total lung capacity.
   b. Teach environmental control of home and child's bedroom (dusting, vacuuming, and cleaning drapes and carpets).
   c. Toys—avoid furry materials that could contain irritants.
   d. Postural drainage to clean mucus from bronchial tree.

5. Skin conditions
A. Tinea capitis (ringworm):

1. Analysis of cause-pathophysiology—
   a. Fungal infection of scalp and hair follicles.
   b. Fungal infection produces an inflammation of the scalp, which causes alopecia and may produce edema and pustules.
2. Assessment—
   a. Pruritus.
   b. Rounded or oval patches covered by scales and broken hairs, disconcerting to child.
3. Nursing goals and implementation—
   a. Recognize lesion and prevent spread of infection through use of sterilized cotton cap.
   b. Administer prescribed medication (griseofulvin, administered orally) and be aware of side effects—headache, nausea, epigastric pain, diarrhea, and itching.
   c. Examine child's family to ascertain if others are infected.
   d. Provide emotional support and stress good hygiene habits—regular shampooing and avoid use of common comb and brush.
   e. Check and treat pets for infestation.

B. Impetigo:
1. Analysis of cause-pathophysiology—
   a. Usually caused by staphylococci or streptococci coupled with poor hygiene.
   b. Infectious disease of superficial layers of skin.
2. Assessment—
   a. Reddish-pink macules, progressing to vesicles.
   b. Progression to pustules, which develop crusts and reddened areas on skin.
3. Nursing goals and implementation—
   a. Be aware of signs and symptoms.
   b. Soften and remove crusts by soaking with 1:20 Burow's solution.
   c. Apply topical bacteriocidal ointment such as Neosporin, NeoPolycin, Garamycin.
   d. Prevent secondary infection by using good hygiene and avoiding scratching.
   e. Maintain adequate nutrition.
   f. Utilize diversional therapy.
   g. Teach good hygiene habits to child and family; explain condition is contagious and child may not attend school until after treatment.

C. Pediculosis (lice infestation):
1. Analysis of cause-pathophysiology—
   a. Infestation by lice.
   b. Eggs or nits attach to hair and clothing.
2. Assessment—

a. Severe itching of infected area.

b. Minute red lesions.

c. Observation of nits (eggs) in hair.

3. Nursing goals and implementation—

a. Prevent spread of infection—isolate child in hospital.

b. Wear gloves and gown when combing or washing child's hair.

c. Inspect skin for infection caused by scratching.

d. Carry out prescribed treatment—Kwell shampoo, use of fine-tooth comb to remove nits.

e. Provide for screening of family, schoolmates.

f. Teach good hygiene habits.

D. Scabies:

1. Analysis of cause-pathophysiology—

a. Caused by parasite—mite.

b. Burrowing parasite causes irritation and formation of vesicles.

2. Assessment—

a. Itching, primarily at night.

b. Burrow lines caused by female mite burrowing into superficial skin to deposit her eggs, most commonly seen between fingers but may occur in any natural folds of body or where elastic on clothing is against skin.

3. Nursing goals and implementation—

a. Prevent spread of infection by medical asepsis.

b. Inspect skin for infection caused by scratching.

c. Carry out prescribed treatment, usually gamma benzene hexachloride (Kwell) baths.

d. Use soothing ointment for pruritus.

e. Provide screening for family.

f. Teach good hygiene habits—regular bathing and clean clothes, washing of linen and clothes to prevent reinfection.

6. *Intestinal parasites (worms)*

A. Analysis of infestation—fecal contamination of food, soil, water, and hands.

B. Analysis of type:

1. Roundworms—

a. Eggs hatch in duodenum, larvae pass through intestinal wall to blood stream, liver, lungs, and epiglottis (swallowed).

b. Develop in small intestine—colicky pain, passed in stool as worm.

c. Treatment—piperazine citrate, two treatments, two days apart.

2. Pinworm—

a. Worm attaches to mucosa of cecum and appendix.

b. Females deposit eggs on perianal and perineum at night—causes anal itching → child scratches → fingers in mouth → reinfection.

c. Treatment—same as for roundworms.

3. Hookworm—

a. Enters body through the skin from contaminated soil.

b. Worms live in small intestine; ova found in fecal smear.

c. Treatment—tetrachloroethylene, single dose.

C. Nursing goals and implementation—prevent reinfection:

1. Wash hands after toileting.

2. Treat entire family, wash all bedding and bedclothes.

3. Dispose of fecal material in safe, hygienic manner (soiled diapers rinsed and disposable diapers in closed container).

4. Avoid putting fingers in mouth.

7. *Juvenile diabetes mellitus*—a disorder of abnormal metabolism of fat, protein, and especially carbohydrates due to inability to produce insulin.

A. Analysis of cause-pathophysiology:

1. Hereditary—recessive disease.

2. Pancreas produces little or no insulin, so body is unable to oxidize glucose properly.

3. Glycosuria—serum level of glucose exceeds renal threshold.

4. Ketones—in blood because of abnormal fat metabolism, excreted in urine.

5. Lower incidence in younger-than-school-age children.

B. Early assessment due to osmotic diuresis:

1. *Three Ps*—polydipsia, polyuria, and polyphagia.

2. Dry skin.

3. Weight loss with nausea and vomiting.

4. Glucose and ketones in urine on testing.

C. Treatment:

1. Diet based on American Diabetes Association exchange method.

2. Subcutaneous administration of insulin (Table 4–14).

D. Complications—arteriosclerosis with hypertension, retinal changes, cataracts, and nephropathy.

TABLE 4–14.   *Insulin therapy**

Type	Onset, peak, and duration	Indications
RAPID		
Crystalline zinc (clear)	Onset 1 hour or less. Peak 2–4 hours. Duration 6–8 hours.	Poorly controlled diabetes, trauma, surgery, and coma.
Prompt insulin zinc suspension (Semilente insulin) (cloudy)	Onset 1 hour. Peak 4–10 hours. Duration 12–16 hours.	Patients allergic to crystalline; and in combination with longer-lasting insulin.
INTERMEDIATE		
Globin zinc insulin injection (clear)	Onset 2–4 hours. Peak 6–12 hours. Duration 18–24 hours.	Rarely used.
NPH insulin (isophane insulin suspension) (cloudy)	Onset 2–4 hours. Peak 6–12 hours. Duration 24–48 hours.	Patients who can be controlled by one dose per day.
Insulin zinc suspension (Lente insulin) (cloudy)	Onset 2–4 hours. Peak 6–12 hours. Duration 24–36 hours.	Patients allergic to NPH.
SLOW-ACTING		
PZI (protamine zinc insulin suspension) (cloudy)	Onset 3–6 hours. Peak 12–20 hours. Duration 24–36 hours.	Rarely used; only if uncontrolled by other types.
Extended insulin zinc suspension (Ultralente insulin) (cloudy)	Onset 2–4 hours. Peak 12–24 hours. Duration 36 hours.	Often mixed with Semilente for 24-hour curve.

*REMINDER: To avoid dangerous error use U-40 syringe with U-40 insulin; U-80 syringe with U-80 insulin; and U-100 syringe with U-100 insulin.

E. Nursing goals and implementation:

1. Recognize signs of diabetic acidosis and teach child and family (refer to Table 4–15).
2. Differentiate between preceding signs and those of insulin reaction; teach child and family (Table 4–15).
3. Be familiar with child's prescribed diet and assist in teaching child and family; increase food intake during physically active times.
4. Assist child and/or family in administering insulin subcutaneously—practice on sponge and progress in steps; be sure to rotate sites.
5. Teach testing of urine—discard first void in A.M.; test second, more accurate than residual urine.
6. Provide good skin and foot care to prevent infection.
7. Promote normal growth and development of child—can participate in activities without feeling different; avoid overprotection.
8. Have child carry lump of sugar or hard candy to use in case of insulin reaction.
9. Teach relationship between extra activity and stress and food-insulin need; decrease food intake during times of inactivity or rest.

TABLE 4–15. *Insulin reaction versus diabetic coma*

	Insulin reaction	Diabetic coma
Definition	Insulin shock is the result of overdose of insulin, reduction of diet, or increase in exercise.	Diabetic coma (acidosis) is result of untreated diabetes, inadequate insulin coverage, failure to follow diet, or chronic or repeated infections.
Onset	Sudden or gradual (minutes to hours).	Slow (days).
Cause	Delayed or missed meal, excessive exercise, or overdose of insulin.	Untreated diabetes, neglect of treatment, infections, or disease process.
Signs	Pallor, shallow respiration, pulse normal, sweating, eyeballs normal, and dilated pupils.	Cherry-red lips; flushed face; increased respiration; loud, labored breathing; rapid pulse; dry skin; and soft, sunken eyeballs.
Symptoms	Nervousness, tremors, abnormal behavior, semiconscious, convulsions, blurred or double vision, and hunger.	Thirst, nausea, vomiting, headache, constipation, dim vision, abdominal pain, and shortness of breath.
Urine	Sugar-free and acetone-free urine.	Sugar and acetone in urine.
Response to treatment	Rapid or slightly delayed.	Slow.

8. Osteomyelitis

A. Analysis of cause-pathophysiology:
1. 90% are associated with *Staphylococcus aureus* infection; in younger children may be *Hemophilus influenzae,* sickle cell anemia, salmonella.
2. Inflammatory process of long bones leading to bone destruction and abscess formation.
3. Incidence usually in boys 5–14 years of age.

B. Assessment:
1. Fever and malaise.
2. Pain in bone at the metaphysis, refusal to move limb, later associated with redness and swelling.
3. May report trauma to afflicted extremity.
4. Irritability.
5. Weakness.
6. Dehydration.
7. Abrupt onset of symptoms.

C. Treatment goals:
1. Prompt institution of IV antibiotic therapy (Penicillin G is often choice).
2. After identification of organism, specific antibiotic.
3. Bedrest for comfort and to prevent movement, which spreads infection.
4. Immobilize limb (splint, cast).
5. If infection does not respond to treatment, dead infected bone may be surgically removed.

D. Nursing goals and implementation:
1. Be aware of signs and symptoms and precipitating primary lesions obtained by history; ask if child had boil or infection recently.
2. Systemic infection—handle discharge material carefully.
3. Monitor vital signs for changes indicating infection—increased pulse, elevated temperature, and increased respiration; and check circulation of affected part or parts.
4. Prepare child and parents for long hospital treatment of IV antibiotics and need for bedrest; provide activities during immobilization appropriate to age and stage of development.
5. Pain—immobilize and support limb and administer analgesics.
6. If in cast, observe extremity for color, swelling,

heat, tenderness, for signs of impaired circulation and/or further infection.

7. If surgery is planned, prepare appropriately for age.

9. Oncology

A. Brain tumors:

1. Analysis of cause-pathophysiology—
   a. Etiology unknown.
   b. Age 5–10 years; males more often than females.
   c. Expanding tumor or lesion, most often (60%) in the posterior fossa, primarily cerebellum or brain stem.
   d. Most frequent types:
      (1) Astrocytoma—slow growing, usually benign; 90% cured by surgical excision.
      (2) Medulloblastoma—fast growing, malignant; radiation and chemotherapy utilized.
      (3) Ependymoma—rate of growth variable, usually involves fourth ventricle, making total excision impossible because of damage to vital control center, irradiation utilized.

2. Assessment—
   a. Headache.
   b. Ataxia.
   c. Abnormal posture of head.
   d. Vomiting without nausea.
   e. Delayed response to commands.
   f. Blurred or double vision.
   g. Change in personality or behavior—lethargy, irritability, hyperactivity, drowsiness, stupor, inattentiveness, or belligerence.
   h. Decreased pulse and respiration, increased blood pressure due to disturbance of regulatory mechanism in cardiorespiratory center.
   i. Papilledema as late sign of increased intracranial pressure (IIP); seizures, changes in EEG.

3. Nursing goals and implementation—
   a. Observe for changes in vital signs, monitor for full minute.
   b. Observe for IIP; slowly falling pulse and respiration with rising blood pressure.
   c. Check pupils—size, equality, reaction to light.
   d. Check level of consciousness—ask older child questions, observe activity, alertness, sleep/wake pattern.
   e. Administer muscle tests—have child grip nurse's hands with both hands and observe any difference in strength; pushing feet against hands to check resistance.
   f. Take convulsive precautions.
   g. Accurately record and report any headaches that indicate IIP; note head circumference or protrusion of eyes/eyelids.
   h. Provide emotional support of child and family.
   i. Prepare for diagnostic tests: lumbar puncture, X-ray procedures.
   j. If surgery is indicated, do preoperative and postoperative preparation, teaching, care (any shaving of hair, types of dressing, no food 24 hours prior to surgery, ICU tour, position flat and on either side).
   k. Play activities—avoid bending of head due to discomfort and increased incidence of headaches.

B. Sarcomas:

1. Analysis of etiology-pathophysiology—
   a. Etiology unknown but heredity may play a part; also question rapid growth rate of osseous tissue.
   b. Peak age 15–19 years old; more often male.
   c. Malignant bone tumor.

2. Osteosarcoma—
   a. Spindle cell; malignant osteoid tissue.
   b. Fifty percent affect femur.
   c. Treatment:
      (1) Radical surgery, usually amputation of affected limb.
      (2) Chemotherapy.

3. Ewing's sarcoma—
   a. Small cell; marrow spaces of bone.
   b. Treatment:
      (1) Irradiation.
      (2) Chemotherapy, usually VAC (Vincristine, actinomycin-C, cyclophosphamide).

4. Assessment—
   a. Localized pain.
   b. Limp.
   c. Palpable mass over site.
   d. Swelling of affected part.

5. Nursing management—
   a. Observe for lung involvement, most common complication.
      (1) Pain in chest.
      (2) Coughing.
      (3) Spitting blood.

b. If limb involved is amputated, prepare child and family postoperatively and give appropriate postoperative care.

c. Provide emotional support to child and family; allow grieving process, particularly if loss of limb.

d. Explain side effects of irradiation and chemotherapy.

10. Epilepsy

A. Analysis of cause-pathophysiology:
   1. Idiopathic.
   2. Organic—trauma, anoxia, infection, degenerative diseases, congenital (PKU and hypoglycemia), and toxic reactions.
   3. Recurrent convulsive disorder marked by sudden and periodic lapses of consciousness; disturbances in electrical discharges in the brain.

B. Assessment:
   1. Aura type—
      a. Small localized seizures; may precede grand mal seizures.
      b. Irritability, headache, and nausea.
      c. May experience sensation of unusual sounds, colors, and sights.
   2. Grand mal—
      a. Abrupt onset.
      b. Tonic phase (20 to 40 seconds):
         (1) Entire body becomes stiff.
         (2) Loses consciousness; may be cyanotic.
         (3) Back arched and head usually to one side.
         (4) Incontinence.
         (5) Pulse weak and irregular.
         (6) Eyes fixed, pupils dilated.
         (7) May bite tongue.
      c. Clonic phase (variable duration):
         (1) Follows tonic stage and becomes generalized.
         (2) Twitching movements of face and extremities.
      d. Sleep follows; feels exhausted or has headache on waking.
      e. Abnormal EEG.
   3. Petit mal (30 seconds)—
      a. Signs—eyes roll, head lowered, and mild twitching.
      b. Will discontinue activity for short period of time and then resume where left off.
   4. Jacksonian-March (focal motor)—seen in infants, progresses to grand mal as child gets older; sudden jerking movements of face, arms, and tongue; may remain conscious; sensory or motor voluntary muscles affected, usually clonic.
   5. Psychomotor—
      a. Brief (one minute).
      b. Purposeful, repetitive movements (chewing or picking at clothes), pale, not tonic or clonic.

C. Treatment:
   1. Aim is to control or reduce number of seizures.
   2. Drugs—phenobarbital, diphenylhydantoin (Dilantin).
   3. Diet—ketogenic, which is high in fats, tends to have tranquilizing effect; reduction of fluids assists this effect.

D. Nursing goals and implementation:
   1. Give medications; side effects—
      a. Phenobarbital—excitement, rash, drowsiness, and vertigo.
      b. Phenytoin (Dilantin)—hypertrophy of gums (suggest daily gum massage).
   2. Observe child for recurrent seizures.
   3. Protect head from injury with pillow during a convulsive episode; place tongue blade or wad of material (towel) between teeth; move furniture or toys out of way; and loosen clothing around neck.
   4. May need to suction and administer O_2 following seizure.
   5. Decrease stressful situations, decrease noise level if loud, and avoid blinking light in order to lessen likelihood of seizure.
   6. Prepare child for diagnostic tests (EEG and blood studies).
   7. Assist parents in raising child as normally as possible; child should attend regular school.
   8. Educate child and parents about epilepsy—child is not insane or retarded; epilepsy can be controlled with medication.
   9. Toys—avoid sharp toys to prevent injury during convulsive episodes.
   10. Encourage use of ID bracelet/Medic Alert.
   11. Refer to Epilepsy Society.

11. Hyperactivity

A. Analysis of cause-pathophysiology:
   1. Often used interchangeably with minimal brain dysfunction and hyperkinetic syndrome; learning disability.
   2. May be due to—
      a. Brain damage or cerebral dysfunction.
      b. Visual problems.
      c. Hearing problems.
      d. Emotional problems.
      e. Limited intellectual capacity.

f. Biochemical etiology; appears sex- and chromosome-linked due to increased incidence of those with Turner's and Klinefelter's syndromes.

3. Occurs more often in males.

B. Assessment:
1. Short attention span.
2. Inability to sit still for long periods of time.
3. Inability to solve problems according to ability of others of same age.
4. Easily distracted.
5. Impulsive.
6. Labile emotions.
7. Poor motor coordination.
8. Perceptual deficits.

C. Treatment:
1. May administer central nervous stimulants.
2. Diet management—no preservatives or food dyes.

D. Nursing goals and implementation:
1. Known side effects of medication—amphetamines—
   a. Anorexia.
   b. Blurred vision.
   c. Sleeplessness.
2. Take a *complete* history of the child; determine when hyperactivity started.
3. Test vision.
4. Test hearing.
5. Assist in decreasing environmental expectations at home, in school, and in hospital.
6. Refer to counselor if parents or teachers are unable to cope with child; to assist and support them in developing workable plan *for child*.

12. Blindness

A. Analysis of cause-pathophysiology:
1. Genetic factors.
2. Rubella in pregnant mother (first trimester).
3. Infections (syphilis).
4. Injury or trauma (retrolental fibroplasia).
5. Inflammatory disease.

B. Assessment:
1. No eye-to-eye contact.
2. Abnormal eye movements.
3. Child does not follow objects.
4. Child bumps into objects.

C. Nursing goals and implementation:
1. Be alert to child's responses to light and objects.
2. Record child's behavior (eye-rubbing and body-rocking).

3. When admitting blind child to hospital, familiarize child with surroundings; learn child's usual routine and self-help capabilities.
4. Utilize other senses when interacting with child—touch, smell, hearing, and taste.
5. Speak to child before touching; let child know you are in the room; say who you are.

13. Impaired eyesight—strabismus— loss of control of eye-movement muscles (intraocular); one or both eyes may deviate rather than function as a unit; untreated condition results in amblyopia, poor vision in affected eye.

A. Detection—must be detected and treated by 6 to 8 years of age or visual loss is irreversible (acute visual development occurs at 1 to 6 years of age).

B. Analysis of cause:
1. Refractive errors.
2. Corneal scarring.
3. Cataracts.
4. Congenital deformities of orbit of eye or extraocular muscles.

C. Treatment goals:
1. Glasses to correct refractive error and control excess accommodation.
2. Occlusion of straight eye to force other eye into activity.
3. Orthoptic training—exercises for eyes.
4. Surgery—
   a. Resection—shortening intraocular muscles.
   b. Recession—lengthening intraocular muscles.

D. Nursing goals and implementation:
1. Encourage early testing of vision—clinics, day-care centers, and nursery schools.
2. Explain that patch over "good" eye must be worn *constantly*.
3. Surgical correction—
   a. Prepare for eye patches after surgery.
   b. *Child should lie flat 24–48 hours after surgery*—restraints may be needed; supply diversion for child, such as familiar tactile and auditory objects in room.
   c. Room quiet and dimly lit—for decreased stimulation and greater comfort.
   d. Advance diet slowly—decrease chance of vomiting, causing increased pressure and movement.
   e. If day-care surgery, prepare child for patches and explain limitations to child and parents when returning home.

f. Use same techniques as for blind child while eyes are patched—speak before touching, explain sounds, and read stories.

14. Impaired hearing

A. Analysis of cause-pathophysiology:
   1. Prenatal factors—rubella and eclampsia.
   2. Prematurity.
   3. Acute infections of middle ear (otitis media), causing perforation of eardrum.
   4. Injury.
B. Assessment:
   1. Infant has little or no interest in environment; begins to coo but then vocalizations cease; no response to noise or voices.
   2. Toddler uses gestures to indicate needs.
   3. School-age child may exhibit intense constant activity, temper tantrums, inattentiveness, and slow learning; speech patterns may be abnormal.
C. Nursing goals and implementation:
   1. Know how long child has had hearing difficulty, how child has adjusted, and how child communicates.
   2. Record observations of behavior during hospitalization.
   3. Interview parents at time of admission to learn child's usual routine and method of communicating.
   4. Refer for testing any child that is suspected of having a hearing difficulty.
   5. Plan activities that will enhance the child's growth and development.

15. Appendicitis— acute condition of inflammation of appendix or blind sac at end of cecum.

A. Incidence—more frequent in spring and in boys (school-age and adolescent).
B. Assessment:
   1. Epigastric pain.
   2. Anorexia with one or two vomiting episodes.
   3. Pain—may become localized after 2 to 12 hours; located in right lower quadrant but remains diffuse in many children; rebound tenderness; pain increases with ambulation.
   4. Constipation.
   5. Mild leukocytosis.
   6. Fever—99 F to 102 F, usual range.
C. Treatment—surgical removal.
D. Nursing goals and implementation:
   1. Prepare child and parent for surgery and explain postoperative course, such as pain, early ambulation, location of scar, and progression from liquid to solid food.
   2. Use ice bag over painful area for comfort—*do not use heat or cathartics,* as these may cause rupture of appendix and peritonitis.

Part D / PREADOLESCENTS AND ADOLES-CENTS

NORMAL GROWTH AND DEVELOPMENT OF PREADOLESCENTS AND ADOLESCENTS

1. Age 12 years, or early adolescence

A. Assessment of physical development (early adolescence):
   1. Eruption of bicuspids and second molars.
   2. Further development of sex characteristics.
B. Assessment of behavior patterns (early adolescence):
   1. Motor development—
      a. Often awkward, uncoordinated.
      b. Displays poor posture.
      c. Tires easily—protein depletion, growth spurt.
   2. Social and mental development—
      a. Increased interest in opposite sex.
      b. Peer group extremely important.
      c. Becomes hostile toward parents.
      d. Forms strong bonds of friendship with one or two peers.
      e. Concerned with morality, ethics, religion, and social customs.
      f. Great variation in academic interest and ability; girls have increased interest in self, cosmetics, etc.; boys have less interest in hygiene and are more interested in sports or team loyalty.
C. Nursing goals and implementation (early adolescence):
   1. Goal: provide appropriate play activities (usual pattern, but any activity may be of interest and appropriate to boy or girl).

a. Girls—social functions, romantic TV shows and movies, makeup, cooking, sewing, art, and poetry.

b. Boys—sports, mechanical and electrical devices, and part-time employment.

2. Goal: provide guidance—

a. Give reassurance and help in accepting changing body image.

b. Understand conflicts as child attempts to deal with social, moral, and intellectual issues.

c. Set realistic but firm limits on expected behavior.

d. Encourage independence, but allow child to turn to adult when there is a need.

e. Provide opportunity to earn own money—paper route, mow lawns, and begin baby-sitting.

2. Late adolescence

A. Assessment of physical development (late adolescence):

1. Completion of sexual development.
2. Appearance of adult.
3. Has 32 permanent teeth.

B. Assessment of behavior patterns (late adolescence):

1. Motor development—
   a. More energy as growth spurt tapers.
   b. Muscular ability and coordination increase.
2. Social and mental development based on Erikson's stages of adolescence (refer to Table 4–1)—early stage, identity versus self-diffusion; later, intimacy versus isolation.
   a. More mature, interdependent relationship with parents.
   b. Romantic love affairs develop as basis for mature relationships.
   c. Ability to balance responsibility and pleasure.
   d. Loosened grasp of peer group; an identity concern about self now and self as an adult.

C. Nursing goals and implementation (late adolescence):

1. Goal: provide appropriate play activities—
   a. Working for altruistic causes.
   b. Sports.
   c. Reading.
   d. Television.
   e. Radio, music, and records.
   f. Challenging mental games (chess).

g. Writing poetry, jokes.

h. Art work.

2. Goal: provide guidance—

a. Provide assistance in selection and preparation for vocation.

b. Provide driver education.

c. Assist in developing healthy attitude—smoking, drinking, drugs, and nutrition.

d. Help parents adjust to loss of their dependent child.

e. Assist in problem-solving.

SPECIAL CONCERNS OF PREADOLESCENTS AND ADOLESCENTS

1. Response to illness and hospitalization—age 12 years to late adolescence.

A. Assessment of discomfort or pain (preadolescence to adolescence):

1. Realizes something is wrong and seeks help.
2. Anxiety is present related to body image and dependency.

B. Assessment of reaction to stage of illness (preadolescence to adolescence):

1. Initial illness or hospitalization—
   a. Expected coping behaviors:
      (1) Resists accepting illness.
      (2) Rebellious against authority.
      (3) Demands control and independence.
      (4) Fearful.
      (5) Temporarily withdraws from social scene.
      (6) Verbalizes how illness has affected life.
   b. Maladaptive behaviors based on loss of self-identity and independence with no hope of redeeming them.
      (1) Tries to manipulate staff.
      (2) Completely dependent and uses denial.
      (3) Denies fear or concern.
      (4) Continues to withdraw.
      (5) Does not verbalize feelings.
2. Prolonged hospitalization and convalescence—
   a. Expected coping or adaptive behaviors:
      (1) Wants to get well.
      (2) Seeks out others.
      (3) Impatient to recover.
      (4) Gives up dependency.
      (5) Concerned about bodily functions and body image.

b. Maladaptive behaviors due to isolation and loss of identity:
   (1) Wants to stay in hospital.
   (2) Childlike and dependent on parents.
c. Nursing goals and implementation (pre-adolescence to adolescence)—
   (1) Allow adolescent as much control as possible—selection of bath time and selection of menu, for example.
   (2) Give independence—let patient chart vital signs and take own medication if possible.
   (3) Offer opportunity for peer contact—room where adolescent can meet others (Peds Pad); have ambulatory patient meet in immobilized patient's room.
   (4) Assist in maintaining identity—dress in own clothes, provide hair-grooming materials, and encourage makeup if worn.
   (5) Listen and validate what you hear from adolescent; encourage patient to discuss feelings.
   (6) Explain hospital rules on admission to ensure cooperation and decrease threat of loss of identity and feelings of isolation.

2. *Nutrition*—age 12 years to late adolescence.
A. Calories:
   1. Age 12 to 14 years—boy, 2700/24 hours; girl, 2300/24 hours.
   2. Age 15 to 16 years—boy, 3000/24 hours; girl, 2300/24 hours.
B. Will select own food and portions; discuss fad diets and eating nonnutritious food.
C. Obesity:
   1. Most common cause is overeating, usually accompanied by reduced activity.
   2. Obese infants tend to become obese older children, who become obese adolescents and adults.
   3. Nursing goals and implementation—
      a. Diet, exercise, and psychologic factors (stress may be a factor, loneliness, "clean plate" award, and food used as a reward for good behavior).
      b. Involve child in selecting weight-reduction method.
      c. Calculate adequate nutritional needs as well as decreased calorie intake.

d. Teach that exercise is more important than diet in child—walking, active play, bicycling, and swimming.
e. Encourage everyone in family to eat regular meals—*not* in front of television or while engaged in some other activity.
f. Administer drugs only as a last resort.
D. Anemia can be a problem in fad diets; nursing goal is to offer acceptable food items high in iron—hamburger, hot dogs, chili with beans, and fortified cereals.

3. *Sex education*
A. Menstruation:
   1. Usually viewed as positive evidence of female sexuality.
   2. Girls should be prepared for onset of menarche.
B. Menstrual disorders:
   1. Amenorrhea—absence of menstruation.
      a. Not unusual when establishing normal cycles.
      b. Primary—delay of menarche after 17 years old.
         (1) Absence or malformation of female genital organs or inability of those organs to respond to hormonal influences.
         (2) Occasionally due to imperforate hymen—treatment is surgical perforation.
      c. Secondary—absence of menstruation for 12 months or more between periods after cycle established.
         (1) Emotional disturbances.
         (2) Pregnancy.
   2. Dysmenorrhea—painful menstruation; usually mild discomfort during first day of period, not uncommon.
   3. Nursing goals and implementation—
      a. Reassure; offer explanation of physiology of menstruation.
      b. Counsel regarding use of mild analgesics and simple exercises.
      c. Stress importance of good hygiene measures, exercise, and balanced diet.
      d. Refer to gynecologist for excessive bleeding, pain.
C. Sexuality:
   1. Assessment of males—
      a. Often appear clumsy with new body and have associated feelings of embarrassment, self-consciousness.

b. Shaving and growth of genitals are equated with male sex role.

c. Sexual feeling are related to genitals and needs are centered on sex act, usually separate from ideas of love.

d. Often use masturbation as means of experimenting and exploring newly developed sexual capacities; relief from pressures in genital organs.

e. Nursing goals and implementation:

   (1) Need reassurance that stage is temporary to strengthen self-concept and maintain self-esteem.

   (2) Need preparation for "wet dreams" (spontaneous ejaculation, usually occurring at night).

   (3) Need reassurance about feelings and practice of masturbation as normal outlet; relieve anxiety and explain myths.

2. Females—

a. Often embarrassed about body changes, especially breast changes and height, which is usually taller than males'.

b. Cultural standards usually cause girls to wish hair removal from legs and underarms; need guidance in proper technique (shaving, depilatories, waxing).

c. May have romantic view of love as opposed to males' view of sex act.

d. May fondle genitals for pleasure but climax is not necessarily all-important or even always desired.

D. Sexual activity:

1. Active teenagers need contraceptive information (see Unit 3 for detailed information); in many states teens may seek advice from free clinic without parents' permission.

2. Increase in sexually transmitted diseases (see *Venereal disease,* p. 379).

3. Number of teenage pregnancies is rising; skilled nurse counselors are necessary to assist in decisions about abortion, adoption, keeping child.

4. Ear-piercing

A. Counsel teens to have ear-piercing done by physician or nurse under sterile conditions rather than by friends or self to minimize side effects, especially in those with diabetes, allergies, skin conditions, other chronic conditions.

B. Culturally determined; popular among U.S. teenagers.

C. Complications include—infection, cyst formation, bleeding, metal allergy, dermatitis.

5. Smoking

A. Prevention is most effective:

1. Posters.

2. Films.

3. Explanations of financial impact, that is, explaining what the cost of cigarettes could purchase.

B. Appeal to newly gained independence *not* to imitate parents or peers who smoke.

CONDITIONS AND DISEASE ENTITIES OF PREADOLESCENTS AND ADOLESCENTS

1. *Juvenile rheumatoid arthritis (Still's disease)*— chronic systemic disease of unknown etiology; there is a wide range of joint involvement; prognosis is good if only one or two joints are involved.

A. Analysis of cause-pathophysiology:

1. Inflammation of joint may be due to virus or postsystemic infection.

2. Growth centers next to inflamed joints may produce premature epiphyseal closure or accelerated epiphyseal growth.

3. Synovial tissues, tendon, and tendon sheaths develop inflammatory changes.

4. Incidence: 9–12 years of age; more often females.

B. Assessment:

1. Stiffness and impaired motion of joints (knees, feet, ankles, wrists, and fingers).

2. Swelling of joints.

3. Spiking fever, malaise, and irritability.

4. Anemia with associated symptoms.

5. Anorexia.

6. Macular rash on trunk and extremities.

7. Hepatosplenomegaly.

8. Lymphadenopathy.

9. Eye inflammation with photophobia, nonreactive pupil, and decreased visual acuity.

10. Joints—deformed, dislocated, and fused.

11. Weak and atrophied muscles near affected joints.

C. Treatment:

1. Goal—to preserve good joint function.

2. Drugs to suppress inflammation of joints.

a. Salicylates—antipyretic, antiinflammatory, and analgesic; given orally or intravenously; side effects are abdominal pain, ringing in ears, hyperventilation in young children, and headaches.

b. Gold salts—exact action unknown; given

intramuscularly; side effects are skin rash, nephritis with hematuria or albuminuria, neurotoxicity, and thrombocytopenia.

   c. Steroids—antiinflammatory given orally, intravenously, intramuscularly, and intraarticularly (in the joint); side effects are masking of infection, peptic ulcer, vascular disorders, hypertension, blurring or dimming of vision, osteoporosis, euphoria, glycosuria, weight gain secondary to water retention, appetite stimulation, round facial contour, and facial hair (Cushing's syndrome).

D. Nursing goals and implementation:
1. Encourage exercise and physical therapy to prevent deformities; night splints for wrists and knees; firm mattress.
2. Administer medications (gold salts, salicylates, and steroids)—explain side effects and reversibility when drug discontinued.
3. Encourage hot tub bath prior to exercises to promote relaxation and decrease pain.
4. Encourage normal activity as tolerated.

2. Scoliosis—lateral curvature of spine.
A. Analysis of etiology-pathophysiology:
1. Most frequently seen in adolescent girls.
2. Cause—idiopathic in 70% of cases.
3. Nonstructural type—
   a. Flexible.
   b. Corrected by bending (lying down, for example).
4. Structural type—
   a. Changes in spine and supporting structures.
   b. Not corrected by side-bending.
B. Assessment:
1. Posterior view of child reveals primary curvature with compensatory curvature, thus child's head is balanced over gluteal fold *or,* if severe, child's head and hips are not in alignment.
2. When child bends over to touch toes, one shoulder is higher than the other; one hand lower than the other.
C. Treatment:
1. Milwaukee brace, steel and leather brace with neck ring and chin pad connected to rods that extend to pelvis and rest on lumbar pads, to halt progression of curvature.
2. Traction—halo pelvic, usually instituted prior to surgical intervention.
3. Surgery—spinal fusion and casting, or imple-

mentation of Harrington metal rod followed by casting.
D. Nursing goals and implementation:
1. Explain type of treatment utilized and prepare for long-term aspects.
   a. Braces may be worn over several years.
   b. Casting following surgery is worn 6–12 months.
2. Suggest clothing styles to "hide" brace/cast such as use of elastic waistband with shirt/blouse worn on outside; tunics for females; measures to encourage positive body image.
3. Explain team approach, orthopedist, physical therapist, orthotist.
4. Assist in discovering alternate ways to care for self: type of shoes, clothing, ways to get in and out of bed; measures to foster independence.

3. Hyperthyroidism (Graves' disease)—endocrine disease manifested by excessive secretion of thyroid hormone.
A. Analysis of cause-pathophysiology:
1. Exact cause unknown.
2. Long-acting thyroid stimulator (LATS) found in serum—causes iodine accumulation and thyroid hyperplasia independent of pituitary.
3. Incidence—mostly females, prior to and during puberty.
B. Assessment:
1. Goiter.
2. Protruding eyeballs, visual disturbances.
3. Hyperactivity.
4. Increased appetite with no weight gain.
5. Increased urination.
6. Skin warm, flushed, moist.
7. Behavior changes; irritability, emotional lability.
C. Diagnosis:
1. Clinical manifestations.
2. Thyroid function tests.
D. Treatment:
1. Diet.
2. Medication.
E. Nursing goals and implementation:
1. Provide calm environment to prevent undue excitement.
2. Encourage high-calorie, high-protein diet because of increased need due to increased activity.
3. Know side effects of medication (propylthiouracil or methimazole) and record any that are noted; toxic effects include fever, rash, headache, nausea, and pain in joints.
4. Provide emotional support of child and family.

4. **Systemic lupus erythematosus**—chronic inflammatory disease of connective tissue that may affect or involve any organ.
A. Analysis of cause-pathophysiology:
   1. Cause unknown but believed to be autoimmune response.
   2. Connective tissue develops fibrinoid change in collagen and cellular infiltration.
   3. Alteration of collagen and thickening of small blood vessel lining obstructs flow of blood.
B. Assessment:
   1. Joints may be painful and swollen.
   2. Anorexia and loss of weight.
   3. Fever.
   4. Butterfly rash across nose and cheeks.
   5. Hematuria and proteinuria.
   6. Weakness.
   7. Nausea and vomiting.
   8. Pleurisy or pericarditis.
   9. Anemia.
   10. Excitability.
C. Treatment:
   1. Aim is to reverse autoimmune and inflammatory process and to prevent complications and exacerbations.
   2. Medications: steroids, immunosuppressants, aspirin.
   3. Activity and diet restrictions to prevent recurrence; diet may be low sodium due to edema and low protein to prevent elevated nitrogen levels.
D. Nursing goals and implementation:
   1. Know side effects of steroid therapy and explain to child and family the expected changes in appearance.
   2. Observe for complications, especially renal involvement (hematuria and proteinuria).
   3. Offer emotional support to child and family.
   4. Use measures to prevent infection.
   5. Avoid exposure to sun—aggravates skin lesions.
   6. Maintain adequate nutrition; offer small portions, as child is anorexic.

5. **Hodgkin's disease**—malignancy of lymphoid system characterized by solid tumors in the lymph nodes.
A. Analysis of cause-pathophysiology:
   1. Etiology unknown.
   2. Malignant cell (Reed-Sternberg cell)—large atypical tumor cell invading spleen, bone marrow, and alimentary tract.
   3. Peak incidence—age 15 to 29 years.
   4. Stages—

   a. Stage I—involvement of single lymph node group, excluding mediastinum and abdomen.
   b. Stage II—involvement of one or more lymph node systems, limited by diaphragm to either upper or lower half of body.
   c. Stage III—involvement above and below diaphragm limited to lymph nodes, spleen, or Waldeyer's throat ring.
   d. Stage IV—systemic involvement of organs other than those listed previously (bone marrow, lungs, kidneys, liver, gastrointestinal tract, and central nervous system).
B. Assessment:
   1. Enlargement of painless, firm, movable lymph nodes.
   2. Fever.
   3. Generalized pruritus.
   4. Night sweats.
   5. Anorexia and weight loss.
   6. General malaise.
   7. Rash.
C. Diagnosis:
   1. Surgical biopsy of affected node.
   2. Lymphangiogram.
D. Treatment:
   1. Based on stage.
   2. Irradiation.
   3. Combination chemotherapy.
E. Nursing goals and implementation:
   1. Prepare for diagnostic tests as appropriate.
   2. Provide symptomatic relief for side effects of chemotherapy (see Appendix D) and/or irradiation.
   3. Maintain adequate nutrition—serve food that child prefers, in pleasant surroundings.
   4. Have change of clothing available to child for night sweats.
   5. Utilize necessary measures, including diversion, to control itching and provide comfort to child.
   6. Provide emotional support to child and family.
   7. Observe for respiratory problems due to airway compression by enlarged lymph glands or organs.
   8. Encourage quiet activities, such as playing musical instruments, art lessons.

6. **Substance abuse**—the addiction to narcotics, experimentation with many drugs, and self-medication.
A. Analysis of cause-pathophysiology:
   1. Taken to promote physical and psychic changes.

2. Physical dependence.
3. Psychic dependence.
4. Self-medication.

B. Assessment:
1. Hallucinogens—
   a. Nausea.
   b. Visual imagery.
   c. Altered and increased sensory awareness.
   d. Anxiety.
   e. Uncoordination, impaired judgement.
2. Narcotics—
   a. CNS depressant.
   b. Euphoria.
   c. Long-term use—loss of weight, constipation, anorexia, and addiction.
3. Sedatives—
   a. Sleep-inducing, drowsiness.
   b. Long-term effects—addiction, irritability, and impaired judgement.
4. Stimulants—
   a. Anorexia.
   b. Insomnia.
   c. Decreased fatigue.
   d. Long-term use—may be habit-forming.
5. Tranquilizers—
   a. Decreased anxiety and tension.
   b. Long-term use—may cause blood dyscrasia, blurred vision, dry mouth, skin rash, and tremors.
6. Miscellaneous—glue or catnip—
   a. Euphoria.
   b. Impaired judgement and coordination.
   c. Long-term use—may cause hallucinations or liver or kidney damage.
7. Cannabis (marijuana)—
   a. Alteration of time perception.
   b. Impaired judgement and coordination.
   c. Euphoria, relaxed state.
   d. Long-term use—habit-forming, decreased sperm count in males, psychologic dependence.

C. Nursing goals and implementation:
1. Teach dangers of drugs.
2. Try to discover why the adolescent is using drugs and refer to counseling resource if appropriate.
3. If overdosed and unconscious, observe for seizures.
4. Stay with child who is experiencing withdrawal symptoms—talk to restore reality, reassurance of care will decrease sense of isolation.
5. Ascertain what was ingested, if possible—ask patient or friend; check pockets for container,

arms for needle marks, and nose for signs of inhalation (sores or foreign substances).
6. Offer support to parents who are experiencing guilt feelings.

7. *Venereal disease*

A. Gonorrhea—inflammation of mucous membrane of genitourinary tract caused by gonococcus, *Neisseria gonorrhoeae;* infection spread by sexual intercourse.
1. Called—GC, clap, gleet, strain, and morning dose.
2. Incubation—two to eight days.
3. Assessment:
   a. Women—may not have any symptoms, but those who do exhibit—
      (1) Light, purulent, yellow vaginal discharge.
      (2) Discomfort, ache in abdomen.
      (3) Bartholin's glands swollen and painful.
      (4) May spread to urethra and bladder with burning, urgency, and urinary frequency.
      (5) Anal area itching, slight discharge.
      (6) Later stage—pelvic inflammatory disease (PID) may be first noticeable symptom (severe pain, high fever, vomiting, and dyspareunia).
   b. Men—
      (1) Thick, purulent discharge from penis.
      (2) Burning on urination.
      (3) Bladder and prostate involvement (penis red, swollen, and sore).
      (4) Inflamed scrotum—hard, swollen, and painful.
4. Can cause sterility in both sexes.
5. One-half of reported cases are under age 25 years.
6. Treatment—aqueous procaine penicillin G, 2.4 million units in one or two doses, IM.

B. Syphilis (syph or lues)—caused by spirochete, *Treponema pallidum,* which enters the body during coitus or through cuts and breaks in skin or mucous membranes.
1. First sign—chancre at site of infection.
2. Incubation period—10 to 60 days, 21 on average.
3. Assessment of stages—
   a. Primary—chancre and enlargement of lymph nodes; most infectious stage.
   b. Secondary—six weeks to six months after primary; skin lesions (macular, papular, fol-

licular, and pustular), arthritic and bone pain, acute iritis, and hoarseness.

   c. Latent—4 to 20 years after primary if developed at all, most serious; destruction of bone tissue, degenerative skin lesions, blindness, heart disease, and severe crippling or paralysis.

  4. Diagnosis—serologic, VDRL.

  5. Treatment—penicillin in first two stages, recovery unpredictable in latent.

C. Herpes simplex virus type II—known as genital herpes; highly contagious.

  1. Incubation: 2–20 days after exposure.

  2. Assessment:

   a. Minor rash, itching in infected area.

   b. Painful, fluid-filled blister(s), often in a group.

   c. Blisters break, forming crusty sore—lasts one to two weeks.

   d. Accompanying symptoms of swollen lymph nodes, fever, aching muscles.

  3. Treatment:

   a. No known effective cure.

   b. Palliative measures such as hot bath or soaks, three times daily; aspirin to relieve pain or topical ointment to relieve itching.

   c. Virus remains in body and may recur any time.

  4. Nursing goals and implementation:

   a. Instruct women to have pap smear every six months, as infection may be related to cervical cancer.

   b. Encourage pregnant women to inform physician; cesarean delivery may be planned, as infection can be passed to infant, with potentially fatal consequences.

   c. Discuss avoidance of sexual activity during active stage of disease.

D. Incidence—increasing due to mobility of population, sexual freedom, promiscuity, and better birth control measures.

E. Nursing goals and implementation for VD in general:

  1. Be specific in history-taking but nonjudgemental and supportive.

  2. Explain necessity of treating partners and ensure confidentiality of contact.

  3. Explain treatment plan.

  4. Educate individuals and groups.

  5. Be aware that most states offer treatment to adolescents without parental consent or knowledge.

8. *Acne vulgaris*—chronic disorder of sebaceous gland activity characterized by glandular secretion of sebum.

A. Analysis of cause-pathophysiology:

  1. Ninety percent of all teenage males and eighty percent of all teenage females are afflicted in some form; mild to severe.

  2. Peak age: 16–20 years old.

  3. Genetic predisposition.

  4. Hormonal changes—production of testosterone or progesterone influences size and activity of sebaceous glands, allowing accumulation and stagnation of sebum.

  5. Predisposing factors—anxiety, stress, and tension, winter weather.

B. Assessment:

  1. Blackheads, whiteheads, pustules, nodules, and cysts.

  2. Lesions block sebaceous glands, causing pustules and scarring.

C. Treatment goals:

  1. Prevent follicular obstruction.

  2. Reduce inflammation.

  3. Prevent secondary infection.

  4. Eliminate predisposing factors.

  5. Noninflammatory (obstructive disease with open and closed comedomes)—

   a. Removal of comedomes.

   b. Use of peeling agent to increase rate of turnover of superficial epithelium.

  6. Inflammatory acne—

   a. Surgical technique (incision and drainage of cyst or nodule).

   b. Chemotherapy with broad-spectrum antibiotic (tetracyclines), corticosteroids (short term), and estrogen (in selected females).

   c. Strict hygiene measures.

D. Nursing goals and implementation:

  1. Have adolescent wash before and after removal of comedomes.

  2. Have patient wash three times a day with mildly abrasive cleaners, shampoo two times a week, and use a brush or rough cloth in bathing.

  3. Instruct in use of peeling agents—

   a. Cleansing agent.

   b. Astringent.

   c. Ultraviolet light.

   d. Topical application of vitamin A acid.

  4. Explain treatment choice.

  5. Instruct in use of comedome extractor.

6. Dispel myths associated with acne; for example, due to masturbation, sexual feelings.

9. Mononucleosis (mono)—an acute infectious disease thought to be viral, self-limiting course.
A. Analysis of cause-pathophysiology:
   1. Often seen at 15 to 25 years of age.
   2. Painful enlargement of cervical lymph nodes.
   3. Spread through oropharyngeal route, mildly contagious.
   4. Incubation period two to six weeks.
B. Positive diagnosis by "spot test"; blood slide test specific for mononucleosis.
C. Assessment:
   1. Fatigue.
   2. Sore throat.
   3. Fever and chills.
   4. Headache.
   5. Lymphadenopathy.
   6. Enlarged spleen.
   7. Difficulty maintaining usual level of activity.
D. Nursing goals and implementation:
   1. Treatment is symptomatic—rest; nutritious, well-balanced diet; and aspirin for fever, chills, and pain.
   2. Avoid exertion, as this may cause rupture of spleen, if enlarged.

Part E / SPECIAL ISSUES

ADMINISTERING MEDICATIONS TO PEDIATRIC PATIENTS

A. Check recommended amount per kilogram of body weight; action of drug being administered; possible side effects; and toxic effects of medication.
B. The following formulas can be used to determine the child's dosage of medications.
   1. The most reliable method is use of *body surface area* as a basis. Use of a nomogram is required (Figure 4–2). If adult dose is known, the following formula is available:

$$\frac{\text{Body surface area of child}}{\text{Body surface area of adult}} \times \text{Adult dose}$$
$$= \text{Estimated child's dose}$$

When the knowledge of average dose per square meter (m^2) of surface area is known, the following formula may be used:

$$\text{Surface area of child } (m^2) \times \text{Dose/m}^2$$
$$= \text{Estimated child's dose}$$

   2. A method for quick computation, particularly for children over age 2 years, is *Clark's Rule* for computation:

$$\frac{\text{Child's weight in pounds}}{150} \times \text{Adult dose}$$
$$= \text{Approximate dose for child}$$

   3. Freid's rule can be used for children under 2 years of age to check a dosage:

$$\frac{\text{Adult dose} \times \text{Age of child (in months)}}{150} = \text{Dose}$$

   4. Another quick computation method for double-checking a dosage for children over age 2 years is Young's rule:

$$\frac{\text{Adult dose} \times \text{Child's age (in years)}}{\text{Child's age} + 12} = \text{Dose}$$

C. Be honest with child; do not bribe or tell child medication is candy.
D. Offer only allowable choices (ask which site child prefers, *not* "Are you ready for an injection?").
E. Do not mix medication with large amounts of food or liquid.
F. Oral medications:
   1. Infant—
      a. Use plastic dropper, syringe, or nipple.
      b. Elevate head and shoulders.
      c. Place thumb on chin to open mouth.
      d. Place dropper on middle of tongue.
   2. Toddler—
      a. May use syringe, straw, medicine cup, or spoon.
      b. Unwise to "hide" medicine in food.
   3. School-age—
      a. Teach child to swallow pill or capsule with fluid.
      b. Offer choice of fluid with medication if appropriate, particularly if taste of medication is unpleasant.
   4. Adolescent—
      a. Allow patient to take own medication if possible.
      b. Explain action of medication to ensure cooperation and to teach health measures.

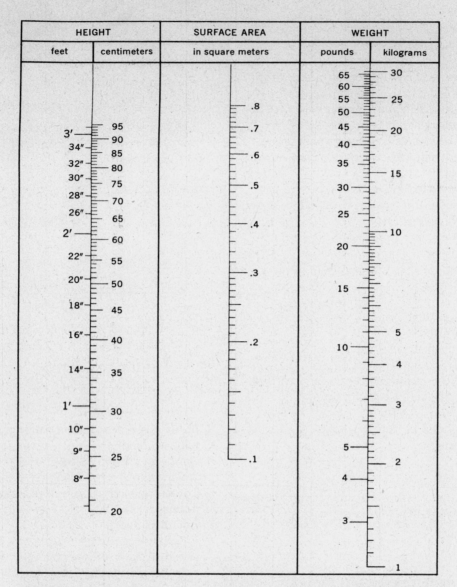

HEIGHT		SURFACE AREA	WEIGHT	
feet	centimeters	in square meters	pounds	kilograms

FIGURE 4–2. Nomogram for estimating surface area of infants and young children
To determine the surface area of the patient, draw a straight line between the point representing his or her height on the left vertical scale to the point representing his or her weight on the right vertical scale. The point at which this line intersects the middle vertical scale represents the patient's surface area in square meters. (Courtesy Abbott Laboratories.)

G. Intramuscular injections (IM):
　1. Infant—
　　a. Lateral and anterior aspect of thigh are preferred sites.
　　b. Insert needle at 90° angle to surface on which child is lying.
　　c. May administer up to 2 cc only in one site.
　2. Toddler, school-age, and adolescent—

　　a. Dorsogluteal, after child has been walking one year or more:
　　　(1) Upper outer quadrant.
　　　(2) Prone position, toes pointed inward.
　　b. Ventrogluteal:
　　　(1) Child on back.
　　　(2) Shield child from observing if upset.
　　c. Deltoid:

(1) Older or larger child.

(2) Bottom of muscle.

H. Subcutaneous injections:

1. To prevent needle from entering the muscle, insert at 45° angle.

2. Commonly used to administer insulin, heparin, and immunizations.

I. Intravenous infusion:

1. Check child hourly to regulate flow, more often if beginning infusion or administering medications; inspect site and record amount and type of fluid given.

2. Regulate flow as necessary to avoid overload of circulatory system; use only mini or micro drops (50–60 drops/cc or ml).

3. A mechanical infusion pump may be used to administer fluid more precisely but should still be checked every hour. *Caution:* pump will continue even if needle becomes dislodged, causing infiltration.

4. Change the bottle and tubing at least every 24 hours.

5. Disconnect the infusion by clamping at site close to needle when ordered, infusion complete, or if infiltrated.

6. Observe for complications—

   a. Fluid overload.

   b. Medication side effects.

   c. Signs of infiltration, phlebitis, or pyrogenic reaction (presence of redness, edema, pain at site).

   d. Nerve damage.

   e. Air embolism.

7. Record essential information—

   a. Time and amount absorbed.

   b. Description of infusion site.

   c. Reaction of child; behaviors.

   d. Rate of infusion.

   e. Intake and output.

   f. Daily weight.

8. Nursing interventions to keep infusion from infiltrating in child—

   a. Tape needle, supported with gauze, firmly in place.

   b. Restrain limb or head if child is very active or nurse is not present; sandbags on either side of head; small, inverted paper cup trimmed and taped to cover site on scalp or foot; arm restraints (clove hitch, elbow sticks, gauze tied to siderails, arm board, foot board).

c. Move or pick up child carefully, supporting intravenous site.

9. Continue to play with and hold child, teach and support parents to hold and comfort child.

J. Ear drops:

1. Warm solution, as cold drops may cause severe pain.

2. Under age 3 years—pull pinna down and back; over age 3 years—pull pinna up and back.

K. Eye medication:

1. Ointments—gently pull lower lid down, forming pocket, and administer in conjunctiva.

2. Drops—place child's head to side so that drops placed in inner cannula flow toward outer cannula.

L. Nose drops:

1. Slightly hyperextend head and administer drops without contacting nasal mucosa with dropper.

2. Administer decongestant drops 20 minutes prior to feeding infant so infant will be able to suck and breathe.

DEATH AND DYING

1. Children's concept of death

A. Evolutionary or progressive, dependent upon cognitive functioning.

B. Stages (ages approximate):

1. Under age 3 years—death itself is not perceived, rather fear of separation and abandonment by parents or caretaker is primary concern.

2. Preschooler, 3–5 years of age, death as an entity is recognized; know it happens to others; viewed as reversible process; may view as punishment.

3. Early school-age, 6–10 years, begins to view death as permanent and universal; questions what happens after death; may express "it isn't fair"; only old people die.

4. Preadolescent and adolescent, over age 10 or 11 years, views death as final, inevitable, personal, and universal; questions the biological process; may ask "What does it feel like?"; concerned about body changes.

2. Nursing goals and implementation

A. Communication:

1. Know the family's concept of life and death; the philosophical, religious, social, and cultural stances.

2. Know own philosophy of life and death and possess ability to determine if you can communicate with child and family.

3. Determine family's and child's past experience with death and emotional response to it.
4. Know of child's concept of death—
   a. Know usual pattern of understanding.
   b. Terminally ill child may be one step ahead of healthy peers in awareness of the facts of death, but is still incapable of understanding death cognitively.
5. Know of process over content in communicating with children; that is, child pays more attention to what nurse *does* and *how* she says something than to *what* is said.
6. Reassure child who is dying that he or she will not be alone at time of death or after death; fearful of abandonment.

B. Comfort:
1. Attend to physical needs of child facing death.
2. Be aware of family, parent and siblings, physical needs; give them permission to eat, sleep, care for self, if necessary.

C. Care:
1. Determine emotional needs of child and devise plan to meet them.
2. Recognize emotional needs and response of family members; assist them to utilize their own resources and offer them support.

MANAGEMENT OF PEDIATRIC EMERGENCIES (TABLE 4–16)

TABLE 4–16. *Management of pediatric emergencies*

Condition	Etiology	Action
Abdominal injury or pain	Ingestion, blow, nausea, vomiting.	Obtain history to determine cause; lie flat; no food intake.
Animal bites: —Bee sting	Stinger may be present or not. Possibility of allergic reaction.	Remove stinger by *scraping,* not pulling out; apply ice or calamine lotion; observe for reaction (hives, asthma). Call First-Aid/Paramedic squad if reaction develops.
—Dog bite	Dog may be ill or victim of teasing.	Wash wound with soap; apply wet dressing; confine dog; and notify Health Dept. and/or police.
—Spider bite	Spiders hide in papers, closets, shoes; some types are potentially harmful to children.	Apply ice. If Black Widow or Brown Recluse, refer small children to physician. Observe for edema, respiratory distress.
—Snake bite	Seen in desert, arid regions beneath rocks; some found in water, temperate climates. Startled snake may bite.	Rinse area; position child so affected area is lower than heart; transport to medical facility for antivenom medication.
Bleeding	Trauma.	Apply pressure to area and elevate. Cover with sterile dressing.
Blisters	Common on feet and hands; from poorly fitting shoes, climbing on ropes, swinging on bars.	Do not puncture; wash with soap and water; Band-aid may be applied to protect from rupture. If rupture, clean with disinfectant and cover with clean dressing to protect from infection.

TABLE 4–16.   *(Continued)*

Condition	Etiology	Action
Bruises, lacerations, abrasions, cuts	Common in all children, usually due to accidents.	Examine extent of injury. Bruise—apply ice for 30 minutes. Wash broken skin with peroxide solution or soap and water; cover with bandage. If deep wound, apply wet, sterile dressing; refer for medical aid.
Burns:		
—Chemical	Due to chemical spill.	Soak in cool water for 30 minutes.
—First-degree	Due to sunburn, hot stove, match head, etc.	Apply ice for 30 minutes; may use dry dressing.
—Second- and third-degree	Severe burns.	Apply ice; transport to medical facility. *No salves or ointments!*
Eye problems:	Types vary with age and activity of child.	
—Blow to eye	Fighting, elbow, knee, racquet sports.	Apply ice; patch eye; *do not irrigate.*
—Chemicals	Burns, chemistry lab.	Rinse with cool, running tap water 20–30 minutes; patch both eyes and transport to medical facility.
—Foreign body	Eyelash, piece of any type material.	If free-floating, attempt removal once with cotton-tipped applicator moistened with water. If unsuccessful or unable to attempt removal, transport to medical facility.
—Penetrating object	Pencil, dart, any object that penetrates eye.	*Do not attempt removal. Do not irrigate.* Patch both eyes and transport to medical facility.
Foreign bodies:		
—Aspiration	Seen in infants and toddlers; usually involves food that child cannot chew (e.g., peanuts, raisins, popcorn), but may be buttons, small toys. Aspiration into bronchial tree or lungs.	Note signs/symptoms of cough, dyspnea, choking, stridor. *Do not attempt digital removal!* If child is coughing or wheezing, leave alone; if *no air* is moving in or out, modified Heimlich maneuver is indicated. Transport *immediately* to medical facility.

(Continued)

TABLE 4–16.   *(Continued)*

Condition	Etiology	Action
—Ingestion	Small infants and toddlers may swallow a nonfood item such as a paperclip or pebble.	Note any painful or difficult swallowing. If object seen in throat, tip child forward, head down, and strike back, or reach in mouth and "hook" object with finger. If swallowed, observe stools for passage *unless* sharp object, in which case transport for X rays and possible surgery.
Fractures	Break in any bone, often seen in athletic accidents. Most common in children over age 6 years is greenstick fracture (incomplete break). Sites commonly seen are clavicle, wrist, forearm, fingers, hands, femur, elbow.	Observe for pain, tenderness, swelling at affected site; immobilize with splint (newspapers, broom handle, towel); use sling for fractured clavicle. Apply cold pack. *Do not move if back or legs involved.* If injury involves chest, have child sit up; call professional aid to transport child.
Head injuries:	Accidents, falls, blows with blunt object.	
—Concussions, subdural hematoma	Most common head injury among children. May be asymptomatic 6–18 hours after injury.	Observe for level of consciousness, vital signs, pupil reactions; keep child calm, quiet, resting; may apply ice bag.
—Skull fracture	Usually accompanied by concussion; confirmed by X ray and fluid in nasal or ear passages; may be line, depressed, or basilar fracture.	Have child lie flat; transport to medical facility. If open wound, cover with light dressing to protect and prevent infection and further trauma.
Nosebleeds	Common occurrence, especially among preadolescent girls. Other causes include trauma, nose-picking, exercise, forcible blowing.	Have child sit with head elevated; apply gentle, firm pressure over bridge of nose. If severe, apply ice pack to nape of neck or to bridge of nose; instruct not to blow nose.
Pencil punctures	Frequently seen in school-age children.	Soak in warm water and antiseptic solution for 30 minutes.

TABLE 4–16.   *(Continued)*

Condition	Etiology	Action
Poisonings, ingestions	1–4 years of age may ingest substances that will cause grave harm to tissues and membranes and seriously impair normal body functions.	Determine *what* was ingested; follow antidotal instructions, if available; call poison control center and/or physician. Dilute substance by giving milk, oil, or water; *do not induce vomiting if child is comatose or substance is corrosive.* Check for chemical burns; rule of thumb: if it burns going down, it will burn coming up.
Sprains	Not frequently seen in small children. May see fingers, elbow, ankle sprains—usually due to sports accidents among older school-age children.	Apply ice for 72 hours; immobilize; heat after 72 hours. May use Ace bandage on sprained joints; tape sprained finger to adjacent finger or use tongue blade.

Questions / NURSING CARE OF CHILDREN AND FAMILIES

1. The developmental theory most widely used by health care professionals is that instituted by:
   1. Freud.
   2. Watson.
   3. Erikson.
   4. Gesell.

2. Project Headstart is administered by:
   1. Department of Health and Human Services.
   2. Children's Bureau.
   3. Family Service.
   4. Local public welfare office.

Mr. and Mrs. Clay have four children, including a new baby, Carrie. Questions 3–20 are based upon the Clay family. You are the nurse/counselor in the Clays' pediatrician's office and have the primary responsibility of counseling the Clays, including anticipatory guidance in growth and development, answering their questions, clarifying the physician's recommendations, and intervening in health crises.

3. As a nurse/counselor in a pediatric setting, the nurse should know that the primary cause of death in children is associated with:
   1. Leukemia.
   2. Suicides.
   3. Accidents.
   4. Congenital heart defects.

4. Mr. Clay is eager to make his house safe for his children. In advising him you explain that when he is considering potential sources of accidents, special consideration should be given to his children's:
   1. Preference of play area.
   2. Intelligence.
   3. Level of development.
   4. Behavior.

5. Mrs. Clay has several questions about her baby, Carrie. She has purchased bibs to keep Carrie's clothes dry when she begins to drool and teethe. The nurse could explain that drooling begins at approximately age:
   1. 1 to 2 months.
   2. 3 to 4 months.
   3. 1 to 3 weeks.
   4. 5 to 6 months.

6. Mrs. Clay questions how she should dress Carrie. In counseling Mrs. Clay on dressing her infant, the nurse should know that normal infants begin to sweat:
   1. Right after birth.
   2. About 1 month of age.
   3. About 3 months of age.
   4. About 6 months of age.

7. Mrs. Clay is also concerned about feeding her baby solid foods. The nurse explains that one should generally follow a certain progression when introducing foods to an infant. The sequence is:
   1. Fruit, vegetables, and cereal.

2. Fruit, meat, and cereal.
3. Cereal, fruit, and vegetables.
4. Cereal, meat, and vegetables.

8. The time for introducing solid foods to an infant's diet should be based on all the following *except:*
1. Infant can sit with support.
2. Stools have more solid characteristics.
3. Infant has demonstrated ability to swallow without tongue protrusion reflex.
4. Point at which infant requires the food nutritionally.

9. Mrs. Clay says her other children drooled and were irritable when they began teething. In reviewing this subject with Mrs. Clay, you recall that the usual pattern of teething is:
1. 2–3 months—lower-central incisors followed by upper incisors.
2. 2–3 months—upper-central incisors followed by lower incisors.
3. 6–7 months—lower-central incisors followed by upper incisors.
4. 6–7 months—upper-central incisors followed by lower incisors.

10. Joe Clay loves to show off his first loose tooth to you when he visits the clinic for his check-up. Joe is probably in which age group?
1. 3–4 years.
2. 5–6 years.
3. 6–7 years.
4. 8–9 years.

11. The Clays also have a daughter, Candy, who is 2 years old. Mrs. Clay is interested in toilet-training her daughter. When discussing toilet-training, the nurse should keep in mind that this is an automatic function that is placed under voluntary control by:
1. Conditioning and reinforcement.
2. Conditioning and maturation.
3. Trial and error.
4. Imitation and learning.

12. As Candy begins to use the toilet, she most likely will have "accidents." The *best* way to handle this is to:
1. Change her clothing and suggest she tell you the next time she has to go.
2. Scold Candy for soiling herself.
3. Praise her for success.
4. Periodically sit her on the potty chair.

13. Mr. Clay tells you that Candy had a temper tantrum while they were visiting some neighbors. He asks your advice as to what he should do when Candy has a tantrum. Your best advice would be:
1. To place Candy in a room by herself.
2. To punish the behavior immediately.
3. To ignore her behavior.
4. To give Candy what she wants.

14. The only other concern that the Clays have about Candy is her unwillingness to go to bed at night. Scolding, pleading, and threatening have not worked. Recalling the normal negativity of this age group, the most effective way to get a 2-year-old child to bed is to:
1. Ask if the child is tired and would like to go to bed.
2. Ask child if she wants you to put her to bed.
3. Tell child that she is a "big girl" and knows it is time to go to bed.
4. Tell child it is time for teddy bear to be put to bed and take child's hand.

15. Nine-year-old Todd Clay has juvenile diabetes mellitus. He is managed by subcutaneous administration of insulin and diet. To effectively counsel and teach Todd and his family about his condition, the nurse must know that the physiologic defect underlying symptom production in diabetes mellitus is:
1. Increased absorption of glucose from the intestine.
2. Increased electrolyte absorption from renal tubule.
3. Increased rate of respiration in the tissue cells.
4. Decreased production of insulin by the pancreas.

16. While teaching Todd about diabetes, the nurse should instruct him to carry the following with him at all times:
1. A piece of hard candy.
2. A bag of salted nuts.
3. Insulin and syringe.
4. A dime to phone parents in case he feels ill.

17. In differentiating between diabetic coma and insulin shock, the nurse needs to know that one of the following is *not* a symptom of insulin shock:
1. Weakness.
2. Pallor.
3. Flushed face.
4. Tremor.

18. Teaching Todd to give his own injections and recording the sites used is your next task. In planning both your presentation and award system, you consider that Todd is mastering Erikson's stage of:
1. Industry versus inferiority.
2. Intimacy versus isolation.
3. Trust versus mistrust.
4. Autonomy versus shame.

19. Joe Clay, the second-grader, comes home with a note that states he has pediculosis. In explaining the treatment to Mrs. Clay, the nurse will include:
1. A discussion on hygiene, as infestation is a direct result of this.
2. The fact that all members of the family must be treated.
3. An explanation of the possibility of hair loss and need for wearing a cap.
4. Reassurance that condition is not contagious.

A general knowledge of immunization is necessary for the pediatric nurse. Questions 20–30 concern this information.

20. Immunizations should be started when child is:
1. Age 6 months.
2. Age 2 months.
3. Age 12 months.
4. Age 2 weeks.

21. Infants do not receive passive immunization against which of the following?
1. Tetanus.
2. Diphtheria.
3. Pertussis.
4. Tetanus and diphtheria.

22. There is no active immunization for:
1. Measles.
2. Smallpox.
3. Chicken pox.
4. Mumps.

23. DPT is used to immunize children against:
1. Diphtheria, polio, and tetanus.
2. Diphtheria, polio, and typhoid.
3. Diphtheria, pertussis, and tetanus.
4. Diphtheria, pertussis, and typhoid.

24. After administering DPT the nurse should:
1. Massage the site and apply a bandage.
2. Avoid massage and apply a bandage.
3. Avoid massage and press sponge on skin over needle.
4. Apply gauze over area and give aspirin for pain.

25. Booster doses of DPT should be given at:
1. Ages 4 months and 12 months.
2. Ages 6 months and 18 months.
3. Ages 18 months and 4 to 6 years.
4. Ages 4 to 6 years and 10 years.

26. The name of the sensitivity test for diphtheria is:
1. Dick.
2. Schick.
3. Babinsky.
4. Schaback.

27. Regular tuberculin testing should be done annually:
1. During the first ten years of life.
2. In the first five years of life.
3. Until the test shows positive results.
4. Until a child graduates from high school.

28. The results of a tuberculin test should be read within:
1. 24 hours.
2. 48 hours.
3. 72 hours.
4. 96 hours.

29. Mumps vaccine is not recommended for the following group:
1. All children 1 to 12 years of age.
2. Pubescent men.
3. Adult men who have not had mumps.
4. Infants 2–6 months of age.

30. Children with scarlet fever display:
1. White spots on skin.
2. White, strawberry tongue.
3. Koplik's spots.
4. Alopecia.

Mary, a 5-month-old infant, is admitted to your unit with diffuse areas of reddened papular lesions on her skin. Her mother states that Mary has never been ill before. Mary is fed pureed foods in addition to breast milk and daily vitamin drops. She is presently irritable and attempts to scratch or rub her lesions. She is admitted with a diagnosis of infantile eczema. Questions 31–35 concern this situation.

31. In response to Mary's mother's questions regarding eczema, you answer that most infants who develop eczema:
1. Have it all their lives.
2. Outgrow it by the time they reach 4 years of age.
3. Outgrow it, but may show allergic reactions or manifestations later in life.
4. Will never have another episode of eczema.

32. Mary will most likely be placed on:
1. A soft diet.
2. A high-protein diet.
3. A regular diet.
4. An elimination diet.

33. To prevent Mary from scratching herself and causing irritation and infection, the best action for the nurse is to:
1. Restrain Mary's limbs using clove-hitch restraints, being certain to change her position frequently.
2. Allow her free motion after trimming her fingernails and toenails.
3. Hold Mary while playing with her, using elbow restraints or mitts as necessary.
4. Ask the doctor to prescribe medication for Mary to stop the itching.

34. Which toys would be best for Mary?
1. Soft, washable toys.
2. Stuffed toys.
3. Puzzles and games.
4. Toy cars.

35. In bathing Mary, the nurse would most likely use the following regimen:
1. Give her a bubble bath.
2. Use mineral oil.
3. Use only Ivory or castile soap.
4. Use baby lotion.

36. As a nurse in the pediatric unit, you should be aware that the following causes the highest incidence of morbidity and mortality in infancy:
1. Rheumatic fever.
2. Infections.

3. Congenital heart defects.

4. Accidents.

Danny, a 2-week-old infant, is suspected to have a congenital heart defect. The tentative diagnosis is patent ductus arteriosus (PDA). Questions 37–40 concern this situation.

37. The most likely symptoms of PDA include:
   1. Becomes cyanotic on exertion.
   2. Becomes cyanotic when lying flat.
   3. Is acyanotic.
   4. Has difficulty breathing.

38. Diagnostic studies have been ordered and you must further explain these tests to Danny's parents. Angiocardiography can best be described as:
   1. A set of chest X rays taken from various angles with the patient in different positions to reveal the surface contour of the heart.
   2. A print-out of sound waves produced by the heart.
   3. An injection of radiopaque dye into a catheter inserted into the chambers of the heart.
   4. A record of the passage of electrical impulses accompanying contraction from the sinoauricular node to all parts of the myocardium.

39. A positive diagnosis is made of PDA and a decision is made to discharge Danny. Your role is to:
   1. Explain comfort measures the parents can provide until Danny dies.
   2. Teach the parents to organize care for Danny.
   3. Reassure his parents that the defect will resolve itself.
   4. Explain that this defect is repaired only if other symptoms develop.

40. An appropriate activity for Danny would be to:
   1. Have a music box played near him.
   2. Hang a mobile in his crib.
   3. Give him pop beads to play with.
   4. Give him a stuffed animal.

Tanya T was born with a cleft lip and palate. The lip was repaired soon after birth, but the palate will be repaired in stages. Questions 41–45 concern this situation.

41. Following repair of the cleft lip, the nurse should:
   1. Use a hard nipple for feeding to exercise muscles used for sucking.
   2. Not allow the mother to care for the child because of the fragile suture line.
   3. Remove the restraints and exercise the child's arms periodically.
   4. Change child's position, rotating from side to abdomen to back.

42. In explaining the cleft palate deformity to Mrs. T, the nurse could explain that one of the following is *not* affected by cleft palate deformities:
   1. Breathing.

2. Swallowing.

3. Neck mobility.

4. Speech.

43. When Tanya is readmitted at age 15 months, she will probably enjoy the following activity:
   1. Playing with her favorite toy.
   2. Constructing a tower of 20 blocks.
   3. Listening to popular tunes on the radio.
   4. Stringing small beads.

44. To prepare Tanya for her cleft palate surgery, the following would be most helpful:
   1. A preadmission tour and movie.
   2. Explaining the postoperative care to Tanya and her parents.
   3. Periodically placing elbow restraints on Tanya.
   4. Recommending a child's book on hospitalization for the parents to read to Tanya.

45. Following the repair, Tanya's parents have questions about future procedures for Tanya. The nurse can best respond:
   1. "You are concerned about your daughter's future."
   2. "There is no need to concern yourself about that now."
   3. "Please discuss that with Tanya's pediatrician."
   4. "The repair is usually done in stages. Would you like to discuss the possible sequence for Tanya?"

Baby Boy Prince was born with hypospadias. Questions 46–47 concern this situation.

46. Hypospadias is a congenital disorder in which:
   1. Genitalia are those of a female but chromosome studies show male genotype.
   2. One or both testes are undescended.
   3. The urinary bladder protrudes from the bladder wall.
   4. The urethral meatus is on the underside of the penis.

47. Mr. Prince is concerned about repairing this defect. Usually this is surgically corrected:
   1. Immediately after birth.
   2. When an infant weighs 10 lb (4.5 kg).
   3. Only if associated problems occur.
   4. Between 2 and 3 years of age.

Mr. and Mrs. C have brought their small child, Cecie, to the emergency department of your hospital. Cecie has a broken arm and head injuries. There are bruises on Cecie's body that are in various stages of healing. Mr. C explains that Cecie fell out of her high chair. The nurse suspects child abuse. Questions 48–51 concern this situation.

48. If a nurse suspects child abuse, her course of action is to:
   1. Tactfully elicit information from parents to prove or disprove abuse.

2. Report suspicion to the physician.

3. Report suspicion to the police.

4. Suggest parenting class to parents.

49. Considering her knowledge of child abuse, the nurse should be aware that most children who are battered:
    1. Are over 6 months of age.
    2. Are preschoolers who misbehave.
    3. Are under the age of 3 years.
    4. Live in underprivileged areas.

50. She also knows that the child *most likely* to be abused in a family is the:
    1. Demanding child.
    2. Oldest child.
    3. Youngest child.
    4. Whining child.

51. Mrs. C appears genuinely concerned about Cecie. In talking with her you discover she and her husband are new to the area and have been unable to meet friends. In general, battering parents exhibit all of the following characteristics, *except:*
    1. Sensitive about ability and general effectiveness as parents.
    2. Like to be alone.
    3. Have unrealistic expectations of child's behavior.
    4. Have no outlet for expression of tension and fear.

Mr. Louis is concerned about Eric, his infant son, who "doesn't look right." The doctor suspects Eric has cerebral palsy. Questions 52–57 concern this situation.

52. A leading diagnostic sign of cerebral palsy is:
    1. Drooling.
    2. Motor function disorder.
    3. Microcephaly.
    4. Scissored lower extremities.

53. When Mr. Louis asks what caused the cerebral palsy, the nurse could explain that possible causes might include any of the following *except:*
    1. Anoxia at birth.
    2. Intrauterine infection.
    3. Prematurity.
    4. Mental retardation.

54. Mr. Louis could also be told that the following is true of cerebral palsy:
    1. It involves a progressive brain lesion.
    2. Motor function is not impaired.
    3. It involves movement and posture due to a defect or lesion of the brain.
    4. It always results in mental retardation.

55. Mr. Louis notices that Eric displays a preference for using his right hand. You interpret this sign as:
    1. Normal behavior.
    2. Abnormal behavior.

3. His imagination.

4. Precocious behavior.

56. Mr. Louis questions whether Eric will be mentally retarded, as his speech is delayed. You know that:
    1. One-third of children with cerebral palsy are mentally retarded.
    2. One-third of children with cerebral palsy are normal.
    3. All children with cerebral palsy are normal.
    4. All children with cerebral palsy are mentally retarded.

57. Home exercises are prescribed as part of Eric's treatment. In assisting the Louis family, you explain that the exercises should be done:
    1. Early in the morning when Eric wakens.
    2. Quickly and often.
    3. After a warm bath.
    4. Slowly and gently.

Mrs. Martinez was instructed to insert a Phenistex strip in Maria's diaper as a routine test for PKU (phenylketonuria). This was done and the strip mailed as requested. Two days later the nurse telephoned Mrs. Martinez and requested an appointment be made for Maria. Questions 58–60 concern this situation.

58. The definitive diagnosis for PKU is accomplished by:
    1. Urine analysis.
    2. Blood test.
    3. Sweat analysis.
    4. Genetic history.

59. The nurse explains the treatment for Maria to Mrs. Martinez, which is a diet free of:
    1. Lactose.
    2. Glutens.
    3. Fats.
    4. Food preservatives.

60. When Maria reaches the toddler stage, she begins refusing certain foods. Mrs. Martinez asks the nurse for some suggestions for this problem. One suggestion for this age is to have Maria:
    1. Eat only when she is hungry.
    2. Have her meal in a location other than the kitchen.
    3. Eat with friends her age.
    4. Feed herself.

Mrs. Kane has noticed that over the past few weeks her 3-year-old son, Patrick, seems to be gaining weight. His clothes fit tighter and his shoes are nearly impossible to get on in the morning. Mr. Kane remarks about Patrick's puffy eyes and suggests a visit to the pediatrician. Following an examination and laboratory tests, the pediatrician's diagnosis of Patrick is nephrotic syndrome. Questions 61–66 concern this situation.

61. For the majority (80%) of patients with nephrotic syndrome, the cause is:

1. Unknown.
2. Autoimmune response.
3. Acute glomerulonephritis.
4. Post-infectious process.

62. While he is undergoing tests, Patrick is admitted to your unit. To help Patrick adjust, you suggest that Mrs. Kane:
    1. Not visit until he is discharged to avoid upsetting him when she leaves.
    2. Spend the night in the hospital.
    3. Bring Fred, Patrick's teddy bear, to him.
    4. Buy him gifts so he won't mind being in the hospital.

63. Patrick is placed on steroid therapy. The aim of this therapy is to prevent:
    1. Diuresis.
    2. Hematuria.
    3. Proteinuria.
    4. Potassium loss.

64. The pediatrician has explained to the Kanes that Patrick will probably require symptomatic treatment for a long period of time. The prognosis for a child with nephrotic syndrome is:
    1. Poor—80% death rate.
    2. Poor—duration is prolonged and death is inevitable.
    3. Good—80% survive.
    4. Good—50% recover.

65. The diet prescribed for Patrick during this acute phase will most likely be:
    1. High protein, high potassium, low sodium.
    2. Low protein, high potassium, low sodium.
    3. High protein, low potassium, low sodium.
    4. Low protein, low potassium, high sodium.

66. When he is at home, Patrick likes to play outside. The following would be *most* appropriate for Patrick:
    1. Two-wheel bike.
    2. Sandbox.
    3. Climbing trees.
    4. Push-toy lawn mower.

Lucas O, a 2-year-old boy, is admitted in sickle cell crisis. Questions 67–73 concern this situation.

67. Sickle cell anemia is:
    1. A type of leukemia.
    2. Curable.
    3. An inherited condition.
    4. A progression of sickle cell trait.

68. Screening for the sickle cell trait or disease in the United States should be done routinely for the following group of persons:
    1. Asians.
    2. Black Americans.
    3. Native Americans (American Indians).
    4. Mexican Americans.

69. In addition to loss of appetite, the nurse would expect to see the following signs exhibited by Lucas:
    1. Fatigue, infection, and paleness.
    2. Alertness, jaundice, and pain in abdomen.
    3. Mental confusion, weakness, and flushing.
    4. Weakness, jaundice, and pain in abdomen, legs, or arms.

70. Lucas has had many tests and painful procedures. Following these, the nurse could best help Lucas by:
    1. Putting him to bed for a nap.
    2. Initiating play with use of a puppet.
    3. Rocking him.
    4. Doing funny tricks for him.

71. Mrs. O states that Lucas has always been a "good" baby but lately has become very headstrong. The nurse should explain that the most likely reason for negative behavior in a 2-year-old child is:
    1. Obstinacy.
    2. Being spoiled.
    3. Seeking independence.
    4. Learning right from wrong.

72. Mrs. O is contemplating having another child but is fearful that the next child will also have sickle cell anemia, although neither she nor her husband has sickle cell anemia. From your knowledge of this inherited condition, you tell Mrs. O:
    1. That it is possible another child will have sickle cell anemia.
    2. That most probably subsequent children will be normal.
    3. That most probably subsequent children will have sickle cell trait only.
    4. That it is sex-dependent; boys have anemia and girls have the trait.

73. If he is following the usual progression of development, Lucas probably has the following number of teeth:
    1. 16.
    2. 8.
    3. 20.
    4. 10.

Questions 74–79 concern Bobby, a 5 year old with hemophilia.

74. Following a bleeding episode the nurse caring for Bobby should:
    1. Promote quiet and rest for Bobby.
    2. Exercise his extremities.
    3. Wrap his joints in cotton batting.
    4. Administer sedatives to Bobby.

75. The nurse should be aware that children with hemophilia often experience the following complication following a bleeding episode:
    1. Hemarthrosis.

2. Bruising scars.
3. Hemangioma.
4. Anemia.

76. Following developmental testing, you determine that Bobby is slightly delayed in some areas for his age. The most likely cause of this is:
    1. Mental retardation.
    2. Overprotection by his parents.
    3. Curtailment of his activities.
    4. Misinterpretation of the results.

77. During his convalescence Bobby draws a picture that is somewhat abstract and shows it to you. The most appropriate verbal response from you is:
    1. "Who is this?"
    2. "Oh, what a lovely picture!"
    3. "What is it?"
    4. "Tell me about your picture."

78. When Bobby returns home, he may display the following behavior to meet his need for love, belongingness, and control:
    1. Participating in parallel play.
    2. Imitating the dress of adults.
    3. Inventing an imaginary companion.
    4. Sympathizing with an injured peer.

79. Bobby's mother tells you that Bobby refuses to take an afternoon nap. You suggest:
    1. A quiet time after lunch in lieu of a nap.
    2. He has outgrown his need for naps.
    3. He needs less sleep at night.
    4. A later time for his nap.

Benjy K, a 5-year-old boy, is admitted with a tentative diagnosis of acute leukemia. He had a cold which seemed to persist. He is pale, apathetic, and losing weight. He also has petechiae on his skin, ulceration of his gums, and large cervical and inguinal lymph nodes. A bone marrow examination to confirm the diagnosis is planned. Questions 80–84 concern this situation.

80. The sites commonly used for bone marrow punctures are:
    1. Humerus, sternum, and femur.
    2. Iliac crest and sternum.
    3. Sternum and femur.
    4. Femur and skull.

81. The diagnosis is confirmed. The changes producing the symptoms of acute leukemia are:
    1. Excessive destruction of red blood cells by the liver.
    2. Abnormal production of white blood cells by the spleen.
    3. Proliferation of abnormal white blood cells.
    4. Decreased production of white blood cells.

82. Benjy's apathy and pallor are an indication of:
    1. Anemia.
    2. Poor nutrition.

3. Renal disease.
4. Infection.

83. The nurse understands that Benjy is especially susceptible to infection because:
    1. Enlarged lymph nodes are not functional.
    2. Immature leukocytes are not capable of normal phagocytosis.
    3. Severe anemia conditions exist.
    4. Liver cannot detoxify toxins.

84. In response to Mrs. K's questions regarding what she could have done to prevent this disease, the nurse should reassure her and explain that the actual etiology of leukemia is:
    1. Viral.
    2. Genetic.
    3. Radiation.
    4. Unknown.

85. Mrs. K is concerned that she did not take Benjy to the doctor when his cold first appeared. The nurse might reply that:
    1. "It is too late to look back."
    2. "Perhaps you should discuss this with your doctor."
    3. "The delay did not have any effect on the course of the disease."
    4. "We'll never know what could have happened if Benjy was treated sooner."

86. Cortisone acetate is one of the drugs Benjy is receiving. The nurse should be alert to possible side effects resulting from cortisone administration. These include:
    1. Increased appetite, edema, and fever.
    2. Tinnitus and nausea.
    3. Anorexia and weight gain.
    4. Hypertension, vomiting, and chills.

87. Benjy is readmitted to the hospital after a six-month remission from his condition. He is now in the terminal stage and seems to feel hopeless and afraid. The nurse could best help Benjy by:
    1. Allowing him to make the decisions for his care.
    2. Making all his decisions for him.
    3. Discussing with him the usual fears of dying children.
    4. Discussing with him the reasons for his fears.

88. Benjy has become unconscious and death appears imminent. The nurse should plan to:
    1. Avoid Benjy and his parents.
    2. Spend the usual amount of time with Benjy in his room.
    3. Remain with Benjy and his parents as much as possible.
    4. Allow Benjy and his parents to have as much time as possible to be alone.

89. To cope effectively with Benjy's death, the nurse must first have:

1. Acquired a firm religious belief.
2. Reached the conclusion that death is for the best.
3. Realized that peace comes with death.
4. Coped with personal feelings about death.

Four-year-old Lisa is scheduled to have a tonsillectomy. Questions 90–94 concern this situation.

90. The *best* form of preparation for Lisa would be:
1. Watching a medical show on television.
2. Preadmission visit by a nurse.
3. Reading a story book.
4. Having Aunt Doris tell the child about her recent hospitalization.

91. In explaining the possible behavioral reactions of this procedure to Lisa's mother, you explain that the primary fear of preschoolers of surgery is:
1. Death.
2. Threat to peer status.
3. Body mutilation.
4. Decreased independence.

92. Following the tonsillectomy, the nurse observes Lisa for possible complications. Which of the following signs should be of concern?
1. Frequent swallowing and vomiting dark red blood.
2. Respiratory rate of 20, frequent swallowing, and dry mouth.
3. Frequent swallowing, noisy respirations, and increased pulse.
4. Refusing liquids and complaining of sore throat.

93. While visiting her, Lisa's grandmother states that she would like to bring Lisa a milkshake. The nurse should:
1. Explain that clear, cool liquids are best right now.
2. Encourage her to do so.
3. Explain that food from outside the hospital is not allowed.
4. Suggest that she wait until Lisa is discharged.

94. Lisa's mother says that prior to hospitalization, Lisa refused to eat anything except peanut butter sandwiches and she is concerned that this might be a recurring problem. You explain Lisa's behavior is:
1. Likely to lead to anemia.
2. Normal for this age group.
3. A sign of a behavior problem.
4. An attention-getting behavior.

Mr. B noticed a mass in his 3-year-old daughter Ellen's abdomen while bathing her. The doctor has tentatively diagnosed her condition as Wilms' tumor. Questions 95–98 concern this situation.

95. The nurse must be aware that the most important aspect of caring for this child preoperatively is:
1. Avoiding palpating the abdomen.
2. Encouraging the child to eat adequately.
3. Supporting the parents emotionally.
4. Keeping the child on strict bedrest.

96. The B family is quite shocked at the diagnosis and wonder if they should seek further testing prior to surgery. The nurse can best help the B's cope with this situation by:
1. Supporting their feelings.
2. Explaining that there will be no difference in the outcome by waiting.
3. Explaining that prognosis is poor and help them prepare for Ellen's death.
4. Encouraging them to consider surgery now as time is of the essence.

97. When Ellen is admitted to the hospital, you would expect her to exhibit the following behavior when her parents leave:
1. Wave goodbye to them.
2. Cry.
3. Hide her head under the covers.
4. Ask to go to the playroom.

98. During Ellen's convalescence, which activity would be appropriate?
1. Reading a book with the nurse.
2. Playing a game with the nurse.
3. Playing house in the playroom.
4. Watching cartoons.

Five-year-old Pete sustained second-degree burns resulting from an accident on his parents' chicken farm when a tub of hot water tipped over on him. Pete is being treated with the open method and is in reverse isolation. Questions 99–103 concern this situation.

99. The nurse must be alert to complications, particularly shock and hypovolemia. The most important sign to observe is:
1. Urine output.
2. Vomiting.
3. Increased pulse.
4. Thirst.

100. Adequate nutrition is essential for healing. The best diet for Pete would be:
1. High caloric, high protein.
2. High carbohydrate, high caloric.
3. High vitamin A and D.
4. High iron, high protein.

101. While caring for Pete the nurse could best prevent contractures by:
1. Maintaining body alignment.
2. Exercising extremities routinely.
3. Allowing free motion.
4. Splinting joints.

102. The best play activity for Pete would be:
1. Watching television.
2. Building a model car.
3. Caring for the ward's goldfish.
4. Puppet play.

103. Pete tells you he wasn't supposed to be in the chicken yard area when he got burned and so he is being punished. You interpret this behavior as:
1. Positive insight into the behavior expected of him.
2. Usual preschooler's view of illness.
3. A maladaptive attitude.
4. Poor parental supervision.

As a school nurse, you are confronted with injuries requiring first-aid action. The following five questions are typical health room situations.

104. Serena comes to the health room with epistaxis (nosebleed). The acceptable first-aid procedure is to have her:
1. Put her head between her knees.
2. Lie down with head tilted back.
3. Sit with head forward.
4. Sit with head elevated, tilted back slightly.

105. Billy comes to the health room after being bumped in the eye by a classmate's elbow. The appropriate action for the nurse after inspecting the eye is to:
1. Apply ice and patch eye.
2. Refer to physician.
3. Rinse with cool solution.
4. Have him lie down for a few minutes.

106. Shirley complains of pain in her index finger after hitting a volleyball "wrong." You suspect a sprain and do the following:
1. Soak her hand in warm water, apply splint.
2. Apply ice and splint the finger.
3. Refer her to emergency department for X rays.
4. Splint the finger.

107. Juan has developed a blister on his heel. The treatment for this is:
1. Puncture blister, apply covering.
2. Puncture blister, advise to keep clean and uncovered.
3. Clean and cover with dressing.
4. Clean and advise him to get new shoes.

108. Sue Li has been stung by a bee and the stinger is still in her arm. Your first action is to:
1. Remove it by scraping maneuver.
2. Remove it with forceps or tweezers.
3. Apply an astringent.
4. Observe her for untoward reaction.

Johnny, an 11-year-old boy, is admitted to the pediatric unit in traction with a fractured femur sustained in a motorcycle accident. Johnny's Uncle Joe, who was driving the cycle when the accident occurred, received only minor injuries. Questions 109–113 concern this situation.

109. When questioning Johnny about the accident, he tells you that his Uncle Joe is not to blame, that he is "the best motorcycle rider in the world." As a nurse, you recognize this as an expression of:

1. Defense mechanisms.
2. Repression.
3. Hero worship.
4. Fantasy.

110. The following activity would be *most* suitable for Johnny while he is immobilized by traction in the hospital:
1. Dramatizing with puppets.
2. Building with Popsicle sticks.
3. Watching television.
4. Coloring with crayons or colored pencils.

111. If you could place Johnny in a room *best* suited for him, you would find him a room with:
1. A 3-year-old child, because Johnny has a 3-year-old sister.
2. Two 11-year-old boys who are ambulatory.
3. A mentally retarded 14-year-old-boy.
4. Another 11-year-old boy who is also confined to bed.

112. You notice that Johnny has been squirting other patients and the staff with a syringe filled with water. Since Johnny has some aggressive feelings, which activity would be *least* helpful for him to release them?
1. Punching a bag.
2. Throwing a bean bag.
3. Cranking a wind-up toy.
4. Pounding clay.

113. According to Erikson, Johnny must develop a sense of industry or he will very likely develop a sense of:
1. Guilt.
2. Inferiority.
3. Shame.
4. Mistrust.

Questions 114–118 concern Tom, an adolescent who has epilepsy.

114. In caring for 12-year-old Tom, the nurse should know that the type of epileptic seizure seen mainly in children is:
1. Grand mal.
2. Petit mal.
3. Jacksonian-March.
4. Myoclonic.

115. Tom's doctor subscribes to dietary control of epilepsy. The type of diet most likely prescribed for Tom would be:
1. Low-salt diet.
2. Soft diet.
3. Ketogenic diet.
4. Low-residue diet.

116. Tom has a convulsive seizure while he is in the playroom. The nurse should:
1. Have everyone else leave the room.
2. Ease Tom to the floor and loosen the clothes around his neck.

3. Hold Tom down to keep him from thrashing about.
4. Put something between his teeth.

117. Tom is on the medication Phenytoin to control his seizures. One of the most important side effects to watch for is:
1. Hypertrophy of the gums.
2. Rash.
3. Hyperactivity.
4. Blurred vision.

118. In selecting an activity for Tom, you could suggest:
1. Soap-carving.
2. Joining the Boy Scouts.
3. Developing his own pictures.
4. Oil painting.

Carla, a 10-year-old girl, has been admitted to the pediatric unit where you work with a diagnosis of rheumatic fever. On admission, Carla has an elevated temperature and complains of joint pains. Carla had been ill only a brief time prior to her admission to the hospital. Questions 119–127 concern this situation.

119. Carla is fortunate that her illness was diagnosed and treated early because:
1. Manifestations of chorea can be prevented.
2. Spread of infection to other members of her family is minimized.
3. Cardiac damage can be minimized or prevented.
4. She will not have to take large amounts of medicine.

120. The most important aspect to which the nurse should adhere in caring for Carla during the acute phase of her illness is:
1. Maintaining contact with Carla's family and friends.
2. Physical and psychologic rest.
3. Continuation of her school work.
4. A nutritious diet.

121. Carla has developed carditis, which may cause transient heart murmurs. The heart valve most often affected in rheumatic fever is:
1. Aortic.
2. Mitral.
3. Tricuspid.
4. Pulmonic.

122. The prognosis for Carla depends primarily on the extent of:
1. Chorea.
2. Cardiac damage.
3. Arthritis.
4. Activity.

123. Treatment for Carla's rheumatic fever includes sodium salicylate. The nurse should be aware of some toxic symptoms, such as:
1. Tinnitus and nausea.
2. Dermatitis and blurred vision.

3. Unconsciousness and acetone odor of breath.
4. Chills and elevation of temperature.

124. Sometimes children with rheumatic fever develop chorea during the convalescent stage. The nurse should be aware that signs of chorea include:
1. Random movements and inappropriate facial expressions.
2. Tachycardia and sudden jerky movements.
3. Pain and fever.
4. Mental confusion, retardation, and pain.

125. Chorea is usually accompanied by:
1. Carditis.
2. Fever.
3. No other signs of inflammation.
4. Tachycardia.

126. According to Erikson's theory of personality development, Carla would have the following core task:
1. Industry versus inferiority.
2. Autonomy versus shame.
3. Initiative versus guilt.
4. Trust versus mistrust.

127. An appropriate activity for Carla while on bedrest would be which of the following?
1. Stringing beads.
2. Pillow-fighting.
3. Knitting or crocheting.
4. Listening to the radio.

Danny, 6 years old, recently recovered from a sore throat caused by a streptococcal infection. Danny has suddenly become acutely ill, displaying hematuria, headache, anorexia, and vomiting, and a high fever (104 F, 40 C). Following an examination, the physician ascertains that Danny also has proteinuria and hypertension. Danny is admitted to your unit with a diagnosis of acute glomerulonephritis. Questions 128–135 concern this situation.

128. When Danny was admitted, the nursing coordinator did *not* place his bed near:
1. Terry, who has leukemia.
2. Tommy, who is mentally retarded.
3. Billy, who has streptococcal tonsillitis.
4. Sean, who has rheumatic fever.

129. Based upon your knowledge of acute glomerulonephritis, you know that the changes in the glomeruli of the kidney are reversible and are the result of:
1. Leakage of protein into the glomerular filtrate.
2. Inflammation.
3. Hypertension.
4. Altered membrane permeability.

130. Danny's treatment would most likely include the following:
1. Bedrest, high-protein diet, limited fluids.
2. Daily weights, bedrest, high-potassium diet.

3. Bedrest, daily weights, low-sodium diet.
4. Activity ad lib, daily weights, low-protein diet.

131. Treatment of Danny's hypertension is an important aspect of treating his acute condition. The drug most likely to be used for this is:
1. Prednisone.
2. Calcium gluconate.
3. Penicillin.
4. Magnesium sulfate.

132. Danny's mother is concerned about her son's convalescence. Unless there are unforeseen complications, you can tell her that the course of this acute phase usually:
1. Recurs over several years.
2. Recurs over several months.
3. Lasts approximately 7–14 days.
4. Lasts 2–3 days.

133. After Danny is discharged, his mother will most likely be instructed to:
1. Allow Danny to return to full activity at school.
2. Restrict Danny to indoor activities.
3. Isolate Danny from contact with other children.
4. Return twice each week for penicillin injections.

134. Based upon his stage of personality development, the following would be an appropriate activity during Danny's convalescence:
1. Practicing magic tricks.
2. Playing catch with a baseball.
3. Putting together a simple puzzle.
4. Constructing a tower of five blocks.

135. As a normal 6-year-old, Danny could be expected to:
1. Dress self, know left and right, and cross street by self.
2. Know left and right, and build a tower of three blocks.
3. Enjoy parallel play and share toys.
4. Select future vocation.

136. Nine-year-old Gloria has cystic fibrosis. When she was undergoing diagnostic tests, the definitive tests done were:
1. Blood and stool tests.
2. Sweat and stool tests.
3. Sweat and blood tests.
4. Sputum and stool tests.

137. All of the following pathophysiologic findings are present in cystic fibrosis, *except:*
1. Excessive secretion of the exocrine glands of the body.
2. Obstruction of air passages in the lungs.
3. Inability to metabolize certain amino acids.
4. Production of excessive amounts of sodium and chloride in the sweat.

138. Gloria must follow a specific diet with vitamin supplements. The usual regimen is:
1. High protein, low fat, fat-soluble vitamins.
2. High calorie, high protein, fat-soluble vitamins.
3. High protein, high carbohydrate, water-soluble vitamins.
4. High protein, low fat, water-soluble vitamins.

139. When administering the pancreatic enzymes, the nurse will give them:
1. With meals.
2. Between meals.
3. Before meals.
4. After meals.

140. In planning some teaching interventions, the nurse must consider Gloria's cognitive development. According to Piaget, the type of thinking that characterizes the child in the middle years of childhood is:
1. Concrete.
2. Preoperational.
3. Formal.
4. Abstract.

141. When Gloria is discharged, a characteristic behavior to satisfy her need for social interaction would be:
1. Rollerskating with a group of girls.
2. Challenging a boy to a game of Monopoly.
3. Telling her parents about her group's activities.
4. Reading a book in her room by herself.

Mrs. Diaz is concerned that her 10-year-old son Pepe's headaches are caused by a brain tumor rather than eye strain, as suggested by the school nurse. Questions 142–145 concern this situation.

142. As a nurse you should know that signs of possible brain tumor in children include:
1. Headache, lethargy, and vomiting.
2. Increased pulse and head-banging behavior.
3. Convulsions and myopia.
4. Vomiting and fever.

143. An astrocytoma is diagnosed and treatment is planned. Based upon your knowledge of brain tumors you know that:
1. This is a fast-growing, malignant tumor.
2. A slow-growing, benign tumor.
3. This tumor is incurable.
4. Radiation is the treatment preferred.

144. Preoperatively, the most likely factor that will upset Pepe is:
1. Having his hair shaved off.
2. Missing school.
3. Spending the night in the hospital.
4. Missing meals for 24 hours.

145. During his convalescence, Pepe is allowed to go to the playroom. He should be encouraged to participate in

activities that avoid bending his head because:
1. His dressing will become dislodged.
2. He will rupture his suture line.
3. This will cause edema of tissues.
4. This will cause discomfort and increased incidence of headache.

Linda, age 15 years, has a diagnosis of hyperthyroidism (Graves' disease). Although she is on medication, Linda refuses to go to school. Questions 146 and 147 concern this situation.

146. You suspect that she is refusing because she is:
1. Failing in school.
2. Spoiled and acting infantile.
3. Upset about her appearance.
4. Too hyperactive to be attentive.

147. In explaining the possible side effects of Linda's medication, propylthiouracil or methimazole, you would include the following group of symptoms to which she should be alert:
1. Fever, rash, nausea, joint pain.
2. Vomiting, lethargy, convulsions.
3. Hypothermia, low blood pressure, rapid pulse.
4. Fever, rash, high blood pressure, slow pulse rate.

Lucia, 13 years old, has a weight problem. She is attending an adolescent obesity clinic to assist her in losing weight and to help her identify those behaviors that led to obesity. Questions 148–150 concern this situation.

148. Lucia has a caloric intake of 3200 per day. To lose one pound per week, she will need to decrease her daily intake to:
1. 3100.
2. 3000.
3. 2700.
4. 2200.

149. All of the following causes of obesity might apply to Lucia, *except:*
1. Giving food as reward for behavior.
2. "Clean plate" award at meal time.
3. Need for attention.
4. Hypothyroidism.

150. Lucia complains that she is "always tired" and doesn't seem to have any energy for exercise. You feel Lucia's complaint is most likely due to:
1. Her poor exercise habits in the past.
2. Normal protein depletion of adolescent period.
3. Her personality.
4. Self-consciousness about her appearance.

Rhonda, 12 years old, suffers from Still's disease (juvenile rheumatoid arthritis). During a visit to her home, you ascertain that Rhonda spends most of her day lying on the couch. Questions 151–153 concern this situation.

151. Since the goal of treatment is to preserve good joint function, you will do which of the following?
1. Support quiet activity.
2. Suggest splinting her joints.
3. Encourage exercises.
4. Perform ROM exercises.

152. Rhonda tells you that she has ringing in her ears. You know the cause of this is most probably:
1. An auditory hallucination.
2. A plea for attention.
3. Side effect of the steroid medication.
4. Side effect of the salicylate medication.

153. Just before you arrived, Rhonda found a dark stain on her underwear and asks you what it could be. Your best response would be:
1. "You found a stain on your underwear?"
2. "Have you discussed the body changes that are taking place in you with anyone?"
3. "Ask your mother about it."
4. "I wouldn't worry about it."

During a routine health screening at school, Katy, 16 years old, was found to have scoliosis. Questions 154–158 concern this situation.

154. The most common type of scoliosis developed by adolescents is:
1. Idiopathic.
2. Psychologic.
3. Postural.
4. Physiologic.

155. Her doctor decides to admit Katy for surgery to insert a Harrington rod. It is necessary for Katy to know what to expect postoperatively. You would teach Katy:
1. To eat lying down.
2. To log roll from side to side.
3. To stoop rather than bend over.
4. To dress herself while in a cast.

156. Katy is a cheerleader at her high school and is eager to resume her activities. In response to her queries about how soon that will be, you explain:
1. She can resume her activities within a week.
2. She will be unable to resume her activities.
3. She will most likely wear her cast 6–12 months.
4. The doctor will tell her when he makes rounds.

157. Katy appears somewhat depressed and spends part of the day daydreaming. Her mother is concerned about Katy and should be counseled by a nurse who is aware that:
1. Her daughter is trying to evade responsibilities.
2. Her daughter is probably schizophrenic.
3. This is typical adolescent behavior.
4. Adolescents tire easily and prefer quiet activity.

158. Katy has been attempting to dc all of her care herself,

declining assistance from the staff. You realize that a "normal" or positive reaction of an adolescent to hospitalization is one that:
1. Holds in feeling about illness.
2. Manipulates staff.
3. Demands control and independence.
4. Shows dependence on parents.

You are working in a drug abuse clinic that sees mostly adolescents. Questions 159–163 relate to drug abuse.

159. In reviewing the history of drugs, you discover that a well-known and long-used mind-altering drug is:
1. Heroin.
2. Marijuana.
3. Mescaline.
4. Nicotine.

160. An adolescent who is admitted with an overdose of "speed" has most likely been using:
1. Barbiturates.
2. Marijuana.
3. Amphetamines.
4. Narcotics.

161. The major sign of barbiturate overdose is:
1. Clammy skin.
2. Pinpoint pupils.
3. Tachycardia.
4. Dilated pupils.

162. A preadolescent boy admitted in a state of mental confusion, ataxic, with red, swollen nasal mucous membranes has probably been using:
1. Marijuana.
2. Glue.
3. LSD.
4. Aspirin.

163. The most significant somatic consequence of drug abuse affecting the heart is:
1. Pericarditis.
2. Endocarditis.
3. Myocarditis.
4. Myocardial infarction.

A nurse working with teenagers in school often encounters the situations presented in Questions 164–168.

164. A high-school group has asked the nurse to lead a discussion on venereal disease. She could point out that a fairly common complication of gonorrhea in women is:
1. Endometriosis.
2. Infertility.
3. Pelvic inflammatory disease (PID).
4. Ovarian cysts.

165. The incubation period of syphilis is:
1. Approximately one week.
2. About three weeks.
3. About three months.
4. Three to six months.

166. The drug of choice for treatment of venereal disease is:
1. Erythromycin.
2. Sulfacetamide sodium.
3. Penicillin.
4. Chlorpromazine hydrochloride.

167. When one of the teens asks if the cold sore on his lip means he will get a cold sore or herpes virus in the genital area, the nurse responds:
1. "Yes, they are caused by the same virus."
2. "Not if you wash your hands before as well as after urinating."
3. "No, they are not caused by the same virus."
4. "We can discuss that privately after class."

168. Sixteen-year-old Burt is quite conscious of his acne. He asks the nurse what causes it. She answers that acne vulgaris is caused primarily by:
1. Erratic diet of the adolescent.
2. Changes in the skin during adolescence.
3. Irritation of the skin due to habit of picking face.
4. Allergy to foods containing chocolate.

Seventeen-year-old Steve has been complaining of fatigue, anorexia, enlarged lymph nodes, and a fever. The physician has considered mononucleosis and Hodgkin's disease as possible diagnoses. Questions 169–171 concern this situation.

169. Before the results of the blood tests are received, one differentiation you consider is that mononucleosis would also present the following:
1. Rash.
2. Generalized pruritus.
3. Night sweats.
4. Painful enlargement of cervical nodes.

170. A diagnosis of Hodgkin's disease is made. Steve's parents are concerned about the prognosis. In helping them understand this condition, you reply:
1. "This is a cancer, and there is no way to predict its prognosis."
2. "Early diagnosis combined with treatment usually means a very good prognosis."
3. "I know several children who are still living with Hodgkin's disease."
4. "You'd better discuss the possibility of death with your son."

171. A lymphangiogram is scheduled for Steve to detect metastatic nodal involvement. To prepare Steve for this procedure, you can best describe it as which of the following?
1. A radiopaque contrast material is injected under

local anesthetic into a vessel in Steve's foot so nodal enlargement can be seen on an X ray.

2. Steve will be asked to swallow a contrast dye in a dark room while a technician watches on an X ray screen.

3. A contrast material will be injected under local anesthetic in Steve's neck so cervical nodes can be visualized.

4. A contrast medium will be injected under general anesthetic into Steve's groin so nodal enlargement can be seen on an X ray.

As team leader of the pediatric unit, the nurse must be knowledgeable about administration of drugs. Questions 172–185 concern drug treatments.

172. The most important responsibility of the nurse when caring for an infant receiving intravenous therapy is to:
1. Remove the needle as soon as the fluid that has been ordered has run into the vein.
2. Change the bed linen promptly if it becomes moistened from the intravenous solution.
3. Frequently check the number of drops of solution running into the vein and regulate the flow of solution as ordered.
4. Add a new bottle of solution when the present one is empty, with or without a physician's order.

173. The most common complication of intravenous therapy in children is:
1. Infiltration.
2. Nerve damage.
3. Phlebitis.
4. Circulatory overload.

174. The preferred site for intravenous infusion in an infant is:
1. Foot.
2. Arm.
3. Scalp.
4. Hand.

175. Two preferred sites for parenteral administration of intramuscular medication in infants are:
1. Deltoid and laterofemoral.
2. Laterofemoral and anteriofemoral.
3. Dorsogluteal and deltoid.
4. Dorsogluteal and ventrogluteal.

176. Eyedrops are instilled by tilting the head so that the drops flow from:
1. Outer to inner canthus.
2. Inner to outer canthus.
3. Upper to lower lid.
4. Lower to upper lid.

177. The nurse should instill eyedrops into the:
1. Center of the eye.
2. Conjunctival sac.

3. Outer corner of the eye.
4. Lower eyelid.

178. Ophthalmic ointments are applied to the:
1. Cornea.
2. Conjunctival sac.
3. Lower eyelid.
4. Upper eyelid.

179. When instilling eardrops in children under 3 years of age, the nurse should hold the earlobe:
1. Up and back.
2. Down and back.
3. Against the head.
4. Straight out.

180. When instilling eardrops in older children, the nurse should hold the earlobe:
1. Up and back.
2. Down and back.
3. Against the head.
4. Straight out.

181. After 4-year-old Pam had received an IM injection, she said to the nurse, "I hate you. Go away." The nurse should answer:
1. "What a naughty girl you are."
2. "You seem angry with me."
3. "I bet your mother would be sad to hear you talk like that."
4. "I'm sorry you hate me. I like you."

182. The adult dose for aspirin is 10 grains. What is the correct amount to order for a 15-lb child? (Use Clark's Rule to compute answer.)
1. 1 grain.
2. 1.5 grains.
3. .15 grains.
4. .05 grains.

183. Ampicillin is ordered for Tony, who weighs 13.6 kg. The adult dosage is 250 mg. The correct dosage for Tony (using Clark's Rule for computation) is:
1. 5 mg.
2. 50 mg.
3. 23 mg.
4. 40 mg.

184. Fifteen milligrams of an antibiotic are ordered for Billy. The medication vial comes 10 mg/cc. You would give:
1. 15 cc.
2. 1.5 cc.
3. .5 cc.
4. .15 cc.

185. A dry drug vial of medication contains 1000 mg. You wish a solution of .5 g/cc, so you add how much diluent?
1. 2 cc.
2. 1 cc.

3. 4 cc.

4. 5 cc.

The nurse in pediatrics also needs a knowledge of cardio-pulmonary resuscitations and needs to be able to administer emergency measures safely and quickly. Questions 186–189 concern emergency procedures.

186. Upon entering his room, you find 2-month-old Kevin unconscious. He does not respond to your shaking him or your loud voice. You open his airway by sliding your hand under his shoulders, causing head tilt. Your next action is to:
1. Begin immediate chest compression.
2. Attempt to feel breath on your face.
3. Clear the mouth.
4. Call the physician.

187. When administering CPR to an infant, a puff of air is sufficient for ventilation. The ratio of ventilation to compression is the same as for two-person rescue in adults, but the number of compressions is increased. The correct ratio and number of compressions is:
1. 1:5; 80–100/minute.
2. 1:5; 60–80/minute.
3. 2:15; 80/minute.
4. 1:5; 100–120/minute.

188. At a family gathering at home, your 13-year-old nephew begins to choke on a piece of meat. He is slightly cyanotic and unable to breathe, cough, or speak. You would do which of the following *first*?
1. Cardiopulmonary resuscitation.
2. Administer four back blows between his shoulder blades.
3. Phone the paramedics.
4. Mouth-to-mouth resuscitation.

189. If CPR is not initiated, brain cell death begins in:
1. 6–8 minutes.
2. 5–10 minutes.
3. 4–6 minutes.
4. 1–3 minutes.

As a nurse in the clinic, you often do nutritional counseling. You must have specific knowledge about foods. Questions 190–195 are based on this knowledge.

190. For children through adolescence, the most essential element of the diet is:
1. Fats.
2. Water.
3. Carbohydrates.
4. Protein.

191. The following foods are highest in calcium:
1. Liver, raisins, and prunes.
2. Milk, leafy vegetables, fish, and cheese.
3. Milk, spaghetti, and prunes.
4. Leafy vegetables, bread, cereal.

192. Foods high in protein are:
1. Spinach, eggs, dried fruit, and apples.
2. Fish, beef, peanut butter, and chicken.
3. Beef, chicken, eggs, dried fruit.
4. Milk, bread, fish, carrots.

193. Foods richest in iodine would be:
1. Fruits.
2. Seafoods.
3. Vegetables.
4. Cereals.

194. Cereal, bread, and macaroni are rich sources of:
1. Minerals.
2. Calcium.
3. Carbohydrates.
4. Fats.

195. Liver, raisins, and prunes are rich sources of:
1. Vitamin C.
2. Protein.
3. Iron.
4. Vitamin A.

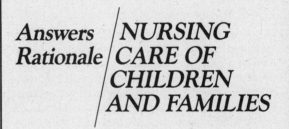

Answers Rationale / NURSING CARE OF CHILDREN AND FAMILIES

1. (3) Erikson's eight stages of man are the most widely utilized developmental theory by the health care profession. His stages incorporate some of (No. 1) Freud's teachings. Nos. 2 and 4 are incorrect because Watson was an early theorist, and Gesell's developmental tool is used in assessing developmental milestones, especially in determining delays.

2. (1) The Department of Health and Human Services now administers Project Headstart, a nursery school for culturally and socioeconomically deprived areas. No. 2, the Children's Bureau, focuses on investigating and reporting upon matters pertaining to the welfare of all children in the United States while No. 3, Family Service, offers counseling aid and No. 4, the local public welfare office, offers financial assistance to needy families.

3. (3) The leading cause of death of children of all ages, excluding the first month, is accidents. No. 1, leukemia, mainly strikes the preschooler, and early diagnosis has removed this disease from the "certain fatality" classification. No. 2, suicide, is rising at an alarming rate in the school-age and adolescent population. No. 4, congenital heart defect, is associated with infant mortality, but newer diagnostic and treatment modalities are reducing the mortality incidence.

4. (3) Level of development is the determining factor in making a house safe for children; toddlers tend to poke objects into electrical outlets, while preschoolers drink caustic agents or get in bicycle/vehicle accidents, etc. Nos. 1, 2, and 4 are incorrect because preference of play area, intelligence, and behavior are associated with the level of development and supervision of the child.

5. (2) Age 3–4 months is when infants begin to drool, and they may do so several months before they learn to swallow their saliva. Nos. 1 and 3 are below the normal age limit while No. 4 may indicate a delay and need for referral.

6. (2) Sweating occurs at approximately 1 month of age as the body attempts to control its temperature. Hence, Nos. 1, 3, and 4 are incorrect. Right after birth the infant's body temperature is very labile. A good rule for dressing infants is to dress them in the same manner in which the majority of persons would be comfortable in the same environment.

7. (3) General progression is cereal, fruit, vegetables, meat, and egg yolk, taking care to introduce only one food at a time. Rice cereal is usually the first food because of the decreased likelihood of allergic reaction. This sequence may vary with individual pediatrician/well-baby care. Vegetables may be introduced before fruit in many instances. Nos. 1 and 2 start with fruit rather than cereal. Nos. 2 and 4 contain meat, which is added later.

8. (2) Stools will not change consistency in an infant who is fed milk only; they become more solid *after* ingestion of solid foods. Nos. 1, 3, and 4 should all be present.

9. (3) The *usual* teething pattern is lower-central incisors erupting at 6–7 months of age. Nos. 1, 2, and 4 may be seen in some children but are considered variations of the usual pattern.

10. (3) Children usually begin losing their primary teeth at age 6–7 years, and usually the lower-central incisors are lost first. No. 1 is considered young while Nos. 2 and 4 may be normal variations.

11. (2) The infant can first be conditioned to perform elimination on the toilet but the *central nervous system must mature* before placing this under voluntary control and assuming responsibility for the action. Nos. 1, 3, and 4 are incorrect because reinforcement should be positive and immediate, trial and error are indicative of a less fully developed child, and imitation may be a factor in proper posture.

12. (1) This action will let Candy know you are not angry and that you understand accidents do happen. It also

offers a gentle reminder to let you know when she has to use the toilet. No. 2 contributes to feelings of shame and doubt (to be avoided). No. 3 reinforces the desired behavior and develops positive self-image. It should be used when Candy is successful. No. 4 is a version of "hit and miss" and will not necessarily prevent accidental soiling.

13. (3) By ignoring her behavior, neither positive nor negative reinforcement is given. Tantrums are a sign of frustration and loss of control, therefore No. 2, punishment, should not be administered. No. 4 is incorrect because the child should not be rewarded for this behavior. No. 1 is inappropriate as the child already feels isolated.

14. (4) Using Candy's favorite sleepmate is most likely to appeal to her sense of autonomy by putting teddy bear to bed (and her with him). By offering a choice, Nos. 1 and 2 automatically elicit the negative response. In No. 3, equating bed with "good" or "big" implies the opposite when child refuses and implies reward if child complies.

15. (4) Decreased production of insulin by the pancreas is the basic defect of juvenile diabetes mellitus, which means that glucose cannot be used by the body without administration of subcutaneous injections of insulin. Hence, Nos. 1, 2, and 3 are incorrect.

16. (1) A piece of hard candy is high in glucose content. In school children, the most likely condition is hyperinsulinism due to increased exercise and growth, which deplete glucose stores. Nos. 2, 4, and 3 are incorrect because salted nuts are not appropriate for this condition; carrying a dime is impractical and phoning home is time-consuming; and even if it were practical to carry insulin and a syringe, Todd is unlikely to need insulin. He will most likely require extra glucose to replace that used during exercise or activity.

17. (3) Flushed face is a symptom of acidosis or diabetic coma. Nos. 1, 2, and 4 are incorrect because weakness, pallor, and tremor are signs of insulin shock.

18. (1) School age is within Erikson's industry-versus-inferiority stage, so the nurse's task is to assist Todd in developing a sense of accomplishment. If the task is too difficult or too fast paced, a sense of inferiority will result. Nos. 2, 3, and 4 are incorrect because intimacy versus isolation is the task of late adolescence, trust versus mistrust is the task of infancy, and autonomy versus shame or doubt is the task of toddlers.

19. (2) The entire family must be treated in cases of pediculosis, or head lice, as chances of family members' infestation is high due to sharing, living together. No. 1 is incorrect because, while hygienic measures are used in controlling pediculosis, they are not its causes; infestation may occur as a result of sharing caps, helmets, combs, etc., which is generally unrelated to hygiene or other factors such as economic status. No.

3, hair loss, may occur in cases of tinea corporis (ringworm), not pediculosis. No. 4 is incorrect because pediculosis can be transmitted as discussed in No. 1.

20. (2) Age 2 months is recommended by the American Academy of Pediatrics, based on acquired protection in utero. Nos. 1, 3, and 4 are incorrect because age 6 months is the usual time for the third series of immunizations (second is at age 4 months); 12 months is the fourth age of immunizations (usually DPT and Tb skin test); and age 2 weeks is considered too young for immunization, since the mother's immunity, acquired in utero, is still effective.

21. (3) Pertussis is not transmitted to the infant, although immunity to tetanus and diphtheria (Nos. 1, 2, and 4) are passed to the infant if the mother is immune and may last up to six months.

22. (3) Chicken pox does not yet have an immunization. Nos. 1, 2, and 4 are incorrect because measles, smallpox, and mumps may all be immunized against, although smallpox vaccine is not given to children who are not at risk (for example, not traveling in a foreign country).

23. (3) DPT are the initials for diphtheria and tetanus toxins with pertussis vaccine. Polio vaccine (Nos. 1 and 2) is given orally, and typhoid vaccine (Nos. 2 and 4) is injected in a series.

24. (3) It is important to avoid massage for best reaction and to press sponge over area to prevent backflow from the needle. Nos. 1, 2, and 4 are incorrect because a bandage is not necessary unless there is some bleeding. Aspirin may be recommended if redness and fever develop.

25. (3) Initial doses are given at ages 2, 4, and 6 months and booster doses at 18 months and 4–6 years (the latter usually upon entering school). Pertussis is contraindicated for children over age 6 years. Hence Nos. 1, 2, and 4 are incorrect.

26. (2) Schick is a toxoid sensitivity test for diphtheria. Nos. 1, 3, and 4 are incorrect because Dick tests for sensitivity to scarlet fever, Babinsky refers to a reflex test for neurologic development, and Schaback tests hearing by using tuning forks.

27. (2) Annual testing in the first five years of life is routine (longer in children who are at risk or who have been exposed). Hence, Nos. 1 and 4 are incorrect. Tb is still an important disease in the United States. Positive results (No. 3) are not the goal, but skin-testing is not continued if results are positive.

28. (3) Within 72 hours. Nos. 1 and 2 are incorrect because a true reading is not possible until the third day. No. 4 is incorrect because the reaction may have resolved in 96 hours.

29. (4) Infants in this age group are immunized because they are not at risk. All other groups listed are high risk. Men who contract mumps run the risk of orchiepididymitis, leading to sterility.

30. (2) White, strawberry tongue is a classic sign that occurs on second to third day. Nos. 1, 3, and 4 are incorrect because white spots may be nonpigmented areas (psitoriasis alba); Koplik's spots are seen inside the mouth as diagnostic of measles (rubeola); and alopecia is loss of hair (baldness).

31. (3) Outgrow it, but may show allergic reactions or manifestations later in life, as eczema is a frequent indication of allergic response. Nos. 1, 2, and 4 are incorrect because there is no reason to believe that she will necessarily have it all her life, that she will outgrow it by the time she is 4 years old, or that she will never have another episode.

32. (4) An elimination diet means first eliminating all foods and then adding them to her diet one food at a time to observe for allergic reaction. Any of the other three diets in Nos. 1, 2, and 3 would be instituted for other conditions as indicated by history, but are not related to Mary's eczema.

33. (3) Holding Mary gives her the security of being held, yet allows some freedom. Play diverts her attention from scratching, and also promotes normal growth and development. No. 1 is incorrect because tying Mary down is unnecessary and undesirable since elbow restraints, properly applied, prevent her from scratching. No. 2, free movement, is inappropriate even with trimmed fingernails. No. 4 is incorrect because medication, though it may be used, is not a substitute for proper nursing measures.

34. (1) Soft, washable toys of smooth, nonallergic material should be used. Nos. 2, 3, and 4 are incorrect because stuffed toys are contraindicated; puzzles and games are inappropriate to Mary's age; and toy cars, also age-inappropriate, could be used for scratching.

35. (2) Mineral oil is nonirritating and promotes softening of crusts and lesions. The other three may produce an allergic reaction, especially bubble bath (No. 1) and baby lotion (No. 4), while Ivory and castile soaps (No. 3) are also very drying, thereby promoting itching. Specific soaks may be prescribed by the physician.

36. (3) Congenital heart defects occur in 5 out of 1000 infants. No. 1, rheumatic fever, is primarily a disease of school-aged children. No. 2, infections, is a cause of concern because of group exposure. No. 4, accidents, is the primary killer of children after age one month.

37. (3) Is acyanotic, but may become short of breath on exertion, develop respiratory infections, and fail to thrive. A murmur is also heard. Nos. 1, 2, and 4 may indicate a different CHD or respiratory problem.

38. (3) An invasive procedure accomplished by an injection of radiopaque dye into a catheter inserted in the chambers of the heart, often preliminary test prior to catheterization, using low-dosage radiation and done in a short time. The other tests are noninvasive: No. 1 is radiography, No. 2 utilizes a transducer to determine exact location of defect, and No. 4 is electrocardiogram/EKG, ECG.

39. (2) Teaching the parents how to organize Danny's care will help him avoid exertion. The defect is usually surgically corrected when a child is 3–10 years of age unless complications arise prior to that time. Hence, Nos. 3 and 4 are incorrect and No. 1 is inappropriate, as this is not a terminal condition.

40. (1) Having a music box near him is age-appropriate (2 weeks) and utilizes an appropriate sensory modality (auditory). Nos. 2, 3, and 4 are not appropriate for a 2-week-old infant. However, a mobile would be the next toy for visual stimulus.

41. (3) Removing restraints and exercising Tanya's arms will improve circulation and allow her some movement. Nos. 1, 2, and 4 are all contraindicated.

42. (3) Neck mobility is not affected by this condition, but Nos. 1, 2, and 4 (breathing, swallowing, and speech) are all involved.

43. (1) Playing with her favorite toy, a familiar object, will help Tanya adjust to the hospital. Nos. 2, 3, and 4 are not appropriate for Tanya.

44. (3) Periodically placing elbow restraints on Tanya prior to hospitalization will help her get used to these restraints. Thus she will have one less new experience to which she must adjust following surgery. No. 1 is incorrect because she is too young to have a movie tour, although this would certainly be advisable for her parents. No. 2, an explanation, is also more appropriate for Tanya's parents than for Tanya. No. 4, a children's book, is also beyond Tanya's complete comprehension, though her parents may be able to use it to help her reach a limited understanding.

45. (4) This response involves giving information about stages of repair, acknowledges her parents' questions, and responds to their concern by offering a discussion. No. 1 avoids answering the parents' questions, No. 2 reflects a judgemental, negative attitude toward them, and No. 3 shirks responsibility, since general questions can be answered by the nurse and references for specifics elicited from the physician.

46. (4) The urethral meatus is on the underside, or ventral aspect, of the penis. No. 1, female genitalia with male genotype, is Turner's syndrome. No. 2 is not unusual, for a newborn's testes may not have descended. No. 3, protrusion of the urinary bladder, is exstrophy of the bladder.

47. (4) The repair is done between 2 and 3 years of age

for function and cosmetic purposes, a bigger area in which to operate, and minimal emotional responses. Hence, Nos. 1 and 2 are incorrect. Associated problems (No. 3) such as chordee may be present and are also corrected by the surgery.

48. (3) The nurse is bound by law to report her suspicion to the police. The exact procedure may be defined by her employing agency and may involve (No. 2) reporting to the physician (with whom she should share her concern). It is not necessary for the nurse to prove or disprove abuse, as stated in No. 1. No. 4, suggesting parenting class, may be appropriate at a later time, but is not the initial course of action.

49. (3) Eighty percent of abused children are under the age of 3 years, and half of those are under six months of age, making No. 1 (over six months of age) grossly inaccurate. Nos. 2 and 4 are incorrect because preschoolers who misbehave are not at greatest risk, and because abusive parents cross economic and social lines.

50. (2) The oldest child is at the highest risk, although any of the other children in Nos. 1, 3, and 4 could certainly be victims of child abuse. The oldest child is often unplanned or conceived out of wedlock, born to parents who lack proper or sufficient parenting skills.

51. (2) Abusive parents are often loners or isolated persons with no support systems, but they do not *like* to be alone. They *do* exhibit the other three behaviors in Nos. 1, 3, and 4.

52. (2) Motor function disorder is due to a static brain lesion. Drooling in infancy (No. 1) is normal but may be of concern if it continues into toddlerhood and beyond. Microcephaly (No. 3) is not indicative of cerebral palsy. Scissored extremities (No. 4) *may* be present in some types of cerebral palsy.

53. (4) Prenatal, perinatal, and postnatal factors can contribute to cerebral palsy. Mental retardation is not a cause of cerebral palsy.

54. (3) Movement and posture are involved. Nos. 1, 2, and 4 are incorrect because the lesion is *not* progressive, motor function *is* impaired, and mental retardation is *not* a given, as many children have normal intelligence or above.

55. (2) Abnormal, but possible, behavior in an infant: hand preference is established after 18 months of age, and children are ambidextrous prior to this. Hence, Nos. 1, 3, and 4 are incorrect.

56. (1) Only one-third of children with cerebral palsy are mentally retarded; speech delay is due to poor muscle control. Hence, Nos. 2, 3, and 4 are incorrect.

57. (4) Slowly and gently, ten times daily, to prevent contractures and deformity. The time of day (No. 1) is not the determining factor in doing the exercises. No. 2 will quickly cause the muscle to block or kickback. No. 3 (after a warm bath) may be nice, but it is only necessary in the case of juvenile rheumatoid arthritis.

58. (2) Blood test for phenylalanine level. When this level rises, phenylketone bodies appear in the urine (No. 1). Sweat analysis (No. 3) is done for cystic fibrosis; genetic history (No. 4) is not a definitive test.

59. (1) Lactose-free diet, which calls for a milk substitute. Nos. 2, 3, and 4 are incorrect because gluten-free is for celiac disease, fat-free is for cystic fibrosis, and food preservative–free is for hyperactivity.

60. (4) Feeding herself would be appropriate to foster independence and self-selection and to have Maria focus on a new skill (such as using a spoon or fork). No. 1, eating only when she is hungry, may reinforce eating patterns that are incompatible with family practices and may still not enforce proper intake. Maria should not be forced to eat, however. No. 2 is incorrect because the environmental change may not change Maria's appetite and because the kitchen may be the only acceptable place for her to eat. No. 3 would not always be practical, especially since friends would probably not eat the same foods as Maria.

61. (1) The cause is unknown in the majority of cases. Nos. 2 and 3 are incorrect because an autoimmune response refers to acute glomerulonephritis, which is not the cause of nephrotic syndrome except in a very small number of patients. Post-infectious process, No. 4, is believed to trigger acute glomerulonephritis.

62. (3) Bringing Patrick's teddy bear will provide him with a sense of security and aid in his adjustment to hospitalization, especially during the times his mother is not there. No. 1 is incorrect because Patrick is displaying a normal reaction to separation when he is upset by his mother's departure. While spending the night in the hospital (No. 2) is an excellent idea, it is unfortunately not always possible and should not be suggested unless it is a definite option. Buying gifts (No. 4) is a form of bribery and should be avoided.

63. (3) The exact mechanism by which steroids prevent proteinuria is unknown, but it is effective. Nos. 2, 4, and 1 are incorrect because steroids do not prevent hematuria or potassium loss, and the aim of therapy is not to prevent diuresis.

64. (3) Prognosis is good, with an 80% survival rate, although the condition is chronic. Hence, Nos. 1, 2, and 4 are incorrect.

65. (1) The diet of high protein, high potassium, and low sodium is appropriate during the acute phase because of the body's loss (through urine) of protein and potassium and retention of sodium in an attempt to establish homeostasis. The other three responses are incorrect because they each include at least one inappropriate choice.

66. (2) Sandbox is age-appropriate for outdoor play. Nos. 1, 3, and 4 are incorrect because Patrick is too young for a two-wheel bike or for climbing a tree without supervision and assistance, and he may be past the stage of pushing a toy lawn mower, which is more appropriate for a toddler.

67. (3) Sickle cell anemia is an inherited trait, not a type of leukemia (No. 1) and not curable (No. 2); neither is it a progression of sickle cell trait (No. 4), which is also inherited but has no symptoms.

68. (2) It is more prevalent among Black Americans. Approximately 10% have the trait and 1:400 have sickle cell anemia. It is also found in those of Mediterranean descent. Nos. 1, 3, and 4 are not prone to this disorder.

69. (4) Weakness, jaundice, and pain in the abdomen, legs, or arms are symptoms of sickling cells flowing through vessels during a dehydrated state. Precipitating factors include extreme fatigue or infectious process. Pain is due to occlusion of small blood vessels by sickled red cells. The victim is neither pale, alert, nor flushed; hence, Nos. 1, 2, and 3 are incorrect.

70. (2) Initiating play with the use of a puppet would be an appropriate way to encourage a 2-year-old child to express his or her feelings about the tests and to provide a healthy outlet, which Nos. 1, 3, and 4 would not do.

71. (3) Seeking independence is his way of distinguishing his own action from that of others. Often obstinacy (No. 1) and being spoiled (No. 2) are labels given this behavior by persons unfamiliar with normal development. Lucas must be taught right from wrong by others (No. 4).

72. (1) Another child could have sickle cell anemia because both parents have the trait. Nos. 2 and 3 are incorrect because the odds have not changed: in each pregnancy there is still a 25% chance that the child will either be normal or will have sickle cell anemia, but a 50% chance that the child will inherit the trait only. No. 4 is incorrect because sex-dependency is associated with hemophilia.

73. (3) Twenty, which is the number of primary teeth if his second molars erupted at 24 months. Nos. 1, 2, and 4 are incorrect because he should have had 16 teeth by 16–18 months, and 10 teeth by 12 months.

74. (1) Promote quiet and rest for Bobby, as anxiety may predispose the child to further bleeding. Exercising his joints (No. 2) is contraindicated. It is not necessary to wrap his joints in cotton batting (No. 3) as a primary measure. Administering sedatives (No. 4) is a prescriptive measure.

75. (1) Hemarthrosis, or bleeding into the joints, is a common complication for these children. While the other three conditions may exist, they are not the best response.

76. (3) Curtailment of his activities is the most likely cause of delayed development, but No. 2, overprotection, may play a part also. Parents and children need suggestions for alternate, acceptable activities that promote normal development. No. 1, mental retardation, is not associated with hemophilia. No. 4, misinterpretation, is unlikely, but retesting can substantiate the results.

77. (4) Asking Bobby to tell you about his picture allows him to express himself without feeling that his drawing must represent something, as he would with Nos. 1 and 3. No. 2 implies that the drawing must have some artistic merit.

78. (3) Inventing an imaginary companion is common in the preschool age group to meet the described needs. No. 1 (parallel play) is common among toddlers, while No. 2 (imitation) and No. 4 (sympathy) would not fulfill these needs now.

79. (1) Providing a quiet time after lunch is an appropriate step toward giving up nap time, which is common for preschoolers to do in preparation for beginning school (No. 2). Less need for sleep at night (No. 3) should not be a substitute for napping, and a later time for napping (No. 4) will interfere with evening bedtime.

80. (2) Iliac crest and sternum are the sites used in children because of their size. Hence, Nos. 1, 3, and 4 are incorrect.

81. (3) Proliferation of abnormal white blood cells that displace or replace normal bone marrow elements. Hence, Nos. 1, 2, and 4 are incorrect.

82. (1) Anemia caused by the decrease in red blood cells carrying hemoglobin. Hence, Nos. 2, 3, and 4 are incorrect.

83. (2) Immature leukocytes are not capable of normal phagocytosis. Infection most frequently occurs in the lungs, gastrointestinal tract, or skin. Hence, Nos. 1, 3, and 4 are incorrect.

84. (4) Although certain factors are felt to be related in some patients, the exact etiology remains unknown. Hence, Nos. 1, 2, and 3 are incorrect.

85. (3) Explaining that the delay did not have any effect upon the course of the disease is realistic. There is no way to predict that Benjy would develop leukemia based on his early symptoms; treatment of a cold will not prevent leukemia or alter the course of the disease. Nos. 1 and 4 are fatalistic responses that leave some doubt in the mother's mind, while No. 2 avoids the question.

86. (1) Increased appetite, edema, and fever are side effects of cortisone and while the first may be a welcome effect in a leukemic patient, discontinuation results in rapid decrease in appetite. Hence, Nos. 2, 3, and 4 are incorrect.

87. (4) By discussing with him the reasons for his fears, it will be easier for Benjy to accept them and not feel abnormal. Nos. 1, 2, and 3 are inappropriate for Benjy.

88. (3) Remain with Benjy and his parents as much as possible, as they need support at this time, not abandonment (No. 1) or an attitude that all is normal (No. 2). If they wish to be alone (No. 4), they will most likely let you know.

89. (4) Coping with personal feelings about death—understanding and acknowledging them—will enable the nurse to help others. This *may* include one of the other three responses, but each person has his or her own beliefs.

90. (3) There are several good children's books that can be used to prepare children for hospitalization, and having parents read these to the children fosters questions and a better understanding. Nos. 1, 2, and 4 are incorrect because medical shows depicted on television are not real and give a false impression of the personnel; a preadmission visit for a tonsillectomy is impractical; and Aunt Doris's story may be interpreted as a fairy tale or horror story.

91. (3) Body mutilation is a common fear due to the child's lack of understanding of physiology, that is, that all the blood in the body will not flow out of a cut and be lost. Nos. 1, 2, and 4 are incorrect because fear of death and threat to peer status are seen in school-age children, while decreased independence is seen in both toddlers and adolescents.

92. (3) Frequent swallowing, noisy respirations, and increased pulse are signs of hemorrhage. No. 1 (vomiting dark red blood) is most likely old blood that was swallowed during surgery. Nos. 2 and 4 are expected behaviors.

93. (1) Explain that clear, cool liquids are best right now, which is the usual protocol for post-surgery patients and will be soothing to Lisa. No. 2 is incorrect; milk products are mucous-producing, which hinders breathing and is also a good medium for bacterial growth. No. 3 is not an honest response that imparts information. While No. 4 may be appropriate, it also does not explain.

94. (2) Normal for this age group and referred to as a food jag, which is best handled by giving her the food but avoiding comment on the continuing request. It will resolve in a short time unless it is allowed to become No. 4, an attention-getter. Because of the self-limiting factor (No. 1), anemia is highly unlikely, and the food jag does not indicate a behavior problem (No. 3).

95. (1) Avoid palpating the abdomen, which can cause metastasis. Hence, Nos. 2 and 4 are incorrect. While the nurse will support the parents (No. 3), it is not the most important function at this time.

96. (4) Immediate surgery after diagnosis leads to the best prognosis, as this tumor is usually encapsulated and can be completely removed at this stage. Therefore, Nos. 2 and 3 are incorrect. While No. 1 is important, it is not the best answer.

97. (2) Crying is normal when a 3-year-old is left in a strange environment. Waving (No. 1) could be expected of an older child who is capable of understanding that the separation is temporary. Covering her head (No. 3) is an abnormal response that needs investigating, while a request to go to the playroom (No. 4) may come later in the hospitalization.

98. (3) Playing house in the playroom affords peer group play, which is necessary and desirable for Ellen's development. The other responses are either solitary activities or involve an adult.

99. (1) Urine output would be the first sign of complications. Nos. 2, 3, and 4 are also signs of shock and hypovolemia, but are not the highest priority.

100. (1) High-caloric (three to four times normal) and high-protein (two to three times normal) diet, due to greatly increased metabolic needs. This combination best meets Pete's nutritional needs. Hence, Nos. 2, 3, and 4 are incorrect.

101. (1) Maintaining body alignment is most important to prevent contractures during the healing stages. No. 4, splinting joints, is inappropriate, although measures to maintain body alignment are important, particularly at night. Nos. 2 and 3 are part of normal nursing care, but should not be viewed as major preventive measures against contracture.

102. (4) Puppet play is appropriate, especially for children who may not be able to play for themselves. The nurse can assume one of the roles and aid the child to express her- or himself. No. 1 may be used with discretion but should not be the primary diversion. Nos. 2 and 3 are not possible for Pete due to his age and condition.

103. (2) Illness as punishment is a usual preschooler's view. It is important for the nurse to dispel this by explaining that the illness was due to an accident. Otherwise, it could become a maladaptive attitude (No. 3). No. 1 is incorrect because the attitude described is more characteristic of older school age children. No. 4 is not known or assumed.

104. (4) Have the child sit with head elevated and tilted back slightly; apply firm pressure over the bridge of the nose. Nos. 1, 2, and 3 are incorrect postures.

105. (1) Apply ice and patch eye to prevent edema and bruising. No. 2 is not indicated unless there is an obvious injury or complication. No. 3 is contraindicated. No. 4 may make Billy more comfortable but is not the first-aid measure.

106. (2) Applying ice and splinting the finger will decrease the edema and prevent further injury. Heat may be applied after 72 hours, but is incorrect now (No. 1). A referral may be appropriate (No. 3) but is not the first-aid measure. Splinting the finger (No. 4) needs to be done in conjunction with ice application.

107. (3) Clean and cover with a dressing to prevent or protect from puncture. Nos. 1 and 2 recommend puncture, which is contraindicated and may lead to infection. No. 4, getting new shoes, may not solve the problem.

108. (1) The scraping maneuver may be accomplished by "flicking" out the stinger with a fingernail, edge of a knife, or other object. No. 2 will release the toxins into the arm. No. 3 should not be applied before removing the stinger. No. 4 is done *after* removing the stinger.

109. (3) Hero worship is very common in this age group. You would not assume No. 1, defense mechanisms, or No. 2, repression, because of the developmental stage; yet Johnny is old enough that fantasy (No. 4) is unlikely.

110. (2) Building with Popsicle sticks will foster Johnny's sense of industry and can be done while he is in bed. Nos. 1 and 4 would be more appropriate for a younger age group. No. 3 will not promote his development, although it can be used as entertainment on occasion.

111. (4) A peer who is also confined to bed would be the most acceptable roommate because of the strong sense of competition in this age group, making two ambulatory peers (No. 2) contribute to a sense of inferiority. A preschooler (No. 1) is inappropriate, but a mentally retarded 14-year-old (No. 3) may be acceptable upon assessment of the boy.

112. (3) Cranking a wind-up toy would not be active enough to release his aggressive feelings. Nos. 1, 2, and 4 would be more appropriate.

113. (2) Inferiority: it is necessary for the school-age child to be successful in his or her tasks, as unrealistic expectations can lead to feelings of inferiority. No. 1 is the antithesis of initiative in the preschooler; No. 3, of autonomy in the toddler; No. 4, of mistrust in the infant.

114. (2) Petit mal; after age 3 years these occur more often in girls than boys; duration is approximately 30 seconds. Grand mal seizures (No. 1) often develop in those children who had Jacksonian-March seizures (No. 3) in infancy. Myoclonic (No. 4) is usually one stage of a seizure.

115. (3) Ketogenic diet, which is high in fats, with a reduction of fluid intake tends to prevent seizures. Hence, Nos. 1, 2, and 4 are incorrect.

116. (2) Ease Tom to the floor and loosen the clothes around his neck accompanied by measures to prevent him from injuring himself, such as moving furniture out of the way. No. 1, having others leave the room, will not help Tom during his seizure. No. 3, restraining Tom's movements, is contraindicated, as is No. 4, putting something between his teeth, both of which may injure Tom or the nurse.

117. (1) Hypertrophy of the gums leads to many complications and is the result of Phenytoin (Dilantin). Recommend daily gum massage. Nos. 2 and 3 may be seen if Tom is also on phenobarbital, while No. 4 could be due to any number of factors.

118. (2) Joining the Scouts or some other youth group will give Tom an outlet to socialize with peers, which he needs. Nos. 2 and 3 are solitary activities. No. 1 should be done under supervision only, as Tom could injure himself with the knife if he had a seizure while carving.

119. (3) Cardiac damage can be minimized or prevented with early detection and treatment. Nos. 1, 2, and 4 are incorrect because the cause of chorea is not known, Carla is not infectious, and early detection does not determine the dosage of medication.

120. (2) Physical and psychologic rest are the main factors in preventing complications and extensive damage during the acute phase. Nos. 3 and 4 will become more important as Carla responds to treatment. No. 1 may be one means of accomplishing the psychologic rest needed.

121. (2) Mitral valve is most often affected. Carditis leads to aortic insufficiency and mitral stenosis, resulting in fibrosis of the mitral valve. Hence, Nos. 1, 3, and 4 are incorrect.

122. (2) Cardiac damage: the younger the child, the poorer the prognosis in those children who develop carditis. No. 1 does not develop until after the rheumatic episode and has no effect on the prognosis. Arthritis (No. 3), or sore, swollen joints, is present during the acute stage and, again, does not determine prognosis. No. 4, activity, is curtailed to help prevent carditis.

123. (1) Tinnitus and nausea may develop, and the physician should then be notified. No. 2 is not a side effect of this drug. No. 3 may be seen in the diabetic patient. No. 4 may signal the onset of an infectious process.

124. (1) Random movements and inappropriate facial expressions are involuntary symptoms, most commonly seen in school-age girls. Nos. 2, 3, and 4 are incorrect.

125. (3) No other sign of inflammation because it occurs after the attack of rheumatic fever symptoms subsides. Therefore Nos. 1, 2, and 4 are incorrect.

126. (1) Industry versus inferiority: successful accomplishment of tasks is necessary for this school-age group.

No. 2 is the task of toddlers, No. 3 is the task of preschoolers, and No. 4 is the task of infants.

127. (3) Knitting or crocheting is appropriate for bedrest for a school-age girl and promotes her sense of industry. No. 1 is for toddlers, No. 2 is too active, and No. 4, while pleasant, does not promote development.

128. (1) Terry, who has leukemia. Danny's primary infection was probably streptococcus, and it is extremely important to isolate Terry from this child because Terry is highly susceptible to infections. Tommy's mental retardation (No. 2) is not a reason for exclusion. Billy's and Sean's conditions (Nos. 3 and 4) share the same organism as Danny's.

129. (2) Inflammation is due to the usual history of prior infection and autoimmune response factors. Hence, Nos. 1, 3, and 4 are incorrect.

130. (3) Bedrest is instituted as well as daily weights to assist in determining fluid retention, and low-sodium diet is indicated because of the hypertension. Hence, Nos. 1, 2, and 4 are incorrect.

131. (4) Magnesium sulfate is the antihypertensive drug in this group. Hence, Nos. 1, 2, and 3 are incorrect.

132. (3) Seven to fourteen days is the usual course. This is not a chronic condition, so Nos. 1 and 2 are incorrect. No. 4 is too short.

133. (2) Restricting Danny to indoor activities until he has fully recovered will prevent complications. He is not yet ready to return to full activity (No. 1), and he is not contagious or infectious, so Nos. 3 and 4 are inappropriate.

134. (1) Practicing magic tricks is age-appropriate for Danny while he is indoors. No. 2 is not an appropriate indoor activity. Nos. 3 and 4 are appropriate for the toddler/preschool age group.

135. (1) Dressing himself, knowing left and right, and crossing the street by himself are appropriate for Danny. Nos. 2 and 3 are appropriate for toddlers; No. 4, for adolescents.

136. (2) A sweat chloride test and stool test for trypsin activity. Blood and sputum are not definitive tests for cystic fibrosis, so Nos. 1, 3, and 4 are incorrect.

137. (3) The inability to metabolize certain amino acids is seen in phenylketonuria. Nos. 1, 2, and 4 are all found in cystic fibrosis.

138. (4) High-protein, low-fat diet with water-soluble vitamins is appropriate because fat digestion is impaired. Hence, Nos. 1, 2, and 3 are incorrect.

139. (1) The pancreatic enzymes are to be taken with meals so they can aid in the digestion of food. They would be ineffective if given at any other time, so Nos. 2, 3, and 4 are incorrect.

140. (1) Concrete thinking is present during the eighth to twelfth year. No. 2 is present during ages 3–7; No. 3, ages 13–16; and No. 4, late adolescence and adulthood.

141. (1) Rollerskating with a group of girls is Gloria's most likely choice of activity to achieve peer contact. No. 2 is in competition with the opposite sex and is a one-to-one activity. No. 3 interacts with adults, not peers. No. 4 is a solitary activity.

142. (1) Headache, lethargy, and vomiting are signs that indicate increased intracranial pressure. Nos. 2, 3, and 4 are incorrect because pulse would be decreased; there would be blurred or double vision; and vomiting without nausea or fever would most likely be present.

143. (2) Slow-growing, benign tumor; 90% are cured by surgical excision. Nos. 1, 3, and 4 are incorrect because it is neither fast-growing nor malignant; it *is* curable; and surgical treatment is preferred.

144. (1) Having his hair shaved off is most likely to upset Pepe. By being different from his peers, he risks losing his sense of self-esteem. No. 2 is incorrect because he may enjoy missing school (though he will probably not like being away from his schoolmates). No. 3 should not be too traumatic at this age, with proper preparation. No. 4 is incorrect because he will be able to miss meals for 24 hours (even though he may not like it); however, he may be anorexic.

145. (4) Discomfort and increased incidence of headache may result from bending his head. Nos. 1, 2, and 3 are unlikely to occur.

146. (3) Linda is upset about her appearance, which would include protrusion of her eyeballs. Nos. 1, 2, and 4 are incorrect because failure in school is an unknown; spoiled and infantile behavior is an erroneous judgement; hyperactivity is being controlled by her medication.

147. (1) Fever, rash, nausea, and joint pain are symptoms of the medication. Hence, Nos. 2, 3, and 4 are incorrect.

148. (3) Her intake should be 2700 calories. To lose one pound per week, intake must be reduced by 500 calories per day. Hence, Nos. 1, 2, and 4 are incorrect.

149. (4) Hypothyroidism would not be a cause unless other signs and symptoms were present, including coarse skin, sluggish, listless behavior, and increased weight gain with no change in eating patterns. Nos. 1, 2, and 3 all contribute to the development of obesity.

150. (2) Normal protein depletion of adolescent period causes many adolescents to complain of "tiredness." Good nutrition is especially important at this time. There is not enough information to assume Nos. 1 or 3; and No. 4 would more likely result from shunning social contact, not exercising.

151. (3) Encourage exercise, explaining that it will be more comfortable after a hot bath. The nurse can perform No. 4 (range-of-motion exercises), but exercising needs to be done more often than the nurse visits. No. 1 is inappropriate. No. 2 is imprecise, as splinting the wrists and knees at night to maintain body alignment would be the only appropriate splinting suggestion.

152. (4) This side effect of the salicylate medication is reversible upon discontinuation of the medication. Nos. 1, 2, and 3 are incorrect.

153. (2) By asking Rhonda if she has discussed body changes, the nurse can determine what information Rhonda possesses and what her response will be. No. 1, repeating Rhonda's question, is an inappropriate response to someone seeking information. No. 3, referring Rhonda to her mother, may be appropriate once the nurse determines what information Rhonda has, from what source. No. 4 is an inappropriate reassurance that stops communication.

154. (1) Idiopathic or unknown; most frequent during rapid periods of growth, usually between 12 and 16 years of age; more often affecting females. Nos. 2, 3, and 4 are possible types, but not the most common among adolescents.

155. (2) She should now learn to log roll from side to side, as that is what she will be required to do following surgery. While she will also need to do the other three, she can be shown how to do No. 1 at any time, and Nos. 3 and 4 are more appropriately taught at a later time.

156. (3) She will most likely wear her cast 6–12 months following insertion of the Harrington rod. Katy should not be given false optimism (No. 1) or pessimism (No. 2), and while she can speak with her physician (No. 4), the nurse can give her information that is general knowledge.

157. (3) This is typical adolescent behavior, as adolescents need time to formulate their philosophies of life, to learn to know themselves, and to plan for their future. Nos. 1, 2, and 4 are incorrect because Katy's personality is unknown, and saying she is trying to evade responsibility is unfair; labeling her schizophrenic is grossly inappropriate; and while tiring easily is typical, the question refers to daydreaming.

158. (3) Demanding control and newly acquired independence is difficult for staff to handle at times but is a normal reaction for a hospitalized adolescent who feels controlled and dependent. Nos. 1, 2, and 4 are all maladaptive behaviors that should be investigated.

159. (3) Mescaline, which comes from the peyote cactus, has been used by some Indian tribes during ceremonies. Nos. 1, 2, and 4 are incorrect.

160. (3) Amphetamines, referred to as speed or uppers, elevate the user's mood. Nos. 1, 2, and 4 would not produce the same symptoms or be called by the same street names.

161. (2) Pinpoint pupils is a classic sign of barbiturate abuse. Nos. 1, 3, and 4 are not.

162. (2) Red, swollen nasal membranes and peculiar odor should alert the nurse to suspect glue-sniffing. Other effects include hallucinations and intense exhilaration. Nos. 1, 3, and 4 have different effects.

163. (2) Endocarditis, or inflammation of the lining membrane of the heart, is usually caused by staphylococci. Drug abusers who inject substances into their blood stream usually pay little attention to the hygiene of their needles and other tools. They tend to be particularly susceptible because their nutritional state is often poor, thereby decreasing their resistance. Nos. 2, 3, and 4 are cardiac complications not associated with drug abuse.

164. (3) PID is a serious complication. Often the symptoms are absent until there is an inflammatory process of great magnitude. It may lead to No. 2. Nos. 1 and 4 are not conditions associated with venereal disease.

165. (2) About three weeks; the limits are 10–60 days. Nos. 1, 3, and 4 are incorrect.

166. (3) The drug of choice is penicillin G procaine. No. 1 is the alternate choice for those with allergies to penicillin; No. 2 is an ophthalmic antiinfective; and No. 4 is usually used as an antipsychotic.

167. (3) They are not caused by the same virus. The common cold sore is herpes virus I, not II. Nos. 1 and 2 presume the virus-causing agent is the same. No. 4 is inappropriate, as it is not necessary to discuss the answer in private.

168. (2) Changes in the skin during adolescence; increased secretion of hormones increase oil gland activity. Diet (Nos. 1 and 4) is now believed to play an insignificant part in causing acne. No. 3 will not cause acne, but should be avoided to prevent infections.

169. (4) Painful enlargement of cervical nodes; these enlarged nodes are painless in Hodgkin's disease. Nos. 1, 2, and 3 are all present in Hodgkin's disease.

170. (2) Explain that early diagnosis combined with treatment offers a good prognosis, as a fact-giving and hope-giving realistic answer to Steve's parents. No. 1 is unnecessary, No. 3 is not reassuring at this time, and No. 4 is inappropriate.

171. (1) A radiopaque contrast material is injected under local anesthetic into a vessel in Steve's foot so nodal enlargement can be seen on X ray. Swallowing dye (No. 2) is referred to as a barium swallow and is used for diagnostic purposes for the upper gastrointestinal system. Nos. 3 and 4 are incorrect.

172. (3) Frequently check the number of drops of solution running into the vein and regulate the flow of solution as ordered. This will help prevent circulatory overload and alert the nurse to ceased flow due to position change or dislodgement of the needle. No. 1 is not correct practice, as the child may require more fluid and will thus be subjected to further trauma by starting a new infusion. No. 4, a new bottle of "standard" fluid, may be hung (check institutional policy) as a "keep-open" until a discontinue order is received. Obviously the bed linen should be changed as it is needed (No. 2), but this is not the most important responsibility.

173. (1) Infiltration is the most common complication due to small veins and physical movement. The nurse *must* check the site often even if the infusion is given via mechanical pump, as the pump will continue to infuse even if infiltration occurs. Nos. 2 and 3 are rare during intravenous infusion in children. No. 4 must be guarded against, but fortunately it is not the most common complication in children.

174. (3) Scalp is the preferred site in infants due to the availability of veins and lessened chance of dislodgement—the infant cannot pull out the needle; hence, it is easier to secure. No. 1 is the second choice; No. 2 is rarely used; and No. 4 may be used only when the other sites are unusable.

175. (2) Laterofemoral and anteriofemoral have adequate muscle for injections. Nos. 1, 3, and 4 are incorrect because the gluteal muscles should not be used until the child has been walking to develop these muscles, and the deltoid is used in older children.

176. (2) Inner to outer canthus is correct to derive the greatest benefit and to avoid infecting the tear ducts, as would occur by instilling them outer to inner (No. 1). Nos. 3 and 4 are also incorrect.

177. (2) The conjunctival sac is the correct place for proper utilization. Hence, Nos. 1, 3, and 4 are incorrect.

178. (3) The lower eyelid is easy to administer to and necessary to ensure correct usage. Nos. 1, 2, and 4 are incorrect.

179. (2) Down and back is necessary because of the immature physiology of the ear canal. Over the age of 3 years the ear should be pulled up and back (No. 1). Nos. 3 and 4 will not accomplish the desired effect.

180. (1) Up and back is correct posture to facilitate passage of fluid onto the tympanic membrane or drum. No. 2 is correct for children under 3 years. Nos. 3 and 4 will not accomplish the desired effect.

181. (4) This response acknowledges the child's feelings, which are normal for a preschooler, without judging her response and reassures her that you like her even when she expresses her feelings. Nos. 1, 2, and 3 are inappropriate for this age group.

182. (1) One grain. Using Clark's Rule:

$$\frac{\text{Child's weight in pounds}}{150} \times \text{Adult dose}$$

$$= \text{Approximate dose for child}$$

$$\frac{15}{150} \times 10 = 1$$

183. (2) Fifty milligrams. Convert Tony's weight to pounds (13.6 × 2.2 = 30), then use Clark's Rule:

$$\frac{30}{150} \times 250 = 50$$

184. (2) 1.5 cc.

$$\frac{\text{Drug available}}{\text{Amount of solution}} = \frac{\text{Dose desired}}{\text{Amount of solution}}$$

$$\frac{10}{1} = \frac{15}{x}, \quad 10x = 15, \quad x = 1.5$$

185. (1) 2 cc. Use formula above and fill in the corresponding numbers. Change .5 g to milligrams so you will be working with like numbers.

$$\frac{500}{1} = \frac{1000}{x}, \quad 500x = 1000, \quad x = 2$$

186. (2) Attempting to feel breath on your face is the next step according to the American Heart Association. You may need to clear the mouth (No. 3). Someone else will hear your shouts and can be instructed to call the physician (No. 4). Chest compression (No. 1) should not begin until you have identified whether he has aspirated or suffered an arrest.

187. (1) 1:5; 80–100/minute according to American Heart Association guidelines. No. 2 is for two-person adult rescue, No. 3 is for one-person adult rescue, and No. 4 is too fast.

188. (2) Administer four back blows between his shoulder blades, which should dislodge the piece of meat. No. 1 is not indicated; No. 3 is a waste of valuable time; and No. 4 may cause aspiration by blowing the meat into the bronchial tree and is, therefore, contraindicated.

189. (3) Brain cell death begins in 4–6 minutes, according to guidelines established by the American Heart Association. Hence, Nos. 1, 2, and 4 are incorrect.

190. (2) Water is actually the most essential element of the diet at any age. It is necessary for a variety of cellular functions, metabolic transport, and regulation of body temperature. Hence, Nos. 1, 3, and 4 are incorrect.

191. (2) Milk, leafy vegetables, fish, and cheese. Calcium needs increase during periods of rapid growth. Nos. 1, 3, and 4 are incorrect lists.

192. (2) Fish, beef, peanut butter, and chicken are high in protein, which is particularly important to the older child. No. 1 would be a good source of iron. Nos. 3 and 4 are incorrect lists of high-protein foods.

193. (2) Seafood is richest in iodine, which is essential for thyroxin production. Hence, Nos. 1, 3, and 4 are incorrect.

194. (3) Carbohydrates are necessary for metabolism of fats and are utilized for energy without depleting protein stores. Hence, Nos. 1, 2, and 4 are incorrect.

195. (3) Iron is necessary to prevent or combat anemia caused by dietary factors. Hence, Nos. 1, 2, and 4 are incorrect.

ANNOTATED BIBLIOGRAPHY

Evans, M., and Hansen, B.: Guide to pediatric nursing: a clinical reference. New York, 1980, Appleton-Century-Crofts. A paperback book that lists topics alphabetically in two sections, general considerations and nursing management. An excellent quick-reference guide with extensive tables, diagrams, and resources included at the back of the book.

Petrillo, M., and Sanger, S.: Emotional care of hospitalized children: an environmental approach, ed. 2. Philadelphia, 1980, J. B. Lippincott Company. A paperback book that discusses behaviors of children who are hospitalized for conditions or procedures. Case studies effectively illustrate certain behaviors. Guidelines for preparing children for specific procedures are easily adaptable to all age groups and procedures. Good theoretical base.

Scipien, G., Bernard, M., Chard, M., Howe, J., and Phillips, P.: Comprehensive pediatric nursing, ed. 2. New York, 1979, McGraw-Hill Book Co. An extensive textbook that includes the nursing process, growth and development, effects of illness on children of each age group, discussion of body systems, and current trends in pediatric nursing practice. A good discussion of pathophysiology.

Whaley, L. F., and Wong, D. L.: Nursing care of infants and children. St. Louis, Missouri, 1979, The C. V. Mosby Co. A voluminous, comprehensive textbook that includes basic and advanced information for the pediatric clinician. A thorough, current discussion of most topics for those desiring in-depth material on pediatric nursing.

SELECTED REFERENCES

American Academy of Pediatrics
  PO Box 1034
  Evanston, IL 60204
Association for the Aid of Crippled Children
  345 East 46th Street
  New York, NY 10017
Association for the Care of Children's Health
  3615 Wisconsin Avenue
  Washington, DC 20036
Epilepsy Foundation of America
  1828 L Street NW
  Washington, DC 20036

National Association for Retarded Children, Inc.
  386 Park Avenue South
  New York, NY 10016
National Cystic Fibrosis Research Foundation
  3379 Peachtree Road, NE
  Atlanta, GA 30326
The National Foundation for Sudden Infant Death
  1501 Broadway
  New York, NY 10036
National Hemophilia Foundation
  25 West 39th Street
  New York, NY 10018

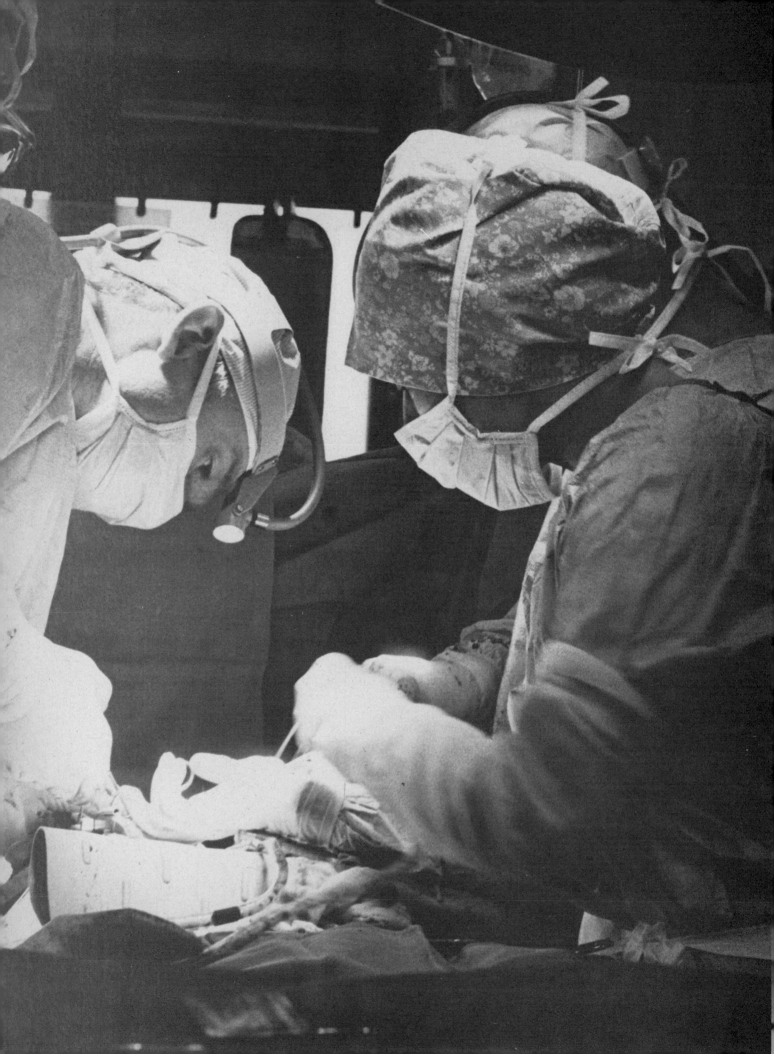

Unit 5 / NURSING CARE OF THE ACUTELY OR CHRONICALLY ILL ADULT

Introduction

This unit is designed to focus on the broad concepts and skills needed to apply the nursing process to the care of the adult patient. To facilitate review, figures and tables supplement and synthesize the material presented in outline format, which is organized into three major sections.

Section I, "Overview," begins with a discussion of stress and adaptation, which forms the overall conceptual framework of the unit, and moves on to guidelines for assessment of the adult, which offers a format for collecting data and identifying nursing problems.

Section II, "Common Medical Problems," is intended to help the student identify common medical problems and to provide a rationale for nursing interventions. The material is organized into six physiologic concepts to present the information in terms of common principles. This organization will facilitate learning through understanding, rather than through memorization of the signs and symptoms of dysfunctions. Common imbalances, discussed under each of these headings, are related to the physiologic dysfunction.

New material for the second edition includes the nursing assessment of tumor reproduction and cancer therapies, a detailed chart on screening assessment, and more information on blood pressure control, serum glucose imbalance, burn care and therapy, lung function, and pharmacology, among other topics.

Section III, "Common Surgical Problems and Emergency Procedures," details the principles of preoperative and postoperative care, surgical complications, and nursing interventions related to specific surgical and emergency procedures. While some specific nursing care procedures have been outlined, the overall intent of this unit is to promote an understanding of the principles and concepts of care that can be applied to the broad spectrum of patients who may be undergoing the same or similar surgical interventions.

New material in Section III includes information on emergency procedures, anesthesia and nursing interventions, updated coverage of the neurologic system, patient education and support, and pharmacology.

Mary Jane Sauvé

Section I / OVERVIEW

Part A / STRESS AND ADAPTATION

The perception of stress is highly individual. Similar situations may be perceived by different people as benign or insignificant, positive and desirable, or negative and undesirable. Negative stressors may be specific or general, ranging from vague physical discomforts and daily hassles in the home, work, or social setting to real or perceived threats to one's physical well-being, self-esteem, or financial or social stability.

A. Responses to stress involve the entire organism.
   1. *Psychologically,* coping strategies are used to reduce the threat, for example, by seeking information, deciding to act or to delay action, instituting palliative modes such as denial or suppression to allay anxiety, or using social supports.
   2. *Physiologically,* the perception of stress elicits the "fight or flight" response, which is mediated through the sympathopituitary-adrenal system. Secretion of norepinephrine at sympathetic peripheral nerve endings produces vasoconstriction, while epinephrine secretion from the adrenal medulla results in tachycardia, increased myocardial contractility, and bronchial dilatation. The adrenal cortex secretes aldosterone, which increases sodium and water retention, and cortisol, which catabolizes proteins and increases serum glucose levels.

B. Adaptation is defined as the temporary or permanent changes in structure, function, behavior, or social milieu of the individual that enable him or her to survive in a particular environment. Like stress, adaptation occurs at all levels of organization, thus it involves the entire organism.

C. Several factors affect the adaptive capacity of the individual.
   1. *Heredity or genetic* potential—limits the growth and development of both structure and function.
   2. The extent to which *needs* have been met in the past—the lack of adequate nutrition, love, acceptance, particularly early in life, seriously reduces the individual's ability to cope with both physical and psychologic stresses.
   3. *Anatomic integrity*—defects in anatomical development, traumas, or diseases may limit physical, intellectual, or psychologic potential.
   4. *Learning*—the degree to which individuals have been able to satisfy their needs, cope with stressors, and adapt to the varying conditions to which they have been exposed affects their flexibility in new situations.
   5. *Age*—physical adaptability is greatest in youth and middle age, least in infancy and old age. Physical immaturity limits the infant, whereas declining reserve capacity of vital organs limits the elderly. Developmental crises may also limit adaptive potential.
      a. *The young adult* (ages 20–40)—intimacy versus self-isolation. The ability to form a commitment to a lasting relationship with another person, cause, institution, or creative effort versus isolation, withdrawal, and avoidance of the issues of life. Developmental tasks of the young adult include establishing personal and financial independence from parents, becoming established in chosen vocation or profession, learning to appraise and express love in a committed manner, and becoming involved in the community.
      b. *The middle-aged adult* (ages 40–65)—generativity versus stagnation. The ability to be as concerned for providing for others as for providing for self versus regression to younger behavior characterized by physical and psychologic self-absorption. Developmental tasks include developing a sense of unity and abiding intimacy with mate; creating a comfortable home consistent with values, time, and resources; balancing work with other roles; adjusting to physical changes; and achieving/maintaining social and civic responsibility.
      c. *The adult in old age* (age > 65)—ego integrity versus despair. The ability to gather together and accept all the previous phases of the life cycle versus a sense of self-disgust and desire to redo life. Developmental tasks of the mature adult include deciding how and where to live remaining life, adjusting living standard to retirement income, maintaining physical health and emotional satisfaction, and adjusting to the death of spouse or significant others.

D. The *nursing process* enables the clinician to:

1. Identify the nature of the stressors—internal, external, or both.
2. Identify the individual's adaptive responses as appropriate, excessive, or deficient.
3. Plan interventions—
   a. *Reduce* stress.
   b. *Support* adaptive behaviors.
   c. *Strengthen* deficient responses.
   d. *Modify* excessive responses.
   e. *Prevent* injury or complications.
4. Reappraise stressors and adaptive responses and modify interventions accordingly.

Part B / ASSESSMENT OF THE ADULT

Assessment is the process of gathering a comprehensive data base about the patient's present and past health problems, as well as a description of the patient as a whole in his or her environment. It includes a comprehensive health history, a physical examination, and laboratory/X-ray data.

1. *Nursing history*—the single most important aspect in establishing a patient's problems.

A. *Chief complaint*—the specific reason prompting the patient to seek professional health care. It is recorded briefly, using the patient's own words.

B. *History of the present health problem*—includes onset, duration, and current status of problem(s) and the reason for seeking care now. Collect quantitative data: (a) location, character, severity, duration, and factors influencing pain, (b) degree of threat patient perceives to physical, psychologic, social, and financial status.

C. *Past health problems*—identify patient's previous illnesses, surgeries, injuries, current medications, allergies, and immunizations. Consists of previously established diagnoses with dates of occurrence, severity, and complications, if any.

D. *Review of systems*—assists in identifying current problems that may be contributing to the present condition, but that have been forgotten or considered insignificant by the patient.
   1. *General:* overall state of health, ability to carry out activities of daily living, fatigue, exercise, spiritual patterns.
   2. *Integument:* rashes, pruritus, unusual hair loss.
   3. *Head:* dental problems, visual problems, speech or hearing problems.
   4. *Respiratory:* shortness of breath, wheezing, cough, sputum.
   5. *Cardiovascular:* chest pain, palpitations, high blood pressure, varicosities.
   6. *Gastrointestinal:* Appetite, food preferences or intolerances, pain, bowel habits.
   7. *Genitourinary:* frequency, urgency, nocturia, venereal diseases.
   8. *Gynecological:* Menarche, painful or heavy menses, vaginal discharge, date of last Pap smear.
   9. *Musculoskeletal:* Weakness, joint or muscle stiffness, pain or swelling.
   10. *Neuropsychiatric:* Orientation to person, place, time; fainting, dizziness, convulsions; decreased or increased peripheral sensation; anxiety, depression.
   11. *Lymphatic and hematologic:* Swollen lymph nodes, excessive bruising, past blood transfusions.
   12. *Endocrine:* Intolerance to heat or cold, sugar in urine, excessive thirst, hunger, sweating.

E. *Family health history*—identifies potential familial or genetic dysfunctions, contact with a communicable disease, and ability to cope with illness or death in the family.

F. *Patient profile*—a summary of the nurse's evaluation of the patient as a whole, psychologically, medically, and socioeconomically.

2. *Physical assessment*—requires knowledge of normal findings and organization (Table 5–1).

A. Inspection—utilizes observations to detect deviations from normal.

B. Palpation—utilized to elicit tenderness and to feel for enlargement of nodes and organs or for tumors and cysts.

C. Percussion—technique utilized to elicit vibrations produced by underlying organ structures.
   1. Flat—normal percussion note over muscle or bone.
   2. Dull—normal percussion note over organs such as liver.
   3. Resonance—normal percussion note over lungs.
   4. Tympany—normal percussion note over stomach or bowel.

D. Auscultation—utilized to perceive and interpret sounds arising from various organs, particularly heart, lungs, and abdomen.

TABLE 5–1. *Screening examination*

Structure	Assessment		Potential nursing diagnoses
	Normal findings	*Abnormal findings*	
Head inspection	Symmetrically developed scalp intact, nontender.	Hematomas, lacerations. Bogginess or bleeding in area of temples or behind ear, cranial crepitations. Tenderness.	Tissue injury potentially related to skull fracture.
Face inspection	Symmetrical structures, skin clear, color consistent with race.	Localized swelling, lesions, trauma.	Tissue injury potentially related to facial fracture. Edema due to local tissue trauma.
Palpation	Sinuses nontender.	Swelling and sinus tenderness.	Sinus congestion and possible infection.
Eyes	Symmetrical, visual fields consistent with examiner's.	Visual fields less than examiner's on confrontation.	Increased dependence due to partial vision loss.
	Lids cover upper iris, lashes full, extend in outward direction.	Lids inflamed, covered with crusty exudate, lashes skimpy, upper eyelid drooping.	Inflammation, potential transmission. Ptosis potentially due to cranial nerve injury, myasthenia gravis.
	Lacrimal ducts patent, conjunctiva pink, sclera white, iris round, borders consistent.	Widened palpebral fissure, infrequent blinking— excessive eye prominence.	Potential vision loss secondary to exposure of eyeball.
		Firm eyeball.	Increased intraocular pressure.
		Soft eyeball.	Inadequate fluid volume.
		Corneal ulcer or haze.	Increased dependence due to partial vision loss.
		Yellow sclera.	Jaundice—potential infectious transmission.
	Pupils round, equal, respond to direct and consensual light, accommodate and converge. Cornea clear, shiny, and convex.	Pupils unequal, reaction to light unilateral.	Increased intracranial pressure potentially due to injury, inflammation, CVA.
		Pupils both dilated and unresponsive.	Cerebral hypoxia potentially due to cardiac arrest, increased intracranial pressures, food or drug poisoning.
		Pupils constricted and unresponsive.	Cerebral hypoxia potentially due to anoxia, mushroom poisoning, morphine reaction.

TABLE 5-1.   *(Continued)*

Structure	Assessment		Potential nursing diagnoses
	Normal findings	*Abnormal findings*	
Ears	Pinna ovoid in shape, nontender. Lobe free or attached.	Lesions, swelling, tenderness.	Tissue injury due to trauma, infection.
	External auditory canal clear, pink, nontender.	Discharge in canal: blood, cerebral spinal fluid.	Tissue injury related to trauma. Potential increase in intracranial pressure.
		Pus or serous drainage.	Earache due to inflammation, infection, foreign body.
	Tympanic membrane pearly grey, malleus clearly visible, light reflex at 5 o'clock right ear, 7 o'clock left ear.	Amber, blue-yellow, bulging, retracted.	Earache due to inflammation, infection, tinnitus.
		Perforated.	Hearing impaired.
Nose	Skin clear, septum straight; nares clear, pink; turbinates pink; no discharge.	External bleeding, swelling, deviated septum.	Tissue injury and inflammation related to trauma.
		Purulent discharge.	Inadequate nasal clearing related to infection.
		Watery nasal discharge.	Inadequate nasal clearing related to allergy, head injury (cerebral spinal fluid).
		Bloody discharge.	Epistaxis potentially related to tissue trauma, hypertension, infection, blood dyscrasias.
		Boggy red turbinates.	Sinus congestion.
		Nasal polyps, foreign bodies, accumulated secretions.	Airway obstruction or potential obstruction.
Oral cavity	Teeth present and in good repair. Tongue pink, moist, symmetrical in shape and strength, mucous membranes moist, pink. Gums pink, fit tightly around teeth. Uvula rises symmetrically on phonation. Tonsils absent or pink, parotid glands patent.	Decayed teeth, accumulation of crusty tartar on teeth margins.	Inadequate or poor oral hygiene.

(Continued)

TABLE 5–1.   *(Continued)*

| Structure | Assessment | | Potential nursing diagnoses |
	Normal findings	Abnormal findings	
		Broken or missing teeth.	Tissue injury related to trauma.
		Bleeding gums.	Tissue injury related to trauma. Gum bleeding related to vitamin deficiency, dental plaque, blood dyscrasia.
		Inflamed, purulent, receding gums.	Chewing difficulty related to infection and inadequate oral hygiene.
		Gum hyperplasia.	Chewing difficulty related to drug toxicity (Dilantin), leukemia.
		Tongue-splitting or denuded tongue.	Oral tenderness related potentially to inadequate hygiene, malnutrition, inadequate fluid intake.
		Ulcerated tongue.	Oral tenderness and chewing difficulty potentially related to inadequate oral hygiene, malnutrition, or infection (herpes simplex, syphilis, tuberculosis).
		Bright red tongue.	Niacin deficiency potentially related to malnutrition.
		Strawberry tongue, beefy red and denuded.	Inflammation related to scarlet fever.
		Poor tongue control, deviates toward paralyzed side, quivers.	Chewing difficulties and impaired swallowing related to cranial nerve dysfunction.
		White, thickened plaques on oral mucosa.	Sore mouth related to monilia infection.
		Pale oral mucosa.	Nutritional deficiency related to malnutrition, excessive blood loss.
		Blue oral mucosa.	Insufficient oxygenation.
		Koplik's spots.	Potential transmission of infection related to measles virus.
		Uvula deviates on phonation.	Potential impairment in swallowing related to 10th cranial nerve dysfunction.

TABLE 5-1. (Continued)

| Structure | Assessment | | |
	Normal findings	Abnormal findings	Potential nursing diagnoses
		Redness, swelling, white or yellow ulcerations on tonsils.	Decreased food and fluid intake related to infectious process.
Neck	Symmetrical, trachea midline, carotid pulses equal, full, with even upstroke and fall.	Trachea deviated.	Inadequate pulmonary ventilation related to pneumothorax, pleural effusion, atelectasis.
		Barely palpable carotid pulses.	Impaired cerebral perfusion due to volume losses, decreased left ventricular contractility.
	Neck veins flat at 45° angle, venous pulsation noted in supine position 2 cm above supersternal notch.	Neck vein distention at 45° angle.	Circulatory overload related to congestive heart failure or excess volume.
		Collapsed neck veins in supine position.	Insufficient volume due to blood loss, fluid losses, inadequate fluid intake.
	Lymph nodes nonpalpable and nontender. Full range of motion.	Painful, tender, swollen lymph nodes.	Edema related to tissue injury, infection, inflammatory process.
		Decreased range of motion.	Tissue injury or painful joint mobility related to trauma or inflammatory process.
		Nucal rigidity.	Decreased range of motion potentially related to cerebral infection.
	Thyroid soft, lobes nonpalpable.	Palpable and enlarged thyroid; thyroid bruit.	Increased basal metabolic rate and decreased stress tolerance related to overactive thyroid function.
Breasts	Symmetrically small or large, round, firm, soft, slightly to very pendulous, one breast may be slightly larger than the other.	Breast asymmetry with dimpling or retraction of nipple, peau d'orange.	Skin retraction potentially related to carcinoma or fat necrosis.
		Localized redness, pain, with limited arm motion.	Inflammation potentially related to infection, abscess, tissue trauma.

(Continued)

TABLE 5–1.   *(Continued)*

Structure	Normal findings	Abnormal findings	Potential nursing diagnoses
	Areolae round, small to large depending upon parity, may be pink to dark brown depending upon overall skin color; nipples erect.	Excoriation or dry scaling of nipple, and areola that bleeds easily on contact.	Skin irritation suggestive of underlying carcinoma (Paget's disease).
		Split in breast nipple tissue.	Cracked nipple potentially related to lactation and nursing.
		Bloody nipple discharge.	Bloody discharge potentially related to ductal disease.
		Yellow or green nipple discharge.	Purulent discharge related to infectious process.
		Breast soreness or tenderness.	Breast tenderness related to premenstrual fullness.
		Nontender, smooth, rubbery mass that is movable and well delineated.	Breast mass suggestive of adenofibroma.
		Nontender, hard, fixed, and poorly delineated mass.	Breast mass suggestive of carcinoma.
		Occasionally tender, multiple movable masses in breast. Round and well delineated.	Multiple breast tumors suggestive of cystic disease.
Chest thorax	Chest wall intact, A-P diameter half lateral diameter. Spinal curvatures not exaggerated. Skin clear, warm, well hydrated.	Increased A-P diameter—barrel chest.	Hyperinflation.
		Kyphosis or scoliosis.	Decreased respiratory excursion related to spinal deformities.
		Increased venous pattern.	Increased collateral circulation potentially related to hepatic congestion.
	No pulsations noted. Respiratory rate 16, unlabored.	Bruising, lacerations, bleeding wounds.	Tissue injury related to trauma.
		Visible apical impulse.	Increased cardiac workload secondary to left ventricular enlargement or contractility.

TABLE 5–1. *(Continued)*

Structure	Normal findings	Abnormal findings	Potential nursing diagnoses
		Visible right ventricular impulse—sternal heave.	Increased cardiac workload secondary to right ventricular enlargement.
		Respiratory rate below 12/min (bradypnea).	Inadequate pulmonary ventilation and potential oxygen deficiency.
		Respiratory rate above 20/min.	Hyperventilation. Distressed respiratory effort.
		Alternate cessation and rapid breathing.	Distressed respiratory pattern, Biot's breathing.
		Increased rate and depth of respirations.	Increased respiratory effort suggestive of metabolic acidosis, Kussmaul's breathing.
		Irregular pattern consisting of apnea, then slowly increased rate and depth, gradually ceasing again.	Distressed respiratory pattern—Cheyne-Stokes.
		Painful breathing.	Painful respirations potentially related to inflammation or trauma.
		Paroxysmal respirations.	Painful, depressed respiratory effort secondary to flail chest (multiple rib fractures).
		Mouth breathing.	Nasal congestion or upper-airway obstruction.
Lungs		Noisy snoring respirations.	Upper-airway obstruction secondary to foreign object, inflammation, edema.
		Use of accessory muscles.	Increased work of breathing secondary to carbon dioxide retention.
		Productive cough with yellow sputum.	Increased pulmonary secretions secondary to infectious process.
	Symmetrical lung expansion.	Unequal chest expansion.	Uneven chest excursion potentially related to infection, trauma, pleural effusions.
	One- to two-inch diaphragmatic excursion.	Decreased diaphragmatic excursion.	Hyperventilation. Abdominal distention.
	Ribs and interspaces nontender.	Tenderness and pain in thorax.	Painful ribs secondary to tissue trauma.

(Continued)

TABLE 5–1. *(Continued)*

Structure	Normal findings	Abnormal findings	Potential nursing diagnoses
		Thoracic skin crepitations (subcutaneous emphysema).	Inadequate ventilation.
	Bilateral resonance.	Dullness to percussion.	Decreased pulmonary ventilation secondary to atelectasis or consolidation.
		Hyperresonance.	Hyperinflation secondary to emphysema. Decreased pulmonary ventilation secondary to pleural effusion or pneumothorax.
	Vesicular breath sounds bilaterally.	Bronchial breath sounds, short inspiration, prolonged expirations in lung fields.	Decreased pulmonary ventilation secondary to atelectasis or consolidation.
	Broncho-vesicular breath sounds between scapula. Bronchial breath sounds over large bronchi or trachea.	Broncho-vesicular breath sounds in lung fields.	Decreased pulmonary ventilation potentially related to pulmonary consolidation.
		Wheezing.	Small airway obstruction.
		Decreased or no breath sounds.	Respiratory arrest. Distressed pulmonary ventilation potentially related to pleural effusion, atelectasis, severe emphysema, pneumothorax.
		Rales.	Decreased alveolar ventilation secondary to pulmonary edema, congestion, embolus, or consolidation.
		Rhonchi.	Airway obstruction secondary to pulmonary edema, congestion, inflammation.
		Pleural friction rub.	Painful respirations secondary to pleurisy.
Heart	Heart sounds regular, between 60–100/min.	Brachycardia rate < 60.	Athletic heart rate. Decreased activity tolerance potentially related to either digitalis toxicity, coronary artery disease, or heart block.

TABLE 5–1.   *(Continued)*

Structure	Assessment — Normal findings	Assessment — Abnormal findings	Potential nursing diagnoses
		Tachycardia rate > 100.	Increased heart rate related to excessive caffeine intake, fever, anxiety. Decreased activity tolerance potentially related either to digitalis toxicity, atrial tachycardia, or shock.
		Irregular rhythms.	Excessive caffeine intake. Digitalis toxicity.
	S_1 louder, longer, and lower-pitched than S_2 at apex.	Accentuated S_1 at apex.	Increased blood pressure potentially related to either anxiety, anemia, or hyperthyroidism.
	S_2 is louder than S_1 at the base.	Decreased S_1 at apex.	Increased body temperature. Potential stenosis of mitral or tricuspid valve. Potential oxygen deficiency related to either delayed AV conduction or complete heart block.
		Accentuated S_2 at base.	Increased systemic or pulmonic blood pressure.
		Decreased S_2 at base.	Potential oxygen deficiency related to either aortic or pulmonic stenosis.
		S_3 or ventricular gallop.	Decreased activity tolerance potentially related to either ventricular failure or valvular insufficiency.
		S_4 or presystolic gallop.	Decreased activity tolerance potentially related to either hypertension, valvular stenosis, anxiety, anemia, or hyperthyroidism.
		Systolic ejection murmur climaxing in early or middle systole.	Functional or innocent murmur. Decreased activity tolerance or potential oxygen deficiency secondary to aortic stenosis, hyperthyroidism, or severe anemia.

(Continued)

TABLE 5–1. *(Continued)*

| Structure | Assessment | | Potential nursing diagnoses |
	Normal findings	Abnormal findings	
		Pansystolic regurgitant murmurs.	Decreased activity tolerance and/or potential oxygen deficiency secondary to mitral regurgitation, tricuspid regurgitation, or ventricular septal defects.
		High-pitched, blowing, pandiastolic murmur.	Decreased activity tolerance and/or potential oxygen insufficiency secondary to either aortic regurgitation or pulmonary regurgitation.
		Mid or late diastolic rumbling murmur.	Decreased activity tolerance and/or potential oxygen insufficiency secondary to either mitral stenosis or tricuspid stenosis.
		Absent heart sounds.	Cardiac arrest.
	PMI—point of maximal impulse in fifth intercostal space inside the left midclavicular line.	Displacement of PMI to the left outside the midclavicular line.	Decreased activity tolerance related to either left ventricular hypertrophy, left ventricular dilatation, right pleural effusion, or pneumothorax. Athletic heart.
	Blood pressure 120/80 (average).	Increased systolic pressure > 140.	Increased blood pressure secondary to hyperthyroidism, anxiety, or severe anemia.
		Increased systolic > 150 and diastolic pressure > 100.	Increased blood pressure secondary to either hypertension, excess epinephrine release, or peripheral vascular disease.
		Systolic pressure < 100 and diastolic < 60.	Decreased arterial pressure secondary to hypovolemia or potential shock states.
		Sudden drop of blood pressure when changing from lying to sitting or standing position.	Orthostatic hypotension secondary to either hypovolemia, impending shock states, or antihypertension therapy.
	Pulse pressure 30–50.	Decreased pulse pressure, < 30.	Decreased stroke volume secondary to either hypovolemia or left ventricular failure.

TABLE 5–1. *(Continued)*

| | Assessment | | |
Structure	Normal findings	Abnormal findings	Potential nursing diagnoses
		Increased pulse pressure, > 50.	Increased stroke volume secondary to hypertension, hyperkinetic states, or valvular insufficiency.
Abdomen: inspection	Flat or rounded, symmetrical. Skin clear, well hydrated. Umbilicus flat or slightly inverted.	Bruising, scars, lacerations.	Tissue injury related to trauma or previous surgery.
		Scaphoid abdomen.	Inadequate nutritional intake.
		Upper abdomen distended.	Gastric distention.
		Lower abdomen distended.	Bladder distention or pregnant uterus.
		Protuberant abdomen. Umbilicus appears sunken.	Obesity.
		Protuberant abdomen with bulging flanks and everted umbilicus.	Abdominal distention secondary to ascitic fluid.
		Silver striae.	Skin-stretching secondary to obesity, abdominal distention, old pregnancy.
		Pink-purple striae.	Skin-stretching secondary to Cushing's syndrome, present pregnancy.
	Peristaltic wave may be seen in very thin people.	Active peristaltic waves.	Increased peristalsis secondary to either intestinal obstruction or ulcerative colitis.
	Slight epigastric pulsation (abdominal aorta).	Strong epigastric pulsation.	Increased abdominal aortic pulsation secondary to either anxiety, hyperthyroidism, or aortic aneurysm.
Abdomen: auscultation	Clicks and gurgles from 5–30/min.	Borborygmi.	Hyperperistalsis secondary either to hunger or diarrhea.
		Increased bowel sounds—high-pitched, tinkling sounds with abdominal cramping.	Bowel distention and/or potential intestinal obstruction.
		Bruits over abdominal aorta, renal artery, or iliac artery.	Bruits secondary either to partial arterial obstruction or aneurysm.

(Continued)

TABLE 5–1.   *(Continued)*

Structure	Assessment		Potential nursing diagnoses
	Normal findings	*Abnormal findings*	*Potential nursing diagnoses*
Percussion	Tympany throughout bowel and over lowest interspace in the left anterior line (spleen).	Dullness.	Enlarging uterus. Ascitic fluid. Potential solid tumor. Splenic enlargement.
		Dullness over suprapubic area.	Bladder distention.
		Dullness below right intercostal margin.	Liver enlargement.
Light palpation	Some voluntary muscle resistance.	Tenderness, involuntary rigidity, and spasm of abdominal muscles.	Potential peritoneal inflammation.
Deep palpation	Some voluntary muscle guarding.	Rebound tenderness.	Peritoneal inflammation.
	Liver edge smooth, firm, nontender.	Tenderness in right upper costal area.	Anorexia, nausea secondary to inflammation of the liver.
		Increased tenderness, rigidity, history of trauma, pain and swelling over ischium.	Decreased motility potentially related to pelvic fracture.
Extremities: inspection	Symmetrical development of arms and legs, equal strength and tone.	Swelling, bruising, lacerations.	Tissue injury related to trauma.
		Deformity, crepitus, point tenderness.	Potential bone fracture.
	Full range of motion all joints, with minor crepitations.	Joint swelling, heat, redness, decreased mobility.	Edema related to local tissue injury or rheumatoid arthritis. Potential dislocation.
	Skin clear, well hydrated.	Differences in muscle size—atrophy of musculature.	Decreased mobility secondary to lower motor neuron lesion.
		Continuous or involuntary muscle contraction.	Muscle spasm. Muscle spasticity limiting range of motion. Potential joint contractures.
		Stiff extension position.	Decerebrate rigidity secondary to either head injury or brain inflammation.
		Stiff flexion or extension position.	Decorticate rigidity secondary to either head injury or brain inflammation.

TABLE 5–1. *(Continued)*

| Structure | Assessment | | Potential nursing diagnoses |
	Normal findings	Abnormal findings	
		Inability to move one side of body, one limb, both lower limbs, or all four limbs.	Impaired mobility. Decreased ability to handle activities of daily living. Alteration in body image.
Inspection and palpation	Peripheral pulses equal.	Unequal peripheral pulses.	Inadequate peripheral circulation secondary to either peripheral vascular disease or trauma.
	Sensory perception equal to light touch, pinprick, and temperature.	Absent peripheral pulses. Unequal sensory perception of light touch, pinprick, and temperature.	Circulatory block. Impaired sensory perception. Increased potential for burn accidents.
	Hand grasps, leg pushes and foot pulls equal bilaterally.	Unequal hand grasps, leg pushes, and foot pulls.	Impaired motor function. Decreased ability to initiate activities of daily living. Alterations in body image.
	Deep-tendon reflexes 2^+ to 3^+.	Diminished or absent deep-tendon reflexes.	Impaired motor function may be secondary to early CVA or lower motor neuron lesion.
		Hyperactive deep-tendon reflexes.	Impaired motor function secondary to upper motor neuron lesion.
	Cervical concavity.		
	Thoracic convexity. Lumbar concavity.	Accentuated-rounded thoracic convexity (kyphosis). Accentuated lumbar concavity (lordosis).	Muscle spasm. Backache. Potential oxygen insufficiency secondary to decreased thoracic compliance.
	Spinous processes aligned horizontally.		Muscle spasm. Low back pain.
	Spinous processes C_7 or T_1 are usually prominent.	Lateral curvature of the spine (scoliosis), iliac crest, and shoulders uneven.	Muscle spasm. Backache.
	Full range of motion.	Muscle tenderness, decreased range of motion.	Muscle spasm. Edema of local tissue secondary to either tissue trauma or inflammation.
		Local deformity, swelling, tenderness.	Tissue injury due to trauma. Potential for spinal shock.

(Continued)

TABLE 5–1. *(Continued)*

Structure	Normal findings	Abnormal findings	Potential nursing diagnoses
Male reproductive system: inspection	Penis is cone-shaped, with or without prepuce.	Prepuce cannot be retracted (phimosis).	Painful urination. Edema to localized tissue trauma possible.
		Penis ulceration (round, dark red, painless, with an indurated base).	Possible infectious transmission secondary to syphilis.
		Nontender indurated nodule or ulcer.	Possible carcinoma.
	Urethra is located ventrally on shaft of penis.	Urethra meatus displaced to the inferior surface of penis.	Difficult sphincter control. Alteration in body image.
		Purulent or nonpurulent urethral discharge.	Painful urination. Possible infectious transmission secondary to gonorrhea or GU infection.
	Testicles are about 4 cm long and left is usually somewhat lower than right.	Painful swelling of testes.	Edema related to local tissue trauma or inflammation.
Female reproductive system: inspection	Labia majora are rounded folds. Labia minora are pink folds extending anteriorly to cover clitoris. Introitus open, semi or completely covered by hymen.	Lacerations and swelling, local swelling.	Tissue injury due to trauma.
		Tenderness and inflammation.	Enlargement of Bartholin's gland.
		Vulva redness, itching, and edema.	Pruritus and tissue injury secondary to poor hygiene.
		Wartlike lesions.	Possible infectious transmission secondary to venereal disease.
	Urethra orifice pink—opening between clitoris and vagina—patent.	Cheesy, frothy white, or yellow discharge.	Possible infectious transmission secondary to Monilia, Trichomonas, or other organism.
		Foul, chocolate-brown discharge.	Inadequate feminine hygiene postmenses. Possible uterine malignancy.
		Profuse vaginal bleeding.	Possible shock secondary to tissue trauma, spontaneous abortion, postpartum bleeding.

E. General survey—provides information on the patient as a whole.
   1. *Race, sex, apparent age* in relation to stated age.
   2. *Nutritional status*—well hydrated and developed, obesity, cachexia.
   3. *Apparent health status*—general good health, mild, moderate, severe debilitation.
   4. *Posture and motor activity*—erect, symmetrical, and balanced gait and muscle development; ataxic, circumducted, scissors, or spastic gait; slumped or bent-over posture; mild, moderate, or hyperactive motor responses.
   5. *Behavior*—alert; oriented to person, time, place; hears and comprehends instructions; tense, anxious, angry; uses abusive language; slightly or largely unresponsive; delusions, hallucinations.
   6. *Odors*—noncontributory, acetone, alcohol, fetid breath, incontinent of urine or feces.
   7. Skin—deviations in color (jaundice, cyanosis, pallor; flushing), temperature (cold, hot), moisture (dry, moist, profuse diaphoresis, oily), texture (rough, scaley, smooth), mobility and turgor (falls back easily, slowly, thick, thin, edema).

3. Routine laboratory studies—see Appendix C for normal ranges.
A. *Hematology:*
   1. Complete blood count—detects presence of anemia, infection, allergy, and leukemia.
   2. Prothrombin time—increase may indicate need for vitamin K therapy.
   3. Serology (VDRL)—determines presence of syphilitic reagin; false positives may indicate collagen dysfunctions.
B. *Urinalysis:*
   1. Specific gravity—measures ability of kidney to concentrate urine. Fixed specific gravity indicates renal tubular dysfunction.
   2. Albumin and pus—indicate renal infection.
   3. Sugar and acetone—presence indicates metabolic disorder.
C. *Chest X ray*—detects tuberculosis or other pulmonary dysfunctions as well as changes in size and/or configuration of heart.
D. *Electrocardiogram* (ECG)—detects rhythm and conduction disturbances, presence of myocardial ischemia or necrosis, and ventricular hypertrophy.
E. *Blood chemistries*—detect deviation in electrolyte balance, presence of tissue damage, and adequacy of glomerular filtration.

Section II / NURSING ACTIONS IN COMMON MEDICAL PROBLEMS

Part A / BLOOD PRESSURE

THE PHYSIOLOGY OF BLOOD PRESSURE

A. Blood pressure is the pressure exerted by blood on the walls of the arterial system.
B. Acts to maintain adequate transport of nutrients to the tissue and to remove waste products.
C. Arterial pressures are measured indirectly with auscultation of the brachial artery after it has been compressed with the inflatable cuff of a sphygmomanometer.
   1. Systolic pressure—first tapping sound.
   2. Diastolic pressure—first muffled sound.
   3. Recorded—*systolic/muffling/disappearance of sound*—120/80/76.
   4. Normal range—100/60 to 140/90.
D. The *systolic pressure* is the maximum pressure of the blood against the artery walls and occurs with left ventricular ejection.
   1. Provides information about the force of left ventricular contraction.
   2. Is influenced by the total blood volume, blood viscosity, and the distensibility of the major arteries.
E. The *diastolic pressure* represents the lowest force exerted against the artery wall and occurs when the heart is relaxing.
   1. Provides information about the condition of peripheral vessels.
      a. Narrowed arterioles increase diastolic pressure.
      b. Dilated arterioles decrease diastolic pressure.
   2. Influenced by kidney function, nervous, and humoral factors.
F. The *mean arterial pressure* is the average pressure circulating the blood volume.

TABLE 5–2.   *Factors controlling blood pressure*

Components	Influencing factors	Homeostatic regulator	Imbalances	Pathophysiologic mechanism
CARDIAC OUTPUT				
Stroke volume	Blood volume.	Endocrine system; ADH-aldosterone, kidney.	**HYPOTENSION**	
			Hemorrhage.	↓ Circulatory volume.
			Burns (1st stage), intestinal obstruction.	Volume shift. Plasma → INS fluid (interstitial).
			Vomiting, diarrhea, excessive sweating.	Excessive loss of fluid and electrolytes.
			Diabetes insipidus.	↓ ADH → ↑ H_2O excretion.
			Addison's disease.	↓ Aldosterone → ↑ Na and H_2O excretion.
			Diabetes mellitus.	Osmotic diuresis.
			HYPERTENSION Hyperaldosteronism.	↑ Aldosterone → ↑ Na^+ and H_2O retention.
			Renal insufficiency, renal or systemic disease, infections, hereditary disease, obstructions, calculi, or tumors.	↓ GFR (glomerular filtration rate) → ↑ retention of fluid, electrolytes, and metabolic waste products → azotemia, acidosis, hypervolemia.
	Venous return.	Local blood flow regulators. Capillary dynamics.	**HYPOTENSION** Severe liver disease with ↓ synthesis of plasma proteins.	↓ Blood colloidal oncotic pressures → plasma-to-INS fluid shift.
			Anaphylaxis, radiation therapy.	↑ Capillary permeability → ↑ interstitial fluid, colloidal oncotic pressures → plasma-to-INS fluid shift.
	Iatrogenic volume overload.	Excessive infusions of colloidal solutions, such as dextran, albumin. INS fluid-to-plasma shift (burns, 2nd stage).	**HYPERTENSION** Burns (2nd stage).	↓ Capillary permeability → INS fluid-to-plasma shift.

TABLE 5–2. *(Continued)*

Components	Influencing factors	Homeostatic regulator	Imbalances	Pathophysiologic mechanism
CARDIAC OUTPUT				
	Strength of cardiac contraction (inatrophic action).	Sympathetic nervous system.	***HYPOTENSION*** Myocardial infarction.	Asynergistic cardiac contraction → ↓ SV (stroke volume) → ↓ CO.
			Pericarditis, tamponade.	Restriction of heart muscle due to fibrosis or effusion.
			Severe valvular defects.	↓ SV → LVF (left ventricular failure) → ↑ pulmonary congestion and capillary pressures → pulmonary hypertension → RVF (right ventricular failure).
			HYPERTENSION Pheochromocytoma.	↑ Epinephrine and norepinephrine → ↑ HR (heart rate) and vasoconstriction.
			Increased intracranial pressure.	Irritation and/or hypoxia to CV medullary centers → ↓ HR/ ↑ SV → systolic hypertension → widening pulse pressure.
Heart rate	Exercise, anxiety, nervous excitement, eating, metabolic rate, sleep.	Autonomic nervous system— sympathetic increases rate and parasympathetic decreases rate.	***HYPOTENSION*** Tachyarrhythmias: atrial with rapid ventricular response; ventricular.	↑ HR → ↓ SV → ↓ CO/min.
			Bradyarrhythmias, atrial, 2° and 3° heart block.	↓ HR → ↑ SV → ↓ CO/min.
			HYPERTENSION Anemia.	↓ Hb/O_2 binding capacity → tissue hypoxia → ↑ HR and ↑ CO.
			Thyrotoxicosis or hyperthyroidism.	↑ Cellular metabolism → ↑ HR and ↑ CO to meet cellular nutritional requirements.

(Continued)

TABLE 5–2.   *(Continued)*

Components	Influencing factors	Homeostatic regulator	Imbalances	Pathophysiologic mechanism
PERIPHERAL VASCULAR RESISTANCE Elasticity of arterial walls	Age, sclerosis, injury, inflammatory process.	Dietary intake, smoking, sympathetic nervous system activity, generalized atherosclerosis.		Unknown: associated with vessel injury due to ↑ pulse pulsations → formation of microthrombi in vessel wall → ↑ plaque formation. Plaque formation greatly increased in presence of ↑ circulating, low-density lipoproteins.
			Arteriosclerosis obliterans.	↑ Fatty deposits in arterial walls, narrowing lumens, ↓ blood flow due to increased resistance → tissue ischemia.
Viscosity of blood	Hematocrit.	Hematopoietic system.	**HYPERTENSION** Anemias.	See above.
			Polycythemia vera.	↑ RBC production → ↑ blood volume → ↑ systolic pressure ↑ viscosity → ↑ resistance to flow → ↑ diastolic pressures.
Caliber of arterioles (vasoconstriction, vasodilation)	Blood volume, cardiac output, arterial oxygen tensions, pH of body fluids, pain, emotional reactions.	Autonomic nervous system—sympathetic nervous system increases vasomotor tone.	**HYPOTENSION** Shock.	
			Anaphylactic.	↑ Histamine → ↑ vasodilation → ↑ venous pooling and plasma-to-INS fluid shift → ↓ VR → ↓ CO.
			Septic.	↑ Endo- or exotoxins → ↑ vasodilation and capillary permeability → ↓ VR → ↓ CO.
			Neurogenic.	Interruption of sympathetic NS outflow → ↓ vasomotor tone → ↓ VR.

TABLE 5–2. *(Continued)*

Components	Influencing factors	Homeostatic regulator	Imbalances	Pathophysiolgoic mechanism
			HYPERTENSION Pheochromocytoma.	As above.
			Renal ischemia: · Obstruction. · Hypovolemia. · Trauma. · Tumor.	↑ Renin → ↑ angiotension II → peripheral and renal vasoconstriction → ↓ GFR → ↑ Na^+ and H_2O retention (aldosterone) → ↓ UO (urinary output).

1. Mean pressure is one-third systolic pressure plus two-thirds diastolic pressure.
2. Normal kidney function requires a mean arterial pressure of 70 mm Hg.
3. Indicates average stress level to which heart and blood vessels are subjected.

G. The *pulse pressure* is the difference between the systolic and diastolic pressure—averages 40 mm Hg.
   1. Diminished with decreased stroke volume or in obstruction of left ventricular output.
   2. Increased with increased stroke volume, abnormally rapid runoff of blood, and aortic rigidity.

H. Blood pressure therefore is essentially a reflection of the relationship between cardiac output (stroke volume × heart rate) and peripheral resistance, BP = CO × PVR (Table 5–2).

IMBALANCES IN BLOOD PRESSURE

There are two basic types of imbalance in blood pressure: hypotension and hypertension (Table 5–3).

1. Hypotension—a condition that develops as a result of a decrease in cardiac output, a decrease in peripheral vascular resistance, or both.

A. *Etiology of decreased cardiac output:*
   1. *Decreased blood volume.*
      a. Hemorrhage.
      b. Plasma loss—burns, intestinal obstruction.
      c. Excessive loss of fluid and electrolytes— vomiting, diarrhea, sweating.
      d. *Angina pectoris*—insufficient coronary blood flow.

(1) Pathophysiology:
   (a) Narrowing of coronary arteries due to atherosclerosis, spasm, or inflammation.
   (b) Decreased coronary blood flow due to hypotension, aortic valve defects, polycythemia.
   (c) Increased need for myocardial oxygenation, as in cardiac hypertrophy and during heavy exertion, or in conditions in which cardiac output is increased, as in anemia and hyperthyroidism.
(2) Assessment findings:
   (a) Subjective data.
      i. Pain:
         • *Type—burning, aching, squeezing.*
         • *Location—substernal; may radiate to left shoulder.*
         • *Duration—5 to 20 minutes.*
         • *Precipitated by exertion, emotional stresses, or cold temperatures.*
         • *Relieved by rest or nitroglycerin.*
      ii. Shortness of breath.
      iii. Indigestion.
      iv. Faintness.
   (b) Objective data—vital signs.
      i. Blood pressure—normal range.
      ii. Pulse—tachycardia.
(3) *Nursing goals* are designed to provide relief during acute attacks, identify pre-

TABLE 5–3. *Imbalances in blood pressure: comparative assessment of hypotension and hypertension*

	Hypotension	Hypertension
Common causes—	Angina pectoris. Myocardial infarction. Acute and chronic pericarditis. Valvular defects. Congestive heart failure.	Essential hypertension. Iron deficiency anemia. Pernicious anemia. Arteriosclerosis obliterans. Polycythemia vera.

ASSESSMENT OF BLOOD PRESSURE IMBALANCES

	Hypotension	Hypertension
Behavior	Anxiety, apprehension, decreasing mentation, confusion.	Nervousness, mood swings, irritability, difficulty with memory, depression, confusion.
Neurologic	Essentially noncontributory.	Decreased vibratory sensations, increased/decreased reflexes, Babinski reflex, changes in coordination.
Head/neck	Distended neck veins, worried expression.	Bruits over carotids, distended neck veins, epistaxis, diplopia, ringing in ears, dull occipital headaches on arising.
Skin	Pale, cool, moist.	Dry, pale, glossy, flakey, cold; decreased or absent hair.
GI	Anorexia, nausea, vomiting, constipation.	Anorexia, flatulence, diarrhea, constipation.
Respiratory	Dyspnea, orthopnea, paroxysmal nocturnal dyspnea, tachypnea, moist rales, cough.	Dyspnea, orthopnea, moist rales.
Cardiovascular	Tires easily, decreased systolic pressure, decreased systolic/diastolic pressure. Pulse—increased/decreased, weak, thready, irregular arrhythmias.	Decreased exercise tolerance, weakness, palpitations. Blood pressure—increased systolic, increased systolic and diastolic. Decreased or absent pedal pulses.
Renal	Oliguria.	Oliguria, nocturia, proteinuria.
Extremities	Dependent edema.	Tingling, numbness, or cold hands and feet, dependent edema, ulcers of legs or feet.

cipitating factors, and promote measures that prevent attacks.

(a) Bedrest until pain subsides.
(b) Oxygen as needed.
(c) Nitroglycerin sublingually, as ordered.
(d) Assist in identifying stressful people, activities, and situations.
(e) Involve patient and family in health teaching.
  i. Review action, effects, dosage, and administration of medication; carry "fresh" nitroglycerin at all times, as it loses potency after six months.
  ii. Encourage weight loss if indicated.
  iii. Devise program of regular exercise and rest to promote coronary circulation.
  iv. Explain need to avoid physical and emotional stress.
    • *Large meals and heavy exercise.*
    • *Extremes in temperature.*
    • *Stimulants—coffee, smoking.*

- *Sexual relations when fatigued.*
2. *Inadequate or inefficient myocardial contractility:*
   a. *Myocardial infarction*—localized necrosis of myocardium due to sudden cessation of coronary blood flow; a leading cause of death in the United States.
      (1) Pathophysiology—
         (a) Coronary occlusion due to thrombosis, embolism, or hemorrhage of atheromatous plaque or insufficient blood flow for muscle mass due to cardiac hypertrophy, hemorrhage, shock, or severe dehydration.
         (b) Asynergic pumping of left ventricle, decreased stroke volume, decreased blood pressure.
      (2) Predisposing factors—family history, sex, age, stressful life style, diet, and chronic diseases such as diabetes mellitus and hypertension.
      (3) Assessment findings—
         (a) Subjective data.
            i. Pain:
               - *Type—severe, crushing, burning.*
               - *Location—precordial or substernal, often radiating to one or both arms, neck, jaw, or back.*
               - *Duration—lasts longer than 30 minutes.*
               - *Precipitating factors—unrelated to exercise or respirations and is not relieved by rest or nitroglycerin.*
            ii. Shortness of breath (dyspnea).
            iii. Sweating.
            iv. Indigestion, nausea.
            v. Severe anxiety—fear of death very strong.
         (b) Objective data.
            i. Vital signs:
               - *Blood pressure—decreased.*
               - *Apical pulse—tachycardia (rate over 100); heart sounds diminished.*
               - *Peripheral pulse—weak, rapid.*
               - *Temperature—elevates within 24 hours (100–103° F).*
               - *Respirations—increased, shallow.*
            ii. Skin—pale, cool, diaphoretic.
            iii. Emotional status—restless.
            iv. Laboratory studies (see Table 5–3 and Appendix C, Diagnostic tests).
               - *Elevated WBC, sedimentation rate.*
               - *Elevated serum enzymes (CPK, SGOT, LDH).*
      (4) *Nursing goals* are designed to reduce the cardiac workload, relieve anxiety and pain, prevent complications, and provide support for patient and family.
         (a) Bedrest in a semi-Fowler's position, avoiding unnecessary nursing functions.
         (b) Humidified oxygen per mask, cannula, or nasal catheter.
         (c) Medications, as ordered (see Table 5–4 and Appendix D, Drugs, for action, side effects, observations).
            i. Analgesics—morphine, meperidine (Demerol) HCl.
            ii. Sedatives—phenobarbital, diazepam (Valium).
            iii. Antiarrhythmics—lidocaine HCl, quinidine HCl, procainamide (Pronestyl), isoproterenol (Isuprel) HCl.
            iv. Anticoagulants—heparin sodium, bishydroxycoumarin, or dicoumarin.
         (d) Institute and maintain parenteral infusions.
         (e) Assist with insertion and continuous monitoring of central venous pressure (CVP).
            i. Reflects the pressure exerted by blood returning to the right atrium from the systemic circulation.
            ii. Measure central venous pressure (CVP).
               - *Position manometer so that zero is at level of right atrium.*
               - *By way of three-way stop-*

TABLE 5–4.   *Drug therapies for imbalances in blood pressure*

Imbalance	Indications	Usual dose	Action	Assessment: side effects
HYPOTENSION 1. *Adrenergics* —*Alpha & beta mimetics*				
Epinephrine (Adrenalin)	Asystole.	1 mg or 0.25–0.5 ml in 1:1,000 solution IV— intercardiac.	Stimulates pacemaker cells.	Ventricular arrhythmias, fear, anxiety, anginal pain, decreased renal blood flow.
Norepinephrine (Levophed)	↓ Blood pressure. Cardiogenic shock.	2–4 µg/min titrated to desired response.	Increases rate and strength of heart beat. Increases vasoconstriction.	Palpitations, pallor, headache, hypertension, anxiety, insomnia, dilated pupils, nausea, vomiting, glycosuria, tissue sloughing.
Metaraminol (Aramine)	↓ Blood pressure.	2–10 mg IM. 15–100 mg in 500 ml O$_5$W titrated to desired response.	Vasoconstriction ↑ myocardial contractility ↓ pulse rate.	Reflex bradycardia, ventricular arrhythmias, tissue sloughing.
—*Beta mimetics*				
Isoproterenol (Isuprel)	Cardiogenic shock, heart block, bronchospasm— asthma, emphysema.	10–15 mg sublingually 0.5–4.0 µg/min in IV solution.	↑ Cardiac contractility, facilitates AV conduction and pacemaker automaticity.	Tachyarrhythmias, hypotension, headache, flushing of skin, nausea, tremor, dizziness.
Dopamine (Intropin)	↓ Cardiac output.	2–5 µg/kg/min titrated to desired response.	↑ Cardiac contractility, ↑ renal blood flow.	Ectopic beats, nausea, vomiting, tachycardia, anginal pain, dyspnea, hypotension.
2. *Antiarrhythmics*				
Atropine	Bradycardia, Stokes-Adams syndrome.	0.3–1.2 mg po, Sub q, IM or IV.	Blocks parasympatho-mimetic effects of acetylcholine on effector organs.	Dry mouth, dysphagic rash, skin flushing, urinary retention. Contraindications: glaucoma and paralytic ileus.

TABLE 5–4. *(Continued)*

Imbalance	Indications	Usual dose	Action	Assessment: side effects
HYPOTENSION				
Quinidine SO$_4$	Atrial fibrillation, PAT, ventricular tachycardia, and PVCs.	Po 0.2–0.6 g q2h loading dose. Maintenance: 400–1,000 mg tid, qid.	Lengthens conduction time in atria and ventricles and blocks vagal stimulation of heart.	Nausea, vomiting, diarrhea, vertigo, tremor, headache, abdominal cramps, AV block, and cardiac arrest.
Procainamide HCl (Pronestyl)	Atrial and ventricular arrhythmias, PVCs, overdose of digitalis, and general anesthesia.	Po, IM 500–1,000 mg 4–6 times qd, IV, 1 g.	Depresses myocardium and lengthens conduction time between atria and ventricles.	Polyarthralgia, fever, chills, urticaria, nausea, vomiting, psychoses, and rapid decrease in BP.
Lidocaine HCl	Ventricular tachycardia, and PVCs.	IV 50–100 mg bolus 1–4 mg/min IV drip.	Depresses myocardial response to abnormally generated impulses.	Drowsiness, dizziness, nervousness, confusion, and paresthesias.
Diphenylhydan-toin (Dilantin)	Digitalis toxicity, ventricular ectopy.	Po 16 mg loading dose, 100 mg qid, IV 50–100 mg over 5–10 min.	Depresses pacemaker activity in SA node and Purkinje tissue without slowing conduction velocity.	Severe pain if administered in small vein. Ataxia, vertigo, nystagmus seizures, confusion, skin eruptions, hypotension if administered too fast.
3. Anticoagulants				
Heparin	Acute thromboembolic emergencies.	Initial dose: 30,000 units.	Prevents thrombin formation.	Hematuria, bleeding gums, and ecchymosis. Antagonist: protamine sulfate.
Warfarin sodium (Coumadin)	Venous thrombosis, atrial fibrillation with embolization, and pulmonary emboli, myocardial infarction.	Initial dose: po, 40–60 mg; po 20–30 mg. Elderly: maintenance dose: po 5–10 mg qd.	Depresses liver synthesis of prothrombin and factors VII, IX, and X.	Minor or major hemorrhage, alopecia, fever, nausea, diarrhea, and dermatitis. Antagonist is vitamin K.

(Continued)

TABLE 5-4. *(Continued)*

Imbalance	Indications	Usual dose	Action	Assessment: side effects
HYPOTENSION 4. *Cardiac glycosides*				
Digitoxin	Congestive heart failure, atrial fibrillation and flutter, and supraventricular tachycardia.	Digitalizing dose: po, 1.2–1.5 mg; IM or IV, 1.2 mg; maintenance dose: po, 1.2 mg qd.	Increases force of cardiac contractility, slows heart rate, decreases right atrial pressures, and promotes diuresis.	Arrhythmias; nausea; vomiting; anorexia; malaise; color vision, yellow or blue. Hold medication if pulse below 60 or over 120.
Digoxin	See digitoxin for use, action, side effects, and nursing implications.	Digitalizing dose: po, 1.5–3.0 mg; IM or IV, 0.75–1 mg; maintenance dose: po, 0.25–0.75 mg qd.		
Lanatoside C (Cedilanid)	See digitoxin for use, action, side effects, and nursing implications	Digitalizing dose: po, 6 mg; maintenance dose: po, 1 mg qd.		
Deslanoside (Cedilanid-D)	See digitoxin for use, action, side effects, and nursing implications.	Digitalizing dose: IV or IM, 1.2–1.8 mg.		
Ouabain	See digitoxin for use, action, side effects, and nursing implications.	Digitalizing dose: IV or IM, 0.25–0.5 mg.		
5. *Vasodilators*				
Nitroglycerin	Angina pectoris.	Subling, 0.3–0.16 mg prn.	Directly relaxes smooth muscle, dilating blood vessels; lowers peripheral vascular resistance; and increases blood flow.	Faintness, throbbing headache, vomiting, flushing, hypotension, and visual disturbances.
Cyclandelate (Cyclospasmol)	Thrombophlebitis, intermittent claudication, frostbite, Raynaud's disease, and peripheral arteriosclerosis.	Po, 100–200 mg qid with meals and hs.	Acts directly on smooth vascular muscle to relax it and enhance blood flow.	Faintness, flushing, and hypotension.

TABLE 5–4. *(Continued)*

Imbalance	Indications	Usual dose	Action	Assessment: side effects
HYPERTENSION				
1. *Antihypertensives*				
Reserpine (Serpasil)	Mild and moderate hypertension.	Po, 0.25 mg qd.	Depletes catecholamines and decreases peripheral vasoconstriction, heart rate, and BP.	Depression, nasal stuffiness, increased gastric secretions, rash, and pruritus.
	Maternal use: preeclampsia/ eclampsia.		CNS depressant, tranquilizer, sedation is major effect; decreases neural transmission to nerves; decreases tone in blood vessels.	Low level of toxicity; nasal stuffiness; weight gain; diarrhea; allergic reactions—dry mouth, itching, skin eruptions.
Guanethidine SO₄ (Ismelin)	Severe to moderately severe hypertension.	Po, 10–150 mg qd in divided doses.	Blocks norepinephrine at postganglionic synapses.	Orthostatic hypotension, diarrhea, and inhibition of ejaculation.
Methyldopa (Aldomet)	Severe to moderately severe hypertension.	Po, 500 mg–2 g in divided doses.	Inhibits formation of dopamine, a precursor of norepinephrine.	Initial drowsiness, depression with feelings of unreality, edema, jaundice, and dry mouth.
Hydralazine HCl (Apresoline)	Moderate hypertension.	Po, 10–50 mg qid.	Dilates peripheral blood vessels, increases renal blood flow.	Palpitations, tachycardia, angina pectoris, tremors, and depression.
Propranolol HCl (Inderal)	Ventricular ectopy, angina unresponsive to nitrites, paroxysmal atrial tachycardia, hypertension.	0.5–1 mg IV push (up to 3 mg), 20–60 mg orally 3 to 4 times daily.	↓ Cardiac contractility, ↓ heart rate, ↓ myocardial oxygen requirements.	Contraindicated in CHF and COPD. Bradycardia, hypotension, vertigo, paresthesia of hands.

cock, allow fluid from infusion bottle to enter the manometer.

- *CVP is recorded after stopcock has been turned to patient and final height of column in manometer has been reached.*
- *Fluid in manometer should fluctuate with patient's respirations.*
- *Normal CVP is 4 to 10 cm water—increase indicates fluid overload or congestive heart failure; decrease indicates low blood volume and more parenteral infusions are needed.*

(f) Check vital signs and apical pulse every one to two hours and prn.
   i. Observe rate, rhythm, and characteristics of pulse.
   ii. Observe for pulse deficit— apical pulse greater than radial pulse.

(g) Monitor ECG pattern, observing for ectopic beats and rhythm changes.

(h) Provide emotional support.
   i. Stay with anxious patients.
   ii. Encourage communication with families.
   iii. Explain procedures and treatments—may be necessary to do frequently with anxious patients.

(i) Maintain tissue nutrition:
   i. Parenteral fluids.
   ii. Diet—liquid, low-sodium, or low-cholesterol (see Appendix A, Diets).

(j) Measure intake and output:
   i. Notify physician if urine output falls below 25 ml/hour or specific gravity exceeds 1.020.
   ii. Weigh daily, as ordered.
   iii. Utilize bedside commode for bowel movements if possible.

(k) Deal with anxiety, loss of body image, sexuality, and fears of dying and death.

b. *Convalescent phase of myocardial infarction*—commences with transfer from acute care unit to progressive unit or floor care.

(1) *Goals of cardiac rehabilitation:*
   (a) To minimize negative physical and psychologic effects of AMI (acute myocardial infarct).
   (b) To prevent deconditioning due to bedrest.
   (c) To provide psychologic support through graduated activity program and educational program.

(2) *Assessment of functional status* of cardiac patients according to American Heart Association:
   (a) Class I—has no unusual tiredness, dyspnea, angina, or palpitations with ordinary physical activity.
   (b) Class II—comfortable at rest but develops symptoms with ordinary activity.
   (c) Class III—comfortable at rest but develops symptoms with less than ordinary activity.
   (d) Class IV—has symptoms at rest, which worsen with any physical activity.

(3) *Assessment of psychologic reactions* and learning readiness:
   (a) Anxiety—mild anxiety increases alertness, motivation, and ability to absorb information. Moderate and severe anxiety reduce the patient's ability to focus and comprehend.
   (b) Denial—patients who deny having a heart attack or who refuse to view its consequences are not yet ready to learn about their health problem or its management.
   (c) Depression—feelings of helplessness and hopelessness interfere with patient's perception of acuteness of illness. These patients need information designed to allay fears and promote realistic perceptions and acceptance of health problems.

(4) *Nursing interventions* designed to promote optimal rehabilitation:
   (a) *Physical activities*—emphasis is on isotonic exercise, which requires alternate degrees of muscle con-

traction (walking), rather than iso-metric exercise, which involves muscle contraction without move-ment (pushing, pulling, lifting).

 i. Continue with activities begun in acute unit such as self-feed-ing, bathing, sitting in chair and up to commode (energy mets 1–2).

 ii. Progress to active range of motion of all extremities, trunk bending and twisting at moderate speed, walking in room, showering, and stand-ing at sink to shave (energy mets 2–4).

 iii. Before discharge patient should be able to walk increasing distances in hospi-tal corridor and to climb stairs (energy mets 4–6).

 iv. Precaution—tachycardia occur-ring ten minutes after exercise indicates lack of cardiac reserve. Activity should be reduced to next lower level at which tachycardia does not occur.

(b) *Cognitive needs:*

 i. Nature and extent of AMI—includes anatomy and physiol-ogy, risk factors, healing process.

 ii. Patient's role—includes indi-vidual risk factor identification and plans for modification, plans for management of diet restriction, exercise program, medications, pulse-monitoring techniques, aid in cessation of smoking.

 iii. Patient should be able to describe:
- *Dosage timing, actions and side effect of medications (Digoxin, nitroglycerin). See Table 5–4.*
- *Progressive activity program and rationale.*
- *Demonstrate pulse-taking techniques and understand significance of tachycardia after exercise.*

- *Demonstrate correct body mechanics and breathing techniques to avoid strain of isotonic exercises.*
- *Foods that are consistent with a low-calorie, low-sodium, low-cholesterol diet.*
- *Techniques used successfully by others to quit smoking.*

(c) *Affective needs*—

 i. Utilize group and individual support to explain plans and promote motivation.

 ii. Reward satisfactory responses and experiences with praise and encouragement.

 iii. Encourage sexual expression—hand-holding, caressing, kissing.
- *Sexual activity can usually be resumed in four to eight weeks postinfarct in uncom-plicated infarcts.*
- *Maximum energy expendi-ture during coitus is approx-imately 5 mets.*
- *Avoid coitus during extremes in temperature, after heavy meals, alcohol ingestion, or fatiguing day.*
- *Utilize less-fatiguing posi-tions—side to side, noncar-diac patient on top.*
- *Onset of dyspnea, angina pain, or palpitations signal to cease or moderate sexual activity.*

c. *Congestive heart failure*—clinical syn-drome in which heart is unable to maintain normal outflow of blood.

d. *Myocarditis*—inflammation of the cardiac muscle.

3. Restriction of heart muscle:

a. *Acute and chronic pericarditis*—inflamma-tion of parietal and/or visceral pericar-dium.

 (1) Pathophysiology—

  (a) Compression of heart pumping action by fibrosis of pericardium or accumulation of fluid in peri-cardium.

  (b) Decreased cardiac output results

in increased systemic and pulmonic venous pressures.

(2) Etiology—

    (a) Bacterial, viral, or fungal infections.

    (b) Tuberculosis.

    (c) Collagen diseases.

    (d) Uremia.

    (e) Transmural myocardial infarction.

    (f) Trauma.

(3) Assessment findings—

    (a) Subjective data.

        i. Pain:

            • *Type—sharp, moderate to severe.*

            • *Location—over wide area of precordium; may radiate down right arm or to jaw and teeth.*

            • *Precipitating factors—may be aggravated with movement and with deep inspiration.*

        ii. Chills with sweating.

        iii. Apprehension, anxiety.

        iv. Fatigue.

        v. Abdominal pain.

        vi. Shortness of breath.

    (b) Objective data.

        i. Vital signs:

            • *Elevated temperature—runs erratic course; may be low grade.*

            • *Decreased pulse pressure, tachycardia.*

            • *Pericardial friction rub—appears on first day and has wide distribution over precordium.*

            • *Pulsus paradoxus—an abnormal drop in systemic blood pressure of more than 8 to 10 mm Hg during inspiration.*

        ii. Increased CVP, distended neck veins.

        iii. Dependent pitting edema, liver engorgement.

        iv. Restlessness.

        v. Serum enzymes—SGOT may elevate slightly; elevated WBC (see Appendix C, Diagnostic tests).

vi. Chest X ray may indicate cardiac enlargement.

(4) *Nursing goals* are designed to reduce discomfort, provide physical and emotional support, and prevent complications.

    (a) Bedrest—semi-Fowler's position.

    (b) Vital signs every two to four hours and prn.

        i. Cooling measures as indicated.

        ii. Apical as well as radial pulse—notify physician if heart sounds decrease in amplitude.

        iii. Notify physician if pulse pressure narrows.

    (c) Parenteral infusions, as ordered.

    (d) Strict intake and output records.

    (e) Low-sodium diet may be ordered—assist with feedings as needed.

    (f) Oxygen, as ordered.

    (g) Medications, as ordered.

        i. Analgesics—aspirin, morphine sulfate.

        ii. Antibiotics.

        iii. Digitalis and diuretics if heart failure present.

    (h) Assist with aspiration of pericardial sac if needed.

    (i) Prepare for pericardectomy (excision of constricting pericardium), as ordered.

    (j) Provide continuous emotional support to patient and family.

b. *Cardiac tamponade*—acute compression of the heart by a rapid accumulation of fluid in the pericardial sac.

4. *Valvular defects:*

a. *Mitral stenosis*—progressive thickening and calcification of mitral leaflets, which narrows orifice and obstructs blood flow between left atrium and left ventricle.

(1) Pathophysiology—

    (a) Blood flow across narrowed orifice; cardiac output is maintained by an elevated atrioventricular pressure gradient.

    (b) Elevated left atrial pressure results in elevated pulmonary venous and capillary pressure.

    (c) Elevation of pulmonary vascular

resistance may result in eventual right-sided heart failure.

(2) Etiology and incidence—
   (a) Most common sequelae of rheumatic heart disease.
   (b) Congenital defects.
   (c) Patients—75% are women under 45 years of age.

(3) Assessment findings—
   (a) Subjective data.
      i. Shortness of breath on exertion.
      ii. Excessive fatigue.
      iii. Cough.
      iv. Bloody sputum (hemoptysis).
      v. Sleeps with two or more pillows (orthopnea).
      vi. Breathlessness in sleep (paroxysmal nocturnal dyspnea).
   (b) Objective data.
      i. Vital signs:
         • *Blood pressure—normal or slightly low.*
         • *Pulse—weak, may be irregular.*
         • *Respirations—increased, shallow.*
      ii. Cardiac palpation, auscultation:
         • *Diastolic thrill (palpable murmur) at apex of heart.*
         • *Presystolic, low-pitched, rumbling murmur, heard best at apex.*
      iii. Severe stenosis with right-side failure:
         • *Facial and peripheral cyanosis.*
         • *Neck vein distention, liver enlargement, dependent edema.*
      iv. Pulmonary function tests (Table 5–5):
         • *Decreased vital capacity.*
         • *Decreased total lung capacity.*
      v. Left heart catheterization—detects extent of stenosis and chamber pressures.
      vi. Ultrasound—detects mobility of mitral valve.

(4) Nursing care is designed to reduce cardiac workload, prevent complications, and prepare the patient for surgical intervention (commissurotomy or prosthetic valve replacement); see nursing care: (a) congestive heart failure and (b) cardiac surgery.

b. *Mitral insufficiency or regurgitation*—distorted or damaged mitral valve is no longer able to approximate during systole.

(1) Pathophysiology—
   (a) During systole, blood regurgitates from the left ventricle into the left atrium.
   (b) Compensation consists of rapid left ventricular decompression into the left atrium during early ejection, reducing ventricular size and tension and resulting in more complete emptying of the left ventricle.
   (c) As the end-diastolic volume (blood in ventricles at end of diastole) increases, left atrial enlargement may occur along with elevation of left atrial pressures and resultant increased pulmonary vascular resistance.
   (d) As larger quantities of blood are regurgitated into the left atrium, the left ventricle deteriorates, decreasing cardiac output.

(2) Etiology and incidence—
   (a) Chronic rheumatic heart disease—in contrast to stenosis, affects men more frequently than women.
   (b) Congenital anomaly.
   (c) Myocardial infarction with ischemia of the papillary muscles.
   (d) Bacterial endocarditis.
   (e) Marked ventricular hypertrophy.

(3) Assessment findings—
   (a) Subjective data:
      i. Fatigue.
      ii. Shortness of breath on exertion.
      iii. Sleeping on two or more pillows (orthopnea).
      iv. Breathlessness during sleep (paroxysmal nocturnal dyspnea, PND).
      v. Weight loss.
   (b) Objective data.

TABLE 5–5.   *Lung volumes—pulmonary function testing*

	Definition	Normal	Abnormalities
Tidal volume (TV)	Volume inspired and expired with a normal breath.	500 ml	Increased: exercise. Decreased: restrictive lung disease.
Inspiratory reserve volume (IRV)	Maximal amount that can be inspired after a normal inspiration.	3000 ml	Increased: athletes. Decreased: COPD, restrictive lung disease.
Expiratory reserve volume (ERV)	Maximal amount that can be exhaled after a normal expiration.	1100 ml	Increased: obstructive disease. Decreased: restrictive lung disease.
Residual volume (RV)	Volume of gas remaining in lungs after maximal exhalation.	1200 ml	Increased: COPD. Decreased: restrictive lung disease.
Vital capacity (VC) (TV + IRV + ERV)	Maximal amount of air that can be expelled after maximal inhalation.	4000–5000 ml	Normal to slightly increased: early COPD. Decreased: late COPD, restrictive lung disease.
Functional residual capacity (FRC) (ERV + RV)	Amount of air left in lungs after a normal expiration.	2300 ml	Increased: COPD. Decreased: restrictive lung disease.
Total lung capacity (TLC) (TV + IRV + ERV + RV)	Amount of air left in lungs after a maximal inspiration.	5500–6000 ml	Increased: obstructive pulmonary disease. Decreased: restrictive lung disease.
Forced expiratory volume (FEV_T)	Percentage of vital capacity that can be expired: one second (FEV_1) two seconds (FEV_2) three seconds (FEV_3)	80–83% 90–94% 95–97%	Decreased values indicate expiratory airway obstruction.
Maximal breathing capacity (MBC)	Maximal amount of air that can be breathed in and out in one minute with maximal rates and depths of respiration.	Best overall measurement of ventilatory ability.	Decreased: restrictive and chronic lung disease.

NOTE: Normals based on young male adult. 20–25% less in females.

i. Vital signs:
  * *Blood pressure, temperature, respirations—usually normal.*
  * *Pulse—regular, characterized by a sharp upstroke.*
ii. Precordial inspection, palpation, and auscultation:
  * *Rocking motion of chest with each cardiac cycle.*
  * *Systolic thrill palpable at apex.*
  * *Holosystolic (throughout systole) murmur, which usually radiates to axilla.*
iii. Chest X ray—extreme left atrial enlargement.
(4) *Nursing goals* are designed to reduce cardiac workload, prevent complications, and prepare patient for surgical intervention if indicated (prosthetic valve replacement); see nursing care: (a) congestive heart failure and (b) cardiac surgery

c. *Aortic stenosis*—fibrosis and calcification of aortic valve resulting in narrowing of orifice between left ventricle and the aorta.
(1) Pathophysiology—
   (a) Blood flow is obstructed by narrowing aortic orifice, increasing left ventricular pressures.
   (b) Increased ventricular pressures result in left ventricular hypertrophy.
   (c) As ventricular compliance decreases, left atrial contractions become more forceful, raising left ventricular end-diastolic volumes to a level necessary to maintain ventricular contraction.
   (d) Cardiac output and stroke volume maintained at rest but fail to rise during exercise.
   (e) Ventricular dilatation and failure.
   (f) Ventricular hypertrophy increases oxygen needs of heart, whereas increasing ventricular pressures compress coronary arteries, decreasing cardiac perfusion—ischemic attacks.
(2) Etiology and incidence—
   (a) Congenital anomaly.
   (b) Rheumatic heart disease.
   (c) Idiopathic in elderly.
   (d) Symptoms usually not manifested until fourth or fifth decade.
(3) Assessment findings—
   (a) Subjective data.
      i. Shortness of breath on exertion.
      ii. Chest pain (angina pectoris).
      iii. Fainting.
   (b) Objective data.
      i. Vital signs:
         • *Blood pressure—usually within normal limits.*
         • *Pulse—slow rise and delayed peak.*
      ii. Precordial examination:
         • *Cardiac apex displaced laterally and inferiorly.*
         • *Systolic thrill at base of heart and along carotid arteries.*
         • *Low-pitched, rasping systolic murmur radiating to carotid arteries.*

iii. Diagnostic tests:
   • *Electrocardiogram—nonspecific.*
   • *Left heart catheterization.*
   • *Angiocardiography.*
(4) *Nursing goals* are designed to reduce cardiac stress, promote comfort, and, if indicated, prepare patient for surgery (valvular prosthesis or aortic valve homograft); see nursing care for (a) angina pectoris, (b) congestive heart failure, and (c) cardiac surgery.
d. *Aortic insufficiency or regurgitation*—aortic valve leaflets fail to close during ventricular diastole.
(1) Pathophysiology—
   (a) As aortic pressures increase and ventricular pressures decrease, blood flows backwards into left ventricle.
   (b) End-diastolic left ventricular volumes are increased.
   (c) Left ventricle dilates and increases its muscle mass to accommodate increased stroke volume and to eject it.
   (d) Reflexly peripheral arterioles relax, lowering diastolic pressures.
(2) Etiology and incidence—
   (a) Rheumatic heart disease.
   (b) Bacterial endocarditis.
   (c) Congenital anomaly.
   (d) Syphilis.
   (e) Ankylosing spondylitis.
   (f) Patients—75% with pure aortic insufficiency are men.
(3) Assessment findings—
   (a) Subjective data.
      i. Palpitations; pounding in head.
      ii. Shortness of breath on exertion.
      iii. Chest pains at rest as well as with exertion (angina pectoris).
      iv. Sleeps with two pillows (orthopnea).
      v. Shortness of breath during sleep (PND).
      vi. Excessive sweating.

(b) Objective data.
　i. Vital signs:
　　• *Blood pressure—elevated systolic pressure (up to 300 mm Hg) and widened pulse pressure.*
　　• *Pulse—rapid rising "water hammer" or "Corrigan's" pulse.*
　ii. Abrupt distention and collapse of larger arteries.
　iii. Head may bob with each heart beat.
　iv. Precordial examination:
　　• *Forceful apical impulse, which may be displaced laterally and inferiorly.*
　　• *Diastolic thrill over left sternal border.*
　　• *High-pitched, blowing, decrescendo diastolic murmur best heard in third intercostal space to left of sternum.*
　v. Diagnostic tests (see Appendix C):
　　• *ECG—nonspecific.*
　　• *Chest X ray—varying degrees of left ventricular enlargement.*
　　• *Angiocardiograms.*
(4) *Nursing goals* are designed to support adaptation, reduce cardiac workload, and prepare the patient for surgery if ordered; see nursing care: (a) congestive heart failure, (b) angina pectoris, and (c) cardiac bypass surgery.

5. Arrhythmias (Figure 5–1, Table 5–6).
　a. *Bradyarrhythmias*—rates below 60.
　　(1) Normal in well-trained athletes.
　　(2) May be secondary to drugs such as digitalis.
　　(3) Third-degree *heart block.*
　　　(a) Pathophysiology—
　　　　i. Wave of excitation begun at the SA node is blocked at the AV node and does not pass down to ventricles.
　　　　ii. Conductive tissues in ventricles establish independent rhythm.

　　　(b) Etiology—
　　　　i. Atherosclerotic heart disease.
　　　　ii. Myocardial infarction.
　　　　iii. Congenital heart disease.
　　　　iv. Myocarditis.
　　　(c) Assessment findings—
　　　　i. Subjective data:
　　　　　• *Dizziness.*
　　　　　• *Fainting.*
　　　　ii. Objective data:
　　　　　• *Disorientation—unaware of person, time, place.*
　　　　　• *Seizures.*
　　　　　• *Vital signs: (a) increased systolic pressure with widened pulse pressure and (b) pulse—25 to 45 beats/minute, full; rate is regular and increases slightly or not at all with exercise.*
　　　(d) Complications—
　　　　i. Heart failure.
　　　　ii. Shock.
　　　　iii. Stokes-Adams attack—intermittent ventricular standstill or ventricular fibrillation.
　　　(e) *Nursing goals* are designed to promote comfort, prevent complications, and prepare the patient for transvenous (permanent) *pacemaker insertion.*
　　　　i. Limited activity or bedrest to decrease tissue oxygen needs.
　　　　ii. Oxygen, as ordered.
　　　　iii. Medications, as ordered (see *Table 5–4*):
　　　　　• *Isoproterenol.*
　　　　　• *Atropine.*
　　　　　• *Epinephrine.*
　　　　iv. Include patient and family in instructions on transvenous pacemaker insertion—pacing catheter is advanced into right ventricle via jugular or subclavian vein; battery pack is placed subcutaneously beneath clavicle or in axilla.
　　　　　• *Outline procedure, its duration, equipment utilized, and importance of postinsertion monitoring.*
　　　　　• *Explain purpose of pacemaker and type: (a) set*

COMPARISON OF CARDIAC RHYTHMS

A. Cardiac Cycle

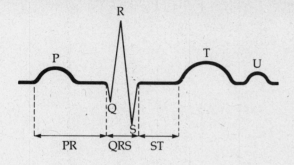

Components	Definition
1. P wave	Atrial depolarization
2. QRS wave	Ventricular depolarization
3. T wave	Ventricular repolarization
4. PR interval (Normal range: 0.12–0.20 seconds)	Start of atrial depolarization to start of ventricular depolarization
5. QRS interval (Normal Range: 0.06–0.10 seconds)	Start to end of ventricular depolarization
6. QT interval	Duration of ventricular depolarization and repolarization
7. ST segment	Interval between the end of ventricular depolarization and the T wave

B. Normal Sinus Rhythm

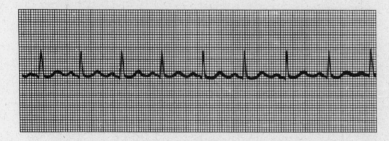

Description

Regularity and rate	
Ventricular	Regular 60–100
Atrial	Same as ventricular
P waves	Rounded, symmetrical
P: QRS ratio	1:1
PR interval	0.12–0.20 seconds
QRS interval	0.06–0.10 seconds

FIGURE 5–1. Comparison of cardiac rhythms
(Adapted from Holloway, N. *Nursing the critically ill adult.* Menlo Park, 1979, Addison-Wesley Publishing Co.)

TABLE 5–6. *Comparison of cardiac arrhythmias*

Arrhythmia	Description	Etiology	Symptoms/ consequences	Treatment
Sinus tachycardia	P waves present followed by QRS. Rhythm regular. Heart rate 100 to 150.	Increased metabolic demands. Decreased oxygen delivery: CHF, shock, hemorrhage, anemia.	May produce palpitations. Prolonged episodes may lead to decreased cardiac output.	Treat underlying cause. Occasionally sedatives.
Sinus bradycardia	P waves present. Rhythm regular. Heart rate less than 60.	Physical fitness. Parasympathetic stimulation (sleep). Brain lesions. Digitalis excess.	Very low rates may cause decreased cardiac output; light-headedness, faintness, chest pain.	Atropine if cardiac output is decreased. Pacemaker.
Complete heart block	Atria and ventricles beat independently. P waves have no relation to QRS. Heart rate 20 to 40.	Digitalis toxicity. Infectious disease. Coronary artery disease. Myocardial infarction.	Very low rates may cause decreased cardiac output: light-headedness, faintness, chest pain.	Pacemaker. Isoproterenol to increase heart rate.
Premature atrial beats (PAB)	Early P wave followed by normal QRS. Rhythm irregular.	Stress, ischemia, atrial enlargement, caffeine, nicotine.	May produce palpitations. Frequent episodes may decrease cardiac output. Is sign of chamber irritability.	Sedation. Quinidine.
Premature ventricular beats	Early wide bizarre QRS, not associated with a P wave. Rhythm irregular.	Stress, acidosis, ventricular enlargement. Electrolyte imbalance. Drug toxicity (digitalis, quinidine). Hypoxemia, hypercapnia.	Same as PAB.	Procainamide (Pronestyl). Lidocaine. Oxygen. Sodium bicarbonate. Potassium. Treat CHF.
Atrial fibrillation	Rapid, irregular waves (over 350/ min). Ventricular rhythm irregularly irregular. Heart rate varies, may be increased to 150 to 170/min.	Rheumatic heart disease. Mitral stenosis. Atrial infarction.	Pulse deficit. Decreased cardiac output if rate is rapid. Promotes thrombus formation in atria.	Digitalis. Quinidine. Cardioversion.

TABLE 5–6. *(Continued)*

Arrhythmia	Description	Etiology	Symptoms/consequences	Treatment
Ventricular fibrillation	Chaotic electrical activity. No recognizable QRS complex.	Myocardial infarction. Electrocution. Freshwater drowning. Drug toxicity.	No cardiac output. Absent pulse or respiration. Cardiac arrest.	Defibrillation. Epinephrine. Sodium bicarbonate.
Ventricular standstill	Can only be distinguished from ventricular fibrillation by ECG. P waves *may* be present. No QRS. "Straight line."	Myocardial infarction. Chronic diseases of conducting system.	Same as ventricular fibrillation.	CPR. Pacemaker. Intracardiac epinephrine.

From Brown, F. R.: Problems of the heart and major blood vessels. In Phipps, Long, Woods, eds.: *Medical/surgical nursing.* St. Louis, 1979, The C. V. Mosby Co.

rate—ventricles stimulated at fixed rate and (b) demand—stimulates ventricles only when patient's heart rate falls below preset time limit.
- *Practice postinsertion ROM exercises.*
v. *Postinsertion goals* are designed to prevent complications and promote comfort and rehabilitation.
  - *Continuous cardiac monitoring.*
  - *Report excessive bleeding or signs of infection at insertion site.*
  - *Bedrest in position of comfort.*
  - *Observe for signs of pacemaker failure: (a) decreased blood pressure, pulse, (b) pallor, cyanosis, fatigue, dyspnea, and (c) ECG, absent or runaway pacemaker blip.*
  - *Avoid electrical hazards by grounding all equipment.*
  - *Provide opportunities for patient and family to verbal-ize feelings about living with pacemaker.*
  - *Postinsertion teaching should include (a) daily pulse taking, (b) avoidance of stimulants such as tea, coffee, cola, and (c) safety factors—electrical hazards (microwave ovens, radar), extensive dental work, over-the-counter medications.*
  b. *Tachyarrhythmias*—rates over 100 (Table 5–6).
B. *Etiology of decreased peripheral vascular resistance:*
  1. *Inadequate tissue perfusion—*
    a. *Congestive heart failure*—combined right- and left-sided heart failure, resulting in decreased tissue perfusion and tissue hypoxia.
    (1) Pathophysiology:
      (a) Increased cardiac workload or decreased effective myocardial contractility results in inefficient ventricular emptying and decreased cardiac output.
      (b) Pulmonic congestion develops due to decreased left ventricular emptying.
      (c) Systemic congestion develops due

to inability of right atria and ventricle to pump blood into pulmonic circulation.

(2) Etiology of decreased myocardial contractility:

    (a) Myocarditis.

    (b) Myocardial infarction.

    (c) Tachyarrhythmias.

    (d) Bacterial endocarditis.

    (e) Acute rheumatic fever.

(3) Etiology of increased cardiac workload:

    (a) Elevated temperature.

    (b) Physical or emotional stress.

    (c) Anemia.

    (d) Thyrotoxicosis (hyperthyroidism).

    (e) Valvular defects.

(4) Assessment findings:

    (a) Subjective data.

        i. Shortness of breath.

        ii. Sleeps on two or more pillows.

        iii. Sudden breathlessness during sleep (PND).

        iv. Swelling of the feet (edema).

        v. Feeling of puffiness (edema).

        vi. Weight gain (edema).

        vii. Fatigue and weakness.

        viii. Chest pain.

    (b) Objective data.

        i. Vital signs:

          • *Blood pressure—decreasing systolic pressure and narrowing pulse pressure.*

          • *Pulse—pulsus alternans (regular rhythm in which there is an alternation between a strong and a weak cardiac contraction) and increased rate.*

          • *Respirations and temperature—nonspecific.*

        ii. Distention of neck veins.

        iii. Lungs—moist inspiratory rales over lung bases.

        iv. Heart sound—pulsus alternans.

        v. Dependent pitting edema.

        vi. Enlarged tender liver.

        vii. Chest X ray.

          • *Cardiac enlargement.*

          • *Dilatation of pulmonary vessels.*

          • *Diffuse interstitial edema in lungs.*

(5) *Nursing goals* are designed to reduce cardiac workload and tissue oxygen needs, increase strength of cardiac contraction, reduce extracellular fluid volumes, and promote physical and mental relaxation.

    (a) Bedrest in a semi- or high-Fowler's position.

        i. Elastic stockings and leg exercises to prevent thrombus formation.

        ii. Skin care.

        iii. Plan periods of rest.

    (b) Oxygen at low flow rate.

        i. Encourage deep breathing.

        ii. Auscultate chest for breath sounds.

    (c) Medications, as ordered (Table 5–4).

        i. Digitalis preparations.

        ii. Diuretics—thiazides, furosemide, and ethacrynic acid, for example (Table 5–12).

        iii. Tranquilizers—phenobarbital, diazepam (Valium), and chlordiazepoxide (Librium) HCl (see Appendix D, Drugs).

        iv. Stool softeners.

    (d) Institute and maintain intake and output records.

        i. Report output of less than 30 ml/hour.

        ii. Estimate insensible water loss in diaphoretic patient.

        iii. Weigh daily—same time, clothes, scale.

        iv. Utilize microdrip for parenteral infusions to avoid circulatory overloading.

    (e) Low-sodium diet, as ordered—restriction depends on severity of failure (see Appendix A, Diets).

        i. Offer small, frequent feedings—large meals increase anorexia.

        ii. Discuss food preferences with patient.

    (f) Involve patient and family in discharge teaching and planning.

i. Diet restrictions and meal preparation.
ii. Activity restrictions, if any, and planned rest periods.
iii. Medication schedules, purpose, dosage, and side effects:
   • *Daily pulse-taking.*
   • *Daily weights.*
   • *Potassium-containing foods (see Appendix A, Diets).*
iv. Refer to community resources as indicated.

b. *Peripheral circulating failure*—circulatory collapse due to a marked fall in cardiac output.

c. *Hemorrhagic shock*—peripheral circulatory collapse due to blood loss.

2. *Loss of vasomotor tone*—

a. Antibody-antigen reaction with histamine release—anaphylactic shock (see *Anaphylactic shock* in Section III, Table 5–21, *Postoperative complications*).
b. Toxin release by bacteria (see *Septic shock* in Section III, Table 5–21).
c. Interruption of sympathetic nervous system outflow.
   (1) Deep anesthesia.
   (2) Brain trauma.
   (3) Spinal cord injuries (see *Spinal shock*).

2. **Hypertension**—a condition that results from abnormal increases in peripheral vascular resistance; systolic and/or diastolic pressures may be elevated.

A. *Essential hypertension*—etiology unknown, affects 90% of hypertensive patients (Table 5–7).

TABLE 5–7. *Five phases of essential hypertension*

Phase	Assessment: indications
Prehypertensive and/or labile hypertension	Blood pressure fluctuates. Elevated during periods of stress. Normal or near normal at rest.
Mild hypertension	Resting diastolic pressure between 90 mm Hg and 110 mm Hg. May demonstrate mild changes in the optic fundi and minor cardiac and renal involvement.
Moderate hypertension	Resting diastolic pressure between 110 mm Hg and 120 mm Hg. May demonstrate narrowing of retinal arterioles, left ventricular enlargement, and a trace of protein in the urine.
Severe hypertension	Resting diastolic pressures between 120 mm Hg and 140 mm Hg. May demonstrate advanced retinal changes such as copper and silver wiring and cardiac and renal decompensation (tachycardia, distended neck veins, proteinuria, oliguria).
Malignant hypertension	Accelerated form of hypertension or one that is unresponsive to therapy. Diastolic blood pressure above 140 mm Hg. Encephalopathy (mental confusion, disorientation, seizures), retinal hemorrhages, exudates, and papilledema; congestive heart failure and kidney failure may be present.

1. Etiology and incidence of essential hypertension—present hypotheses include:
   a. Hypersensitivity to sympathetic system stimulation.
   b. Increased renin-angiotensin release by the kidneys.
   c. Failure of kidney to release a vasodepressor substance.
   d. Genetic or family predisposition.
   e. Higher incidence among Americans and Europeans than among Asians and Africans.
   f. Higher incidence among American Blacks than among Whites.
   g. Onset after 30 years of age; more women than men.
2. Assessment findings:
   a. Subjective data—
      (1) Dull, pounding occipital headache on awakening, wears off during day or is relieved by vomiting.
      (2) Dizziness.
      (3) Weakness.
      (4) Palpitations.
      (5) Nervousness, mood swings.
      (6) Flatulence.
      (7) Ringing in the ears.
      (8) Nose bleeds (epistaxis).
      (9) Double vision (diplopia).
   b. Objective data—
      (1) Vital signs:
         (a) Blood pressure—elevated systolic and diastolic.
         (b) Pulse, respirations, temperature—noncontributory unless complications present.
      (2) Cardiac, cerebral, and renal changes.
      (3) Diagnostic tests (see Appendix C):
         (a) Blood tests—complete blood cell count (CBC), hemoglobin, hematocrit, blood urea nitrogen (BUN), serum electrolytes and creatinine, and uric acid; abnormalities may indicate underlying causes or severity of organ involvement.
         (b) Urinalysis and urine culture—screen for kidney dysfunction.
         (c) 24-hour urine collections—vanillylmandelic acid (VMA) and 17-ketosteroids and 17-hydroxysteroids; screen for pheochromocytoma.
         (d) X ray, intravenous pyelogram (IVP)—detects sclerosis of renal artery.
3. *Nursing goals* are designed to encourage patient to cooperate with the therapy regimen, to increase understanding of lifestyle modifications, and to reduce physical and emotional stress, anxiety, and feelings of insecurity.
   a. Individualize nursing approaches.
      (1) Provide consistency in nursing procedures.
      (2) Reduce situations that increase physical stress and raise blood pressure.
      (3) Identify patient's misconceptions of hypertension and institute measures to clarify.
         (a) Repeat explanations of nature of disease, stressing its chronicity as necessary.
         (b) Review purpose, side effects, and administration of drugs; time consistent with patient's daily activities.
         (c) Stress importance of reporting even minor symptoms to physician to regulate treatment.
         (d) Discuss effects of excess weight on blood pressure and include family in diet instructions.
         (e) Discuss value of exercise; encourage walking.
   b. Antihypertensive therapy as ordered (see Table 5–4).
      (1) Antihypertensives—reserpine, methyldopa (Aldomet), guanethidine (Ismelin) SO_4, hydralazine (Apresoline).
      (2) Diuretics—thiazides (Diuril, Hydrodiuril), chlorthalidone (Hygroton), furosemide (Lasix), ethacrynic acid (Edecrin), spironolactone (Aldactone).
      (3) Sedation—phenobarbital, diazepam (Valium), chlordiazepoxide (Librium) HCl.
   c. Diet, as ordered, explaining dietary restrictions and determining food preferences.
      (1) Low calorie—weight reduction.
      (2) Low fat—indicated with elevated serum cholesterol or obvious atherosclerotic disease.
      (3) Sodium restricted—decreases blood volumes; occasionally not ordered if on diuretics.
      (4) Potassium sources—indicated particu-

larly with thiazide, furosemide, or ethacrynic acid therapy.

d. Include patient and family in teaching and discharge planning.

(1) Importance of not smoking.

(2) Medication scheduling, side effects.

(3) Dietary restrictions.

(4) Exercise and rest.

(5) Taking own blood pressures if ordered.

(6) Causes and symptoms of intermittent hypotension:

(a) Antihypertensive medications—caution patient not to rise quickly from a lying or sitting position; to sit down if feeling dizzy; to avoid stooping.

(b) Alcoholic intake, hot weather, and exercise cause vasodilation.

(c) Vomiting and diarrhea deplete blood volumes.

e. Refer to appropriate community resources for follow-up care.

B. *Secondary hypertension*—affects 10% of hypertensive patients.

1. *Systolic hypertension:*

a. Decreased aortic distensibility—aortic calcification.

b. Increased cardiac output—anemia, thyrotoxicosis, anxiety, fever.

(1) *Iron deficiency anemia* (hypochromic microcytic anemia)—inadequate production of red blood cells due to the lack of heme (iron).

(a) Pathophysiology—

i. Decreased dietary intake, impaired absorption or increased utilization of iron decreases the amount of iron bound to plasma transferrin and transported to bone marrow for hemoglobin synthesis.

ii. Decreased hemoglobin in erythrocytes decreases amount of oxygen delivered to tissues.

(b) Etiology and incidence—

i. Excessive menstruation.

ii. Gastrointestinal (GI) bleeding—peptic ulcer, hookworms, tumors.

iii. Inadequate diet—anorexia, diet fads, cultural practices.

iv. Deficiencies most common in infants, pregnant women, and premenopausal women.

(c) Assessment findings—

i. Subjective data:

- *Increasing fatigue.*
- *Headache.*
- *Decreased or increased appetite.*
- *Heartburn.*
- *Palpitations.*
- *Shortness of breath on exertion.*
- *Ankle edema.*
- *Numb, tingling extremities.*
- *Flatulence.*
- *Menorrhagia.*

ii. Objective data:

- *Vital signs: (a) blood pressure—increased systolic, widened pulse pressure, (b) pulse—tachycardia, (c) respirations—tachypnea, and (d) temperature—normal or subnormal.*
- *Skin and mucous membranes—pale, dry.*
- *Pearly white sclera.*
- *Nails—flattened, longitudinally ridged, brittle.*
- *Diagnostic tests: Blood—decreased hemoglobin, mean corpuscular volume (MCV), mean corpuscular hemoglobin concentration (MCHC), and mean corpuscular hemoglobin (MCHb) and increased iron-binding capacity.*

(d) *Nursing goals* are designed to relieve iron deficiency and promote physical and mental equilibrium.

i. Activity to tolerance.

ii. Iron therapy, as ordered:

- *Oral therapy—ferrous sulfate: (a) single dose initially, building to three to four tablets daily and (b) give with meals.*

- *Intramuscular therapy—
iron dextran: (a) utilize second needle for administration after withdrawal from ampule,
(b) use Z-tract method, and (c) inject 0.5 cc of air before removing needle (prevents tissue necrosis).*
  - iii. Include patient and family in teaching plan.
    - *Diet—food preferences which are high in iron (see Appendix A).*
    - *Iron therapy—purpose, dosage, side effects: (a) black or green stools, (b) constipation, diarrhea, and (c) take with meals to avoid gastric upsets.*
    - *Exercise to tolerance with planned rest periods.*

(2) *Pernicious anemia* (hyperchromic macrocytic anemia).

(a) Pathophysiology—
  i. Lack of intrinsic factor in gastric mucosa leads to vitamin B_{12} deficiency.
  ii. Vitamin B_{12} deficiency alters DNA synthesis needed for cell division.
  iii. Delayed cellular division results in an alteration of the nuclear pattern and increases the size of red blood cells (megaloblast).
  iv. Hemoglobin formation proceeds normally in greatly enlarged cell.
  v. Ineffective erythropoiesis accounts for increased serum bilirubin and urobilinogen excretion.
  vi. The vitamin B_{12} deficiency affects tissues in the mouth, stomach, vagina, and the myelin sheath covering central and peripheral nerve tracts.

(b) Etiology and incidence—
  i. Gastric resection.
  ii. Atrophy of gastric mucosa.
  iii. Gastritis or extensive neoplasia.

  iv. Rarely occurs before age 35 years.
  v. Affects both sexes equally.
  vi. More common in blue-eyed, fair-skinned blonds who gray prematurely.

(c) Assessment findings—
  i. Subjective data:
    - *Tingling and numbing of hands and feet.*
    - *Weakness and fatigue.*
    - *Sore tongue.*
    - *Anorexia.*
    - *Diarrhea.*
    - *Shortness of breath.*
    - *Palpitations.*
    - *Difficulties with memory and balance.*
    - *Complaints of irritability or mild depression.*
  ii. Objective data:
    - *Skin—pale, flabby, jaundice.*
    - *Sclera—icterus (yellow).*
    - *Tongue—smooth, glossy, red.*
    - *Vital signs: (a) blood pressure—normal or elevated systolic, (b) pulse—tachycardia, and (c) respirations and temperature—nonspecific.*
    - *Nervous system—decreased vibratory sense in lower extremities, loss of coordination; Babinski reflex (flaring of toes with stimulation of sole of foot); positive Romberg (lose balance when eyes closed); increased or diminished reflexes.*
    - *Diagnostic tests (see Appendix E): (a) blood—increased Hb, MCV, MCHC, MCHb; reduced RBCs and platelets; increased bilirubin, (b) gastric analysis—decreased secretions, (c) urine and feces—increased urobilinogen, and (d) Shilling test—decreased.*

(d) *Nursing goals* are designed to promote relief of symptoms and emotional and physical comfort.
  i. Bedrest or activities to toler-

ance—plan care activities with patient and avoid inconsistency.

ii. Vitamin B_{12} therapy, as ordered.

iii. Nutritious diet in six small feedings.

iv. Allow for verbalization of feelings regarding lifelong medical therapy, mood changes, and nervous system changes.

v. Involve family in patient teaching:
- *Teach importance of diet, rest, and exercise to tolerance.*
- *Assure medical therapy will relieve most symptoms.*
- *Teach injection techniques if medication is to be given at home.*

2. Systolic-diastolic hypertension—

a. *Kidney disorders*—pyelonephritis, glomerulonephritis, sclerosis of renal artery. (See Part F, *Metabolic acidosis.*)

b. *Adrenal gland disorders:*

(1) *Pheochromocytoma*—excess release of epinephrine and norepinephrine → vasoconstriction → increased peripheral vascular resistance → increased blood pressure.

(2) *Primary hyperaldosteronism*—excess aldosterone secretion → sodium and water retention → hyperchloremia → increased blood pressure.

c. Central nervous system dysfunction—*increased intracranial pressure.* (See Part G, *Hypertonia.*)

d. *Decreased elasticity of systemic arterial walls.*

(1) *Arteriosclerosis obliterans*—a degenerative and occlusive disorder of the arterial system in the lower extremities.

(a) Pathophysiology:

i. Fatty deposits in the intimal and medial layer of the arterial walls result in plaque formation that narrows arterial lumens and decreases arterial distensibility.

ii. Decreased blood flow through a narrowed and obstructed artery results in ischemic changes in the tissues supplied by that artery.

(b) Etiology and incidence:

i. Age—more frequent after 50 years of age.

ii. Sex—men more commonly affected.

iii. Diabetes mellitus.

iv. Hyperlipemia—obesity.

v. Cigarette smoking.

vi. Hypertension.

vii. Polycythemia vera.

(c) Assessment findings.

i. Subjective data:
- *Pain: (a) type—cramplike, (b) location—foot, calf, thigh, and buttocks, (c) duration—variable, may be relieved with rest, and (d) precipitating causes—on exercise (intermittent claudication) and occasionally even at rest.*
- *Cold feet and hands.*
- *Tingling and numbness in toes and feet.*

ii. Objective data:
- *Diminished or absent pedal pulses.*
- *Lower extremities—shiny, glossy, dry, cold, chalky white skin, decreased or absent hair, ulcers, gangrene.*
- *Diagnostic tests: (a) blood—increased serum cholesterol, triglycerides, CBC, platelets and (b) angiography—delineates location and nature of occlusion.*

(d) *Nursing goals* are designed to decrease discomfort, promote circulation, and prevent infection.

i. Head of bed elevated on blocks, 3 to 6 inches high, gravity aids in perfusion of legs and thighs.

ii. Protect extremity from injury with bed cradle, sheepskin, heel pads.

iii. Keep extremity warm and avoid chilling; avoid heating pads.

iv. Skin care techniques:
- *Use mild soap, dry thoroughly.*
- *Apply lotions but do not massage as this could release thrombus.*

v. Check pedal pulses, skin color, and temperature qid.

vi. Medications, as ordered:
- *Vasodilators.*
- *Anticoagulants—heparin sodium, dicumarol, ASA.*
- *Antihyperlipemias—clofibrate, cholestyramine resin, nicotinic acid.*

vii. Diet high in vitamins B and C (see Appendix A).

viii. Patient teaching:
- *Skin care.*
- *Balanced exercise and rest program—exercise increases collateral circulation.*
- *Elevate legs when seated.*
- *Diet—low fat, high vitamins B and C.*
- *Avoid smoking.*

e. *Increased blood volume.*
(1) *Polycythemia vera*—abnormal increase in circulating red blood cells.
(a) Pathophysiology:
i. Increased viscosity of blood increases peripheral vascular resistance and reduces blood flow.
ii. Reduced flow and increased platelet formation result in frequent intravascular thrombosis.
(b) Etiology and incidence:
i. Unknown etiology.
ii. Occurs in middle age, affecting men more frequently than women.
(c) Assessment findings.
i. Subjective data:
- *Headache.*
- *Dizziness.*
- *Ringing in the ears.*
- *Weakness, loss of interest.*
- *Feelings of abdominal fullness.*
- *Frequent belching or constipation.*
- *Weight loss.*
- *Pain or swelling in the legs.*
- *Difficulty in breathing.*
- *Pruritus.*
- *Frequent nose bleeds.*
ii. Objective data:
- *Skin—face is deep red, particularly lips, cheeks, and tips of nose, ears.*
- *Ecchymoses, gum bleeding.*
- *Blood pressure—normal, elevated.*
- *Enlarged liver and spleen.*
- *Diagnostic tests—blood: increased hemoglobin, hematocrit, RBC.*
(d) *Nursing goals* are designed to promote comfort and prevent complications.
i. Observe for signs of bleeding and thrombosis and employ care which reduces occurrence of injury:
- *Avoid prolonged sitting, knee gatch.*
- *Assist with ambulation.*
- *Utilize cool water in baths—decreases pruritus.*
- *Observe stools, urine, and gums for bleeding, skin for ecchymosis, extremities for color and temperature.*
ii. Assist with venesection (phlebotomy) as ordered, explaining procedure and rationale to patient.
iii. Encourage patient to verbalize feelings about condition, its process and outcomes.
iv. Push fluids as ordered—helps to reduce blood viscosity and promote urine excretion.
v. Maintain diet as ordered—foods high in iron such as oysters, liver, and legumes are contraindicated unless frequent phlebotomies are being done.

Part B | SERUM GLUCOSE LEVELS

PHYSIOLOGY

A. The physiologic and chemical processes carried out by our body cells require energy; energy for cellular metabolism is supplied by a compound called adenosine triphosphate (ATP).
   1. ATP can be utilized to:
      a. Synthesize cellular components such as proteins.
      b. Facilitate muscle contraction.
      c. Transport ions across membranes, as in active reabsorption in the kidney tubule and transmission of nerve impulses.
         (1) ATP can also be synthesized from proteins and fats.
         (2) The most important source for ATP synthesis is carbohydrates.
B. Carbohydrates are absorbed from the gut in the form of the monosaccharides, fructose, glucose, and galactose.
   1. These sugars are transported to the liver via portal circulation.
   2. Fructose and galactose are converted into glucose in the liver.
   3. Glucose is the only sugar of the blood.
C. The levels of blood glucose are homeostatically balanced between the energy needs of the body tissues and the sources of glucose in the body— most tissues can shift to fats or proteins for energy, but glucose is the only nutrient that can be utilized for energy by the central nervous system and the red blood cells.
D. Normal range of fasting blood glucose is 60 mg–120 mg/100 ml of blood.

MECHANISMS REGULATING BLOOD GLUCOSE CONCENTRATION

1. Glucose-buffer function of the liver
A. Excess glucose is stored in liver as glycogen.
B. Deficient serum glucose activates:
   1. Glycogenolysis, or breakdown of glycogen in liver, to replenish serum glucose levels.
   2. Gluconeogenesis—formation of glucose from amino acids and fats.

2. Hormonal regulators
A. Pancreatic hormones:
   1. Insulin—produced by the beta cells of the islets of Langerhans.
      a. Increases rate of oxidation of glucose in tissues.
      b. Increases rate of glycogen formation in the liver.
      c. Increases rate of glucose conversion into fat and its storage in adipose tissue.
      d. Lowers serum glucose levels.
   2. Glucagon—probably produced by the alpha cells in islets of Langerhans.
      a. Increases glycogenolysis in liver.
      b. Promotes lipolysis in adipose tissue.
      c. Increases serum glucose concentration.
B. Adrenal hormones:
   1. Glucocorticoids—
      a. Increase gluconeogenesis.
      b. Decrease tissue utilization of glucose.
      c. Increase serum glucose levels.
   2. Epinephrine—
      a. Effects rapid glycogenolysis in liver.
      b. Increases utilization of muscle glycogen.
      c. May produce transient hyperglycemia.
C. Pituitary hormones:
   1. Somatotropin (growth hormone)—
      a. Increases gluconeogenesis.
      b. Antagonizes action of insulin.
      c. Stimulates release of glucogen.
      d. Increases serum glucose levels.
   2. Adrenocorticotropic hormone (ACTH) or corticotropin—
      a. Stimulates adrenal cortex to increase secretion of glucocorticoids.
      b. Increases serum glucose level.
   3. Thyroid hormone—
      a. Increases rate of glucose absorption from intestine.
      b. Increases tissue utilization of glucose.

IMBALANCES IN SERUM GLUCOSE LEVELS

The two basic types of imbalance in serum glucose levels are hypoglycemia and hyperglycemia (Table 5–8).

1. Hypoglycemia—fasting serum glucose levels below 60 mg/100 ml of blood.

A. *Functional hypoglycemias*—decreased serum glucose without demonstrable disease process.

TABLE 5–8. *Assessment: imbalances in serum glucose*

Assessment	Hypoglycemia	Hyperglycemia
Common causes	Functional hypoglycemia. Insulin reaction.	Diabetes mellitus. Acute pancreatitis.
Behavior	Anxiety, apprehension, irritability. Difficulty concentrating, psychoses.	Irritability, confusion, lethargy, coma.
Neurologic	Muscle tremors, hyperreflexia. Temperature normal, decreased.	Decreased reflexia, loss of strength, tingling or loss of sensation in extremities, elevated temperature.
Head/neck	Headache, numbness of lips, tongue, diplopia.	Acetone breath, blurring or decreasing vision.
Skin	Pale, cool, moist, profuse, diaphoresis.	Warm, dry, flushed, loss of skin turgor, sunken eyeballs.
GI	Excessive hunger, nausea, vomiting.	Sudden weight loss, excessive hunger, excessive thirst, vomiting, abdominal pain.
Respiratory	Normal, slightly increased rate.	Hyperpnea—increased rate and depth (Kussmaul respirations).
Cardiovascular	Increased blood pressure, pulse—tachycardia, forceful, weakness, fatigue, fainting.	Decreased—may be in hypovolemic shock. Pulse—normal, increased, fatigue.
Renal	Decreased, normal—may be positive for sugar and acetone, then negative in insulin reactions.	Excessive output, positive for sugar and acetone, vulvar pruritus.
Extremities	Noncontributory.	Tingling, loss of sensations, foot ulcers.

1. Pathophysiology:
   a. Excessive beta cell secretion of insulin.
   b. Abnormally high blood insulin level depletes nutrients (glucose, amino acids, fatty acids) in blood stream by facilitating entry into skeletal muscle, fat, and other tissue cells.
   c. Insulin does not facilitate entry of glucose into brain cells, rather their metabolism is dependent on adequate serum glucose levels.
   d. Decreasing levels of serum glucose result in depression of cerebral function.
   e. Sympathetic nervous system elicits alarm mechanism, which stimulates glycogenolysis in liver to raise serum glucose levels.
2. Etiology and incidence:
   a. Reactive functional—excess insulin release in response to normal rises in blood sugar following meals.
   b. Reactive secondary to mild diabetes—insulin first delayed, then excessive response.
   c. Alimentary hypoinsulinism—excessive insulin release due to rapid emptying of carbohydrates into intestines (dumping syndrome).

d. Alcohol ingestion and poor nutrition—decreased gluconeogenesis and glycogenolysis.

B. *Organic hypoglycemias*—decreased serum glucose levels due to disease processes.

1. Decreased glycogen stores:
   a. Extensive liver disease, cirrhosis, carcinoma.
   b. Hepatic enzyme deficiencies.
2. Hyperinsulinism:
   a. Islet cell adenoma.
   b. Complication of insulin therapy in diabetes mellitus.
3. Decreased gluconeogenesis:
   a. Adrenal cortical hypofunction—
      (1) Addison's disease.
      (2) Adrenal hemorrhage.
      (3) Rapid withdrawal of steroid therapy in septicemia.
   b. Hypopituitarism.
4. *Nursing goals* are designed to reduce underlying metabolic disorder and promote adaptive behaviors.
   a. Administer and explain rationale for low-carbohydrate, high-protein, and adequate-fat diet divided into six equal feedings.
   b. Monitor vital signs and check for neurologic changes—frequent hypoglycemic attacks can result in permanent neurologic changes:
      (1) Diplopia.
      (2) Babinski reflex.
      (3) Hyperreflexia.
      (4) Decreased ability to concentrate.
   c. Support and promote adaptive behaviors:
      (1) Discuss factors predisposing to recurrence of symptoms—large carbohydrate ingestion and stressful situations or people.
      (2) Discuss nature of dysfunction and importance of diet therapy.
      (3) Provide the patient and family with opportunities to verbalize feelings and concerns—behavior changes and mood swings exhibited by patient before therapy may have strained or disrupted communication lines.
      (4) Discuss dosage, action, and side effects of medications ordered (see Appendix D).
         (a) Phenobarbital.
         (b) Diazepam (Valium).
         (c) Chlordiazepoxide (Librium) HCl.
      (5) Refer patient and family to appropriate community resource as indicated.

2. *Hyperglycemia*—fasting serum glucose levels above 120 mg/100 ml blood.
A. *Functional hyperglycemia:*
   1. Excessive intake of carbohydrates at a given meal.
   2. Increased glucose formation due to epinephrine.
      a. Stress—alarm reaction.
      b. Epinephrine administration.
   3. Parenteral infusions of glucose.
B. *Organic hyperglycemia:*
   1. Endogenous overproduction of glucose.
      a. Increased epinephrine release due to hyperactivity of adrenal medulla—pheochromocytoma.
      b. Increased release of ACTH from anterior pituitary—Cushing's syndrome.
      c. Increased production of growth hormone—acromegaly.
   2. Failure of mechanisms for lowering serum glucose.
      a. *Diabetes mellitus*—decreased or absent insulin production resulting in hyperglycemia and in alterations of protein and fat metabolism.
         (1) Pathophysiology:
            (a) Deficient beta cell activity leads to inadequate blood levels of insulin.
            (b) Glucose fails to enter muscle cells, resulting in decreased glucose utilization and hyperglycemia.
            (c) Other sources of energy—fats and proteins—are utilized by cells, causing excess production of keto acids and metabolic acidosis ($\downarrow$ HCO_3^-) $\rightarrow$ increased ventilation ($\downarrow$ Pco_2).
            (d) Increased glomerular filtration of glucose results in osmotic diuresis as transport mechanism for glucose is exceeded $\rightarrow$ sodium depletion $\rightarrow$ dehydration $\rightarrow$ circulatory failure.
         (2) Etiology and incidence:
            (a) Inherited disorder.
            (b) Worldwide distribution.

(3) Assessment findings:
  (a) Subjective data—
    i. Growth onset:
      • *Excessive hunger (poly-phagia).*
      • *Excessive thirst (polydipsia).*
      • *Excessive urination (poly-uria).*
      • *Sudden weight loss.*
      • *Loss of strength.*
      • *Increased irritability.*
    ii. Maturity onset:
      • *Weight loss or gain.*
      • *Nighttime urination (noctu-ria).*
      • *Vulvar itching (pruritus).*
      • *Blurring or decreasing vision.*
      • *Fatigue.*
      • *Tingling or loss of sensation in extremities.*
      • *Impotence.*
      • *Foot ulcer.*
  (b) Objective data—
    i. Vital signs:
      • *Blood pressure—normal, decreased.*
      • *Pulse—normal, increased.*
      • *Temperature—normal, increased.*
      • *Respirations—increased rate and depth; acetone breath, Kussmaul respirations.*
    ii. Diagnostic tests (see Appendix C).
      • *Blood: (a) fasting blood sugar—increased, (b) glucose tolerance test—blood glucose elevated after 180 minutes, (c) postprandial blood glucose—elevated blood glucose after 150 minutes, (d) serum ketones—elevated, and (e) CO_2 combining power—decreased.*
      • *Urine—positive for sugar and acetone.*

(4) *Nursing goals* are designed to reduce underlying metabolic dysfunction, attain and/or maintain normal weight, and prevent or delay renal, vascular, and neurologic complications.

  (a) Institute and explain diet therapy as ordered (check a diabetic exchange list):
    i. Diet based on patient's ideal weight, age, and activity level.
    ii. Foods may be interchanged within each list but not switched between lists.
    iii. Involve patient and family in planning meals that are varied and contain preference foods.
    iv. Discuss coordination of meals with hypoglycemic medica-tion.
  (b) Hypoglycemic medications as ordered (Tables 5–9 and 5–10).
  (c) Assess patient closely to avoid complications.
    i. Vital signs frequently.
    ii. Intake and output:
      • *Administer parenteral fluids as ordered (see Appendix B)—normal saline, electro-lytes, sodium bicarbonate.*
      • *Push fluids, as ordered.*
      • *Check urine for sugar, ace-tone, and specific gravity.*
    iii. Check for neurologic changes:
      • *Blurring of vision, increas-ing irritability, and confu-sion indicate ketoacidosis.*
      • *Diaphoresis, trembling, headache, and fainting indi-cate insulin reaction (hypo-glycemia).*
  (d) Provide comfort measures.
    i. Skin care with position changes.
    ii. Avoid exposure to cold.
    iii. Oral hygiene—keep mouth and lips moist.
  (e) Support and promote adaptive behaviors.
    i. Encourage patient and family to verbalize concerns, fears— deal with feelings of loss of body image, denial, anger.
    ii. Discuss nature of diabetes and purpose of treatment with patient and family:
      • *Factors that may precipitate recurrence of symptoms— infection, concentrated car-*

TABLE 5–9. *Insulin therapy*

Type	Onset, peak, and duration	Indications
RAPID		
Crystalline zinc (clear)	Onset 1 hour or less. Peak 2–4 hours. Duration 6–8 hours.	Poorly controlled diabetes, trauma, surgery, and coma.
Prompt insulin zinc suspension (Semilente insulin) (cloudy)	Onset 1 hour. Peak 4–10 hours. Duration 12–16 hours.	Patients allergic to crystalline; and in combination with longer-lasting insulin.
INTERMEDIATE		
Globin zinc insulin injection (clear)	Onset 2–4 hours. Peak 6–12 hours. Duration 18–24 hours.	Rarely used.
NPH insulin (isophane insulin suspension) (cloudy)	Onset 2–4 hours. Peak 6–12 hours. Duration 24–48 hours.	Patients who can be controlled by one dose per day.
Insulin zinc suspension (Lente insulin) (cloudy)	Onset 2–4 hours. Peak 6–12 hours. Duration 24–36 hours.	Patients allergic to NPH.
SLOW-ACTING		
PZI (protamine zinc insulin suspension) (cloudy)	Onset 3–6 hours. Peak 12–20 hours. Duration 24–36 hours.	Rarely used; only if uncontrolled by other types.
Extended insulin zinc suspension (Ultralente insulin) (cloudy)	Onset 2–4 hours. Peak 12–24 hours. Duration 36 hours.	Often mixed with Semilente for 24-hour curve.

Reminder: To avoid dangerous error, use U-40 syringe with U-40 insulin, U-80 syringe with U-80 insulin, and U-100 syringe with U-100 insulin.

bohydrate ingestion, skipped medication.
- Signs of hypoglycemia and precipitating causes—missed meals, heavy exercise.
- Importance of diet and regular exercise.
- Methods of regular urine-testing.
- Importance of hygiene measures and foot care.

- Medications—dosage, purpose, side effects: (a) rotation of injection sites and (b) calculation, scheduling, injection techniques.
  iii. Refer patient and family to appropriate community resource.
b. *Acute pancreatitis*—inflammation of the pancreas.
  (1) Pathophysiology:

TABLE 5–10. *Oral hyperglycemic agents*

Type	Dose/duration	Action/side effects (all classes)
SULFONYLAREAS		
Acetohexamide (Dymelor)	200–1500 mg qd. 1–2 per day. Duration 8–10 hours.	Action: lowers blood glucose by stimulating insulin release from beta cells. Effective only if pancreas has ability to produce insulin.
Chlorpropamide (Diabinese)	100–500 mg. 1 per day. Duration 30–60 hours.	Side effects: hypoglycemia, GI upset, skin rashes, bone marrow depression, liver toxicity.
Tolazamide (Tolinase)	100–750 mg. 1 per day. Duration 10–14 hours.	Contraindications: liver disease, renal disease.
Tolbutamide (Orinase)	500–3,000 mg. 2–3 per day. Duration 6–12 hours.	
BIGUANIDES		
Phenformin (DBI)	25–150 mg. 2 per day. Duration 4–6 hours.	Action: inhibits glucose absorption from gut; increases peripheral utilization of glucose; decreases gluconeogenesis.
Phenformin—timed release (DBI-TD)	50–150 mg. 1 per day. Duration 8–14 hours.	Side effects: lactic acidosis, nausea, vomiting, metallic aftertaste. Contraindications: hepatic and renal disease.

(a) Escape of activated pancreatic enzymes into interstitial tissue.
(b) Chemical irritant produces edema and vascular engorgement.
(c) Edema may subside spontaneously or progress to hemorrhage and tissue necrosis.
(d) Necrosis is result of ischemia due to pancreatic congestion and also of activation of powerful pancreatic enzymes in the ducts, which attack pancreatic and surrounding tissue.
(e) Effusion of blood, digested tissue, and pancreatic enzymes into the peritoneal cavity results in peritonitis with ascitic fluid and decreased intestinal motility (paralytic ileus).
(2) Etiology and incidence:

(a) Gallstones obstructing sphincter of Oddi.
(b) Alcohol ingestion.
(c) Trauma.
(d) Hypercalcemia.
(e) Infections.
(3) Assessment findings:
  (a) Subjective data.
    i. Pain:
      • *Type—sudden, severe, and constant.*
      • *Location—epigastric, abdominal; may radiate to back, substernal area and flanks.*
      • *Precipitating factors—more intense when in supine position; may be relieved somewhat by lying on side with spine flexed.*

    ii. Nausea and vomiting.

    iii. Fever.

(b) Objective data.

    i. Patient appears acutely ill.

    ii. Vital signs:

- *Blood pressure—slightly elevated, decreased in shock.*
- *Pulse and respirations—tachycardia, tachypnea.*
- *Temperature—elevated, subnormal in shock.*

    iii. Skin: pale, moist, cold, may become cyanotic, jaundiced.

    iv. Abdomen—distended, tenderness with guarding.

    v. Diagnostic tests (see Appendix C, Lab Values).

- *Blood: (a) serum amylase—usually elevated, (b) serum Ca^{++}, Na^+, K^+—decreased, (c) glucose tolerance test—hyperglycemia, (d) serum lipids—elevated, (e) CBC—RBCs and hemoglobin normal unless hemorrhage occurs, leukocytosis.*
- *Urine: (a) 24-hour urine amylase—elevated, (b) positive for sugar.*
- *Abdominal X ray—may demonstrate paralytic ileus, regional calcification of pancreas.*

(4) *Nursing goals* are designed to control pain and shock, maintain fluid and electrolyte balance, and prevent complications.

(a) Place in position of comfort or in semi-Fowler's.

(b) Administer meperidine (Demerol) 75 to 100 mgm every 4–6 hours as ordered.

    i. Reduces pain and does not cause spasm of sphincter of Oddi as do morphine and codeine.

    ii. Note length of pain relief and observe for side effects—hypotension, nausea, and vomiting.

(c) Administer parenteral transfusions as ordered to maintain blood volume and electrolyte balance (see Appendix B, IV Therapy).

    i. Whole blood, plasma, albumin, dextran.

    ii. Normal saline with supplemental potassium chloride and calcium gluconate—glucose administered cautiously as may aggravate hyperglycemia.

    iii. Drugs—prophylactic antibiotics (see Appendix D, Drugs), penicillin, cephalothin (Keflin), tetracyclines.

(d) Institute measures designed to reduce pancreatic activity.

    i. NPO.

    ii. Insert nasogastric tube and attach to low intermittent suction.

    iii. Administer enzyme inhibitors as ordered (Diamox).

(e) Monitor physical and emotional parameters closely and employ measures to prevent complications.

    i. Vital signs.

    ii. Central venous pressure.

    iii. Urine output.

    iv. Check urine for sugar and acetone qid.

    v. Oral care—prevents parotitis.

    vi. Turning, coughing, and deep breathing—prevents atelectasis, infection.

    vii. Positive Chvostek's sign, muscular twitching—signs of hypocalcemia.

    viii. Restlessness, tremors of hands and face, insomnia, extreme fear—indications of alcohol withdrawal.

(f) Involve patient and family in teaching and discharge planning.

    i. Importance of diet (see Appendix A, Diets).

- *Low fat; increase amounts gradually.*
- *Avoidance of alcohol, spicy foods, skipped meals, coffee, tea.*

    ii. Instruct in urine-testing procedures.

    iii. Maintain stool observations—frothy, foul-smelling stools indicate steatorrhea and should be reported to physician.

    iv. Purpose, dosage, and side effects of medications:
- *Anticholinergics—Banthine, Pro-Banthine.*
- *Antacids—Maalox, Gelusil.*
- *Enzymes—Viokase, pancreatin.*

  (g) Refer to appropriate community agency for follow-up care.

Part C / FLUID AND ELECTROLYTES

PHYSIOLOGY

1. Composition of body fluids

A. Water constitutes 60% to 70% of the total body weight.

B. Electrolytes are substances that dissociate and form electrically charged particles, called ions, when dissolved in water.

2. Body fluids separated by cell membranes into two compartments

A. Intracellular fluids:
1. Constitute 55% of total body fluids.
2. Primary electrolytes—
    a. Potassium.
    b. Phosphate.
    c. Magnesium.
    d. Proteinase.
3. Provide medium for chemical reactions within the cell.

B. Extracellular fluids:
1. Constitute 45% of total body fluids.
2. Primary electrolytes—
    a. Sodium.
    b. Calcium.
    c. Chloride.
    d. Bicarbonate and plasma proteins.
3. Serve as transport media for cellular nutrition and excretion.

3. Body fluids in state of dynamic equilibrium—fluid composition of each compartment remains relatively stable despite a constant interchange of body fluids from one compartment to another.

A. Dynamic equilibrium is dependent on the osmolarity of the fluid compartment and the active transport of ions across the cellular membrane.
1. Osmolarity—the total number of dissolved particles (electrolytes and colloids) per liter of fluid.
    a. Affected by electrolyte concentrations, electrolyte shifts, and movement of water from one compartment to the other.
      (1) Diffusion—movement of substances from high to low concentrations.
      (2) Osmosis—movement of water from high to low concentrations through a semipermeable membrane.
2. Active transport moves substances against concentration, electrical and pressure gradients, that is, from an area of low concentration to one of high concentration.
    a. Maintains intracellular potassium concentration and extracellular sodium concentrations.
    b. Facilitates active reabsorption of some substances such as sodium in the renal tubules.

4. Concentration gradients—interchange of body fluid between the intracellular and extracellular compartments is due to concentration gradients.

5. Pressure gradients—interchange or transport of body fluids between the vascular compartment and the interstitial fluid compartment is due to pressure gradients.

A. Capillary hydrostatic pressures (Figure 5–2):
1. Pressure of blood within capillary.
2. Dependent on blood pressure, blood flow, and venous pressure.
3. Favors outward flow of fluids.

B. Interstitial fluid pressures:
1. A negative pressure due to lymphatic drainage of fluid and proteins from interstitial spaces.
2. Favors outward flow of fluid plasma.

C. Colloid osmotic pressures:
1. Results from large quantity of plasma proteins in blood.
2. Favors inward flow of fluids.

D. Filtration pressures:
1. Difference between capillary hydrostatic pressure and plasma colloidal pressure.
2. Greater at arterial end of capillary—fluid moves outward from capillary to interstitial space.
3. Decreased significantly at venule end—facili-

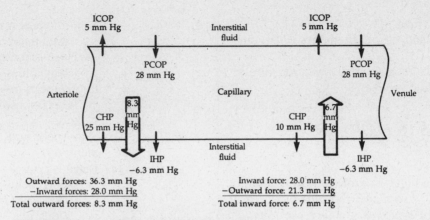

FIGURE 5–2. Capillary fluid dynamics
ICOP, interstitial colloid osmotic pressure; *PCOP*, plasma colloid osmotic pressure; *CHP*, capillary hydrostatic pressure; *IHP*, interstitial hydrostatic pressure. (From Holloway, N. *Nursing the critically ill adult.* Menlo Park, 1979, Addison-Wesley Publishing Co. Values from Guyton, *Textbook of medical physiology,* 5th Ed. Philadelphia, 1980, W. B. Saunders Co.)

tates movement of fluid from interstitial space back into capillary.

6. **Fluid transport between the vascular compartment and the interstitial fluid compartment—** designed to keep interstitial fluid pressures negative.
A. A change of interstitial fluid pressure from negative to positive results in edema formation.
B. Interstitial fluid pressures are kept negative by:
   1. Reabsorption of fluid into the circulatory system.
   2. Diffusion of excess fluid and protein (net filtration) from interstitial spaces into the lymphatics.

HOMEOSTATIC MECHANISMS CONTROLLING FLUID AND ELECTROLYTE BALANCE

1. **The kidney**—a complex organ that has the responsibility of regulating water, sodium, and hydrogen-ion concentrations.
A. Actively excretes or reabsorbs Na^+ and H_2O.
B. Excretes nitrogenous wastes, drugs, and toxins.
C. Excretes excess hydrogen ions to maintain normal pH of body fluids.
D. Maintains extracellular fluid osmolarity by:
   1. Selective filtration.
   2. Active reabsorption of electrolytes.

2. **The endocrine system**—secretes hormones that act to conserve various ions and total body water.

A. Antidiuretic hormone (ADH):

   1. Synthesized in hypothalamus and secreted by pituitary gland.
   2. Acts on distal tubules and collecting ducts of kidney nephron.
      a. Promotes water reabsorption.
      b. Decreases urine output.
   3. Release stimulated by hyperosmolarity of extracellular fluid.
B. Aldosterone:
   1. Synthesized and secreted by adrenal cortex.
   2. Increases the rate of sodium reabsorption in all segments of the renal tubule system.
      a. Actively conserves sodium—passively conserves water.
      b. Regulates blood and extracellular fluid volume.
      c. Decreases urine output.
   3. Stimulated by sodium depletion.

3. **The cardiovascular system**
A. Maintains optimum environment for cells through capillary exchange mechanism.
B. Glomerular filtration determined by renal blood flow.
   1. Normally increased with increased blood pressure.
   2. Decreased blood pressure decreases renal blood flow.

4. **The gastrointestinal system**
A. Primary route of fluid and electrolyte intake.
B. Conducts fluid and electrolytes rapidly across intestinal mucosa in both directions.

5. The nervous system
A. Manufactures and stores hormones (ADH and ACTH).
B. These hormones decrease urine output and increase extracellular fluid volume.

IMBALANCES IN FLUID AND ELECTROLYTES

Imbalances in fluid and electrolytes may be due to *changes in the total quantity of either substance* (deficit or excess), *protein deficiencies,* and/or *extracellular fluid volume shifts* (Table 5–11).

1. Changes in total quantity of fluid and electrolytes
A. Decreased quantities of fluid and electrolytes may be caused by deficient intake (poor dietary habits, anorexia, and nausea) or excessive output (vomiting, nasogastric suction, and prolonged diarrhea).
  1. *Addison's disease*—adrenocortical insufficiency.
    a. Pathophysiology—
      (1) Decreased adrenal cortical secretions of glucocorticoids, mineralocorticoids, and androgenic hormones.
        (a) Decreased or absent physiologic stress response (vascular insufficiency and hypoglycemia).
        (b) Decreased aldosterone secretion (sodium depletion, dehydration).
        (c) Decreased axillary and pubic hair.
      (2) Increased ACTH release—excessive skin pigmentation.
    b. Etiology and incidence—
      (1) Tuberculosis.
      (2) Fungal infections.
      (3) Autoimmune response.
      (4) Iatrogenic (surgical removal).
    c. Assessment findings—
      (1) Subjective data:
        (a) Muscle weakness.
        (b) Fatigue—most evident toward end of day.
        (c) Dizziness, fainting.
        (d) Weight loss.
        (e) Nausea, vomiting, food idiosyncrasies.
        (f) Abdominal pain, diarrhea.
      (2) Objective data:
        (a) Vital signs—
          i. Blood pressure—decreased, orthostatic hypotension, narrowed pulse pressure.
          ii. Pulse—increased, collapsing, irregularities.
          iii. Temperature—subnormal.
          iv. Respirations—noncontributory.
        (b) Skin—poor turgor, excessive pigmentation.
        (c) Diagnostic tests—
          i. Blood chemistry:
            • Decreased Na^+, Cl^-, and HCO_3^-.
            • Increased K^+.
            • Decreased serum glucose.
            • Increased hematocrit.
          ii. Urine—decreased or absent 17-ketosteroids and 17-hydroxycorticosteroids.
    d. *Nursing goals* are designed to reduce stress and provide physical and emotional comfort—
      (1) Provide quiet, nondemanding care schedule.
      (2) High-sodium, low-potassium diet; frequent carbohydrate nourishment to prevent hypoglycemia.
      (3) Force fluids—weighing daily to assess fluid balance.
      (4) Medications, as ordered (see Appendix D).
        (a) Glucocorticoids (cortisone acetate).
        (b) Mineralocorticoids (fludrocortisone acetate).
      (5) Involve patient and family in teaching and discharge planning.
        (a) Purpose, dosage, and side effects of medications—how to use emergency kit of injectable steroids, sudden withdrawal of steroid therapy may precipitate adrenal crisis.
        (b) Importance of avoiding stress and need to report to physician conditions that increase stress (flu, dental extractions, fever).
  2. *Cholelithiasis and cholecystitis*—gallstones and inflammation of the gallbladder:
    a. Pathophysiology—
      (1) Liver secretes bile that is supersaturated with cholesterol.

TABLE 5–11.   *Imbalances in fluid and electrolytes*

	Deficits	*Excesses*
EXAMPLES	Addison's disease, cholelithiasis, ulcerative colitis, hyperthyroidism.	Cushing's syndrome, pyelonephritis, hepatitis, cirrhosis.
FLUID SHIFTS	Burns, phase 1.	Burns, phase 2.
ASSESSMENT OF IMBALANCES		
Behavior	Apprehension, restlessness, apathy, coma in severe cases, shock.	Irritability, disorientation, apathy, convulsions, coma.
Neurologic	Elevated temperature, muscle twitch, tingling, tetany.	Muscle twitching.
Head/neck	Eyeballs soft, shrunken; circle under eyes. Flattened neck veins in supine position. Shrunken tongue, sticky mucous membranes.	Periorbital edema, distended neck veins, facial edema.
Skin	Cool, pale, doughy, dry, decreased turgor.	Warm, moist, taut, cool in areas of edema.
GI	Anorexia, nausea, vomiting, abdominal distention, cramps, diarrhea.	Anorexia, nausea, vomiting, ascites, abdominal fluid wave.
Respiratory	Increased rate and depth of breathing.	Dyspnea, orthopnea, tachypnea, moist rales, productive cough.
Cardiovascular	Decreased blood pressure, changes in pulse rate, lowered venous pressures, arrhythmias.	Fatigue, changes in pulse rate.
Renal	Oliguria, anuria in severe cases, concentrated urine, high specific gravity.	Polyuria if kidneys healthy, oliguria if diseased, nocturia.
Extremities	Pretibial edema, tingling and numbness of hands and feet.	Dependent pitting edema.

(2) Cholesterol crystals precipitate in bile, aggregating with other matter to become stones.

(3) Stones may then occlude duct, which results in distention of gallbladder, with edema, hyperemia, and tissue necrosis.

b. Etiology and incidence—

(1) Etiology of gallstones unknown.

(2) Gallstones most frequent cause of cholecystitis.

(3) Wide incidence particularly among Caucasians, Chinese, and Native Indians (American Indians).

(4) Highest incidence between ages 40 and 60 years.

(5) Affects more women than men.

c. Assessment findings—

(1) Subjective data:
 (a) Pain—
  i. Type—moderate to severe.
  ii. Location—upper right quadrant—may radiate to right shoulder.
  iii. Precipitating factors—may be accentuated with deep inspiration.
 (b) Anorexia, nausea, vomiting.
(2) Objective data:
 (a) Vital signs—
  i. Pulse—increased.
  ii. Temperature—elevated.
 (b) Abdomen—moderate rebound tenderness.
 (c) Icterus (yellow sclera).
 (d) Skin—jaundiced.
 (e) Diagnostic studies—
  i. Blood—leukocytosis.
  ii. Urine—urobilin.
  iii. X-ray studies—failure of the gallbladder to visualize after either oral or intravenous administration of radiopaque dye (see Appendix C, Diagnostic Tests).
d. *Nursing goals* are designed to reduce pain, provide support during diagnostic workup, and prepare patient for surgery (see Section III, under *Cholecystectomy*).

3. *Ulcerative colitis*—inflammation of mucosa and submucosa of the colon characterized by remissions and exacerbations.
 a. Pathophysiology—
  (1) Specific physiologic response to emotional trauma.
  (2) Edema and hyperemia of colonic mucous membrane → superficial bleeding with peristalsis → shallow ulcerations → abscesses → bowel wall thins and shortens → loses sacculation.
  (3) Increased rate of flow of liquid ileal contents → decreased water absorption → diarrhea.
 b. Etiology and incidence—
  (1) Genetic predisposition.
  (2) Autoimmune response.
  (3) Infections.
  (4) Greatest occurrence in young adults, ages 20 to 40 years.
  (5) More common in urban areas, upper-middle incomes, and groups with better educational backgrounds.
 c. Assessment findings—
  (1) Subjective data:
   (a) Frequent diarrhea (10 to 20 times daily).
   (b) Stools contain mucus, blood, pus.
   (c) Urgency to defecate, particularly when standing (*tenesmus*).
   (d) Loss of appetite, nausea, vomiting.
   (e) Colic-like stomach pains.
   (f) Weight loss.
   (g) Influenza-like symptoms (malaise, low-grade fever).
  (2) Objective data:
   (a) Temperature—elevated.
   (b) Stools—small amount of fecal matter, mainly blood, pus, mucus.
   (c) Diagnostic tests—
    i. Sigmoidoscopy—extent of rectal involvement.
    ii. Barium enema—detects lesions in proximal bowel.
    iii. Blood chemistries—increased hematocrit (hemoconcentration—decreased water and excess sodium), decreased potassium.
 d. *Nursing goals* are designed to reduce psychologic stresses, relieve symptoms, promote physical and psychologic equilibrium, prevent complications, and facilitate remission.
  (1) Provide quiet, supportive environment, encouraging patient to verbalize worries—decrease anxiety.
  (2) Institute measures designed to control diarrhea, abdominal pain, and tenesmus.
   (a) Medications (see Appendix D):
    i. Codeine PO_4 (intramuscular) or codeine SO_4 (oral).
    ii. Camphorated tincture of opium (paregoric).
    iii. Tincture of belladonna.
    iv. Phenobarbital sodium.
    v. Atropine (Lomotil) SO_4.
   (b) Avoid coarse residue foods, whole milk, cold beverages—stimulate bowel activity.
  (3) Institute measures designed to improve nutritional and electrolyte balance:

(a) Parenteral hyperalimentation (see Appendix B).

(b) High-calorie, high-protein, low-residue diet.

(c) Parenteral, intramuscular, or oral vitamin and mineral supplements—potassium, iron, vitamins C and B.

(d) Push fluids to 3000 ml/day.

(4) Provide comfort measures—skin care, rest periods, diversional activities, sitz baths.

(5) Institute and maintain steroid therapy as ordered to facilitate remission.

(6) Patient and family teaching should include diet, medications, and importance of avoiding stress and maintenance of emotional stability.

(7) Refer to appropriate community resource as indicated.

(8) If exacerbation continues, assist in preparation for surgery (*Ileostomy,* see Section III).

4. Excessive output also occurs due to:

a. Increased insensible water loss—fever, bronchiectasis.

b. Lack of ADH production by pituitary—diabetes insipidus.

c. Osmotic diuresis—diabetes mellitus.

d. Draining fistulas, large wounds, extensive surgery.

B. Excessive quantities of fluid and electrolytes may be due to increased ingestion, tube feedings, intravenous infusions, enemas, or an inability to excrete excesses.

1. *Acute and chronic renal dysfunctions:*

a. *Acute glomerulonephritis*—inflammation of glomeruli characterized by increased glomerular permeability; results in proteinuria, cylindruria, hematuria, azotemia, hypertension, and anemia (also see Unit 4, Nursing Care of Children and Families).

b. *Pyelonephritis*—acute or chronic inflammation due to bacterial infection of the parenchyma and the pelvis of the kidney.

(1) Pathophysiology—

(a) Inflammation of renal medulla or diffuse inflammation of the lining of the renal pelvis.

(b) Nephrons are destroyed, resulting in hypertrophy of intact nephrons needed to maintain urine output.

(c) Dilatation of tubules may result in defects in sodium reabsorption and inability of the kidney to concentrate urine.

(2) Etiology and incidence—

(a) 95% caused by gram-negative enteric bacilli (*Escherichia coli*).

(b) Occurs more frequently in young women and older men.

(c) Predisposing factors include obstruction, hypertension, hypokalemia, diabetes mellitus, pregnancy, catheterization.

(3) Assessment findings—

(a) Subjective data:

i. Flank pain.

ii. Chills and fever.

iii. Loss of appetite.

iv. Night sweats.

v. Pain on urination.

(b) Objective data:

i. Costovertebral angle tenderness.

ii. Diagnostic tests (see Appendix C):

• *Blood—polymorphonuclear leukocytosis.*

• *Urine—leukocytosis, hematuria, white blood cell casts, proteinuria (less than 3 gm in 24 hours), positive cultures.*

• *Intravenous pyelogram (IVP)—may manifest structural changes.*

(4) *Nursing goals* are designed to alleviate symptoms, identify predisposing factors, and prevent recurrence.

(a) Relieve pain and fever—

i. Administer analgesics—pentazocine lactate (Talwin) and meperidine (Demerol) HCl.

ii. Administer acetaminophen (Tylenol) to reduce fever.

iii. Institute cooling measures as indicated.

(b) Administer sulfonamides and/or antibiotics to support body defense mechanisms.

(c) Prevent complications—

i. Maintain intake and output—observe urine characteristics.

TABLE 5–12. *Drug therapies in fluid/electrolyte imbalances (diuretics)*

Drug and dosage	Use	Action	Side effects	Nursing implications
Thiazides (Diuril, Hydrodiuril, and Esidrix)—po, 0.5–1 g qd	Edema, congestive heart failure, Na⁺ retention in steroid therapy, hypertension.	Inhibits sodium chloride and water reabsorption in the proximal tubules of the kidneys.	Hypokalemia, nausea, vomiting, diarrhea, dizziness, and paresthesias; may accentuate diabetes.	Watch for muscle weakness; give well-diluted potassium chloride supplement; monitor urine for changes in sugar and acetone.
	Maternal use: preeclampsia-eclampsia.	Decrease fluid retention, eliminate Na⁺, control BP, and no acidosis.	All diuretics must be used with caution since they produce fluid-electrolyte imbalance in mother-fetus; may cause allergic reaction.	Weigh daily, accurate I & O, assess edema, and replace electrolytes per order; less electrolyte imbalance with proper precautions (replace K⁺ with orange juice, banana, etc.).
Spironolactone (Aldactone)—po, 25 mg bid-qid	Cirrhosis of liver and when other diuretics are ineffective.	Inhibits effects of aldosterone in distal tubules of kidney.	Headache, lethargy, diarrhea, ataxia, skin rash, gynecomastia.	Potassium-sparing drug; *do not* give supplemental KCl; monitor for signs of electrolyte imbalance.
Furosemide (Lasix)—po, 40–80 mg qd in divided doses	Edema and associated heart failure, cirrhosis, renal disease, nephrotic syndrome, and hypertension.	Inhibits Na⁺ and Cl⁻ reabsorption in the Loop of Henle, the distal and proximal renal tubule.	Dermatitis, pruritus, paresthesia, blurring of vision, postural hypotension, nausea, vomiting, and diarrhea.	Assess for weakness, lethargy, leg cramps, anorexia; peak action in 1–2 hours; duration 6–8 hours; do not give at bed time; supplementary KCl indicated; may induce digitalis toxicity.
Ethacrynic acid (Edecrin)—po, 50–200 mg qd in divided doses	Pulmonary edema, ascites, edema of congestive heart failure.	Inhibits the reabsorption of Na⁺ in the ascending Loop of Henle.	Nausea, vomiting, diarrhea, hypokalemia, hypotension, gout, dehydration, deafness, and metabolic acidosis.	Assess for dehydration—skin turgor, neck veins; hypotension; KCl supplement.

TABLE 5–12. *(Continued)*

Drug and dosage	Use	Action	Side effects	Nursing implications
Meralluride (Mercuhydrin)—IM, 1–2 ml; mercaptomerin (Thiomerin)—IM, 1–2 ml; mercurophylline (Mercuzanthin)—IM, 1–2 ml	Acute edematous states.	Enhances sodium excretion in proximal renal tubules.	Metabolic alkalosis due to hypochloremia or bone marrow depression.	Closely observe urine output—mercurial salts may cause tubular necrosis and renal failure; watch for signs of chloride depletion—apathy, somnolence, weakness, and disorientation.
Osmotic diuretic 30% urea, 10% invert sugar, 20% mannitol	Cerebral edema.	Hypertonic solution that kidney tubules cannot reabsorb and thus causes obligatory water loss.		
Acetazolamide (Diamox)	*Maternal use:* preeclampsia-eclampsia.	Potent diuretic; produces acidosis; self-limiting effect.	Electrolyte depletion symptomatology—lassitude, apathy, decreased urinary output, and mental confusion; may be fetotoxic.	Weigh daily; I & O; assess edema; give early in day to allow sleep at night; observe for side effects; replace electrolytes as ordered.
Ammonium Cl	*Maternal use:* preeclampsia-eclampsia.	Promote Na^+ excretion; may lead to acidosis; self-limiting effect.	See *Acetazolamide.*	See *Acetazolamide.*

ii. Monitor vital signs q4h.

iii. Maintain bedrest or activity to tolerance.

iv. Push fluids unless contraindicated—prevents stasis of urine.

v. Avoid tub baths.

(d) Provide emotional support—

  i. Include family in care and teaching plans.

  ii. Provide diversional activities.

  iii. Encourage activities of daily living as tolerated.

  iv. Answer patient's questions and discuss concerns.

2. *Edema and transudation of fluids* (Table 5–12):

  a. *Cushing's syndrome*—increased cortisol secretion by the adrenal gland.

    (1) Pathophysiology—

      (a) Excess glucocorticoid production increases gluconeogenesis raising serum glucose levels → glucose in urine and increased fat deposition in face and trunk.

      (b) Gluconeogenesis also decreases amino acids, leading to protein deficiencies → muscle wasting → poor antibody response → lack of collagen.

    (2) Etiology and incidence—

(a) Adrenal hyperplasia due to dysfunction of hypothalamus or pituitary tumor.

(b) Adrenal adenoma.

(c) Adrenal carcinoma.

(d) Prolonged steroid therapy.

(3) Assessment findings—

   (a) Subjective data.

     i. Muscle weakness—decreasing work capacity.

     ii. Backache.

     iii. Weight gain—obesity.

     iv. Impotence.

     v. Cessation of menstrual flow, clitoral enlargement.

     vi. Frequent mood changes—nervousness, depression.

   (b) Objective data.

     i. Vital signs—elevated blood pressure.

     ii. Skin—thin, purple striae over obese areas, red face, ecchymoses, pitting edema of ankles.

     iii. Truncal obesity with thin extremities—moon face, buffalo hump.

     iv. Hirsutism—fine downy hair over face, forehead, upper trunk.

     v. Diagnostic tests:

      • *Blood—increased 17-hydroxycorticosteroid levels, decreased eosinophils, increased neutrophils, decreased potassium chlorides, metabolic alkalosis.*

      • *Urine—increased 17-hydroxycorticosteroids, glucosuria.*

      • *X rays—osteoporosis particularly of spine and pelvis, adrenal enlargement.*

(4) *Nursing goals* are designed to prevent complications, promote patient relaxation, and prepare patient for surgery (see *Adrenalectomy* in Section III).

b. *Hepatitis*—inflammation of the liver.

(1) Pathophysiology:

   (a) Infection with either hepatitis A (infectious hepatitis) or hepatitis B (serum hepatitis)—produces inflammation, necrosis, and regeneration of liver parenchyma.

   (b) Hepatocellular injury impairs clearance of urobilinogen → elevated urinary urobilinogen and, as injury increases → conjugated bilirubin does not reach the intestines → decreased urine and fecal urobilinogen → increased serum bilirubin → jaundice.

   (c) Failure of liver to detoxify products → increased toxic products of protein metabolism → gastritis and duodenitis.

(2) Etiology, incidence, and epidemiologic comparison between infectious and serum hepatitis:

   (a) Infectious hepatitis A—

     i. Incubation—two to six weeks.

     ii. Transmission—fecal-oral.

     iii. Sources—crowding; contaminated food, milk or water; asymptomatic carriers.

     iv. HB antigen—not present.

     v. Incidence—sporadic epidemics.

   (b) Serum hepatitis B—

     i. Incubation—six weeks to six months.

     ii. Transmission—parenteral.

     iii. Sources—contaminated needles, syringes, surgical instruments, blood plasma, or transfusions.

     iv. HB antigen—present.

     v. Incidence—increased in ages 15 to 29 years, particularly in heroin addiction; occupational hazard for laboratory workers, nurses, physicians.

(3) Assessment findings:

   (a) Subjective data—

     i. Influenza-like aches (malaise).

     ii. Loss of appetite.

     iii. Nausea, vomiting.

     iv. Repugnance to food, cigarette smoke, strong odors, alcohol.

     v. Dull ache in upper right quadrant.

     vi. Headache, fever.

     vii. Rash.

   (b) Objective data—

i. Liver—enlarged, tender, smooth.

ii. Skin—icterus in sclera of eyes, jaundice.

iii. Urine—normal, dark.

iv. Stools—normal, clay-colored, loose.

v. Diagnostic tests:

- *Blood—leukocytosis, increased SGOT, SGPT, and bilirubin levels, alkaline phosphatase.*
- *Urine—increased urobilinogen.*

(4) *Nursing goals* are designed to reduce discomforts and promote conditions favorable to liver functioning.

(a) Bedrest and precaution or isolation techniques.

(b) Diet as tolerated.

i. NPO with parenteral infusions.

ii. High-protein, high-carbohydrate, low-fat diet offered in frequent small meals.

iii. Push fluids if not contraindicated.

(c) Assess physical and emotional parameters and employ comfort measures.

i. Intake and output; observation for urine and stool changes; weigh daily.

ii. Observe for increasing jaundice—if pruritus is present, use mild, oil-based lotions to reduce itching.

iii. Provide oral hygiene q1h to q2h and institute ROM exercises.

iv. Provide opportunities for patient to express concerns and questions.

(d) Discharge planning and teaching—

i. Instructions on diet and fluid intake to promote liver regeneration.

ii. Importance of rest and limited activity to reduce metabolic workload of liver.

iii. Personal hygiene practices to prevent contamination.

iv. Avoidance of alcohol, blood donations, and individuals with communicable infections.

v. Refer to appropriate community resource for follow-up care.

c. *Cirrhosis*—chronic progressive liver disease characterized by degeneration and disorganized regeneration of liver tissue resulting in fibrosis.

(1) Pathophysiology:

(a) Decreased cellular function → impaired detoxification → bad breath → abnormal behavior → peripheral vasodilatation → sodium retention → increased sensitivity to drugs.

(b) Impaired protein synthesis → fall in plasma proteins → decreased oncotic pressures → edema and ascites → decreased clotting factors → increased bleeding tendency.

(c) Decreased glycogenolysis → hypoglycemia.

(d) Decreased bile secretion → malabsorption of fats → deficiencies in fat-soluble vitamins (A, D, and K).

(e) Impaired bilirubin conjugations → jaundice.

(f) Portal hypertension, causing enlarged spleen → excessive red and white blood cell breakdown → diversion of portal blood → esophageal and rectal varices.

(2) Etiology and incidence:

(a) Toxins, including alcohol and drugs.

(b) Hepatitis.

(c) Obstruction of common bile duct.

(d) Malnutrition.

(e) Incidence parallels increased alcohol consumption.

(f) Ages 45 to 65 years, more men than women, more non-Whites than Whites.

(3) Assessment findings:

(a) Subjective data—

i. Anorexia, nausea, vomiting, foul breath.

ii. Weight loss.

  iii. Distended abdomen.
  iv. Low-grade fever.
  v. Flatulence, diarrhea, constipation.
  vi. Impotence, cessation of menstrual flow.
 (b) Objective data—
  i. Enlargement of liver and frequently spleen, ascites.
  ii. Skin—jaundice, spider angiomas, palmar erythema, breast enlargement in males, testicular atrophy and sparse body hair.
  iii. Diagnostic studies (see Appendix C): blood—moderate red blood cells, decreased clotting times and serum albumin, increased bromsulphalein (BSP) retention, serum bilirubin, SGOT and SGPT, positive cephalin-cholesterol flocculation test.
(4) *Nursing goals* are designed to reduce metabolic activity, provide substitutes for decreased liver function, promote comfort, and prevent or delay liver failure.
 (a) Bedrest in position of comfort—turning, coughing, and deep breathing q2h to promote ventilation and prevent venous stasis.
 (b) Provide for maintenance of nutrition and fluid and electrolyte balance.
  i. NPO—nasogastric suction may be ordered, parenteral infusions with electrolytes and vitamins, as ordered.
  ii. No- or low-protein, moderate-carbohydrate-and-fat diet; liver unable to detoxify proteins.
  iii. Low-sodium diet and fluid restrictions if ascites present.
  iv. Small frequent meals to avoid anorexia.
  v. Diuretics and serum albumin, as ordered—to establish normal fluid volumes (Table 5–12).
 (c) Observe closely for signs of complications—
  i. Monitor intake and output, noting character of urine and stools; report urine output of less than 25–30 ml/hour.
  ii. Check vital signs—institute cooling measures if necessary, observe for signs of cardiac decompensation.
  iii. Assess neurologic status—awareness of time and place, confusion, decreased response to verbal commands, tremors; report changes to physician immediately.
  iv. Check gums and injection sites for bleeding.
 (d) Assist with paracentesis, as ordered (see Appendix B).
 (e) Promote comfort measures and emotional support—rest, skin care, quiet environment, verbalization of concerns.
 (f) Patient teaching includes diet; avoidance of stress, alcohol, and exposure to infections; and referral to appropriate community agencies.
 (g) Complications of cirrhosis—
  i. Bleeding esophageal varices:
   • *Sengstaken-Blakemore tube with esophagogastric balloon is utilized to control bleeding.*
   • *Gastric lavage with ice water may also be employed to encourage vasoconstriction.*
  ii. Hepatic coma—changes in consciousness, flapping tremor, grimacing, and sweet, musty breath odor.

2. *Protein deficiencies*

A. Proteins are basic constituents of living cells and are essential for body growth and maintenance and repair of tissue. Deficiency may result from:
1. Inadequate intake.
2. Severe loss, as in burns or hemorrhage.
3. Increased utilization by the body, as in wound-healing or severe injury.
4. Increased catabolism as in hyperthyroidism, fever, infection, and malignancy.
5. *Thyrotoxicosis (hyperthyroidism or Graves' disease)*—excessive thyroid hormone in the blood.
 a. Assessment:
  (1) Pathophysiology—

(a) Diffuse hyperplasia of thyroid gland results in overproduction of thyroid hormone and increased blood serum levels.

(b) Hormone stimulates mitochondria to increase energy for cellular activities and heat production.

(c) As metabolic rate increases, fat reserves are depleted despite increased appetite and food intake.

(d) Cardiac output is increased to meet increased tissue metabolic needs and peripheral vasodilation occurs in response to increased heat production.

(e) Neuromuscular hyperactivity results in accentuation of reflexes, anxiety, and increased alimentary tract mobility.

(2) Etiology and incidence—

(a) Possible autoimmune response resulting in increase of a gamma globulin called *long-acting thyroid stimulator* (LATS).

(b) Occurs generally in third and fourth decade.

(c) Affects women more frequently than men.

(3) Symptomatology—

(a) Subjective data:

i. Complaints of nervousness, mood swings.

ii. Increased sweating.

iii. Palpitations.

iv. Heat intolerance.

v. Weight loss despite appetite increase.

vi. Fatigue, muscle weakness, tremors.

vii. Frequent bowel movements.

(b) Objective data:

i. Vital signs: (a) blood pressure—increased systolic pressure and widened pulse pressure; (b) pulse—tachycardia; and (c) temperature, respirations—nonspecific.

ii. Skin—warm, moist, velvety, increased melanin pigmentation.

iii. Eyes—characteristic stare with widened palpebral fissures, lid lag, and failure to wrinkle brow with upward gaze.

iv. Pretibial edema with thickened skin and color changes.

v. Goiter.

vi. Diagnostic tests (see Appendix C): (a) blood—increased protein-bound iodine (PBI), T_4 and T_3 resin uptake and thyroid uptake of radioiodine and (b) basal metabolic rate (BMR)—increased.

b. Interventions

(1) *Nursing goals* are designed to protect patient from stress, promote physical and emotional equilibrium, and prevent complications.

(a) Provide quiet environment that is cool and well ventilated—reduces stimulation and lessens diaphoresis.

(b) Maintain unhurried appearance and avoid discrepancies in treatments and procedures—lessens patient's nervousness.

i. Accept mood swings.

ii. Restrict activities and visitors—prevents undue fatigue.

(c) Provide eye care as indicated:

i. Sunglasses to protect from photophobia, wind, dust.

ii. Instill protective drops such as methylcellulose to soothe exposed cornea.

iii. Tape eyelids that do not close in sleep.

iv. Apply cold compresses for comfort.

(d) High-caloric, high-protein, high–vitamin B diet:

i. Six full meals per day, as needed.

ii. Weigh daily.

iii. Avoid stimulants (coffee, tea, colas).

(e) Observe for complications:

i. Heart failure (hypotension, pulmonary edema).

ii. Thyroid storm (crisis)—hyperthermia, extreme tachycardia, extreme restlessness, weakness, and delirium.

(f) Medications, as ordered:

      i. Antithyroid preparations: (a) propylthiouracil—blocks thyroid synthesis; usual dosage 100 mg q8h, initially; patients should be instructed to report rashes, sore throat, or fever to physicians immediately and (b) methimazole—similar action and side effects; utilized for patients allergic to propylthiouracil.

      ii. Iodine preparations—reduce vascularity of thyroid gland; used in treatment of thyroid storm: (a) SSKI—5 gm in H_2O q 3 to 4 times daily and (b) Lugol's solution.

  (2) Prepare for thyroidectomy, as ordered (see Section III).

  (3) Prepare for oral radioiodine therapy (iodine 131), as ordered.

B. Blood proteins (albumin, fibrinogen, globulin) are essential for maintenance of oncotic pressures.

  1. Deficiencies result from decreased liver function as in cirrhosis or renal dysfunction (glomerulonephritis).

3. Extracellular fluid volume shifts

A. Plasma-to-interstitial fluid shift:

  1. Fluid shifts from injured areas to noninjured areas.

  2. Fluid shifts from plasma into peritoneum or pleural space.

  3. Shift results in—

    a. Decreased blood volume.

    b. Edema of noninjured areas.

    c. Dehydration of injured areas.

B. Interstitial fluid-to-plasma shifts:

  1. Shift of fluid and electrolytes to vascular compartment, usually after a plasma-to-interstitial fluid shift.

  2. *Burns*—wounds caused by exposure to excessive heat, chemicals, fire, steam, radiation, or electricity.

    a. Pathophysiology:

      (1) Shock due to pain, fright, or terror → fatigue and failure of vasoconstrictor mechanisms → hypotension.

      (2) Capillary dilatation and increased permeability → plasma loss creating blisters and edema → hemoconcentration → hypovolemia → hypotension → decreased renal perfusion → renal shutdown.

      (3) Interstitial-to-plasma fluid shift → hemodilution → hypervolemia → heart failure → pulmonary edema.

    b. Incidence:

      (1) Two million annually in the United States.

      (2) Most occur in home owing to carelessness or ignorance.

      (3) 8000 deaths annually.

      (4) Survival best in ages 15 to 45 years and in burns covering less than 20% of the total body surface.

    c. Assessment findings:

      (1) Utilize "rule of nine" to ascertain extent of body surface involved—head and both upper extremities, 9% each; front and back of trunk, 18% each; lower extremities, 18% each; and perineum, 1%.

        (a) Repeat on second and third days.

        (b) Facial, perineal, and hand and foot burns have greater fatality rates.

      (2) Estimate depth of burn.

        (a) First degree—epidermal tissue only.

          i. Usually red.

          ii. Not serious unless large areas involved.

        (b) Second degree—epidermal and dermal tissue.

          i. Blisters formed.

          ii. Hospitalization required if over 30% of body (major burn).

        (c) Third degree—destruction of all skin layers and, frequently, fat, muscle, and bone.

          i. Requires immediate hospitalization.

          ii. 10% of body surface considered major burn.

    d. *Nursing goals* in the case of the burned patient are designed to institute measures to save life, reduce discomfort, prevent disability and deformities, and promote rehabilitation and safety measures.

      (1) Institute *emergency* measures:

        (a) Apply cold to burn and get patient to hospital.

        (b) Cover burn with clean or sterile towel to protect from contamination and reduce pain from contact

with air—do not use ointment of any kind.
   (c) Irrigate chemical burns with copious amounts of water.
   (d) Roll victim whose clothes are on fire on ground and douse with cold water when flames are extinguished.
(2) Alleviate pain, relieve shock, and institute measures to maintain fluid and electrolyte balance.
   (a) Administer narcotic while physical examination is being completed; remove burned clothing.
   (b) Weigh patient if possible to establish baseline data for fluid therapy.
   (c) Institute parenteral therapy (see IV therapy in Appendix B), as ordered, and insert indwelling catheter.
      i. Maintain strict intake and output records.
      ii. Weigh daily.
   (d) Observe physical and emotional parameters and employ measures to prevent complications.
      i. Vital signs hourly.
      ii. Utilize hematocrit, CVP, and urinary output to determine cardiovascular status.
      iii. Administer medications as ordered:
         • *Tetanus booster.*
         • *Antibiotics—prevent infections.*
         • *Sedatives and analgesics.*
         • *Steroids.*
         • *Antipyretics—avoid aspirin.*
      iv. Prevent contractures by utilizing anatomic positioning.
         • *Stryker frame or circle bed if circumferential trunk burns present.*
         • *Head and neck burns—no pillows.*
         • *Hand burns—use towel rolls or sandbags to align hands.*
         • *Upper-body burns—keep arms at 90° angle from body and slightly above shoulders.*
         • *Ankles and feet—allow feet to hang at 90° angle from ankles in prone position; utilize footboards to maintain 90° angle in supine position.*
         • *Utilize traction and splints to maintain positions.*
         • *Utilize passive and active ROM exercises.*
      v. Control gastrointestinal disturbances:
         • *Initial NPO, then juices or carbonated beverages; do not give ice chips or plain water as these may contribute to electrolyte imbalance.*
         • *As food is tolerated—high-protein, high-calorie diet for energy and tissue repair.*
         • *Observe for Curling's (stress) ulcer—sudden drop in hemoglobin.*
      vi. Observe for emotional reactions and provide supportive therapy:
         • *Loss of body image, threat of pain, repeated operations, long convalescence, dependency conflicts.*
         • *Care by same personnel as much as possible.*
         • *Involve patient in care plans.*
         • *Answer questions clearly and accurately.*
         • *Encourage contact with family and/or significant person.*
         • *Provide diversional activities and change furnishings or room adornments when possible to prevent perceptual deprivation.*
         • *Encourage self-care to tolerance.*
e. Burn therapies:
   (1) *Open method*—exposure of burns to drying effect of air.
      (a) Advantages—
         i. Useful in treating burns of neck, face, trunk, and perineum.

TABLE 5–13. *Dressing materials for burn care today*

Dressing	Description	Actions	Advantages
Silver sulfadiazine (Silvadene)	A nontoxic salt of silver sulfadiazine in a water-based cream.	Binds to bacteria cell membranes and interferes with DNA.	Doesn't cause hypochloremia, hyponatremia, electrolyte imbalance, or kidney disease. Has a wide-spectrum antimicrobial action against both gram-negative and gram-positive organisms. Its action is long lasting (up to 48 hours). Has a long shelf life. Delays eschar separation less than many other topicals.
Mafenide acetate (Sulfamylon)	A soft, white, nonstaining water-based cream.	Exerts a bacteriostatic action against many gram-negative and gram-positive organisms.	Effective against *Pseudomonas*. Long shelf life. Excellent for treating electrical burns. Penetrates thick eschar.
Bismuth tribromphenate (Xeroform)	A yellow substance used on Vaseline gauze.	Debrides and protects donor sites and grafts.	Conforms to wound. Nontoxic and nonsensitizing. Has a long shelf life.
Scarlet red	A red dye in an oil base on gauze.	Promotes healing of wound, but has no antiseptic effect.	Protects donor site. Long shelf life.
Sodium hypochlorite (Dakin's solution)	A 10% aqueous sodium hypochlorite solution.	Bactericidal.	Helps dry wounds that have become soupy. Aids debridement.
Povidone-iodine (Betadine)	Iodine complex, available as solution, ointment, and foam.	Microbicidal against gram-positive and gram-negative organisms.	Is effective against many infections not well controlled by Silvadene. Is available in a wide assortment of forms.
Nitrofurazone (Furacin)	Antibiotic available as cream, solution, and water-soluble powder.	Wide-spectrum antibacterial.	Is effective against *Staphylococcus aureus* and some antibiotic-resistant organisms. Not absorbed systemically. Causes neither pain nor maceration. Available in a wide assortment of forms.
Silver nitrate	10% silver salt solution, diluted to 0.5% for application.	Antimicrobial.	Is inexpensive. Applies easily.
Gentamicin sulfate (Garamycin)	Wide-spectrum antibiotic, available as a cream or solution for topical use.	Exerts antibiotic action against many organisms that do not respond to other topical antibiotics.	Effective against many organisms, including *Pseudomonas*. Does not cause pain.

TABLE 5–13.   *(Continued)*

Disadvantages	Nursing considerations
Absorbed into eschar less than mafenide acetate (Sulfamylon). May cause rash, pruritus, and burning. Not consistently effective for burns covering more than 60% of patient's body or against some bacteria and yeasts. Depresses granulocyte formation.	Watch for signs of infection, such as soupiness.
May lead to superinfection. May cause metabolic acidosis, hyperpnea, and rash. Causes pain when applied. (Pain usually lasts 30–40 minutes.) Slows eschar separation.	Premedicate patient for pain before application. Monitor blood gases and serum electrolytes if patient develops hyperpnea in response to metabolic acidosis. Don't use in cases of sulfa drug allergy, or respiratory or kidney disease.
Sticks to wound so that removal is very painful. Neither antiseptic nor antibacterial.	Apply carefully so that sheets don't overlap. Observe patient closely for signs of infection.
Stains clothing and temporarily stains skin. Irritates skin. Causes pain when patient moves. May cause systemic effects.	Apply to donor sites at time of harvest; leave until site heals and scarlet red gauze sloughs. Watch closely for signs of infection beneath gauze. If needed to dry site, use a heat lamp for a few minutes every 4 hours.
Dissolves blood clots and may inhibit clotting. May irritate skin.	Change dressings every 4–12 hours. Observe site carefully for signs of irritation.
May cause metabolic acidosis and elevated serum iodine levels. May form crusts if burns are not cleaned properly. Causes rash and burning with some patients. Stains clothing and linen.	Check serum electrolytes and serum iodine levels frequently.
May cause contact dermatitis (rare). Is messy to apply in cream form.	Observe patient carefully for signs of allergic reaction and for evidence of a superinfection.
Penetrates wound only 1–2 mm, so it acts only on surface organisms. Stains and stings. May cause hyponatremia, hypochloremia, and hypocalcemia.	Keep dressings wet with solution. Check serum electrolytes daily.
May cause ototoxicity and nephrotoxicity. Organisms may become resistant.	Use with caution in patients with decreased renal function, because of possible nephrotoxicity. Order serum creatinine and urine creatinine clearance studies before treatment and weekly during treatment to monitor renal function.

(Continued)

TABLE 5–13.   *(Continued)*

Dressing	Description	Actions	Advantages
Third's	Solution of ⅓ 3% hydrogen peroxide, ⅓ 0.25% acetic acid, and ⅓ normal saline.	Inhibits bacteria growth by oxidizing constituents and lowering pH. Effervescence cleans wounds.	Provides good cleansing action. Causes no known side effects. Is inexpensive.
Neomycin sulfate (Neomycin)	Wide-spectrum antibiotic in a 0.1% to 0.5% aqueous solution.	Bactericide used to decrease organisms before debridement and grafting.	Effectively combats most organisms. Can be applied easily. Is inexpensive.
Bacitracin with polymyxin B (Polysporin, Polycin)	Combination bactericidal ointment, effective on small burn areas.	Bactericidal for gram-positive and gram-negative organisms.	Is capable of minimal systemic absorption. Is aesthetically suitable for use on the face. Does not cause pain.
Merbromin (Mercurochrome)	Organic mercurial compound available as a solution or tincture.	Acts as a desiccating agent which promotes epithelialization.	Is not expensive. Aids epithelialization of small areas. Dries wound.
Sutilains ointment (Travase)	Proteolytic enzymes developed from *Bacillus subtilis* in a petroleum base.	Digests necrotic tissue, aiding escharotomies and debridement.	Aids initial debridement, before patient can tolerate surgical debridement. Can be easily applied.
Fibrinolysin and desoxyribonuclease, combined (bovine) (Elase)	Two lytic enzymes combined in a petroleum base.	Digests necrotic tissue, aiding escharotomies and debridement.	Doesn't require refrigeration. Has long shelf life.
Amniotic membrane	Biologic dressings from healthy mothers with normal deliveries.	Temporary wound dressing that helps reduce heat and water loss, eases pain.	Is not expensive. Can be prepared relatively easily. Prepares wound for grafting.
Pig skin	Split-thickness skin available in several useful forms.	Temporary wound dressing that helps reduce heat and water loss, eases pain.	Is easily applied. Is available in fresh, lyophilized, frozen, or freeze-irradiated forms. Prepares wound for grafting.
Cadaver skin	Human skin.	Temporary wound dressing that helps reduce heat and water loss, ease pain.	Easy to apply. Can be meshed so that it covers a greater area. Prepares wound for grafting.
Poly 2-hydroxyethyl methacrylate (Hydron Burn Dressing Kit)	Spray-on powder.	Establishes an environmental barrier to protect against exogenous microbial contamination.	Conforms precisely to the wound. Is flexible enough to permit moderate patient mobility. Does not support bacterial growth, yet permits fluid transmission. Causes no pain on application.

TABLE 5–13.   *(Continued)*

Disadvantages	Nursing considerations
Decomposes quickly and is short acting. Exerts limited antimicrobial action.	Add new solution to the dressings or change the dressings every 4–6 hours.
May cause ototoxicity and nephrotoxicity. Is absorbed systemically. Must be refrigerated and applied to patient ice cold.	Remove from wound after 24 hours to decrease systemic absorption. Monitor patient's temperature after application of cold solution. Order serum and urine creatinine tests to watch for signs of nephrotoxicity.
May cause itching, burning, or inflammation. Cannot be used for full-thickness burns.	Observe patient closely for signs of sensitivity, such as rash. Wash ointment off and reapply it every 8 hours.
Causes stains. Is not antibacterial or antiseptic.	Cover wound with nonadherent dressing to prevent sticking.
Increases fluid loss. Requires refrigeration. May cause bleeding. Irritates wound and sometimes surrounding skin. Is not bactericidal.	Patient must be stable enough for surgery after a few days so that digested wounds can be covered with membranes or grafted. Use with Silvadene, Sulfamylon, bacitracin, Neomycin, or Garamycin. Don't use with hexachlorophene, iodine, Furacin, or silver nitrate. Observe patient closely for signs of infection; change every 8 hours. Use on no more than 15% of the total burn surface at one time.
Causes sensitivity in patients allergic to bovine materials. Causes itching and burning. Requires preparation immediately before application.	Wait for the doctor to remove any thick, dry eschar before applying Elase. Observe patient closely for signs of infection. Change dressings daily.
May be difficult and time-consuming to apply properly.	Observe patient closely for signs of infection.
Is expensive. Not recommended for use on donor sites. May cause sensitivity reaction.	Observe patient closely for signs of infection and rejection.
Expensive. Unpredictable availability.	Observe patient closely for signs of infection.
Does not prevent oozing, so burn wound remains wet because of fluid loss. Does not prevent clothes and linen from sticking to the wound.	First spray the cleaned burn wound with a thin layer of polyethylene glycol 400 (PEG-400); then cover with thin layer of Hydron powder. Repeat above process two or three times; allow to set for 30 minutes. To remove, soak or peel off Hydron dressing.

From Schumann, L., and Gaston, S., Commonsense guide to topical burn therapy. Reprinted with permission from the March issue of *Nursing 79.* Copyright © 1979, Intermed Communications, Inc.

ii. Eliminates painful dressing changes.

(b) Disadvantage—patient must be placed in isolation.

(2) *Closed method*—pressure dressings applied to burned areas, particularly extremities. Table 5–13 shows an overview of current therapies, their advantages, and their disadvantages.

f. *Convalescent burn therapy:*

(1) *Tubbing and debridement*—

(a) Tub bath or Hubbard tank used to cleanse wound and remove soiled dressing.

i. Bath water body temperature.

ii. Loosen dressings so they will float off.

iii. Soak for 15–20 minutes.

iv. Encourage limb exercises.

v. Do not leave unattended.

(b) Removal of eschar (debridement) is done with forceps and curved scissors.

i. Sterile technique.

ii. Only loose eschar removed to prevent bleeding.

iii. Examine wound for infection, color changes, decreased granulation— report these changes immediately.

(2) *Wound coverage*—decreases chances of infection.

(a) Biological dressings:

i. Homograft—skin from another person (cadaver).

ii. Xenograft—animal skin applied with sterile technique after tubbing.

(b) Autograft—patient donates skin for wound coverage.

i. Types—free (unattached to donor site) and pedicle grafts (attached to donor site).

ii. Operative procedure performed under general anesthesia.

iii. Donor sites shaved and prepared in OR.

iv. Graft applied to granulation bed.

v. When several grafting procedures required, face, hands, and arms usually grafted first.

vi. Post–skin graft care includes:

• Rolling graft with cotton-tipped applicator to remove excess exudate, maintaining dressings, and aseptic technique using heat lamps to dry donor sites.

• On third to fifth day—graft should take on pink appearance if it has taken.

vii. To prevent contractures following grafting procedures, skeletal traction may be used.

viii. Elasticized bandages may be applied for six months to one year to wound site to prevent hypertrophy of scar tissue.

(3) *Psychologic assessment and interventions*—

(a) *Acute period*—severe anxiety, mental confusion.

i. Orient frequently to person, time, place.

ii. Maintain eye contact to help patient focus.

iii. Explain all procedures.

(b) *Intermediate period*—reactions associated with pain, dependency, depression, anger.

i. Use narcotics and sedatives to decrease pain.

ii. Explain reasons for various procedures.

iii. Use other patients as models.

iv. Maintain open, nonjudgemental attitude.

v. Maintain consistent approaches to care.

vi. Establish contract with patient regarding division of responsibilities.

vii. Encourage as much self-care as possible.

(c) *Recuperative period*—grief process reactivated. Anxiety, depression, anger, bargaining, as patient tries to deal with altered body image, leaving security of hospital, finances.

i. Encourage verbalization regarding changes in body image.

ii. Utilize psychiatric nurse practitioner, burn recovery group, to assist adaptation.

(4) *Follow-up care*—
  (a) Evaluate physical and psychologic parameters.
      i. Examine wounds for breakdown or contractures.
      ii. Make adjustments in braces, splints.
      iii. Physical therapy may be necessary for several months.
      iv. Interview patient privately—providing emotional support—refer as appropriate for more in-depth counseling.

Part D / HYDROGEN ION CONCENTRATION

PHYSIOLOGY

1. **Normal hydrogen ion concentration**—hydrogen ions (H^+) are normally present in body fluids but in far lower concentrations than other ions (0.00004 mEq/liter).

2. **Sources of hydrogen ion in the body**
A. Volatile H^+ of carbonic acid, which is formed during tissue metabolism.
   1. Circulates in body fluids as CO_2 and water.
   2. Excreted by the lungs.
B. Nonvolatile H^+, which is formed from oxidation of sulfur-containing amino acids and phosphoprotein residue or the production of organic acid.
   1. Daily dietary intake of balanced diet produces 50 to 100 mEq of nonvolatile H^+.
   2. Excreted by the kidneys.

3. **pH**—the *negative logarithm* of the hydrogen ion (H^+) concentration is usually represented by the symbol pH.
A. Increases in H^+ concentrations therefore reduce pH—*acidemia*.
B. Decreases in H^+ concentration therefore increase pH—*alkalemia*.
C. pH scale extends from 0 to 14, with 7 being neutral; that is, exact balance between number of hydrogen ions (H^+) and hydroxyl ions (OH^-).
D. pH of body fluids range from 1.0 (gastric juice) to 8.2 (pancreatic juice).
E. pH of blood is 7.4—slightly alkalotic (normal range 7.35 to 7.45).

4. **Biochemical reactions**—the basis for physiologic activity of the cell; dependent on optimum pH (hydrogen ion concentration).
A. Facilitates the function of enzyme systems.
B. Essential for the binding of oxygen to hemoglobin.

HOMEOSTATIC MECHANISMS THAT REGULATE H^+ CONCENTRATIONS IN THE BODY

1. **Buffers**—solutions of two or more chemical compounds that minimize changes in pH by combining with a strong acid or a strong base to form a weak acid or a weak base.
A. Provide the body's first means of regulation of hydrogen ion concentration.
B. Buffer systems of the body are composed of a weak acid and the salt of that acid.
   1. Bicarbonate buffer system:
      a. Consists of carbonic acid (H_2CO_3) and its salt, sodium bicarbonate ($NaHCO_3$).
      b. Buffers up to 90% of H^+ in the extracellular fluid.
      c. Concentration of these two chemicals is regulated by the lungs and kidneys.
         (1) CO_2 excreted by respiratory system.
         (2) HCO_3 excreted by the kidneys.
         (3) pH of blood can therefore be shifted up or down by the respiratory and renal systems.
         (4) Acid base status ultimately depends on maintenance of a 20:1 ratio of bicarbonate ions to dissolved CO_2.
   2. Phosphate buffer system:
      a. Composed of sodium diphosphate (NaH_2PO_4) and disodium phosphate (Na_2HPO_4).
      b. Abundant in cells and kidney tubules.
      c. Acts primarily in intracellular fluid.

2. **Respiratory regulation of hydrogen ion concentration**—the body's second line of defense against alterations in pH.
A. Carbon dioxide is constantly being formed by cellular metabolism; it is transported to the lungs in three forms:
   1. As dissolved CO_2 in the plasma.
   2. As sodium bicarbonate.
   3. As carbaminohemoglobin.
B. Increases in carbon dioxide concentrations in the body fluids lower the pH toward the acidic side.
   1. The respiratory center in the medulla is stimulated to increase the rate and depth of respirations.
   2. Increased rate and depth of respiration increases pulmonary ventilation, thereby decreasing carbon dioxide and returning pH toward optimum.
C. Decreases in carbon dioxide concentrations result in decreased pulmonary ventilation.
D. Respiratory system is limited in its control of hydrogen ion balance.

1. Can retain or excrete only carbon dioxide.
2. Can compensate only for temporary changes in hydrogen ion concentrations.
3. Can only partially correct deviations in pH.

3. Basis of kidney regulation of hydrogen ion concentration

A. Hydrogen ions are secreted by the proximal and distal tubules of the kidney.
B. Sodium reabsorption by the kidney tubules:
   1. For each sodium ion reabsorbed, a hydrogen ion or potassium ion is excreted.
   2. An increase in the concentration of hydrogen ions results in more hydrogen ions than potassium ions being exchanged for sodium.
C. Bicarbonate ion secretion:
   1. An increase in hydrogen ions (acidity) increases bicarbonate reabsorption in the kidney tubules.
   2. When relatively more bicarbonate is available than hydrogen ions (alkalinity), $NaHCO_3$ is excreted in the urine.

D. Ammonia—synthesized by cells of the proximal and distal renal tubules and collecting ducts.
   1. Ammonia (NH_3) diffuses into tubular lumen and combines with excess hydrogen ions to form ammonium (NH_4).
   2. Ammonium (NH_4) combines with chloride (Cl^-) or sulfate ions (SO^-_4) to form a neutral salt.
   3. Ammonia mechanism responds quickly to changes in pH and is capable of buffering large amounts of excess acid in a short period of time.
   4. Helps prevent tubular pH from falling below 4.5; hydrogen ion secretion ceases below this critical value.

IMBALANCES IN HYDROGEN ION CONCENTRATION

Table 5–14 provides an overview assessment of acid/base imbalances. Table 5–15 outlines how to interpret arterial blood gas values.

TABLE 5–14. *Assessment: imbalances in acid/base*

	Acidemia	*Alkalemia*
EXAMPLES	Acute renal failure, chronic renal failure, emphysema, tuberculosis, pulmonary edema.	Gastric/duodenal ulcers, hyperventilation.
ASSESSMENT OF ACID-BASE IMBALANCES		
Behavior	Lethargy, disorientation, delirium, stupor, coma.	Giddiness, belligerence, dizziness, convulsions, coma.
Neurologic	Hyporeflexia, muscle weakness, flaccidity ($\uparrow$ K).	Hyperreflexia, paresthesias ($\downarrow$ K). Carpopedal spasms, tetany ($\downarrow$ Ca).
Head/neck	Facial edema.	
Skin	Dry, flushed.	Pale, cool, moist.
GI	Anorexia, nausea, vomiting.	Paralytic ileus.
Respiratory	Decreased rate and depth ($\uparrow$ CO_2). Compensatory increase in rate and depth ($\downarrow$ HCO_3), distant breath sounds, rales, rhonchi.	Increased rate and depth ($\downarrow$ CO_2). Compensatory decrease in rate and depth ($\uparrow$ HCO_3).
Cardiovascular	Severe arrhythmias, cardiac arrest.	Irregular pulse, cardiac arrest.
Renal	Oliguria, anuria, acidic urine.	Alkalotic urine.
Extremities	Dependent edema, nail-clubbing.	Numbness and tingling in lips, feet, hands.

TABLE 5–15.   *Arterial blood gas interpretation*

1. If only the pH and one other parameter are abnormal, an uncompensated single disorder is present.

pH	PCO_2	HCO_3^-	Disorder
↓	↑	normal	Uncompensated respiratory acidosis.
↓	normal	↓	Uncompensated metabolic acidosis.
↑	↓	normal	Uncompensated respiratory alkalosis.
↑	normal	↑	Uncompensated metabolic alkalosis.

2. If the pH is normal but both the PCO_2 and HCO_3^- are abnormal, the values indicate a compensated single disorder.

pH	PCO_2	HCO_3	Disorder
Acid normal	↑	↑	Compensated respiratory acidosis.
Acid normal	↓	↓	Compensated metabolic acidosis.
Alkaline normal	↓	↓	Compensated respiratory alkalosis.
Alkaline normal	↑	↑	Compensated metabolic alkalosis.

3. If the pH, PCO_2, and HCO_3^- all are abnormal, they indicate an inadequately compensated single disorder or a mixed disorder.

pH	PCO_2	HCO_3	Disorder
↓	↑	↑	Inadequately compensated respiratory acidosis.
↓	↓	↓	Inadequately compensated metabolic acidosis.
↑	↓	↓	Inadequately compensated respiratory alkalosis.
↑	↑	↑	Inadequately compensated metabolic alkalosis.
Very ↓	↑	Slightly ↑ or ↓	Mixed respiratory and metabolic acidosis.
Very ↑	↓	Slightly ↑ or ↓	Mixed respiratory and metabolic alkalosis.

(Continued)

TABLE 5–15. *(Continued)*

3. If the pH, PCO$_2$, and HCO$_3^-$ are all abnormal, they indicate an inadequately compensated single disorder or a mixed disorder.

Slightly ↑ or ↓	↑	↑	Mixed respiratory acidosis and metabolic alkalosis.
Slightly ↑ or ↓	↓	↓	Mixed respiratory alkalosis and metabolic acidosis.

Key: ↑ denotes an increased value; ↓ denotes a decreased value.
From Holloway, N. *Nursing the critically ill adult.* Menlo Park, 1979, Addison-Wesley Publishing Co.

1. **Metabolic acidosis**—result of excess metabolic acid formation or abnormal loss of alkali (sodium bicarbonate) and is partially compensated for by respiratory hyperventilation.
   A. Loss of pancreatic, biliary, and lower bowel secretions—*severe diarrhea, draining fistulas.*
   B. Utilization of stored fats for energy—*diabetes mellitus, starvation.*
   C. Increased cellular metabolism—*hyperthyroidism, fever, tissue repair.*
   D. Severe tissue hypoxia—*congestive heart failure, shock.*
   E. Decreased excretion of metabolic wastes:
      1. *Acute renal failure*—broadly defined as rapid onset of oliguria accompanied by a rising BUN and serum creatinine.
         a. Pathophysiology—
            (1) Acute renal ischemia → tubular necrosis → decreased urine output.
            (2) Renal blood flow remains reduced after an acute attack due to:
               (a) Vasoconstriction mediated by juxtaglomerular apparatus, which reduces glomerular filtration.
               (b) Interstitial edema in kidney, which reduces filtration rate and collapses tubules by increasing the pressures in the interstitial spaces.
            (3) During the oliguric phase, waste products are retained → metabolic acidosis → water and electrolyte imbalances → anemia.
            (4) Recovery phase is marked by rapid diuresis → diluted urine → rapid depletion of sodium, chloride, and water → dehydration.
         b. Etiology—
            (1) *Prerenal*—occurs due to factors outside of kidney; usually circulatory collapse—
               (a) Hemorrhage, severe dehydration.
               (b) Myocardial infarction.
               (c) Septicemia.
            (2) *Intrinsic renal*—parenchymal disease of kidney.
               (a) Nephrotoxic agents:
                  i. Poisons, such as carbon tetrachloride.
                  ii. Heavy metals—arsenic, mercury.
                  iii. Antibiotics—kanamycin SO$_4$, neomycin SO$_4$.
                  iv. Incompatible blood transfusion.
                  v. Alcohol myopathies.
               (b) Acute renal disease:
                  i. Acute glomerulonephritis.
                  ii. Systemic lupus erythematosus.
            (3) *Postrenal*—obstruction in collecting system.
               (a) Renal or bladder calculi.
               (b) Tumors of bladder, prostate, or renal pelvis.
               (c) Gynecologic or urologic surgery in which ureters are accidentally ligated.
         c. Assessment findings—

(1) Subjective data:
  (a) Sudden decrease or cessation of urine output.
  (b) Anorexia, nausea, vomiting.
  (c) Abdominal bloating, hiccoughs.
  (d) Sudden weight gain.
(2) Objective data:
  (a) Vital signs—
    i. Blood pressure—decreased, elevated.
    ii. Pulse—tachycardia, irregularities.
    iii. Respirations—increased rate and depth, rales, rhonchi.
    iv. Temperature—normal, subnormal, elevated.
  (b) Central venous pressure—decreased, elevated.
  (c) Neurologic—decreasing mentation, unresponsive to verbal or painful stimuli, psychoses, convulsions.
  (d) Skin—dry, rashes, purpura.
  (e) Diagnostic studies—
    i. Blood—increased potassium, BUN, creatinine; decreased pH, bicarbonate, hematocrit, hemoglobin.
    ii. Urine—decreased volume and specific gravity, proteinuria, casts, red and white blood cells.
d. *Nursing goals* are designed to continually assess physical parameters and to provide emotional support.
  (1) Assessment of fluid and electrolyte balance and maintenance of nutrition:
    (a) Weigh daily.
    (b) Frequent monitoring of vital signs, CVP, and blood chemistries.
    (c) Parenteral infusions, as ordered—
      i. Blood: plasma, packed cells, electrolyte solutions to replace losses.
      ii. Restricted fluids if hypertension is present.
    (d) High-calorie, low-protein diet if tolerated.
      i. Hypertonic glucose solutions if oral feedings are not toler-

ated—prevent ketosis from fat metabolism.
      ii. Intravenous L-amino acids and glucose.
    (e) Control of hyperkalemia—
      i. Infusions of hypertonic glucose and insulin—forces potassium into cells.
      ii. Calcium gluconate (IV)—reduces myocardial irritability.
      iii. Sodium bicarbonate (IV)—corrects acidosis.
      iv. Polystyrene sodium sulfonate (Kayexalate) or other exchange resins, orally or rectally (enema)—removes excess potassium.
      v. Peritoneal or hemodialysis.
  (2) Utilize assessment and comfort measures to reduce occurrence of complications.
    (a) Respiratory system—
      i. Monitor rate and depth of respirations, breath sounds, arterial blood gases.
      ii. Encourage turning, coughing, and deep breathing.
      iii. Utilize IPPB as indicated.
    (b) Provide frequent oral care to prevent stomatitis.
    (c) Observe for signs of infection—elevated temperature, localized redness, swelling, heat, or drainage.
  (3) Maintain continuous emotional support.
    (a) Same care givers, consistency in procedures.
    (b) Give opportunities to express concerns, fears.
    (c) Allow family interactions.
2. *Chronic renal failure*—as a result of progressive destruction of kidney tissue, the kidneys are no longer able to maintain their homeostatic functions.
  a. Pathophysiology—
    (1) Destruction of glomeruli → reduced glomerular filtration rate → retention of metabolic waste products → increased serum urea → osmotic

diuresis and release of ammonia in skin and alimentary tract by bacterial interaction with urea → inflammation of mucous membranes.

(2) Retention of phosphate → decreased serum calcium → muscle spasms, tetany and increased parathormone release → demineralization of bone.

(3) Failure of tubular mechanisms to regulate blood bicarbonate → metabolic acidosis → hyperventilation.

(4) Urea osmotic diuresis → flushing effect on tubules → decreased reabsorption of sodium → excess sodium loss → depletion.

(5) Waste-product retention → depressed bone marrow function → decreased circulating RBCs → renal tissue hypoxia → decreased erythropoietin production → further depression of bone marrow → anemia.

b. Etiology—
(1) Polycystic kidney disease.
(2) Chronic glomerulonephritis.
(3) Chronic urinary obstruction, ureteral stricture, calculi, neoplasms.
(4) Chronic pyelonephritis.
(5) Severe hypertension.
(6) Congenital or acquired renal artery stenosis.
(7) Systemic lupus erythematosus.

c. Assessment findings as previously given, only gradual in onset and including ammonia breath, bronze-colored skin, and excessive fatigue and weakness.

d. *Nursing goals* in conservative management of chronic renal failure are designed to preserve renal function, reduce fluid and electrolyte imbalances, provide comfort, and postpone or eliminate the need for dialysis.

(1) See preceding guidelines monitoring fluid and electrolyte balance and maintaining nutrition and serum potassium levels—administer diuretics, as ordered—to reduce excess fluid volumes (Table 5–12).

(2) Employ comfort measures that reduce distress and support physical function.
(a) Bedrest in position that facilitates ventilation.
(b) Oral hygiene to prevent stomatitis

and reduce discomfort from mouth ulcers.
(c) Turn, cough, and deep breath q2h.
(d) Passive and active ROM exercises—promote venous return and prevents thrombi.
(e) Skin care with soothing lotions—reduces pruritus.
(f) Perineal care each shift.
(g) Encourage communication of concerns.

3. *Dialysis*—differential diffusion of solute through a semipermeable membrane that separates two solutions (Table 5–16).

a. Indications—
(1) Acute poisonings.
(2) Acute or chronic renal failure.
(3) Hepatic coma.
(4) Metabolic acidosis.
(5) Extensive burns with azotemia.

b. *Peritoneal dialysis*—involves introduction of a dialysate solution into the abdomen, where the peritoneum acts as the semipermeable membrane between the solution and blood in abdominal vessels.

(1) Procedures:
(a) Area around umbilicus is prepped, anesthetized with local anesthetic, and a catheter is inserted into the peritoneal cavity through a trocar; the catheter is then sutured into place to prevent displacement.
(b) Dialysate is then allowed to flow into the peritoneal cavity.
    i. Inflow time—10 to 20 minutes.
    ii. Two liters of solution are used in each cycle in the adult.
    iii. Solutions contain glucose, Na^+, Ca^{++}, Mg^{++}, K^+, Cl^-, and lactate or acetate.
(c) When solution bottle is empty, dwell time or exchange time begins.
    i. Dwell time—15 to 45 minutes.
    ii. Processes of diffusion, osmosis, and filtration begin to move waste products from blood stream into peritoneal cavity.

TABLE 5–16.   *Comparison of hemodialysis and peritoneal dialysis*

	Hemodialysis	*Peritoneal dialysis*
Speed	Rapid—up to 8 hours per treatment.	Slow—up to 72 hours initially, up to 12 hours per treatment thereafter. Can be advantage in patients who cannot tolerate rapid fluid and electrolyte changes.
Cost	Expensive.	Manual—relatively inexpensive; automated—expensive.
Equipment	Complex.	Manual—simply and readily available; automated—complex.
Vascular access	Required.	Not necessary, so suitable for patients with vascular problems.
Heparinization	Required; systemic or regional.	Little or no heparin necessary, so suitable for patients with bleeding problems.
Technical nursing skill necessary	High degree.	Manual—moderate degree; automated—high degree.
Complications (other than fluid and electrolyte imbalances common to both)	Dialysis disequilibrium syndrome (preventable). Mechanical dysfunctions of dialyzer.	Peritonitis. Protein loss (0.5 g/liter of dialysate). Bowel or bladder perforation.

From Holloway, N. *Nursing the critically ill adult.* Menlo Park, 1979, Addison-Wesley Publishing Co.

(d) Draining of the dialysate begins with the unclamping of the outflow clamp.

c. *Hemodialysis*—circulation of patient's blood through a compartment formed of a semipermeable membrane (cellophane or cuprophane) surrounded by dialysate fluid.

(1) Advantages:
  (a) Rapid and efficient procedure.
  (b) Long-term treatment feasible.

(2) Disadvantages:
  (a) Fluid and electrolyte derangement.
  (b) Requires specialized equipment and staff.
  (c) Requires heparinization and maintenance of a shunt.
  (d) May necessitate blood transfusions.

(3) Types of dialyzers:
  (a) Coil-type.
  (b) Parallel-plate.
  (c) Hollow-fiber.

(4) Types of venous access for hemodialysis:
  (a) External shunt (Figure 5–3).
    i. Cannula is placed in large vein and a large artery that approximate each other.
    ii. Shunt care:
      • *Daily cleansing and application of a sterile dressing.*
      • *Prevention of physical trauma and avoidance of some activities, such as swimming.*
    iii. External shunts, while providing easy and painless access to blood stream, are prone to infection and clotting and

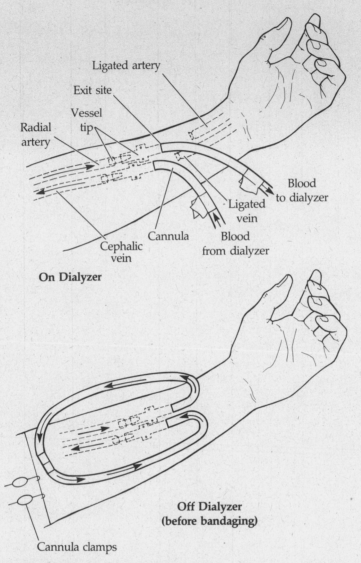

Ligated artery

Exit site

Vessel tip

Radial artery

Cephalic vein

Cannula

Ligated vein

Blood to dialyzer

Blood from dialyzer

On Dialyzer

**Off Dialyzer
(before bandaging)**

Cannula clamps

FIGURE 5–3. AV shunt (cannulae)
(From Holloway, N. *Nursing the critically ill adult.* Menlo Park, 1979, Addison-Wesley Publishing Co. Adapted. Used by permission of Ann Holmes, RN, Head Nurse, West Contra Costa Dialysis Clinic, San Pablo, California.)

cause erosion of the skin around insertion area.

(b) Arteriovenous fistulas (Figure 5–4).

   i. Large artery and vein are sewn together (anastamosed) below the surface of the skin.

   ii. Purpose is to create blood vessel that can relieve and receive blood.

   iii. Advantages of fistulas include greater activity range and no protective asepsis.

   iv. Disadvantage is necessity of

two venipunctures with each dialysis.

(5) Complications during hemodialysis:

(a) Disequilibrium syndrome—rapid removal of urea from blood → reverse osmosis with water moving into brain cells → cerebral edema → may cause headache, nausea, vomiting, confusion, and convulsions.

(b) *Hypotension*—results from excessive ultrafiltration or excessive antihypertensive medications.

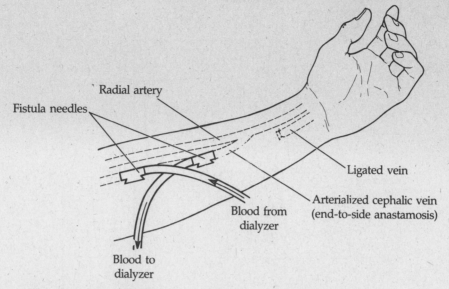

FIGURE 5–4. *AV fistula*
(From Holloway, N. *Nursing the critically ill adult.* Menlo Park, 1979, Addison-Wesley Publishing Co. Adapted. Used by permission of Ann Holmes, RN, Head Nurse Contra Costa Dialysis Clinic, San Pablo, California.)

(c) *Hypertension*—results from volume overload—water and/or sodium, causing disequilibrium syndrome or anxiety.

(d) Transfusion reactions (see Appendix B).

(e) *Arrhythmias*—occur due to hypotension, fluid overloads, or rapid removal of potassium.

(f) *Psychologic problems*—
  i. Patients react to dependency on hemodialysis in varying ways.
  ii. The nurse needs to identify patient reactions and defense mechanisms, and to employ supportive behaviors.
   • *Include patient in care, helping patient and family understand illness and treatment as much as possible; continuous repetition and reinforcement.*
   • *Do not interpret patient's behavior for them—for example, do not say, "You're being hostile" or "You're acting like a child."*
   • *Answer questions honestly regarding the quality and length of life with dialysis and/or transplantation.*
   • *Encourage independence as much as possible.*
   • *Identify family interactions and encourage family to verbalize concerns, fears, anger.*

2. **Respiratory acidosis**—result of alveolar hypoventilation; compensated for by increased hydrogen ion excretion by the kidneys (acidification of urine) and retention of bicarbonate (metabolic alkalosis). For the effects of abnormalities in lung volumes and capacities, see Table 5–5 and Figure 5–5.

A. *Chronic obstructive pulmonary disease (COPD):*
  1. Characteristics—
   a. Persistent obstruction of bronchial air flow.
   b. Chronic or recurrent productive cough.
  2. *Bronchitis*—inflammatory mononuclear infiltration in bronchial walls, which results in hypertrophy of mucus-producing globlet cells and destruction of cilia (see Section III for signs and symptoms, nursing care).
  3. *Asthma*—hypersensitive response of trachea and bronchi to various allergens; stimulates contraction of smooth muscle and increases bronchial secretions, which results in narrowed air-

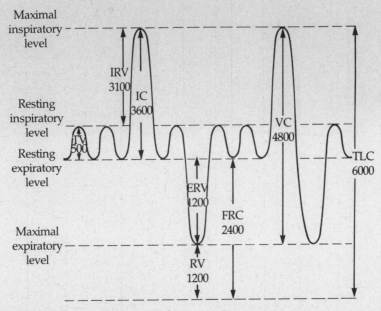

FIGURE 5–5. Lung volumes and capacities
ERV, expiratory reserve volume; *FRC,* functional residual capacity; *IC,* inspiratory capacity; *IRV,* inspiratory reserve volume; *RV,* residual volume; *TLC,* total lung capacity; *TV,* tidal volume; *VC,* vital capacity. (Based on data from Comroe, J.H., Jr., et al. *The lung: clinical physiology and pulmonary function tests,* 2nd ed. Chicago, 1962, Copyright © by Year Book Medical Publishers, Inc. Used by permission.)

ways filled with tenacious mucus (see Unit 4 for signs, symptoms, and nursing care).

4. *Emphysema*—enlargement of air sacs distal to terminal bronchioles with destruction of septum between alveoli.
   a. Pathophysiology—
      (1) Increased airway resistance during expiration results in air trapping and hyperinflation → increased residual volumes.
      (2) Increased dead space → unequal ventilation → perfusion of poorly ventilated alveoli → hypoxia, carbon dioxide retention (hypercapnia).
      (3) Chronic hypercapnia reduces sensitivity of respiratory center → chemoreceptions in aortic arch and carotid sinus become principle regulators of respiratory drive (respond to hypoxia).
      (4) Obliteration of capillaries owing to unequal ventilation, hypoxia, and acidosis → increased pulmonary vascular resistance → hypertrophy of the right ventricle → cor pulmonale.
   b. Etiology and incidence—
      (1) Smoking.
      (2) Air pollution.
      (3) Occupational hazards—fumes, dust.
      (4) More common among men than women.
   c. Assessment findings—
      (1) Subjective data:
         (a) Shortness of breath on exertion or exposure to cold air.
         (b) Wheezing.
         (c) Cough, may be productive.
         (d) Weakness.
         (e) Loss of appetite.
         (f) Weight loss.
         (g) Feelings of anxiousness.
      (2) Objective data:
         (a) Vital signs—
            i. Blood pressure—normal, elevated.
            ii. Pulse—tachycardia.
            iii. Respirations—tachypnea.
            iv. Temperature—normal, elevated.

(b) Respiratory system—
   i. Increased AP diameter of chest.
   ii. Diminished chest expansion.
   iii. Use of accessory muscles of respirations (pectorals) on inspiration.
   iv. Palpation—decreased tactile fremitus.
   v. Percussion—hyperresonance.
   vi. Auscultation—distant breath sounds, rales, rhonchi, wheezes.
(c) Skin—pale, cyanosis, nail clubbing.
(d) Diagnostic studies—
   i. Blood gases—decreased PO_2 (hypoxia), increased PCO_2 (hypercapnia) and bicarbonate levels (metabolic compensation).
   ii. Decreased chlorides.
d. *Nursing goals* are designed to promote optimal ventilation, reduce hypercapnia, and provide physical and psychologic comfort.
(1) Institute measures designed to decrease airway resistance and enhance gas exchange.
   (a) Semi-Fowler's position.
   (b) Oxygen with humidification—no more than 2 liters per minute to prevent depression of hypoxic respiratory drive (see Appendix E, Oxygen therapy).
   (c) Intermittent positive-pressure breathing (IPPB) with nebulization.

   (d) Assisted ventilation.
   (e) Postural drainage.
   (f) Instruction in breathing exercises, such as pursed-lip breathing and diaphragmatic breathing.
   (g) Medications, as ordered (Table 5–17).
      i. *Bronchodilators*—aminophylline, isoetharine (Bronkosol), isoproterenol HCl.
      ii. *Antibiotics*—determined by sputum cultures and sensitivity.
      iii. *Steroids*—methylprednisolone sodium succinate (Solu-Medrol), dexamethasone (Decadron).
      iv. *Expectorants*—acetylcysteine (Mucomyst), glyceryl guaiacolate (Robitussin).
(2) Employ comfort measures and support other body systems.
   (a) Oral hygiene prn.
   (b) High-protein, high-calorie diet to prevent negative nitrogen balance.
      i. Give small, frequent meals if patient fatigues easily.
      ii. Supplement diet with high-calorie drinks.
   (c) Push fluids to 3000 ml per day, unless contraindicated—helps moisten secretions.
   (d) Skin care—water bed, air mattress, foam pads to prevent skin breakdown.
   (e) Active and passive ROM exercises to prevent thrombus formation.

TABLE 5–17. *Drug therapies for respiratory acidosis*

Drug and dosage	Use	Action	Assessment: side effects	Nursing implications
BRONCHODILATORS				
Aminophylline— po, 250 mg, bid–qid; R, 250–500 mg; IV, 250–500 mg over 10–20 min.	Rapid relief of bronchospasm; asthma; and pulmonary edema.	Relaxes smooth muscles and increases cardiac contractility; interferes with reabsorption of Na^+ and Cl^- in proximal tubules.	Nausea, vomiting, cardiac arrhythmias, intestinal bleeding, insomnia, and restlessness.	Give oral with or after meals; monitor vital signs for changes in BP and pulse; and weigh daily.

(Continued)

TABLE 5–17.   *(Continued)*

Drug and dosage	Use	Action	Assessment: side effects	Nursing implications
Ephedrine SO₄— po, subq, or IM, 25 mg tid–qid.	Asthma, allergies, bradycardia, and nasal decongestant.	Relaxes hypertonic muscles in bronchioles and GI tract.	Wakefulness, nervousness, dizziness, palpitations, and hypertension.	Monitor vital signs; avoid giving dose near bed time; check urine output in older adults.
Isoproterenol HCl (Isuprel)— inhalation of 1:100 or 1:200 sol.	Mild to moderately severe asthma attack, bronchitis, and pulmonary emphysema.	Relaxes hypertonic bronchioles.	Nervousness, tachycardia, hypertension, and insomnia.	Monitor vital signs before and after treatment; teach patient how to use nebulizer.
ANTIBIOTICS				
Dia-mer-sulfonamides (Sulfonamides duplex), sulfisoxazole (Gantrisin), sulfamethizole (Thiosulfil), and sulfisomidine (Elkosin)	Acute, chronic, and recurrent urinary tract infections.	Bacteriostatic and bactericidal.	Nausea, vomiting, oliguria, anuria, anemia, leukopenia, dizziness, jaundice, and skin rashes.	Maintenance of blood levels very important; encourage fluids to prevent crystal formation in kidney tubules— push up to 3000 ml/day.
Penicillin— penicillin G, penicillin G potassium, and penicillin G procaine	*Streptococcus, Staphylococcus, Pneumococcus, Gonococcus,* and *Treponema pallidum.*	Primarily bactericidal.	Dermatitis and delayed or immediate anaphylaxis.	Outpatients should be observed for 20 minutes postinjection; hospitalized patients should be observed at frequent intervals for 20 minutes after injection.
Tetracyclines— chlortetracycline (Aureomycin), doxycyline (Vibramycin hyclate), oxytetracycline (Terramycin), and tetracycline HCl (Sumycin)	Wide-spectrum antibiotic.	Primarily bacteriostatic.	GI upsets as diarrhea, nausea, and vomiting; sore throat; black, hairy tongue; glossitis; and inflammatory lesions in anogenital region.	Phototoxic reactions have been reported; patients should be advised to stay out of direct sunlight and medication should not be given with milk or snacks, as food interferes with absorption of tetracyclines.

TABLE 5–17.   *(Continued)*

Drug and dosage	Use	Action	Assessment: side effects	Nursing implications
MUCOLYTIC AGENTS				
Entex—po 1 cap qid or adult 2 tsp qid	Bronchitis, bronchial asthma, sinusitis.	Decongests swollen mucous membranes, enhances flow of respiratory tract fluid, promotes ciliary action.	CNS stimulation with overdose.	Monitor vital signs, particularly in patients with hypertension, heart disease, diabetes. Contraindicated in patients receiving MAO inhibitors.
Acetylcysteine (Mucomyst)—1–10 ml of 20% solution per nebulizer tid	Emphysema, pneumonia, tracheostomy care, atelectasis.	Lowers viscosity of respiratory secretions by opening disulfide linkages in mucus.	Stomatitis, nausea, rhinorrhea, bronchospasm.	Observe respiratory rate; maintain open airway with suctioning as necessary. Observe asthmatics carefully for increased bronchospasm. Discontinue treatment immediately if this occurs.
EXPECTORANTS				
Ammonium Cl— po, 300 mg	Stimulate secretory activity of respiratory tract; diuretic	NH_4 ions cause gastric irritation, which reflexly stimulates respiratory tract secretions.	Nausea, vomiting, and bradycardia.	Monitor respirations; keep IV record to avoid dehydration and metabolic acidosis.
Ipecac—po, 0.5–1 ml, for cough; po, 15–30 ml for emesis	Bronchitis, bronchiectasis, emergency emetic for poison ingestion.	See *Ammonium Cl.*	Violent emesis, tachycardia, decreased BP, and dyspnea.	Contraindicated in liver and renal disease; if given for emesis, follow dose with as much water as patient will drink.
Potassium iodide— po, 300 mg tid–qid	Bronchial asthma, bronchitis, actinomycosis, blastomycosis, and sporotrichosis.	Reduces viscosity of bronchial secretions by stimulating flow of respiratory tract fluids.	Sore mouth, throat, conjunctivitis, headache, mental depression, ataxia, fever, and sexual impotence.	Administer diluted in milk or juice to decrease gastric irritation; observe for side effects and teach patient signs.
Terpin hydrate— po, 5–10 ml q3–4h	Bronchitis, emphysema.	Liquifies bronchial secretions.	Nausea, vomiting, and gastric irritation.	Administer undiluted; push fluids.

      i. Antiembolic stockings or Ace bandages may also be applied.

      ii. Increase activities to tolerance.

  (f) Provide rest and sleep periods—prevents mental disturbances due to sleep deprivation and reduces metabolic rate.

  (g) Provide emotional support for patient and family.

      i. Identify factors that increase anxiety:

- *Machines that take over bodily functions, fears of mechanical failure.*
- *Loss of body image, fears of dying.*
- *Families who deny illness or react with exceptional concern.*

      ii. Do not reinforce denial or encourage over-concern—give accurate, up-to-date information on patient's condition.

      iii. Be open to questioning and ascertain answers if possible.

      iv. Encourage patient-family communication.

      v. Provide appropriate diversional activities.

B. Decreased lung expansion—restrictive lung disease:

1. Characteristics—
   a. Decreased or asymmetrical lung expansion.
   b. Rapid, shallow respirations.

2. *Pulmonary consolidation (pneumonias)*—inflammation of lung parenchyma—results in air being replaced by exudates in the alveoli (see Section III, *Surgical Complications,* for patho-physiology, assessment findings, and nursing care).
   a. Etiology:
      (1) Gram-positive and gram-negative bacteria.
      (2) Viruses.
      (3) Fungi.
      (4) Protozoa.
      (5) Cancer.

3. *Pulmonary fibrosis*—excessive amount of connective tissue in all or part of the lung due to infections, noxious fumes, or aspirations, which cause inflammation and necrosis of tissue.

4. *Pulmonary abscess and cavitation*—tuberculosis invasion of lung tissue by tubercle bacillus.

  a. Pathophysiology:
    (1) Inhalation of *Mycobacterium tuberculosis* results in invasion of tissue and localized consolidation.
    (2) Infection spreads by way of lymphatics to hilus → antibodies are released → fibrosis → calcification or
    (3) Inflammation → exudate formation → caseous necrosis → liquification of caseous material → cavitation.

  b. Etiology and incidence:
    (1) *Mycobacterium tuberculosis.*
    (2) Greatly declined since beginning of century, although decline less rapid in past ten years.
    (3) Occurs more frequently in urban areas.

  c. Assessment findings:
    (1) Subjective data—
      (a) Loss of appetite.
      (b) Weight loss.
      (c) Weakness, fatigue, loss of energy.
      (d) Night sweats.
      (e) Fever—low-grade, frequently in late afternoon.
      (f) Cough—green or yellow sputum, bloody.
      (g) Knifelike chest pain (pleuritic).
    (2) Objective data—
      (a) Vital signs:
        i. Blood pressure—noncontributory.
        ii. Pulse—tachycardia.
        iii. Temperature—normal, elevated.
        iv. Respiration—normal rate and depth, increased rate.
      (b) Respiratory exam:
        i. Asymmetrical lung expansion.
        ii. Increased tactile fremitus over area of lesion.
        iii. Dullness to percussion.
        iv. Auscultation—rales following short cough.
      (c) Diagnostic studies:
        i. Chest X ray—infiltration, cavitations.
        ii. Blood—decreased RBCs, WBC within normal limits, elevated sedimentation rate.
        iii. Sputum—positive acid-fast smear and cultures.

iv. Positive tuberculin test.
d. *Nursing goals* are designed to reduce spread of the bacteria and to promote the patient's physical and psychologic equilibrium.
(1) Respiratory precautions—isolation may be ordered.
  (a) Avoid direct contact with sputum.
  (b) Teach cough and tissue techniques.
    i. Cough into tissue.
    ii. Place tissues in disposable container.
    iii. Have patient wear mask if unable to follow directions.
(2) Administer drug therapy (Table 5–18).
(3) Promote physical equilibrium.
  (a) Provide high-protein, high-calorie diet in frequent small feedings.
  (b) Force fluids.
  (c) Exercise to tolerance—avoid fatigue.
(4) Provide emotional support.
  (a) Include patient and family in teaching plan about disease process, diagnostic and treatment program, and communicability.
  (b) Encourage patient and family to verbalize concerns—many people still believe tuberculosis is a deadly disease.
  (c) Provide diversional activities and encourage communications with family.
(5) Refer to appropriate community health agency for follow-up.
C. Disturbances in pulmonary vascularity:
1. Characteristics—
  a. Exertional dyspnea, dyspnea, weakness.
  b. Chest pain may or may not be present.
2. *Pulmonary emboli and infarction*—occlusion of a pulmonary artery or arteriole by a substance, usually a blood clot, resulting in obstruction of blood flow and tissue necrosis (see Section III, *Surgical Complications*).
3. *Pulmonary edema*—sudden transudation of fluid from pulmonary capillaries into alveoli.
  a. Pathophysiology:
  (1) Increased blood hydrostatic pressures or increased pulmonary capillary permeability → increased filtration of fluids into interstitial space.

(2) As interstitial fluid pressures become positive, fluid begins to move into alveoli.
(3) Fluid accumulation in alveoli increases air-fluid interface → decreases compliance → decreases diffusion of gases → hypoxia and hypercapnia.
b. Etiology and incidence:
(1) Left ventricular heart failure due to hypertension, aortic valve disease, or myocardial infarction.
(2) Overinfusion of blood, dextran, saline.
(3) Renal shutdown.
(4) High altitudes.
(5) Silo-filler's disease (inhalation of corn gas).
(6) Transfusion reaction.
(7) Drug sensitivities.
c. Assessment findings:
(1) Subjective data—
  (a) Extreme shortness of breath.
  (b) Feelings of smothering.
  (c) Palpitations.
  (d) Sweating.
(2) Objective data—
  (a) Vital signs:
    i. Blood pressure—elevated, hypotension.
    ii. Temperature—normal, subnormal.
    iii. Pulse—tachycardia, pounding, thready.
    iv. Respiration—tachypnea, moist, bubbly, wheezing.
  (b) Skin—pale, cool, diaphoretic, cyanotic.
  (c) Respiratory auscultation—rales, coarse rhonchi.
  (d) Productive cough—frothy, pink-tinged sputum.
  (e) Distended neck veins and engorged peripheral veins.
  (f) Mental status—restless, anxious, confused, stuporous.
d. *Nursing goals* are designed to promote physical and psychologic relaxation, relieve hypoxia, retard venous return, and improve cardiac function.
(1) Institute measures to relieve anxiety and slow respirations.
  (a) Administer morphine sulfate, as ordered—reduces muscular and

TABLE 5–18. *Treatment of mycobacterial disease in adults and children*

Drugs	Dosage		Most common side effects	Tests for side effects	Remarks
	Daily	Twice weekly			
FIRST-LINE DRUGS					
Isoniazid	5–10 mg/kg up to 300 mg po or IM.	15 mg/kg po or IM.	Peripheral neuritis, hepatitis, hypersensitivity.	SGOT/SGPT (not as a routine).	Bactericidal; pyridoxine 10 mg as prophylaxis for neuritis; 50–100 mg as treatment.
Ethambutol	15–25 mg/kg po.	50 mg/kg po.	Optic neuritis (reversible with discontinuation of drug; very rare at 15 mg/kg), skin rash.	Red-green color discrimination and visual acuity.	Use with caution with renal disease or when eye testing is not feasible.
Rifampin	10–20 mg/kg up to 600 mg po.	Not recommended.	Hepatitis, febrile reaction, purpura (rare).	SGOT/SGPT (not as a routine).	Bactericidal; orange urine color; negates effect of birth control pills.
Streptomycin	15–20 mg/kg up to 1 g IM.	25–30 mg/kg.	Eighth cranial nerve damage, nephrotoxicity.	Vestibular function, audiograms; BUN and creatinine.	Use with caution in older patients or those with renal disease.
SECOND-LINE DRUGS					
Viomycin	15–30 mg/kg up to 1 g IM.		Auditory toxicity, nephrotoxicity, vestibular toxicity (rare).	Vestibular function, audiograms; BUN and creatinine.	Use with caution in older patients; rarely used with renal disease.
Capreomycin	15–30 mg/kg up to 1 g IM.		Eighth cranial nerve damage, nephrotoxicity.	Vestibular function, audiograms; BUN and creatinine.	Use with caution in older patients; rarely used with renal disease.
Kanamycin	15–30 mg/kg up to 1 g IM.		Auditory toxicity, nephrotoxicity, vestibular toxicity (rare).	Vestibular function, audiograms; BUN and creatinine.	Use with caution in older patients; rarely used with renal disease.
Ethionamide	15–30 mg/kg up to 1 g po.		GI disturbance, hepatotoxicity, hypersensitivity.	SGOT/SGPT.	Divided dose may help GI side effects.
Pyrazinamide	15–30 mg/kg up to 2 g po.		Hyperuricemia, hepatotoxicity.	Uric acid, SGOT/SGPT.	Combination with an aminoglycoside is bactericidal.

TABLE 5–18. *(Continued)*

Drugs	Dosage		Most common side effects	Tests for side effects	Remarks
	Daily	Twice weekly			
Para-aminosalicylic acid (aminosalicylic acid)	150 mg/kg up to 12 g po.		GI disturbance, hypersensitivity, hepatotoxicity, sodium load.	SGOT/SGPT.	GI side effects very frequent, making cooperation difficult.
Cycloserine	10–20 mg/kg up to 1 g po.		Psychosis, personality changes, convulsions, rash.	Psychologic testing.	Very difficult drug to use; side effects may be blocked by pyridoxine, ataractic agents, or anticonvulsant drugs.

*From Phipps, Long, Woods, eds.: *Medical/surgical nursing,* St. Louis, 1979, The C. V. Mosby Co.
Adapted from American Thoracic Society: Treatment of mycobacterial disease, ATS statement, Am. Rev. Respir. Dis. **115:**185–187, 1977.

respiratory activity; provides sedation.
  (b) Remain with patient and encourage slow, deep breathing; assist with coughing.
(2) Institute measures to relieve hypoxia.
  (a) Apply oxygen with mask.
  (b) Utilize IPPB with 100% oxygen.
    i. Reduces ventilatory rate.
    ii. Provides uniform ventilation.
    iii. Reduces venous return by replacing negative intrathoracic pressures with positive pressure.
  (c) Administer aminophylline, as ordered.
    i. Increases cardiac output.
    ii. Lowers venous pressures.
(3) Institute measures to retard venous return.
  (a) Rotating tourniquets.
  (b) High-Fowler's position with extremities in dependent positions.
  (c) Assist with phlebotomy, as ordered.
(4) Institute measures to improve cardiac function.
  (a) Digitalis, as ordered.
  (b) Diuretics, as ordered.
    i. Ethacrynic acid (Edecrin).
    ii. Furosemide (Lasix).
(5) Continuously monitor physical and psychologic parameters to assess effectiveness of therapies.
  (a) Vital signs.
  (b) Auscultate breath sounds.
  (c) Weigh daily.
  (d) Intake and output.
  (e) Mentation—restless, aware of time and place, not responding.
(6) Institute measures to support adaptive mechanisms.
  (a) Low-sodium diet (see Appendix A, Diets).
  (b) Fluid restriction, as ordered.
  (c) Exercise to tolerance.
  (d) Breathing exercises, oral hygiene.
  (e) Frequent rest periods.
  (f) Patient teaching.
    i. Involve family or significant other.
    ii. Medications—digitalis, diuretics:
      • *Pulse-taking.*
      • *Side effects.*
      • *Potassium supplements if indicated.*
    iii. Exercise and rest.
    iv. Low-sodium diet.

v. Symptoms of edema that should be reported to physician.

D. Disturbances of neurologic innervation of respiratory musculature:

1. *Poliomyelitis*—acute viral infection that attacks anterior horn cells in spinal cord and motor cells in brain stem and cortical levels; results in muscular fasciculations, painful tender muscles, and paralysis.

2. *Myasthenia gravis*—impaired transmission of nerve impulses at myoneural junction results in excessive muscular fatigability (see Part E, *Lower motor neuron lesions*).

3. *Tetanus (lockjaw)*—an infectious disease characterized by extreme stiffness of the body.

3. *Metabolic alkalosis*—result of an abnormal increase in bicarbonate or a decrease in hydrogen ion concentration; compensated for by hypoventilation and excretion of large amounts of sodium and potassium bicarbonate in the urine (alkaline urine).

A. Loss of hydrogen ion:
1. Vomiting.
2. Gastric suctioning (particularly with plain-water irrigation).

B. Increase in bicarbonate—excessive ingestion of alkaline drugs.

1. *Gastric and duodenal ulcers*—circumscribed loss of mucosa, submucosa, and muscle layer in areas of the digestive tract exposed to acid-pepsin gastric juice.

   a. Pathophysiology:
      (1) Imbalance develops between resistance of mucous membrane lining digestive tract and the secretion of acid-pepsin.
      (2) Increased vagal stimulation due to emotional factors (anger, resentment) or stimulants, such as alcohol, increase hydrochloric acid secretion and pepsin formation.
      (3) Increased sympathetic nervous system responses to emotional factors or stimulants, such as tobacco, decrease blood supply to gastric mucosa, thereby reducing its resistance to effects of acid-pepsin.

   b. Etiology and incidence:
      (1) Duodenal ulcer—
         (a) Stress and responsibility.
         (b) Competitive jobs.
         (c) Usually between 25 and 50 years of age.
         (d) Twice as many men as women.
         (e) Usually well nourished.
         (f) Increased acid secretion.
         (g) More frequently are in type O blood group.
      (2) Gastric ulcer—
         (a) Endocrine factors.
         (b) Emotional stress.
         (c) Usually over 50 years of age.
         (d) Four times as many men as women.
         (e) Often malnourished.
         (f) Normal to decreased acid production.
         (g) No differentiation in blood groups.

   c. Assessment findings:
      (1) Subjective data—
         (a) Pain:
            i. Type—dull, gnawing.
            ii. Location—midepigastric, back, may be to right or left upper abdominal area.
            iii. Duration—intermittent, continuous one to three hours after eating.
            iv. Relieved by ingestion of food or alkali.
         (b) Heartburn, belching.
         (c) Nausea, vomiting.
         (d) Tarry stools.
      (2) Objective data—
         (a) Diagnostic studies:
            i. Stools—positive for occult blood.
            ii. Upper GI series—outlines ulcerations in stomach or duodenum.
            iii. Gastric analysis—hyperchlorhydria or hypochlorhydria.

   d. *Nursing goals* are directed toward reducing stress and controlling gastric acidity.
      (1) Institute measures to reduce emotional and physical stress.
         (a) Bedrest—position of comfort.
         (b) Quiet, nonstimulating environment.
         (c) Plan procedure times with patient.
         (d) Allow time for verbalization of

concerns and encourage communication with family.

    (e) Restrict visitors who upset patient.

(2) Institute measures to control gastric acidity.

    (a) Insert nasogastric tube and attach to low intermittent suction—for nausea and vomiting.

    (b) Medications, as ordered (Table 5–19).

        i. Sedatives—phenobarbital, diazepam (Valium), chlordiazepoxide (Librium) HCl.

        ii. Anticholinergics—atropine SO_4, propantheline (Pro-Banthine) Br.

        iii. Antacids—magnesium and aluminum hydroxide mixture (Maalox), magnesium trisilicate and aluminum hydroxide (Gelusil), Mylanta, aluminum hydroxide gel (Amphojel).

    (c) Bland diet (see Appendix A, Diets).

    (d) Milk and cream therapy (Sippy diet) may still be ordered but is no longer considered central to therapy due to increase in serum lipids.

(3) Monitor effectiveness of therapy and observe for complication of ulcers (hemorrhage, perforation, pyloric obstruction).

    (a) Vital signs.

    (b) Stools for blood after each movement.

    (c) Hemoglobin levels.

(4) Promote emotional support through patient teaching.

    (a) Involve family and patient in diet-teaching and meal-planning.

    (b) Stress need to avoid stimulants, such as tobacco, alcohol, coffee, tea.

TABLE 5–19. *Antacids*

Drug and dosage	Use	Goals: action	Assessment: side effects	Nursing implication
Aluminum hydroxide gel (Amphojel)—po, 5–10 ml q2–4h or 1h pc	Gastric acidity, peptic ulcer, and phosphatic urinary calculi.	Buffers HCl in gastric juices without interfering with electrolyte balance.	Constipation and fecal impaction.	Shake well before administering; encourage fluids to prevent impaction and milk-alkali syndrome.
Calcium carbonate (Titralac, Ducon) —po, 1–2 gm taken with H_2O pc and hs	Peptic ulcer and chronic gastritis.	Reduces hyperacidity.	None known.	
Aluminum hydroxide and magnesium trisilicate (Gelusil)—po, 5–30 ml pc and hs	Peptic acid gastritis, heartburn, and esophagitis.	Neutralizes and absorbs excess acid.	Diarrhea and hypermagnesemia.	Avoid prolonged administration to patients with renal insufficiency.
Magnesium and aluminum hydroxides (Maalox suspension)—po, 5–30 ml pc and hs	Gastric hyperacidity, peptic ulcer, and heartburn.	Neutralizes and binds acids.	Constipation and fecal impaction.	Encourage fluid intake; contraindicated for debilitated patients or those with renal insufficiency.

(c) Encourage expression of feelings.
(d) Plan exercise and rest periods.
(e) Stress importance of ongoing medical care.

4. **Respiratory alkalosis**—occurs with excessive secretion of carbon dioxide and is compensated for by respiratory hypoventilation and retention of hydrogen ions by the kidney.
A. Hyperventilation—anxiety, hysteria, high altitudes, fever.
B. Aspirin poisoning—salicylates have a direct stimulating effect on the respiratory system, which results in hyperventilation and loss of carbon dioxide.

Part E/MUSCLE TONE

PHYSIOLOGY

A. Muscle tone is a state of continuous mild contractions of muscles—it is dependent on an intact nervous system and the inherent contractility and elasticity of muscle.
B. Muscle tone is clinically manifested by:
   1. Muscles that are resilient, not flabby, at rest.
   2. Muscles that will offer some resistance when passively stretched by a joint movement.

FACTORS AFFECTING MAINTENANCE AND CONTROL OF MUSCLE TONE

1. **The idiomuscular system**—the inherent elasticity, contractility, and extensibility of muscles themselves.

2. **The spinal cord**—lowest level of sensory integration is in the grey matter of the spinal cord.
A. Simple stretch reflexes, such as the knee-jerk, are mitigated through spinal-cord centers.
B. The spinal cord is capable of eliciting almost all the muscle movements required for posture and locomotion.
C. Coordination of these patterns, however, requires neuronal control by higher centers in the central nervous system.

3. **The reticular formation of the brain stem**—contains both excitatory and inhibitory centers.
A. Excitatory centers, when stimulated, increase muscle tone throughout the body or in localized areas.
B. Inhibitory centers, when stimulated, decrease muscle tone.
C. The excitatory impulses transmitted in conjunction with impulses from the vestibular nuclei provide the muscle tone needed by limb muscles to support the body against gravity.

4. **The basal ganglia**—consist of the striate bodies and the globus pallidus.
A. Have numerous nerve pathways to the cerebral cortex and reticular formation and among themselves.
B. Generally have an inhibitory effect on muscle tone through stimulation of specific areas; can elicit muscle contraction and patterns of movement.

5. **The cerebellum**—a deeply fissured structure located behind the brain stem.
A. It receives sensory fibers from the spinal cord and thalamus and has motor fibers to the basal ganglia, reticular formation, and cerebral cortex.
B. The cerebellum is principally responsible for the coordination and timing of movements.

6. **The cerebral cortex**—the highest level for control of muscle tone.
A. Frontal lobe of cerebral cortex gives rise to two motor tracts.
B. The corticospinal or direct motor pathway from the cortex to the spinal cord:
   1. Projects fibers down through the internal capsule to the medulla, where the fibers collect in bundles (pyramids).
   2. Prior to entering the cord, 75% to 90% of the fibers cross over and descend the lateral funiculus on the opposite side of the cord—control of limb musculature is largely contralateral.
   3. Initiates and controls discrete muscle movements; also facilitates or lowers the thresholds of anterior motor neurons.
C. The extrapyramidal tract—a functional rather than anatomic unit consisting of those motor nuclei and their fibers outside the corticospinal tract.
   1. Nerve fibers reach segmental levels in the cord after making a number of neuronal connections in the basal ganglia, subcortical ganglia, and reticular formation.

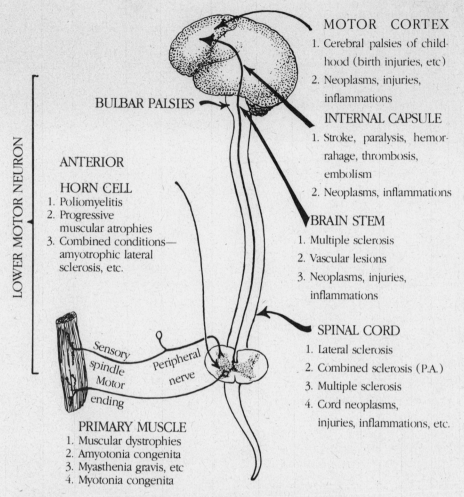

FIGURE 5–6. *Upper and lower motor neuron regions*
(From Chusik, J.G., *Correlative neuroanatomy and functional neurology,* 15th ed. Los Altos, Calif., 1973, Lange Medical Publications. Reprinted from Physiotherapy Review 16(2): 35–42, 1936, with permission of the American Physical Therapy Association.

2. Principally concerned with associated movements, postural adjustments, and autonomic integration.

IMBALANCES IN MUSCLE TONE

The two basic types of imbalance in muscle tone are hypertonia and hypotonia (Table 5–20).

1. ***Hypertonia (upper motor neuron lesions)***—rigid, spastic muscles that offer resistance to passive movement (Figure 5–6).
A. *Lesions of the cerebral cortex:*
   1. Electrical disturbances (*dysrhythmias*)—

a. *Epilepsies*—abnormal electrical activity that produces involuntary muscular contractions and disturbances of consciousness.
   (1) Pathophysiology:
      (a) Increased excitability of a neuron → may activate adjacent neurons → synchronous discharge of impulses → vigorous involuntary sustained muscle spasms (tonic contractions).
      (b) Onset of neuronal fatigue → intermittent muscle spasms (clonic contractions) → cessation of muscle spasms → sleep.

TABLE 5–20. *Assessment: imbalances in muscle tone*

	Hypertonia	*Hypotonia*
EXAMPLES	*Upper motor neuron lesions:* epilepsies, head traumas, increased intracranial pressures, encephalitis, cerebral vascular accidents, Parkinson's disease, multiple sclerosis.	*Lower motor neuron lesions:* spinal shock, myasthenia gravis.
ASSESSMENT OF MUSCLE TONE IMBALANCES		
Behavior	Alert, aware, mood alterations, confusion and disorientation, restlessness, irritability, stupor, semicoma, coma.	Alert and aware, mood swings.
Neurologic	Altered level of consciousness, pupils round, equal, react to light; unequal ipsalateral dilatation, bilateral dilatation, unresponsive. Hyporeflexia in acute situations, hyperreflexia, Babinski reflex, spastic, rigid muscles, nuchal rigidity, decerebrate posturing.	Weak, flaccid muscles, muscle atrophy. Depressed or absent reflexes. Decreased or absent pinprick, pressure and vibratory sensations.
Head/neck	Impaired or double vision, slowed, slurred speech, decreased expression.	Ptosis, diplopia (intermittent). Difficulties with mastication, decreased or absent facial expressions, high-pitched, nasal voice tones.
Skin	Noncontributory.	Absence of sweating.
GI	Nausea, vomiting.	Anorexia, abdominal distention.
Respiratory	Altered pattern, tachypnea, deep, sonorous, Cheyne-Stokes, bradycardia.	Tachypnea, shallow.
Cardiovascular	Gradual or rapid elevation of blood pressure, widened pulse pressure.	Normal, decreased (loss of vasomotor tone with decreased venous return).
Renal	Oliguria.	Urinary retention.
Extremities	Spasticity, gaits: ataxia, scissors, circumduction, propulsive paresis or paralysis.	Flaccidity, flaccid paralysis.

(2) Etiology and incidence:
   (a) Idiopathic or functional.
   (b) Brain injury.
   (c) Infection (meningitis, encephalitis).
   (d) Water and electrolyte disturbances.
   (e) Hypoglycemia.
   (f) Tumors.
   (g) Vascular disorders (hypoxia or hypocapnia).
(3) Assessment findings:

   (a) *Grand mal seizures—*
     i. *Aura*—flash of light, peculiar smell, sound, feelings of fear, euphoria.
     ii. *Convulsive stage*—tonic and clonic muscle spasms, loss of consciousness, breath-holding, frothing at mouth, biting of tongue, urinary or fecal incontinence.
     iii. *Postconvulsion*—headache, malaise, nausea, vomiting,

sore muscles, choking on secretions, aspiration.

(b) *Petit mal seizures*—

  i. *Momentary loss* of consciousness (10 to 90 seconds), fixation of gaze, blank facial expression.

  ii. *Loss of motor tone*—flickering of eyelids, jerking of facial muscle or arm.

  iii. *Postconvulsion*—patient resumes action previously being performed.

(4) *Nursing goals* in seizure conditions are designed to prevent injury, prevent recurrences, and assist patient in understanding condition and treatment.

  (a) Institute measures during seizure to prevent injury.

    i. Place soft object, such as padded tongue blade or handkerchief, between teeth—*Do not force* jaws open during convulsion.

    ii. Do *not* restrict limbs—support head, turn to side if possible.

    iii. Loosen constrictive clothing.

    iv. Note time, level of consciousness, and type and duration of muscle spasms.

    v. Postseizure care:
      • *Oropharyngeal suction as necessary.*
      • *Orient to time and place.*
      • *Oral hygiene if tongue or cheek injury.*
      • *Check vital signs, pupils, level of consciousness.*

  (b) Prevent or reduce recurrences of seizure activity.

    i. Encourage patient to identify factors that precipitate seizures.

    ii. Involve family in instructions, stressing moderation in diet and exercise.

    iii. Medications, actions, side effects (see Appendix D, Drugs):
      • *Phenobarbital.*
      • *Diphenylhydantoin (Dilantin) sodium.*
      • *Primidone (Mysoline).*
      • *Trimethadione (Tridione).*

    iv. Encourage patient to stay on medications and to have follow-up urinalysis and blood studies.

  (c) Assist patient in understanding condition:

    i. Encourage positive attitude toward life and treatment.

    ii. Attempt to clarify misconceptions and fears—especially about insanity, bad genes.

    iii. Encourage maintenance of activities, interests—avoiding stress.

    iv. Encourage use of Medic Alert band or tag.

    v. Refer to appropriate community resource.

2. *Traumatic injuries:*

  a. Types—

    (1) *Concussion*—transient disorder due to injury in which there is a brief loss of consciousness due to paralysis of neuronal function; recovery is usually total.

    (2) *Contusion*—structural alteration of brain tissue characterized by extravasation of blood cells (bruising); injury may occur on side of impact or on opposite side (opposite side when the cranial contents shift forcibly within the skull with impact).

    (3) *Laceration*—tearing of brain tissue or blood vessels due to a sharp bone fragment or object or a shearing force.

  b. Pathophysiology of impaired central nervous system function—

    (1) Depressed neuronal activity in cerebral cortex → impaired mental ability → inability to concentrate → forgetfulness → emotional instability → inability to interpret significance of sensations (agnosia) → loss of learned motor responses (apraxia).

    (2) Depressed neuronal activity in reticular activating system → depressed consciousness (Table 5–21).

    (3) Depressed neuronal function in lower brain stem and spinal cord → depres-

TABLE 5–21. *Levels of consciousness*

Stage	Characteristics
Alertness	Aware of time and place.
Automatism	Aware of time and place but demonstrates abnormality of mood (euphoria to irritability).
Confusion	Inability to think and speak in coherent manner; responds to verbal requests but is unaware of time and place.
Delirium	Restless and violent activity; may not comply with verbal instructions.
Stupor	Quiet and uncommunicative; may appear conscious—sits or lies with glazed look; unable to respond to verbal instructions; bladder and rectal incontinence may occur.
Semicoma	Unresponsive to verbal instructions but responds to vigorous or painful stimuli.
Coma	Unresponsive to vigorous or painful stimuli.

sion of reflex activity → decreased eye movements, unequal pupils → gradual dilation → decreased response to light stimuli → widely dilated and fixed pupils.

(a) Superficial and deep reflexes decrease → disappear → absent corneal reflex (eye does not close when touched) → decreased vasoconstriction → decreased blood pressure → circulatory collapse.

(b) Decreased muscle activity → vasomotor collapse → decreased body temperature → skin pale and cool.

(c) Depression of respiratory center → altered respiratory pattern (Cheyne-Stokes) → decreased rate → respiratory arrest.

c. Etiology and incidence—
   (1) Automobile accidents.
   (2) Industrial and home accidents.
   (3) Motorcycle accidents.
   (4) Military accidents.
   (5) Affects people of all ages.

d. Assessment findings—
   (1) Subjective data:
      (a) Headache.
      (b) Dizziness, loss of balance.
      (c) Double vision.

Nausea, vomiting.

(2) Objective data:
   (a) Lacerations or abrasion around face and head.
   (b) Drainage from ears or nose.
   (c) Projectile vomiting, hematemesis.
   (d) Vital signs—
      i. Blood pressure—elevated, decreased.
      ii. Temperature—elevated, decreased.
      iii. Pulse—bradycardia, tachycardia.
      iv. Respiration—tachypnea, bradypnea, Cheyne-Stokes.
   (e) Neurologic exam—
      i. Altered level of consciousness.
      ii. Pupils—equal, round, react to light; unequal, dilated, unresponsive to light.
      iii. Extremities—paresis or paralysis.
      iv. Reflexes—hypo- or hypertonia, Babinski's.
   (f) Inability to handle respiratory secretions.

e. *Nursing goals* are designed to monitor physical and mental status continuously and to employ measures to sustain vital functions and minimize or prevent complications.

(1) Respiratory system:
  (a) Maintain patent airway—endotracheal tube or tracheostomy may be ordered.
  (b) Oxygen, IPPB, as ordered—hypoxia increases dysfunction and promotes development of cerebral edema.
  (c) Position patient in semiprone or prone position with head level—improves gaseous exchange and prevents aspiration—*keep off back*.
  (d) Turn from side to side—prevents stasis of secretions in lungs.
(2) Neurologic system:
  (a) Vital signs.
  (b) Neurologic check—pupils, level of consciousness, muscle strength.
  (c) Report changes to physicians.
  (d) Maintain seizure precautions—padded tongue blade at bedside, padded siderails.
  (e) Medications, as ordered—
    i. Steroids—to reduce inflammation.
    ii. Phenobarbital or diphenylhydantoin (Dilantin) sodium to control seizures.
    iii. Analgesic—to reduce discomfort; morphine contraindicated.
  (f) Institute cooling measures or hypothermia for elevated temperature.
  (g) Assist with diagnostic tests—
    i. Lumbar puncture.
    ii. Electroencephalogram (EEG).
(3) Nutritional balance:
  (a) NPO for 24 hours, progressing to clear liquids if awake.
  (b) Maintain unconscious patients with parenteral infusions, nasogastric tube feedings.
  (c) Strict intake and output.
  (d) Monitor blood chemistries—disturbances of sodium balance not uncommon with head injuries.
(4) Provide emotional support and utilize comfort measures.
  (a) Skin care, oral hygiene, sheepskins, wrinkle-free linen.
  (b) Lubricate eyes, if periocular edema present, q4h.
  (c) Institute passive and active ROM exercise, physical therapy as tolerated.
  (d) Support during periods of restlessness—avoid restraints.
  (e) Encourage verbalization of concerns about changes in body image, limitations.
  (f) Encourage family communication.
f. Complications of head injuries—
  (1) *Increased intracranial pressures:*
    (a) Etiology—
      i. Cerebral edema.
      ii. Abscess or inflammation.
      iii. Tumor or other space-occupying lesion.
      iv. Increased production or blockage of cerebrospinal fluid.
      v. Hemorrhage.
    (b) Clinical indications—
      i. Altered level of consciousness.
      ii. Pupillary changes—unequal, dilated, and unresponsive to light.
      iii. Vital signs—changes variable:
        • *Blood pressure—gradual or rapid elevation, widened pulse pressure.*
        • *Pulse—bradycardia, tachycardia, significant sign is slowing of pulse as blood pressure rises.*
        • *Respirations—pattern changes, deep and sonorous to Cheyne-Stokes.*
        • *Temperature—moderate elevation.*
      iv. Complaints of headache, nausea.
    (c) *Nursing actions:*
      i. Report changes to physician at once.
      ii. Administer medications, as ordered:
        • *Hyperosmolar diuretics (mannitol and urea)—reduce brain swelling.*
        • *Steroids—antiinflammatory.*
        • *Antacids—prevent stress ulcer.*

- *Anticholinergics—prevent stress ulcer.*
  iii. Utilize cooling measures to reduce temperature elevations.
  iv. Prepare for surgical intervention as indicated.
  (2) *Subdural hematoma*—occurs as a result of torn or ruptured veins between the dura and brain.
3. *Inflammation of brain tissue:*
  a. *Meningitis*—acute inflammation of meninges characterized by severe headache, nuchal rigidity, irritability and restlessness (see Unit 4).
  b. *Encephalitis*—inflammation of the brain and its coverings.
    (1) Pathophysiology:
      (a) Brain tissue injury → release of enzymes increases vascular dilatation and capillary permeability → edema formation.
      (b) Edema formation in cerebral tissues increases intracranial pressures → depression of central nervous system function.
    (2) Etiology:
      (a) Syphilis.
      (b) Lead or arsenic poison.
      (c) Carbon monoxide.
      (d) Typhoid fever.
      (e) Measles, chicken pox.
      (f) Viruses.
    (3) Assessment findings:
      (a) Subjective data—
        i. Severe headache.
        ii. Sudden fever.
        iii. Nausea, vomiting.
        iv. Sensitivity to light (photophobia).
        v. Difficulty concentrating.
      (b) Objective data—
        i. Altered levels of consciousness.
        ii. Nuchal rigidity.
        iii. Tremors.
        iv. Facial weakness.
        v. Nystagmus.
        vi. Elevated temperature.
        vii. Diagnostic studies:
          - *Blood—slight to moderate leukocytosis.*

- *Cerebrospinal fluid— cloudy, increased neutrophils.*
    (4) *Nursing goals* are designed to support physical and emotional relaxation.
      (a) Vital signs and neurologic checks.
      (b) Institute seizure precautions.
      (c) Cooling measures as necessary.
      (d) Isolation is not necessary.
      (e) Administer mannitol or urea, as ordered—to reduce cerebral edema.
B. Lesions of the internal capsule, basal ganglia, pons, and medulla (Figure 5–6):
  1. Vascular lesions—
    a. *Cerebral vascular accident*—interference of cerebral blood flow; this ultimately results in ischemia and necrosis of tissue.
      (1) Pathophysiology:
        (a) Reduced or interrupted blood flow → interruption of nerve impulses down corticospinal tract → decreased or absent voluntary movement on one side of the body → fine movements are more affected than coarse movement.
        (b) Initially reflex activity that is normally facilitated by cortical centers is lost → later reflex centers begin to act autonomously → exaggerated tendon reflexes → increased muscle tone due to gamma efferent neuron activity → spasticity and rigidity of muscles.
      (2) Etiology and incidence:
        (a) Cerebral thrombosis.
        (b) Intracerebral hemorrhage.
        (c) Cerebral embolism.
        (d) Vascular insufficiency.
        (e) Highest incidence in elderly.
      (3) Assessment findings:
        (a) Subjective data—
          i. Weakness.
          ii. Sudden or gradual loss of movement of extremities on one side.
          iii. Difficulty forming words.
          iv. Difficulty swallowing (dysphagia).
          v. Nausea, vomiting.

(b) Objective data—
   i. Vital signs:
- *Blood pressure—elevated, widened pulse pressure.*
- *Temperature—elevated.*
- *Pulse—normal, slow.*
- *Respirations—tachypnea, altered pattern, deep, sonorous, Cheyne-Stokes.*

   ii. Neurologic:
- *Altered level of consciousness.*
- *Pupil inequality.*
- *Ptosis of eyelid, drooping mouth.*
- *Paresis or paralysis.*
- *Loss of sensation and reflexes.*
- *Incontinence of urine or feces.*
- *Aphasia.*

(4) *Nursing goals* are directed toward reducing cerebral anoxia, supporting vital functions, and promoting rehabilitation.

(a) Institute measures to reduce hypoxia.
   i. Maintain patent airway.
   ii. Oxygen therapy, IPPB, as ordered.
   iii. Bedrest—position to optimize ventilation.
   iv. Naso-oral suctioning as needed to remove secretions and prevent aspiration.
   v. Turn, cough, and deep breathe q2h.

(b) Institute measures that promote cardiovascular function and maintain cerebral perfusion.
   i. Vital signs.
   ii. Medications, as ordered:
- *Antihypertensives—prevent rupture.*
- *Anticoagulants—prevent thrombus.*

   iii. Parenteral infusions to prevent hemoconcentration:
- *Intake and output.*
- *Weigh daily.*

(c) Monitor neurologic parameters.
   i. Orient to time and place prn.

   ii. Identify grief reaction to changes in body image.
   iii. Maintain ROM exercises—prevent contractures, muscle atrophy, and phlebitis.

(d) Employ comfort measures to provide for physical and emotional relaxation.
   i. Skin care, assist with feedings, support with pillows when on side, utilize hand rolls and arm slings as ordered.
   ii. Involve patient and family, in establishing care plan:
- *Exercise routines.*
- *Diet and rest.*
- *Encourage resumption of care activities.*
- *Use of supportive devices.*

   iii. Encourage expression of feelings and concerns.

b. *Transient ischemic attacks*—temporary, complete or relatively complete cessation of cerebral blood flow to a localized area of brain, producing symptoms ranging from weakness and numbness to monocular blindness; an important precursor to CVA.

2. Degenerative diseases—
a. *Parkinson's disease.*
(1) Pathophysiology:
(a) Degeneration of basal ganglia and/or substantia nigra → decreased dopamine (neurotransmitter) → decreased and slowed voluntary movement → wooden facies → difficulty initiating ambulation.
(b) Decreased inhibition of alpha-motoneurons → increased muscle tone → rigidity both of flexor and extensor muscles → development of tremor at rest.

(2) Etiology and incidence:
(a) Unknown cause.
(b) Occurs in ages 50 to 65 years.
(c) Affects both sexes and all races.

(3) Assessment findings:
(a) Subjective data—
   i. Tremors of hands and feet.
   ii. Stiffness in legs and shoulders.
   iii. Loss of coordination—such as in writing.

    iv. Insomnia.

    v. Weight loss.

  (b) Objective data—

    i. Neurologic:

- *Gait—initiated slowly, then propulsive.*
- *Speech—slowed, slurred.*
- *Facies—wide-eyed, decreased expression, eye-blinking, excessive salivation, drooling.*
- *Limbs—stiff, offer resistance throughout to passive rotation.*
- *Tremor—pill-rolling of fingers, head movement to and fro.*

(4) *Nursing goals* are designed to be supportive and to promote maintenance of daily activities.

  (a) Levodopa therapy, as ordered.

    i. Given in increasing doses until patient's tolerance is reached.

    ii. Not a cure—decreases rigidity and dyskinesia (jagged, incomplete movement).

    iii. Take vitamin B_6 out of diet—it cancels effect of levodopa.

    iv. Side effects include nausea, vomiting, postural hypotension, mental confusion, arrhythmias.

  (b) Provide emotional and physical support.

    i. Encourage activity, physical therapy, warm baths, massage to relax muscles—avoid sitting for long periods of time.

    ii. Identify reaction to changing body image; allow for verbalization of feelings; encourage social activities.

    iii. High-protein, high-calorie, soft diet; assist with cutting of food if necessary; push fluids, small frequent feedings.

  b. *Huntington's chorea*—hereditary disease characterized by progressive dementia and bizarre involuntary movements.

3. Demyelinating diseases—

  a. *Multiple sclerosis*—progressive neurologic disease characterized by demyelination of the brain and spinal cord.

  (1) Pathophysiology (see CVA for pathologic description of corticospinal tract interference).

  (2) Etiology and incidence:

    (a) Unknown cause.

    (b) Affects males and females equally.

    (c) Onset between 20 and 40 years of age.

    (d) Greater incidence in northern latitudes.

  (3) Assessment findings:

    (a) Subjective data—

      i. Weakness.

      ii. Impaired, blurred, or double vision.

      iii. Difficulty in coordination.

      iv. Numbness in extremities.

    (b) Objective data—

      i. Motor system—decreased strength in muscles of lower extremities.

      ii. Decreased visual acuity, nystagmus, weakness of eye muscles.

      iii. Gait—ataxic-spastic.

      iv. Sensory—decreased sensation to pressure and pinprick, impaired vibratory sense.

      v. Mental status: emotionally labile, alteration in consciousness.

      vi. Marked by exacerbations, remissions over period of years.

      vii. Cerebrospinal fluid—protein count normal or slightly elevated, gamma globulin elevated.

  (4) *Nursing goals* are designed to maintain function as long as possible and to relieve symptoms.

    (a) Institute measures designed to maintain mobility.

      i. Muscle-stretching exercises.

      ii. Avoidance of fatigue, stress.

      iii. Encourage to sleep prone to minimize flexor spasms of knees and hips.

      iv. Encourage walking to tolerance.

v. Diazepam to relax muscles, as ordered.
(b) Institute measures to avoid injury due to loss of sensation.
i. Avoid temperature extremes.
ii. Teach to walk with feet wide apart to maintain balance.
(c) Institute *bladder training* to avoid urinary retention and infection—voiding schedule and manual massage if needed over pubic symphysis.
(d) Establish *bowel program*—
i. Regular meals and evacuation time.
ii. Glycerin suppository 30 minutes before scheduled evacuation time.
iii. Instruct to assume normal position bearing down with abdominal muscles—apply pressure with hand as indicated.
(e) Steroids during exacerbations, as ordered.
(f) Involve patient and family in care plans.
(g) Identify patient's defense mechanisms and assist with dealing with fears.
(h) Refer to appropriate community resource for follow-up care.
b. *Encephalomyelitis*—an acute process, characterized by symptoms related to damage of the white matter of the brain or spinal cord; may occur following such childhood diseases as measles or chicken pox or following vaccination for rabies or smallpox.

2. **Hypotonia**—weak, flaccid muscles that offer less than normal resistance to passive movement.
A. Lesions/injuries of the spinal cord (Figure 5–6):
1. *Spinal shock*—temporary flaccid paralysis and areflexia following a severe injury to the spinal cord.
a. Pathophysiology—
(1) Squeezing or shearing of the cord due to fractures or dislocation of vertebrae → interruption of sensory tracts → loss of conscious sensation.
(2) Interruption of motor tracts → loss of

voluntary movement → loss of facilitation → loss of reflex activity.
(3) Loss of reflex activity → loss of muscle tone → stretch reflexes → urine and fecal retention.
(4) If injury between *T*-1 and *L*-2 → loss of sympathetic tone → decreased blood pressure.
b. Etiology and incidence—
(1) Trauma—automobile or motorcycle accidents, falls.
(2) Inflammation in the cord (myelitis).
(3) Local restricted blood flow; tumor or protrusion of an intervertebral disk.
c. Assessment findings—
(1) Subjective data:
(a) Loss of sensation below level of injury.
(b) Inability to move extremities.
(c) Pain at level of injury.
(2) Objective data:
(a) Neurologic exam—
i. Absent pinprick, pressure, and vibratory sensations below level of injury.
ii. Absent reflexes below injury.
iii. Muscles—flaccid.
(b) Vital signs—
i. Blood pressure—decreased (loss of vasomotor tone below injury).
ii. Pulse—tachycardia.
iii. Respiration—increased rate.
iv. Temperature—elevated.
(c) Absence of sweating below injury.
(d) Urinary retention.
(e) Abdominal (bowel) distention.
d. *Nursing goals* are designed to support body functions until shock is reduced or relieved.
(1) Maintain patent airway—intubation and mechanical ventilation may be necessary with cervical-cord injuries.
(2) Monitor vital signs—administer blood transfusions and parenteral infusions, as ordered.
(3) Relieve bladder distention by inserting catheter that is attached to closed drainage.
(4) Relieve bowel distention with colon lavage or enemas.
(5) Maintain nutrition as tolerated; NPO

with intravenous infusions—high-protein, high-calorie, high-vitamin diet.
   (6) Prevent contractures—maintain proper body alignment.
   (7) Frequent skin care, turning (Stryker frame).
 2. *Amyotrophic lateral sclerosis* (Lou Gehrig's disease)—degenerative disease of anterior motor neurons.
B. Lesions in the muscle or disturbances in synaptic transmission:
 1. *Polymyositis.*
 2. *Dystrophies* (muscular).
 3. *Myasthenia gravis*—disease characterized by weakness and easy fatigability of facial, oculomotor, pharyngeal, and respiratory muscles.
   a. Pathophysiology—inadequate acetylcholine or excessive or altered cholinesterase → impaired transmission of motor impulses at myoneural junction.
   b. Etiology and incidence—
      (1) Possible autoimmune reaction.
      (2) Affects women predominantly, 20 to 40 years of age.
   c. Assessment findings—
      (1) Subjective data:
         (a) Drooping of an eyelid.
         (b) Double vision (intermittent).
         (c) Difficulty chewing food.
         (d) Choking on food.
      (2) Objective data:
         (a) Expressionless facies.
         (b) Easy fatigability of muscles.
         (c) Abnormal speech pattern with high-pitched nasal voice.
         (d) Respiratory studies (see Table 5–5)—
            i. Decreased vital capacity.
            ii. Decreased ability to deep breathe and cough.
   d. *Nursing goals* are designed to promote muscle function and provide physical and emotional relaxation.
      (1) Institute measures to promote motor function.
         (a) Anticholinesterase drugs, as ordered—neostigmine Br (Prostigmin), edrophonium Cl (Tensilon).
            i. Give with milk or crackers.
            ii. Always give at scheduled

time—20 to 30 minutes before meals (ac).
            iii. Side effects—nausea, vomiting, excessive salivation, increased muscle weakness.
         (b) Passive and active ROM exercises, increasing activity to tolerance.
         (c) Suction excessive oral secretions and keep tracheostomy set at bedside.
      (2) Institute comfort and safety measures.
         (a) Medications—
            i. Keep atropine SO_4 at bedside.
            ii. Morphine contraindicated.
         (b) Diet as tolerated—tube feedings, pureed, soft.
         (c) Oral hygiene after meals (pc) and prn.
         (d) Vital signs—check respirations q2h.
         (e) Keep call bell within reach—utilize paper and pencil for voice difficulties.
         (f) Skin care—sheepskins, back rubs.
         (g) Eye care—remove crusts, patch for affected eye, eyedrops.
         (h) Encourage independence and provide opportunities to express feelings.
      (3) Institute preoperative care if thymectomy is ordered.

Part F/SPECIAL SENSES

EYES

1. The blind patient

A. Blindness is legally defined as vision less than 20/200 with the use of corrective lenses or a visual field of no greater than 20 degrees.
B. Etiology and incidence:
 1. Glaucoma.
 2. Cataracts.
 3. Diabetic retinopathy.
 4. Atherosclerosis.
 5. Traumas.
 6. Greatest incidence after age 65 years.
C. *Rehabilitation goals:*

1. Institute measures that are designed to promote independence and provide emotional support.
   a. Familiarize patient with surroundings; encourage use of touch.
   b. Establish communication lines.
   c. Deal with feelings of loss and overprotectiveness by family members.
   d. Answer patient's and family's questions and make suggestions that can prevent accidents in the home.
   e. Provide appropriate diversional activities.
   f. Encourage self-care activities and allow patients to vent frustrations when unable to complete activities to their satisfaction.
2. Institute referrals to appropriate community resources.
   a. Voluntary agencies—
      (1) American Foundation for the Blind—provides catalogs of devices for visually handicapped.
      (2) National Society for the Prevention of Blindness—comprehensive educational program and research.
      (3) Recording for the Blind, Inc.—provides recorded educational books free on loan.
      (4) Lion's Club.
      (5) Catholic charities.
      (6) Salvation Army.
   b. Official agencies—
      (1) Social and Rehabilitation Service—counseling and placement services.
      (2) Veterans Administration—screening and pensions.
      (3) State Welfare Department, Division for the Blind—vocational.

2. **Acute and chronic glaucoma**—increased intraocular pressure.
A. Pathophysiology:
   1. Impaired passage of aqueous humor into the circular canal of Schlemm due to closure of the angle between the cornea and the iris (acute or closed-angle glaucoma) or local obstruction of aqueous between the anterior chamber and the canal (chronic or open-angle glaucoma).
   2. Imbalance between rate of secretion of intraocular fluids and rate of absorption of aqueous → increased aqueous humor pressures → decreased peripheral vision → corneal edema → halos and blurring of vision → blindness.

B. Etiology and incidence:
   1. Unknown, but associated with—
      a. Emotional disturbances.
      b. Hereditary factors.
      c. Allergies.
      d. Vasomotor disturbances.
   2. Affects 2% of the population over 40 years of age.
C. Assessment findings:
   1. Subjective data—
      a. Acute:
         (1) Severe pain in or around eyes.
         (2) Headache.
         (3) Halos of lights.
         (4) Blurring of vision.
         (5) Nausea and vomiting.
      b. Chronic:
         (1) Eyes tire easily.
         (2) Loss of peripheral vision.
   2. Objective data—
      a. Corneal edema.
      b. Decreased peripheral vision.
      c. Increased cupping of optic disc.
      d. Tonometry—pressures over 22 mm Hg.
      e. Dilated pupils.
D. *Nursing goals* are directed toward implementation of therapies designed to reduce intraocular pressures and toward patient education.
   1. Institute measures designed to reduce intraocular pressures.
      a. Bedrest—semi-Fowler's position; physical activity tends to increase pressures.
      b. Medications (see Appendix D, Drugs):
         (1) Miotics—pilocarpine HCl, carbachol.
         (2) Carbonic anhydrase inhibitors—acetazolamide (Diamox).
         (3) Anticholinesterase—demecarium Br (Humorsol); facilitates outflow of aqueous humor.
         (4) Contraindicated drugs—atropine—dilates pupils, obstructing aqueous flow.
      c. Provide emotional support:
         (1) Place patient's personal objects within field of vision.
         (2) Assist patient with activities.
         (3) Allow opportunities for patient and family to verbalize concerns, fears of blindness, loss of independence.
      d. Institute preoperative measures for iridec-

tomy (surgical removal of part of iris), as
ordered.

e. Involve patient and family in discharge
planning and teaching.

(1) Avoid activities and stresses that
increase intraocular pressures:

(a) Anger, excitement, worry.

(b) Constrictive clothing.

(c) Heavy lifting.

(d) Excessive fluid intake.

(e) Atropine or other mydriatics.

(2) Encourage activities that reduce intraocular pressures:

(a) Medications—purpose, dosage,
frequency: (*a*) teach eyedrop
installation and (*b*) caution to
have extra bottle in case of loss or
breakage.

(b) Moderate use of eyes.

(c) Moderate exercise—walking.

(d) Regular diet and elimination patterns; straining increases pressures.

(3) Safety measures:

(a) Medic Alert wrist band or tag.

(b) Ongoing outpatient care—refer to
community resources as necessary.

(c) Use other eye medications or
washes only with consent of physician.

EARS

1. The deaf patient

A. Hard of hearing—slight or moderate hearing loss
that is serviceable for activities of daily living.

B. Deafness—hearing that is nonfunctional for activities of daily living.

C. Etiology and incidence:

1. Conductive hearing losses:

a. Impacted cerumen (wax).

b. Foreign body in external auditory canal.

c. Defects (thickening, scarring) of eardrum.

d. Otosclerosis of ossicles.

2. Sensory hearing losses—

a. Arteriosclerosis.

b. Infectious diseases—mumps, measles,
meningitis.

c. Drug toxicities—quinine, streptomycin,
neomycin SO_4.

d. Tumors.

e. Head traumas.

f. High-intensity noises.

3. Greatest incidence over age 65 years.

D. Indications of hearing loss:

1. Inattentive or strained facial expression.

2. Excessive loudness or softness of speech.

3. Frequent need to clarify content of conversation
or inappropriate responses.

4. Tilting of the head while listening.

5. Lack of response when spoken to.

E. Rehabilitation goals:

1. Institute measures to maximize hearing ability,
support adaptive mechanisms, and provide
emotional support.

a. Evaluative studies—audiogram.

b. Establish communication system—

(1) Speech (lip) reading.

(2) Sign language.

(3) Hearing aid.

(4) Paper and pencil.

c. Provide a supportive, nonstressful environment.

d. Refer to appropriate community
resource—

(1) National Association of Hearing and
Speech Agencies—counseling services.

(2) National Association for the Deaf—
assists with employment, education,
and legislation.

(3) Alexander Graham Bell Association for
the Deaf, Inc.—serves as information
center for those working with the deaf.

(4) American Hearing Society—educational information, employment services, and social clubs.

Part G/CELLULAR MATU-RATION AND REPRODUCTION

PHYSIOLOGY

A. The process of cellular multiplication is called
mitosis.

B. Begins with duplication of genes and chromosomes.

C. Ends with the formation of two new or daughter
cells.

D. Phases of mitosis:
1. Duplication of centrioles—centrioles move apart and form spindles, which penetrate nucleus.
2. Prophase—dissolution of nuclear envelope.
3. Metaphase—chromosomes pulled to the center of cell.
4. Anaphase—chromosomes broken apart.
5. Telophase—two sets of chromosomes pulled completely apart and new nuclear membrane develops around each set; cells pinch in two, midway between the two new nuclei.
E. Homeostatic mechanisms controlling cell reproduction have not been specifically identified.

NORMAL CELL GROWTH AND REPRODUCTION

1. **Causes of cell growth and reproduction**—as a result of either an intrinsic or extrinsic stimulus.
A. Hemorrhage stimulates increased erythrocyte production.
B. Physical exercise stimulates increased skeletal muscle mass.

2. **Needs of the body**—cell growth and reproduction must be sufficient to meet the needs of the body.
A. Continuous replacement of worn-out cells.
B. Increased erythrocyte production at high altitudes.
C. Increased leukocytosis in response to infection and tissue destruction.
1. Venereal diseases—diseases that are acquired through sexual contact or congenitally.
a. *Syphilis*—
(1) Pathophysiology:
(a) Spirochete enters blood through mucous membrane via the lymphatics.
(b) Incubation 10–90 days.
(c) *Primary* lesion, chancre, occurs at site of entry and heals spontaneously in two to six weeks.
(d) *Secondary* phase, rash, appears about six weeks later and heals in two to six weeks.
(e) *Tertiary* phase is detectable only with serology testing.
(2) Etiology and incidence:
(a) Peak age group 20 to 24 years.
(b) Incidence higher in men.
(c) Caused by spirochete, *Treponema pallidum.*

(3) Assessment findings:
(a) Subjective data—
i. Chancre on genitals.
ii. Rash.
iii. Fever.
iv. Headache.
v. Weight loss.
(b) Objective data—
i. Primary:
- *Chancre—a painless, indurated ulcer on mouth or genitals.*
- *Lymphadenopathy.*
- *Positive VDRL.*
- *Spirochete visualized on dark-field examination.*
ii. Secondary:
- *Rash.*
- *Hair loss.*
- *Condyloma latum (moist, pink or gray-white lesion, highly infectious).*
- *Elevated temperature.*
iii. Tertiary:
- *80% asymptomatic.*
- *Ulcers in heart, lungs, bones, liver, and CNS from breakdown of gummas.*
(4) *Nursing goals* are designed to relieve symptoms, secure treatment for all infected persons, and educate the public.
(a) Case-finding and interviewing infected persons and their contacts.
(b) Nurse must maintain a nonjudgemental attitude to be effective.
(c) Education of the public:
i. Syphilis is a reportable disease.
ii. Prevention is the best way of combating the spread.
iii. It is important to obtain and continue treatment.
iv. The signs and symptoms of possible infection.
(d) Administer appropriate drug therapy:
i. Penicillin.
ii. Tetracycline.
iii. Erythromycin.
b. *Gonorrhea*—

(1) Pathophysiology:
   (a) Begins with local infection after three days' to two weeks' incubation period.
   (b) Bacteria can penetrate intact mucous membrane and set up inflammatory response (edema, redness).
   (c) If untreated, the bacteria spread throughout the reproductive system, causing strictures and adhesions in the recovery phase (which can lead to sterility).
   (d) Bacteria is drained off by the lymph system and into the blood stream, causing septicemia and spreading the disease to all areas of the body.
(2) Etiology and incidence:
   (a) Most common venereal disease.
   (b) Over 200,000 cases reported annually.
   (c) Caused by bacteria, *Neisseria gonorrhoeae.*
(3) Assessment findings:
   (a) Subjective data—
      i. Burning and pain on urination.
      ii. Yellowish discharge from urethra.
      iii. Fever, chills, and abdominal pain in women.
   (b) Objective data—
      i. Abscessed Skene's or Bartholin's glands.
      ii. Visualization of bacteria on gram stain or in culture.
      iii. Visualization of bacteria by means of immunofluorescence.
      iv. Elevated temperature, salpingitis.
(4) *Nursing goals* (see *Syphilis,* nursing goals.

2. Infectious diseases—diseases acquired from human, animal, or insect carriers.
   a. *Measles* and *chickenpox.*
   b. *Malaria*—chronic protozoan disease transmitted by *Anopheles* mosquito.
      (1) Pathophysiology:
         (a) Bite of *Anopheles* mosquito introduces the malarial parasite into blood stream.
         (b) Parasite invades, alters, and destroys red blood cells.
      (2) Etiology and incidence:
         (a) Protozoa of species *Plasmodium* are causative organism.
         (b) Incubation period of ten days to six weeks.
         (c) Endemic in many areas of the world.
      (3) Assessment findings:
         (a) Subjective data—
            i. Chills.
            ii. Fever.
            iii. Headache.
            iv. Muscle pains.
            v. Profuse sweating.
         (b) Objective data—
            i. Vital signs:
               • *Blood pressure—noncontributory.*
               • *Pulse—tachycardia.*
               • *Respirations—tachypnea.*
               • *Temperature—elevated.*
            ii. Splenomegaly, hepatomegaly.
            iii. Skin—urticaria; moist.
            iv. Attacks occur in paroxysms:
               • *Cold stage—rigor that lasts 20 to 60 minutes.*
               • *Hot stage—temperature of 104 to 107 F for three to eight hours.*
               • *Wet stage—profuse diaphoresis.*
            v. Diagnostic tests:
               • *Elevated sedimentation rate.*
               • *Demonstrable protozoa in peripheral smear.*
            vi. Decreased Hb, Hct.
      (4) *Nursing goals* are designed to eradicate the disease and provide symptomatic relief.
         (a) Assist with administration of chemotherapy.
            i. Chloroquine PO_4 (quinine).
            ii. Pyrimethamine.
            iii. Sulfisoxazole or sulfadiazine.
         (b) Provide warmth with blankets and clothing during the cold phase.
         (c) Provide linen and clothing change during the wet phase.

3. *The nature of cell growth*—cells produced should mature into normal functioning tissue.

4. *Decrease in cell production*—cell production should decrease when the demand or need for the cells ceases.
A. A decrease in adipose tissue results in a decrease in capillary beds.
B. Immobilization results in decreased muscle mass.

IMBALANCES IN CELLULAR GROWTH AND REPRODUCTION

1. *Inappropriate cellular production in response to intrinsic or extrinsic stimuli*
A. Intrinsic stimuli:
  1. Hormones—
    a. *Acromegaly*—a disease of excessive body growth.
      (1) Pathophysiology:
        (a) Tumor stimulates increased production of the growth hormone, causing continued growth and expansion of bones and soft tissue.
      (2) Etiology and incidence:
        (a) Eosinophilic adenomas of the posterior pituitary.
        (b) Rare disease.
        (c) Usually begins about third or fourth decade of life.
      (3) Assessment findings:
        (a) Subjective—
          i. Excessive growth.
        (b) Objective data—
          i. Coarse, heavy features.
          ii. Enlargement and broadening of hands, feet, and head.
          iii. Frontal sinuses become particularly pronounced.
          iv. Diagnostic tests:
            • *Increased basal metabolic rate.*
            • *Impaired glucose tolerance test.*
            • *Elevated plasma growth hormone.*
            • *Elevated serum inorganic phosphorus and alkaline phosphatase.*
      (4) *Nursing goals* are designed to alleviate the discomfort of therapy, prepare the patient for surgery, and provide emotional support.
        (a) Radiation therapy.
        (b) Pre- and postoperative nursing care (see Section III).
        (c) Physical changes are irreversible even with removal of the tumor, and patients need a great deal of support to accept their altered body images.
    b. *Dwarfism*—deficient thyroid, or growth hormone.
  2. Immunologic excesses—
    a. *Systemic lupus erythematosus.*
    b. *Glomerulonephritis.*
    c. *Hodgkin's disease*—believed to be an infectious or neoplastic disease of the lymph system.
    d. *Rheumatoid arthritis*—chronic inflammatory disease.
      (1) Pathophysiology:
        (a) Synovitis, which causes edema.
        (b) Various blood materials proliferate and form a pannus.
        (c) Pannus invades joint cartilage, destroys it, and replaces it with fibrous tissue (fibrous ankylosis).
        (d) Calcification of fibrous tissue (osseous ankylosis).
        (e) Follows a course of exacerbations and remissions.
      (2) Etiology and incidence:
        (a) Etiology unknown.
        (b) Onset at 20 to 40 years of age.
        (c) Seen more in women than men.
        (d) 2% to 3% of total population.
      (3) Assessment findings:
        (a) Subjective data—
          i. Vague pain or stiffness in joints.
          ii. Intermittent joint swelling.
          iii. Limited function.
          iv. Tires easily.
        (b) Objective data—
          i. Bilateral symmetrical involvement of joints.
          ii. Subcutaneous nodules over bony prominences.
          iii. Contractures.
          iv. Sjögren's syndrome, dry eyes and mouth and patchy hair loss.

(4) *Nursing goals:*
(a) Prevent or correct deformities.
   i. Active and passive ROM exercises; exercise even during acute phase.
   ii. Low-sodium, high-protein, high-calcium diet.
(b) Prevent complication from drug therapy.
   i. Instruct patients to report any tarry stools, since aspirin and steroids are an integral part of therapy.
   ii. Suggest antacids or milk as necessary for GI upsets.
   iii. Instruct patient to drink at least 1500 ml liquid daily to avoid renal calculi.
(c) Assist the patient in dealing with the psychosocial aspects of chronic illness.
   i. Altered self-image may lead to exaggeration or denial of disease.
   ii. Altered functioning may lead to change in life style.
   iii. Disease may necessitate retirement and cause financial hardships.
   iv. Loss of libido and/or satisfactory sexual relations.

B. Extrinsic stimuli:
1. Carcinogenic agents, such as nickle, ultraviolet light, viruses, cigarette smoking.
2. Habits and customs—
   a. Peptic ulcer disease.
   b. Hypertension.
   c. Chronic obstructive pulmonary disease (COPD).
   d. Black lung—coal miners.
   e. Byssinosis—textile workers.
3. Allergens—
   a. Asthma (see Unit 4).
   b. Migraine headaches.
   c. Contact dermatitis—acute skin inflammation caused by contact with external irritating factors.

2. Cellular production that is insufficient or excessive in relation to body's need

A. Anemia.
B. Polycythemia.

3. Nonhomogeneous cellular production that results in abnormal growth of new tissue

A. *Benign tumors:*
1. Neoplastic cells that resemble healthy cells.
2. Tumors that are well differentiated.
3. Papilloma, fibroma, adenoma, lipoma, and astrocytoma are examples.

B. *Malignant tumors:*
1. Bear little or no resemblance to tissue from which they arise.
2. Tend to be primitive.
3. Disorganized, poorly differentiated cellular growth.
4. Drain the nutritional resources of the host tissue.
5. Able to metastasize through lymph channels to other sites favorable to multiplication.
6. Adenocarcinoma, malignant melanoma, and fibrosarcoma are examples.

4. Nursing care in tumor reproduction

A. *Early assessment*—specific symptoms depend upon the anatomical and functional characteristics of the organ or structure involved.
1. *Mechanical effects:*
   a. *Pressure*—tumors growing in confined areas such as bone produce pain early, whereas abdominal tumors may go undetected for some time.
   b. *Obstruction*—tumors that compress tubular structures such as the esophagus, bronchi, or lymph channels may cause symptoms such as swallowing difficulties, shortness of breath, edema.
   c. *Interruptions* of blood supply—compression of blood vessels or diversion of blood supply into highly vascular masses may cause necrosis or ulceration or may precipitate hemorrhage.
2. *Systemic effects:*
   a. Anorexia, weakness, weight loss.
   b. Metabolic disturbances—malabsorption syndrome.
   c. Fluid and electrolyte imbalances.
   d. Hormonal imbalances—increased ADH, ACTH, TSH, or PTH.
3. Seven danger signals of cancer:
   a. Any sore that does not heal.
   b. Lump or retraction of skin in the breast or elsewhere.
   c. Chronic indigestion or swallowing difficulties.

d. Changes in color or texture of nevi.
e. Unusual bleeding or discharge.
f. Chronic hoarseness or cough.
g. Change in bowel habits.
4. Diagnostic procedures:
    a. Biopsy—excision of part of tumor mass.
    b. Needle biopsy—aspiration of cells from subcutaneous masses or organs such as liver.
    c. Exfoliative cytology—scraping of any endothelium (cervix, mucous membranes) and applying to slide.
    d. X rays, blood and urine samples.
        (1) X rays—detect tumor growth in GI, respiratory, and renal systems.
        (2) Alkaline phosphatase—greatly increased in osteogenic carcinoma.
        (3) Calcium—elevated in multiple myeloma, bone metastases.
        (4) Sodium—decreased in bronchogenic carcinoma.
        (5) Potassium—decreased in extensive liver carcinoma.
        (6) Serum gastrin—measures gastric secretions. Decreased in gastric carcinoma. Normal value—40–150 pg/ml.
        (7) CBC—complete blood count. Decreased Hct and Hb, increased white cell count.
            (a) Neutrophilic leukocytosis—tumors.
            (b) Eosinophilic leukocytosis—brain tumors, Hodgkin's disease.
            (c) Lymphocytosis—chronic lymphocytic anemia.
5. *Nursing goals and priorities:*
    a. Assist with diagnostic work-ups by providing psychologic support and information and by assisting with procedures when appropriate.
    b. Decrease anemia by providing well-balanced, iron-rich, small, frequent meals, administering supplemental vitamins and iron, and administering packed cells as ordered.
    c. Prevent hemorrhage by monitoring platelet count and maintaining platelet infusions.
    d. Prevent infection by observing for signs of sepsis (changes in vital signs, temperature of skin, mentation, urinary output, or pain) and administer antibiotics as ordered.
    e. Enhance nutrition by providing nutritional

supplements or maintaining hyperalimentation.
    f. Alleviate pain and discomfort by frequent position changes, diversions, conversations, back rubs, and narcotics as ordered.
    g. Reduce anxiety by listening to patient, referring special problems, supplying information, or correcting misinformation as appropriate.
B. *Nursing responsibilities in specific therapies:*
    1. Surgery—may be curative (lesion localized or minimal metastases to lymph nodes) or palliative (decreases symptomatology). (See Section III for individual surgeries.)
        a. *Preoperative nursing goals* are designed to reduce apprehension and support optimal outcomes.
            (1) Provide for nutritional deficiencies (diet, blood transfusions, vitamin and mineral supplements, hyperalimentation).
            (2) Assess learning readiness and provide emotional support.
                (a) Deep breathing techniques, care of ostomies or tubes, postoperative expectations.
                (b) Clarify questions for patient.
        b. *Postoperative goals* are designed to maintain optimal physiologic and psychologic functioning.
            (1) Monitor respiratory and hemodynamic status.
            (2) Prevent postoperative complications—wound care, passive exercises, respiratory hygiene.
            (3) Alleviate pain and discomfort.
            (4) Encourage early ambulation.
            (5) Maintain nutritional status.
            (6) Involve patient in rehabilitation program.
            (7) Prepare for further therapies such as radiation or chemotherapy.
    2. Radiation therapy—used in high doses to kill cancer cells.
        a. Types:
            (1) Electromagnetic—
                (a) X rays and gamma rays.
                (b) Substances such as Cobalt-60.
                (c) Products interact with cellular DNA, producing widespread disruption and damage.
            (2) Particulate—

(a) Alpha and beta particles and neutrons.

(b) Used where it can be directed into localized areas.

(c) Substances such as radium, radon.

(d) Causes more tissue damage than X rays or gamma rays.

b. Side effects of radiation therapy include nausea, vomiting, diarrhea, depression of bone marrow, suppression of immune response, decreased life span, and sterility.

c. External radiation:

(1) Usually cobalt or cesium.

(2) Patient placed in room alone during treatment.

(3) Patient told to lie still.

(4) Marks are made on skin to delineate area of treatment.

(5) *Nursing responsibilities*—

(a) Do not wash off marks; keep skin dry with baby powder or cornstarch.

(b) Reduce skin friction by avoiding constricting bedclothes or clothing. Use electric shaver.

(c) Instruct patient to avoid strong sunlight, extremes in temperature, synthetic clothes that are nonporous.

(d) Dress areas of skin breakdown with nonadherent dressing and paper tape.

(e) Provide meticulous oral hygiene.

(f) If diarrhea occurs—IV infusions may be needed.

(g) Monitor vital signs, particularly respiratory function.

(h) Monitor hematologic status—bone marrow depression can cause fatal toxicosis.

(i) Institute reverse isolation as necessary to prevent infections.

d. Internal radiation:

(1) Sealed—

(a) Usually radium or iridium applicators, seeds, molds, needles.

(b) Used for localized masses—mouth and cervix common sites.

(c) Exposure from source only—none from contact with patient, excretions, or linens.

(d) *General nursing responsibilities:*

i. Forewarn patient that nursing care will be limited to essential activities in postinsertion period.

ii. Maintain partial isolation, such as private room or room with patient with radium implant or patient who is past the childbearing age.

iii. Minimize exposure of self, patient's family, and other health professionals by maintaining distance and limiting exposure.

(e) Patient with *cervical radium implantation:*

i. *Prior to insertion*—give douche, enema, perineal prep; insert Foley.

ii. *After implantation*—check position of applicator q24h, keep patient on bedrest in flat or semi-Fowler's position to avoid displacing applicator (may turn to side for eating); notify physician if temperature elevates or nausea, vomiting develop (indicates radiation reaction or infection).

iii. Never handle radium directly—if applicators should accidentally be removed, pick up applicator by strings with long-handled forceps—notify radiation officer.

iv. After removal of implant (48–144 hours) patient given bath, douche and catheter removed.

(2) Unsealed radiation (radioisotope/radionuclide):

(a) Given orally, intravenously, or instilled into a cavity as a liquid.

(b) Patient's excretions now a source of exposure.

(c) Includes gold, iodine, phosphorus.

(d) *General nursing responsibilities:*

i. Know half-life, mode of administration, type of radiation emitted and manner of excretion of specific radionuclide.

ii. Isolate patient and tag room with radioactivity symbol.

iii. Specific precautions should be posted in chart and on door of patient's room.

iv. Personnel are rotated through patient care activities to avoid overexposure of individual staff members.

v. Maintain emotional support by encouraging family telephone contact, using intercom, planning diversional activities.

(e) *Specific precautions:*

i. Iodine—excreted in urine, saliva, perspiration, vomitus, feces. Wear rubber gloves and isolation gowns. Paper plates, eating utensils, and linen collected in impermeable bags and checked for contamination prior to disposal. *All urine* collected in shielded container and sent to lab to monitor excretion rate and disposal.

ii. Phosphorus—injected into cavity, turn patient q 10–15 minutes for two hours to assure distribution. Beta radiation, therefore no radiation hazard unless leakage from installation site. Seepage will stain linens blue—wear gloves when handling contaminated linens, dressings.

iii. Gold—usually injected into pleural or abdominal cavity. May seep from instillation site or drainage tubes in cavity. Prepared so it stains purple. Precautions as above.

3. Chemotherapy—used as single treatment or in combination with surgery and radiation, early and advanced diseases.

a. Types:

(1) *Alkylating agents*—act on DNA in the cell nucleus, hindering cell growth and mitosis.

(2) *Antimetabolites*—pyrine or pyrimidine analogs or folic acid antagonists, which interfere with the metabolic processes and protein manufacture in cancer cells.

(3) *Antibiotics*—interfere with RNA synthesis.

(4) *Plant alkaloids*—act by interfering with mitosis.

(5) *Enzymes*—deplete supply of essential amino acids in cancer cells.

(6) *Hormones*—alter hormonal imbalances that support hormone-dependent cancers.

b. Major problem of chemotherapeutic agents is that they lack specificity, thus affecting normal as well as malignant cells.

c. Major side effects include bone marrow depression, stomatitis, nausea and vomiting, gastrointestinal ulcerations, diarrhea, and alopecia.

d. *Nursing responsibilities:*

(1) Prior to therapy, establish baseline data on hematologic and nutritional status.

(2) Orient patient and family to purpose of proposed drug regimen and anticipated side effects.

(3) Advise that frequent checks on hematologic status will be necessary.

(4) Assist with treatment of specific side effects.

(a) Nausea and vomiting—small, frequent, high-calorie, high-protein meals; carbonated drinks; IV therapy; nasogastric tube; antiemetic drugs.

(b) Diarrhea—low-residue diet, Lomotil or Kaopectate.

(c) Stomatitis (painful mouth)—soft toothbrushes, mouth care q 2–4 hours, viscous Xylocaine.

(d) Alopecia—tourniquet around forehead for 10–15 minutes during and after infusion of drug; avoid hairbrushing; wigs, night caps, scarves should be used with caution.

(e) Monitor hematologic status—if WBC falls below 2000 ml^3, institute reverse isolation to prevent infection, install laminar air flow unit.

4. Immunotherapy:

a. Relatively new treatment modality whose goal is to stimulate the body's defense mechanism to attack and reject malignant cells.

   b. Immuno-surveys used to assess patient's immune status (serum antibody blocking titer and/or hypersensitive skin reactions).

   c. Used with small tumor masses and cancer cells.

   d. BCG (Bacille Calmette-Guérin) vaccine has been used with some patients.

      (1) Administered intravenously or more commonly by scarification.

      (2) Skin deeply lacerated five times and BCG dropped into open skin and covered with plastic film.

      (3) Area kept dry and covered for 24 hours, after which it may be gently washed.

      (4) Side effects include influenza-like symptoms—aching, fever, malaise.

      (5) Watch specifically for anaphylactic reactions.

C. Terminal or late phase of malignancy—treatment modalities have been ineffective in the control of disease process, and symptoms increase in severity.

   1. Physical findings:

      a. Cachexia—progressive weakness, wasting, and weight loss.

      b. Anemia, leukopenia, thrombocytopenia.

      c. Anorexia, gastrointestinal disturbances, constipation.

      d. Tissue breakdown leading to decubiti, seeping wounds.

      e. Urine retention, incontinence, renal calculi.

      f. Hypercalcemia occurs in 10% to 30% of patients.

      g. Pain due to tumor growth or secondarily to complications such as decubiti, stiffened joints, stomatitis.

   2. *Nursing management* of the terminally ill patient is directed toward making the patient physically and psychologically as comfortable as possible.

      a. Nutrition—high-calorie, high-protein diet; small, frequent meals; blenderized or strained commercial protein supplements (Vivomex, Sustagen).

      b. Assist patient to engage in self-care to tolerance.

      c. Prevent tissue breakdown and vascular complications by frequent turning, skin massage, air mattresses, active and passive range-of-motion exercises.

   d. Observe for toxic reactions to therapy, particularly diarrhea.

   e. Utilize supportive measures and drugs for pain relief:

      (1) Codeine, Percodan, Talwin, morphine.

      (2) Brompton mixture.

      (3) Diamorphine.

   f. Maintain open communication with patient and family.

      (1) Listen and observe nonverbal communication.

      (2) Assist patient to maintain self-esteem and identity.

      (3) Encourage active patient participation in aspects of care.

Section III / NURSING ACTIONS IN COMMON SURGICAL PROBLEMS AND EMERGENCY PROCEDURES

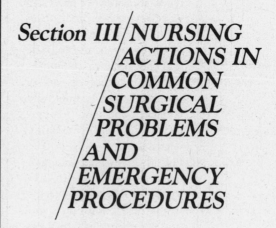

Part A / PREPARING THE PATIENT FOR SURGERY

PHYSICAL AND MENTAL ASSESSMENT

1. **Legal aspects**—all surgical procedures, however minor, cannot proceed without the voluntary, informed, and written consent of the patient.

A. Surgical permits are witnessed by the physician, nurse, or other authorized person.

B. Surgical permits protect the patient against unsanctioned surgery and also protect the surgeon and hospital staff against claims of unauthorized operations.

C. Informed consent means that the operation has been fully explained to the patient, including possible complications and disfigurements, as well as whether any organ or parts of the body are to be removed.

D. Adults and emancipated minors may sign their own operative permits if they are mentally competent; permission for surgery of minor children and incompetent or unconscious adults must be obtained from a responsible family member or guardian.

E. The signed operative permit is placed in a prominent place on the patient's chart and accompanies the patient to the operating room.

2. **Preparatory and preventive teaching**—purpose is to reduce preoperative and intraoperative anxiety as well as to prevent postoperative complications.

A. *Preoperative teaching assessment:*

1. Understanding of proposed surgery—site, type, extent of hospitalization, postoperative limitations, diagnostic tests prior to surgery.
   a. Provide information about hospital and nursing routines—reduce fear of the unknown.
   b. Explain purpose of diagnostic procedures—knowledge enhances patient's ability to cooperate with and tolerate uncomfortable procedures.
2. Previous experiences with hospitalization—type, nature of dysfunction, length of time.
3. Concerns or feelings about surgery—encourage patient to ask questions and express concerns. Allows nurse to assess and intervene in common misconceptions and fears:
   a. Exaggerated ideas of surgical risk and disability, such as fear of colostomy when none is being considered.
   b. Nature of anesthesia, such as fears of going to sleep and not waking up, of saying or revealing things of a personal nature, or of postoperative nausea and vomiting.
   c. Degree of pain, such as fear that pain may be incapacitating or that patient will not be able to handle it well.
   d. Misunderstandings regarding prognosis—patient may read into physician's statements or gestures and assume the worst.
4. Identification of significant others—may also be included in preoperative teaching plan as a source of patient support and/or may have major care responsibilities in postdischarge period.

B. *Preoperative teaching strategies and content:*

1. Provide rationale for preoperative teaching of how surgery will affect patient in postoperative period. Keep explanations simple.
2. Tell patient what will occur and what will be expected of him or her in the postoperative period:
   a. Will be returned to room, recovery room or intensive-care unit.
   b. Special equipment—monitors, tubes, suction equipment.
3. Instruct in exercises to reduce complications.
   a. Diaphragmatic breathing—refers to flattening of diaphragm during inspiration, which results in enlargement of upper abdomen; during expiration the abdominal muscles are contracted, along with the diaphragm.
      (1) The patient should be in a flat, semi-Fowler's, or side position with knees flexed and hands on the midabdomen.
      (2) Have the patient take a deep breath through the nose and mouth, letting the abdomen rise.
      (3) Have the patient exhale through the nose and mouth, squeezing out all the air by contracting the abdominal muscles.
      (4) Repeat 10 to 15 times with a short rest after each five to prevent hyperventilation.
      (5) Inform the patient that this exercise will be repeated five to ten times every hour postoperatively.
   b. Coughing—helps clear chest of secretions and, although uncomfortable, will not harm incision site.
      (1) Have the patient lean forward slightly from a sitting position and place the patient's hands over the incisional site; this acts as a splint during coughing.
      (2) Have the patient inhale and exhale several times.
      (3) Have the patient inhale deeply and cough sharply three times—the patient's mouth should be slightly open.
      (4) Tell the patient to inhale again and to cough deeply once or twice.
   c. Turning and leg exercises—help prevent circulatory stasis, which may lead to thrombus formation and postoperative flatus or "gas pains" as well as respiratory problems.
      (1) Tell the patient to turn on one side

with the upper-most leg flexed; use siderails to facilitate the movement.

(2) In a supine position, have the patient bend the knee and lift the foot; this position should be held for a few seconds, then the leg should be extended and lowered; repeat five times, and do the same with the other leg.

(3) Teach the patient to move each foot through full range of motion.

C. Outcome criteria for preoperative teaching:
1. Patient is able to relate events that will occur.
2. Patient is able to identify concerns; is less apprehensive.
3. Patient is able to explain and demonstrate postoperative exercises.
4. Significant other is able to relate events, explain postoperative exercises, identify own concerns.

3. **Preparing the patient's skin**—the purpose of the bath and skin preparation is to reduce the number of bacteria on the skin so as to eliminate the transference of these bacteria into the incision.

A. The area of the skin prep is always wider and longer than the proposed incision in case a larger incision is necessary.

B. The area is gently scrubbed with an antiseptic agent such as Betadine.
1. Soap containing hexachlorophene should be left on the skin for five to ten minutes.
2. When benzalkonium (Zephiran) Cl solution is ordered, do not soap the skin prior to use; soap reduces the effectiveness of Zephiran by causing it to precipitate.

C. A clean safety razor with a new blade should be used; shave against the grain of the hair shaft.

D. Any nicks, cuts, or irritations should be noted; these are potential infection sites.

E. Depilatory creams may also be employed—these are left on the skin for ten minutes, then washed off along with the hair; transient rashes are an occasional side effect with their use.

4. **Preparing the patient's gastrointestinal tract**—the purpose of this preparation is to reduce the risk of vomiting and aspiration during anesthesia and to prevent contamination of abdominal operative sites by fecal material.

A. *Food and fluid restriction:*
1. Food generally remains in the stomach for six hours after ingestion.
2. Fluids pass far more quickly into the duodenum;

but to ensure an empty stomach, fluids are withheld for at least four hours prior to surgery.

3. *Nursing measures* include—
a. Telling the patient why no food or fluid is allowed.
b. Removing food and water from the bedside.
c. Placing NPO signs on patient's bed or door.
d. Informing the kitchen and the oncoming nursing staff that the patient is NPO in preparation for surgery.

4. Patients who are dehydrated or malnourished may receive IV infusions up to the time of surgery.

B. *Enemas:*
1. An empty bowel is essential to prevent contamination when the proposed surgery involves the intestinal tract and colon; generally two or three enemas are given the evening prior to surgery.
2. Enemas may also be ordered preoperatively if the surgical procedure involves a pelvic organ— an empty bowel enhances the exposure of the operative field and reduces the possibility of injury to the bowel.
3. Surgeries involving the large intestine are usually preceded by three days of bowel cleansing and antibiotic therapy to reduce the colonic flora.
4. *Nursing measures* are designed to maximize the effectiveness of bowel-cleansing and to minimize the physiologic and psychologic discomfort to the patient.

C. *Gastric or intestinal intubation:*
1. Gastric or intestinal tubes may be inserted the evening prior to major abdominal surgery to remove stomach and intestinal contents or to reduce intestinal dilatation.
2. Decompression is accomplished by these tubes when suction is applied.
a. A single-lumen Levin tube is sufficient to remove fluids and gas from the stomach.
b. A long single- or double-lumen tube (Miller-Abbott) is required to remove the contents of the jejunum or ileum.
3. Abdominal suction pressures should not exceed 1.5 pounds of negative pressure—excessive pressures will result in injury to the mucosal lining of the intestine or stomach.

5. **Sleep and relaxation**—the evening prior to surgery a barbiturate such as pentobarbital sodium (Nembutal) 0.05 to 0.1 g or secobarbital (Seconal)

sodium 0.1 to 0.2 g are ordered by the physician to ensure that the patient sleeps well and to facilitate reduction of apprehension.

Part B | THE DAY OF SURGERY

1. The staff nurse's responsibilities

A. Be sure that the operative permit has been signed.
B. Have the patient shower or bathe or see that it is done.
   1. Dress the patient in hospital pajamas.
   2. Remove hair pins and cover hair.
   3. Remove nail polish—facilitates observation of peripheral perfusion.
   4. Remove all jewelry and tape wedding bands securely.
   5. Remove pierced earrings and contact lenses.
   6. Remove and store dentures and give mouth care.
C. Check to see that the patient is wearing the proper identification.
D. Identify relatives or friends who will be awaiting information during the procedure.
E. Take the patient's vital signs.
F. Have the patient void—prevents distention and possible injury to the bladder.
G. Administer the preoperative medication—purpose is to reduce patient anxiety to ensure smooth induction and maintenance of anesthesia.
   1. Should be administered 45 to 75 minutes before anesthetic induction.
   2. Siderails should be raised, as the patient will begin to feel drowsy and lightheaded.
   3. Tell the patient that it is normal for the mouth to feel dry if atropine SO_4 has been given.
   4. Observe for side effects of medication—morphine SO_4 and meperidine (Demerol) HCl may cause nausea and vomiting or drop in blood pressure.
   5. Maintain quiet environment until patient is transported to operating room.
H. Note the completeness of the chart:
   1. Vital signs.
   2. Routine laboratory reports.
   3. Administration of preoperative medication.
   4. Significant patient observations.
I. Assist the patient's family in finding the proper waiting room.

1. Inform them that the surgeon will contact them after the procedure is over.
2. Explain the length of time the patient is expected to be in the recovery room.
3. Prepare the family for any special equipment or devices that may be needed to care for the patient postoperatively—oxygen, monitoring equipment, or blood transfusions.

2. Anesthesia—purpose is to block transmission of nerve impulses, suppress reflexes, promote muscular relaxation, and in some instances, achieve unconsciousness.

A. *Regional anesthesia*—purpose is to block pain reception and transmission in a specified area.
   1. Agents used in regional anesthesia act by preventing action potentials or impulse formation by inhibiting the movement of sodium into the neuron and preventing potassium from moving out of the neuron.
   2. Commonly used drugs are lidocaine HCl, tetracaine HCl, cocaine HCl, and procaine HCl.
   3. Types of regional anesthetics:
      a. *Topical*—applied to mucous membranes or skin; the drug anesthetizes the nerves immediately below the area. May be utilized for bronchoscopic or laryngoscopic examinations. Side effects: rare anaphylaxis.
      b. *Local infiltration*—used for minor procedures; the anesthetic drug is injected directly into the area to be incised, manipulated, or sutured. Side effects: rare anaphylaxis.
      c. *Peripheral nerve block*—regional anesthesia is achieved by injecting the drug into or around a nerve after it passes from the vertebral column; the procedure is named for the nerve involved, such as brachial-plexus block. Requires a high degree of anatomical knowledge. Side effects: may be absorbed into the blood stream. Observe for signs of excitability, twitching, changes in vital signs, or respiratory difficulties.
      d. *Field block*—a group of nerves are injected with anesthetic as they branch from a major or main nerve trunk. May be used for dental procedures, plastic surgery. Side effects: rare.
      e. *Epidural anesthesia*—the anesthetizing drug is injected into the epidural space of the vertebral canal; produces a bandlike

anesthesia around body. Frequently used in obstetrics. Rare complications.

   f. *Spinal anesthesia*—the anesthetizing drug is injected into the subarachnoid space and mixes with the spinal fluid; the drug acts on the nerves as they emerge from the spinal cord, thereby inhibiting conduction in the autonomic, sensory, and motor systems.

    (1) Advantages: Rapid onset; produces excellent muscle relaxation.

    (2) Utilization: Surgery on lower limbs, perineum, and lower abdomen.

    (3) Disadvantages—

      (a) Loss of sensation below point of injection for two to eight hours—watch for signs of bladder distention; prevent injuries by maintaining alignment, keeping bedclothes straightened.

      (b) Patient awake during surgical procedure—avoid light or upsetting conversations.

      (c) Leakage of spinal fluid from puncture site—keep flat in bed for eight hours. Keep well hydrated—aids in spinal-fluid replacement. Depression of vasomotor responses—frequent checks of vital signs.

   g. *Intravenous regional anesthesia*—utilized on an extremity whose circulation has been interrupted by a tourniquet; the anesthetic is injected into the vein and blockage is presumed to be achieved from the extravascular leakage of anesthetic near a major nerve trunk. Precautions as for peripheral nerve block.

B. *General anesthesia*—a reversible state in which the patient loses consciousness due to the inhibition of neuronal impulses in the brain by a variety of chemical agents.

  1. General anesthesia may be administered intravenously, by inhalation, or rectally.

  2. *Intravenous anesthetics:*

   a. Thiopental (Pentothal) SO_4—a rapid-acting barbiturate; most frequently used drug for induction of anesthesia. *Major side effects:* laryngospasm and bronchospasm, hypotension, and respiratory depression.

   b. Droperidol (Inapsine) and fentanyl (Innovar and Sublimaze)—combine a potent tranquilizer and an analgesic to produce a rapid anesthesia. *Major side effects:* respiratory depression, muscle rigidity, and hypotension. *Note:* most patients receiving Innovar should not need narcotic analgesics in the immediate postoperative period. If narcotic analgesics are required, they should be reduced to as low as ¼ to ⅓ the usual amount.

   c. Ketamine HCl—chemically related to the hallucinogens, it produces an anesthesia characterized by a patient who appears awake but who will have no awareness or recollection of the procedure.

  3. *Inhalation anesthesia*—produced by inhalation of the vapors of certain gases or volatile liquids.

   a. *Ether*—a volatile, flammable liquid that, while irritating to the mucous membranes, provides excellent muscle relaxation and a wider margin of safety than other anesthetic agents.

   b. *Nitrous oxide*—although irritating to the mucous membranes, it is the most widely used of the gases; it is nonflammable and is frequently combined with oxygen and halothane (side effect—severe liver damage).

   c. *Cyclopropane*—more potent than nitrous oxide; it is highly flammable but quickly produces unconsciousness and good muscle relaxation.

   d. *Halothane*—a volatile, nonflammable liquid that quickly produces anesthesia and allows for rapid emergence from anesthesia; it has a low incidence of postoperative nausea and vomiting.

  4. *Precaution:* concomitant medications—to prevent hazardous drug interactions, notify the anesthesiologist if the patient is taking any of the following drugs:

   a. *Antibiotics* such as neomycin SO_4, streptomycin SO_4, polymyxin A and B SO_4, colistin SO_4, and kanamycin SO_4—when mixed with curariform muscle relaxant they interrupt nerve transmission and may cause respiratory paralysis and apnea.

   b. *Antidepressants*—particularly MAO (monoamine oxidase) inhibitors, which increase hypotensive effects of anesthetic agents.

   c. *Diuretics*—particularly thiazide diuretics, which may induce potassium depletion; a potassium deficit may lead to respiratory depression during anesthesia.

d. *Antihypertensives* such as reserpine, hydralazine, and methyldopa—potentiate the hypotensive effects of anesthetic agents.

e. *Anticoagulants* such as heparin dicoumarol—increase bleeding times, which may result in excessive blood loss and/or hemorrhage.

f. *Aspirin*—decreases platelet aggregation and may result in increased bleeding.

g. *Steroids* such as cortisone—antiinflammatory effect may delay wound-healing.

5. *Stages of anesthesia and nursing interventions:*

   a. Stage I—extends from beginning of induction to loss of consciousness.

      (1) Sensory functions dulled; reflexes intact; skin pink or flushed; pupils equal and react to light; blood pressure may increase; respirations irregular.

      (2) *Nursing goals* are designed to reduce external stimuli, as all movement and noises are exaggerated for the patient and can be highly distressing.

   b. Stage II—extends from loss of consciousness to relaxation.

      (1) Stage of delirium and excitement; skeletal tone is increased; respirations are exaggerated and irregular; pupils are dilated but react to light; blood pressure and pulse rate increase.

      (2) *Nursing goals* are designed to prevent injury by assisting anesthesiologist to restrain patient if necessary and by maintaining a quiet, nonstimulating environment.

   c. Stage III—extends from loss of lid reflex to cessation of voluntary respirations.

      (1) Patient is unconscious; muscles are relaxed; reflexes are absent; pupils are small but react to light; respirations are regular; blood pressure normal; pulse slow and steady; skin pink or slightly flushed.

      (2) *Nursing goals* during the period include preparing the operative site, assisting with procedures, and observing for signs of complications.

   d. Stage IV—indicates overdose and consists of respiratory arrest and vasomotor collapse due to medullary paralysis.

      (1) Death will ensue unless artificial respirations are given and anesthetic discontinued; respirations are shallow; pulse thready, decreased blood pressure, pupils are dilated and do not react to light; cyanosis develops gradually.

      (2) *Nursing goals* are designed to promote restoration of ventilation and vasomotor tone by assisting with cardiac arrest procedures and by administering cardiac stimulants or narcotic antagonists as ordered.

C. *Muscle relaxants*—drugs such as curare and succinylcholine (Anectine) Cl are given to supplement general anesthetic agents.

   1. Facilitate endotracheal intubation.

   2. Provide relaxation of abdominal muscles.

   3. Facilitate the administration of lower doses of potent general anesthetic.

   4. May cause respiratory depression.

D. *Hypothermia*—a specialized procedure in which the patient's body temperature is lowered to 28 to 30 C (82 to 86 F).

   1. Reduces tissue metabolism and oxygen requirements.

   2. Employed in heart surgery, brain surgery, and surgery on major blood vessels.

   3. Complications—respiratory depression, cardiac arrest, fat necrosis, edema, and fluid imbalances.

   4. *Nursing goals* are designed to prevent complications.

      a. Monitor vital signs.

      b. Note levels of consciousness.

      c. Record intake and output accurately.

      d. Maintain good body alignment.

3. **Immediate postanesthesia nursing care**—purpose is to maintain the patient's physiologic and psychologic equilibrium.

A. *Maintenance of physiologic equilibrium:*

   1. Position patient on side or on back with head turned to side—prevents obstruction of airway by tongue and allows secretions to drain from mouth.

   2. Collect *operative* data—

      a. General condition of patient.

      b. Type of operation performed.

      c. Pathologic findings.

      d. Anesthesia and medications received.

      e. Any problems that arose that will affect postoperative course.

f. Amount of intravenous infusion or transfusions received.

g. Any symptoms or complications to observe.

h. Any symptoms that should be reported immediately.

i. Whether or not the patient needs to be attached to a drainage or suction apparatus.

3. *Observations*—
   a. Note patient's level of consciousness.
   b. Vital signs.
   c. Skin color and dryness.
   d. Presence of airway.
   e. Status of reflexes.
   f. Dressings.
   g. Type and rate of intravenous infusion and blood transfusion.
   h. Rate, depth, and regularity of respirations.
   i. Presence of urinary catheter and, if present, color and amount of urine.

4. Promote a quiet, nonstressful *environment*—patients need to have siderails up at all times and a nurse in constant attendance.

5. Maintain *respiratory* function—
   a. Leave the oropharyngeal or nasopharyngeal airway in place until patient awakens and begins to eject it—leaving airway in after pharyngeal reflex has returned may initiate gagging and vomiting.
   b. After airway is removed, turn patient on side in a lateral position; support upper arm with a pillow—promotes lung expansion and reduces risk of aspiration.
   c. Suction excessive secretions from mouth and pharynx—prevents aspiration and obstruction of airway.
   d. Encourage cough and deep breathing—increases lung expansion and promotes gaseous exchange, aids in upward movement of secretions, and prevents atelectasis.
   e. Administer humidified oxygen as necessary—humidification reduces respiratory irritation and keeps bronchotracheal secretions soft and moist.
   f. Utilize mechanical ventilation, such as Bird or Bennet respirator, if needed.

6. Maintain *cardiovascular* function—
   a. Take vital signs.
      (1) Compare with preoperative vital signs.
      (2) Immediately report a systolic blood pressure that drops 20 mm Hg or more, a pressure below 80 mm Hg, or a pressure that continually drops 5 to 10 mm Hg over several readings.
      (3) Immediately report pulse rates under 60 or over 110 beats per minute or that are, or become, irregular.
      (4) Report respirations over 30 per minute or those that become shallow, quiet, slow, and in which the patient uses neck and diaphragmatic muscles—these are symptoms of *respiratory depression* and artificial respiration is indicated.
   b. Observe for other alterations in circulatory function—pallor; thready pulse; cold, moist skin; decreased urine output; and restlessness.
      (1) Decreased blood volume → decreased venous return → decreased cardiac output → decreased blood pressure → increased peripheral vascular constriction → decreased tissue perfusion and oxygenation.
      (2) Immediately report to physician, initiate oxygen therapy, and place patient in shock position unless contraindicated—feet elevated, legs straight, head slightly elevated. Increases venous return and prevents reflex hypotension associated with Trendelenburg position.
   c. Check time and rate of intravenous infusions and whether any medications have been ordered.
   d. Monitor blood transfusions and observe for signs of reaction, such as chills, elevated temperature, urticaria, laryngeal edema, and wheezing.
   e. If reaction occurs, stop transfusion immediately and notify physician. Send STAT urine to lab.

B. *Maintenance of psychologic equilibrium:*
   1. Reassure patient on awakening—orient frequently.
   2. Explain procedures even though patient does not appear alert.
   3. Answer patient's questions briefly and accurately.
   4. Maintain quiet, restful environment.
   5. Institute comfort measures.
      a. Maintain good body alignment.
      b. Support dependent extremities to avoid pressure areas and possible nerve damage.

c. Check dressings, clothing, and bedding for constriction.

d. Protect arm with intravenous infusion and check frequently for patency and signs of infiltration.

C. *Maintain proper function of tubes and apparatus* (Table 5–22).

4. *General postoperative nursing care*—purpose is to prevent complications and promote recovery of normal function (Table 5–23).

A. *Promote lung expansion, gaseous exchange, and elimination of bronchotracheal secretions.*
1. Turn, cough, and deep breathe every two hours.
2. Utilize blow bottles, as ordered—enables patient to observe depth of ventilation.
3. Administer IPPB, as ordered—increases ventilation and helps mobilize secretions.
4. Encourage hydration—thins mucus secretions.
5. Assist in ambulation as soon as allowed.

B. *Maintain body alignment*—promotes functioning of all body organs and enhances drainage from body cavities.

C. *Provide relief of pain:*
1. Assess type, location, intensity, and duration of pain as well as possible causative factors, such as poor body alignment or restrictive bandages.
2. Observe and evaluate patient's reaction to discomfort.
3. Utilize comfort measures, such as back rubs and proper ventilation, staying with patient and encouraging verbalization.
4. Reduce incidence of pain by changing position frequently; supporting dependent extremities with pillows, sandbags, and footboards, and keeping bedding dry and straight.
5. Administer analgesics or tranquilizers, as ordered, with verbal assurance that it will help.
6. Observe for desired and untoward effects of medication.

D. Assist in the promotion of adequate nutrition and fluid and electrolyte balance.
1. Administer parenteral fluids, as ordered—monitor blood pressure and intake and output to assess adequate, deficient, or excessive extracellular fluid volume.
2. Encourage liquid diet when nausea and vomiting stops and bowel sounds established, as ordered.
   a. Stimulates gastric juices and promotes gastric motility and peristalsis.
   b. Promotes vitamin, mineral, and nitrogen balance.

E. Assist patient with *elimination*:
1. Patient should void eight to ten hours after surgery.
2. Aid voiding by allowing patient to stand or use commode, if not contraindicated; use other means such as running tap water or soaking feet in warm water to promote micturition.
3. Avoid catheterization when possible but utilize if bladder is distended and conservative treatments have failed.
4. Maintain accurate intake and output records.
5. Expect bowel function to return in two to three days.

F. Facilitate *would-healing and prevent infection.*
1. Avoid pressure on or around incisional site—enhances venous drainage and prevents edema.
2. Elevate injured extremities to reduce swelling and promote venous return.
3. Support or splint incision when patient coughs.
4. Check dressings every two hours for drainage.
5. Change dressings on draining wounds prn and utilize protective ointments to reduce skin irritation.
6. If suction is applied to a draining wound, observe carefully for kinking or twisting of the tubes.

G. Promote *comfort and rest.*
1. Recognize factors that may cause restlessness—fear, anxiety, pain, oxygen lack, and wet dressings.
2. Utilize analgesics or barbiturates or apply oxygen as indicated.
3. Change positions, encourage deep breathing, or massage back to reduce restlessness.
4. Perform as many care activities at one time as possible, allowing patient to rest in between.
5. Administer antiemetic for relief of nausea and vomiting, as ordered.

H. Encourage early *movement and ambulation*—prevents complications of immobilization.
1. Assist in turning, coughing, and deep breathing.
2. Institute passive and active ROM exercises.
3. Encourage leg exercises.
4. Assist with standing or use of commode if allowed.
5. Encourage resumption of personal care as soon as possible.
6. Assist with ambulation as soon as allowed—note ambulation does not mean getting up and sitting in chair; chair-sitting should be avoided as it enhances venous pooling and may predispose to thrombophlebitis; patients should ambulate in room and then return to bed.

TABLE 5-22.   *Review of the use of common tubes in postoperative patients*

Tube or Apparatus	Purpose	Examples of Surgical Use	Key Points in Nursing Care
Note: Focus of this review is on the care of the tubes—not on the total patient, as is essential in the actual clinical area!			
Chest tubes	Anterior tube drains mostly air from pleural space Posterior tube drains mostly fluid from pleural space Removal of fluid and air from pleural space is necessary to reestablish negative intrapleural pressure	*Thoractomy Open heart surgery Spontaneous pneumothorax Traumatic pneumothorax*	See Key Points under each of the three components of chest drainage. Sterile technique is used when changing dressings around the tube insertions
A Bottle #1 Drainage bottle or compartment #1 if PleuroVac is used	Collects drainage		Mark level in bottle each shift so can keep accurate record—*not* routinely emptied each shift Never raise bottle above the level of the chest or back flow will occur
B Bottle #2 Water seal bottle or chamber	Water seal prevents flow of atmospheric air into pleural space. Essential to prevent recollapse of the lung		Air bubbles from post-operative residual air will continue for 24–48 hours Persistent large amounts of air bubbles in this compartment indicate an air leak between the alveoli and the pleural space Keep clamps handy in case the water seal is disconnected If air leak is present clamping the tube for very long may cause a tension pneumothorax Fluctuation of the fluid level in this bottle is expected (when the suction is turned off) because respiration changes the pleural pressure If there is no fluctuation of the fluid in the tube of this bottle (when the suction is turned off) then either the lung is fully expanded or the tube is blocked by kinking or by a clot Milking or stripping the tubes is necessary to prevent blockage from clots

TABLE 5–22. *(Continued)*

Tube or Apparatus	Purpose	Examples of Surgical Use	Key Points in Nursing Care
Bottle #3 Suction Control or Breaker bottle— connected to wall suction	Level of the column of water (i.e. 15–20 cm) is used to control the amount of suction applied to the chest tube—if the water evaporates to only 10 cm depth then this will be the maximum of suction generated by the wall suction		Air should continuously bubble through this compartment when the suction is on. The bubbles are from the atmosphere—not the patient. When the wall suction is turned higher the bubbling will be increased but the increased pulling of air is from the atmosphere and not from the pleural space. Since the level of H_2O determines the maximum negative pressure that can be obtained, make sure the water does not evaporate—keep filling the bottle to keep the ordered level. If there is no bubbling of air through this bottle the wall suction is too low.
Heimlich Flutter valve	Has a one-way valve so fluids and air can drain out of the pleural space but cannot flow back Eliminates the need for a water seal—no danger when tube is unclamped below the valve	Same conditions as other chest tubes	Can be connected to suction if ordered. Sometimes can just drain into portable bag so patient more mobile.
Tracheostomy tube	Maintain patent airway and promote better O_2–CO_2 exchange Makes removal of secretions by suctioning easier Cuff on trach is necessary if need air tight fit for an assisted ventilation	*Acute respiratory distress* due to poor ventilation *Severe burns of head and neck Laryngectomy* (trach is permanent)	Use oxygen before and after each suctioning. Humidify oxygen. Sterile technique in suctioning. Cleanse inner cannula as needed— only leave out 5–10 minutes. Hemostat handy if outer cannula is expelled—have obturator taped to bed and another trach set handy Cuff must be deflated periodically to prevent necrosis of mucosa
Central venous pressure	To measure the venous pressure at the right atrium—useful in determining circulatory overload (increase in CVP) or hypovolemia (decrease in CVP)	*Open heart surgery* Any situation where *fluid balance* is of critical concern.	Mark the area on the chest so the manometer will be held at the level of the right atrium Fluid in the manometer should fluctuate with respirations Trends are more important than just a one time measurement
Penrose drains	Soft collapsible rubber drain inserted to drain serosanguineous fluid from a surgical site. Usually brought out to the skin via a stab wound	Cholecystectomy	Expect drainage to progress from serosanguineous to more serous Sterile technique when changing dressing—do often Physician will advance tube a little each day

(Continued)

TABLE 5–22. *(Continued)*

Tube or Apparatus	Purpose	Examples of Surgical Use	Key Points in Nursing Care
Nasogastric tubes— Levin tubes	Inserted into stomach to decompress by removing gastric contents and air— prevents any buildup of gastric secretions which are continuous Used when stomach needs to be washed out (lavaged) Used for feedings when patient is unable to swallow	Any abdominal or other *surgery where peristalsis is absent* for a few days. *Overdoses* *Gastrointestinal hemorrhage* *Cancer of the esophagus* *Early post-operative laryngectomy patient or radical neck dissection*	Connected to low intermittent suction. Irrigated prn with normal saline Clean procedure but not sterile Mouthcare needed Report "coffee ground" material (digested blood) For overdose, stomach is pumped out as rapidly as possible. For hemorrhage, iced normal saline is usually used to lavage. Critical to make sure tube still in stomach before beginning feeding Follow feeding with some water to rinse out the tube.
Miller-Abbott tubes Cantor tubes	Longer than nasogastric tubes—have mercury in bags so tube can be used to decompress the lower intestinal tract	*Small bowel obstructions* *Intussusception* *Volvulus*	Care similar to N/G tube— irrigated—connected to suction, not sterile technique Orders will be written on how to advance the tube, gently pushing tube a few inches each hour, patient position may affect advancement of the tube X rays determine the desired location of the tube
Gastrostomy tubes	Inserted into stomach via abdominal wall—may be for decompression but used long term for feedings	Conditions affecting esophagus where it is impossible to insert a nasogastric tube	Principles of tube feedings much as with nasogastric tube except no danger that tube may be near trachea If permanent, tube may be replaceable
T-Tube	To drain bile from the common bile duct until edema has subsided	Cholecystectomy when a CDE (common duct exploration) or choledochostomy was also done	Bile drainage is controlled by the height of the drainage bag Clamp tube as ordered to see if bile will flow into duodenum normally
Hemovac	A type of closed wound drainage connected to suction—used to drain a large amount of serosanguineous drainage from under an incision.	*Mastectomy* *Total hip procedures* *Total knee procedures*	May compress unit and have portable vacuum or connect to wall suction Small drainage tubes may get clogged—physician may irrigate these at times
Three-way Foley	To provide avenues for constant irrigation and constant drainage of the urinary bladder	Transurethral resection (TUR) Bladder infections	Watch for blocking by clots—will cause bladder spasms Irrigant solution often has antibiotic added to the normal saline

TABLE 5–22. *(Continued)*

Tube or Apparatus	Purpose	Examples of Surgical Use	Key Points in Nursing Care
Suprapubic catheter	To drain bladder via an opening through the abdominal wall above the pubic bone	Suprapubic prostatectomy	May have orders to irrigate prn May have continuous irrigation
Ureteral catheters	To drain urine from the pelvis of one kidney, or for splinting ureter	*Cystoscopy* for diagnostic work-ups *Ureteral surgery* *Pyelotomy*	Never clamp tube—pelvis of kidney only holds 4–8 cc Use only 5 cc sterile normal saline if order to irrigate

Source: Jane Vincent Corbett, RN, MS, Assistant Professor, School of Nursing, University of San Francisco. Used with permission.

TABLE 5–23. *Postoperative complications*

Condition and etiology	Pathophysiology	Assessment: signs and symptoms	Nursing interventions
RESPIRATORY COMPLICATIONS—MOST COMMON ARE ATELECTASIS, BRONCHITIS, PNEUMONIAS (LOBAR, BRONCHIAL, AND HYPOSTATIC), AND PLEURISY; OTHER COMPLICATIONS ARE HEMOTHORAX AND PNEUMOTHORAX			
Atelectasis—Undetected preoperative upper respiratory infections, aspiration of vomitus; irritation of the tracheobronchial tree with increased mucus secretions due to intubation and inhalation anesthesia, a history of heavy smoking or chronic obstructive pulmonary disease; severe postoperative pain or high abdominal or thoracic surgery, which inhibits deep breathing; and debilitation or old age, which lowers the patient's resistance	Clogged bronchi → removal of air from entrapped alveoli by capillaries → collapse of alveoli—may affect all or part of lung	Dyspnea, elevated temperature, absent or diminished breath sounds over affected area, asymmetrical chest expansion, increased respirations and pulse rate, anxiety, and restlessness	1. Position on unaffected side 2. Turn, cough, and deep breathe 3. Postural drainage 4. Nebulization 5. Force fluids if not contraindicated
Bronchitis—see *Atelectasis* for etiology	Inflammation or infection of mucous membrane lining and/or bronchi → local hyperemia → edema → leukocytic infiltration of submucosa → increased tenacious mucopurulent secretions	Elevated temperature, chills, malaise, nonproductive cough that gradually becomes productive, wheezes, and moist rales	1. Position of comfort—semi-Fowler's 2. Provide humidified air 3. Force fluids to 3000 ml/day 4. Avoid iced drinks 5. Frequent oral hygiene if cough productive 6. Avoid fatigue and chilling 7. Administer bronchodilators, as ordered
Pneumonia—see *Atelectasis* for etiology	Acute inflammation of alveoli → exudate fill alveoli → consolidation of lung tissue → decreased gaseous exchange	Rapid, shallow, painful respirations; rales; ronchi; diminished or absent breath sounds; asymmetrical lung expansion; chills and fever; productive cough, rust-colored sputum; and circumoral and nailbed cyanosis	1. Position of comfort—semi- to high-Fowler's 2. Force fluids to 3000 ml/day 3. Provide humidification of air and oxygen therapy 4. Oropharyngeal suction prn 5. Assist during coughing 6. Administer antibiotics and analgesics, as ordered 7. Maintain high-calorie diet as tolerated 8. Provide proper disposal of secretions and oral hygiene

TABLE 5–23. *(Continued)*

Condition and etiology	Pathophysiology	Assessment: signs and symptoms	Nursing interventions
Pleurisy—see *Atelectasis* for etiology	Inflammation of the pleura	Knifelike chest pain on inspiration; intercostal tenderness; splinting of chest by patient; rapid, shallow respirations; pleural friction rub; elevated temperature; malaise	1. Position patient on affected side to splint the chest 2. Manually splint patient's chest during cough 3. Apply binder or adhesive strapping, as ordered 4. Administer analgesics, as ordered
Hemothorax—chest surgery, gunshot or knife wounds, and multiple fractures of chest wall	Blood from torn vessel fills pleural space inhibiting lobular or total lung expansion → decreased alveolar ventilation → decreased PO_2	Chest pain, increased respiratory rate, dyspnea, decreased or absent breath sounds, decreased blood pressure, tachycardia, and mediastinal shift may occur (heart, trachea, and esophagus great vessels are pushed toward unaffected side)	1. Observe vital signs closely for signs of shock and respiratory distress 2. Assist with thoracentesis (needle aspiration of fluid) 3. Assist with insertion of thoracostomy tube to closed chest drainage (see care of water-sealed drainage system)
(Pneumothorax, open—see also Sucking chest wound)			
Pneumothorax, closed or tension—thoracentesis (needle nicks the lung), rupture of alveoli or bronchi due to accidental injury, and chronic obstructive lung disease	Air enters pleural space with each inspiration and is trapped; intrapleural pressures become positive, inhibiting lung expansion and decreasing alveolar ventilation; pressure may collapse lung and cause mediastinal shift, which may result in compression of unaffected lung and great vessels → decreasing venous return and cardiac output	Marked dyspnea, sudden sharp chest pain, subcutaneous emphysema (air in chest wall tissue), cyanosis, tracheal shift to unaffected side, hyperresonance on percussion, decreased or absent breath sounds, increased respiratory rate, tachycardia, asymmetrical chest expansion, feeling of pressure within chest; *mediastinal shift*—severe dyspnea and cyanosis, deviation of larynx and trachea toward unaffected side, deviation either medially or laterally of apex of heart, decreased blood pressure, distended neck veins, and increased pulse and respirations	1. Remain with patient—keep as calm and quiet as possible 2. Place in high-Fowler's (sitting) position 3. Notify physician through another nurse and have thoracentesis equipment brought to bedside 4. Administer oxygen as necessary 5. Take vital signs to evaluate respiratory and cardiac function 6. Assist with thoracentesis 7. Assist with initiation and maintenance of closed-chest drainage

(Continued)

TABLE 5–23.   *(Continued)*

Condition and etiology	Pathophysiology	Assessment: signs and symptoms	Nursing interventions
CIRCULATORY COMPLICATIONS—SHOCK, THROMBOPHLEBITIS, PULMONARY EMBOLISM, AND DISSEMINATED INTRAVASCULAR COAGULATION			
Shock, hypovolemic—hemorrhage, sepsis, decreased cardiac contractility (myocardial infarction, cardiac failure, tamponade), drug sensitivities, transfusion reactions, pulmonary embolism, and emotional reaction to pain or deep fear	Decreased venous return due to diminished blood volume (hemorrhage) or plasma loss (intestinal obstruction, burns, or dehydration) → decreased cardiac output → decreased mean systemic pressures → decreased tissue perfusion and oxygenation	Dizziness; fainting; restlessness; anxiety; decreased or falling blood pressure; weak, thready pulse; shallow, rapid respirations; pallor; cool, clammy, pale to cyanotic skin; decreased temperature; thirst; oliguria; and CVP below 5 cm water	1. Position patient with foot of bed raised 20°, keeping knees straight, trunk horizontal, and head slightly elevated; avoid Trendelenburg's position 2. Administer blood transfusions, plasma expanders, and intravenous infusions, as ordered 3. Check vital signs, CVP, and temperature 4. Insert urinary catheter to monitor hourly urine output 5. Administer oxygen, as ordered
Shock, septic—see *Hypovolemic shock* for etiology	Local or generalized infection → vasodilation, locally then generally → increased cardiac output in response to vasodilation and increased metabolic rate due to fever → red cell agglutination with sludging of blood → decreased venous return → decreased cardiac output → circulatory collapse	As hypovolemic shock, except temperature may be elevated; CVP may elevate over 15 cm water	1. Position as for hypovolemic shock 2. Institute cooling measures if indicated 3. Administer antibiotics, steroids, and intravenous infusions, as ordered 4. Monitor vital signs, CVP, temperature, and urinary output as for hypovolemic shock
Shock, anaphylactic—see *Hypovolemic shock* for etiology	Antigen-antibody reaction → cellular damage → release of histamine and histaminelike substance → venous dilatation → increased vascular capacity → dilatation of arteriolae → decreased mean systemic blood pressure → decreased venous return → cardiac failure	Flushing; sneezing; itching; urticaria; asthmatic wheezing; decreased or falling blood pressure; edema, particularly laryngeal edema; and weak, thready pulse	1. If patient is receiving a blood transfusion, stop immediately 2. Administer antihistamines and steroids, as ordered 3. Prepare epinephrine in event of respiratory distress 4. Maintain intravenous infusions, as ordered 5. Monitor vital signs, CVP, temperature, and urinary output 6. If transfusion reaction suspected, send blood and urine samples to lab for hemoglobin

TABLE 5–23. *(Continued)*

Condition and etiology	Pathophysiology	Assessment: signs and symptoms	Nursing interventions
Shock, cardiogenic—see *Hypovolemic shock* for etiology	Myocardial infarction → decreased cardiac output → decreased cardiac perfusion → decreased peripheral perfusion → tissue ischemia → release of toxins → increased capillary permeability and vascular dilatation → decreased blood volume and venous pooling → decreased venous return → cardiac depression.	As for hypovolemic shock, with orthopnea, irregular or absent peripheral pulses, cardiac arrhythmias, CVP above 15 cm water, heart failure, and pulmonary edema	1. Position for optimal ventilation, semi- or high-Fowler's 2. Avoid routine nursing functions 3. Monitor ECG continuously 4. Administer parenteral infusions, as ordered 5. Administer vasopressors, vasodilators, digitalis preparations, steroids, and narcotics, as ordered 6. Monitor vital signs, CVP, and urine output—axilla for temperature determinations 7. Administer oxygen, as ordered
Thrombophlebitis—injury to vein wall by tight leg straps or leg holders during gynecologic surgery; hemoconcentration due to dehydration or fluid loss; and stasis of blood in extremities due to postoperative circulatory depression	Roughened endothelial surface of vessel due to trauma → formation of platelet plug—activation of prothrombin into thrombin, which converts fibrinogen into fibrin threads, which enmesh red blood cells and plasma to form blood clot; slow blood flow → increased concentrations of procoagulants (prothrombin, etc.) in local areas → initiation of clotting mechanism	Calf pain or cramping, redness and swelling (the left leg is affected more frequently than the right), slight fever, chills, Homans' sign, and tenderness over the anteromedian surface of thigh	1. Maintain complete bedrest, avoiding positions that restrict venous return 2. Apply elastic stockings or wrap legs from toes to groin with elastic bandages—prevents swelling and pooling of venous blood 3. Apply warm moist soaks to area, as ordered 4. Administer anticoagulants, as ordered 5. Use bed cradle over affected limb 6. Provide active and passive ROM exercises in unaffected limb
Pulmonary embolism—obstruction of a pulmonary artery by a foreign body in the blood stream, usually a blood clot that has been dislodged from its original site	Embolus, usually from systemic vein, travels to right side of heart → pumped to lungs → total or partial obstruction of pulmonary blood flow → decreased venous return to left side of heart → peripheral circulatory failure may occur; dammed up blood in lungs causes dilatation of right side of heart and engorgement of systemic veins	Sudden, severe stabbing chest pain; severe dyspnea; cyanosis; rapid pulse; anxiety and apprehension; pupillary dilatation; profuse diaphoresis; and loss of consciousness	1. Administer oxygen and inhalants with the patient sitting upright 2. Maintain bedrest and frequently reassure patient 3. Administer heparin sodium, as ordered 4. Administer analgesics, such as morphine SO_4, to reduce pain and apprehension

(Continued)

TABLE 5–23.   *(Continued)*

Condition and etiology	Pathophysiology	Assessment: signs and symptoms	Nursing interventions
Disseminated intravascular coagulation (DIC)—septicemia (gram-negative), severe and prolonged hypotension (shock), toxemia of pregnancy, carcinoma of the prostate, chemotherapy for cancer, acidosis, and liver damage	Tissue injury → activation of coagulation system → thrombin formation reacts with fibrinogen to form fibrin → fibrin clots deposited throughout microcirculation in kidneys, brain, and lungs → microinfarcts and tissue necrosis → red blood cells are trapped in fibrin and destroyed → excessive clotting causes consumption of fibrinogen, platelets, and other clotting factors and results in formation of fibrin split products, which inhibit clotting and lead to bleeding	Petechiae and ecchymoses on skin and mucous membranes, cyanosis of fingers, toes, and limbs; wound and venipuncture bleeding; subcutaneous hematomas; severe uncontrollable hemorrhage during surgery and childbirth or from ulcer; oliguria; anuria; convulsions; coma; abnormal coagulation tests (prothrombin time, platelet count, and fibrinogen level)	1. Carry out nursing measures designed to alleviate basic problem (shock, septicemia, and cancer) 2. Administer heparin SO_4, q4–6h, as ordered, to reverse abnormal clotting 3. Monitor and record intake and output, vital signs (oral and axillary temperature), and central venous pressure; report changes to physician 4. Administer blood or plasma, as ordered 5. Avoid administering parenteral medications if possible; this further irritates vein walls and may increase thrombus formation

WOUND COMPLICATIONS—INFECTION, DEHISCENCE, AND EVISCERATION

Condition and etiology	Pathophysiology	Assessment: signs and symptoms	Nursing interventions
Wound infection—obesity or undernutrition, particularly protein and vitamin deficiencies; decreased antibody production in aged; decreased phagocytosis in newborn; metabolic disorder, such as diabetes mellitus, Cushing's syndrome, malignancies, and shock; breakdown in aseptic technique	Tissue necrosis or decreased local tissue perfusion provide medium for pathogenic growth, eliciting inflammatory response; blood vessels dilate → rapid blood flow → increased filtration pressures → edema; slowing of blood flow → migration of leukocytes to area → phagocytosis	Redness, tenderness, and heat in area of incision; wound drainage; elevated temperature; and increased pulse rate	1. Assist in the cleansing and irrigation of the wound and insertion of a drain 2. Apply hot wet dressings, as ordered 3. Administer antibiotics, as ordered, and observe responses
Wound dehiscence and evisceration—obesity and undernutrition, particularly protein and vitamin C deficiencies; metabolic disorders; cancer; liver disease; common site is midline abdominal incision, frequently about seven days postoperatively; and precipitating factors include abdominal distention, retching, coughing, hiccups and uncontrolled motor activity	Inadequate tissue nutrition → decreased formation of new or scar tissue → inadequate wound approximation → increased intra-abdominal pressures due to flatus, retching, etc. → splitting of incisional site	Slow parting of wound edges with a gush of pinkish serous drainage or rapid parting with coils of intestines escaping onto the abdominal wall; the latter is accompanied by pain and, often, vomiting	1. Maintain bedrest in a low-Fowler's or horizontal position 2. Notify physician immediately 3. Cover exposed coils of intestines with sterile towels or dressing and keep moist with sterile normal saline 4. Monitor vital signs frequently 5. Remain with the patient, and reassure patient that physician is coming

TABLE 5–23. *(Continued)*

Condition and etiology	Pathophysiology	Assessment: signs and symptoms	Nursing interventions
			6. Prepare for physician's arrival by setting up IV equipment, suction equipment, and nasogastric tube and by obtaining sterile gown, mask, gloves, towels, and warmed normal saline 7. Notify surgery that patient will be returning to operating room

URINARY COMPLICATIONS—RETENTION AND INFECTIONS

Condition and etiology	Pathophysiology	Assessment: signs and symptoms	Nursing interventions
Urinary retention—obstruction in the bladder or urethra; neurologic disease; mechanical trauma as in childbirth or gynecological surgery; psychologic conditioning that inhibits voiding in bed; and prolonged bedrest	Depression of urinary reflex by general anesthetic and anticholinergic drugs (atropine SO_4) given before surgery → blockage of parasympathetic stimulation → failure of bladder to empty	Inability to void in 10 to 18 hours postsurgery, despite adequate fluid replacement, palpable bladder, frequent voiding of small amounts of urine or dribbling, and suprapubic pain	1. Assist patient to stand or use bedside commode if not contraindicated 2. Provide privacy 3. Reduce tension and provide psychologic support 4. Use warm bedpan 5. Run tap water 6. Place patient's feet in warm water. 7. Pour warm water over vulva 8. Catheterize if conservative measures fail
Urinary infections—urinary retention, bladder distention, repeated or prolonged catheterization	Slowing of urinary flow and/or presence of foreign body in normally sterile bladder → decreased resistance → increased susceptibility to infection → bladder trigone may show increased vascularity, generalized edema, and ulceration; chronic cystitis → bladder may become thick-walled and contracted	Burning and frequency of urination, low-back or flank pain, pyuria, hematuria, elevated temperature, chills, anorexia, and positive urine culture	1. Push fluids to 3000 ml daily unless contraindicated 2. Avoid stimulants such as coffee, tea, and cola beverages 3. Administer antibiotics, sulfonamides, or acidifying agents, as ordered 4. Maintain meticulous perineal care 5. Administer perianal care after each bowel movement

(Continued)

TABLE 5–23.   *(Continued)*

Condition and etiology	Pathophysiology	Assessment: signs and symptoms	Nursing interventions
GASTROINTESTINAL COMPLICATIONS—GASTRIC DILATATION, PARALYTIC ILEUS, AND INTESTINAL OBSTRUCTION			
Gastric dilatation—depressed gastric motility due to sympathoadrenal stress response, idiosyncrasy to drugs, emotions, pain, shock, and fluid and electrolyte imbalances	Failure of neuromuscular innervation → decreased motor function (peristalsis) → abdominal distention → thinning of gastric mucosa → decreased blood supply → further decrease in gastric motility	Feeling of fullness, hiccups, overflow vomiting of dark foul-smelling liquid; severe retention leads to decreased blood pressure (due to pressure on vagus nerve) and other symptoms of shock syndrome	1. Report signs to physician immediately 2. Insert or assist in the insertion of a nasogastric tube and attach to intermittent suction 3. Irrigate nasogastric tube with saline (using water will deplete electrolytes and result in metabolic alkalosis) 4. Administer IV infusions with electrolytes, as ordered
Paralytic ileus—see *Gastric dilatation*	Decreased motor activity (due to toxic or traumatic disturbance of the autonomic nervous system) → decreased peristalsis → increased intestinal retention	Greatly decreased or absent bowel sounds, failure of either gas or feces to be passed by rectum, nausea and vomiting, abdominal tenderness and distention, fever, dehydration	1. Notify physician 2. Insert or assist with insertion of nasogastric tube and attach to intermittent suction 3. Insert rectal tube 4. Administer IV infusion with electrolytes, as ordered 5. Irrigate nasogastric tube with saline 6. Assist with insertion of Miller-Abbott tube if indicated 7. Administer medications to increase peristalsis, as ordered
Intestinal obstruction—poorly functioning anastomosis, hernia, adhesions, and fecal impaction	Moderate obstruction → increased peristalsis above obstruction → stretching of mesentery → severe pain and occasionally reflex vomiting → increased secretion and distention of gut → intestinal paralysis → vascular to intestinal fluid shift due to failure to reabsorb excessive secretions → accumulation of fluids → dehydration → decreased blood volume → increased pulse rate and falling blood pressure	Severe, colicky abdominal pains, mild to severe abdominal distention, nausea and vomiting, anorexia and malaise, fever, lack of bowel movement, electrolyte imbalance, and high-pitched tinkling bowel sounds	1. Assist with insertion of nasoenteric tube and attach to intermittent suction 2. Maintain IV infusions with electrolytes 3. Encourage nasal breathing to avoid air swallowing 4. Check abdomen for distention and bowel sounds every two hours 5. Encourage verbalization 6. Plan rest periods for patient 7. Administer oral hygiene frequently

TABLE 5–23. *(Continued)*

Condition and etiology	Pathophysiology	Assessment: signs and symptoms	Nursing interventions
TRANSFUSION REACTIONS—ALLERGIC, FEBRILE, AND HEMOLYTIC			
Allergic and febrile reactions—unidentified antigen or antigens in donor blood or transfusion equipment; previous reaction to transfusions; small thrombi; bacteria; and lysed red cells	Unknown antigen → formation of antibodies → cellular damage → release of histamine and histaminelike substances → vascular dilatation → edema of tissue.	Fever to 103 F, may have sudden onset; chills; itching; erythema; urticaria; nausea; vomiting; and dyspnea and wheezing, occasionally	1. Stop transfusion and notify physician 2. Administer antihistamines, as ordered 3. Send STAT urine to lab for analysis 4. Institute cooling measures if indicated 5. Maintain strict input and output records. 6. Send remaining blood to lab for analysis and order recipient blood sample for analysis.
Hemolytic reaction—infusion of incompatible blood.	Infusion of incompatible blood → hemolysis (rupture of RBC) of erythrocytes by isoagglutinins in recipient → release of cellular contents → microemboli → decreased blood volume → decreased cardiac output → shock.	Early chills and fever; feeling of burning in face; hypotension; tachycardia; chest, back, or flank pain; nausea; vomiting; feeling of doom; spontaneous and diffuse bleeding; icterus; oliguria; anuria; and hemoglobinuria.	1. Stop infusion immediately, take vital signs, and notify physician. 2. Send patient blood sample and unused blood to lab for analysis. 3. Send STAT urine to lab 4. Save all urine for observation of discoloration 5. Administer parenteral infusions to combat shock, as ordered 6. Administer medications, as ordered—diuretics, sodium bicarbonate, hydrocortisone, and vasopressors
EMOTIONAL COMPLICATIONS			
Emotional disturbances—grief associated with loss of body part or loss of body image; previous emotional problems; decreased sensory and perceptual input; sensory overload; fear and pain; decreased resistance to stress as a result of age, exhaustion, or debilitation	Unknown	Restlessness, insomnia, depression, hallucinations, delusions, agitation, and suicidal thoughts	1. Report symptoms to physician 2. Encourage verbalization of feelings and give realistic assurance 3. Orient to time and place as necessary 4. Provide safety measures, such as siderails 5. Keep room well lighted to reduce incidence of visual hallucinations 6. Administer tranquilizers, as ordered 7. Use restraints as a last resort

Part C / SPECIFIC NURSING OBSERVATIONS AND INTERVENTIONS IN COMMON SURGICAL PROCEDURES

RESPIRATORY SYSTEM

1. **Tonsillectomy and adenoidectomy**—removal of tonsils and adenoids.
A. Rationale—chronic tonsillitis and/or adenoiditis, adenoiditis with recurrent episodes of otitis media, severe tonsillar hypertrophy with obstruction of the pharynx.
B. *Preoperative nursing observations* are designed to prevent postoperative complications:
   1. Bleeding time.
   2. Signs of upper-respiratory infection.
C. *Postoperative nursing goals* are designed to reduce incidence of postoperative bleeding, maintain fluid and electrolyte balance, and promote physical and psychologic relaxation.
   1. Signs of bleeding—emesis of large amount of bright red or brown liquid, frequent swallowing, increased pulse rate, decreased blood pressure, pallor, and restlessness.
   2. Provide ice collar—minimizes bleeding and reduces discomfort.
   3. Administer fluids when tolerated, ice chips, water, popsicles, sherbet.
   4. Rinse mouth frequently with water to aid in eliminating thick oral mucus.
D. *Outcome criteria*—the patient, parent, or guardian will be able to:
   1. State rationale for preventing coughing, excessive clearing of the throat, and nose-blowing until healing occurs.
   2. Relate dietary restrictions: citrus juices; hot, rough, or spicy foods.
   3. Describe signs of possible complications, such as bleeding, persistent fever.
   4. State plans for maintaining activity restrictions for two to three days postdischarge.

2. **Tracheostomy**—an opening into the trachea, temporary or permanent.

A. Rationale—indicated in airway obstruction due to foreign body, edema, tumor, excessive tracheobronchial secretions, respiratory depression, decreased gaseous diffusion at alveolar membrane, or increased dead space as in severe emphysema.
B. *Preoperative nursing observations and procedures* are designed to relieve anxiety and fear.
   1. Explain purpose of procedure and equipment.
   2. Demonstrate suctioning procedure.
   3. Establish a means of postoperative communication—paper and pencil, magic slate, picture cards, and call bell.
   4. Remain with patient as much as possible.
C. *Postoperative nursing goals* are designed to maintain a patent airway and alleviate apprehension.
   1. Administer mist to tracheostomy—natural humidifying oropharynx pathways have been eliminated.
   2. Place patient in a semi-Fowler's position—prevent forward flexion of neck; facilitates respiration, promotes drainage, and minimizes edema.
   3. Suction each hour or prn—increased respirations; moist, noisy respirations; or nonproductive coughing indicate need for suctioning.
      a. Secretions may be slightly blood-tinged at first.
      b. Strict aseptic technique and sterile suctioning catheters with each aspiration.
         (1) Prevent hypoxia by administering 100% oxygen before suctioning unless contraindicated.
         (2) Do not suction when inserting suction catheter.
         (3) Turn patient's head to right to facilitate suctioning of left bronchus; turn patient's head to left to facilitate suctioning of right bronchus.
         (4) If patient coughs during suctioning, gently remove catheter to permit ejection and suction of mucus.
         (5) Apply suction intermittently for no longer than 10 to 15 seconds—prolonged suction decreases arterial oxygen concentrations.
         (6) If tracheostomy cuff is used, deflate for five minutes every hour to prevent damage to trachea.
         (7) Clean inner cannula of silver tracheostomy tube every two to eight hours or as needed, depending on amount and consistency of secretions (aseptic procedure).

(a) Soak in detergent solution or solution of half-strength hydrogen peroxide if secretions are congealed.

(b) Remove adhering secretions with pipe cleaners or small test-tube brush.

(c) Rinse in sterile water.

(d) Run gauze through lumen to remove excess secretions and solution.

(e) Suction outer tube before reinserting inner cannula.

c. Remain with patient as much as possible.

d. Encourage patient to communicate feelings, using preestablished communication system.

3. **Laryngectomy (radical neck dissection)**—consists of removal of entire larynx, lymph nodes, sternomastoid muscle, and jugular vein on the same side as the lesion.

A. Rationale—cancer of the larynx that extends beyond the vocal cords.

B. *Preoperative nursing goals* are designed to provide emotional support and optimal physical preparation.

1. Encourage verbalization of fears and answer all questions honestly, particularly about having no voice after surgery.

2. Preoperative care before tracheostomy.

3. If possible, plan to have a person who has successfully adapted to laryngectomy visit patient. (Information about local chapters can be obtained from International Association of Laryngectomees.)

4. Emphasize the life-saving aspects of the surgery and that it is possible to learn other means to speak again.

C. *Postoperative nursing goals* are designed to maintain a patent airway, maintain fluid and electrolyte balance, prevent aspiration, and promote optimal postoperative physical and psychologic functioning.

1. Place in semi-Fowler's position—preventing forward flexion of neck; reduces edema and maintains open airway.

2. Observe for respiratory embarrassment—*early signs:* increased respiratory and pulse rate, apprehension, restlessness. *Late signs:* dyspnea, cyanosis.

3. Institute laryngectomy tube care:

a. Observe for presence of stridor (coarse, high-pitched inspiratory sound)—report to physician immediately.

b. Have stand-by laryngectomy tube available at bedside.

4. If pressure dressings are used, note color and amount of drainage and reinforce as ordered.

5. If Hemovac is used (Figure 5–7), expect 80 to 120 ml of serosanguineous drainage the first postoperative day.

a. Drainage should decrease daily.

b. Observe patency of drainage tubes.

6. Prevent infection by maintaining clean surgical technique.

7. Answer patient's call bell immediately, utilizing preestablished means of communication.

8. Reexplain all procedures while giving care.

9. Observe for swallowing difficulties—teach patient to chew food well and to swallow each bite with water to facilitate movement of food to stomach.

10. Speech rehabilitation is begun as soon as esophageal suture is healed.

a. Information on laryngeal speech can be obtained from

(1) International Association of Laryngectomees

(2) American Cancer Society

(3) American Speech and Hearing Association

b. Esophageal speech generally learned best at a speech clinic

(1) To learn, person must first practice burping—provides column of air needed for sound.

(2) Person learns to coordinate articulation with column of air.

(3) New voice sounds are natural but somewhat hoarse.

(4) Other surgical and prosthetic devices are being tested.

11. Patient Teaching:

a. Instruct to cover opening with scarf or shirt of a porous material—material substitutes for nasal passage to warm and screen out dust and other air pollutants.

b. Exercise caution while bathing or taking shower—decreases likelihood of aspiration.

c. Swimming and boating may be contraindicated.

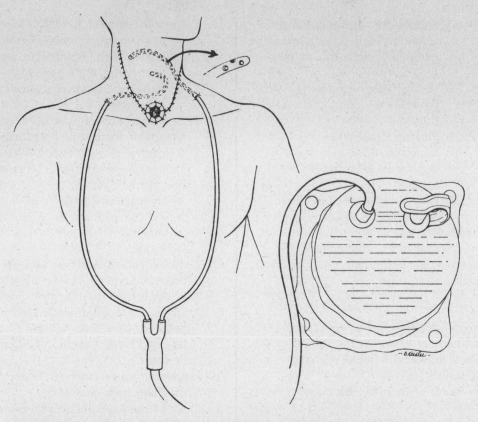

FIGURE 5–7. Hemovac apparatus for constant closed suction
In this system of wound drainage, suction is maintained by plastic container with spring inside that tries to force apart lids and thereby produces suction that is transmitted through plastic tubing. Neck skin is pulled down tight, and no external dressing is required. Container serves as both suction source and receptacle for blood. It is emptied as required, and drainage tubes are left in neck for three days. (From DeWeese, D.D.; and Saunders, W.H.: 1977. *Textbook of otolaryngology,* Fifth ed. St. Louis, The C. V. Mosby Co.)

d. Instruct in simple range of motion exercises of neck and how to support head.

D. Outcome Criteria—the patient and/or significant other will be able to:
1. Verbalize feelings about surgery.
2. State plans for speech therapy and resource agencies in the community.
3. State rationale for covering stoma.
4. Identify signs and symptoms necessitating immediate medical attention, i.e. respiratory infectious block.

4. ***Thoracic surgeries***—*thoracotomy* (incision in the chest wall to examine lung tissue and secure biopsy), *lobectomy* (removal of a lobe of the lung), *pneumonectomy* (removal of an entire lung).

A. Rationale—bronchogenic and lung carcinomas, lung abscess, tuberculosis, bronchiectasis, emphysematous blebs, and benign tumors.

B. *Preoperative nursing goals* are designed to provide optimal physical and psychologic preparation for the surgical procedure.
1. Minimize pulmonary secretions:
   a. Humidify air to moisten secretions.
   b. Teach patient to cough against a closed glottis—increases intrapulmonary pressure.
   c. Utilize IPPB as ordered to improve ventilation.
   d. Administer bronchodilators, expectorants, and antibiotics, as ordered.
   e. Utilize postural drainage, cupping, and vibration to mobilize secretions.

2. Instruct in diaphragmatic breathing and coughing.

3. Instruct and supervise practice of postoperative arm exercises—flexion, abduction, and rotation of shoulder prevents ankylosis and stiffness of the arm on operative side.

4. Explain to the patient that there will be chest tubes, intravenous infusion, and oxygen therapy postoperatively.

C. *Postoperative nursing goals* are designed to maintain a patent airway, promote ventilation and gaseous exchange, maintain fluid and electrolyte balance, prevent complications, and provide physical and mental relaxation.

1. High-Fowler's position—promotes greater ventilation.

2. Turn, cough, and deep breathe.

  a. Pad area around chest tube when turning on operative side—reduces incisional stress and discomfort.

  b. Do not turn pneumonectomy to unaffected side, as it inhibits lung expansion and interferes with drainage of secretions.

  c. Splint chest during coughing.

    (1) Support incision—reduces discomfort and incisional stress.

    (2) Coughing up sputum is the single most important activity the thoracic patient performs postoperatively.

3. Attach chest tubes to water-seal drainage system (Figure 5–8).

  a. Insert to drain off excess fluid and air, speed reinflation of lungs, and reestablish normal negative intrapleural pressures.

  b. Mark original fluid level on drainage bottle to facilitate calculation of drainage; mark level, time, and date each time drainage is measured.

  c. Keep drainage bottles below chest level to prevent backflow of fluid and air into intrapleural space.

  d. Milk tubing in the direction of drainage bottle each hour to maintain patency and prevent plugging, as ordered.

  e. Observe fluctuation of fluid level in the glass tubing—will stop when lung reexpanded or plugged by fibrin or clot.

  f. Observe and report leaks in the system—constant bubbling in water-seal bottle, leaking trapped air can result in tension pneumothorax.

  g. Observe and report *immediately* crepitations, labored or shallow breathing, tachypnea, cyanosis, tracheal deviation, and symptoms of hemorrhage.

  h. Keep two hemostats at the bedside at all times—if water-seal drainage bottle is broken, *immediately* clamp chest tube to prevent air from entering chest cavity.

4. Auscultate chest for breath sounds—report diminished or absent breath sounds on unaffected side; indicates decreased ventilation and may lead to respiratory embarrassment.

5. Check patient who has had pneumonectomy for *mediastinal shift*—trachea should always be midline—movement toward either side indicates shift. Notify physician immediately.

6. Administer parenteral infusions slowly—greater threat of pulmonary edema in these patients due to decrease in pulmonary vasculature with removal of lung lobe or whole lung.

7. Institute passive and active range of motion of operative arm and ambulate as condition permits—prevents ankylosis of shoulder.

D. *Outcome criteria*—the patient and/or significant other will be able to:

1. Explain rationale for activity restrictions as well as demonstrate prescribed exercises.

2. Identify name, dosage, side effects, and schedule of prescribed medications.

3. State plans for necessary modifications in life style, home.

4. Identify support systems (family, friends, community health nurse).

5. Chest injuries

A. *Flail chest*—multiple rib fractures resulting in instability of the chest wall with subsequent paradoxical breathing (portion of lung under injured chest wall moves in on inspiration while remaining lung expands; on expiration it expands while unaffected lung tissue contracts).

1. *Assessment*—pain, dyspnea, cyanosis, uneven chest expansion, tachypnea, pneumothorax, hemothorax, and shock.

2. Complications of severe chest injuries include hemothorax (blood in pleural cavity) and pneumothorax (air in pleural cavity).

3. Nursing measures are designed to stabilize chest wall and promote ventilation.

  a. Internal stabilization—use of volume-controlled ventilator to control patient's respi-

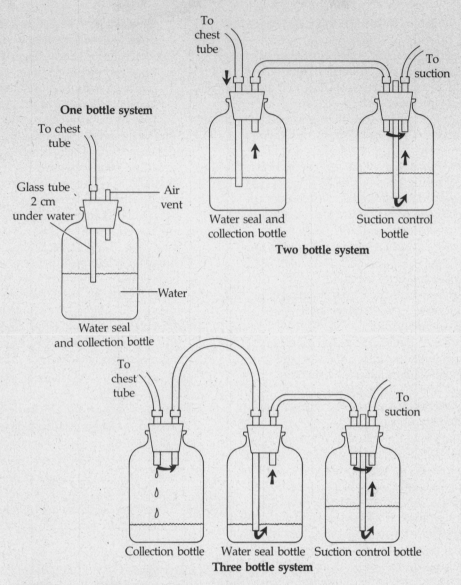

FIGURE 5–8. Bottle chest drainage systems
(a) One-bottle system. (b) Two-bottle system. (c) Three-bottle system. (From Holloway, N. *Nursing the critically ill adult*. Menlo Park, 1979, Addison-Wesley Publishing Co.)

rations → decreases movement of fractured ribs.
  b. External stabilization—achieved by skeletal traction applied to broken portion of ribs.
  c. Assist with chest-tube insertion, as ordered.
B. *Sucking chest wound*—penetrating wound of chest wall with hemothorax and pneumothorax, resulting in collapse of lung and mediastinal shift toward the unaffected lung.
  1. *Assessment*—severe dyspnea; weak, rapid pulse;

clammy, cold skin; hypotension; and rush of air through hole in chest with respiration.
  2. *Nursing goals* are designed to eliminate positive intrapleural pressures and to restore adequate ventilation.
    a. Apply pressure bandage over wound as patient exhales forcefully against a closed glottis (Valsalva movement).
      (1) Prevents further air from entering pleural cavity.

(2) Valsalva movement aids in expanding collapsed lung by creating positive intrapulmonary pressures.
   b. Assist with insertion of endotracheal tube if needed.
   c. Assist with thoracentesis and insertion of chest tubes with connection to water-seal drainage as needed.

CARDIOVASCULAR SYSTEM

1. Cardiac catheterization

A. Rationale—obtain pressure measurements in cardiac chambers; obtain blood samples from chambers for analysis of oxygen content; determine presence and location of vascular lesions.

B. Procedures:
   1. *Right heart catheterization*—utilizes venous approach (brachial or femoral vein). Catheter advanced through vena cava → right atrium → right ventricle → pulmonary artery.
   2. *Left heart catheterization*—
      a. Venous approach (femoral vein) → inferior vena cava → right atrium → interatrial septum → left atrium → left ventricle.
      b. Arterial approach (femoral or brachial artery) → aorta → left ventricle.
   3. *Coronary arteriography*—utilizes arterial approach (femoral or brachial) → aorta → coronary artery → multiple injections of contrast material.

C. *Precatheterization nursing care:*
   1. *Assessment*—
      a. Vital signs—baseline measures.
      b. Allergies—particularly to iodine.
      c. Skin test—detect potential reactions to iodine-based contrast medium.
      d. Level of anxiety.
   2. *Patient teaching*—
      a. Procedure done in catheterization laboratory; contains X-ray table, fluoroscope, monitors, and resuscitation equipment.
      b. Requires one to three hours—will need to lie still.
      c. Catheter inserted in blood vessel and contrast dye instilled—may have hot, flushed feeling.
      d. Will be strapped to table for safety reasons during changes in position.
      e. Nose clip will be applied during oxygen consumption measurements.
      f. Explanations will be provided during procedure.
   3. Other measures—
      a. Signed informed consent.
      b. NPO except for medications six to eight hours prior to procedure—prevents vomiting, aspiration; ensures basal metabolic rate.
      c. Administer sedative as ordered.
      d. Have patient urinate before going to lab.

D. *Postcatheterization nursing care:*
   1. *Assessment*—observe for potential complications.
      a. Check pressure dressing over puncture site—bleeding, pain.
      b. Monitor ECG—arrhythmias due to catheter manipulations, myocardial infarction.
      c. Vital signs—observe for shock, respiratory distress (pulmonary emboli, allergic reactions), complaints of palpitations.
      d. Palpate peripheral pulses—assures patency of artery.
      e. Check extremity used for catheter insertion for color, temperature, pain, tingling, numbness—symptoms indicate vascular trauma and should be reported to physician at once.
   2. *Nursing interventions*—
      a. Bedrest three to six hours in supine position—prevents stress on puncture site.
      b. Administer medications as ordered—sedatives, mild narcotics, antiarrhythmics.
      c. Provide emotional support and brief, accurate explanations to patient's questions/concerns.
      d. Refer for counseling as indicated.

2. Cardiopulmonary bypass—blood from cardiac chambers and great vessels is deviated into a pump oxygenator that allows surgical repair of the heart with full visualization and maintains perfusion and function of the body.

A. Rationale—repair of atrial and ventricular septal defects, transposition of great vessels, tetralogy of Fallot, pulmonary and aortic stenosis, coronary artery bypass, and mitral and aortic valve replacement.

B. *Preoperative nursing goals* for the cardiac patient are designed to promote optimal physical functioning, reduce anxiety, and enhance coping mechanisms.

1. Preoperative teaching:
   a. Customary procedures as cough, deep breathe, and turn.
   b. Tour of the intensive-care unit.
   c. Introduction to personnel.
   d. Demonstration of postoperative equipment that will be utilized.
2. Encourage verbalization and questions—fear, depression, and overwhelming despair are frequent feelings.
3. Supportive measures:
   a. Provide opportunity for family to visit patient on morning of surgery.
   b. Provide for religious consultation if desired.
   c. Explain to the patient that medication will be given to reduce pain and that patients are awakened frequently postoperatively for vital signs, deep breathing, coughing, and turning.
C. *Postoperative nursing goals* are designed to promote physiologic function of all body systems, maintain fluid and electrolyte balance, provide comfort and relief from pain, and prevent postoperative complications.
D. *Postoperative assessment:*
   1. *Neurologic observations*—
      a. Levels of consciousness.
      b. Pupillary reactions—dilatation of the pupils occurs when the blood contains excess carbon dioxide.
      c. Movement of limbs and temperature—failure of patient to awaken, hemiplegia, and disorientation may be due to cerebral emboli.
   2. *Respiratory observations*—
      a. Rate, depth, and symmetry of respirations.
         (1) Respirations *increase* in airway obstruction, pain.
         (2) Respirations *decrease* in extreme carbon dioxide retention.
         (3) Respirations *are shallow* and uneven with pain and atelectasis.
      b. Skin color.
      c. Patency and drainage from chest tubes.
      d. Amount and color of sputum.
   3. *Cardiovascular observations*—
      a. Blood pressure:
         (1) Decrease may indicate low cardiac output, tamponade, hemorrhage, arrhythmias, and thrombosis.

(2) Increase may indicate anxiety or hypervolemia.
   b. Radial, apical, and pedal pulses:
      (1) Check for rate, rhythm, and quality.
      (2) *Increased* pulse rate (> 100)—shock, fear, fever, hypoxia, arrhythmias.
      (3) Pulse *deficit*—atrial fibrillation, ectopic beats.
      (4) *Absent* pedal pulse—peripheral emboli.
   c. Central venous pressure (CVP).
   d. Temperature—normal to two- or three-degree elevation during first and second postoperative day.
   4. *Gastrointestinal observations*—presence of nausea, vomiting, or abdominal distention (abdominal distention restricts pulmonary expansion and may indicate electrolyte imbalances).
   5. *Renal system observation*—
      a. Observe volume, color, and specific gravity of urine.
         (1) Report decreased urinary output *below* 25 ml/hour to physician.
         (2) *Lowered* specific gravity—lower than 1.010:
            (a) Overhydration.
            (b) Renal tubular dysfunction.
         (3) *Elevated* specific gravity—greater than 1.020:
            (a) Dehydration.
            (b) Oliguria.
            (c) Presence of blood in urine.
   6. Employ comfort measures and the judicious administration of narcotics to relieve pain.
   7. Utilize passive and active range-of-motion exercises to prevent complications—patient having coronary artery surgery should be positioned in supine position for 48 hours to prevent hypotension; after this period, the patient may be turned from back to right side every two hours.

3. **Splenectomy**—removal of the spleen.
A. Rationale—rupture due to trauma, tumor, idiopathic thrombocytopenic purpura, and acquired hemolytic anemia.
B. *Preoperative nursing goals:*
   1. Administer whole blood, as ordered.
   2. Insert nasogastric tube to decrease postoperative abdominal distention, as ordered.
C. *Postoperative nursing goals* are designed to prevent complications.

1. Observe for signs of hemorrhage—increased bleeding tendency in patients with thrombocytopenia purpura due to decreased platelet counts.
2. Observe for gastrointestinal distention—removal of enlarged spleen may result in distention of stomach and intestines to fill void.
3. Recognize that temperature elevation up to 101 F is not unusual for ten or more days after splenectomy.
4. Manually splint incision when patient coughs—high incidence of atelectasis and pneumonia due to tendency to decrease diaphragmatic excursion with upper abdominal surgery.

4. Vein ligation and stripping

A. Rationale—advancing varicosities, stasis ulcerations, and cosmetic needs of patient.
B. *Postoperative nursing goals* are designed to prevent complications and to promote health habits that help decrease recurrence of varicosities.
   1. Assist with early and frequent ambulation. No chair-sitting. Patient ambulates and then returns to bed. Prevents venous pooling and thrombus formation.
   2. Check elastic bandages and dressings frequently for signs of bleeding.
   3. Review health practices that *prevent* venous stasis:
      a. Weight reduction.
      b. Avoid garments that constrict venous flow, such as garters and girdles.
      c. Frequent changes of position.
         (1) If sitting—walk several minutes each hour to promote circulation.
         (2) If standing—sit and elevate legs when they become tired.
      d. Utilize support hose or elastic stockings to enhance venous return.

GASTROINTESTINAL SYSTEM

1. **Gastrostomy**—the surgical establishment of a fistulous opening between the stomach and the skin to establish a route for administration of food and fluid to the patient.

2. **Gastric surgeries to relieve complications of peptic ulcers**—hemorrhage, perforation, pyloric stenosis or obstruction and/or failure of medical management to promote healing.

A. *Vagotomy with gastrojejunostomy or pyloroplasty:*
   1. Ligation of vagus nerve results in decreased secretions and atonicity of stomach muscle, necessitating an additional drainage procedure.
   2. Gastrojejunostomy provides a second outlet for gastric contents through the anastomosis of jejunum to stomach—treatment of choice for elderly patients who cannot tolerate extensive surgery.
   3. Pyloroplasty divides the pylorus on gastric and duodenal sides transversely, thus providing a larger opening from the stomach to the duodenum—one of the most common procedures.
B. *Vagotomy and antrectomy:*
   1. Resection of vagus nerve and removal of the antral portion of the stomach.
   2. Antral portion of stomach produces gastrin, which stimulates acid secretion.
   3. Procedure removes more of stomach and prevents later duodenal ulceration due to antral stasis.
C. *Partial gastrectomy (Billroth I):*
   1. Distal one-third to one-half of stomach is removed, and the duodenum is anastomosed to remaining portion.
   2. May be done with or without vagotomy.
D. *Hemigastrectomy and vagotomy (Billroth II):*
   1. First part of duodenum, the pylorus, and up to one-half of the stomach are removed.
   2. The duodenal stump is closed, and the jejunum is anastomosed to the remaining stomach.
E. *Preoperative nursing goals* are designed to relieve anxiety and to physically prepare the gastrointestinal system for surgery.
   1. Allow for verbalization of feelings and fears—aids in identifying factors that produce stress and predispose to ulcer formation.
   2. Insert nasogastric tube on morning of surgery to decompress stomach and intestines.
      a. Prevents vomiting and flatulence.
      b. Reduces stress on suture line.
      c. Prevents secretions from infiltrating site of the anastomosis.
   3. Enemas, as ordered.
F. *Postoperative nursing goals* are designed to promote comfort, wound-healing, and nutrition and to prevent complications.
   1. Administer analgesics, as ordered—assures deep

breathing, coughing, and turning, preventing vascular and pulmonary complications.

2. Initiate nasogastric suction:
   a. Check drainage—report excessive bleeding to physician; drainage normally bloody for first 10 to 14 hours postsurgery, then turns dark green.
   b. Irrigate nasogastric tube with saline, as ordered.
   c. Relieve discomfort of nasogastric tube with frequent mouth care, applying water-base lubricant or lotion around nostril and properly taping tube to face.
   d. Maintain low suction to prevent damage to gastric mucosa or suture line.

3. Administer parenteral infusions, as ordered— patient remains NPO one to three days. IV infusions to 3500 ml/day to maintain adequate hydration.

4. Check dressings for bleeding.

5. Check for bowel sounds beginning second postoperative day.
   a. Oral fluids are begun after bowel sounds return and adequate healing of suture line has taken place.
   b. Feedings progress from 30 ml water to bland diet divided into six feedings with 120 ml of fluid every hour between feedings.
   c. Observe for nausea, vomiting, and distention. Regurgitation may be due to eating too fast, eating too much, or to postoperative edema.

6. Instruct the patient in diet modifications to avoid *dumping syndrome:*
   a. Dumping syndrome is a hypoglycemic-type attack that occurs when high osmotic fluids pass quickly into the jejunum, producing hypovolemia and initiating the sympathoadrenal response; symptoms include fainting, dizziness, sweating, and increased pulse rate.
   b. Treatment of dumping syndrome—
      (1) Avoid foods high in salt and carbohydrates.
      (2) Eat frequent, small meals.
      (3) Take fluids between rather than with meals.
      (4) Eat regularly and slowly.
      (5) Rest after meals.

G. *Outcome criteria*—patient and family will be able to:

1. Discuss specific diet modifications following discharge.
   a. Select foods appropriate to a high-protein, high-fat, low-carbohydrate diet.
   b. Set up a pattern of six small feedings a day.
   c. List foods and fluids to be avoided—concentrated sweets such as pastries, soft drinks.
   d. Determine appropriate times for fluid ingestion—if symptoms of dumping syndrome severe, at least two hours after meals.

2. Name drugs, dosage, side effects, and any special precautions in administration (sedatives, antispasmodics, vitamin and mineral replacements, antacids).

3. Identify symptoms that necessitate medical follow-up (vomiting, increasing abdominal distention, hematemesis, tarry stools, pain, diarrhea, elevated temperature).

4. Verbalize plans for reducing stress in home or work environment.

3. *Gastric resection*—treatment of choice for cancer of the stomach.

A. Total gastric resection involves complete removal of the stomach and anastomosis of the esophagus and jejunum.

1. *Nursing interventions* are as given previously for other gastric surgeries, plus measures designed for chest surgery, since the chest cavity is usually entered.

2. Meals are frequent and small to allow absorption in the intestinal tract.

3. Vitamins, particularly vitamin B_{12} and iron, are administered to prevent pernicious anemia.
   a. Removal of stomach halts secretion of "intrinsic factor" needed for absorption of vitamin B_{12}.
   b. Decreased levels of hydrochloric acid inhibit iron absorption.

4. Primary goal of supportive care is to assist patient to maintain the activities of daily living as long as possible with comfort.

B. Partial or subtotal gastric resection is the same as the gastrectomy for ulcer (Billroth II).

4. *Appendectomy*—removal of the appendix.

A. Rationale—acute appendicitis.
   1. *Assessment:*
      a. Generalized abdominal pain that localizes

gradually in right lower quadrant of abdomen.
  b. Low-grade fever.
  c. Rebound tenderness and some rigidity in lower right quadrant.
  d. Moderate leukocytosis.
  e. Anorexia, nausea, and vomiting.
B. *Preoperative nursing goals* are designed to prevent rupture of the appendix.
  1. Laxatives and enemas are contraindicated.
  2. Utilize conservative nursing measures to relieve pain until diagnosis is made—lying with right knee flexed occasionally relieves pain.
C. *Postoperative nursing goals* are designed to promote comfort and prevent complications (see postoperative care).

5. **Herniorrhaphy**—surgical repair of hernia (protrusion of abdominal contents through a weakened area of abdominal cavity).
A. Types:
  1. Inguinal—site is usually posterior inguinal wall. More common in men. Most difficult to repair and more likely to recur after surgery.
  2. Femoral—may result from pregnancy or obesity. More common in women. High incidence of strangulation of intestines.
  3. Umbilical—may result from pregnancy, intestinal obstruction, chronic cough or COPD. Seen most frequently in elderly, obese women.
B. Rationale—prevention of strangulation or incarceration of intestines.
C. See preoperative care.
D. *Postoperative nursing goals* are designed to prevent disruption of the repair.
  1. Encourage deep breathing and turning more than coughing.
    a. Coughing increases intraabdominal pressures, placing stress on incision.
    b. Assist patient to splint incision when coughing.
  2. Administer mild cathartics, as ordered—straining during defecation increases intraabdominal pressures.
  3. Should swelling of scrotum occur, utilize ice bags and elevate scrotum on rolled towel to reduce edema.
  4. Check for voiding. Usually permitted to stand to void. Catheterize if necessary.
  5. Check for abdominal distention. Report to physician. A nasogastric or rectal tube may be ordered.

  6. *Postoperative teaching:*
    a. Encourage patient to stand up straight, as stooping will shorten abdominal muscles, making later posture corrections difficult.
    b. Remind patient not to lift anything heavy and that strenuous activity must be avoided for three to six weeks.

6. **Ileostomy**—surgical formation of a fistula, or artificial anus, between the abdominal wall and ileum (Figure 5–9).
A. Rationale—in ulcerative colitis when the patient's condition does not respond to medical regimen or in which there is profuse bleeding, stricture, or perforation of the bowel or carcinoma is suspected.
B. *Preoperative nursing goals* are designed to relieve anxiety and promote a positive self-image in the patient.
  1. Provide accurate, brief, and reassuring explanations of all procedures.
    a. Allow time for patient to assimilate information emotionally.
    b. Plan to repeat explanations as necessary.
  2. Allow for verbalizations of fears, fantasies, and questions.
  3. Introduce patient to a member of an "Ostomy Club" if possible—provides model for patient of someone who has successfully mastered or adjusted to ileostomy.
  4. Additional physical preparation for surgery includes:
    a. Fluid, electrolyte, and blood replacement.
    b. Low-residue or clear-liquid diet.
    c. Neomycin SO_4 or sulfonamides to reduce intestinal flora.
    d. Enemas until clear.
    e. Insertion of nasogastric tube.
C. *Postoperative nursing goals* are designed to maintain fluid, electrolyte, and nutritional balance, to promote physical and psychologic comfort, and to assist patient in assuming self-care activities.
  1. Administer parenteral fluids with electrolytes and vitamins, as ordered.
    a. Large amounts of fluid and electrolytes may be lost through ileostomy.
    b. Maintain strict intake and output records, as deficits can develop quickly.
  2. Initiate ostomy care.
    a. Apply temporary ileostomy appliance.
      (1) Ileostomy drainage contains digestive enzymes, which can excoriate skin.
      (2) Appliance must be worn at all times.

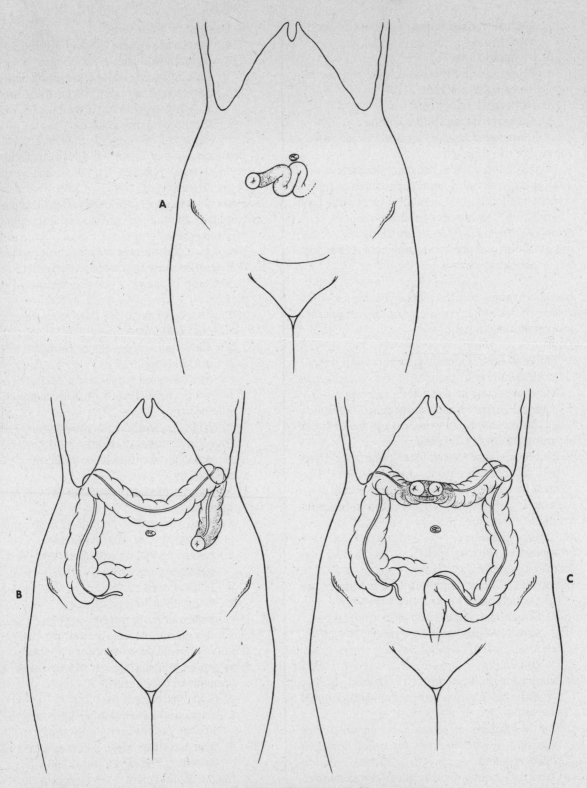

FIGURE 5–9. A. Ileostomy. B. Permanent colostomy. C. Transverse colostomy.
(From Nivinsky, J., Durham, N., and Miller, P. L.: Management of the person with impaired elimination. In Phipps, Long, Woods, eds.: *Medical/surgical nursing*. St. Louis, 1979, The C. V. Mosby Co.)

b. Change appliance prn.
  (1) Observe color, consistency, and amount of drainage.
  (2) Avoid damaging skin by gently peeling appliance from outside toward midline.
c. Keep skin around stoma clean and dry, applying soothing ointments as necessary.
d. Control odors:
  (1) Frequently empty and rinse bag.
  (2) Add deodorizing drops to bag.
  (3) Administer bismuth or chlorophyll preparation, as ordered.
  (4) Ventilate and deodorize room.
e. Recognize that loss of anatomical integrity initiates grieving process.
  (1) Accept feelings of depression, silence, apathy, or disinterest.
  (2) Assist family in understanding patient's behavior.
f. Assist in learning self-management by explaining procedures and why they are done.
  (1) Slowly involve patient in procedures as they are being performed.
  (2) Encourage movement toward independence in bowel care.
  (3) Provide for practice sessions with nursing supervision.
3. Assist patient to identify fears and concerns in home situation—refer patient to community health nurse for follow-up home care.
4. Inform patient of the importance of diet management.
  a. Encourage food high in sodium and potassium—bananas, bouillon, and citrus juices.
  b. Avoid gas-producing, highly seasoned foods; also nuts, raisins, and raw fruits.
5. Advise patient of possible complications that require medical intervention.
  a. Nausea, vomiting, and diarrhea—may lead to fluid and electrolyte imbalance.
  b. Abdominal cramps, vomiting, and watery or no discharge—signs of intestinal obstruction.

7. **Colostomy**—the surgical formation of an artificial anus between the surface of the abdominal wall and the colon.
A. Rationale—intestinal obstruction, cancer of the colon or rectum, severe diverticulitis, infection, perforation, or trauma.

B. Types of colostomies:
1. *Single-barrel*—only one loop of bowel is opened to abdominal surface.
  a. Permanent if bowel distal to it has been resected.
  b. Permanent colostomy usually done close to the end of the descending colon.
2. *Double-barreled*—consists of two loops of bowel, a proximal and a distal portion, opened to abdominal wall.
  a. May be temporary or permanent.
  b. Temporary colostomy usually located at midpoint in descending colon or in the transverse colon.
C. *Preoperative nursing goals* are designed to alleviate fears and promote a positive self-image in the patient (see preoperative ileostomy care).
D. *Postoperative nursing goals* are designed to promote physiologic and psychologic equilibrium and to assist patient in assuming self-care of the colostomy.
1. Initiate ostomy care:
  a. Apply appliance as soon as possible.
  b. Measure stoma each day for current appliance size.
  c. Change appliance prn.
  d. Keep skin around stoma clean and dry, applying protective creams as indicated.
  e. Control odors.
2. Institute colostomy irrigations seven to ten days after surgery.
  a. Aids in controlling elimination and establishing pattern of evacuation.
  b. Prevents intestinal obstruction and reduces excoriation of skin.
3. Explain irrigation procedure and equipment in a concise, reassuring manner.
  a. Involve patient and family with procedure as soon as they are emotionally able.
  b. Encourage return demonstrations.
4. Observe the following precautions during colostomy irrigation:
  a. Place patient in a sitting position in bed or on commode—facilitates the flow of expelled drainage into receptacle or toilet; also some patients find it helps stimulate straining, as if having anal elimination.
  b. Insert lubricated catheter gently 4 to 6 inches (10 to 15 cm) allowing solution to flow into colon slowly—slow-flowing solution relaxes the bowel and facilitates insertion of the tube.

c. Clamp tubing and allow patient to rest if cramping occurs—cramps generally occur due to rapid flow or too much solution.

d. Allow 25 to 45 minutes for return of flow—abdominal massage or position change may assist slow return.

5. Allow patient to verbalize feelings and reassure that radical changes in life style are not necessary.

   a. Involve in colostomy club if one is available.

   b. Refer to community health nurse for follow-up at home.

6. Inform patient of foods that might increase flatulence—corn, beans, cabbage, broccoli, and cauliflower.

7. Inform patient of signs indicating obstruction—abdominal cramps, vomiting, and watery or no discharge.

8. **Gallbladder surgeries**—removal of stones, bile, or pus in the gallbladder itself (*cholecystostomy*) or in the common duct (*choledochostomy*), or complete removal of the gallbladder (*cholecystectomy*).

A. Rationale—acute or chronic cholecystitis, cholelithiasis, or obstruction of the bile duct.

B. *Preoperative nursing goals* are designed to prepare the patient physically and psychologically for surgical procedure.

1. Explain and assist patient with presurgical diagnostic evaluation.

   a. *Cholecystography*—purpose is to estimate the ability of gallbladder to fill, concentrate, and excrete normally.

     (1) Types:

       (a) Oral—2–3 g radiopaque iodine dye (Telepaque [iopanoic acid], Priodax [iodoalphionic acid]) given 10–15 hours before X ray.

       (b) Intravenous—administration of iodide approximately ten minutes before X ray. Allergic responses include nausea, urticaria, dyspnea, chills, faintness.

     (2) Patient preparation—oral:

       (a) Explain procedure and assess for allergies to iodine or seafood.

       (b) One hour after low-fat evening meal, administer prescribed number of tablets (usually six).

       (c) Tablets taken one at a time at

three- to five-minute intervals with at least 8 oz of water.

       (d) Nothing by mouth except water for remainder of evening. NPO after midnight.

       (e) Observe for and report to physician any nausea, vomiting, or diarrhea.

       (f) In morning, after initial X ray, patient given a fatty meal and re-X-rayed in order to observe contractility of gallbladder.

   b. Blood, urine, and stool specimens.

     (1) Leukocyte count may be elevated.

     (2) Blood and urine bilirubin elevated.

     (3) Clay-colored stools.

2. Initiate preoperative instructions.

C. *Postoperative nursing goals* are designed to provide for T-tube or cholecystostomy-tube drainage, prevent complications, and promote physiologic and psychologic equilibrium.

1. Connect nasogastric tube to intermittent suction, as ordered.

2. Connect T-tube to closed-gravity drainage—preserves patency of edematous common duct and ensures bile drainage.

   a. Maintain low- to semi-Fowler's position if not contraindicated—facilitates gravity drainage.

   b. Provide enough tubing to allow turning without tension.

   c. Record bile output every eight hours—initially 300–500 ml and then decreasing amounts—and report increases.

   d. Keep dressings clean and dry—apply protective ointment as necessary to protect skin.

   e. Clamp T-tube, as ordered.

     (1) Observe for abdominal distention, pain, nausea, chills, or fever.

     (2) If symptoms appear, unclamp T-tube and report to physician.

3. Observe skin, sclera, urine, and bowel movements for indication of jaundice.

4. Ambulate early—prevents flatus and respiratory complications.

5. *Outcome criteria*—the patient will be able to:

   a. Discuss diet modifications and identify those foods to be avoided initially (whole milk, cream, fried foods, ham and pork, avocados, etc.).

   b. Recognize that after two to three months,

he/she may begin to add fatty food to tolerance.

   c. Identify drugs, dosage, side effects and any special precautions in administration: vitamin supplements (A, D, E, and K), anticholinergics, antispasmodics.

   d. State plans for follow-up care and symptoms necessitating medical interventions (pain, fever, jaundice, dark urine, clay-colored stools, itching).

9. *Hemorrhoidectomy*—removal of all internal and external hemorrhoids by ligation and excision, clamping and cauterization, or other procedure.

A. Rationale—bleeding, prolapsed, strangulated, or thrombosed hemorrhoids.

B. *Preoperative nursing goals* are designed to promote comfort and physical equilibrium.

  1. Administer low-residue diet—reduces stool formation.

  2. Administer cleansing tap-water enemas, as ordered.

C. *Postoperative nursing goals* are designed to reduce pain, promote gastrointestinal function, and prevent complications.

  1. Administer ice packs, warm compresses, sitz baths, analgesic ointments, or narcotics to relieve discomfort and pain, as ordered.

  2. Assist patient in assuming a position of comfort.

  3. Assist with voiding to reduce bladder distention and urinary retention.

   a. Assist male patients in standing.

   b. Utilize bedside commode for women.

   c. Encourage fluids.

   d. Administer bethanechol (Urecholine) Cl, as ordered (see Appendix D, Drugs).

   e. Catheterize if necessary.

  4. Assist with the reestablishment of normal bowel patterns.

   a. Liquid or low-residue diet until successful defecation:

    (1) Prevents bowel movement until some healing has taken place.

    (2) Modifies consistency of stool.

   b. Mineral oil or psyllium (Metamucil) to facilitate elimination, as ordered.

   c. Low oil-retention enema, as ordered, usually third postoperative day.

   d. Reduce discomfort of first defecation by administering analgesic 30 minutes before patient attempts defecation.

    (1) Provide privacy but remain with patient and observe for dizziness or fainting.

    (2) Utilize moist cotton rather than toilet paper to cleanse area.

   e. Follow each defecation with a warm sitz bath—promotes healing and reduces discomfort.

  5. Observe for signs of hemorrhage—may occur immediately or four to ten days after surgery.

  6. Should hemorrhage occur:

   a. Place patient on bedrest.

   b. Record vital signs.

   c. Note amount and color of drainage.

   d. Apply pressure dressing and ice pack.

   e. Notify physician.

  7. *Outcome criteria*—the patient will be able to:

   a. State rationale for diet modifications (enhanced evacuation of soft stools).

    (1) Bulk-producing foods.

    (2) Sufficient fluid intake.

   b. Plan for regular exercise periods daily.

   c. Demonstrate cleansing techniques of rectal area and explain importance of utilizing until healing has occurred.

   d. Identify symptoms requiring prompt medical follow-up—bleeding, continued pain on defecation, foul drainage, constipation.

GENITOURINARY SYSTEM

1. *Cystoscopy*—see Appendix C.

2. *Prostatectomies*

A. Types:

  1. *Transurethral resection* of prostate (TUR)—removal of obstructive prostatic tissue by an electric wire (resectoscope) introduced through the urethra.

  2. *Suprapubic* prostatectomy—low midline incision is made directly over the bladder; bladder is opened and prostatic tissue is removed through incision in urethral mucosa.

  3. *Retropubic* prostatectomy—removal of hypertrophied prostatic tissue through a low abdominal incision; bladder is not opened.

  4. *Perineal* prostatectomy—removal of prostatic tissue is accomplished through an incision made between the scrotum and the rectum; usually results in impotency.

B. Rationale—to relieve urinary retention and frequency caused by benign prostatic hypertrophy or cancer of the prostate.

C. *Preoperative nursing goals* are designed to facilitate optimal kidney function.

   1. Sterile insertion of indwelling urinary catheter or suprapubic cystostomy—to reestablish urinary drainage.
   2. Antibiotics, as ordered—to prevent and control infection.
   3. Push fluids to ensure adequate hydration—patients often limit their own fluid intake because of urinary frequency.
      a. Monitor intake and output.
      b. Weigh daily.
   4. Assist with renal function studies—determine if backflow has damaged kidneys.
   5. Assist with hematologic studies—to identify any clotting defects, as hemorrhage is a major postoperative complication.
   6. Provide diet high in protein, vitamins, and iron.

D. *Postoperative nursing goals* are designed to promote optimal bladder drainage, prevent complications, promote comfort, and assist in rehabilitation.

   1. Utilize sterile closed-gravity system for urinary drainage—maintain external traction, as ordered.
   2. In suprapubic prostatectomy, connect suprapubic catheter to closed-gravity drainage system—observe character, amount, and flow of urethral and suprapubic catheters.
   3. Check dressings:
      a. Keep dry and clean.
      b. Reinforce if necessary.
      c. Notify physician of excess bleeding.
   4. Maintain continuous bladder irrigation, as ordered.
      a. Helpful in controlling bleeding and keeping clots from forming.
      b. Observe frequently for bladder distention:
         (1) Distinct mound over pubis.
         (2) Slow drop in collecting bottle.
         (3) Irrigate catheter, as ordered.
      c. Observe for signs of increased bleeding:
         (1) Bright red drainage and clots.
         (2) Cool, clammy skin, pallor, and increased pulse rate.
   5. Explain purpose of catheter to patient.
      a. Urge to void due to bladder spasm.
      b. Pulling on catheter will increase bleeding and clot formation.

   6. Administer anticholinergic medications to reduce bladder spasms (see Appendix D, Drugs).
   7. Diet—clear-liquid to regular diet as tolerated.
   8. Force fluids to 3000 ml per day unless contraindicated.
   9. After removal of suprapubic catheter, observe for urinary drainage q4h for 24 hours.
      a. Administer skin care.
      b. Report excessive drainage to physician.
   10. Ambulate, as ordered, keeping urinary drainage bag dependent.
   11. Deal with fears of incontinence and loss of male identity.
   12. After urinary catheter is removed:
       a. Note time and amount of each voiding.
       b. Begin perineal exercises—buttocks are pressed together and held in that position as long as possible; 10 to 20 times each hour; assist patient in regaining urinary control.
       c. Inform patient he can expect "dribbling" following catheter removal.
   13. Postoperative instructions include avoiding:
       a. Long automobile trips—increases tendency to bleed.
       b. Alcoholic beverages—causes burning on urination.
       c. Tub baths—increases possibility of infections.

3. *Nephrectomy*—removal of a kidney; may be done through a flank, retroperitoneal, abdominal, thoracic, or thoracic-abdominal approach.

A. Rationale—malignant tumor or severe trauma resulting in nonfunctioning organ.

B. *Preoperative nursing goals* are designed to optimize physical and psychologic function (see general preoperative assessment).

   1. Assist in diagnostic studies designed to evaluate renal function.
      a. Serum electrolytes, BUN, creatinine, and phenolsulfonphthalein.
      b. Intravenous urography.

C. *Postoperative nursing goals* are designed to promote comfort and prevent complications.

   1. Observe for signs of paralytic ileus—a fairly common complication following renal surgery.
   2. Assess fluid and electrolyte balance by weighing

patient daily—maintain within 2% of preoperative levels.

3. Observe carefully for signs of hemorrhage.

4. *Ureterolithotomy*—key points similar to nephrectomy.

5. *Kidney transplantation*—placement of a donor (sibling, parent, cadaver) kidney into the iliac fossa of a recipient and the anastomosis of its ureter to the bladder of the recipient.

A. Rationale—end stage of renal disease.

B. Donor selection:

1. Sibling or parent donor—survival rate of kidney is greater and is preferred procedure for transplantation.

2. Cadaver—greater rate of rejection following transplantation, but the majority of transplants are with cadaver kidneys.

C. *Preoperative nursing goals* are designed to promote optimal physical and emotional support for patient and family.

1. Patient teaching should include:

   a. Nature of surgery and placement of kidney.

   b. Possibility of postoperative dialysis.

   c. Purpose and effects of immunosuppressive therapy.

   d. Rationale for employing reverse isolation and its techniques.

   e. Drainage tubes that will be inserted during surgery.

   f. Postoperative turning, coughing, and deep breathing exercises.

   g. Assurance that medication will be given for relief of pain.

2. Identify and deal with the fears and anxieties of patient and family.

3. Support patient who needs continued dialysis prior to surgery—optimal preoperative physical condition requires removal of waste products and fluid, important to electrolyte and acid-base balance.

4. Begin administration of immunosuppressive drugs.

   a. Azathioprine—an antimetabolite that interferes with cellular division:

      (1) Results in dysfunction and death of immunologic and other body cells.

      (2) Side effects—

         (a) Gastrointestinal bleeding.

         (b) Bone marrow depression.

         (c) Development of malignant neoplasms.

         (d) Infection.

         (e) Liver damage.

   b. Glucocorticoids—believed to effect lymphocyte production by inhibiting nucleic acid synthesis.

      (1) Antiinflammatory action helps prevent tissue damage if rejection occurs.

      (2) Side effects—

         (a) Stress ulcer with bleeding.

         (b) Decreased glucose tolerance.

         (c) Muscle weakness.

         (d) Osteoporosis.

         (e) Moon facies.

         (f) Acne and striae.

         (g) Depression and hallucinations.

D. *Postoperative nursing goals* are designed to maintain urinary output and fluid and electrolyte balance, observe for signs of rejection, prevent infections, and promote physical and emotional comfort.

1. Institute reverse isolation techniques.

2. Attach indwelling catheter to closed drainage system.

   a. Monitor color, characteristics, and amount of urinary output.

      (1) Kidney may begin to function immediately, putting out large amount of urine.

      (2) If kidney does not function within 24 to 48 hours, hemodialysis is instituted.

      (3) Kidney may not function for a week or more.

      (4) Gross hematuria or clots in urine should be reported immediately to physician.

      (5) Carry out perineal care each shift—prevents bacteria from entering meatus and bladder.

3. Institute and maintain respiratory hygiene procedures:

   a. Coughing and deep breathing.

   b. Clapping.

   c. Blow bottles.

   d. IPPB.

   e. Mouth care.

4. Observe for fluid and electrolyte disturbances.

   a. Hypovolemia:

      (1) Decreased blood pressure.

      (2) Increased pulse rate.

    (3) Increased hematocrit (hemoconcentration).

    (4) Confusion, hallucinations, and delirium.

  b. Hypervolemia:

    (1) Hypertension.

    (2) Peripheral and pulmonary edema.

    (3) Puffy face.

    (4) Distended neck veins.

    (5) Tachycardia.

    (6) Increased CVP.

  c. Hyperkalemia:

    (1) Intestinal colic and diarrhea.

    (2) Muscle weakness.

    (3) Flaccid paralysis.

  d. Azotemia and acidosis:

    (1) Increased rate and depth of respirations.

    (2) Irritability, lethargy.

    (3) Decreasing ability to carry on a conversation.

5. Observe for early signs and symptoms of rejection.

  a. In functioning and nonfunctioning kidneys:

    (1) Low-grade fever.

    (2) Tenderness and/or pain over graft site.

  b. In functioning kidneys:

    (1) Decreasing urine output.

    (2) Decreased creatinine clearance.

    (3) Increasing serum potassium and BUN.

    (4) Decreasing urinary sodium.

    (5) Increased proteinuria.

6. Observe for side effects of immunosuppressive therapy.

7. Promote psychosocial adjustment.

  a. Assure patient that feelings of depression may be drug-related.

  b. Allow verbalization of fears.

  c. Deal with feelings due to transition from chronically ill state to relative state of wellness.

    (1) Reassumption of role responsibilities.

    (2) Alteration of dependent habits and life style.

    (3) Sexual adjustments:

      (a) Problems of contraception.

      (b) Normal sexual development and attendant confusion in adolescents.

    (4) Bodily changes due to steroid therapy—moon facies, weight gain (truncal obesity).

    (5) Reemployment or new employment.

8. *Outcome criteria*—the patient and/or family member will be able to:

  a. Explain diet modifications if ordered and develop a meal plan consistent with prescribed diet.

  b. Identify each drug prescribed and explain dosage, timing, and side effects of each.

  c. Demonstrate taking and recording of oral temperature, daily weight, intake and output, and means of collecting 24-hour urine specimens.

  d. Explain rationale for preventive health care practices—

    (1) Measures to avoid infections.

    (2) Plans for dental and gynecologic care.

    (3) Need to avoid immunization with live-virus vaccines.

  e. Identify signs and symptoms of rejection, infections that require prompt medical intervention.

  f. Name community resources available for assistance with illness and/or rehabilitation.

SURGERIES OF FEMALE REPRODUCTIVE SYSTEM

1. **Hysterectomy**—removal of the uterus.

A. Types:

  1. Total hysterectomy—removal of entire uterus, may be done abdominally or vaginally.

  2. Panhysterectomy—removal of uterus, tubes, and ovaries.

B. Rationale—cancer of the cervix, severe endometritis, cancer of the uterus, uterine prolapse, and fibroid tumors.

C. *Preoperative nursing goals* are designed to reduce anxiety and depression and promote optimal physical and psychologic functions.

  1. Allow verbalization of feelings.

    a. Many women fear the loss of femininity and changes in secondary sex characteristics.

    b. Patient may fear cancer or the discovery of venereal disease.

    c. Disappointment may be acute if woman has not had children.

  2. Assess relationships with husband, family, and significant others.

  3. Administer vaginal douche or enemas, as ordered.

D. *Postoperative nursing goals* are designed to prevent complications and support coping mechanisms.
  1. Catheter care—temporary bladder atony may be present as a result of edema or nerve trauma; occurs primarily when vaginal approach is utilized.
  2. Observe for abdominal distention.
     a. Utilize rectal tube to decrease flatus.
     b. Auscultate abdomen for bowel sounds.
     c. Encourage early ambulation.
  3. Utilize measures to decrease pelvic congestion and prevent venous stasis.
     a. Avoid high-Fowler's position.
     b. Apply antiembolic stockings, as ordered.
     c. Institute passive leg exercises.
  4. Apply abdominal support, as ordered.
  5. Allow for verbalization of feelings.
  6. *Discharge teaching plan* includes:
     a. Avoidance of coitus or vaginal douching until advised by physician.
     b. Avoidance of heavy lifting for at least two months.
     c. Explanation of hormonal replacement therapy if applicable.
     d. Avoidance of sitting for long periods of time wearing constrictive clothing, which tends to increase pelvic congestion.
     e. Understanding that menstruation will no longer occur.
     f. Importance of reporting symptoms such as fever, increased or bloody vaginal discharge, and hot flashes to physician.

2. *Radical mastectomy*—surgical removal of the entire breast; subclavicular, apical, pectoral, and axillary nodes; and the pectoralis major and minor muscles. There are several modifications to this procedure.

A. Rationale—carcinoma of the breast, intraductal papillomas, and Paget's disease.

B. *Preoperative nursing goals* are designed to support the patient and family.
  1. Allow for verbalization of fears and feelings and dispelling misconceptions.
  2. Answer all questions clearly and concisely.
  3. Institute preoperative instruction.

C. *Postoperative nursing goals* are designed to minimize complications and facilitate physical and psychologic functioning (see postoperative care).

  1. Observe pressure dressings, axilla and under shoulder, for bleeding.
     a. Report excessive drainage or bloody drainage.
     b. Do not remove dressings but reinforce if necessary.
  2. Connect drainage tubes to suction machine or portable suction (Hemovac)—drains serum and blood, allowing skin flap to adhere to chest wall.
  3. Facilitate venous and lymphatic drainage.
     a. Place patient in semi-Fowler's position.
     b. Elevate arm above right atrium with pillows.
  4. Maintain joint mobility.
     a. Flexion and extension of fingers and elbows.
     b. Initiate active ROM exercises as soon as ordered to prevent ankylosis—exercises should not be painful.
     c. Encourage self-care activities, as ordered.
  5. If skin graft has been performed, check donor site every four hours—limit active arm exercises.
  6. Assist with emotional response to changes in body image.
     a. Encourage patient to look at scar.
     b. Involve patient in incision care as tolerated.
     c. Refer to "Reach for Recovery" program of American Cancer Society.
  7. Inform patient about occurrences of postoperative edema and importance of avoiding even minor injury to the arm, since removal of lymph nodes decreases the body's ability to combat infection.
  8. *Outcome criteria*—the patient will be able to:
     a. Identify her feelings regarding loss of breast.
     b. Demonstrate postmastectomy arm exercises (Figure 5–10) and explain necessity for continuance until full range of motion in affected shoulder returns.
     c. Describe rationale for avoiding fatigue and constricting garments, and means for avoiding minor injuries to the arm while carrying out activities of daily living.
     d. Describe symptoms indicating need for prompt medical attention (increased edema in affected arm, redness or signs of infection in or around incision, mass in unaffected breast).
     e. Describe procedure and demonstrate breast self-examination on unaffected breast.

Exercise: Climbing the wall
1. Stand facing wall with toes close to wall.
2. Bend elbows and place palms of hands against wall at shoulder level.
3. Move both hands parallel to each other up the wall as far as possible until incisional pull or pain occurs.
4. Move both hands down to starting position.
5. Goal: complete extension with elbow straight.
6. Activities that utilize the same action: reaching top shelves, hanging out clothes, washing windows, hanging curtains, setting hair.

Exercise: Arm swinging
1. Bend forward from waist, permitting both arms to relax and hang naturally.
2. Swing arms together left to right (motion comes from shoulder).
3. Swing arms in circles parallel to floor, clockwise and counterclockwise.
4. Stand up slowly.

Exercise: Rope pull
1. Attach a rope over a shower rod or hook.
2. Grasp each end of rope, alternately pulling on each end, raising affected arm to a point of incisional pull or pain.
3. Shorten rope over time until affected arm is raised almost directly overhead.

Exercise: Elbow spread
1. Clasp hands behind neck.
2. Raise elbows to chin level, holding head erect. Move slowly and rest when incisional pull or pain occurs.
3. Gradually spread elbows apart. Rest when pull or pain occurs.

FIGURE 5–10. Postmastectomy arm exercises
(From Long, B. C.: Problems of the breast. In Phipps, Long, Woods, eds.: *Medical/ surgical nursing.* St. Louis, 1979. The C. V. Mosby Co.)

ENDOCRINE SYSTEM

1. **Thyroidectomy**—partial or total removal of the thyroid gland.
A. Rationale—total removal if malignancy is present; partial removal (five-sixths) to correct hyperthyroidism.
B. *Preoperative nursing goals* are designed to promote normal thyroid function and reduce side effects of thyrotoxicosis. (See Part C: Blood Pressure, for assessment of findings in hyperthyroidism.)
   1. Provide quiet, nonstimulating, stable environment.
      a. Avoid discrepancies in timing and performance of procedures.
      b. Restrict visitors if indicated.
      c. Assist with activities that are difficult due to tremors—pouring beverages or tying shoes.
   2. Provide high-protein, high-carbohydrate, high–vitamin B diet—to rebuild lost tissue and meet increased energy needs.
      a. Avoid stimulating beverages such as coffee, tea, and colas.
      b. Provide food choices when possible.
   3. Administer medications, as ordered.
      a. Antithyroid preparations—propylthiouracil and methimazole (Tapazole):
         (1) Slow-acting chemicals that inhibit synthesis of thyroxine.
         (2) Important to time and space dosages to maintain therapeutic levels.
         (3) Side effects—
            (a) Sore throat.
            (b) Fever.
            (c) Rash.
            (d) Jaundice.
      b. Iodine preparations—Lugol's solution:
         (1) Iodine preparations reduce thyroid vascularity and help prevent postoperative hemorrhage.
         (2) Measure solution accurately.
         (3) Add drops to fruit juice or milk to disguise unpleasant taste.
C. *Postoperative nursing goals* are designed to promote physical and emotional equilibrium and to prevent complications.
   1. Place patient in semi-Fowler's position, immobilizing head with pillows or sandbags.

a. Prevents flexion or hyperextension of neck, thus reducing stress on sutures.

b. Reduces edema and promotes venous return.

2. Support patient's neck by placing a hand on either side during position changes.

   a. As soon as patients are able, teach them to support weight of the head by placing their hands at back of the neck while moving in bed.

   b. After sutures are removed, institute ROM exercises (flexion, lateral movement, and hyperextension), as ordered—prevents contractures.

3. Prevent or relieve complications.

   a. Hemorrhage:
      (1) Check vital signs.
      (2) Check dressings for drainage.
      (3) Reinforce dressing as needed.
      (4) Report excess drainage to physician.

   b. Respiratory obstruction:
      (1) Turn, cough, and deep breathe.
      (2) Apply ice packs to incision, as ordered—to promote comfort and reduce edema.

   c. Hoarseness and weakness of voice due to laryngeal nerve damage:
      (1) Check quality of voice.
      (2) Avoid unnecessary talking.
      (3) Establish alternate means of communication—pencil and paper.

   d. Hypocalcemia and tetany due to accidental removal of parathyroid gland:
      (1) Check reflexes q2h and report any muscle twitching immediately.
         (a) Chvostek's sign—tapping of the face in front of the ear produces spasm of ipsilateral facial muscles.
         (b) Trousseau's sign—compression of upper arm elicits carpal (wrist) spasm.

4. Promote comfort measures:
   a. Administer narcotics, as ordered.
   b. Offer iced fluids (if preferred and tolerated)—soothes sore throat.

5. Ambulation and diet as tolerated.

2. *Adrenalectomy*—surgical excision of adrenal tumor.

A. Rationale—pheochromocytoma, primary aldosteronism, and Cushing's syndrome; bilateral adrenalectomy may be done for cancer of the breast or prostate with metastasis.

B. *Preoperative nursing goals* are designed to reduce risk of postoperative complications.

1. Steroid therapy is discontinued to prevent postoperative infection.

2. Antihypertensive drugs are discontinued as surgery may result in severe hypotension.

3. Administer phenobarbital for sedation, as ordered.

4. Institute general preoperative care.

C. *Postoperative nursing goals* are designed to promote hormonal balance and prevent postoperative complications.

1. Administer hydrocortisone parenteral therapy, as ordered—rate dictated by fluid and electrolyte balance, blood sugar, and blood pressure.

2. Monitor vital signs per protocol and prn for 48 hours or until stability is regained.

3. If on vasopressor drugs such as metaraminol (Aramine) bitartrate, check vital signs every 15 minutes.

   a. Maintain flow rate, as ordered.
   b. Notify physician of significant changes.
   c. Readings that are normotensive for some may be hypotensive for patient who has been hypertensive.
   d. Observe for signs of decreased perfusion—confusion, oliguria, tachycardia, and increased pulse and respiratory rates.

4. NPO—attach nasogastric tube to intermittent suction; abdominal distention is common side effect of this surgery.

5. Promote respiratory hygiene and prevent complications.

   a. Turn, cough, and deep breathe.
   b. Splint flank incision when coughing.
   c. Administer narcotic 30 minutes before coughing—as flank incision is close to diaphragm, coughing may be extremely painful.
   d. Place in flat or semi-Fowler's position.
   e. Auscultate breath sounds q2h—decreased or absent breath sounds, sudden chest pain, and dyspnea should be reported immediately, as spontaneous pneumothorax can occur.
   f. Administer frequent mouth care.

6. Check dressings, reinforcing as needed.

7. Ambulate, as ordered.

   a. Check blood pressure every 15 minutes when ambulation is first attempted.
   b. Apply elastic stockings to lower extremities to enhance stability of vascular system.

8. Maintain diet as tolerated after nasogastric tube is removed.
9. *Postoperative teachings* should include:
    a. Signs and symptoms of adrenal crisis—
       (1) Rapid, weak, or thready pulse.
       (2) Elevated temperature.
       (3) Restlessness.
       (4) Severe weakness and lethargy.
       (5) Headache.
       (6) Convulsions.
    b. Importance of maintaining steroid therapy schedule—to ensure therapeutic serum level:
       (1) Weigh daily.
       (2) Clinitest daily.
       (3) Report undesirable side effects to physician.
    c. Importance of avoiding persons with infections—decreased resistance.
    d. Importance of adequate rest, moderate exercise, and good nutrition.

3. Hypophysectomy—complete removal of hypophysis or pituitary gland.

SPECIAL SENSES—EYE AND EAR

1. Cataract removal—removal of opacified lens; opacity may be due to degeneration with age, or to toxic, metabolic, or traumatic injuries.

A. Rationale—loss of vision.
B. *Preoperative nursing goals* are designed to reduce patient's anxiety.
   1. *Preoperative teaching:*
      a. Instruct patient not to rub, touch, or squeeze eyes shut after surgery.
      b. Inform patient that eye patches will be on after surgery.
      c. Reassure patient that assistance will be given for needs.
   2. Administer mydriatic eye drops prior to surgery (see Appendix D, Drugs).
      a. Note dilatation of pupils.
      b. Avoid glaring lights.
   3. Determine degree of sight by testing visual fields and acuity.
C. *Postoperative nursing goals* are designed to reduce stress on the sutures, prevent hemorrhage, and promote psychologic well-being.
   1. Maintain bedrest up to 24 hours in a flat or low-Fowler's position.

2. Patient may lie on back and turn to *unoperated* side—turning to operative side increases pressures.
3. Avoid activities that may increase intraocular pressures:
    a. Antiemetic for nausea, avoid vomiting if possible.
    b. Deep breathe but avoid coughing.
    c. Brushing teeth, hair, shaving, bending, and stooping are usually forbidden.
       (1) Provide mouth wash.
       (2) Provide hair care.
       (3) Place equipment and personal items within easy reach.
       (4) Utilize "step-in" slippers.
4. Provide frequent contacts with elderly to prevent development of emotional disturbances associated with sensory deprivation.
5. Diet and ambulation, as ordered.
6. Assist patient in adjusting to temporary cataract spectacle lenses.
    a. Explain about magnification of objects, perceptual distortion, and blind areas in peripheral vision.
    b. Guide patients through some activities with glasses on to help them adjust to distortions and spatial relationships.
    c. To decrease distortion, instruct patient to look through the central portion of the lens and to turn head to the side when looking to the side.
7. Involve patient and family in *postoperative teaching:*
    a. Instillation of eye drops.
    b. Signs and symptoms of infections—
       (1) Redness and pain.
       (2) Edema and drainage.
    c. Need to continue wearing eye shield at night to prevent injury.
    d. Avoidance of heavy lifting.
    e. Encouraging independence in the performance of self-care activities.

2. Retinal detachment—separation of retina from choroid as the result of trauma or degeneration; vision becomes blurred, patchy, and may be totally lost.

A. Surgical interventions:
   1. Electrodiathermy—electrode needle is passed through sclera, draining the subretinal fluid; retina will then adhere to the choroid.
   2. Cryosurgery—supercooled probe is applied to

the sclera, causing a scar, which pulls the choroid and retina together.

3. Laser beam—a beam of intense light from a carbon arc is directed through the dilated pupil onto the retina; effect is the same as in electrodiathermy.

4. Sclera buckling—the sclera is resected or shortened to enhance the contact between the choroid and retina.

B. *Preoperative nursing goals* are designed to orient the patient to environment and to reduce anxiety.

1. Encourage verbalization of feelings and answer all questions, reinforce physician's explanation of surgical procedures.

2. Prevent further detachment by keeping patient quiet in bed.
   a. Eyes are usually covered to reduce stress and provide rest.
   b. Position so that retinal hole is in the lowest position.

3. Administer medications, as ordered:
   a. Cycloplegic or mydriatics.
   b. Keep pupils widely dilated.

C. *Postoperative nursing goals* are designed to reduce intraocular stress, prevent hemorrhage, and support the patient's coping mechanisms.

1. Bedrest in flat or low-Fowler's position—sandbags may be used to position head.

2. Movements that increase intraocular pressures are usually restricted.

3. Administer medications, as ordered (see Appendix D, Drugs).
   a. Mydriatics.
   b. Antibiotics—prevent infections.
   c. Corticosteroids—reduce inflammation.

4. Employ ROM exercises and apply elastic stockings to legs to avoid thrombus formation during period of bedrest.

5. To allay anxiety, plan all care with the patient.
   a. Allow patient to verbalize feelings and fears.
   b. Encourage family interaction and diversional activities.

3. **Stapedectomy**—removal of the stapes and its replacement with a prosthesis.

A. Rationale—deafness due to otosclerosis, which fixes the stapes, preventing it from oscillating and transmitting vibrations to the fluids in the inner ear.

B. *Preoperative nursing goals* are designed to provide emotional support and to assist patient in understanding the nature of the procedure.

1. Preoperative teaching includes:
   a. Informing patient of the importance of keeping head in position ordered by physician postoperatively.
   b. Necessity of avoiding activities such as sneezing, blowing the nose, and vomiting, which increase pressure in eustachian tubes.
   c. Breathing exercises.

C. *Postoperative nursing goals* are designed to promote physical and psychologic equilibrium.

1. Place patient in position ordered by physician—this varies according to preference.

2. Raise siderails as vertigo is a common experience.

3. Check ear dressings frequently.

4. Administer medications, as ordered.
   a. Antiemetic to control vomiting.
   b. Analgesics to control pain.
   c. Antibiotics to control infection.

5. Provide emotional support to patient and family—reassure patient that reduction in hearing is normal and that hearing may not immediately improve following surgery.

6. Assist with ambulation and avoid rapid turning—reduces vertigo.

7. *Postoperative teaching principles:*
   a. Keep ear covered outdoors.
   b. Keep outer ear plug clean, dry, and changed.
   c. Avoid washing hair for two weeks.
   d. Avoid air travel and swimming for six months.
   e. Avoid individuals with upper respiratory infections.
   f. Avoid heavy lifting.

NEUROLOGIC SYSTEM

1. **Craniotomy**—excision of a part of the skull (burr hole to several centimeters) in order to treat disease or dysfunction with minimal neurologic deficit.

A. Rationale—for exploratory purposes and biopsy; to remove neoplasms, evacuate hematomas or excess fluid, control hemorrhage, repair skull fractures, remove scar tissue, repair or excise aneurysms, and drain abscesses.

B. *Preoperative nursing care:*

1. *Assessment*—obtain baseline measures—
   a. Vital signs.
   b. Levels of consciousness.

    c. Mental and emotional status.
    d. Pupillary reactions.
    e. Motor strength and functioning.
    f. Facial-muscle integrity and symmetry.
  2. *Interventions*—
    a. Provide psychologic support—listening; accurate, brief explanations.
    b. Cut hair and shave scalp (P.M. or A.M. of surgery).
    c. Cover scalp with clean towel.
    d. Enema and/or cathartics, as ordered.
    e. Insert indwelling Foley catheter, as ordered.

C. *Postoperative nursing care:*
  1. *Assessment*—observe for changes indicating complications.
    a. Vital signs—
      (1) Decreased blood pressure—shock.
      (2) Widened pulse pressure—increased intracranial pressure.
      (3) Respiratory failure—compression of medullary respiratory centers.
      (4) Hyperthermia—disturbance of heat-regulating mechanism—infection.
    b. Neurologic—
      (1) Pupils—ipsilateral dilation (increased intracranial pressure), visual disturbances.
      (2) Altered levels of consciousness.
      (3) Altered cognitive or emotional status—disorientation common.
      (4) Motor function and strength—hypertonia, hypotonia, seizures.
    c. Blood gases—adequacy of ventilation.
    d. Check dressings frequently.
      (1) Maintain asepsis.
      (2) Reinforce as necessary.
      (3) Report CSF leakage immediately.
    e. Check eyes for periorbital edema.
      (1) Apply light ice compresses as necessary.
      (2) Remove crusts from eyelids.
    f. Check integrity of seventh cranial nerve (facial).
  2. *Interventions:*
    a. Supratentorial surgery (cerebrum)—
      (1) Semi-Fowler's position.
      (2) May not lie on operative side.
    b. Infratentorial (brain stem, cerebellum)—
      (1) Flat in bed.
      (2) May turn to either side but not on back.

      (3) NPO for 24 to 48 hours.
      (4) Administer antiemetic to avoid vomiting—increases intracranial pressures.
    c. Administer medications to reduce intracranial pressures as ordered (osmotic diuretics—mannitol), corticosteroids (Decadron).
    d. Orient patient frequently to person, time, place—reduces restlessness and confusion.
    e. Keep siderails up for safety.
    f. Avoid restraints—increases agitation and intracranial pressures.
    g. Ice bags to head—reduces headache.
    h. Administer mild analgesics for pain—narcotics and sedatives avoided or given judiciously to prevent masking of neurologic signs and/or respiratory depression.
    i. Provide coverage (scarves, wigs) for scalp once dressings removed.
    j. Assist with ambulation.
    k. Deal realistically with neurological deficits—facilitate acceptance, adjustment, independence.

2. **Laminectomy and spinal fusion**—excision of the dorsal arch of the vertebra, with fusion of two or more vertebrae with a bone graft (from iliac crest) to stabilize the spine.

A. Rationale—excision of herniated intervertebral disks, removal of neoplasms, abscesses, and/or dissection of anterolateral spinothalmic tracts for relief of intractable pain.

B. *Preoperative nursing care:*
  1. *Assessment*—baseline data—
    a. Vital signs.
    b. Muscle strength and function.
    c. Sensory integrity.
    d. Cognitive and emotional responses.
  2. *Interventions*—
    a. Bedrest on firm mattress (herniated disk).
    b. Edemas or cathartics, as ordered.
    c. Insert Foley retention catheter as ordered.
    d. Administer analgesics, muscle relaxants, as ordered.
    e. Surgical prep, as ordered.

C. *Postoperative nursing care:*
  1. *Assessment*—
    a. Vital signs—after cervical laminectomy, observe for respiratory distress.
    b. Motor function—flexion and extension of feet, hands.

c. Sensory function—sensations of tingling, numbing should be reported to physician.

d. Observe for abdominal distention—rectal tube as indicated, listen for bowel sounds, NPO until established and patient has passed flatus or stool.

2. *Interventions*—
   a. Keep flat for at least four hours.
   b. Turn every two to three hours—log roll keeping back straight.
   c. When on side, pillow between knees, knees flexed.
   d. Flat in bed if cervical laminectomy.
   e. Maintain intravenous infusion until diet as tolerated.
   f. Ambulate as ordered, avoid sitting position.
   g. Apply brace or corset as ordered.

SKELETAL SYSTEM

1. *Fractures*—A disruption in the continuity of bone as the result of trauma or various disease processes, such as Cushing's syndrome, which weaken the bone structure.

A. Types of fractures:
   1. *Open or compound*—the fractured bone extends through to the skin and mucous membranes; increased potential for infection.
   2. *Closed or simple fracture*—fractured bone does not protrude through the skin.
   3. *Complete fracture*—fracture extends through the entire bone, disrupting the periosteum on both sides of the bone.
   4. *Incomplete fracture*—fracture extends only part way through the bone; bone continuity is not totally interrupted.
   5. *Greenstick or willow-, hickory-stick*—fracture of one side of bone, the other side merely bends.
   6. *Impacted or telescoped*—fracture in which bone fragments are forcibly driven into other or adjacent bone structures.
   7. *Comminuted*—fracture having more than one fracture line and bone fragments broken into several pieces.
   8. *Depressed*—fractures in which bone or bone fragments are driven inward, as in skull or facial fractures.

B. *Assessment* of bone fracture:
   1. Deformity.
   2. Pain.

3. Swelling and bruising.
4. Abnormal or impaired mobility.
5. Crepitus—grating sensations heard or felt as bone fragments rub against each other.

C. *Treatment goals* for fractures are designed to restore function to the affected part, prevent complications, and obtain normal (cosmetic) appearance.

1. Reduction or setting of the bone—restores bone alignment as nearly as possible.
   a. *Closed reduction*—manual traction or manipulation.
      (1) Usually done under general anesthesia to reduce pain and muscle spasm.
      (2) Maintenance of reduction and immobilization is accomplished by casting.
   b. *Open reduction*—operative procedure utilized to achieve bone alignment; pins, wire, nails, or rods may be used to secure bone fragments in position.
   c. *Traction reduction*—force is applied in two directions to obtain alignment.
      (1) Used for fractures of long bones.
      (2) May be applied by:
         (a) *Skin* traction—secured by adhesive or moleskin strips.
         (b) *Skeletal* traction—secured by wires, pins, or tongs placed through the bone.

2. Immobilization—maintains reduction and promotes healing of bone fragments.
   a. External fixation or immobilization is achieved by application of casts, splints, or continuous traction.
   b. Internal fixation is achieved by utilizing nails, rods, and wires in joining bone fragments.

3. Complications of fractures (Tables 5–23 and 5–24):
   a. Shock.
   b. Fat embolism.
   c. Thrombophlebitis.
   d. Infection.
   e. Peripheral nerve damage.
   f. Nonunion and avascular necrosis.

D. Purpose, types, and complications of casting:
   1. Main purpose of cast is immobilization, but it is also used to support body tissues and to prevent or correct deformities—in fractures, the joint above and the joint below the injury are immobilized.
   2. Types of casts—

TABLE 5–24. *Complications of fractures*

Condition and etiology	Pathophysiology	Signs and symptoms	Nursing interventions
CARDIOVASCULAR COMPLICATIONS—SHOCK, THROMBOPHLEBITIS, AND FAT EMBOLI			
Fat emboli—multiple injuries, fracture of long bones, severe burns, soft tissue injury, and orthopedic procedures.	Fat released from marrow of fractured bones → alteration of fat emulsion due to catecholamines → minute globules of fat carried in blood stream → embolization in vascular system in vital organs.	*Respiratory*—dyspnea, cyanosis (in black patients, skin becomes slate gray), tachypnea, and severe chest pain. *Cerebral*—pupillary changes, muscle twitching, change from alertness to confusion, agitation, and loss of consciousness. *Skin*—petechiae over chest and shoulders, axilla, and soft palate. *Extremity*—pale, cold, numb, and cold to touch; nausea; vomiting; faintness; and shock.	1. Place in high-Fowler's position to relieve respiratory symptoms. 2. Administer oxygen at once—relieves anoxia and reduces surface tension of fat globules. 3. Institute respiratory support measures, as ordered—IPPB and respirator. 4. Observe closely for heart failure and shock. 5. Administer parenteral fluids, as ordered: (a) IV alcohol and (b) blood and fluid replacement. 6. Administer medications, as ordered: (a) corticosteroids, (b) digitalis, (c) aminophylline, and (d) heparin sodium.

a. Spica—applied to immobilize hip or shoulder joints.
b. Body cast—applied to trunk.
c. Short leg cast—applied to lower leg, ankle, and foot.
d. Long leg cast—applied to midthigh, leg, and foot.
e. Short arm cast—applied from forearm to palmar crease, may include thumb.
f. Long arm cast—applied from upper level of axillary fold to palmar crease, immobilizing elbow at right angle.
3. *Assessment*—complications of pressure and immobility:
a. Circulatory impairment—reduced blood flow and venous return.
   (1) Weak or absent pulse.
   (2) Color, temperature, or sensation changes.
   (3) Swelling and numbness.
b. Decreased innervation—
   (1) Decreased mobility of toes and fingers.
   (2) Increasing or constant pain.

(3) Smarting or burning sensation under cast.
(4) Numbness.
c. Tissue necrosis—
   (1) Foul odor from cast.
   (2) Drainage through the cast.
   (3) Decubitus formation around edges of cast.
   (4) Elevated temperature.
d. For patient in spica cast—observe for duodenal distress: anorexia, nausea, and abdominal pain.
   (1) Report to physician immediately.
   (2) Place patient in prone position to relieve pressure.
   (3) Have cast-cutters and nasogastric suction available.
E. Principles of cast care:
1. Expose cast to air until dry—avoid the use of plastic or disposable diapers (Chux) containing plastic, which inhibit drying. Cast will feel hot and moist for several hours.
2. Casts on extremities should be elevated on pil-

lows, each joint higher than preceding joint, to promote venous return and reduce swelling.

3. Patients with spica casts should remain supine until cast is dry.
   a. Mattress firm and level; bed boards may be used—reduces muscle spasm.
   b. Maintain warmth by covering uncasted areas only.
   c. Avoid turning for eight hours.
   d. When turning is allowed, utilize enough personnel so that patient is entirely turned at one time—log rolling.
   e. Support chest and cast with pillows.
   f. Observe for signs of *respiratory distress*—increased respiratory rate, apprehension.

4. If blood or drainage appears on cast, mark the spot with a circle.
   a. Note date and time and continue observations.
   b. Report further drainage to physician.

5. Promote skin care—
   a. Apply lotion or cornstarch—no powders.
   b. Tape edges of cast to reduce irritation.
   c. Inspect skin under cast frequently for signs of irritation.
   d. Caution patient not to stick anything down cast in an effort to scratch—skin abrasion may lead to decubitus ulcer.

6. Promote motor function by initiating active range-of-motion exercises to unaffected extremities.
   a. Use footboard to prevent footdrop.
   b. Encourage use of trapeze if applicable.
   c. Isometric exercises, as ordered.
   d. Flex hand or foot of affected extremity—passive and active.

7. Ambulate patients in extremity casts.
   a. Support arm cast as needed.
   b. Allow no weight bearing on leg cast unless ordered.

8. Instruct in crutch-walking techniques if applicable.
   a. When one leg only can bear weight—
      (1) *Swing-to gait*—crutches forward, swing body to crutches.
      (2) *Swing-through gait*—crutches forward, swing body through crutches.
      (3) *Three-point gait* (Figure 5–11)—crutches and affected extremity forward; swing forward placing good foot ahead or between crutches.

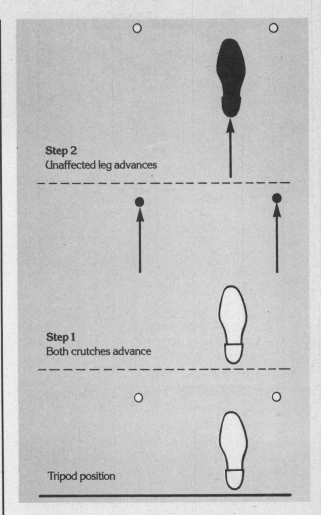

FIGURE 5–11. *Three-point crutch gait*
(From Kozier, B., and Erb, G. L.: *Fundamentals of Nursing.* Menlo Park, Calif. 1979. Addison-Wesley Publishing Co.)

   b. When both legs can move separately and bear some weight—
      (1) *Four-point gait*—right crutch forward, left foot forward; swing weight to right side while bringing left crutch forward, then right foot forward; gait simulates normal walking.
      (2) *Two-point gait*—as four-point gait but faster; one crutch and opposite leg moving forward at same time.
   c. Utilize *tripod gait* when the patient is unable to walk—crutches forward at a wide distance, drag legs to point just behind crutches, balance, and repeat.
   d. Measure crutches accurately.
      (1) Subtract 16 inches from total height.

Top of the crutch should be two inches below the axilla.

   (2) Complete extension of the elbows should be possible without pressure of axillary bar into the axilla.

   (3) Handgrip should be adjusted so that complete wrist extension is possible.

  e. Instruct in body alignment—

   (1) Head erect.

   (2) Back straight.

   (3) Chest forward.

   (4) Feet 6 to 8 inches apart—wide base for support.

  f. Instruct in safety measures—

   (1) Weight bearing on hands, not axilla.

   (2) Position crutches 4 inches to side and 4 inches to front.

   (3) Use short strides, looking ahead, not at feet.

   (4) If patient should begin to fall, crutches should be thrown to the side to prevent falling on them.

   (5) If patient should begin to fall, the body should be relaxed, "go limp," to prevent injury.

   (6) Check floors for potential hazards—water, oil spots, extension cords, and throw rugs.

F. Traction—purpose, types, general nursing approaches:

  1. Purpose—utilizing a system of ropes, pulleys, and weights, force is applied in two directions to—

   a. Obtain and maintain normal alignment.

   b. Reduce fractures and decrease muscle spasm.

   c. Prevent deformities.

  2. Types of traction—

   a. Continuous—used with fracture or dislocation of bones or joints.

   b. Intermittent—employed to reduce flexion contractures or lessen pain and muscle spasms.

   c. *Skin*—traction applied to the skin by using adhesive, plastic, or moleskin strip bound to the extremity by elastic bandage.

    (1) Exerts indirect traction on muscles and bone.

    (2) *Nursing* measures include:

     (a) Shave extremity and apply tincture of benzoin—improves adher-ence of strip and reduces skin itching.

     (b) Check all bony prominences for evidence of pressure.

     (c) Check bandage for slippage, bunching, and replace prn.

   d. *Skeletal*—direct traction applied to bone using pins (*Steinmann*), wires (*Kirschner*), or tongs (*Crutchfield*), which are inserted through the bone in or close to the involved area.

    (1) Most effective traction.

    (2) Utilized for fractures of long bones.

  3. *General traction care and precautions*—

   a. Maintain straight line—ropes taut and riding freely over pulleys.

   b. Never remove or lift weights.

   c. Add trapeze to bed if upper extremities are unaffected.

   d. Initiate active range of motion of unaffected limbs and isometric exercises in affected limb.

   e. Administer diet high in protein and moderate in carbohydrates—improves tissue repair but prevents weight gain.

   f. Encourage fluids—long immobilization increases occurrence of kidney stones.

   g. Provide activities to reduce perceptual deprivation—reading, handcrafts, model-building. Encourage social contacts.

  4. Methods of applying traction—

   a. *Cervical traction*—direct traction applied to cervical vertebrae using Crutchfield and Vinke tongs that are inserted into the skull.

    (1) Traction is increased with weights until vertebrae move into position and alignment is regained.

    (2) After reduction is obtained, weights are decreased to the amount needed to maintain reduction.

    (3) *Nursing measures:*

     (a) Elevate head of bed—patient's body serves as a counterweight to traction weight.

     (b) Keep tongs free from bed and keep weight hanging freely.

   b. *Balanced-suspension traction*—countertraction produced by a force other than the patient's body weight; the extremity is suspended in a traction apparatus that maintains the line of traction despite changes in

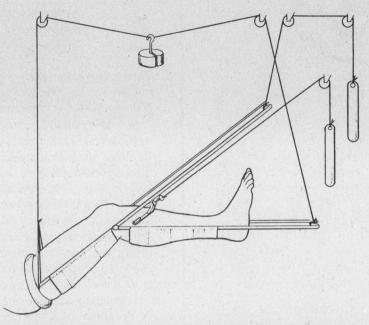

FIGURE 5–12. *Balanced suspension used in conjunction with skeletal traction*
(From Buergin, P. Management of the person with motor problems. In Phipps, Long, Woods, eds.: *Medical/surgical nursing.* St. Louis, 1979. The C. V. Mosby Co.)

the patient's position, for example, *Russell's leg traction,* the *Thomas splint,* and *Pearson's attachment.*

(1) Patient may move as desired, turn slightly (no more than 30° to unaffected side), and may have head of bed elevated.

(2) The heel of the affected leg must remain free of the bed.

(3) *Nursing goals* are designed to maintain alignment and countertraction.

  (a) 20° angle between thigh and bed.

  (b) Check for pressure from sling in popliteal area.

  (c) Provide foot support to prevent footdrop.

  (d) Maintain abduction of extremity.

  (e) Check for sign of infection at sites of pin insertion.

c. *Running traction*—traction that exerts a pull in one plane; countertraction is supplied by the weight of the patient's body or can be increased through the use of weights and pulleys in the opposite direction (Figure 5–12). Examples: *Buck's extension* (Figure 5–13) and *Russell's traction.*

(1) Patient must be kept well centered in the bed.

(2) Head of bed can only be elevated to the point of countertraction.

(3) Patient may not turn from side to side, as this will result in rubbing of the bony fragments.

(4) Check toes or fingers frequently for decreased circulation.

(5) Provide regular back care.

d. *Halo traction and cast*—an apparatus that employs both a plaster cast and a metal frame. The cast extends from the axillae to the iliac crest and houses a metal frame. The struts of the frame extend to the skull and attach to a round metal (halo) device. The halo is attached to the skull by four pins—two located anterolaterally and two located posterolaterally—that are inserted into the external *cortex* of the cranium.

(1) Halo cast and traction may be utilized to:

  (a) Immobilize the cervical spine following cervical spinal fusion.

  (b) Give some correction to scoliosis prior to spinal fusion.

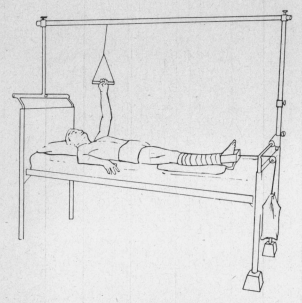

FIGURE 5–13. Buck's extension
Note that limb is not raised but lies parallel with bed. Note also blocks to raise foot of bed to provide countertraction and to help keep patient from moving to foot of bed. (From Phipps, Long, Woods, eds.: *Medical/surgical nursing.* St. Louis, 1979, The C. V. Mosby Co.)

   (2) *Nursing measures:*
      (a) Explain and show patient apparatus before application.
      (b) Allow patient to verbalize fears about having screws placed in skull.
      (c) Postapplication measures are same as for patient in spica cast.
      (d) Check screws to the head and screws that hold upper portion of the frame several times each day to be sure they are tight.
      (e) Pin sites cleaned once daily with a solution of hydrogen peroxide, Phisohex, or Zephiran Cl—prevents granulation formation and cellulitis.
      (f) Position patient as any other patient in a body cast except no pressure is allowed to rest on halo—pillows may be placed under abdomen and chest when patient is prone.
      (g) Institute range-of-motion exercises to prevent contractures.

      (h) Turn frequently to prevent development of pressure areas.

  2. **Total hip replacement**—femoral head and acetabulum are replaced by a prosthesis, which is cemented into the bone with plastic cement.
  A. Rationale—painful degenerative joint disease, such as rheumatoid arthritis and osteoarthritis; may also be done for complications of femoral neck fractures and congenital hip disease.
  B. Purpose—to restore or improve mobilization of the hip joint that has limited and painful function due to bony ankylosis.
  C. *Preoperative nursing goals* are designed to optimize physical and psychologic functioning and prevent postoperative complications.
    1. Fit patient with antiembolic stockings—thrombophlebitis and pulmonary emboli are frequent complications of this type of surgery.
    2. Administer antibiotics, as ordered—commonly given prophylactically.
    3. *Patient teachings* include:
      a. Isometric exercises—gluteal, abdominal, and quadricep setting.
      b. Dorsiflexion and plantar flexion of the feet.
      c. Use of trapeze.
      d. Explanation of positioning of the operative leg and hip postoperatively to prevent adduction and flexion.
      e. Transfer techniques—bed to chair and chair to crutches.
    4. Assist patient with skin scrubs with antibacterial soap.
  D. *Postoperative nursing goals* are designed to maintain abduction of the affected joint (prevents dislocation of the prosthesis), promote physical and mental comfort, and prevent complications (see general postoperative care and care of the patient in casts or traction).
    1. Maintain abduction of affected leg:
      a. Buck's extension or Russell's traction may be applied.
      b. Plaster booties with an abduction bar may be utilized.
      c. Place Charnley wedge pillow between the knees and lower legs.
      d. Place two to three pillows or sandbags between patient's legs.
    2. Avoid external hip rotation by placing sandbags along upper outer aspects of thigh.

3. Initiate skin care:
   a. Alternating-pressure mattress.
   b. Back care q2h.
   c. Sheepskin when supine.
4. Check dressings, drainage tubes (Hemovac), and vital signs.
5. Elevate head of bed and turn per individual physician's orders—if turning is allowed, turn to unaffected side with pillows between legs to maintain abduction.
6. Initiate isometric exercises and dorsiflexion and plantar flexion of foot as soon as allowed.
7. Initiate progressive ambulation, as ordered.
8. Be sure patient lies flat in bed several times each day—prevents hip flexion contractures and strengthens hip muscles.
9. *Postoperative and discharge teachings* include:
   a. Detailed exercise program and list of activity restrictions.
   b. Placing pillow between legs when in bed for several weeks—to prevent hip adduction when turning.
   c. Avoidance of sitting for more than an hour—patient should stand, stretch, and walk frequently to prevent hip flexion contractures.
   d. Informing patient that hip flexion should not exceed 90° or dislocation may occur.
      (1) May need assistance putting on shoes and stockings.
      (2) Sit in straight-back chairs only.
      (3) Use raised toilet seat.
      (4) Avoid crossing legs.
      (5) Avoid driving car for at least six weeks.
   e. Continue to wear support hose for at least six weeks to enhance venous return and avoid thrombus formation.

3. *Above-the-knee amputation*—severance of a portion of the leg through surgery.
A. Rationale—peripheral vascular disease, malignant bone tumors, bone infections, complications from diabetes mellitus, traumas, and thermal, chemical, or electrical injuries.
B. *Preoperative nursing goals* are designed to promote psychologic adjustment to changes in body image and to optimize physical condition of patient.
   1. *Preoperative teachings* include:
      a. Reiterating explanations of operative procedures.
      b. Explaining phantom-limb sensation.
      c. Utilization of prosthesis.
      d. Preparation for rehabilitation.
         (1) Crutch-walking.
         (2) Exercises to increase upper-body strength, such as push-ups, using weights while flexing and extending arms, and isometric sitting exercises.
         (3) Use of overhead trapeze.
   2. Allow for verbalization of feelings about changes in body image.
      a. Identify behaviors associated with grieving process (denial, aggression, anger, and hostility).
      b. Involve patient and family in preoperative teaching to facilitate understanding.
      c. Stress the importance of patient's remaining capabilities.
      d. Clarify for the patient and family that, following surgery and rehabilitation, the patient should still be able to carry out the activities of daily living and maintain independence.
C. *Postoperative nursing goals* are designed to prevent complications, provide physical and emotional support, and promote rehabilitation.
   1. Elevate stump on pillow for first 24 to 48 hours to reduce edema and prevent hemorrhage; remove after 24 to 48 hours as prolonged elevation may lead to hip flexion contractures.
   2. Observe for signs of hemorrhage frequently.
      a. Outline any drainage on dressing, marking date and time.
      b. Reinforce dressing prn.
      c. Have heavy tourniquet on bed at all times to apply in case of sudden hemorrhage.
   3. If open amputation has been done, maintain Buck's traction.
      a. Traction prevents skin retraction and flexion contractures.
      b. Pulley should be centered to permit turning to abdomen.
   4. Avoid external rotation of hip by placing sandbags or trochanter roll along outer side of stump.
   5. Initiate cast care if plaster dressing has been applied—report any slippage to physician.
   6. Administer pain medications, as ordered.
   7. Initiate active range-of-motion exercises on unaffected limb and provide footboard to prevent footdrop.

8. Reposition patient every two hours while on bedrest, turning to the prone position several hours each day—prevents flexion contractures.
9. Initiate range-of-motion bed, chair, and stand-up exercises as ordered to prevent abduction and flexion contractures.
10. Apply elastic bandage to stump after healed to produce shrinkage and conical shape.
11. Begin stump-strengthening exercises, as ordered.
    a. Push stump against pillow.
    b. Push stump against harder surface.
    c. Massage stump (toward suture line)—decreases tenderness, improves vascularity, and aids in "toughening" stump.
12. Encourage patient and family to verbalize their feelings—recognize that it will take the patient time to adjust to altered body image and modifications in activities.
13. Keep patient as active as possible during post-operative and rehabilitative phases, as activity tends to reduce occurrence of phantom-limb pain.

4. Total knee replacement—replacement of articular surfaces of both tibia and femur with single-unit, hinge-type or polycentric prosthesis.
A. Rationale—inflammation or destruction of joint tissue secondary to arthritis, trauma.
B. *Preoperative nursing goals* are designed to evaluate range of motion and muscle strength and to reduce anxiety.
   1. *Assessment:*
      a. Range of motion of affected versus unaffected joint.
      b. Muscle strength and function.
      c. Level of anxiety and understanding of dysfunction.
      d. Vital signs and other laboratory baseline data.
   2. *Interventions:*
      a. Continue muscle exercises begun before admission, as ordered.
      b. Surgical scrub of affected joint, as ordered.
      c. Administer prophylactic antibiotics, as ordered.
      d. Instruct in postoperative breathing, coughing, quadricep setting, leg and ankle exercises.
C. *Postoperative nursing goals* are directed toward promoting physical and psychologic equilibrium.

   1. *Assessment:*
      a. Vital signs.
      b. Check peripheral pulses below compression dressing as well as color and skin temperature—circulatory integrity.
      c. Check muscle tone and tendon reflexes below compression bandages—neurologic integrity.
      d. Maintain intravenous infusions as ordered, then diet as tolerated.
      e. Administer analgesics, as ordered.
      f. Maintain anticoagulant therapy (two weeks) as ordered to reduce occurrence of thromboemboli.
      g. Assist with removal of compression dressing on day 4 or 5.
      h. Assist with application of elastic bandage or light cast postdressing removal.
      i. Ambulate—walker, crutches, cane.
      j. Maintain exercise program—quadriceps setting, range of motion, leg lifts—goal is 90° knee flexion by discharge.

Part D/EMERGENCY NURSING PROCEDURES

A. Purpose—to initiate assessment and intervention procedures that will speed total care of the patient toward a successful outcome.
B. Emergency nursing procedures for adults are detailed in Table 5–25.
C. Legal issues in the emergency room:
   1. Record-keeping plays an essential role in both the prevention and defense of malpractice suits. Detailed documentation not only provides for continuity of care, but also perpetuates evidence that care was appropriately given. Records should:
      a. Be written legibly.
      b. Clearly note events and time of occurrence.
      c. Contain all lab slips and results of other tests.
      d. Describe events and patient objectively.
      e. Clearly note physician's parting instructions to the patient.
      f. Be signed where appropriate, such as with doctor's orders.

TABLE 5–25. *Nursing care of the adult in medical and surgical emergencies*

Condition	Assessment: signs and symptoms	Prehospitalization nursing care	In-hospital nursing care
CARDIOVASCULAR EMERGENCIES			
Myocardial infarction— ischemia and necrosis of cardiac muscle secondary to insufficient or obstructed coronary blood flow.	*Prehospital:* Chest pain—vise-like choking, unrelieved by rest or nitroglycerin. Skin—ashen, cold, clammy. Vital signs: pulse—rapid, weak, thready; increased rate and depth of respirations; dyspnea. Behavior: restless, anxious. *In hospital:* C/V: blood pressure and pulse pressure decreased. Heart sounds soft, S_3 may be present. Resp.: fine basilar rales. Lab: ECG consistent with tissue necrosis (Q waves) and injury (ST seg. elevation). Serum enzymes elevated.	If suspect coronary, call physician, paramedic service, or emergency ambulance. Calm and reassure patient that help is coming. Place in semi-Fowler's position. Keep patient warm but not hot.	Rapidly assess hemodynamic and respiratory status. Start IV of 5% D/W per microdrip—establishes lifeline for emergency drug treatment. Draw blood for electrolytes, enzymes, and SMA panel. Place on cardiac monitor. Relieve pain—morphine SO_4 IV of 5 min. Take 12-lead ECG. Once patient is stable, transfer to CCU.
Cardiac arrest—cardiac stenosis or ventricular fibrillation secondary to rapid administration or overdose of anesthetics or narcotic drugs, obstruction of the respiratory tract (mucus, vomitus, foreign body), acute anxiety, cardiac disease, dehydration, shock, electric shock, or emboli.	Cyanosis, gasping. Respirations: rapid, shallow. Pulse weak, thready > 120. Pulse weak, slow < 50. Muscular twitching. Pupillary dilatation. Cold, clammy skin. Absent respiration. Absent pulse. Loss of consciousness.	*CPR* Lay patient flat on back. Tilt head back. Clear throat if indicated. Check for breathing. *No breathing* Kneel close to head. Place hand under neck, bringing lower jaw forward and opening airway. Pinch nostrils shut and blow four quick, full breaths into patient's mouth. Lips must form airtight seal. Watch chest for adequate expansion. Check pulse—if present, breathe into mouth every four to five seconds.	*Monitored arrest—one-person rescue:* Palpate carotid for 5–10 seconds. Note cardiac rhythm on monitor—ventricular standstill, ventricular fibrillation, ventricular tachycardia. Thump chest once with fleshy part of fist. Palpate carotid and note monitor rhythm. If arrest continues—call for help and note time. Countershock if rhythm is ventricular fibrillation or ventricular tachycardia. If countershock unsuccessful, begin CPR.

(Continued)

TABLE 5–25. *(Continued)*

Condition	Assessment: signs and symptoms	Prehospitalization nursing care	In-hospital nursing care
CARDIOVASCULAR EMERGENCIES			
		No heartbeat Two-person CPR: 60 chest compressions per minute with one breath between every 5 compressions.	Remove pillows, open airway by hyperextending neck and bringing lower jaw forward.
		One-person CPR: 80 chest compressions per minute with two quick breaths between every 15 compressions.	Check pupils.
			Start mouth-to-mouth resuscitation.
		Check pulse at neck after one minute and every few minutes thereafter.	Deliver four quick breaths—watch for rising of the chest.
		Check pupils to determine effectiveness of CPR—should begin to constrict.	If unable to ventilate, check for airway obstruction. Attempt to dislodge obstruction with back blows, manual thrusts, or finger probes.
		If heartbeat returns: Assist respiration and monitor pulse. Continue CPR until help arrives.	Once ventilation established, begin chest compression.
			Compress 80 times per minute with two ventilations between each 15 compressions.
			Check after one minute and then every 5 min. for spontaneous return of pulse and/or respirations.
			Unmonitored arrest—one-person rescue: Shake patient vigorously and call name—establishes unconsciousness.
			Call for help and note time.
			Roll on back, remove pillows.
			Tilt head back and lift lower jaw to open airway and check pupils.
			Check for breathing—look at chest, listen at mouth. If no breathing, give four quick breaths.

TABLE 5–25. (Continued)

Condition	Assessment: signs and symptoms	Prehospitalization nursing care	In-hospital nursing care
CARDIOVASCULAR EMERGENCIES			
			Palpate carotids for 5–10 seconds. If absent, proceed with chest compression at 80/min with two quick breaths between each 15 compressions.
			Two-person rescue: First person begins CPR as described above.
			Second person: Pages arrest team. Brings defibrillator to bedside and counter shocks if indicated by rhythm. Brings emergency cart to bedside. Suctions airway if indicated due to vomitus or secretions. Bags patient with 100% O_2. Assists with intubation when arrest team arrives. Establishes intravenous line if one is not available.
Shock—cellular hypoxia and impairment of cellular function secondary to: trauma, hemorrhage, fright, dehydration, cardiac insufficiency, allergic reactions, septicemia, impairment of nervous system, poisons.	*Early shock* Conscious, apprehensive and restless, some slurring of speech. Pupils dull but reactive to light. Pulse rate < 140/min. Amplitude full to mildly decreased. Blood pressure: normal to slightly decreased. Neck veins: normal to slightly flat in supine position. May be full in septic shock or grossly distended in cardiogenic shock.	Check breathing—clear airway if necessary. If no breathing, give artificial respirations. If breathing, irregular or labored—raise head and shoulders. Control bleeding by placing pressure on the wound or at pressure points (proximal artery). Make comfortable and reassure. Cover lightly to prevent heat loss, but don't bundle up. If you suspect neck or spine injury—do not move, unless victim in danger of more injury.	Check vital signs rapidly— pulse, pupils, respirations. Check airway, clear if necessary. PaO_2 should be maintained above 60 mm Hg. Elevated $PaCO_2$ indicates need for intubation and ventilatory assistance. Control gross bleeding. Insert intravenous line and central lines—if abdominal injuries present. Peripheral line should be placed in upper extremity if fluids being lost in abdomen.

(Continued)

TABLE 5–25. *(Continued)*

Condition	Assessment: Signs and symptoms	Prehospitalization nursing care	In-hospital nursing care
CARDIOVASCULAR EMERGENCIES			
	Skin: cool, clammy, pale. Respirations: rapid, shallow. GI: nausea, vomiting, thirst. Renal: urine output 20–40 cc/hour.	If patient unconscious or has wounds of the lower face and jaw—place on side to promote drainage of fluids. Position patient on back unless otherwise indicated.	Draw blood for specimens Hb, Hct, CBC, glucose, CO_2, sodium amylase, BUN, K^+, type and cross-match, blood gases, enzymes, prothrombin times. Start infusion of 5% D/NS unless hypernatremia suspected. Dextran if blood loss.
	Severe or Late Shock Sensorium: confused, disoriented, apathetic, unresponsive, slow, slurred speech, often incoherent. *Pupils:* dilating, dilated, slow or nonreactive to light. *Pulse:* rate > 150/min, thready, weak. *Blood pressure:* 80 mm Hg or unobtainable. *Neck veins:* flat in a supine position—no filling. Full to distended in septic or cardiogenic shock. *Skin:* cold, clammy, mottled, circumoral cyanosis, dusky, cyanotic. *Eyes:* sunken—vacant expression. *Renal:* urine output < 20 cc/hr.	Raise feet 6–8 inches unless patient has head or chest injuries. If victim becomes less comfortable, lower feet. If patient complains of thirst, do not give fluids unless you are more than six hours away from professional medical help. Under no conditions give water to unconscious patients, ones having seizures or vomiting, ones appearing to need general anesthetic, or ones with a stomach, chest, or skull injury. Be calm and confident; reassure patient help is on the way.	Assessment and initial interventions as above, then obtain information as to onset and past history. Catheterize and monitor urine output. Take 12-lead EKG. Insert nasogastric tube and assess aspirate for volume, color, and blood. Save specimen if poison or drug overdose suspected. If CVP low—infuse 200–300 ml over 5–10 min. If CVP rises sharply, fluid restriction necessary. If remains low hypovolemia present. If patient febrile, take blood cultures and wound cultures. If urine output scanty or absent, administer mannitol as ordered.
RESPIRATORY EMERGENCIES			
Choking—obstruction of airway secondary to aspiration of a foreign object.	Gasping, wheezing. Looks panicky, but can still breathe, talk, cough. Cough weak and ineffective, breathing sounds like high-pitched crowing, color—white, gray, blue.	Do not interfere, watch closely, call for assistance. *Victim standing, sitting and conscious:* Strike sharply on back four times with heel of hand between shoulder blades. Blows must be hard.	As in prehospital care. Do not slap on back.

TABLE 5–25. *(Continued)*

Condition	Assessment: Signs and symptoms	Prehospitalization nursing care	In-hospital nursing care
RESPIRATORY EMERGENCIES			
	Difficulty speaking, clutches throat.	If distress continues, give four quick abdominal thrusts. Stand behind victim, wrap arms around waist, place fist against abdomen and with your other hand, press it into the victim's abdomen with a quick upward thrust, four times (Heimlich maneuver).	
		Victim lying down: Kneel beside victim. Roll toward you, supporting victim against your thighs with one hand. Strike four rapid blows between shoulder blades with the heel of your other hand.	As in prehospital care.
		Roll on back. Place heel of hand in the middle of abdomen. Place other hand on top of the first, stiffen arms and deliver four sharp thrusts.	
		Unconscious victim: Try to ventilate. If unsuccessful, give four sharp blows to back and four abdominal thrusts using technique described in above. Probe mouth for foreign objects.	As in prehospital care. When probing mouth for foreign object, turn head to side, unless patient has neck injury. In event of neck injury, raise the arm opposite you and roll the head and shoulders as a unit, so that head ends up supported on the arm.
		Keep repeating above procedure until ventilation occurs. As victim becomes more deprived of air, muscles will relax and maneuvers that were previously unsuccessful will begin to work.	
		When successful in removing obstruction, give four quick breaths. Check pulse. Start CPR if indicated.	

(Continued)

TABLE 5–25. *(Continued)*

Condition	Assessment: signs and symptoms	Prehospitalization nursing care	In-hospital nursing care
RESPIRATORY EMERGENCIES			
		On obese or pregnant victims, use chest thrusts instead of abdominal thrusts.	
		You are victim and alone: Place your two fists for abdominal thrusts. Bend over back of chair, sink, etc. and exert hard, repeated pressure on abdomen to force object up. Push fingers down your throat to encourage regurgitation.	
Acute respiratory failure—sudden onset of an abnormally low PO_2 (< 60 mm Hg) and/or high pCO_2 (> 60 mm Hg) secondary to lung disease or trauma, peripheral or central nervous system depression, cardiac failure, severe obesity, airway obstruction, environmental abnormality.	*Hypoxia* *Sensorium:* acute apprehension. *Respiration:* dyspnea, shallow, rapid respirations. *Skin:* circumoral cyanosis, pale, dusky skin, nailbeds. *C/V:* slight hypertension and tachycardia or hypotension and bradycardia. *Hypercardia* *Sensorium:* decreasing mentation, headache. *Skin:* flushed, warm, moist. *C/V:* hypertension, tachycardia.	If you suspect respiratory distress, call physician. Calm and reassure patient. Place in a chair or semi-sitting position. Keep warm but not hot. Phone for ambulance. If respirations cease or patient becomes unconscious: clear airway and commence respiratory resuscitation. Check pulse: initiate CPR if necessary. Continue resuscitation until help arrives.	Check patient's ability to speak. Maintain airway by placing in high-Fowler's position. Check vital signs: B/P, pulse rate and rhythm, temperature, skin color, rate and depth of respirations. Prepare for intubation if: 1. Patient has flail chest. 2. Patient is comatose without gag reflex. 3. Has respiratory arrest. Maintain mouth to mouth until intubation. 4. PCO_2 is > 55 mm Hg. 5. PO_2 is < 60 mm Hg. 6. F_1O_2 is $> 50\%$ using nasal cannula, catheter or mask. 7. Respiratory rate > 36. *After intubation:* Check bilateral lung sounds. Observe for symmetrical lung expansion. Maintain humidified oxygen at lowest F_1O_2 possible to achieve PO_2 of 60 mm Hg.

TABLE 5-25. *(Continued)*

Condition	Assessment: signs and symptoms	Prehospitalization nursing care	In-hospital nursing care
RESPIRATORY EMERGENCIES			
			Improve ventilation (decreased PCO_2) by: 1. Liquifying secretions—oral and parenteral fluids. —if intubated, frequent installations of normal saline or sodium bicarbonate. 2. Frequent suctioning. 3. Utilizing IPPB and 4. Chest physiotherapy. Administer drugs as ordered: sympathomimetics, xanthines, antibiotics, and steroids. Monitor arterial blood gases, electrolytes, Hct, Hb, and WBC. *Do not:* 1. Administer sedatives. 2. Correct acid-base problems without monitoring electrolytes. 3. Overcorrect PO_2. 4. Leave patient alone while oxygen therapy is initiated. Once patient is stable, transfer to ICU.
Drowning—death by asphyxiation due to immersion or submersion in a fluid or liquid medium.	*Conscious victim* Acute anxiety, panic. Increased rate of respirations. Pale, dusky.	*Conscious victim* Try to talk victim out of panic so he can find footing and way to shore.	*Nonsymptomatic near-drowning victim* Draw blood for arterial blood gases with patient breathing room air.

(Continued)

TABLE 5–25. *(Continued)*

Condition	Assessment: signs and symptoms	Prehospitalization nursing care	In-hospital nursing care
RESPIRATORY EMERGENCIES			
Near-drowning— asphyxiation or partial asphyxiation due to immersion or submersion in a fluid or liquid medium.	*Unconscious victim* Shallow or no respirations. Weak or no pulse. If victim not breathing, as soon as you have firm support begin mouth-to-mouth resuscitation. Tilt head back, place hand under neck, bring jaw forward, pinch nostril shut, give four quick breaths.	Utilize devices such as poles, rings, clothing to extend to victim. Do not let panicked victim grab you. Do not attempt swimming rescue unless specially trained. If you suspect head or neck injury, handle carefully, floating victim back to shore with body and head as straight as possible. Endeavor not to turn head or bend back. *On shore:* Check breathing. Lay victim flat on back. Cover and keep warm. Calm and reassure victim. Do not give food or water. Get to medical assistance as soon as possible. When on shore, turn victim on stomach, put your hands under abdomen and lift forcefully—helps force water and air from bloated stomach. Turn to back and resume respiratory resuscitation. If airway obstructed, wipe foreign matter from mouth. Turn to side and deliver four sharp blows between shoulder blades. Wipe out mouth. Attempt ventilation again. Once ventilation established, check pulse. If absent, begin chest compressions as in CPR. One-person or two-person rescue.	PA and lateral chest X ray. Auscultate lungs. Admit to hospital for further evaluation if: $PO_2 < 80$ mm Hg. pH < 7.35. Pulmonary infiltrates present or auscultation reveals rales. Victim inhaled fluids containing chlorine, hydrocarbons, sewerage, or hypotonic or fresh water. *Symptomatic near-drowning victim* Provide basic or advanced cardiac life support. Provide clear airway and adequate ventilation by: 1. Suctioning airway. 2. Inserting artificial airway and attach to ventilator as indicated. 3. Inserting nasogastric tube to suction to minimize aspiration of vomitus. Monitor ECG continuously. Start IV infusion 5% D/W at keep-open rate for *fresh water near-drowning.* 5% D/NS in *salt water near-drowning.* Insert CVP and Swan-Ganz catheter to guide subsequent infusion rates. Administer drugs as ordered: anticonvulsants; steroids, antibiotics, stimulants, antiarrhythmics. Provide rewarming if hypothermia present.

TABLE 5–25.   *(Continued)*

Condition	Assessment: signs and symptoms	Prehospitalization nursing care	In-hospital nursing care
RESPIRATORY EMERGENCIES			
		Continue CPR until victim revives or help arrives. If victim revives, cover and keep warm. Reassure victim help is on the way. Rescue personnel can further assist emergency room personnel by: 1. Documenting prehospital resuscitation methods used. 2. Immobilizing victims suspected of cervical spine injuries. 3. Utilizing a sterile container to take a sample of immersion fluid. 4. Take on-scene arterial blood gas sample for later analysis.	Insert Foley to assess kidney output—fresh water near-drowning causes renal tubular necrosis due to RBC hemolysis. Transfer to ICU when stabilized.
SYSTEMIC INJURIES *Multiple traumas*	*Sensorium:* alert, disoriented, stuporous, coma. *Respirations:* increased rate, depth, shallow, asymmetrical, paradoxical breathing, mediastinal shift, gasping, blowing. *C/V:* signs of shock (see above). *Abdomen:* contusions, pain, abrasions, open wounds, rigidity, increasing distention. *Skeletal system:* pain, swelling, deformity, inappropriate or no movement.	Don't move patient unless you must to prevent further injury. Send for help. Check breathing—give mouth-to-mouth resuscitation if indicated. Check for bleeding. Control bleeding by applying pressure on wound or on pressure points (artery proximal to wound). Use tourniquet only if above pressure techniques fail to stop severe bleeding. Check for shock (pulse, pupils, skin color) and other injuries. Fractures: keep open fracture area clean.	Assess vital functions. Establish airway; ventilate with ambu-bag, volume-cycled ventilator. Draw arterial blood gases. Control bleeding. Support circulation by closed chest massage. Infusions of dextran, blood, crystalloids. Assess for other injuries: head injuries—suspect cervical neck injury with all head injuries. Place sandbags to immobilize head and neck. Do mini neuro exam: level of consciousness, pupils, bilateral movement and sensation.

(Continued)

TABLE 5–25. *(Continued)*

Condition	Assessment: signs and symptoms	Prehospitalization nursing care	In-hospital nursing care
SYSTEMIC INJURIES			
	Neuro: pupils round, equal, react to light. Ipsilateral dilatation and unresponsive. Fixed and dilated bilaterally. Alert oriented to time and place. Momentary loss of consciousness. Alert, drowsy, stupor, coma.	Stop bleeding, observe for shock.	Get history—time of injury. Any loss of consciousness, any drug ingestion.
		Do not try to set bone.	Stop bleeding on or about head.
		If patient must be moved—splint broken bones with splints that extend past the limb joints.	Apply ice to contusions and hematomas.
	Bilateral movement and sensation in all extremities.	Tie splints on snugly but not so tight as to cut off circulation.	Check for bleeding from nose, pharynx, ears.
	Progressive contralateral weakness.	Check peripheral pulses.	Check for cerebrospinal fluid from ears or nose.
	Loss of voluntary motor function.	If suspect head or back injury—keep body straight. Move only with help.	Assist with spinal tap if ordered.
		Reassure patient help is on the way.	Keep accurate I & O.
			Protect from injury if restless, seizures; orient to time, place, person.
			Administer steroids, diuretics, as ordered.
			Check for signs of increasing intracranial pressure: increased temperature, slowing pulse and respiration, widened pulse pressure, decreasing mentation.
			Spinal injuries: Assess and support vital functions as above.
			Immobilize—no flexion or extension allowed.
			If in respiratory distress—nasotracheal intubation or tracheostomy to avoid hyperextending neck.

TABLE 5–25.   (Continued)

Condition	Assessment: signs and symptoms	Prehospitalization nursing care	In-hospital nursing care
SYSTEMIC INJURIES			
			Check for level of injury and function asking patient to:
			1. Lift elbow up to shoulder height (C5).
			2. Bend elbow (C6).
			3. Straighten elbow (C7).
			4. Grip your hand (C8–T1).
			5. Lift leg (L3).
			6. Straighten knee (L4, L5).
			7. Wiggle toes (L5).
			8. Push toes down (S1).
			If patient comatose:
			1. Rub sternum with knuckles.
			2. If all extremities move, severe injury unlikely.
			3. If one side moves and other does not, potential hemiplegia.
			4. If arms move, legs don't, lower spinal cord injury.
			Administer steroids as ordered.
			Assist with application of skull tongs—Vinke or Crutchfield.
			Maintain IV infusions.
			Insert Foley as indicated.
			Assist with dressing of open wounds.
			Chest injuries (see *Surgery*). Note color and pattern of respirations, position of trachea.
			Auscultate lungs and palpate chest for crepitus, pain, tenderness, and position of trachea.
			Chest tubes if pneumothorax or hemothorax present.

(Continued)

TABLE 5–25.   *(Continued)*

Condition	Assessment: signs and symptoms	Prehospitalization nursing care	In-hospital nursing care
SYSTEMIC INJURIES			
			Place gauze soaked in petroleum jelly over open pneumothorax (sucking chest wound) to seal hole and decrease respiratory distress.
			Assist with tracheostomy if indicated.
			Abdominal injuries: Observe for rigidity.
			Check for hematuria.
			Auscultate for bowel sounds.
			Assist with paracentesis to confirm bleeding in abdominal cavity.
			Prepare for exploratory laparotomy.
			Insert nasogastric tube— detects presence of UGI bleeding.
			Monitor vital signs.
			If organs protruding: 1. Flex patient's knees. 2. Cover intestines with sterile towel soaked in saline. 3. Do not attempt to replace organs.
			Administer tetanus toxoid as ordered.
			Fractures: Observe for pain, peripheral pulses, pallor, loss of sensation and/or movement.
			Assist with wound cleansing, casting, X rays, reduction.
			Prepare for surgery if indicated.
			Monitor vital signs.

TABLE 5–25. *(Continued)*

Condition	Assessment: signs and symptoms	Prehospitalization nursing care	In-hospital nursing care
SYSTEMIC INJURIES			
Burns—tissue trauma secondary to scalding (fluid or flame), chemicals, or electricity.	*First degree:* Erythema and tenderness. Usually sunburn.	Relieve pain by applying cold, wet towel or cold water (not iced).	Cleanse thoroughly with mild detergent followed with soap and water.
			Apply petroleum gauze or sterile towel.
			Administer sedatives and narcotics as ordered.
			Arrange for follow-up care or prepare for admission if burn ambulatory care impractical.
	Second degree: Swelling, blisters. Moisture due to escaping plasma.	Douse with cold water until pain relieved.	Check tetanus immunization status.
		Blot skin dry and cover with clean towel.	Administer sedatives or narcotics as ordered.
		Do not break blisters, remove pieces of skin or apply antiseptic ointments.	Assess respiratory and hemodynamic status: oxygen or ventilatory assist as indicated, intravenous infusions as ordered to combat shock.
		If arm or leg burned, keep elevated.	
		Seek medical attention if second degree burns: 1. Cover 15% of body surface in adult. 2. Cover 10% of body surface in children. 3. Involve hands, feet, or face.	Remove all clothing from burn area. Using aseptic technique, cleanse burns with antiseptic followed by soap and water, and irrigate with normal saline.
	Third degree: White, charred areas.	Don't remove charred clothing.	Do not break blebs or attempt debridement.
		Cover burned area with clean towel, sheet.	Assist with application of dressings as ordered.
		Elevate burned extremities.	Maintain frequent checks of vital signs, urine output.
		Apply cold pack to hand, face, or feet.	
		Sit patient with face or chest wound up to assist respirations.	Provide psychologic support—explain procedures, orient, etc.
		Maintain airway.	Assist with application of splints as ordered.
		Observe for shock.	Administer tetanus immune globulin or toxoid as ordered.

(Continued)

TABLE 5–25. *(Continued)*

Condition	Assessment: signs and symptoms	Prehospitalization nursing care	In-hospital nursing care
SYSTEMIC INJURIES			
		Do not: 1. Put ice water on burns or immerse wounds in ice water—increases shock. 2. Apply ointments. Calm and reassure victim. Get to medical assistance promptly. If patient conscious, not vomiting, and medical assistance is more than six hours away, may give sips of weak solution of salt, soda, and water.	Assist with transfer to hospital unit.
	Chemical burns	Flush with copious amounts of water.	Flush with copious amounts of water.
		Get rid of clothing over burned area.	Administer sedation or narcotics as ordered.
	Burns of the eye Acid	Flush eye with water for at least 15 minutes.	Irrigate with water. Never use neutralizing solution.
		Pour water from inside to outside of eye to avoid contaminating unaffected eye.	Instill 0.5% tetracaine as ordered. Apply patch.
		Cover—seek medical attention at once.	Get ophthalmologic consult.
	Alkali (laundry detergent or cleaning solvent)	Don't allow patient to rub eye.	As above for acid.
		Flush eye with water for at least 30 minutes.	
		Cover—seek medical attention at once.	
ABDOMINAL EMERGENCIES			
Aortic aneurysm—rupture or dissection	Primarily males over 60.	Notify physician.	Assess respiratory and hemodynamic status.
	Sudden onset of excruciating abdominal, lumbosacral, groin or rectal pain.	Lay patient flat or raise head if in respiratory distress.	Institute shock measures as above if indicated.
	Orthopnea, dyspnea.	Cover—keep warm but not hot.	Evaluate and compare peripheral pulses.

TABLE 5–25. *(Continued)*

Condition	Assessment: signs and symptoms	Prehospitalization nursing care	In-hospital nursing care
ABDOMINAL EMERGENCIES			
	Fainting, hypotension. If dissecting, marked hypertension may be present.	Institute shock measures as above.	Assist with X rays.
		· Calm, reassure help is on the way.	Assist with emergency preoperative treatment.
	Palpable, tender pulsating mass in umbilical area.		
	Femoral pulse present. Dorsalis pedes—weak or absent.		
Blunt injuries—Spleen	Left upper quadrant pain, tenderness and moderate rigidity. Left shoulder pain (Kehr's sign).	Lay patient flat. Institute shock measures as above.	Assess respiratory and hemodynamic status. —Maintain airway and ventilation as indicated. —Institute infusions of colloids and/or crystalloids as ordered. —Insert both CVP and arterial monitoring lines. —Insert Foley catheter. —Prepare for splenectomy.
	Hypotension, weak thready pulse, increased respirations (shock).		
EYE AND EAR EMERGENCIES			
Chemical burns		See burns.	See burns.
Blunt injuries secondary to flying missiles such as balls, striking face against car dashboard.	Decreased visual acuity, diplopia, blood in anterior chamber.	Prevent victim from rubbing eye.	Test visual acuity of each eye using Snellen or Jaeger chart.
	Pain, conjunctiva reddened, edema of eyelids.	Cover eye with patch. Seek medical assistance immediately.	Assist with fluorescein administration—facilitates identifying breaks in cornea.
			Call for ophthalmologic consult.
Sharp ocular trauma—secondary to small or larger foreign bodies.	History of feeling as if something were hitting eye.	Keep victim from rubbing eye.	Check visual acuity in both eyes.
	Pain, tearing, reddened conjunctiva.	Cover very lightly—do not apply pressure.	Check pupils.
	Blurring of vision.		Instill 1% tetracaine HCl as ordered to relieve pain.
	Foreign object may be visible.		Administer antibiotic drops or ointment as ordered.
			Call for ophthalmologic consult.

(Continued)

TABLE 5–25. *(Continued)*

Condition	Assessment: signs and symptoms	Prehospitalization nursing care	In-hospital nursing care
EYE AND EAR EMERGENCIES			
			Apply eye patch.
			Provide instructions for subsequent care and follow-up.
Conjunctivitis—inflammation of conjunctiva secondary to infection, allergy.	Vision normal, moderate to copious discharge, eye discomfort, cornea clear; pupil: round, equal, responsive to light; ocular pressures normal.	Flush eye or eyes with water to remove crusting and excess secretions. Seek medical attention.	Check visual acuity. Check pupils. Irrigate eyes thoroughly. Instill antibiotic ointment or drops as ordered. Instruct to see ophthalmologist if symptoms persist more than 48 hours.
Acute glaucoma—sudden increase in intraocular pressures secondary to closure of canal of Schlemm.	Blurring of vision. Severe eye pain. Reddened eye. Cornea hazy. Pupil semidilated with poor or no response to light. Eyeball hard. Intraocular pressures > 20 mm Hg. Nausea, vomiting.	Notify physician at once. Calm and reassure patient. Cover eye if bright daylight. Get to medical assistance at once.	Calm, reassure patient. Notify ophthalmologist at once. Assist with tonometry. Administer pilocarpine eyedrops as ordered. Transfer to hospital unit when stabilized.
Foreign bodies in ears—beans, peas, candy, foxtails, insects.	Decreased hearing, pulling, poking at ear and ear canal, buzzing, discomfort.	Do not attempt to remove object. Seek medical assistance.	Inspect ear canal. Assist with sedating children—restraint may be necessary. Assist with procedures to remove object. Forceps or curved probe for foxtails, irregularly shaped objects. #10 or #12 French catheter with tip cut squarely off and attached to suction to remove round object.

TABLE 5–25. *(Continued)*

Condition	Assessment: signs and symptoms	Prehospitalization nursing care	In-hospital nursing care
EYE AND EAR EMERGENCIES			
Otitis media—inflammation of middle ear secondary to infection; common in children and divers.	Pain, earache, fever, malaise. Tympanic membrane reddened and inflamed—may be bulging.	Aspirin or aspirin substitutes for relief of pain and fever. Seek medical attention to prevent permanent damage.	Irrigate external auditory canal to flush out insects, materials which do not absorb water—do not irrigate if danger of perforation. Assess vital signs. Assist with otoscopic examination. Administer antibiotics as ordered. Apply hot compresses as ordered. Administer aspirin or narcotic for relief of pain as ordered. Culture any ear drainage. Instruct patient or parents concerning the necessity of completing antibiotic regimen.

g. Contain descriptions of every event that might lead to a lawsuit, such as fights, injuries, equipment failures.

2. Consent—while there is no law requiring written consent before performing medical treatment, all elective procedures can only be performed if the patient has been fully informed and voluntarily consents to the procedure.

   a. If informed consent cannot be obtained because of the patient's condition and immediate treatment is necessary to save life or safeguard health, the emergency rule can be applied. This rule implies consent. However, if time allows, it is advisable to obtain either oral or written informed consent from someone who has authority to act for the patient.

   b. Verbal consents should be recorded in detail, witnessed and signed by *two* individuals.

   c. Written or verbal consent can be given by alert, coherent, or otherwise competent adults, by parents, legal guardian, or person in loco parentis (one standing in for the parent with the parent's rights, duties, and responsibilities) of minors or incompetent adults.

   d. If the minor is 14 years old or older, consent must be acquired from the minor as well as from the parent or legal guardian. Emancipated minors can consent for themselves.

Questions / NURSING CARE OF THE ACUTELY OR CHRONICALLY ILL ADULT

Mr. Marks is a 65-year-old man admitted with a complaint of increasing weakness and episodes of fainting with minimal exertion. His vital signs at rest are B/P 140/70; HR 40, RR 16, skin warm and dry. On getting Mr. Marks up to the commode, you observed that he suddenly became dizzy, turning ashen and diaphoretic. On returning Mr. Marks to bed, you note his vital signs are now B/P 128/60, HR 42, RR 24. Continuous EKG monitoring is ordered and reveals a pattern of complete heart block.

1. The EKG pattern of complete heart block is characterized by:
   1. Two P waves to every QRS wave without antecedent lengthening of the PR interval.
   2. A gradual lengthening of PR interval until an impulse is blocked.
   3. Independent pacemakers controlling the atria and ventricles.
   4. Wide, bizarre QRS complexes following each atrial contraction.

2. What are the two most common causes of atrioventricular heart block?
   1. Coronary artery disease and potassium depletion.
   2. Hypokalemia and myocardial infarction.
   3. Digitalis toxicity and other electrolyte disturbances.
   4. Degenerative cardiac disease and digitalis toxicity.

3. Which of the following physiologic phenomena explain Mr. Marks's signs and symptoms?
   1. Inability of heart to increase its rate to meet metabolic needs during exercise.
   2. Insufficient blood flow to the coronary arteries.
   3. Increased stroke volume.
   4. Inability of the circulatory reflexes to increase venous return.

4. Mr. Marks's physician orders the insertion of a permanent pacemaker. In preparing a preoperative teaching plan for Mr. Marks, you would initially:
   1. Assess Mr. Marks's interest in learning about the procedure and his current understanding of all or some of the information.
   2. Invite Mrs. Marks to join the preoperative teaching session.
   3. Ascertain from the physician the amount of information she or he has given the patient.
   4. Have the operative permit signed, then institute your teaching plan.

5. Which of the following nursing-care procedures is least important during the period prior to insertion of the pacemaker?
   1. Providing sedation to relieve anxiety and promote relaxation as needed.
   2. Instituting arm and leg range-of-motion exercises to prevent postinsertion complications.
   3. Establishing an intravenous line and having emergency equipment and medications available.
   4. Weighing the patient and instituting strict intake and output records.

6. Which of the following is a medication that should be kept available during Mr. Marks's preoperative period?
   1. Lidocaine.
   2. Isoproterenol.
   3. Digoxin.
   4. Propranolol hydrochloride.

7. This drug is categorized as a:
   1. Beta mimetic.
   2. Cardiac glycoside.
   3. Anticholinergic.
   4. Beta blocker.

8. Besides enhancing pacemaker automaticity and facilitating AV conduction during heart block, this drug also:
   1. Increases peripheral vascular resistance.
   2. Decreases automaticity of Purkinje fibers.
   3. Decreases bronchoconstriction.
   4. Decreases oral secretion.

Mr. Marks's demand pacemaker was inserted under fluoroscopy and local anesthesia in the cardiac catheterization laboratory. The pacing catheter was inserted into the right external jugular vein and positioned in the right ventricle. The pulse generator was implanted in the right anterior chest below the clavicle.

9. Which of the following nursing-care activities is your first priority in the *early* postimplantation period?
   1. Restricting activity to prevent pacing catheter displacement.
   2. Monitoring the ECG continuously, noting rhythm, rate, appearance, and amplitude of pacing spike.
   3. Implementing passive range-of-motion exercise to the right arm to prevent "frozen shoulder."
   4. Maintaining sterile dressings over the operative site to prevent infection.

10. Which of the following would receive the least emphasis in your predischarge education plan?
    1. Rationale for pacemaker implantation.
    2. Pacemaker function and signs indicating malfunction.
    3. Therapeutic program including medication, diet, activity schedule, and safety precautions.
    4. Necessity for periodic follow-up visits to physician.

11. Mr. Marks will be restricted from continuing which of his following hobbies?
1. Swimming.
2. Fashioning lamps from driftwood and metal.
3. Operating ham radio.
4. Playing golf.

12. Outcome criteria for Mr. Marks included the goal that he and his wife should be able to describe signs of pacemaker malfunction. Which of the following behaviors would indicate that this goal had been met?
1. Counts pulse correctly and identifies need to monitor rate daily.
2. Counts pulse correctly and identifies the significance of drainage or discoloration around the battery insertion site.
3. Counts pulse correctly and states the estimated life of the battery and understands need of prophylactic replacement.
4. Counts pulse correctly and identifies need to report rate changes and symptoms such as dizziness, palpitations and hiccoughs.

Mr. Smith is a 50-year-old man who owns and operates a small business. He is married and has four children. He is a member of two fraternal organizations and has held a seat on several community advisory councils and commissions. Six years ago he developed mild hypertension (B/P 144/96), which his physician treated by instructing him to lose weight. Mr. Smith lost 25 lb, but has since regained and lost this weight several times. On presenting himself to his private physician for his yearly physical, Mr. Smith complained of increasing shortness of breath on exertion. Physical exam revealed a moderately overweight (20 lb) male, head and neck unremarkable, lung field resonant, fine basilar rales in both lung fields, PMI (point of maximal impulse) shifted to the left and down by 1.5 cm, heart rate regular, no extra cardiac sounds or murmurs, abdominal and neuromuscular exam noncontributory. B/P 152/120, HR 82, RR 16.

13. Which of the following statements correctly characterizes essential hypertension?
1. Forty percent of the American adult population is affected by hypertension.
2. Essential hypertension is more severe in men than women.
3. American Blacks develop hypertension at an earlier age than Caucasians but have a lower mortality rate.
4. Given newer screening devices most hypertensive persons are now being detected.

14. Shifting of the PMI to the left and down in Mr. Smith indicates:
1. Compensatory left ventricular enlargement in the face of increasing peripheral resistance.
2. Left ventricular decompensation and/or failure.
3. A normal finding in middle-aged and older adults.
4. Compensatory right ventricular enlargement due to increased pulmonary artery pressures.

15. Of the following, which physiologic phenomenon best explains Mr. Smith's increasing shortness of breath with exercise?
1. Pulmonary venous congestion due to decreased left ventricular efficiency.
2. Decreased venous return to right heart due to peripheral vasodilation.
3. Asynergistic pumping of the left ventricle.
4. Obesity and sedentary life style.

16. Essential hypertension *does not* have the following effect on the cardiovascular system:
1. Cardiomegaly.
2. Sclerosis of vessels.
3. Increased tissue perfusion.
4. Decreased glomerular filtration rate.

17. Arterial pressures are highest:
1. Between the first and second heart sound.
2. During the QRS wave.
3. Just before the first heart sound.
4. During ventricular diastole.

Initial medical therapy for Mr. Smith included:
Hydrochlorothiazide (HydroDiuril) 50 mgm bid
Hydrazaline (Apresoline) 25 mgm bid
1500 cal reducing diet.

18. Hydrochlorothiazide is classified as:
1. An aldosterone inhibitor.
2. A carbonic anhydrase inhibitor.
3. A potassium-sparing drug.
4. A potassium-wasting drug.

19. Hydrochlorothiazide exerts its primary effect on:
1. The proximal and distal tubules of the kidney.
2. The distal tubule of the kidney only.
3. The ascending loop of Henle and the distal tubule of the kidney.
4. The descending loop of Henle and the proximal tubule of the kidney.

20. Side effects of this drug include all of the following *except:*
1. Hyponatremia.
2. Hypokalemia.
3. Hyperchloremic acidosis.
4. Hyperuricemia.

21. The antihypertensive effects of hydralazine are believed due to:
1. Decreased renal blood flow and decreased venous capacitance.
2. Direct vasodilation of the vascular smooth muscle and increased renal blood flow.
3. Increased methylation of norepinephrine at the sympathetic synapses of vascular smooth muscle.
4. Inhibition of cardioaccelerator and vasoconstrictor centers in the medullary vasomotor center.

22. If Mr. Smith's therapy is effective you would expect:

1. A greater decrease in systolic than diastolic pressure.
2. A greater decrease in diastolic than systolic pressure.
3. An approximately equal decrease in both systolic and diastolic pressure.
4. An approximately equal increase in both systolic and diastolic pressure.

Terry Adams is a 30-year-old advertising executive with a history of ulcerative colitis since age 22. She has been admitted to your unit for an acute exacerbation of her condition. Her chief complaint is severe abdominal cramping and diarrhea. She states that she has had 18–20 stools a day for four days. The stools consisted mostly of mucus and blood; very little fecal material was present. Physical examination revealed a thin, pale, obviously fatigued and physically weak young woman: (a) Abdomen was scaffold and very tender to palpation; rapid peristaltic waves were evident on inspection. Bowel sounds were hyperactive. Sacral/anal area was red and excoriative. (b) Neuromuscular exam revealed decreased muscle tone and deep-tendon reflexes. Wrists and knee joints tender, warm, and slightly swollen. Decreased abduction and extension of wrist joints. (c) Cardiopulmonary: B/P 110/78 (supine), P 88, RR 22, T 102.2 F. Heart sounds unremarkable and lung fields clear to auscultation.

23. Blood and fluid loss from frequent diarrhea may cause hypovolemia. You can quickly assess volume depletion in Ms. Adams by:
    1. Measuring the quantity and specific gravity of her urine output.
    2. Taking her blood pressure first supine, then sitting; noting any changes.
    3. Comparing the patient's present weight with her weight on her last admission.
    4. Administering the oral water test.

24. Other signs of hypovolemia include all of the following *except:*
    1. Dry mucous membranes and soft eyeballs.
    2. Increased hematocrit and hemoglobin.
    3. Decreased pulse rate and widened pulse pressure.
    4. Increased lethargy and confusion.

25. With severe diarrhea, electrolytes as well as fluids are lost. What electrolyte imbalance is indicated by Ms. Adams's decreased muscle tone and deep-tendon reflexes?
    1. Hypernatremia.
    2. Hypokalemia.
    3. Hyperchloremia.
    4. Hypocalcemia.

26. Ms. Adams's laboratory values indicate hemoconcentration secondary to fluid loss. Which of the following intravenous solutions would be most appropriate during *initial* fluid replacement therapy?
    1. 10% dextrose and saline.

2. 5% dextrose and water with 60 mEq KCl.
3. 5% dextrose and water only.
4. Distilled water.

27. Three days after admission Ms. Adams continued to have frequent stools. Her oral intake of both fluids and solids was poor. Her physician ordered parenteral hyperalimentation. Hyperalimentation solutions are:
    1. Hypotonic solutions used primarily for hydration when hemoconcentration is present.
    2. Hypertonic solutions used primarily to increase osmotic pressure of blood plasma.
    3. Alkalyzing solutions used to treat metabolic acidosis, thus reducing cellular swelling.
    4. Hyperosmolar solutions used primarily to reverse negative nitrogen balance.

28. Maintaining the infusion rate of hyperalimentation solutions is a nursing responsibility. What side effects would you anticipate from too rapid an infusion rate?
    1. Cellular dehydration and potassium depletion.
    2. Circulatory overload and hypoglycemia.
    3. Hypoglycemia and hypovolemia.
    4. Potassium excess and congestive heart failure.

29. Which of the following statements regarding nursing care of the patient on hyperalimentation is *not true?*
    1. The patient's urine should be tested for glucose-acetone every 4–6 hours.
    2. The hyperalimentation subclavian line may not be utilized for CVP readings and/or blood withdrawal.
    3. Occlusive dressings at the catheter insertion site are changed every 48 hours using the clean technique.
    4. Records of intake and output and daily weights should be kept.

After ten days of therapy, Ms. Adams's physician decided to perform an ileostomy. For three days prior to surgery she was given neomycin. On the morning of surgery she was catheterized and a nasogastric tube was inserted.

30. Which of the following nursing interventions would be the most beneficial in preparing Ms. Adams psychologically for this surgery?
    1. Include her family in preoperative teaching sessions.
    2. Encourage her to express her concerns and to ask questions regarding the management of the ileostomy.
    3. Thorough, brief explanation of all preoperative and postoperative procedures.
    4. Have a member of an "Ostomy Club" visit her.

31. Neomycin was administered preoperatively:
    1. To decrease the incidence of postoperative atelectasis due to decreased depth of respirations.
    2. To increase the effectiveness of the body's immunologic response following surgical trauma.
    3. To reduce the incidence of wound infections by decreasing the number of intestinal organisms.

4. To prevent postoperative bladder atony due to catheterization.

32. Following ileostomy, the drainage appliance is applied to the stoma:
    1. 24 hours later, when edema has subsided.
    2. In the operating room.
    3. After the ileostomy begins to function.
    4. When the patient is able to begin self-care procedures.

33. Which of the following goals would you give as your highest postoperative nursing priority?
    1. Relief of pain to promote rest and relaxation.
    2. Assisting the patient with self-care activities.
    3. Maintenance of fluid, electrolyte, and nutritional balance.
    4. Skin care and control of odors.

34. Two days postoperatively, Ms. Adams begins to refuse care and repeatedly says to the staff "Leave me alone, I just want to sleep." What would be your first nursing action?
    1. Provide accurate, brief, and reassuring explanations of all procedures.
    2. Encourage ambulation in the hall with other patients.
    3. Invite a member of an "Ostomy Club" to visit Ms. Adams.
    4. Encourage Ms. Adams to verbalize her feelings, fears, and questions.

35. During the early postoperative period you initiate ileostomy care. The primary objective of this procedure is:
    1. To facilitate maintenance of intake and output records.
    2. To control unpleasant odors.
    3. To prevent excoriation of the skin around the stoma.
    4. To reduce the risk of postoperative wound infection.

36. After discharge, Ms. Adams calls you at the hospital to report the sudden onset of abdominal cramps, vomiting, and watery discharge from her ileostomy. What would you advise?
    1. Call the physician if symptoms persist for 24 hours.
    2. Take 30 cc of m.o.m. (milk of magnesia).
    3. NPO until vomiting stops.
    4. Call physician immediately.

Mrs. Washington is a 42-year-old housewife admitted for right breast biopsy and possible modified radical mastectomy. She had noted a small lump in the upper outer quadrant of her right breast two months ago. She had delayed seeking medical consultation until ten days ago because she had a history of breast cysts and thought it might go away. Family history revealed an aunt who had died of breast carcinoma 15 years previously. During the interview, Mrs. Washington answered questions in a rushed, breathless manner. She constantly straightened the bedclothes. On examination,

Mrs. Washington appeared to be a well-nourished female, who looked younger than her stated age. Breast exam revealed no dimpling, but a small, firm, nontender, non-movable mass was palpable in the right upper quadrant. Lungs were clear to auscultation. Apical heart sounds were rapid, regular, and accentuated. Vital signs were B/P 186/110, pulse 90, respirations 22, temperature 98.4 F.

37. Breast self-examinations are best carried out:
    1. During the middle of the menstrual cycle.
    2. On the first day of each month.
    3. One week after the onset of menses.
    4. The week before the onset of menses.

38. Patients who tend to delay seeking medical advice after discovering a lump in the breast are displaying what common defense mechanism?
    1. Suppression.
    2. Denial.
    3. Repression.
    4. Intellectualization.

39. Given Mrs. Washington's behavior and vital signs, what is your first nursing action?
    1. Notify the physician immediately.
    2. Check pupils for size and responsiveness to light and extremities for edema.
    3. Reassure Mrs. Washington that the breast biopsy may be negative and she should not jump to conclusions.
    4. Sit down and encourage Mrs. Washington to talk about her feelings and ask questions.

40. A half-hour later you retake Mrs. Washington's vital signs. They are now B/P 132/86, pulse 80, and respirations 16. Mrs. Washington's elevated blood pressure indicates:
    1. She may be an individual who is highly sensitive to sympathetic nervous system stimulation.
    2. She is emotionally labile and will need to be assessed closely in the postoperative period.
    3. She is psychologically unprepared for surgery and a psych consult is in order.
    4. She is denying the possible loss of her breast.

41. Preoperative teaching for Mrs. Washington included deep breathing and coughing. Which of the following is not a desired outcome of your teaching plan? Mrs. Washington:
    1. States the rationale for repeating these exercises every one to two hours postoperatively.
    2. Demonstrates coughing technique.
    3. Inhales through both nose and mouth and raises abdomen with each respiration.
    4. States she recognizes the need to repeat exercises until she is feeling light-headed.

42. In preparation for surgery, Mrs. Washington's right upper chest, right upper arm and axilla were cleansed with Betadine and shaved. The primary objective of a skin prep is:

1. To clean the skin of excess oils and hair.
2. To prevent postoperative infection by sterilizing the skin.
3. To prevent postoperative infection by reducing the number of microorganisms normally on the skin.
4. To provide a clear field for the incision.

43. On the morning of surgery you are assigned to assist Mrs. Washington in the final preparations before going to surgery. Before going in to see Mrs. Washington, your first action is to:
1. Prepare her preoperative medication.
2. Check to be sure the operative permit has been signed.
3. Check to see if the preoperative laboratory reports have been placed in the chart.
4. Check the diet orders to be sure she has been placed on the NPO list.

44. In assisting Mrs. Washington to prepare herself for surgery, you would do all of the following *except:*
1. Tape wedding band securely to her finger.
2. Begin exploring her fears and anxieties toward surgery.
3. Assist in removing hairpins and nail polish.
4. Remind her to void prior to receiving preoperative medication.

45. The preoperative medication ordered for Mrs. Washington by the anesthesiologist is morphine sulfate 15 mg and atropine SO_4 0.4 mg, subcutaneously. This medication should be given:
1. Right before the patient leaves for surgery.
2. 45–60 minutes before anesthetic induction.
3. 20–30 minutes before anesthetic induction.
4. 10–15 minutes before anesthetic induction.

46. While preparing Mrs. Washington's preoperative medication, you note that the atropine SO_4 you have on hand is in a strength of 0.6 mg per ml. The correct amount of atropine to administer is:
1. 1.5 milliliters.
2. 1 milliliter.
3. 10 minims.
4. 8 minims.

47. The desired effect of morphine SO_4 and atropine SO_4 administration is:
1. Pain relief and reduction of anxiety.
2. Reduced sensitivity to stimuli and decreased oral and respiratory secretions.
3. Induction of sleep and reduced oral secretion.
4. Reduced sensitivity to pain and muscular relaxation.

48. Side effects of morphine and atropine administration are:
1. Bradycardia, anorexia, and decreased urine output.
2. Hypertension, nausea, vomiting, tachycardia.
3. Hypotension, cotton-mouth, nausea, and vomiting.
4. Dryness, cotton-mouth, constricted pupils, and bradycardia.

49. Following administration of Mrs. Washington's preoperative medication, you should do all of the following *except:*
1. Raise the siderails to prevent injury from restlessness.
2. Let her know she may not be asleep when she leaves the unit.
3. Tell her that you or another nurse will be here when she returns to assist with turning, coughing, and deep breathing.
4. Get her up to the bathroom when she complains of bladder fullness.

50. Mr. Washington has arrived early to be with his wife before surgery. After his wife leaves for the operating room, you would initially:
1. Tell him to go on to work and come back in the early evening when his wife is likely to be more responsive.
2. Explain that following surgery his wife will be taken to the recovery room, but that the surgeon will contact him when the procedure is over.
3. Get him a cup of coffee and tell him to make himself comfortable, as it will be some time before his wife returns to her room.
4. Encourage him to express his feelings and concerns so as to plan for postoperative family teaching.

51. Mrs. Washington's frozen section is positive for carcinoma and the surgeon performs a modified radical mastectomy. This procedure involves removal of:
1. The right breast only.
2. The right breast and axillary nodes.
3. The right breast, pectoralis major muscle, and axillary lymph nodes.
4. The right breast, underlying chest muscle, axillary lymph nodes, and internal mammary lymph nodes.

52. On admission to the recovery room, Mrs. Washington is very restless. Her respirations are deep and somewhat irregular; she startles easily and moans when you touch her. Your nursing action is:
1. Continue to stimulate her by telling her the operation is over.
2. Raise the siderails and remain quietly in attendance.
3. Administer meperidine (Demerol) HCl 100 mg IM.
4. Check her nail beds for cyanosis.

53. Mrs. Washington has an airway in place and is in a supine position. To prevent airway obstruction you should:
1. Leave the airway in and turn her head to the side.
2. Maintain her present position.
3. Remove the airway and turn her head to the side.
4. Remove the airway and maintain a prone position.

54. You are monitoring Mrs. Washington's vital signs every 15 minutes. Which of the following changes should be reported immediately to the surgeon?
1. Dry, cool skin.

2. A systolic blood pressure that drops 20 mm Hg or more.
3. A diastolic pressure below 70.
4. A pulse rate that increases and decreases with respirations.

55. A unit of blood is ordered for Mrs. Washington when her BP drops to 90/60. Which of the following is the most important safeguard prior to administering blood?
1. Refrigerate until used.
2. Agitate the blood so it is well mixed.
3. With another nurse, carefully check the label on the blood bag with the patient's wrist band.
4. Infuse through a blood warmer.

56. Mrs. Washington has a unit of whole blood transfusing in her left arm. The earliest signs of transfusion reaction are:
1. Headache, chills, and elevated temperature.
2. Hypertension and flushing.
3. Urticaria and wheezing.
4. Oliguria and jaundice.

57. Mrs. Washington's incision is covered with a pressure dressing and she has two drains attached to a Hemovac pump. Nursing observations and care of the patient with a Hemovac include all of the following *except:*
1. Observing and recording the amount and color of the drainage.
2. Maintaining suction by emptying and recompressing the apparatus regularly.
3. Increasing suction by attaching Hemovac to wall suction as the drainage increases.
4. Preventing traction on the drainage tubes by repositioning the Hemovac each time the patient is repositioned.

58. What is the primary advantage of Hemovac wound suction?
1. Exerts high, even suction.
2. Lightweight, allows easy mobility.
3. Speeds wound-healing by removing excess fluids.
4. Reduces the occurrence of postoperative infection.

59. The pressure dressing encircles Mrs. Washington's chest and fits very snugly. You can anticipate difficulty in which of the following postoperative nursing functions?
1. Maintaining good body alignment.
2. Initiating arm exercises.
3. Promoting deep breathing and coughing.
4. Taking vital signs.

60. On turning Mrs. Washington to her left side, you note a moderately large amount of serosanguineous drainage on the bedsheets. You should:
1. Remove the dressing to ascertain the origin of the bleeding.
2. Milk the Hemovac tubing using a downward motion.
3. Note vital signs, reinforce the dressing, and notify the surgeon immediately.

4. Recognize that this is a frequent occurrence with this type of surgery.

61. If Mrs. Washington begins to demonstrate some early signs of shock, such as increased pulse, cool, clammy skin, and restlessness you could enhance venous return by:
1. Administering oxygen to reduce restlessness.
2. Raising the foot of the bed 20°, keeping her knees straight, trunk horizontal, and head slightly elevated.
3. Placing her in Trendelenburg's position.
4. Wrapping her in blankets.

62. Which of the following arm positions will best facilitate venous return on the operative side and reduce the occurrence of lymphedema?
1. Semi-Fowler's position with the elbow flexed and the arm across the chest.
2. Low-Fowler's position with the arm elevated so that the hand and elbow are slightly higher than the shoulder.
3. High-Fowler's position with the elbow flexed and the right hand positioned next to the head.
4. Adduction of the shoulder, extension of the elbow, and flexion of the wrist.

63. Depending on the extent of surgery and the physician's orders, it is possible to initiate arm exercises as early as 24 hours after surgery. Which of the following is appropriate initial therapy for Mrs. Washington?
1. Encouraging self-feeding and hair-combing.
2. Passive/active flexion and extension of the elbow and pronation and supination of the wrist.
3. Abduction and external rotation of the right shoulder.
4. Early ambulation and active extension and flexion of the elbow.

64. Mrs. Washington has meperidine 75 mg every 3–4 hours prn ordered for postoperative pain. Prior to administering this narcotic, the nurse should:
1. Take vital signs, noting rate and depth of respirations.
2. Assess the type, location, and intensity of discomfort.
3. Evaluate whether the pain is real.
4. Try other measures, such as position change, to relieve discomfort.

65. To which of the following postoperative complications is Mrs. Washington predisposed due to the nature of her surgery?
1. Peripheral thrombophlebitis.
2. Wound dehiscence.
3. Atelectasis.
4. Paralytic ileus.

66. On the third postoperative day, Mrs. Washington voiced concern about her husband's reaction to her surgery. Of the following approaches, which is most likely to minimize Mrs. Washington's concern?

1. Emphasizing the life-saving aspects of her surgery.
2. Explaining that depression and anxiety are common behaviors following radical surgery.
3. Interviewing Mr. Washington to ascertain his real reaction.
4. Encouraging Mrs. Washington to elaborate on her concerns and to identify the strengths in her relationship with her husband.

67. In planning for discharge, Mrs. Washington should be informed of actions that may increase lymphedema. Which of the following activities is *most likely* to increase symptoms?
   1. Wearing gloves for household tasks or gardening.
   2. Carrying groceries.
   3. Wearing dresses with elasticized sleeves.
   4. Driving to and from work.

Mr. Chen is a 63-year-old electrician admitted to the hospital for bronchoscopy. He has a smoking history of two packs per day for 30 years, although he has not smoked for the last six months. Ten days ago he developed an upper respiratory infection with runny nose, cough, and slight fever, which he treated with aspirins and fluids. Six days ago, his fever increased and his cough was productive of greenish sputum. He decided to see his physician, who ordered a chest X ray. The chest X ray was positive for pneumonia, but the physician also noted an abnormality in the left lower lobe. On admission to his room, Mr. Chen stated he was in the hospital because he was short of breath and had not been able to shake off his cold. During your assessment he mentions casually that his doctor also thought there was something funny in his left lung. Vital signs: B/P 140/90, pulse 78, respirations 22, temperature 99 F.

68. Physical assessment of Mr. Chen revealed a thin muscular man with rhonchi and wheezes in the left lung and some wheezes in the right lower lobe. Rhonchi and wheezes occur due to:
   1. Total obstruction of small bronchioles.
   2. Partial obstruction of bronchi and bronchioles.
   3. Fluid in the alveoli.
   4. Inflammation of the pleura.

69. Bronchoscopy is:
   1. An X-ray procedure that allows for multiple views of the lungs.
   2. A procedure utilizing a lighted mirror lens to observe the walls of the trachea, mainstem bronchus, and major bronchial tubes.
   3. A diagnostic test during which a radiopaque substance is inserted into the tracheobronchial tree for clear visualization.
   4. A needle puncture of the lung mass, identified on an X ray with aspiration of cells for microscopic examination.

70. Following bronchoscopy, what is your most important nursing observation?

1. Blood pressure, pulse, and temperature.
2. Color and consistency of sputum.
3. Function of the tenth cranial nerve.
4. Presence of urticaria.

71. Dyspnea is best defined as:
   1. Increased awareness of respiratory effort.
   2. Decreased alveolar ventilation.
   3. Increased rate and depth of respiration.
   4. Decreased oxygen saturation of venous blood.

72. Bronchoscopy revealed a squamous cell carcinoma. The lesion appeared fairly localized and Mr. Chen's surgeon decided to do a lower left lobectomy. Preoperative teaching for Mr. Chen includes coughing, deep breathing, and arm exercises. The most important postoperative activity the thoracic patient performs is:
   1. Arm exercises to prevent shoulder ankylosis.
   2. Deep breathing and coughing up of sputum to prevent airway obstruction.
   3. Leg exercises to prevent thrombophlebitis due to prolonged bedrest.
   4. Deep breathing only to prevent undue suture stress while maintaining ventilation.

73. In preparing Mr. Chen psychologically for his surgery and postoperative care you should include all of the following *except:*
   1. Explain to him that he will be surrounded by equipment, such as chest tubes, oxygen, and IV infusions, and that these are routine.
   2. Tell him he will have periods of rest, but will be awakened approximately every two hours for turning, coughing, and deep breathing.
   3. Assure him he will receive medication that will assist in relieving his discomfort.
   4. Assure him that anesthesia will not have any untoward effects on his respiratory status.

74. Prior to surgery, pulmonary function tests are done and arterial blood gases are drawn to establish baseline data. Given Mr. Chen's respiratory symptomatology, you would expect which of the following outcomes?
   1. Increased vital capacity and respiratory acidosis.
   2. Decreased vital capacity and respiratory alkalosis.
   3. Increased total lung capacity and metabolic acidosis.
   4. Decreased FEV_1 and respiratory acidosis.

75. Prior to surgery Mr. Chen was instructed in the use of an incentive spirometer. The primary purpose of this activity is:
   1. To encourage coughing.
   2. To arouse and stimulate the patient.
   3. To encourage deep breathing.
   4. To measure tidal volume and expiratory reserve volume.

On returning from the recovery room, Mr. Chen has a chest tube to a two-bottle, water-sealed drainage system and oxygen per nasal cannula. Postoperative orders included:

Meperidine 100 mg IM every 3–4 hours prn for pain.
1000 mL 5% dextrose/water every 10 hours.
Ampicillin 500 mg IM every 6 hours.
Tigan 200 mg IM every 3–4 hours prn nausea and vomiting.
IPPB with normal saline qid.
Incentive spirometer qid.

76. The essential purpose of the water-sealed drainage system is to:
1. Prevent early precipitous reinflation of the lung.
2. Drain off excess fluid and air, thereby promoting reestablishment of negative intrapleural pressures.
3. Drain off excess fluid and air, thereby promoting reestablishment of positive intrapleural pressures.
4. Decrease atelectasis in unaffected lung tissue and to monitor blood loss.

77. In a two-bottle, water-sealed drainage system:
1. The first bottle establishes the suction pressure and the second bottle collects the drainage.
2. The first bottle establishes the suction pressure and the second bottle is attached to motor suction.
3. The first bottle collects the drainage and the second bottle provides easy access for removing drainage specimens.
4. The first bottle collects the drainage and the second bottle establishes the suction pressure.

78. After making Mr. Chen comfortable in bed, your first nursing measure concerning the water-seal drainage is:
1. Milking the tubing to prevent accumulation of fibrin and clots.
2. Raising the bottle to bed height to accurately assess the meniscus level.
3. Attaching the chest tubes to the bed linen to assure that airflow and drainage are unhindered by kinks.
4. Marking the time and amount of drainage in the collection bottle.

79. On the second postoperative day, the fluid in the suction bottle's glass tube ceases to fluctuate. This most likely indicates:
1. The chest tube is plugged by fibrin or a clot.
2. There is an air leak in the system.
3. Pulmonary edema has occurred due to increased blood volumes in remaining lung tissue.
4. The patient's position needs to change to facilitate drainage.

80. Humidification is given with oxygen administration because:
1. Oxygen is highly permeable in water, thereby increasing gaseous diffusion.
2. Oxygen is very drying to the mucous membranes.
3. The partial pressures of oxygen are increased by water dilution, allowing more oxygen to reach the alveoli.

4. Water acts as a carrier substance facilitating movement of oxygen across the respiratory membrane.

81. To correctly administer 1000 mL of 5% dextrose/water in 10 hours using a standard 12-drop administration set, you would adjust Mr. Chen's infusion rate to:
1. 32 drops per minute.
2. 25 drops per minute.
3. 20 drops per minute.
4. 15 drops per minute.

82. The purpose of IPPB with normal saline is to maintain patent airways and to mobilize secretions. To accomplish this, IPPB exerts:
1. Positive pressures on inspiration.
2. Negative pressures on inspiration.
3. Positive pressures on expiration.
4. Negative pressures on expiration.

83. Passive arm exercises are instituted on Mr. Chen's left arm four hours after surgery. These exercises are designed to prevent which of the following dysfunctions?
1. Hyperflexion of the wrist.
2. Ankylosis of the shoulder.
3. Flexion of the elbow.
4. Spasticity of the intercostal muscles.

84. On the fifth postoperative day, fluctuation in the water-sealed bottle again ceased. Auscultation of Mr. Chen's upper left chest indicated the lung had reexpanded. The physician ordered a chest X ray to assess the degree of reexpansion. To safely transport Mr. Chen to X ray you would:
1. Remove the chest tubes, immediately covering the incision site with a sterile vaseline gauze to prevent air from entering the chest.
2. Disconnect the drainage bottles from the chest tubes, covering the catheter tip with a sterile dressing to prevent contamination.
3. Send Mr. Chen to X ray with his chest tube clamped but still attached to the drainage system to prevent air from entering the chest wall if the bottles are accidentally broken.
4. Send Mr. Chen to X ray with his chest tube attached to the drainage system, taking precautions to prevent breakage.

Miss Marble is a 21-year-old woman admitted to the hospital for an arthrotomy. Vital signs are B/P 120/78, pulse 78, respirations 18. She has had diabetes mellitus for two years. On admission her blood sugar, pH, and electrolytes were normal. Her urine was negative for glucose and acetone. She is on NPH insulin, 40 units, which she administers to herself every A.M. This dose was ordered for the day of surgery as well as rainbow coverage with regular insulin on the following scale:

0   —none
1 +—none

2 +—6 units
3 +—10 units
4 +—14 units
On the morning of surgery her urine was 1 + for sugar and acetone.

85. The basic pathology of diabetes mellitus is:
    1. Osmotic diuresis with sodium depletion.
    2. Inadequate glucagon production by the alpha cells in the islets of Langerhans.
    3. Decreased insulin production by beta cells of the islets of Langerhans.
    4. Decreased renal tubular transport of glucose.

86. If glucose fails to cross cell membrane for the enzymatic synthesis of ATP, fats and proteins are converted into a source of energy. This process is known as:
    1. Glycogenolysis.
    2. Gluconeogenesis.
    3. Glycosuria.
    4. Ketogenesis.

87. What is the most likely mechanism behind Miss Marble's elevation of urine glucose and acetone on the morning of surgery?
    1. Increased glycogenolysis due to psychologic stress.
    2. Early morning urines are usually elevated.
    3. Her insulin dose needs to be reevaluated.
    4. Increased glomerulo-filtration rate.

88. Normal fasting serum glucose levels are:
    1. 30–60 mg/100 ml of blood.
    2. 60–100 mg/100 ml of blood.
    3. 120–140 mg/100 ml of blood.
    4. 140–200 mg/100 ml of blood.

89. Acetonuria develops in diabetes due to:
    1. Excessive oxidation of fatty acids for energy, which increases ketones in glomerular filtrate.
    2. Osmotic diuresis, accompanying elevation in serum glucose levels, which decreases exchange of electrolytes in renal tubules.
    3. Failure of sodium-hydrogen ion exchange mechanism in the renal tubules to secrete excess hydrogen ions.
    4. Increased volatile H^+ ions and decreased nonvolatile H^+ ions in the glomerular filtrate.

On the evening of her first postop day, Miss Marble began to complain of increasing nausea. Her face was flushed, she appeared lethargic, and her vital signs were B/P 108/78, pulse 100, RR 24 and deep. Intake 2100 cc/IV. Urine output 2000 cc.

90. What is your first nursing action?
    1. Call the attending physician.
    2. Check her urine for sugar and acetone.
    3. Administer an antiemetic.
    4. Decrease her IV infusion rate.

91. Miss Marble's vital signs and urine output reflect:

1. Increased ADH release in response to physiologic stress of surgery.
2. Decreased ECF volume due to osmotic diuresis.
3. A hypo-osmolar fluid imbalance.
4. Circulatory overload.

92. Regular or crystalline insulin is utilized as an adjunct to Miss Marble's NPH therapy because:
    1. There is increased tissue metabolism with surgery.
    2. Insulin production is decreased even further with the stress of surgery.
    3. Physiologic and psychologic stress increases serum glucose levels via sympathetic nervous system stimulation.
    4. An increased insulin load is necessary to prevent hyperkalemia.

93. NPH insulin reaches its peak action:
    1. 4 hours after injection.
    2. 6–12 hours after injection.
    3. 12–14 hours after injection.
    4. 15–18 hours after injection.

94. When is the patient receiving NPH insulin *most* likely to have a hypoglycemic reaction?
    1. Before lunch (10–11 A.M.).
    2. Early afternoon (1–3 P.M.).
    3. Late afternoon (4–7 P.M.).
    4. After supper (8–10 P.M.).

95. Symptoms of a hypoglycemic reaction include:
    1. Irritability, confusion, and lethargy.
    2. Increased temperature and flushing of skin.
    3. Muscle tremors and hyperreflexia.
    4. Decreased blood pressure and fatigue.

96. Which of the following statements correctly differentiates ketoacidosis from insulin shock?
    1. Deep and rapid respirations are characteristic of ketoacidosis, whereas slow, shallow respirations are characteristic of insulin shock.
    2. Acetone breath characterizes ketoacidosis, whereas the breath of the patient in insulin shock is frequently fetid.
    3. Warm, dry, flushed skin and loss of turgor characterize the patient with ketoacidosis, while the skin of the patient with insulin shock is usually pale, cool, and diaphoretic.
    4. Apprehension, irritability, and combative behavior occur with ketoacidosis, while the patient in insulin shock is more likely to be confused, lethargic, or comatose.

97. The laboratory test that measures serum and urine glucose levels before and after ingestion of a glucose load is called:
    1. Fasting blood sugar.
    2. Glucose tolerance test.
    3. Postprandial blood glucose.
    4. Tolbutamide response test.

98. In the above test, blood glucose levels should return to normal in about how many hours?
1. One.
2. Two.
3. Three.
4. Four.

Diet and weight control are the foundation of diabetic management. In discussing Miss Marble's diet with her before her discharge, you go over possible food exchanges. She has been placed on an 1800-calorie diet. A typical lunch includes two meat exchanges, two bread exchanges, one vegetable exchange, one fruit exchange, one fat exchange, and one milk exchange.

99. Miss Marble states she is a "peanut butter" freak. What may she exchange for 2 Tbsp. peanut butter?
1. Eight ounces of whole milk.
2. Two Tbsp. of butter.
3. One quarter cup cottage cheese.
4. Two Tbsp. cream cheese.

100. Given her allowances, Miss Marble can eat all of the following at her birthday luncheon except:
1. A piece of plain sponge cake.
2. Eight-ounce glass of coca cola.
3. A taco (tortilla, meat, cheddar cheese, lettuce).
4. Avocado and orange salad.

Mrs. Jones, a 35-year-old mother, was admitted with dysmenorrhea and excessive vaginal bleeding. A diagnostic D & C discovered uterine fibroid tumors. A hysterectomy was discussed, and a decision to go home was made for child care arrangements. That night she experienced excessive vaginal bleeding and feelings of extreme weakness. She was readmitted at 2:00 A.M. after being examined by the ER physician. Upon admission to the general floor, the nurses discovered a friendly, very apprehensive, slightly pale female. The nursing assessment revealed a soft, tender abdomen with normal bowel sounds and a saturated kotex pad. Her chest was clear to auscultation and cardiac sounds normal with a rapid apical. Extremities were slightly cool and pale, and nail beds were pale. Following a physical examination, the physician decided to perform an emergency hysterectomy. Her vital signs were: B/P 94/60, AP 126, RR 28. Laboratory data: Hct 30% Hgb 8.5, CBC 5.

101. Emergency surgical procedures are those that must be performed:
1. Upon completion of the necessary surgical preparation.
2. Within 24 hours.
3. Immediately.
4. At the start of the next surgical day.

102. The surgical treatment most often implemented for excessive vaginal bleeding due to uterine fibroids is:
1. Panabdominal hysterectomy.
2. Vaginal hysterectomy.
3. Dilatation and curettage.
4. Abdominal hysterectomy.

103. Emergency procedures such as this increase the surgical risk to the patient because:
1. The surgery is performed immediately.
2. There is little time for psychologic/physical preparation.
3. There is decreased physiologic stress.
4. The anesthesia of choice is different for emergency surgery.

104. Assessing past medical history and use of medications is always necessary for any surgical candidate. Which of the following drugs can negatively interfere with anesthesia or contribute to postoperative complications?
1. Anticoagulants and antihypertensives.
2. Anticoagulants and insulin.
3. Digoxin and thiazide diuretics.
4. Vitamins and mineral replacements.

105. The laboratory data recorded a Hgb of 8.5. What is your nursing responsibility?
1. To attach the lab report to the chart.
2. To hang a unit of blood.
3. To notify the physician immediately.
4. To chart the report in the nurses' notes.

106. One potential complication of an abdominal hysterectomy is abdominal distention. Postoperative nursing measures designed to *avoid* abdominal distention are:
1. Auscultation of the abdomen for bowel sounds.
2. Abdominal massage and bedrest.
3. Insertion of nasogastric and rectal tubes, and early ambulation.
4. Progression of postoperative diet.

107. During discharge teaching the nurse should include the following instructions:
1. Avoid sitting for long periods of time.
2. Evacuate bowels daily.
3. Restrict sexual activity for six months after hysterectomy.
4. Avoid all household chores for two months.

108. Other postoperative instructions would include all of the following *except:*
1. Monitor vaginal drainage and report any color changes.
2. Expect that vaginal discharge will diminish and cease gradually.
3. Plan on contraception, considering her ovaries are still intact.
4. Expect that menses will no longer occur.

109. On the morning of discharge, Mrs. Jones is found sitting with her back to the door staring out the window. She says that she no longer feels like a real woman. Your response should be to:

1. Ask her if she would like her Valium.
2. Notify the physician.
3. Ask "Can you tell me what makes you feel that way?"
4. Reassure her that this is a common reaction.

Mr. Noble sustained second-degree burns on his left leg and thigh when his pants caught fire while he was burning leaves. His left ankle was charred and dry. On arrival at the hospital he was given morphine sulfate for his severe pain and an IV of lactated Ringer's was started via cut down. Unburned areas were pale and felt cold to the touch. Vital signs were B/P 96/70, pulse 116, respirations 26. Mr. Noble was also restless and disoriented.

110. Burns are classified according to the depth of tissue destruction. Second-degree burns:
1. Involve the epidermis only.
2. Extend to the dermis and are very painful.
3. Extend to subcutaneous tissues and are rarely painful.
4. Extend to muscle and bone and are very painful.

111. Equally important in determining severity of burns is the total body surface involved. Management of fluid and electrolyte balance is critical when burns:
1. Are first-degree and cover 20% of the body surface.
2. Are second-degree and cover 15% of the body surface.
3. Are third-degree and cover 10% of the body surface.
4. Are fourth-degree and cover 5% of the body surface.

112. Besides assessing size and depth of the burn, which of the following physical parameters are also important baseline data for fluid replacement therapy?
1. Age, sex, and vital signs.
2. Age, weight, vital signs, and skin turgor.
3. Vital signs, level of mentation, and urine output.
4. Vital signs and quantity and specific gravity of urine.

113. The physiologic response to the stress of extensive burns may result in which of the following complications in the postburn period?
1. Curling's ulcer due to elevated serum cortisol.
2. Positive nitrogen balance due to mobilization of body proteins.
3. Decreased hematocrit due to red blood cell agglutination by epinephrine.
4. Hypo- and hyperthermia due to failure of hypothalamic temperature regulators.

114. Admission ER lab values for Mr. Noble were: Hematocrit 50%, hemoglobin 17.2 g, serum sodium 140 mEq/liter, serum potassium 7.6 mEq/liter. Serum sodium levels are within normal limits at this time because:
1. The pituitary has increased ADH release.
2. Vascular fluid losses due to exudate and edema formation have resulted in hemoconcentration.
3. Sodium has diffused from disrupted cells into the vascular compartment.

4. Increased serum potassium depresses aldosterone secretion by the adrenal cortex.

115. Sodium and potassium levels are affected by severe burns. Hyponatremia may develop in burn patients due to:
1. Displacement of sodium in edema fluids and loss through denuded areas of skin.
2. Increased aldosterone secretion.
3. Inadequate fluid replacement.
4. Metabolic acidosis.

116. Hyperkalemia develops following burn damage due to:
1. Increased exudate formation at the burn site.
2. Disruption of cell membrane integrity, allowing intracellular electrolytes to diffuse into the vascular compartment.
3. Decreased aldosterone secretion, increasing sodium excretion and retention of potassium.
4. Hyperbilirubinemia secondary to red blood cell destruction.

117. The treatment of choice to reduce hyperkalemia in Mr. Noble is:
1. Morphine sulfate.
2. Kayexalate.
3. Insulin and 50% glucose solution.
4. Synthetic aldosterone.

118. During the initial stages of burns, the primary fluid imbalance occurs due to a shift of fluids from:
1. The cell to the interstitial space.
2. The interstitial space into the cell.
3. The interstitial space to the plasma.
4. The plasma to the interstitial space.

119. Nursing care in the immediate 24 hours postburn are directed toward monitoring adequacy of fluid therapy. Initial intravenous therapy may include both colloidal and crystalloid solutions. Which of the following replacement fluids is least often administered?
1. Ringer's lactate.
2. Whole blood.
3. Dextran.
4. Dextrose and water.

120. Adequacy of fluid volume replacement in the early postburn period is best reflected by:
1. Blood pressure, pulse rates, and daily weights.
2. Quantity of urinary output and vital signs.
3. Hemoglobin and hematocrit levels.
4. Serum electrolyte levels and urinary output.

121. Fifty-four hours after Mr. Noble sustained his burns his urine output increased from 1020 ml/24 hours to 2300 ml/24 hours. Laboratory values were serum sodium 136 mEq/liter, serum potassium 4 mEq/liter; hematocrit 34%. The changes in Mr. Noble's urinary output and lab studies indicate:

1. Beginning of interstitial-to-plasma fluid shift phase of burns.
2. Kidney failure.
3. Circulatory overload due to rapid IV infusion rate.
4. Hyponatremia.

122. The hematocrit is reduced due to:
1. Lack of erythropoietin factor.
2. Hemodilution and volume overload.
3. Metabolic acidosis.
4. Hypoalbuminemia.

123. Mr. Noble's burns are treated by the closed method. His left leg was cleaned and the left ankle debrided. Mafenide 1% (Sulfamylon) was applied and his left leg was wrapped in fine mesh gauze. Nursing measures when this approach is used include:
1. Cleansing of the wound daily and maintenance of strict isolation to prevent air contamination.
2. Cleansing of the wound daily or more often if needed and application of new dressings using clean technique.
3. Cleansing the wound one or more times each day and application of new dressing using sterile technique.
4. Cleansing of the wound daily and utilization of heat lamps to help maintain normal body temperature.

124. A side effect of mafenide 1% (Sulfamylon) application is:
1. Severe electrolyte disturbances.
2. Metabolic acidosis.
3. Metabolic alkalosis.
4. Staining of linen.

125. As Mr. Noble's nurse, you can help prevent contractures in the burned leg by:
1. Maintaining abduction of the left leg, extension of the left knee, and flexion of the left ankle.
2. Maintaining adduction of the left leg and extension of the left knee and ankle.
3. Maintaining abduction of the left leg and flexion of the left knee and ankle.
4. Maintaining adduction of the left leg, flexion of the left knee, and extension of the left ankle.

126. Which of the following behaviors is least likely to occur during Mr. Noble's recovery period?
1. Anxiety with mild confusion.
2. Desperation and panic.
3. Withdrawal and depression.
4. Dependency and regression.

127. Psychologic reactions during the recuperation stage of a burn are related primarily to:
1. Pain and immobility.
2. Changes in body image.
3. Financial concerns.
4. Anger.

Mr. Swenson is a 48-year-old man admitted to the hospital by his private physician with complaints of increasing dyspepsia, intermittent bouts of diarrhea, increasing fatigue, and weight loss. Past medical history included pneumonia, viral hepatitis, and low back syndrome. Examination revealed abdominal distention, enlarged liver and spleen, and scleral icterus. Vital signs B/P 110/80, pulse 106, respirations 20. Laboratory results: Decreased Bromsulphalein (BSP) excretion, increased serum alkaline phosphatase, increased SGOT and SGPT, serum sodium 135 mEq/liter, serum potassium 3.6 mEq/liter, total serum proteins 4.8 g/100, A/G ratio— albumin 3.0, globulin 5.2, Hct 32%, Hb 9.4 g. Following a liver biopsy, diagnosis was postnecrotic cirrhosis.

128. Of the following, which is *not* a metabolic function of the liver?
1. Detoxification of chemicals.
2. Glycogen synthesis and storage.
3. Erythrocyte and leukocyte breakdown.
4. Bile synthesis and secretion.

129. The main pathophysiologic effect of decreased total serum proteins and a reversal of the A/G ratio is:
1. Increased aldosterone and ADH production.
2. Decreased plasma oncotic pressures.
3. Increased blood hydrostatic pressure.
4. Decreased interstitial oncotic pressures.

130. Spontaneous bleeding (ecchymoses) may occur in cirrhosis due to:
1. Rupture of esophageal varices.
2. Decreased synthesis of blood-clotting factors by the liver.
3. Failure of the gut to absorb water-soluble vitamins needed to promote coagulation.
4. Decreased venous pressures and slow blood flow.

131. Of the following, which is *not* a factor in the development of ascites in cirrhosis of the liver?
1. Portal hypertension, venous dilatation, and stasis.
2. Hypoproteinemia.
3. Decreased blood volume resulting in increased serum levels of aldosterone and ADH.
4. Increased blood volume causing increased blood hydrostatic pressures in the capillary bed.

132. Mr. Swenson's anemia is the result of:
1. Increased RBC fragility due to folic acid deficiencies from inadequate dietary intake.
2. Decreased efficiency of Kupffer cells in the liver.
3. Increased blood ammonia levels.
4. Decreased amino acid breakdown and synthesis.

Mr. Swenson was placed on a moderate-protein, high-carbohydrate, high-calorie, low-salt diet. Medications included water- and fat-soluble vitamin supplements and the diuretic spironolactone (Aldactone).

133. The rationale for Mr. Swenson's diet is:
1. Since the liver may not be able to detoxify proteins,

carbohydrates are substituted to meet his metabolic and nutritional needs.
2. Proteins are given in sufficient amount to facilitate tissue repair. High-carbohydrate ingestion prevents further weight loss and spares proteins from energy metabolism. Sodium restriction facilitates management of fluid imbalances.
3. High-protein foods are harder to digest and also have a high sodium content. Carbohydrates are more palatable and will more quickly correct Mr. Swenson's weight loss.
4. High-carbohydrate diets, particularly if they contain adequate fiber, are more likely to decrease dyspepsia and diarrhea. Sodium is always restricted when the patient is edematous.

134. Spironolactone (Aldactone) is classified as:
1. An aldosterone antagonist.
2. A carbonic anhydrase inhibitor.
3. A thiazide.
4. An osmotic diuretic.

135. Which of the following supplements would not ordinarily be administered to the patient receiving spironolactone?
1. Vitamin B_6.
2. Potassium chloride.
3. Ascorbic acid.
4. Calcium carbonate.

136. One nursing measure that might increase Mr. Swenson's compliance with his diet is to:
1. Sit with him until he has eaten everything.
2. Give his wife the responsibility of seeing that he eats.
3. Feed him yourself.
4. Offer frequent small feedings instead of three large ones.

137. Paracentesis is a minor surgical procedure done at the bedside whose purpose is to remove ascitic fluid. After explaining the procedure to Mr. Swenson, your next nursing action would be to:
1. Position the patient in a chair or high-Fowler's position.
2. Instruct the patient to void.
3. Take vital signs.
4. Drape the abdomen with sterile towels.

138. Since ascitic fluids are rich in serum proteins, which of the following complications is most common with this procedure?
1. Disequilibrium.
2. Hypotension.
3. Hypoalbuminuria.
4. Paralytic ileus.

139. Generally the amount of ascitic fluid removed rarely exceeds:
1. 500 ml.
2. 1000 ml.
3. 2000 ml.
4. 3000 ml.

140. Four days after admission Mr. Swenson began to bleed from an esophageal varices. The earliest indications of bleeding in this patient would include:
1. Tachycardia, restlessness, and pallor.
2. Tachycardia, lethargy, and flushing.
3. Sudden drop in blood pressure of 10 mm Hg or more.
4. Increasing combativeness and widening pulse pressure.

141. Initially Mr. Swenson's bleeding was controlled by an ice-cold saline lavage. Later a Sengstaken-Blakemore tube was inserted. The primary purpose of this tube is:
1. To prevent bleeding by applying pressure to the esophageal varices.
2. To prevent accumulation of blood in the GI tract, which could precipitate hepatic coma.
3. To stop bleeding by applying pressure to the cardiac portion of the stomach and against the esophageal varices.
4. To reduce transfusion requirements.

142. The physician has left orders to deflate the tubes every 12 hours for 5 minutes to prevent esophageal erosion. Two hours following the second reinflation, Mr. Swenson suddenly became severely dyspneic and dusky. You should:
1. Call a code blue (cardiac arrest).
2. Cut the tube, thus deflating the balloons.
3. Decrease the traction on the tube where it enters the nose.
4. Irrigate the tube with ice-cold saline to facilitate movement of the balloons into the stomach.

143. 24 hours after the above incident, Mr. Swenson became increasingly confused and disoriented. The physician diagnosed hepatic coma. Which of the following nursing actions is designed to reduce ammonia intoxication in this patient?
1. Active and passive range-of-motion exercises to prevent venous stasis.
2. Tap water enemas to remove blood that may still be in the gut from the bleeding esophageal varices.
3. Administration of insulin and glucagon to reduce serum potassium levels.
4. Holding all antibiotic medications so that the action of the intestinal bacteria on protein is enhanced.

144. Mr. Swenson's prognosis is guarded. His prognosis will improve markedly if his hepatic coma lasts no longer than:
1. 24 hours.
2. 36 hours.
3. 48 hours.
4. 72 hours.

Mrs. Kate Logan is a 41-year-old housewife and mother who works approximately 20 hours a week as a salesperson in a local boutique. She has had varicose veins in both legs since the birth of her first child 15 years ago. Currently she is experiencing increased muscle fatigue and ankle swelling, particularly after being on her feet for more than two or three hours. She states, "I've been planning to have these veins fixed for years because I think they make my legs look ugly, but something else was always more important. Now I want them fixed so I can continue to work at my job, which I really enjoy." Vital signs and preoperative lab work are within normal limits.

145. Routine preoperative laboratory studies may include:
1. VDRL, NA, K, Cl.
2. Prothrombin time, SGOT, VDRL.
3. UA, CBC, prothrombin time.
4. WBC, VDRL, serum glucose.

146. The Trendelenburg test is frequently used to evaluate the competence of venous valves. This test consists of:
1. Having the patient walk up and down the room to observe venous changes during walking.
2. Injecting a contrast medium into the veins and taking multiple X rays as the dye flows in the veins.
3. Stripping a superficial vein, occluding flow, then releasing the vein and observing the direction of filling.
4. Having the patient elevate the involved leg to empty the veins, applying a tourniquet to the upper thigh, having the patient stand, then removing the tourniquet to observe the filling of the superficial veins.

147. Indications for vein-stripping include:
1. Advancing varicosities and cosmetic reasons.
2. Stasis ulceration and thrombophlebitis.
3. Lymphedema and Reynaud's disease.
4. Advancing varicosities only.

148. Vein-stripping is usually done under what type of anesthesia?
1. Local.
2. Topical.
3. Regional.
4. General.

149. Postoperative measures would *not* include which of the following?
1. Administration of analgesics for discomfort.
2. Elastic stockings from toe to groin.
3. Sitting in a chair.
4. Ambulation on the day of surgery.

150. Elevation of the foot of the bed postoperatively is utilized to:
1. Decrease pain.
2. Aid venous return.
3. Increase blood supply to feet.
4. Make the patient more comfortable.

151. During a predischarge teaching session, you tell Mrs. Logan that elastic stockings are best applied:
1. Before rising in the morning to prevent pooling of blood in the lower extremities.
2. After showering and application of skin care to the legs to prevent undue dermal irritation.
3. After 15 minutes of vigorous leg exercises designed to increase blood flow.
4. Only when she plans to be on her feet for an extended period of time because undue constriction of the veins can cause a recurrence of varicosities.

Mrs. Arturri is a 55-year-old lawyer admitted to the hospital with a diagnosis of bacterial pneumonia. On admission she was pale to dusky in color. Her respiratory rate was 32, temperature 103 F, pulse 100. Auscultation revealed decreased or absent lung sounds in both bases, and rales and rhonchi in both upper lung fields. She was oriented to person, time, and place, but her responses were brief due to her increased respiratory work and obvious fatigue. An IV infusion of 1000 ml 5% dextrose/water with 1,000,000 units of penicillin was started in her left arm. Arterial blood gases were PO_2 65, Pco_2 36, HCO_3^- 22, pH 7.37 (normals PO_2 85–100 mm Hg, Pco_2 40 mm Hg, HCO_3^- 24 mEq/L, pH 7.35–7.45). Oxygen per nasal cannula is administered at 7 L/minute.

152. While checking Mrs. Arturri one hour after admission, you note that she is less responsive, answering only yes or no to questions. Her vital signs are basically unchanged, though her respirations seem somewhat more shallow and have decreased to 27/minute. Your first nursing action is to:
1. Increase the IV infusion rate in order to increase the amount of circulating antibiotics.
2. Notify the physician of Mrs. Arturri's changed mental status and await further orders.
3. Increase the oxygen flow rate to 10 liters/minute.
4. Continue to stimulate Mrs. Arturri until she responds appropriately.

153. A second blood gas is drawn, and results indicate increasing hypoxemia (PO_2 58) and hypercapnia (Pco_2 45). What physiologic mechanism explains Mrs. Arturri's initial Pco_2?
1. Carbon dioxide diffuses across the respiratory membrane 20 times faster than oxygen, thus a patient can be hypoxic without being hypercapnic.
2. Increased rate and depth of respirations facilitates CO_2 exchange more than O_2 exchange.
3. Exhalation requires less work of breathing than inhalation.
4. Carbon dioxide is more permeable in water than oxygen, which enables it to move rapidly through respiratory secretions in the airways.

154. Mrs. Arturri's physician decides to perform a tracheostomy. The purpose of a tracheostomy is to:

1. Decrease patient's anxiety by increasing the size of the airway.
2. Provide more controlled ventilation and ease removal of secretions the patient is unable to handle.
3. Provide increased cerebral oxygenation, thereby preventing further respiratory depression.
4. Facilitate nursing care, since tracheal tubes have fewer side effects than nasotracheal tubes.

155. A preoperative *nursing priority* for Mrs. Arturri is:
1. Establishing means of postoperative communication.
2. Drawing blood for serum electrolytes and blood gases.
3. Inserting a foley catheter and attaching it to dependent drainage.
4. Doing a surgical prep of her neck and upper chest wall.

Following insertion of the tracheostomy tube, Mrs. Arturri appears less distressed. Oxygen therapy was reinstituted with nebulization, as well as previous medication orders. The tracheostomy was to be suctioned every hour and prn. Questions 156–163 pertain to this situation.

156. One of the most sensitive and effective indicators of increased tracheobronchial secretions is:
1. Increased rate and depth of respirations.
2. Increased or decreased systolic and diastolic blood pressure.
3. Coarse, prolonged expiratory sounds.
4. High-pitched, crowing inspiratory sounds.

157. Which of the following nursing actions is essential to prevent hypoxemia during tracheal suctioning?
1. Removal of oral and nasal secretions.
2. Encouraging the patient to deep breathe and cough to facilitate removal of upper-airway secretions.
3. Administer 100% oxygen to reduce the effects of airway obstruction during suctioning.
4. Auscultate the lungs to determine the baseline data to assess the effectiveness of suctioning.

158. Turning the patient's head from side to side when suctioning:
1. Provides passive exercise for the sternocleidomastoid and trapezius muscles.
2. Prevents nuchal rigidity.
3. Facilitates entry into the main right and left bronchi.
4. Decreases tissue resistance, making catheter insertion easier.

159. The proper method of suctioning includes:
1. Suctioning only while inserting the catheter.
2. Suctioning only while withdrawing the catheter.
3. Suctioning during both insertion and withdrawal of the catheter.
4. Suctioning on insertion only if secretions are copious.

160. What is the current maximum cuff pressure acceptable in a tracheostomy tube?
1. 150 mm Hg.
2. 20 mm Hg.
3. 80 mm Hg.
4. 40 mm Hg.

161. If a double-lumen tracheostomy tube is used, the inner cannula should be removed and cleansed with hydrogen peroxide and normal saline:
1. Only as necessary.
2. Every two to four hours.
3. Once a day.
4. Do not remove the inner cannula for any reason.

162. The rationale for using humidified oxygen with tracheal tubes is:
1. It is a traditional procedure.
2. It is a means of providing fluid intake.
3. It decreases insensible water loss.
4. The natural humidifying pathway has been bypassed.

163. Crepitus in Mrs. Arturri's neck and upper chest is a sign of:
1. Subcutaneous emphysema from displaced trachea tube.
2. An inadequately inflated cuff.
3. An overinflated cuff.
4. Edema from the trauma of surgery.

Mr. Langley is a 51-year-old auto salesman admitted to your unit for recurrent complaints of burning epigastric pain, nausea and vomiting, and one episode of hemoptysis. He has been treated medically for gastric ulcer for the past year with antacids, antispasmodics, and an ulcer diet. On admission you note Mr. Langley appears tense and is holding his hand over his stomach. Vital signs are B/P 124/78, pulse 96, respirations 18, and temperature 99.4 F. His skin is pale and moist. He states he has had black stools two or three times in the past week, but he didn't really worry about it until he threw up blood this morning. A nasogastric tube was passed and attached to low intermittent suction. Gastric drainage resembles coffee grounds with a small amount of red blood.

164. What is believed to be the basic emotional issue underlying or contributing to the development of ulcers?
1. Anxiety neurosis.
2. Dependence-independence conflict.
3. Repressed anger and hostility.
4. Compulsive time orientation.

165. Forty-eight hours after admission, Mr. Langley is scheduled for an upper GI series. Nursing preparation for this procedure includes all of the following *except:*
1. Holding the patient NPO from six to eight hours before the procedure.
2. Administering an enema or cathartic to enhance visualization.

3. Discouraging the patient from smoking the morning of the procedure because smoking can stimulate gastric motility.
4. Forewarning the patient that he will be placed in a variety of positions on a tilt table during the procedure.

166. Mr. Langley's barium X ray revealed a large cavitation in the antral portion of the stomach and scarring of the pyloric sphincter. The physician ordered a gastroscopy for the following day. Nursing preparations for this procedure include all the following *except:*
1. Holding the patient NPO from six to eight hours before the procedure.
2. Having an operative or procedure permit signed.
3. Reassuring the patient that gastroscopy is not an uncomfortable procedure, though he will need to lie quietly.
4. Removing dentures and administering a sedative prior to the procedure.

167. Following the gastroscopy the patient may begin oral intake:
1. As soon as he returns to the room.
2. One hour later or after he is fully alert.
3. Three to four hours later or when the gag reflex returns.
4. Six to eight hours later to prevent the electrolyte imbalance that may occur with this procedure.

Following these diagnostic tests, Mr. Langley's physician discussed possible therapies with him. It was decided that a partial gastrectomy, vagotomy, and gastrojejunostomy would be performed. Preoperative laboratory work was completed and was within normal range.

168. A vagotomy is done in conjunction with a subtotal gastrectomy because the vagus nerve:
1. Stimulates increased gastric motility.
2. Decreases gastric motility, thereby preventing the movement of HCl out of the stomach.
3. Stimulates both increased gastric secretion and gastric motility.
4. Stimulates decreased gastric secretion, thereby increasing nausea and vomiting.

169. Which of the following is *not* a preoperative nursing measure prior to Mr. Langley's surgery?
1. Insertion of a nasogastric tube on the morning of surgery.
2. NPO for 6–12 hours prior to surgery.
3. Sippy diet for one week before surgery.
4. Assurance that he will receive pain medication to reduce his discomfort.

170. Which of the following complications would you primarily anticipate in Mr. Langley's postoperative period?
1. Thrombophlebitis from decreased mobility.
2. Abdominal distention due to air-swallowing.

3. Atelectasis due to shallow breathing.
4. Urinary retention due to prolonged use of anticholinergic medications.

171. Drainage of blood from the nasogastric tube after surgery is abnormal if:
1. It continues after 6 hours.
2. It continues for a period greater than 12 hours.
3. It turns greenish yellow in less than 24 hours.
4. It is dark red in the immediate postoperative period.

172. Which of the following statements is *not true* regarding nasogastric-tube irrigation?
1. Nasogastric tubes should be irrigated with normal saline, never plain water.
2. Irrigating fluids should be instilled with minimum pressure.
3. If you meet resistance when you are irrigating the tube, the physician should be notified.
4. If instilled irrigating fluids fail to return, the physician should be notified.

173. Which of the following imbalances may occur with prolonged nasogastric suctioning?
1. Hypernatremia.
2. Hyperkalemia.
3. Metabolic alkalosis.
4. Hypoproteinemia.

174. Of the following mouth care measures, which one should be utilized with caution when a patient has a nasogastric tube?
1. Brushing teeth and tongue with soft brush regularly.
2. Sucking on ice chips to relieve dryness.
3. Occasionally rinsing mouth with a nonastringent substance and massaging gums.
4. Application of lemon juice and glycerine swabs to the lips.

175. The nasogastric tube is removed:
1. Standardly on the fourth postoperative day.
2. When bowel sounds are established and the patient has passed flatus or stool.
3. Thirty-six hours after the cessation of bloody drainage.
4. After two days of alternate clamping and unclamping of the tube.

176. Pernicious anemia may be a problem after gastrectomy because:
1. The extrinsic factor is produced in the stomach.
2. The extrinsic factor is absorbed in the antral portion of the stomach.
3. The intrinsic factor is produced in the stomach.
4. Decreased hydrochloric acid production inhibits vitamin B_{12} reabsorption.

177. Ambulation of the postgastrectomy patient usually begins:
1. The day after surgery.

2. Three to four days after surgery.
3. After four days' bedrest.
4. Immediately upon awakening.

178. Dumping syndrome is a significant problem for:
1. 70% to 80% of patients having gastrectomies.
2. 50% of patients having gastrectomies.
3. 25% of patients having gastrectomies.
4. 5% to 10% of patients having gastrectomies.

179. Small, frequent feedings of which type of diet are recommended for patients experiencing dumping syndrome?
1. Low-protein, high-fat, low-carbohydrate diet.
2. High-protein, high-fat, high-carbohydrate diet.
3. High-protein, high-fat, low-carbohydrate diet.
4. Low-protein, low-fat, high-carbohydrate diet.

180. Patients suffering from dumping syndrome should be advised to:
1. Drink liquids between meals.
2. Drink liquids only with meals.
3. Drink liquids any time they want.
4. Restrict fluid intake to 1200 cc per day.

181. Which of the following is not a symptom of dumping syndrome?
1. Dizziness.
2. Perfuse perspiration.
3. Epigastric fullness.
4. Hunger.

182. Which of the following foods should be avoided by the patient experiencing dumping syndrome?
1. Liver and bacon.
2. Orange and avocado salad.
3. Creamed chicken.
4. Glazed donuts and coffee.

183. Before discharge Mr. Langley asks you pointedly, "How long will it be before I can eat three meals a day like the rest of my family?" You respond:
1. "Eating six meals a day can be a bother, can't it?"
2. "Some patients can tolerate three meals a day by the time they leave the hospital. It seems it will be a little longer for you."
3. "You will probably have to eat six meals a day for the rest of your life."
4. "It varies with patients, but generally in six to twelve months most patients can return to their previous meal patterns."

Mr. Davis is a 49-year-old man admitted to CCU with an anterior MI. Past health history reveals occasional substernal chest pains lasting approximately 15 minutes that were relieved by rest. Mr. Davis explained he believed that the pains were related to indigestion since they generally occurred after a heavy meal.

184. Angina pectoris, which occurs after eating, may be due to:

1. Incomplete digestion of fats due to a decrease in pancreatic enzyme, thereby increasing reflux.
2. Local blood flow regulators that shunt blood to gut during digestion, thereby decreasing coronary artery perfusion pressures.
3. Abdominal distention from air-swallowing during eating, thereby decreasing diaphragmatic excursion and arterial PO_2.
4. Decreased heart rate and blood pressure resulting in increased myocardial oxygen consumption.

The nursing notes on admission gave the following assessment data: B/P 124/92/84, apical pulse 100 and regular, RR 24, skin cool, pale, and slightly diaphoretic. Blood gases PO_2 85, Pco_2 37, pH 7.36, HCO_3 19.

185. Given that Mr. Davis's normal B/P is 140/90/86 and his average pulse is 72, which of the following mechanisms might explain his present vital signs?
1. Increased vagal stimulation of SA node.
2. Arrhythmias.
3. Cardiogenic shock.
4. Sympathetic nervous system response to decreased cardiac output.

186. Circulatory reflexes, which follow coronary occlusion, are designed to:
1. Increase peripheral perfusion.
2. Increase glomerular filtration rate.
3. Increase venous return.
4. Increase venous capacitance.

187. Which of the following coronary vessels is involved in an anterior MI?
1. Left circumflex artery.
2. Right coronary artery.
3. Left coronary artery.
4. Left anterior descending artery.

188. Mr. Davis's blood gases indicate:
1. Compensated metabolic acidosis.
2. Hyperventilation.
3. Uncompensated metabolic acidosis.
4. Alveolar hypoventilation.

189. Mr. Davis's electrocardiogram shows ischemia, injury, and necrosis. Which of the following EKG changes would you *not* expect to find?
1. Appearance of abnormal Q waves.
2. ST segment elevation in the leads overlying the injured area.
3. ST segment depression in the leads overlying the injured area.
4. Peaked T waves in the precordial leads.

190. Morphine sulfate 0.6 mg has been ordered to relieve Mr. Davis's chest pain. This narcotic is utilized because it:
1. Increases the threshold for pain tolerance and decreases arterial resistance.

2. Increases arterial resistance and reduces apprehension and anxiety as well as pain.
3. Relieves apprehension, anxiety, and pain and stimulates medullary respiratory centers.
4. Reduces venous capacitance and reduces pain threshold.

191. Before administering morphine sulfate, the nurse should check Mr. Davis's:
1. Apical and radial pulse.
2. Respiratory rate.
3. Urinary output.
4. Skin color and turgor.

192. Three hours after admission to the CCU, Mr. Davis develops increasing ventricular ectopy, followed by a short burst of ventricular tachycardia. Your first nursing action is to:
1. Notify the attending physician.
2. Increase the flow of O_2 from 4 to 8 L.
3. Administer a bolus of lidocaine.
4. Repeat the morphine sulfate.

193. Your intervention terminates Mr. Davis's ventricular tachycardia, but he continues to have frequent PVCs (> 5/min). Your next nursing action is to:
1. Notify the attending physician.
2. Begin a lidocaine drip.
3. Ascertain if Mr. Davis is having more chest pain.
4. Do a partial physical assessment.

194. An early indicator of the extent of tissue necrosis in Mr. Davis's heart is:
1. The duration of sinus tachycardia.
2. CPK and SGOT enzyme measures.
3. The duration of his chest pain.
4. The occurrence of primary ventricular fibrillation.

On the third day of hospitalization, Mr. Davis becomes increasingly restless. You note that his pulse rate displayed on the cardiac monitor has increased to 126 beats per minute. Questions 195–203 refer to this situation.

195. Your first nursing action is to:
1. Do a partial physical assessment, which includes vital signs, pulmonary auscultation, and cognitive functions.
2. Ask Mr. Davis if he is upset, since depression is common on the third day of hospitalization.
3. Readminister oxygen per nasal tongs at 6 liters, as restlessness is an early sign of cerebral hypoxia.
4. Decrease the rate of Mr. Davis's intravenous infusion to prevent fluid volume overload.

196. Tachycardia may result in increased restlessness because:
1. Decreased ventricular filling time results in decreased venous return and cerebral edema.
2. Palpitations result in anxiety.
3. Decreased ventricular filling time always results in decreased cardiac output and tissue perfusion.

4. Decreased ventricular filling time may cause a significant decrease in stroke volume, which results in decreased cardiac output and tissue perfusion.

197. Mr. Davis states that he can hardly get his breath. His vital signs are B/P 100/70, apical pulse 126, RR 26. Pulmonary rales and rhonchi are heard halfway up his chest. Your first nursing action is to:
1. Administer morphine sulfate to allay Mr. Davis's apprehension.
2. Assist Mr. Davis into a sitting position and lower his legs to pool blood in the periphery.
3. Remove excess pulmonary secretions with suction.
4. Administer oxygen at 10 L per mask instead of nasal prongs.

198. Mr. Davis's dyspnea is *not* the result of:
1. Decreased lung compliance due to mechanical congestion.
2. Increased CO_2 retention.
3. Decreased venous return.
4. Blood volume shift from systemic circulation to lungs.

199. The physician has ordered rotating tourniquets to be applied to Mr. Davis. You have applied the tourniquets correctly if:
1. You have wrapped the cuffs low on each extremity.
2. After applying pressure to the cuffs, you are still able to palpate the peripheral pulse distal to the cuff.
3. You have applied sufficient pressure in each extremity to occlude the peripheral pulses.
4. You have wrapped the cuffs high on each extremity except the limb with the intravenous line, which is cuffed below the insertion site.

200. Therapy goals for Mr. Davis included strengthening cardiac contraction and increasing glomerular filtration rate. Which of the following medications can frequently accomplish both goals?
1. Epinephrine.
2. Digoxin.
3. Lasix.
4. Hydralazine.

201. Which of the following outcomes is the best indicator that therapy goals have been met?
1. Increased systolic and diastolic pressure.
2. Unlabored respirations and increased urinary output.
3. Decreased pulse rate and increased urinary output.
4. Increased blood pressure and decreased pulse rate.

202. In order to monitor Mr. Davis's fluid volumes more closely, a CVP line has been inserted via the right subclavian vein. CVP reflects the pressure in:
1. The left atrium.
2. The right atrium.
3. The left ventricle.
4. The right ventricle.

203. Normal CVP pressures are:
1. 4–10 cm H_2O.
2. 20–30 mm Hg.
3. 10–20 cm H_2O.
4. 7–14 mm Hg.

Ten days after admission, his physician decides that Mr. Davis has stabilized sufficiently to be transferred to floor care. You are the evening nurse on this unit. Mrs. Davis has stopped by the nurses' station on her way out after visiting hours. She states, "Keep an eye on Mr. Davis, will you? He doesn't seem himself tonight." Because of her worried expression you decide to check Mr. Davis immediately and find him slumped on the siderails of his bed. He does not respond when you shake his shoulder or loudly call his name. Questions 204–208 refer to this situation.

204. In an unmonitored arrest in the hospital, when you are the only person present, your first action is to:
1. Call for help and note the time.
2. Clear the airway.
3. Give two sharp thumps to the precordium.
4. Administer two quick breaths.

205. Your second nursing action is to:
1. Clear the airway.
2. Position the patient for possible resuscitation—roll on back, remove pillows.
3. Administer two sharp thumps to precordium.
4. Call for help and note the time.

206. Your next nursing action in the arrest procedure is to:
1. Clear airway and check pupils.
2. Check for breathing by placing your ear within an inch of the patient's mouth.
3. Check the carotid pulse for 5–10 seconds.
4. Summon help.

207. Following the above, you would next:
1. Bag the patient.
2. Deliver two sharp blows to the precordium.
3. Check for breathing and initiate mouth-to-mouth resuscitation if the patient is not breathing.
4. Palpate the carotid pulse for 5–10 seconds and, if absent, initiate closed-chest massage.

208. To complete this sequence you would:
1. Monitor vital signs.
2. Palpate the carotid pulse and, if absent, give closed-chest cardiac massage.
3. Increase IV infusion rate to prevent hypovolemia.
4. Continue with mouth-to-mouth resuscitation until arrest team arrives.

209. Three days after successful resuscitation, Mr. Davis states to you, "I'm all washed up. I don't think I'll ever be the same man again." You respond:
1. "Most patients who have been as ill as you have feel that way, Mr. Davis."

2. "How do you feel you have changed from before you were ill?"
3. "Getting depressed won't help you get better."
4. "Tell me more."

210. During a predischarge teaching session, Mrs. Davis states, "Don't worry, I'll be sure that he obeys the doctor's orders to the letter." You respond:
1. "Mrs. Davis, I can see that with your help, Mr. Davis should do just fine."
2. "Are you worried?"
3. "I'm not worried, you both have a lot of common sense."
4. "This has been a difficult period for both of you. Can you foresee any problems with these instructions?"

Mr. Lawson is a 38-year-old, married executive for an electronics firm who is admitted to a small community hospital for diagnostic evaluation. Recent complaints include increasing fatigue and nocturia. Past history includes a fractured tibia at age 9 and acute glomerulonephritis at age 13. Vital signs: B/P 150/100, pulse 78, RR 22.

211. Acute glomerular nephritis is the result of:
1. Acute infection of the kidney by gram negative bacteria.
2. An immune response of the glomerular membrane to protein of the beta-hemolytic streptococcus.
3. Destruction of the glomerular membrane by gram positive streptococci.
4. Ischemia of glomerular capillary and vasa recta.

Several tests were ordered by the physician to evaluate Mr. Lawson's present kidney function. Results of the urine test included: 24-hr creatinine clearance .8 g/24 hr (normal: 1.0–1.6 g/24 hr), protein + 1 (normal: neg.), multiple casts (normal: neg.).

212. A 24-hour urine-for-creatinine clearance measures which of the following kidney functions?
1. Filtration fraction.
2. Glomerular filtration rate.
3. Renal blood flow.
4. Quantity and specific gravity of urinary output.

213. Proteinuria has the following effect on the rate of fluid volume excretion:
1. Increases glomerular oncotic pressures, thereby decreasing urine output.
2. Increases the arterial pressure, thereby decreasing urine output.
3. Increases the osmotic pressure of the tubular fluid, thereby creating an osmotic diuresis.
4. Increases the amount of aldosterone; thereby decreasing sodium and water retention.

The results of Mr. Lawson's blood chemistries were as follows: Hct 38%, Hb 10, BUN 40 mg/100 ml (normal: 10–20 mg/

100 ml), potassium 5.0 mEq/L (normal 3.5–5.0 mEq/L), sodium 139 mEq/L (normal: 138–146 mEq/L), albumin 3.0 mg/dl (normal: 3.2–4.5 mg/dl). Total bicarbonate 22 mEq/L (normal: 24–28 mEq/L).

214. Hematocrit is decreased in chronic renal failure due to:
1. Decreased secretion of erythropoietin factor by the diseased kidney.
2. Chronic hypertension, which tends to suppress bone marrow centers.
3. Metabolic alkalosis, which tends to increase red blood cell fragility.
4. Increased excretion of red blood cells in the urine.

215. Hyperkalemia tends to occur in chronic renal dysfunction because:
1. As metabolic acidosis increases, the kidneys selectively secrete more H^+ than K^+ in exchange for Na^+
2. As edema forms, sodium diffuses into the interstitial space and is balanced by increased serum potassium.
3. Respiratory compensation for metabolic acidosis tends to increase K^+ reabsorption by the kidneys.
4. The nausea and vomiting that occur with metabolic acidosis tend to increase serum potassium to compensate for chloride losses.

216. Mr. Lawson has been NPO for the last 21 hours in preparation for an IVP (intravenous pyelogram). He has been complaining of thirst. The specific gravity of his urine has been averaging 1.008. The best physiologic explanation for these signs and symptoms is:
1. The hypothalamus is stimulating increased secretion of ADH.
2. Extracellular fluid hypoosmolarity.
3. The kidneys are no longer able to concentrate urine, making the extracellular fluid hyperosmolar.
4. Most patients complain of thirst after fluid restriction.

217. Besides omission of food and fluids by mouth, preparation for IVP generally includes:
1. Ingestion of dye the night before the procedure.
2. Administration of cathartics or enemas to improve visualization of contrast medium in renal structures.
3. A low-protein and low-salt diet the evening before to increase hyperosmolarity of ECF.
4. Institution of an intravenous line to maintain fluid and electrolyte balance.

218. In assessing Mr. Lawson's acid/base status, you would be alert to the following signs of metabolic acidosis:
1. Hyperreflexia, paresthesias, and tetany.
2. Giddiness, irregular respiratory pattern, and moist, cool skin.
3. Muscle weakness and numbness and tingling in the extremities.

4. Lethargy, disorientation, and increased rate and depth of respirations.

Mr. Lawson's physician ordered: bedrest with commode privileges, methyldopa (Aldomet) 250 mg every 6 hours, and diazepam (Valium) 5 mg tid and a 40 g protein diet.

219. Methyldopa acts to decrease hypertension by:
1. Dilating peripheral blood vessels and increasing renal blood flow.
2. Depleting norepinephrine at postganglionic synapses.
3. Inhibiting formation of dopamine, a precursor of norepinephrine.
4. Depressing the reticular activating system activity.

220. The following is the best single measure of Mr. Lawson's fluid volume status:
1. Skin turgor and oral mucous membranes.
2. Vital signs.
3. Daily weights.
4. Intake and output.

221. Dietary restriction of protein in chronic renal failure is utilized to prevent the accumulation of nitrogenous wastes and resulting azotemia. Which of the following foods containing amino acids would be allowed on Mr. Lawson's diet?
1. Roast beef.
2. Milk and eggs.
3. Chicken and turkey.
4. Shellfish.

Mr. Lawson was discharged on a low-protein, low-salt diet and the above medication. Four weeks later he was readmitted to the hospital with complaints of joint pain, weight gain (15 lb), oliguria, muscle cramps, and lethargy. Vital signs: B/P 152/102, pulse 86, RR 24. Laboratory values: BUN 76 mg/100 L, serum potassium 6.5 mEq/L, serum creatinine 8 mg (normal: 1–2 mg). Blood gases: pH 7.36, PO_2 90, pCO_2 34, serum bicarbonate 20 mEq/L (normals: PO_2 80–100, pCO_2 40, pH 7.35–7.45, HCO_3^- 22–26 mEq/L).

222. Mr. Lawson's signs and symptoms can be related to:
1. Renal ischemia due to increase in circulating toxins and chronic hypertension.
2. A decrease in the number of functioning nephrons, which further decreases glomerular filtration.
3. Increased water and salt loss due to flushing effect in the diseased kidney tubules.
4. Water and salt retention due to insufficient renal blood flow.

223. Mr. Lawson's complaints of joint pain can be explained by:
1. An increase in blood phosphate levels that occurs with renal failure.
2. An increase in serum creatinine levels.
3. His decreased activity level.

4. An increase in plasma of the end products of purine metabolism.

224. What ECG changes would you anticipate Mr. Lawson to demonstrate given his potassium level?
1. Peaked T waves.
2. Flattened T waves.
3. ST segment depression.
4. ST segment elevation.

225. Mr. Lawson's blood gases could be described as:
1. Metabolic acidosis.
2. Compensated metabolic acidosis.
3. Respiratory alkalosis with metabolic compensation.
4. Metabolic acidosis with minimal respiratory compensation.

226. Which of the following blood buffers is regulated by both the kidneys and the lungs?
1. Bicarbonate.
2. Protein.
3. Phosphate.
4. Hemoglobin.

227. Symptoms of circulatory overload in this patient would include:
1. Neck vein distention, apprehension, soft eyeballs.
2. Periorbital edema, distended neck veins, moist rales.
3. Increased blood pressure, flattened neck veins, shock.
4. Decreased pulse pressure, cool, dry skin, and decreased skin turgor.

Mr. Lauson's physician ordered complete bedrest, Kayexalate 15 g tid, furosemide 40 mg bid and Aldomet 500 mg qid.

228. Kayexalate reduces hyperkalemia by:
1. Exchanging sodium ions for potassium ions in the GI tract, thereby increasing potassium excretion in the feces.
2. Inhibiting potassium absorption sites in the GI tract.
3. Promoting diarrhea, thereby decreasing potassium absorption from the gut.
4. Altering the effects of aldosterone in the kidney tubules.

229. The peak action of furosemide (Lasix) is:
1. 30–60 minutes.
2. 1–2 hours.
3. 3–4 hours.
4. 6–8 hours.

230. After three days of the above therapy, Mr. Lawson's physician decides to institute peritoneal dialysis to decrease Mr. Lawson's increasing symptoms of azotemia. After explaining the procedures to Mr. Lawson and his wife and obtaining a signed operative permit, your next nursing action is to:
1. Have the patient empty his bladder.

2. Position the patient in a comfortable supine position.
3. Weigh the patient and record vital signs.
4. Cleanse and drape the abdomen.

231. Following the insertion of the catheter into the abdominal cavity, the warmed dialyzing solution is allowed to run rapidly (10–20 minutes) into the abdominal cavity. The solution is warmed to body temperature to prevent abdominal pain and to:
1. Expand the molecules and increase the osmotic gradient.
2. Increase dilation of the peritoneal vessels, thereby increasing urea clearance.
3. Decrease the likelihood of peritonitis due to constriction of peritoneal vessels.
4. Explicate the movement of the dialyzing solute into the abdomen.

232. The dwell time or equilibration period of the dialyzing fluid is normally:
1. 10–15 minutes.
2. 30–45 minutes.
3. 50–60 minutes.
4. More than one hour.

233. The drainage period generally takes 20 minutes, though this may vary with patients. If fluid is not draining properly you can facilitate return by:
1. Turning the patient to a prone position.
2. Manipulating the indwelling catheter.
3. Elevating the head of the bed, thereby increasing intraabdominal pressures.
4. Elevating the foot of the bed, thereby increasing abdominal pressures and gravity flow.

234. Which of the following signs and symptoms is *least likely* to occur if fluid drainage is inadequate?
1. A negative balance between the amount drained and the amount instilled.
2. Confusion, lethargy, and coma.
3. Moist rales and rhonchi.
4. Flattened neck veins in a supine position.

235. Outcome criteria for Mr. Lawson would include:
1. Serum potassium less than 3.5 mEq/L and serum sodium greater than 148 mEq/L.
2. Quantity and specific gravity of urine unchanged.
3. BUN less than 20 mg%, serum creatinine less than 1.2 mg%.
4. Abdomen moderately soft and percussion note dull.

Mr. Victor Cloutier is a 34-year-old male admitted to your unit with a complaint of intermittent hematuria. He states he started having blood in his urine about a month ago and that two days ago he developed a continuous dull pain in his left side. Initial examination revealed a well-developed muscular male with moderate discomfort. Lungs clear to auscultation, heart sounds regular, marked left flank ten-

derness. Vital signs B/P 150/100, P 70, RR 16, temperature 101.6 F. Physician orders include:
> *Diet as tolerated.*
> *Demerol 50 mg every 3–4 hours prn pain.*
> *Intravenous pyelogram in the A.M.*

236. Intravenous pyelogram (IVP) is utilized to:
1. Determine the size, shape, and placement of the kidneys.
2. Test renal tubular function and the patency of the urinary tract.
3. Measure renal blood flow.
4. Outline the kidney vasculature.

237. Preparation for IVP includes all of the following *except:*
1. Warning the patient that the dye may produce a warm, flushing feeling and a salty taste in the mouth.
2. Bowel-cleansing to provide for better visualization.
3. Ascertaining whether or not the patient has any allergies to iodine.
4. Pushing fluids until two hours before the test to prevent dehydration.

Results from the IVP indicate the presence of a small mass in the left renal parenchyma. To differentiate the mass from a cyst, a renal angiogram is ordered.

238. The angiogram is performed using a catheter inserted into the left femoral artery. Which of the following nursing actions is your first priority following this procedure?
1. Monitoring vital signs until stable.
2. Frequently checking the puncture site for fresh bleeding, swelling, or increasing tenderness.
3. Measuring the quantity and specific gravity of urinary output.
4. Checking the peripheral pulses distal to the femoral puncture site.

Following the angiogram a diagnosis of probable carcinoma of the left kidney was made and the patient was scheduled for a left nephrectomy. Preoperative blood work indicated a mild polycythemia.

239. Polycythemia may occur with renal carcinoma because:
1. The tumor infringes on renal blood flow, thereby increasing renin release.
2. Some renal tumors enhance the production of erythropoietin factor by the kidney.
3. Polyuria tends to give a false high red blood count due to dehydration.
4. Bone marrow is stimulated to overproduce red blood cells with recurrent blood losses (hematuria).

240. Postoperatively, Mr. Cloutier has a large flank incision. In order to facilitate deep breathing and coughing, you should:
1. Have the patient lie on the unaffected side.
2. Coordinate breathing and coughing exercises with administration of analgesics.
3. Maintain the patient in a high-Fowler's position.
4. Push fluid administration to loosen respiratory secretions.

241. Urinary output is assessed closely after nephrectomy. Which of the following assessment findings is an early indicator of fluid retention in the postoperative period?
1. Increased specific gravity of urine.
2. Daily weight gain of two or more pounds.
3. A urinary output of 50 ml/hr.
4. Periorbital edema.

242. The postoperative nephrectomy patient should also be closely observed for:
1. Hemorrhage.
2. Hyperkalemia.
3. Respiratory alkalosis and tetany.
4. Polyuria.

243. Forty-eight hours after surgery, Mr. Cloutier complains of increasing nausea. You note his upper abdomen appears distended and bowel sounds have not returned. Your first nursing action is to:
1. Change the patient's position to relieve abdominal pressure.
2. Notify the physician of Mr. Cloutier's complaints and your assessment findings.
3. Insert a rectal tube to relieve flatus.
4. Administer morphine SO_4 6 mg as ordered for the relief of discomfort.

244. Mr. Cloutier has developed paralytic ileus. This dysfunction is characterized by:
1. Edema of the intestinal mucosa.
2. Acute dilatation of the colon.
3. Absent, diminished, or uncoordinated autonomic stimulation of peristalsis.
4. High, tinkling bowel sounds over the area of obstruction.

245. Mr. Cloutier's physician decides to insert a Miller-Abbott tube to decompress the abdomen. Which of the following statements accurately describes the Miller-Abbott tube?
1. A double-lumen tube with one lumen leading to the inflatable balloon and the other entirely independent tube used for aspiration.
2. A plastic or rubber tube with holes near its tip facilitating withdrawal of fluids from the stomach.
3. A single-lumen, mercury-weighted tube approximately six feet long.
4. A ten-foot long rubber tube with a mercury bag at its end.

246. Before insertion of the Miller-Abbott tube, the balloon is tested for patency and capacity and then deflated. Which of the following nursing measures will ease the insertion of the nasoenteric tube?
1. Chilling the tube well before insertion.
2. Administering a sedative to reduce anxiety.

3. Warming the tube before insertion.
4. Positioning the patient in a low-Fowler's position.

247. What nursing actions would facilitate the passage of the nasoenteric tube through the pylorus and into the duodenum?
    1. Gently advancing the tube 2 to 3 inches at regular intervals.
    2. Positioning the patient on his right side for two hours after insertion.
    3. Maintaining strict bedrest and avoiding all unnecessary movement.
    4. Positioning the patient in a flat supine position.

248. Two days before discharge Mr. Cloutier expresses renewed concern over his ability to continue many of his activities with only one kidney. You respond:
    1. "You seem depressed. Actually you are very lucky since the path reports indicate your tumor was encapsulated."
    2. "Lots of people do quite well with only one kidney."
    3. "Would you like me to call the doctor so you can discuss it with him?"
    4. "I can understand your concern, but your remaining kidney is sufficient to maintain normal renal functions."

Mr. Dobson is a moderately overweight 58-year-old retired policeman admitted to your unit for repair of bilateral indirect inguinal hernias. He reports to you that he has worn a truss for several years but since he and his wife were planning a long-awaited vacation together, he had decided to have the hernias taken care of now. Mr. Dobson also reveals that he had the right hernia repaired five years ago, but that it returned after he helped a fellow officer move into his new home. He further states he has had several operations without complications, and does not feel unduly anxious about this surgery if for no other reason than that he has a high pain tolerance. He has smoked one pack of cigarettes a day for 25 years and has what he calls a smoker's cough.

249. Indirect inguinal hernias occur when a loop of intestine:
    1. Passes through the femoral ring and down the femoral canal.
    2. Passes through the abdominal ring and follows the course of the spermatic cord into the inguinal canal.
    3. Passes through the posterior inguinal wall.
    4. Passes through the umbilical ring into the inguinal canal.

250. What are the most likely causes for herniation in Mr. Dobson?
    1. Intestinal obstruction.
    2. Failure of resected muscles in previous operations to heal properly.
    3. Chronic cough and vigorous exercise.
    4. Obesity.

251. A truss is a pad of firm material which is placed over the hernial opening and held in place with a belt. A truss should be applied:
    1. After getting out of bed but before engaging in strenuous activity.
    2. After the hernia has been reduced by lying down with the feet elevated.
    3. Whether or not the hernia has been reduced to prevent further extrusion of the bowel.
    4. Physicians no longer recommend the use of a truss because athletic supporters are sufficient in preventing further herniation.

252. Given Mr. Dobson's medical history and the surgery he is about to have, which of the following preoperative nursing actions will be a priority?
    1. Explanation of the surgical procedure.
    2. Respiratory hygiene measures and instructions in deep breathing.
    3. Discussion of postoperative nursing-care measures.
    4. Assurance that pain medication will be available whenever he needs it.

253. Again considering the above nursing history data, which type of surgical anesthesia may be most appropriate in this situation?
    1. General.
    2. Intravenous.
    3. Spinal.
    4. Local infiltration.

The following preoperative orders were written by Mr. Dobson's physician:
    NPO after midnight.
    Abdominal surgical prep.
    CBC and UA.
    Chest X ray.
    Pulmonary ventilation testing this P.M.

254. Pulmonary function testing revealed a vital capacity within normal limits but a reduced forced expiratory volume (FEV_1). This indicates that:
    1. Mr. Dobson has difficulty moving air in and out of his lungs.
    2. Mr. Dobson may have some airway obstruction.
    3. Mr. Dobson has weakened expiratory muscles of respirations.
    4. Mr. Dobson may have some areas of atelectasis in his lungs.

255. The surgical prep for Mr. Dobson would include cleansing and shaving of:
    1. The entire abdomen from just below the nipple line to the midthigh.
    2. The entire abdomen from the axilla to the pubis.
    3. From the waistline of the abdomen to below both knees.
    4. Lower abdomen, the pubic area, perineum, and inner sides of thighs and buttocks.

256. Mr. Dobson has a spinal anesthetic. In the recovery room, it will be important that the nurse immediately position him:
1. On his side to prevent obstruction of airway by tongue.
2. Flat on his back.
3. On his back with knees flexed 15°.
4. Flat on his stomach with head turned to side.

257. After positioning the patient, which of the following observations should the recovery room nurse initially make?
1. Status of reflexes.
2. Vital signs.
3. Patient's level of consciousness.
4. Integrity of airway.

Postoperative orders include:
Flat in bed for 8 hours.
Vital signs till stable and then every hour for 4 hours and every 2 hours for 4 hours.
Meperidine 100 mg IM every 3–4 hours prn pain.
Diet as tolerated.

258. Shortly after Mr. Dobson returns to the surgical unit, the nurse observes that his scrotum is quite swollen. Your first nursing action is to:
1. Notify the surgeon stat.
2. Elevate the scrotum on a rolled towel and apply ice bags.
3. Administer prn pain medication.
4. Encourage vigorous deep breathing and coughing.

259. Mr. Dobson became extremely lethargic following administration of meperidine HCl 100 mg IM for pain. What is your most appropriate nursing action?
1. Give only 50 mg of meperidine next time pain medication is required.
2. Administer an oral preparation of meperidine instead of intramuscular preparation.
3. Consult with physician about decreasing amount of pain medication ordered.
4. Endeavor to prolong the time between medication dosages by employing alternate pain relief strategies.

260. Ten hours after surgery and despite repeated efforts, Mr. Dobson has still not been able to void. He states he feels like he could void but just can't seem to get his stream started. You should:
1. Try getting him up in a standing position once again.
2. Insert a Foley catheter stat.
3. Run water while he attempts to use the urinal.
4. Consult with his physician to obtain either a medication or catheterization order.

261. Urinary retention may be a problem after spinal anesthesia because:
1. Conduction of autonomic nervous system impulses

is inhibited as well as central nervous system impulses.
2. Sensation and motor responses are decreased.
3. Patients tend to secrete less ADH with spinal anesthesia than they do with general anesthesia.
4. Vasomotor depression, which occurs with spinal anesthesia, reduces the glomerulo-filtration rate.

262. Prostigmin 0.5 mg subcutaneously stat is ordered by Mr. Dobson's physician to relieve urinary retention. This drug is classified as:
1. A cholinergic.
2. An anticholinesterase.
3. An anticholinergic.
4. A beta blocker.

263. On the sixth postoperative day, Mr. Dobson complains of a "giving" sensation around his wound when he is walking about. After assisting him back in bed, you note that the dressing covering the right incision is saturated with clear, pink drainage. You suspect:
1. Late hemorrhage.
2. Dehiscence.
3. Infection.
4. Evisceration.

264. On lifting the edges of Mr. Dobson's dressings, you note the wound edges are entirely separated. What is your next nursing action?
1. Tell the patient to remain quiet and not to cough.
2. Offer the patient a warm drink to relax him.
3. Position the patient in a chair with his feet elevated.
4. Apply a Scultetus bandage.

265. Of the following activities of daily living, which should Mr. Dobson avoid after discharge?
1. Driving to and from work.
2. Walking three miles a day.
3. Washing and polishing his car.
4. Carrying out the garbage cans.

Mrs. Jane Klein is a 41-year-old administrative assistant. She has been admitted to your unit for severe pain in her right upper quadrant. During your nursing interview, she relates a history of increasing gastric discomfort and heartburn after meals. Approximately two hours after a business luncheon today, she experienced an abrupt stabbing pain in her upper abdomen that tended to radiate to her right shoulder. She became very nauseated and felt weak and sweaty. On inspection you note a moderately overweight female who appears in moderate distress. Skin is pale, moist, and cool. Slight icterus is present in both eyes. Palpation of the abdomen reveals increased guarding with tenderness in the upper right abdomen that increases with respirations. Vital signs are B/P 140/90, P 88, RR 22, T 100.6 F. Physician's orders were:
NPO.
ProBanthine 30 mg IM every 6 hours.
Papaverine HCl 30 mg IM every 3–4 hours prn for pain.

Tetracycline.
Schedule for IV cholangiogram in A.M.

266. The function of the gallbladder is to:
1. Synthesize and manufacture bile.
2. Collect, concentrate, and store bile.
3. Collect and dilute bile.
4. Regulate bile flow into the duodenum.

267. If bile flow into the duodenum is obstructed, absorption of fat-soluble vitamins is reduced. Which of the following complications would you therefore observe for?
1. Peripheral neuritis.
2. Scurvy.
3. Increased bleeding tendencies.
4. Macrocytic anemia.

268. Besides the assessment of the sclera and skin for jaundice, what other clinical parameters might indicate biliary obstruction in the patient?
1. Increased systolic and diastolic pressures.
2. Frequent eructation between meals.
3. Darkened urine and clay-colored stools.
4. Longitudinal ridging of the fingernails.

269. Probanthine bromide is used in this situation because it:
1. Reduces gastric secretions and intestinal hypermobility.
2. Decreases bile secretion by the liver and gallbladder.
3. Slows the emptying of the stomach, thereby reducing chyme in the duodenum.
4. Inhibits contraction of the gallbladder and the bile duct.

270. Papaverine HCl is given to Mrs. Klein for pain relief rather than morphine SO_4 because:
1. Morphine depresses gallbladder contractions, thereby decreasing bile secretions.
2. Opiates tend to mask symptoms in patients with acute abdomens.
3. Morphine tends to increase contractions of the sphincter of Oddi, thereby increasing intraductal pressures.
4. Morphine relaxes smooth muscles, thereby increasing bile production.

271. In preparing Mrs. Klein for her IV cholangiogram, it is important to ascertain:
1. If she has ever had the procedure before.
2. If she has any known allergies, particularly to fish or other iodine-containing substances.
3. If her epigastric discomfort only occurs with fatty-food ingestion.
4. If there is a family history of gallstones.

272. Preparation of the patient undergoing IV cholangiogram includes all of the following *except:*

1. Cleansing enemas or oral cathartic the evening before the examination.
2. A fatty meal the evening before examination.
3. Food and fluid restriction for 6 to 8 hours before examination.
4. Informing the patient he/she may experience a feeling of warmth, flushing of face, and/or a salty taste when the dye is injected.

273. Which of the following nursing actions is inappropriate in the preparation of a patient for *oral* cholecystography?
1. Administering a fat-free diet the evening before the test.
2. Administering Telepaque tablets in five-minute intervals one hour after supper.
3. Administering at least 6 oz of water with each Telepaque tablet.
4. Allowing the patient to have water until midnight after ingesting the tablets, then NPO.

Following Mrs. Klein's cholecystogram, a diagnosis of cholelithiasis and cholecystitis is made and arrangements are made for surgery in three days.

274. Preoperative nursing measures for Mrs. Klein include all of the following *except:*
1. Observing for bruising or easy bleeding due to potential prothrombin deficiency.
2. Informing Mrs. Klein of the purpose of the postoperative T-tube.
3. Providing relief for abdominal discomfort by placing a heating pad on the upper abdomen.
4. Providing a high-carbohydrate diet in order to build up glycogen stores in the liver.

275. Postoperative coughing and deep breathing may become a nursing problem following cholecystectomy because:
1. Patients having abdominal surgery are prone to pulmonary complications.
2. Patients with biliary surgery tend to breathe shallowly to prevent pain and discomfort.
3. Women tend to be thoracic rather than diaphragmatic breathers.
4. Patients with upper abdominal surgery usually have a nasogastric tube in place, which inhibits deep breathing.

276. Mrs. Klein refuses to cough "because it hurts." Your action would be to:
1. Administer an analgesic and wait a few minutes.
2. Assist Mrs. Klein to sit up on the side of the bed and splint her incision with a pillow during coughing.
3. Allow Mrs. Klein to rest this time but inform her she will be expected to cough the next time.
4. Increase fluid intake so as to loosen secretions and ease expectoration.

277. Mrs. Klein has a T-tube to dependent drainage. The purpose of the T-tube is to:

1. Maintain patency of the common bile duct.
2. Reduce the occurrence of postoperative hemorrhage.
3. Prevent infection.
4. Reduce bile flow into the duodenum.

278. In observing the drainage from the T-tube during Mrs. Klein's early postoperative period, you would notify the physician if:
    1. The drainage contained blood during the first two to four hours postsurgery.
    2. The drainage was less than 500 ml on the first postoperative day.
    3. The drainage turned greenish-brown in color.
    4. The drainage was more than 500 ml on the fourth postoperative day.

279. On the fourth postoperative day, the surgeon orders Mrs. Klein's T-tube clamped for one hour prior to her first solid meal. The purpose of clamping the T-tube is to:
    1. Inhibit excessive bile drainage during meals.
    2. Allow bile to flow into the duodenum and aid digestion.
    3. Relieve abdominal distention and promote normal peristalsis.
    4. Assess the patency of the common bile duct.

280. While the T-tube is clamped, the nurse should observe Mrs. Klein for signs of:
    1. Abdominal discomfort or pain.
    2. Eructation.
    3. Jaundice.
    4. Increased respiratory rate.

281. While instructing Mrs. Klein about her diet, you inform her that:
    1. She will not be able to include fatty food in her diet for at least one year.
    2. After approximately three months she will be able to begin to add polyunsaturated fats to her diet.
    3. There are no specific dietary restrictions in the postoperative period, but she will be more comfortable if she avoids large, fatty meals.
    4. Her diet will be limited to 20 g of fat per day.

282. Of the following foods, which would you advise Mrs. Klein to delete from her normal diet?
    1. Whole milk.
    2. Cottage cheese.
    3. Whole-grain breads.
    4. Eggs.

Mr. Sam Gold is a 68-year-old retired engineer who has been in consistent good health since childhood. He jogs two miles per day, has never smoked, drinks only on social occasions, and has many outside interests. Lately he has been having problems with intermittent diarrhea and constipation. Two weeks ago he noted blood in the stool and on the tissue wipes

after defecation. Because he was concerned about this new development, he went to see his family physician. Manual examination of the rectum and anal canal revealed no abnormalities. Mr. Gold's physician then ordered a lower GI series on an outpatient basis. Three days later, Mr. Gold's physician called and explained he would like Mr. Gold to enter the hospital for further testing. A sigmoidoscopy was ordered for the morning.

283. Sigmoidoscopy involves:
    1. Instillation of a radiopaque dye into the lower gastrointestinal tract.
    2. Insertion of a rigid instrument that allows for direct visual examination of the anal canal, rectum, and sigmoid colon.
    3. Insertion of a fiber-optic scope that allows for direct visualization of the sigmoid colon, transverse colon, and neocecal valve.
    4. Surgical removal of polyps and biopsy of suspicious gastrointestinal mucosa.

Proctoscopy reveals severe diverticulitis of the upper sigmoid colon. The physician decides to do a temporary colostomy to prevent perforation of the bowel.

284. Preoperative preparation of Mr. Gold included administration of neomycin SO_4. This antibiotic acts to:
    1. Combat postoperative wound infection.
    2. Decrease bacterial count of the colon.
    3. Reduce the size of the tumor before surgery.
    4. Stimulate peristalsis and facilitate action of cleansing enemas.

285. Which of the following is a side effect of neomycin administration?
    1. Deafness.
    2. Nausea and vomiting.
    3. Diarrhea.
    4. Anaphylaxis.

Postoperatively Mr. Gold had a double-barrel transverse colostomy. Postoperative orders were:
    1000 cc 5% D/Ringer's every 8 hours.
    Meperidine 100 mg IM every 4 hours prn for pain.
    IPPB with normal saline 15 min tid.
    Attach nasogastric tube to low intermittent suction.
    Out of bed tonight times one.

286. Which of the following statements correctly describes a double-barrel colostomy?
    1. It is the least common type of colostomy and discharges liquid or unformed stool.
    2. A single loop of the transverse colon is exteriorized and supported by a glass rod. There are two openings, a proximal loop and a distal loop.
    3. It has two stomas. A proximal loop discharges feces and a distal loop discharges mucus.
    4. It is most often permanent and is done to treat disorders of the sigmoid colon.

287. A colostomy begins functioning:
1. Immediately.
2. Two to three days postoperatively.
3. One week postoperatively.
4. Two weeks postoperatively.

288. Colostomy irrigations should be done:
1. Before breakfast.
2. Before lunch.
3. Before dinner.
4. At the time closest to the patient's normal defecation pattern.

289. The purpose of colostomy irrigations is to:
1. Stimulate peristalsis.
2. Relieve constipation.
3. Relieve diarrhea.
4. Remove bacteria.

290. Which of the following foods should be avoided by the colostomy patient?
1. Carbonated drinks.
2. Fresh-cooked green beans.
3. Liver and bacon.
4. Cooked cereals.

John Collins is a 56-year-old man admitted to the hospital with increasing breathlessness for the past five days. He reported that ten days previously he had a runny nose and sneezing with a nonproductive cough. Five days later, the cough became productive of yellowish sputum and shortness of breath became more prominent. He has no fever, chills, or chest pain. Past history included frequent bronchitis. He has smoked 2 packs of cigarettes a day since age 25 and has had a productive cough on rising for the past 15 years. Physical examination reveals a short, stocky, barrel-chested male, blood pressure 150/96, pulse 88, respirations 16, temperature 98 F. Percussion note hyperresonant, breath sounds soft and flat, medium-pitched rhonchi and wheezes heard in right upper lobe and both lower lung lobes.

291. Bronchitis is characterized by:
1. Hypertrophy of the bronchial mucous glands and the production of mucoid sputum sometimes difficult to expectorate.
2. Bronchoconstriction and edema of the wall of the bronchioles.
3. Exudate in the alveoli.
4. Increasing lung stiffness.

292. A wheeze:
1. Is a high-pitched musical sound produced by airflow in narrowed bronchioles.
2. Is rarely considered an indication of pathology.
3. Is a medium-pitched sonorous sound produced by airflow in narrowed or obstructed bronchi.
4. Is a high-pitched crowing sound produced by edema in the trachea.

Mr. Collins's laboratory work reveals: Hct 50%, Hb 17, Na^+ 144, K^+ 4.2, ^-Cl 92, $^-HCO_3$ 32. Arterial blood gases: pH 7.38, PO_2 65, pCO_2 55.

293. Mr. Collins's low chloride can be attributed to:
1. Increased kidney reabsorption of bicarbonate.
2. Increased reversal of the chloride shift in the capillary bed.
3. Increased hemoglobin levels for buffering serum hydrogen ions.
4. Increased serum osmolarity.

294. Mr. Collins's blood gases indicate that he has:
1. Uncompensated respiratory acidosis.
2. Compensated respiratory acidosis.
3. Uncompensated metabolic alkalosis.
4. Compensated metabolic alkalosis.

295. Mr. Collins demonstrates the "increased work of breathing" during this acute period by:
1. Increasing the rate and depth of his respirations.
2. Utilizing pursed-lip exhalations.
3. Increasing diaphragmatic excursion.
4. Utilizing accessory muscles for ventilation.

Pulmonary function data were also collected on Mr. Collins. The results were:

	TLC	FRC	RV	VC	FEV_1
Predicted	6000	3000	2000	4000	3000
Observed	7000	5000	4200	2800	2000

296. These data indicate:
1. Hyperinflation.
2. Hyperventilation.
3. Hyperpnea.
4. Hypercapnia.

297. The pattern of pulmonary dysfunction reflected by these lung volumes is:
1. Restrictive lung disease.
2. Obstructive lung disease.
3. Vascular lung disease.
4. A combination of restrictive and obstructive lung disease.

298. After a nebulizer treatment with isoproterenol (Isuprel) the following measurements were obtained:

	TLC	FRC	RV	VC	FEV_1
Observed	7000	4000	3000	3800	2500

The data indicate what kind of change in lung volumes?
1. Improvement.
2. Deterioration.
3. No change.
4. Inadequate data to decide.

299. The pathophysiologic changes in this patient would include:
1. A decrease in anatomical dead-space air.

2. An increase in anatomical dead-space air.

3. A decrease in physiologic dead-space air.

4. An increase in physiologic dead-space air.

Physician orders for Mr. Collins included:
IPPB tid with Mucomyst (acetylcysteine).
Postural drainage with percussion and vibration for 30 min bid.
Theophylline elixir 1 Tbsp. every 6 hours.
Sputum for culture and sensitivity.

300. The most important effect of intermittent positive-pressure breathing (IPPB) is:
1. Mobilization of bronchial secretions.
2. Increased alveolar ventilation.
3. Prevention of atelectasis.
4. Decreased airway resistance.

301. Side effects of theophylline administration are:
1. Tachycardia and palpitations.
2. Anorexia, nausea, and gastritis.
3. Restlessness and tremors.
4. Headache and nausea.

302. Nursing actions that will facilitate Mr. Collins's medical therapy include:
1. Limiting fluid intake to prevent volume overload and right-sided heart failure.
2. Oral and endotracheal suctioning as necessary.
3. Instructing the patient in deep breathing and coughing techniques as well as pursed-lip exhalations.
4. Maintenance of bedrest and activity restrictions to reduce acidosis.

303. The nurse can also increase Mr. Collins's ventilatory efficiency by positioning him as follows:
1. High-Fowler's.
2. Prone.
3. Sitting up and leaning slightly forward.
4. Trendelenburg.

304. Mr. Collins's teaching plan should emphasize:
1. Smoking and alcohol restrictions.
2. Nutrition, fluid balance, and ways to stop smoking.
3. Vocational rehabilitation programs available in the community.
4. Activity restrictions and pulmonary physiology.

Mrs. Thomas is a 44-year-old public health nurse admitted to the hospital with complaints of increasing fatigue, loss of appetite, and night sweats. She is tall, thin, and pale. She states she has recently returned from a Peace Corps assignment in India. Vital signs: B/P 110/80, pulse 100, respirations 28. Temperature 102.2 F rectally. A skin test (Mantoux) is ordered as well as sputum specimens for acidfast bacilli and chest X ray.

305. In order to administer the Mantoux test correctly, you would inject 5 TU (tuberculin units) of PPD (purified protein derivative) of tuberculin:

1. Intradermally.
2. Subcutaneously.
3. Intramuscularly.
4. Subdermally.

306. The Mantoux test is read in:
1. 6–12 hours.
2. 12–24 hours.
3. 24–48 hours.
4. 48–72 hours.

307. A positive Mantoux test exhibits:
1. An induration of 10 mm or more.
2. An induration of 10 cm or more.
3. An induration of 5–9 mm.
4. A hivelike vesicle.

308. Skin test and sputum culture are positive. The chest X ray demonstrated four small lesions and one of moderate density. Diagnosis—tuberculosis. Respiratory isolation was initiated. This is defined as:
1. Both patient and attending nurse must wear masks at all times.
2. Full isolation; that is, caps and gowns required during the period of contagion.
3. Nurse and visitors must wear masks until chemotherapy is begun. Patient instructed in cough and tissue techniques.
4. Gloves are worn when handling patient's tissues, excretions, and linen.

309. Mrs. Thomas is treated with INH (isoniazid) 300 mg p.o., and RMP (rifampin). Which of the following vitamins is also frequently prescribed to prevent the peripheral neuritis that may occur with INH therapy?
1. Ascorbic acid (vitamin C).
2. Pyridoxine (vitamin B_6).
3. Vitamin E.
4. Vitamin B_{12}.

310. While chemotherapy renders the patient noninfectious within days to a few weeks, barring side effects, Mrs. Thomas will need to continue INH therapy for:
1. Six months.
2. One year.
3. Two years.
4. The rest of her life.

Deanna Thomas, a 36-year-old OR nurse, is admitted for a thyroid scan. Ms. Thomas, who is a part-time student working toward her baccalaureate degree in nursing, had discovered a nodule on her thyroid while practicing the neck exam for a physical-assessment class she was taking. Her instructor had suggested she have it checked by a physician. On inspection, Ms. Thomas was a well-developed and -nourished female who looked younger than her stated age. Blood pressure was 132/68, pulse 72, respirations 16.

311. A thyroid scan:
     1. Assists in differentiating between primary and secondary hypothyroidism.
     2. Demonstrates increased uptake of radioactive iodine in areas of possible malignancy.
     3. Demonstrates decreased uptake of radioactive iodine in areas of possible malignancy.
     4. Measures the effect of TSH on thyroid function.

312. Following a thyroid scan with ^{131}I:
     1. No radiation precautions are necessary.
     2. Full radiation precautions are instituted, including segregating the patient in a private room.
     3. Radiation precautions are limited to urine and feces.
     4. Full radiation precautions are instituted for 8 hours or the extent of half-life of ^{131}I.

Ms. Thomas's thyroid scan revealed a positive cold nodule and a total thyroidectomy was planned. Preoperative orders included:
     Routine CBC and urinalysis.
     Type and cross-match for three units of blood.
     Electrocardiogram.
     200 mg Seconal hs.
     NPO after midnight.

313. A total thyroidectomy is ordered following discovery of a cold nodule. In the case of hyperthyroidism versus malignancy, the appropriate treatment is:
     1. Complete thyroidectomy also.
     2. Partial thyroidectomy (approximately 1/2 of the thyroid is removed).
     3. Partial thyroidectomy (approximately 5/6 of the thyroid is removed).
     4. Administration of thyroid medication.

314. Preoperative teaching measures unique to the patient having a thyroidectomy should encompass:
     1. Active flexion exercise of the neck, special coughing instructions, voice rest, and antithyroid medications postoperatively.
     2. Active flexion and extension neck exercises, deep breathing and coughing, and thyroid replacement when necessary.
     3. Instruction on supporting the back of the neck when repositioning and/or ambulating; avoiding hyperextension and flexion of the neck when coughing.
     4. Instructions on supporting the back of the neck when ambulating and/or repositioning and active flexion exercises to the neck.

315. Complications of a thyroidectomy can be extremely serious if they are not recognized and treated immediately. These complications include all of the following *except:*
     1. Hemorrhage.
     2. Respiratory obstruction.
     3. Tetany and hypercalcemia.
     4. Paralytic ileus.

316. Muscular twitching and hyperirritability of the nervous system indicate tetany (hypocalcemia). This complication can be monitored by:
     1. Checking the urine calcium.
     2. Palpating the calf muscle with the ankle hyperflexed.
     3. Tapping the facial nerve just proximal to the ear.
     4. Checking for ankle clonus.

317. Measures taken to decrease the incidence of hemorrhage postthyroidectomy are:
     1. Frequent checking of dressing, semi-Fowler's position, and ice packs to neck.
     2. Frequent checking of dressing, supine position, and ice packs to neck.
     3. Frequent checking of dressing, coughing every two hours, and moist packs to neck.
     4. Frequent checking of dressings and maintenance of neck flexion.

318. In anticipation of emergency complications, which of the following nursing measures is essential in the postoperative period?
     1. Having calcium gluconate available for possible tetany.
     2. Having a thoracentesis tray available to reduce edema.
     3. Having a tracheostomy tray available for possible airway obstruction.
     4. Having pressure dressings available for possible hemorrhage.

319. Signs and/or symptoms of respiratory obstruction vary with the degree of severity. Early warnings might manifest as:
     1. Hoarseness and weakness of the voice.
     2. Stridor and cyanosis.
     3. Vague feeling of choking, difficulty swallowing, and fullness of the throat.
     4. Pale nail beds, disorientation, and combative behavior.

320. Upon returning from the recovery room, Ms. Thomas begins to complain of a choking sensation. Your immediate nursing action is to:
     1. Elevate the head to high-Fowler's.
     2. Suggest she suck on some ice chips.
     3. Assess the wound and dressing for increased swelling and loosen dressing if necessary.
     4. Call the physician.

321. On her first postoperative evening, while assisting Ms. Thomas to dangle at the bedside, you would:
     1. Support her under the axilla while bringing her feet over the bedside.
     2. Bring her feet to the side of the bed and support the back of her neck while assisting her to assume a sitting position.
     3. Allow her to assume the sitting position at her own pace, unassisted unless necessary.

4. Bring her feet to the side of the bed, then pull her forward.

Mr. Robert Mackey, a 19-year-old college sophomore, sustained a transverse fracture of his right tibia and fibula when he tripped playing football. His fractures were reduced in the emergency room and his right leg immobilized in a long leg cast, which extended from his groin to his toes, with the knee slightly flexed.

322. On his admission to the orthopedic unit, Mr. Mackey's cast is damp and he is complaining that it feels very hot. You should:
1. Explain to Mr. Mackey that the cast will feel hot for several hours as the moisture evaporates and the cast hardens.
2. Recognize that this is a sign of excessive pressure on the soft tissues and notify the physician.
3. Tell Mr. Mackey not to worry, as this is a common complaint.
4. Administer meperidine (Demerol) HCl 50 mg IM to relieve his discomfort.

323. After elevating Mr. Mackey's leg, you check his toes for circulation and motor activity. Which of the following indicates circulatory constriction?
1. Tingling and numbness of toes.
2. Inability to move toes.
3. Blanching or cyanosis of toes.
4. Complaints of pressure or tightness of the cast.

324. Several hours after Mr. Mackey is admitted, you notice his toes have become edematous. The physician decides to bivalve the cast. This procedure:
1. Requires recasting after 24 hours.
2. Includes splitting and spreading the cast down the middle to relieve constriction.
3. Includes splitting and spreading the cast on each side and cutting the underlying padding.
4. Should be followed by placing the patient's leg in a dependent position.

325. Which of the following is *not* an appropriate exercise for Mr. Mackey to engage in to prevent complications of immobility?
1. Wiggling his toes.
3. Quadriceps setting.
3. Active range of motion of hip.
4. Flexion of the right knee.

326. On entering Mr. Mackey's room two days later, you find he is using a long pencil to scratch the skin under his cast. You should:
1. Ask the physician for a medication order to relieve itching.
2. Explain to the patient that scratching under the cast should be avoided, as it may break the skin and cause an infection.

3. Assist Mr. Mackey by gently rolling the casted leg in the palmar surfaces of your hand.
4. Take the pencil away from Mr. Mackey.

327. The doctor has ordered ambulation on crutches with no weight bearing on the affected limb. An appropriate crutch gait for you to teach Mr. Mackey would be:
1. Two-point gait.
2. Three-point gait.
3. Four-point gait.
4. Tripod gait.

328. Which of the following instructions is *not* appropriate when teaching a patient to use crutches?
1. Utilize axilla to help carry weight.
2. Use short strides to maintain maximum mobility.
3. Keep feet 6–8 inches apart to provide a wide base for support.
4. If he should begin to fall, throw crutches to the side to prevent falling on them.

Mr. John Edwards, a 70-year-old retired engineer, is admitted to the hospital for the removal of a cataract from his left eye. Nursing history and physical assessment reveal a wiry, well-nourished man who states he has always enjoyed good health. Preoperative orders for Mr. Edwards include:
Routine lab work.
Regular diet.
500 mg chloral hydrate at bedtime.
NPO after midnight.

329. Nursing measures for Mr. Edwards preoperatively include:
1. Keeping him flat in bed.
2. Applying eye patches to both eyes.
3. Orienting him to his environment and nursing personnel.
4. Teaching him eye-drop instillation.

330. Cataract surgery is generally performed under which kind of anesthesia?
1. Local.
2. General.
3. Intravenous.
4. Rectal.

331. During the procedure to remove the opacified lens, an iridectomy is also performed. This procedure is done:
1. To prevent secondary glaucoma from developing in the postoperative period.
2. To increase pupillary dilatation postoperatively.
3. To facilitate circulation and postoperative healing.
4. To prevent corneal scarring during the procedure.

332. Postoperatively Mr. Edwards should be positioned:
1. In a semi-Fowler's position.
2. In a prone position only.
3. On his back or on the unoperated side.
4. On his operative side.

333. Which of the following activities of daily living must Mr. Edwards avoid to prevent complications in the early postoperative period?
1. Self-feeding.
2. Bathroom privileges.
3. Brushing his teeth.
4. Ambulating.

334. One week after his surgery, Mr. Edwards was fitted with cataract glasses. Which of the following nursing statements would best prepare Mr. Edwards for adjusting to these glasses?
1. "The cataract lenses magnify objects so that they will seem closer to you than they really are."
2. "While your central vision may be somewhat distorted, you will be able to see well peripherally."
3. "These lenses will enable you to see as well as you did before the cataract formed."
4. "The lenses on these glasses are quite narrow, and therefore you may have some double vision."

Melissa Sue is a 29-year-old woman admitted to the emergency room with repetitive seizures characterized by tonic and clonic contractions. She was unconscious and had been incontinent of both urine and feces. She has a history of epilepsy since age 5. The current episode began 30 minutes prior to admission. Vital signs: Blood pressure 165/110, pulse 90, respiration rate 12–32, rectal temperature 102 F. The attending physician diagnosed status epilepticus and instituted emergency measures to end the seizures.

335. Epileptic seizures or convulsions result from:
1. Excessive exercise with lactic acid accumulation.
2. Excessive, simultaneous, disordered neuronal discharge.
3. Excessive cerebral metabolism with local K^+ increased.
4. Excessive circulating cerebrospinal fluid increasing cerebral pressures.

336. Which of the following characterizes grand mal seizures?
1. Brief, abrupt loss of consciousness lasting 10–20 seconds.
2. Loss of consciousness for several minutes, with tonic and clonic contractions of all motor muscle groups.
3. Tonic and clonic contractions of selected motor groups in a somewhat confined area.
4. Twitching of facial muscles.

337. The drug of choice for long-term control of grand mal seizures is:
1. Phenobarbital.
2. Diazepam (Valium).
3. Diphenylhydantoin (Dilantin) sodium.
4. Trimethadione (Tridione).

338. Which of the following nursing actions is *not* indicated during a grand mal seizure episode?

1. Observe and record all events that occur prior to, during, and after the seizure.
2. Maintain a patent airway by inserting a padded tongue depressor between teeth.
3. Protect the patient from injury.
4. Monitor vital signs with special attention directed toward respiratory status.

339. Emergency drug intervention for Melissa Sue included diazepam 10 mg intravenously and diphenylhydantoin .15 g IV in .05 g increments. Diphenylhydantoin given intravenously must be given slowly and in small increments to prevent:
1. Respiratory depression and/or arrest.
2. Vasodepression and circulatory shock.
3. Irritation and/or necrosis of the vein and surrounding tissue.
4. Vasomotor stimulation with a sudden, malignant increase in blood pressure.

Donald Lee is a 70-year-old retired businessman. He went to his ophthalmologist with complaints of decreasing peripheral vision, which he felt was hindering his mobility. He had had a lens changed in his glasses six months previously and was very irritated by the necessity for another change so soon. Tonometry revealed increased intraocular pressures, and cupping of the disc in the left eye was noted on inspection of the inner eye. Mr. Lee was admitted to the hospital with a diagnosis of wide-angle glaucoma. He was placed on bedrest and the following medications were ordered: pilocarpine hydrochloride 2%, gtts i, tid both eyes; acetazolamide (Diamox) 250 mg qd.

340. Glaucoma is defined as:
1. An imbalance between the rate of secretion of intraocular fluids and the rate of absorption of aqueous humor.
2. A degenerative disease characterized by narrowing of the arterioles of the retina and areas of ischemia.
3. An infectious process that causes clouding and scarring of the cornea.
4. A dysfunction of aging in which the retina of the eye buckles from inadequate fluid pressures.

341. Increased cupping of the optic disc means that:
1. The margins of the optic disc are blurred and indistinct.
2. The disc appears pale and white either in part or throughout.
3. The pressure on the disc changes the course of the merging blood vessels so that they disappear from sight at the disc rim and reappear at a slightly different site just past the rim.
4. The disc rim is outlined by a black crescent.

342. Normal intraocular pressures as measured by tonometry are:
1. 5–10 mm Hg.
2. 12–22 mm Hg.

3. 10–20 cm H_2O.

4. 20–30 mm Hg.

343. While taking Mr. Lee's history you would be alerted to a sudden increase in intraocular pressure if he complained of:

1. Generalized decrease in peripheral vision over the past year.

2. Difficulty with close vision.

3. Increasing discomfort in the left eye with radiation to his forehead and left temple.

4. Halos around lights.

344. Wide-angle or chronic glaucoma differs from closed-angle or acute glaucoma in that:

1. Wide-angle glaucoma occurs less frequently than closed-angle glaucoma.

2. Wide-angle glaucoma's symptomatology includes pain, severe headache, nausea, and vomiting; whereas closed-angle glaucoma has a slow, silent, and generally painless onset.

3. The obstruction to aqueous flow in wide-angle glaucoma generally occurs somewhere in Schlemm's canal or aqueous veins. It does not narrow or close the angle of the anterior chamber, as in closed-angle glaucoma.

4. Wide-angle glaucoma rarely occurs in families, however, there is a hereditary predisposition for closed-angle glaucoma.

345. Pilocarpine is the drug of choice in the treatment of wide-angle glaucoma because it:

1. Blocks the action of cholinesterase at the cholinergic nerve endings, thereby increasing pupil size.

2. Constricts the pupil, thereby widening the outflow channels and increasing the flow of aqueous fluid.

3. Decreases the production of aqueous humor.

4. Constricts aqueous veins, thereby decreasing venous pooling in the eye.

346. Pilocarpine is classified as a:

1. Parasympathomimetic.

2. Sympathomimetic.

3. Beta blocker.

4. Anticholinesterase.

347. Bedrest is ordered for Mr. Lee because activity tends to increase intraocular pressure. Which of the following activities of daily living would be discouraged?

1. Watching television.

2. Brushing teeth and hair.

3. Self-feeding.

4. Passive range-of-motion exercises.

348. To correctly instill pilocarpine in Mr. Lee's eyes, the nurse should gently pull down the lower lid of the eye and instill the drops:

1. Directly on the central surface of the cornea.

2. On the inner canthus of the eye.

3. Into the conjunctival sac.

4. Directly on the dilated pupil.

349. Which of the following aspects of wide-angle glaucoma and its medical treatment is the most frequent cause of patient noncompliance?

1. Loss of mobility due to severe driving restrictions.

2. The painful and insidious progression of this type of glaucoma.

3. Decreased light and near-vision accommodation due to miotic effects of pilocarpine.

4. The frequent nausea and vomiting accompanying use of miotic drugs.

350. The legal definition of blindness is:

1. Vision of 20/400 without corrective lenses.

2. Vision of 20/200 with corrective lenses.

3. Vision of 20/100 with corrective lenses.

4. Total loss of peripheral vision (bilateral hemianopsia).

Miss Ann Martin is a 23-year-old secretary readmitted to the hospital with pronounced weakness of the left facial muscles and difficulty swallowing. Physical examination reveals a small, slightly pale female with ptosis of the right eyelid, a snarllike smile, and very nasal voice tones. Miss Martin was diagnosed 14 months ago as having myasthenia gravis. She was doing well until two weeks ago when she developed some nausea and diarrhea and decided to discontinue her medications.

351. Myasthenia gravis is a:

1. Degenerative dysfunction of the basal ganglia.

2. Transmission dysfunction at the myoneural junction.

3. Hypertrophic reaction in the anterior motor neurons of the spinal cord.

4. Hereditary condition of cranial nerves VII, IX, and X.

352. Which of the following statements is *not* true of myasthenia gravis?

1. Thymectomies rarely produce remissions in myasthenia gravis.

2. Myasthenia gravis may be an autoimmune disease.

3. Like rheumatoid arthritis, some families seem to be predisposed to myasthenia gravis.

4. Generally myasthenia gravis runs a chronic, progressive course with occasional spontaneous remissions.

353. Diagnosis of myasthenia gravis is frequently based on the patient's response to an intravenous injection of edrophonium (Tensilon). If the patient responds positively to this drug, you would expect:

1. Exacerbation of symptomatology.

2. Relief of ptosis but not of weakness in other facial muscles.

3. A prompt and dramatic increase in muscle strength.

4. A slight increase in muscle strength that is countered by an increase in muscle fatigability.

The attending physician has ordered the following medical regimen for Miss Martin:

Pyridostigmine bromide (Mestinon) 180 mg bid.
Neostigmine bromide (Prostigmin) .05 mg sub q tid, ac.
Ephedrine sulfate 25 mg tid.
Potassium chloride tablets bid.

354. Which of the following categories of drugs provides the backbone of treatment for patients with myasthenia gravis?
1. Adrenergic drugs.
2. Anticholinergic drugs.
3. Anticholinesterase drugs.
4. Cholinergic drugs.

355. The most common patient problems arising from the use of Mestinon and Prostigmin are:
1. Gastric distress—nausea, anorexia, diarrhea.
2. Elimination problems—urinary retention.
3. Central nervous system excitation—flushing, irritability.
4. Cardiac arrhythmias—palpitations, PVCs.

356. Which of the following nursing interventions can aid in reducing the side effects of these drugs?
1. Give oral medications with milk, soda crackers, or antacids.
2. Push fluids and encourage ambulation.
3. Keep room cool and discourage visitors.
4. Encourage food high in potassium.

357. In order to take full advantage of the effects of pyridostigmine bromide and neostigmine bromide in reducing dysphagia, how long should they be administered before meals?
1. Two hours.
2. 45–60 minutes.
3. 20–30 minutes.
4. 10–15 minutes.

358. Because Miss Martin's medications have been increased, it is important that the nurse observe for signs of "cholinergic crisis." These include:
1. Dilated pupils, profuse diaphoresis, and trembling.
2. Constricted pupils, hypersalivation, and hypotension.
3. Dilated pupils, nausea, and tachycardia.
4. Constricted pupils, dry mucous membranes, and bradycardia.

359. If "cholinergic crisis" is established, all anticholinesterase drugs are withdrawn. To reduce symptoms, which of the following drugs is administered?
1. Atropine.
2. Ephedrine sulfate.
3. Potassium chloride.
4. Neostigmine bromide.

360. In order to assess Miss Martin's functional and vocational rehabilitation potential, you first need to ascertain:
1. The degree of physical and emotional stress in her present occupation.
2. The activities of daily living that cause the greatest degree of muscle weakness and fatigue.
3. Miss Martin's understanding of and attitude toward myasthenia gravis, as well as her ability to cope with activity restrictions.
4. Whether or not Miss Martin will be allowed to sit down and rest when necessary in her current occupation.

361. On evaluating Miss Martin's dysfunction, you decide she has:
1. An upper motor neuron lesion.
2. A lower motor neuron lesion.
3. A combined upper and lower motor neuron lesion.
4. A genetic dysfunction.

Ms. Kim Landry is a 32-year-old teacher and mother of four school-age children. She has complaints of increasing fatigue, weight gain, periorbital edema, and menorrhagia. She states, "I feel foolish coming to see the doctor, but my husband is concerned because I fall asleep so frequently." On the basis of blood chemistries, a diagnosis of hypothyroidism is made.

362. Two common causes of primary hypothyroidism are:
1. Destruction of thyroid tissue by radioactive iodine during therapy for hyperthyroidism, and spontaneous atrophy due to autoimmune response.
2. Spontaneous atrophy due to autoimmune response, and surgical removal of the thyroid gland.
3. Surgical removal of the thyroid gland, and tumors of the pituitary gland that decrease the amount of circulating thyroxine.
4. Tumors of the pituitary gland and/or large doses of antithyroid drugs.

363. The most common clinical manifestations of hypothyroidism are:
1. Increased body temperature, tachycardia, and fatigue.
2. Decreased exercise tolerance, facial and pitting edema.
3. Increased sluggishness, increased cold intolerance, and puffy eyelids, hands, and feet.
4. Decreased facial expression, diarrhea, and weight gain.

364. If treatment with thyroid hormone is effective, you would expect:
1. Diuresis, a decrease in pulse rate, and an increase in blood pressure.
2. Diuresis, a widening pulse pressure, and an increase in both temperature and respiratory rate.
3. Increased pulse rate, decreased respiratory rate, and decreased puffiness.
4. Weight loss, increased diastolic blood pressure, and decreased pulse rate.

365. In contrast to hypothyroidism, hyperthyroidism is due to excessive levels of thyroxine in the plasma. Clinical manifestations of this endocrine dysfunction are:
1. Systolic hypertension and heat intolerance.
2. Diastolic hypertension and widened pulse pressure.
3. Heat intolerance and weight gain.
4. Emotional hyperexcitability and anorexia.

366. Which of the following is not a method of treating hyperthyroidism?
1. Subtotal thyroidectomy.
2. Administration of propylthiouracil.
3. Radioiodine therapy.
4. Administration of thyroglobulin.

367. In contrast to patients with hypothyroidism, patients with hyperthyroidism have:
1. An increased serum cholesterol.
2. An increased basal metabolic rate and serum T_3 and T_4.
3. An increased serum TSH (thyroid stimulating hormone).
4. An increase in menstrual volume.

368. Of the following, which is the "cardinal sign" that heralds the onset of thyroid storm?
1. Fever.
2. Tachycardia.
3. Hypertension.
4. Tremulousness and restlessness.

369. Both Cushing's syndrome and Addison's disease are due to dysfunction of the adrenal cortex. In Cushing's syndrome the primary pathology is:
1. Increased cortisol secretion.
2. Increased epinephrine secretion.
3. Decreased aldosterone secretion.
4. Decreased ACTH secretion.

370. Because this hormone is a glucocorticoid, you would expect:
1. Hypoglycemia due to increased insulin production.
2. Skeletal-muscle wasting because glucocorticoids promote protein and fat mobilization.
3. Dependent edema and severe hypokalemia due to abnormal aldosterone secretion.
4. Discoloration or hyperpigmentation of the skin due to increased pituitary secretion of ACTH.

371. In Addison's disease glucocorticoids, mineral corticoids, and androgenic hormones are all reduced. Therefore, in contrast to Cushing's syndrome, you would expect to find:
1. Hypotension, weight loss, and physical and mental exhaustion.
2. Hypertension, moon facies, and masculinization in females.
3. Hypotension, hyperglycemia, and weight gain.
4. Hypertension, male impotency, and menstrual disturbances.

372. Since aldosterone is the major mineral corticoid secreted by the adrenal cortex, which of the following fluid and electrolyte imbalances would you anticipate with decreased secretion of this hormone?
1. Hyperkalemia.
2. Hypernatremia.
3. Hypervolemia.
4. Hypercalcemia.

373. Nursing actions in caring for patients with Addison's disease will include all of the following *except*:
1. Daily weights.
2. Restriction of fluids to 1500 cc/day.
3. Administering hormone replacement therapy.
4. Reducing physical and emotional stress by providing a quiet, nondemanding care schedule.

374. Iron deficiency anemia is best described as:
1. Hypochromic microcytic.
2. Hyperchromic macrocytic.
3. Hyperchromic microcytic.
4. Hypochromic macrocytic.

375. Oral iron preparations should be given:
1. With meals to decrease gastric upset.
2. One hour before eating to enhance absorption.
3. One hour after eating to slow absorption.
4. At bedtime.

Mrs. Rhonda Sanches is a 32-year-old flight attendant admitted to the hospital with acute rheumatoid arthritis. She has pain and swelling in her hands and severe pain in her left hip. She has been under treatment for this condition for five years. Mrs. Sanches tells you she also has a sister and a cousin with this problem. She thinks the flare-up of her condition, which had been fairly well controlled with salicylates, is due to the fact that her mother recently moved in with her. She states her mother has been treating her as if she were a teenager again. Vital signs are: temperature 101 F orally, B/P 102/68, pulse 88, respirations 22. Medical therapy includes: bedrest, aspirin g X qid, prednisone 10 mg every A.M., diazepam 20 mg qid, passive ROM exercises twice daily.

376. While salicylates are given to relieve pain in rheumatoid arthritis, they also function as an:
1. Analgesic.
2. Antiinflammatory.
3. Anticholinergic.
4. Antiadrenergic.

377. Mrs. Sanches's temperature and pulse are elevated due to:
1. Increased fluid losses.
2. Inflammation of her hand and hip joints.
3. Stress response.
4. Side effect of salicylate therapy.

378. The primary purpose of the nurse's doing passive range-of-motion exercises to Mrs. Sanches's affected limbs is to:

1. Prevent contractures and limited range of motion.
2. Continuously evaluate her functional abilities.
3. Assess her pain tolerance.
4. Evaluate the effectiveness of drug therapy.

379. Which of the following serum factors are increased in acute rheumatoid arthritis?
1. Hemoglobin and hematocrit.
2. Sedimentation rate and C-reactive protein.
3. Wasserman test.
4. Platelet count.

380. To reduce symptoms of early-morning stiffness, the nurse can encourage the patient to:
1. Take a hot tub bath or shower in the morning.
2. Put joints through passive ROM before trying to move them actively.
3. Sleep with a hot pad.
4. Take two aspirins before arising and wait 15 minutes before attempting locomotion.

381. The primary objective in giving prednisone along with aspirin is:
1. To inhibit the autoimmune factors associated with rheumatoid arthritis.
2. To prevent further joint destruction.
3. To decrease inflammation and suppress symptomatology.
4. To increase glucose levels for tissue repair.

382. An indication of prednisone toxicity would be:
1. Tinnitus.
2. Exfoliative dermatitis.
3. Glucosuria.
4. Nausea and vomiting.

383. Which of the following precautions should the nurse advise the patient of during predischarge teaching?
1. Take oral preparations of prednisone before meals.
2. Never stop or change the amount of the medication without medical advice.
3. Have periodic complete blood counts while on the medication.
4. Wear sunglasses if exposed to bright light for an extended period of time.

384. Which of the following is a reliable index of Mrs. Sanches's exercise tolerance?
1. Pulse and respiratory rate.
2. Occurrence and duration of pain in the affected joint.
3. Mobility of joints.
4. Decreased redness and swelling of joints.

385. Mrs. Sanches's emotional responses to her condition will primarily be dependent upon:
1. Her self-concept, body image, and usual affective coping strategies.
2. Her relationship with her mother.

3. Her usual affective or palliative coping strategies only.
4. Economic status and work history.

Mrs. Ryan, a 50-year-old history professor at the local university, is admitted to the hospital with complaints of postmenopausal bleeding. Following a D & C a diagnosis of adenocarcinoma is made. Internal radiation therapy is initiated.

386. Mrs. Ryan has cobalt (^{60}Co) seeds implanted. On returning to the unit, she has a vaginal packing and a urinary catheter to dependent drainage. To prevent displacement of the radioactive substance, the patient should be positioned:
1. With the foot of the bed elevated.
2. Flat in bed.
3. With her head elevated 45° (semi-Fowler's).
4. On her side only.

387. Which of the following are precautionary measures to be utilized when caring for a patient being treated with internal radioisotopes?
1. Maintain strict patient isolation and limit professional contact with patient.
2. Limit exposure and maximize distance between patient, professional, and/or family.
3. Position the patient in a prone position and restrict turning to mealtimes only.
4. Maintain the legs in a flexed position to decrease the likelihood of dislodgement.

388. Which of the following nursing problems would you expect following uterine isotope insertion?
1. Bladder atony.
2. Constipation.
3. Foul-smelling vaginal discharge.
4. Loss of sexual libido.

389. Mrs. Ryan complains of nausea and a general feeling of weakness. Her stools are loose. You might suspect:
1. Extension of her cancer to the abdominal contents.
2. Radiation syndrome.
3. Electrolyte imbalances.
4. Depression.

Frank Henry, a 65-year-old retired merchant seaman, has been hospitalized for two weeks for severe vascular insufficiency and gangrene of the left foot. His response to medical management is poor. Frank is scheduled for an above-the-knee amputation in four days. The nursing assessment revealed a history of insulin-dependent diabetes for 20 years.

390. The majority of amputations are attributed to:
1. Chemical burns.
2. Diabetic ulcers.
3. Arteriosclerosis obliterans.
4. Bone tumors.

391. Mr. Henry is verbalizing feelings of decreased self-

worth and of being less of a man. His acceptance of the surgery is largely dependent upon:
1. What his doctor says.
2. How his family is reacting.
3. How the nursing staff react and respond to his behavior.
4. His ability to grieve.

392. Two days before surgery Frank expresses a desire to learn more about the surgery and outcome. Preoperative teaching is directed toward:
1. Discussing the possibility of another vocation.
2. Learning crutch-walking.
3. Instruction in postoperative exercises.
4. Encouraging the patient to verbalize fears and concerns.

393. The type of anesthesia generally used for an amputation is:
1. IV regional.
2. Spinal.
3. General intravenous and inhalation anesthesia.
4. Muscle relaxant.

394. Above-the-knee (AK) amputations are usually necessary because:
1. Of the degree of vascular insufficiency.
2. The AK amputations are better suited for a prosthesis.
3. The higher the amputation, the less energy required for rehabilitation of balance and walking.
4. The below-the-knee amputation heals less successfully.

395. Because Mr. Henry is NPO prior to surgery, an appropriate nursing measure on the day of surgery is:
1. To withhold the daily insulin dose.
2. To administer the daily insulin dose.
3. To administer the insulin and request Frank to drink a glass of juice.
4. The night before, request specific orders from the anesthetist regarding insulin administration.

396. Despite the occurrence of gangrene, Mr. Henry's physician chooses to do a flap amputation in order to avoid the necessity of another surgery. Immediately upon returning to the recovery room, Mr. Henry's stump should be:
1. Elevated on a pillow to reduce occurrence of edema and hemorrhage.
2. Placed in Buck's traction to prevent skin and muscle retraction.
3. Firmly bandaged to a padded board to prevent contractures.
4. Wrapped in an ace bandage to reduce edema formation.

397. Which of the following is the most common postoperative complication in the elderly after amputation?
1. Hemorrhage and shock.
2. Pulmonary embolus.
3. Disseminated intravascular clotting.
4. Thrombophlebitis.

398. The first postoperative day, Frank's vital signs are stable, his IV is discontinued, and he is getting solid foods. The surgeon has ordered rehabilitation exercises to begin. Which is most important to initiate?
1. External rotation of the stump.
2. Hyperextension of the thigh and stump.
3. Lifting the buttock and stump off the bed while lying flat on back.
4. Arm exercises to prepare for crutch-walking.

399. While you initiate Frank's repositioning onto his abdomen, he states that he can't turn because his "left foot is causing him too much pain." Your first response is:
1. To insist he lie on his abdomen.
2. To ignore his comment and state you will return later.
3. To discuss the principle of phantom pain postamputation.
4. To offer some form of pain control.

400. A measure to help reduce the size of the stump once the surgical wound is healed is:
1. Elevation of the stump on a pillow when reclining.
2. Pushing the stump against hard surfaces.
3. Wrapping moist, warm soaks on the thigh.
4. Applying an elastic bandage.

Answers—Rationale
NURSING CARE OF THE ACUTELY OR CHRONICALLY ILL ADULT

1. (3) In complete heart block the SA node continues to pace the atria and an independent pacemaker arises in the bundles or Purkinje fibers of the ventricles. This results in an EKG pattern in which P waves occur at a regular rate without reference to the QRS waves. QRS waves are usually wide and bizarre, with T waves sloping in the opposite direction of the major deflection. No. 1 is an example of second-degree heart block, No. 2 describes first-degree block, and No. 4 is a pattern seen frequently with bundle branch block.

2. (4) The two most common causes of AV block are degenerative cardiac disease, such as coronary artery disease and fibrosis, which produce anatomical or electrical disruption in or around the AV node, and digitalis toxicity, which commonly causes first-degree heart block and occasionally a second-degree Mobitz type I heart block. In potassium depletion, as in hypokalemia, the S-T segment becomes depressed, a U wave occurs and the T wave loses amplitude. Clinical hypokalemia and other electrolyte imbalances less commonly cause AV block. Inferior myocardial infarction may result in bradycardia and varying degrees of heart block due to ischemia of the AV node; anterior myocardial infarction is more likely to affect transmission of impulses in the bundle branches. However, since myocardial infarction is a type of degenerative cardiac disease, the most comprehensive answer to this question is No. 4.

3. (1) The inherent rate of ventricular excitable tissue is between 20 and 40 and does not increase significantly with exercise in complete heart block. This phenomenon results in decreased cardiac output despite increased diastolic filling time and stroke volume with each ventricular contraction. The decrease in cardiac output results in decreased cerebral perfusion, causing dizziness and fainting. Likewise, the decreased cardiac output results in stimulation of circulatory reflexes to increase venous return; that is, peripheral vasoconstriction, which is the cause of Mr. Marks's pallor and diaphoresis. However, even though these reflexes are intact, the inability of the heart to increase its rate during exercise is the significant factor in his symptomatology. Hence Nos. 2, 3, and 4 are incorrect.

4. (1) Before beginning any teaching plan, you must assess the patient's current understanding of the procedure as well as his interest and ability to comprehend different facets of it. The physician has generally given the patient an outline of the facts as to why the procedure is necessary. However, several intervening variables such as anxiety or decreased cerebral perfusion may be affecting the patient's ability to absorb information. Therefore, it is frequently necessary not only to reinforce information given by the physician (No. 3) but to reexplain the procedure. The patient's husband, wife, or significant others may be invited to join the teaching session if the clinical situation allows (No. 2); otherwise they should be informed separately. Following explanations of the procedure, the operative permit is signed, thereby assuring informed consent (No. 4).

5. (4) The patient's weight and institution of intake and output records are admission procedures. While these procedures provide important baseline data for evaluation of postinsertion outcomes, the nursing actions described in Nos. 1, 2, and 3 are priorities in the immediate preinsertion period.

6. (2) Both isoproterenol (Isuprel) and atropine are kept available in the preoperative period as drugs of choice should the ventricular rate decrease further. Isoproterenol enhances pacemaker automaticity and facilitates AV conduction in heart block. Atropine acts to enhance AV conduction by inhibiting parasympathetic nervous system innervation of the AV node. Lidocaine (No. 1) is an antiarrhythmic utilized to depress myocardial automaticity. Digoxin (No. 3) enhances vagal stimulation of the AV node, decreasing conduction through the node. Propranolol (No. 4) is a beta blocker that depresses cardiac contractility and heart rate. Therefore, these latter three drugs would not be indicated should Mr. Marks's ventricular rate decrease in the preinsertion period.

7. (1) Isoproterenol is categorized as a beta mimetic in that its action simulates beta adrenergic discharge. Actions include increased strength of cardiac contraction, increased heart rate, and decreased venous pooling, which increases venous return. Other actions of isoproterenol include relaxation of smooth muscles in the bronchi, skeletal-muscle vasculature, and alimentary tract. Digoxin is an example of a cardiac glycocide; atropine, an anticholinergic; and propranolol, a beta blocker. Hence Nos. 2, 3, and 4 are incorrect.

8. (3) See question 7 above. An additional effect of isoproterenol is increased myocardial consumption resulting from increased rate and contractility.

9. (1) Each of these activities is a priority in the early postinsertion period. However, since a transvenous approach was used with Mr. Marks, it is essential that his activities be restricted for the first few days to reduce the risk of catheter dislodgement. To monitor for this complication, periodic comparisons of his current rhythm strip should be made, with the tracing taken at the time of insertion. Changes in either the pacemaker artifact or pacemaker-initiated QRS indicate a change in position. While this may not always be significant, it becomes so if the pacemaker fails to capture, causing a decrease in heart rate and cardiac output. Hence Nos. 2, 3, and 4 are incorrect.

10. (1) The rationale for pacemaker implantation is presented in the preinsertion period and is reinforced in the postinsertion period. Nos. 2, 3, and 4 are essential components of a predischarge teaching plan.

11. (3) Patients with permanent pacemakers are cautioned to avoid all sources of high electronic output because they may cause pacemaker malfunction. Other sources of high electronic output include microwave ovens, running car engines, and dental drills. Activities such as swimming, walking, and golf should be encouraged to patient tolerance (Nos. 1 and 4). Creative hobbies such as fashioning lamps (No. 2) are indicated as long as precautions are taken to avoid electrical shocks.

12. (4) Periodic checks on pacemaker function are essential and may be accomplished by pulse-taking, frequent ECGs, or telephone transmission of ECG. Generally rate changes greater than ± 10 beats should be

reported to the physician as well as symptoms such as syncope, dizziness, hiccoughs (diaphragmatic stimulation), dyspnea, chest pain, or fluid retention. No. 1 is incomplete. The second part of No. 2 refers to indicators of infection, and the second part of No. 3 indicates that the patient understands the battery pack has a limited life expectancy.

13. (2) Hypertension is considerably more severe in men than women and tends to occur more frequently at an earlier age. Currently it is estimated that 20 to 25 million Americans have hypertension, many of whom are undetected and untreated. This is due largely to the slow onset and lack of specific symptoms in its early stages. The prevalence of hypertension in every age group is higher for American blacks than whites. Likewise the severity of hypertension in black men is three times that in white men and the severity in black women is almost six times that experienced by white women. Mortality rates for the American black population with hypertension are twice that of the white hypertensive population. Hence Nos. 1, 3, and 4 are incorrect.

14. (1) Left ventricular enlargement is the physiologic adaptation to increasing peripheral resistance. As systemic pressures increase, the muscle mass increases in response to the excessive work load. This tends to displace the PMI to the left and inferiorly. Furthermore, prolonged hypertension may eventually cause deterioration and dilation of the left ventricle with increasing signs of cardiac failure, such as dyspnea on exertion, paroxysmal nocturnal dyspnea, tachycardia, and dependent edema. However, the shift itself is not indicative of cardiac decompensation since it is a normal finding for well-trained athletes. It is not a normal finding in less-active individuals. Right ventricular enlargement would shift the PMI toward the sternum. Hence Nos. 2, 3, and 4 are incorrect.

15. (1) During exercise there is a general increase in vasomotor tone, which increases venous return. To meet the increased metabolic needs of the body, the heart normally increases its rate and stroke volume. In Mr. Smith's case, left ventricular hypertrophy has compromised his heart's ability to increase its efficiency during exercise. Therefore, even though its rate is increased, the stroke volume does not increase sufficiently and the increased venous return tends to back up into the pulmonary vasculature. This results in the perception of increased work of breathing or shortness of breath. No. 2 is incorrect because venous return is increased with exercise. No. 3 is incorrect because asynergistic cardiac contractions occur when a portion of the heart is noncontractile, as with myocardial infarction with ventricular aneurysm. Mr. Smith's obesity and sedentary life style (No. 4) are *contributing* factors to physiologic phenomena underlying his symptoms.

16. (3) While local blood flow regulators (such as precapillary sphincters and tissue metabolism) tend to regulate blood flow over a period of time despite wide variations in pressure, in prolonged hypertension like Mr. Smith's, sclerosis of the arterial vasculature as well as venous congestion tend to decrease tissue perfusion as well as renal blood flow with resultant drop in glomerular filtration. These phenomena tend to increase interstitial edema in both the pulmonary and the systemic circulation. Cardiomegaly refers to cardiac enlargement as discussed in the earlier responses. Hence Nos. 1, 2, and 4 are incorrect.

17. (1) Arterial pressures are highest during systole or ejection phase of the cardiac cycle. This occurs between the closure of the AV valves (first heart sound) and closure of the semilunar valves (second heart sound). The QRS wave precedes or occurs concurrently with AV valve closure. It stimulates the isovolumetric phase of the cardiac cycle, which allows pressure to build in the ventricles until it overcomes the pressure in the aorta and pulmonary artery. During ventricular diastole, the relaxation phase between cardiac contractions, the pressures in both the aorta and pulmonary artery are at their lowest. Hence Nos. 2, 3, and 4 are incorrect.

18. (4) Hydrochlorothiazide is a thiazide diuretic that promotes the excretion of water, sodium, and chloride by inhibiting the reabsorption of sodium ions in the ascending limb of the loop of Henle and in the distal tubule of the nephron. Natriuresis promotes the secondary loss of potassium, thereby classifying this drug as potassium-wasting. Spironolactone is an example of an aldosterone inhibitor and is a potassium-sparing diuretic. Diamox is the most frequently employed carbonic anhydrase inhibitor. Hence Nos. 1, 2, and 3 are incorrect.

19. (3) See question 18 for the site of hydrochlorothiazide action in the kidney.

20. (3) Thiazide diuretics promote the excretion of sodium, chloride, bicarbonate, and potassium. However, chloride excretion tends to be proportionately greater than bicarbonate excretion so that therapy may result in hypochloremic alkalosis, not hyperchloremic acidosis. Hypokalemia may develop, especially with brisk diuresis. Supplemental KCl therapy and/or increased dietary intake of potassium is indicated with thiazide therapy. Other electrolyte imbalances include hyponatremia as well as hyperuricemia, which may precipitate frank gout. Nos. 1, 2, and 4 are known side effects.

21. (2) While the exact mechanisms of hydralazine activity is not known, its primary effect is the relaxation and dilation of arteriolar smooth muscle. A secondary effect of this vasodilation is increased renal blood flow and maintenance of glomerular filtration rate. In some

instances a marked increase in renal function has been noted, decreasing hypervolemia and blood pressure. No. 1 is incorrect because decreased renal blood flow and venous capacitance are circulatory mechanisms for maintaining blood pressure, as in hypovolemic shock. No. 3 is incorrect because it describes the action of reserpine (Serpasil). No. 4 describes the action of clonidine HCl (Catapres).

22. (3) Both systolic and diastolic pressure should decrease as the result of the pharmacologic interventions. Both the vasodilation and decrease in fluid volumes decrease peripheral resistance, thereby lowering the diastolic pressure. Systolic pressures should have a concomitant drop because the left ventricle is delivering its stroke volume at considerably less resistance. Hence Nos. 1, 2, and 4 are incorrect.

23. (2) Postural blood pressure readings are an excellent mode for assessing volume depletion. If the systolic blood pressure decreases more than 10 mm Hg and there is a concurrent increase in the pulse rate, a volume depletion problem is indicated. Urine output and specific gravity (No. 1) are better measures of the adequacy of fluid volume replacement than of fluid volume depletion. Comparing the prior and present weight of the patient (No. 3) will give you an estimate of the slow catabolism of body stores that occurs with this disease. There is no oral water test (No. 4).

24. (3) Decreased pulse rate and widened pulse pressure are not findings consistent with hypovolemia. While a widened pulse pressure might be expected with hypervolemia, pulse rates do not generally decrease. Decreased pulse rate and widened pulse pressure occur together with increased intracranial pressure. Nos. 1, 2, and 4 are consistent with hypovolemia.

25. (2) Weak, flaccid muscles and decreased and/or absent deep-tendon reflexes are findings consistent with hypokalemia or low potassium. Hypernatremia and hyperchloremia (Nos. 1 and 3) do not exert specific effects on the muscles. Hypernatremia is characterized by dry mucous membranes, confusion, and poor skin turgor. Hypocalcemia (No. 4) is characterized by increased muscle twitching, hyperactive reflexes, and tetany.

26. (3) Initial fluid therapy is directed toward increasing fluid volume and urine output. Once adequate urinary output has been established, potassium salts are added (No. 2) to relieve hypokalemia. The amount of added potassium chloride depends upon the extent of hypokalemia. No. 1 is a hypertonic solution that would act to increase intracellular dehydration and is therefore contraindicated. No. 4, distilled water, is a hypotonic solution; that is, it does not contain any additional electrolytes. Hypotonic solutions, such as 0.45% sodium chloride, are frequently given to relieve hypertonic

syndromes. However, distilled water is never given in fluid replacement therapy.

27. (4) Parenteral hyperalimentation solutions are hyperosmolar solutions containing amino acids, 10% to 25% glucose, multivitamins, and electrolytes. These solutions are administered through large veins such as the subclavian to avoid the inflammation or thrombosis that these hyperosmolar solutions tend to cause in peripheral veins. These solutions are given to patients with disturbances of ingestion, digestion or absorption that are combined with excessive catabolism. Nos. 1 and 3 are incorrect because they are not hyperosmolar fluids. No. 2 is partially correct in that hyperalimentation solutions are hypertonic; that is, they have an osmolarity greater than the plasma. However, the goal of hyperalimentation is not to reduce cellular swelling but to reverse negative nitrogen balance. Hypertonic solutions utilized to reduce cellular swelling are indicated in water intoxication and/or severe sodium depletion. Rapid infusion of hyperalimentation solution, however, will cause cellular dehydration.

28. (1) The primary effects of rapid infusion of hyperalimentation solutions are cellular dehydration due to osmosis of water from the cell in response to vascular hyperosmolarity; potassium depletion, hyperglycemia, and occasionally circulatory overload. When infusion rates are rapid, supplementary insulin should be administered to prevent the effects of hyperglycemia. Hypoglycemia may occur if the infusion rate is suddenly decreased because the body generally adapts to hyperosmolar solutions by increasing insulin release from the pancreas. Hence Nos. 2, 3, and 4 are incorrect.

29. (3) If the catheter insertion site remains dry, dressings are changed every 48 hours utilizing strict aseptic technique. Gloves and masks are used during the dressing change and while the IV tubing and filter are changed. Urine-testing is done to detect glycosuria. In the event glycosuria occurs, the physician should be notified. He/she may order insulin coverage or a decrease in the flow rate. Blood withdrawal and CVP readings are contraindicated because infusion rates must be kept constant in order to avoid the formation of clots in the catheter. Intake and output records as well as daily weights provide important measures of the effectiveness of the treatment and are good monitors of fluid balance. Hence Nos. 1, 2, and 4 are incorrect.

30. (2) Each of these interventions is appropriate in the preoperative period. However, research indicates that the best postoperative outcomes are related to the patient's preoperative anxiety levels. Patients who deny apprehension and refuse information as well as those who are highly anxious and who are unable to ask and/or assimilate information have the most difficult postsurgical course. Patients who are able to express their concerns and who are given emotional support as well as accurate, brief explanations tend to have less pain and fewer postoperative complications. Hence Nos. 1, 3, and 4 are incorrect.

31. (3) Neomycin is administered preoperatively because it is a poorly absorbed antibiotic and therefore is effective in reducing the number of intestinal organisms which may cause infection of the suture line. Neomycin is not effective in reducing postoperative atelectasis (No. 1). Prevention of atelectasis is dependent upon adequate pulmonary hygiene (deep breathing and coughing up of secretions) in the postoperative period. No. 2 is correct but not the *best* answer because the ability of the body to ward off infection is a result of the decrease in intestinal organisms. No. 4 is incorrect because bladder atony is generally due to decreased parasympathetic outflow and bladder tone secondary to anesthesia.

32. (2) The stoma drainage bag is applied in the operating room. Drainage from the ileostomy contains secretions that are rich in digestive enzymes and highly irritating to the skin. Protection of the skin from the effects of these enzymes is begun at once. Skin exposed to these enzymes even for a short time becomes reddened, painful, and excoriated. Hence Nos. 1, 3, and 4 are incorrect.

33. (3) Postoperatively the potential for severe fluid and electrolyte imbalances exists for several reasons: (a) the ileostomy drainage contains large amounts of sodium and water; (b) postsurgical diuresis increases both water and potassium excretion; and (c) nasogastric suction further decreases fluid and electrolytes by preventing their normal reabsorption. Nos. 1, 2, and 4 are also important measures in this patient's postoperative care; however, maintenance of fluid and electrolyte balance is most critical.

34. (4) It is important to recognize that the loss of anatomical integrity initiates a grieving process. Allowing the patient to express feelings of depression, apathy, or disinterest indicates that such feelings are acceptable and not uncommon. No. 1 is always appropriate and should be consistently carried out. However, in the situation depicted it would follow the verbalization of feelings. Nos. 2 and 3 are also alternatives that you may wish to employ after assessing the patient's major concerns.

35. (3) The primary objective of stoma care is to prevent skin irritation and excoriation. The stoma and surrounding skin should be washed with mild soap and water, rinsed thoroughly, and patted dry. The ostomy appliance should be fitted close to the stoma to further prevent skin irritation. A tight-fitting seal on the drainage bag and well-ventilated room will decrease odor problems. Likewise, a tight-fitting appliance will prevent contamination of the abdominal incision. While

fecal material is measured as output, this procedure is secondary to control of skin damage. Hence Nos. 1, 2, and 4 are incorrect.

36. (4) Abdominal cramps, vomiting, and watery or no discharge are signs of intestinal obstruction, a complication that requires immediate medical intervention. Nos. 1, 2, and 3 are incorrect not only because they can delay appropriate medical intervention, but because they also increase the risk of severe fluid and electrolyte imbalance. While obstruction of an ileostomy is a rare problem, a very small stoma or one that is contracted may need to be dilated regularly so that the little finger can be inserted easily.

37. (3) Breast self-examinations are best done the week following onset of menses. The breasts are then the softest and any lumps not associated with hormonal changes are more evident. Nos. 1 and 4 are incorrect because breast changes due to hormonal changes, such as fullness or tenderness, may occur at these times, obscuring possible pathology. No. 2 is a good idea (that is, having a regular time or pattern for examination) but does not take into account the normal breast tissue changes during the menstrual cycle.

38. (2) Denial is a very strong defense mechanism utilized to allay the emotional effects of discovering a potential threat. While denial has been found to be an effective mechanism for survival in some instances, such as during natural disasters, it may result in greater pathology in a woman with potential breast carcinoma. Nos. 1, 3, and 4 are also defense mechanisms; suppression occurs when the individual recognizes the threat but consciously refuses to think about it, repression is an unconscious mechanism that keeps the knowledge of the threat from coming to one's conscious awareness, and intellectualization occurs when the individual attempts to consciously allay anxiety by attributing symptoms to possible other causes such as cystic breast disease. However, the patient who intellectualizes does not attempt to deny the possibility that a more serious pathology may be present.

39. (4) It is not unusual for surgical patients, particularly those with tentative disfiguring surgeries, to be anxious on admission. Patients who are moderately to severely anxious need support in allaying their fears and in refocusing on the situation. Sitting down with the patient and establishing eye contact in a nonhurried, relaxed manner may enable the patient to verbalize these concerns and gives the nurse an opportunity to clarify misconceptions, assess particular needs, and begin planning appropriate interventions, such as a visit from a member of the ostomy club. Nos. 1, 2, and 3 are incorrect because these are approaches that may be utilized by a nurse who is in fact denying her own fears about this surgery and defending herself against becoming too involved.

40. (1) Anxiety, like pain, glucose imbalance, or changes in blood pressure, stimulates discharge of the sympathetic nervous system. In some patients this increased adrenergic discharge results in moderate to severe increases in systolic and diastolic pressures that decrease to normal levels when emotional equilibrium is restored. Mrs. Washington may be emotionally labile (No. 2), but at this time there is insufficient data to make this judgement. Mrs. Washington is fearful, but that does not mean she is unprepared for this surgery (No. 3). Should her anxiety remain high, however, the attending physician should be notified. While Mrs. Washington may be attempting to employ denial ("I only have a cyst") her emotional response (restlessness and increased blood pressure) indicates this defense mechanism is ineffective in allaying her present anxieties (No. 4).

41. (4) Repeating breathing exercises until light-headed is inappropriate. It indicates hyperventilation, which may lead to tetany due to loss of volatile hydrogen ions. Patients should, however, be able to supply a rationale for deep breathing and coughing techniques as well as demonstrate them correctly. Nos. 1, 2, and 3 are desirable outcomes.

42. (3) Skin preps are designed primarily to reduce the occurrence of postoperative infections by reducing the number of microorganisms on the skin and by removing any hair that may tend to harbor these organisms. Skin preps do not sterilize the skin or kill all the microorganisms (No. 2). Nos. 1 and 4 are secondary objectives of a skin prep.

43. (2) Before any operative procedure can proceed, however minor, a voluntary, informed consent must be given. Before initiating preoperative care, charts should be checked first for operative consent, second for laboratory results (noting any abnormalities), and third for the time and type of preoperative medication. Finally, check to be sure the patient has been placed on the NPO list and follow this up by checking for the sign on her bed when you go to assist her in preparing for surgery. Hence Nos. 1, 3, and 4 are incorrect.

44. (2) In the short time available before surgery, the patient should be allowed to voice her concerns and should be given any needed support. However, time will not permit an extensive exploration of the basis of her concerns. Nos. 1, 3, and 4 are standard preoperative nursing procedures.

45. (2) To reduce anxiety and ensure ease of induction, a preoperative medication should be administered 45 to 60 minutes prior to anesthesia. Siderails should be raised after administration of medication, as the patient will begin to feel drowsy and light-headed. Giving medication earlier, as in Nos. 1, 3, and 4, would not allow sufficient time for the medication to reach its peak effect.

46. (3) Correct medication administration is exceedingly important. When the medication order is of a different strength from the supplies at hand, employing the following formula will be helpful in determining the correct dose.

$$\frac{\text{Desired}}{\text{Available}} \times \text{Quantity} = \frac{.04}{.06} \times \frac{15\,\text{minims}}{1}$$

$$= \frac{2}{3} \times \frac{15}{1}$$

$$= \frac{30}{3}$$

$$= 10\,\text{minims}$$

47. (2) The desired effect of morphine in this situation is to reduce sensitivity to stimuli in order to allay apprehension and in some cases to induce drowsiness. Atropine acts to dry oral and bronchial secretions, reducing the hazards of aspirations during anesthetic induction. While morphine effectively relieves pain, pain relief is usually not an objective in administering a preoperative medication. Hence Nos. 1, 3, and 4 are incorrect.

48. (3) Morphine sulfate acts not only to reduce pain and anxiety by blocking the activity of the reticular substance in the brain stem, but it also relaxes vascular smooth muscle, thereby decreasing blood pressure (not increasing it as in No. 2). Nausea and vomiting are common adverse side effects of this medication. Atropine is an anticholinergic whose drying effects tend to cause the patient to complain that his mouth feels like cotton. Atropine also blocks vagal effects on the heart, increasing pulse rate (not decreasing it as in Nos. 1 and 4). Atropine also causes pupillary dilatation, not constriction.

49. (4) The patient should be encouraged to void before administration of the preoperative medication. Once the medication has been given, safety needs of the patient dictate the use of a bedpan if the patient again needs to void. Nos. 1, 2, and 3 are all proper safety procedures after administration of medication.

50. (2) After the patient has left for surgery, family members should be told the approximate time the patient will be in surgery and that from there the patient will go to the recovery room until awake and all vital signs are stable. Clarify that delays may occur and that the induction of as well as the emergence from anesthesia take time. Allow family members to decide whether they will stay or go and come back later. If family members decide to wait, direct them to a waiting area where they can be comfortable. Assure them that you will direct the surgeon to them after the surgery is finished. Answer any questions and/or concerns the family members may have, being as supportive as possible. Hence Nos. 1, 3, and 4 are incorrect.

51. (2) Modified radical mastectomies consist of removal of the breast and all or selected lymph nodes and, on rare occasions, partial removal of muscle. No. 1 is an example of a simple mastectomy, No. 3, of the classical radical mastectomy, and No. 4, of a supraradical mastectomy.

52. (2) Anesthesia is divided into four stages. Most surgical procedures are carried out in Stage III, during which time the patient is unconscious and her reflexes are depressed. As the patient eliminates the anesthetic agent, she goes into Stage II, which is the stage of delirium or excitement. Respirations are exaggerated and irregular, and muscle tone is increased. To prevent injury during this stage, nursing measures are designed to reduce stimulation by maintaining a quiet, well-regulated environment. No. 1 is incorrect because continued stimulation will only increase restlessness. Pain medication as in No. 3 may delay elimination of the anesthetic secondary to decreased respiratory excursion. While nail beds should always be checked for signs of hypoxia, cyanosis (No. 4) only occurs with severe respiratory depression.

53. (1) The airway should remain in place and the patient's head turned to the side to prevent obstruction of the airway by the tongue and to allow secretions to drain from the mouth. The airway should never be removed until the patient is alert enough to begin attempting to eject it herself. Leaving the airway in after this point may cause vomiting due to stimulation of the gag reflex. Hence Nos. 2, 3, and 4 are incorrect.

54. (2) A drop in the systolic blood pressure of 20 mm Hg or more below preoperative blood pressure readings is indicative of impending shock. Shock may be due to hemorrhage, vasodilation caused by anesthesia, insufficient fluid replacement, or abnormal clotting. Skin may be dry and cool (No. 1) in the immediate postoperative period because of normal temperature-regulating mechanisms, that is, vasoconstriction due to skin exposure in the operating room. A diastolic reading below 70 mm Hg (No. 3) is significant only if it is abnormal for the patient and is accompanied by a drop in systolic or a narrowing pulse pressure. Pulse rates normally increase and decrease with respirations to some extent (No. 4) because changes in intrathoracic pressures affect venous return. This phenomenon, however, is more evident in children.

55. (3) Some of the most serious reactions occurring with blood transfusions are the result of human error. To reduce human error, it is essential for two nurses to verify that the patient's name and hospital number on the blood bag correspond *exactly* to that on her wrist band. Nos. 1, 2, and 4, while all proper safeguards, are not first in priority.

56. (1) The earliest indications of blood transfusion reactions are headache, chills, and elevation of temperature. The skin may also become pale and cool, and hypotension may develop quickly. Respirations gen-

erally increase in rate and depth. Wheezing and urticaria (No. 3) may occur. Late signs of transfusion reaction are oliguria and jaundice (No. 4) secondary to hemolysis of red blood cells. Should symptoms occur, stop transfusion, notify physician, and send a STAT urine specimen to the lab for analysis. Hypertension and flushing are not indicators of a transfusion reaction (No. 2).

57. (3) The Hemovac is a portable suction that provides low negative pressure (30–45 mm Hg) to gently remove excess fluid and debris from the wound. It does not require attachment to any other suction system. Nos. 1, 2, and 4 are standard nursing measures.

58. (3) The primary advantage of Hemovac suction is that it removes excess fluid and debris from the wound site that could retard tissue granulation and healing. If serum is allowed to accumulate under the skin, the pressure can cause sloughing of tissue flaps. The Hemovac exerts low, even pressure, which makes No. 1 incorrect. The Hemovac is also lightweight (No. 2), which is an advantage in postoperative ambulation, but not its primary advantage. Likewise, the removal of excess sera reduces the likelihood of postoperative infection (No. 4), but this is a secondary advantage.

59. (3) Tight pressure dressing, discomfort, and fear of tearing the incision tend to limit chest expansion and the patient's willingness to cough. The nurse can assist the patient in this procedure by helping her sit upright and by supporting both the anterior and posterior chest wall at the incisional site with her hand. Frequent turning will also facilitate mobilization of secretion and the prevention of atelectasis. Hence Nos. 1, 2, and 4 are incorrect.

60. (3) Pressure dressings are never removed but, if saturated, should be reinforced with sterile dressings. The possibility of hemorrhage is everpresent, and signs of increased bleeding should be immediately reported to the surgeon. This is not a normal occurrence. Vital signs and Hemovac drainage and function should also be assessed. Hence Nos. 1, 2, and 4 are incorrect.

61. (2) The head slightly elevated, the legs elevated in a straight line, and the trunk horizontal improve venous return to the heart and prevent abdominal viscera from impinging on the diaphragm. The Trendelenburg position (No. 3), after initially increasing blood flow to the brain, initiates a reflex mechanism that causes cerebral vasoconstriction. Wrapping the patient in blankets (No. 4) will cause dilatation of the peripheral vasculature, which will further decrease venous return. Oxygen administration (No. 1) may have a palliative effect but does not affect venous return.

62. (2) Low- to semi-Fowler's position with the arm elevated on pillows so that the wrist and elbow are slightly higher than the shoulder best facilitates venous return, reducing the occurrence of edema. Some physicians may order that the patient be positioned so that the hand is raised above the head. Nos. 1, 3, and 4 are either incorrect or less desirable because venous return is not enhanced or possible muscle contractures may develop.

63. (2) The earliest exercises initiated are passive range of motion of the elbow, wrist, and hand, which are begun on the first postoperative day. As the patient is able, she is encouraged to put these joints through active range of motion. These exercises assist in maintaining function and in reducing lymphedema. Progression to other exercises such as hair-combing and wall-reaching is dependent upon wound-healing, grafts, presence of drainage tubes, and the patient's tolerance. Nos. 1, 3, and 4 are exercises implemented after radical mastectomy, but are not appropriate initial therapy.

64. (2) Prior to administering any narcotic, the nurse should assess the type, location, and intensity of pain as well as factors that seem to precipitate or relieve it. Based on this information, it is then possible to decide whether the patient needs supportive measures (such as a back rub or position change as in No. 4), the bedpan, and/or the administration of a narcotic. Meperidine, like morphine, does have a hypotensive effect. However, it is not a respiratory depressant like morphine. Generally it is not necessary to take vital signs before administering narcotics (No. 1). Pain and discomfort are subjective symptoms that are always real to the patient (No. 3).

65. (3) Splinting of the incision as well as tight pressure dressings tend to reduce lung expansion and ventilation. As a result, mucus can block off small bronchioles causing atelectasis or collapse of distal alveoli. Peripheral thrombophlebitis (No. 1) is always a threat if the patient's legs are not exercised. In most patients early ambulation prevents its occurrence. Wound dehiscence and paralytic ileus are more likely to occur with abdominal surgeries though paralytic ileus (Nos. 2 and 4) may occur as the result of the effects of anesthesia on autonomic nervous system function or hypokalemia.

66. (4) Initial intervention when patients are reacting to the loss of a significant body part is to encourage verbalization of their fears and to assist them in identifying how they see the change in their body image as well as how it may affect their marriage relationship. One of the most important factors in the mastectomy patient's response to surgery is the reaction of her husband or the man with whom she is intimately involved. Many men are very supportive, others are not. It is therefore also important to assist the male to acknowledge his feelings and concerns (No. 3). The patient needs the reassurance of his love and support to work through her own emotional reaction and begin the work of recovery. Nos. 1 and 2 tend to cut off communication in this instance.

67. (2) Carrying any heavy object such as groceries or even a purse on the affected side may increase the occurrence of lymphedema. Wearing gloves for household tasks or gardening (No. 1) is encouraged to prevent lymphedema and/or possible infection if the skin is broken. Elasticized sleeves (No. 3) may be worn if they are not tight. However, any constricting garment or jewelry should be avoided. Driving (No. 4), particularly if the affected arm is kept high on the steering wheel, should not increase lymphedema.

68. (2) Rhonchi and wheezes occur when there is partial obstruction of the bronchi or bronchioles. These sounds occur due to the increased vibration of air molecules as they pass over these obstructions. No. 1 is incorrect because total obstruction would produce no sounds. No. 3 is incorrect because the sounds produced by fluid in the alveoli are finer, less harsh sounds generally referred to as rales. No. 4 is incorrect because inflammation of the pleura creates a grating sound referred to as a friction rub.

69. (2) Bronchoscopy provides direct visualization of the airways by utilizing a long, slender, hollow instrument through which a light is reflected. Bronchoscopy can be utilized for diagnostic purposes, for removal of foreign objects, for removal of mucus plugs, and/or for obtaining a biopsy or bronchial washings for cytology. No. 1 is an example of a fluoroscopic exam. No. 3 characterizes a bronchogram and No. 4, a lung biopsy.

70. (2) After bronchoscopy the patient generally produces a large amount of sputum that must be observed carefully for signs of hemorrhage, particularly if a biopsy has been taken during the procedure. While the sputum is generally blood-streaked, any pronounced bleeding should be reported immediately. Nos. 1 and 3 are also observations made after a bronchoscopy. Vital signs are observed until stable, and food and fluids are withheld until the gag reflex returns. No. 4, urticaria, does not occur following bronchoscopy, though it may after a bronchogram if the patient reacts to the iodine-based dye.

71. (1) Dyspnea is a term utilized to describe the patient's subjective awareness of increased respiratory effort. The increased work of breathing may indeed be related to alveolar hypoventilation (No. 2) and/or exercise (No. 4), which result in an increased rate and depth of respiration (No. 3).

72. (2) Postoperatively, deep breathing and particularly coughing up of sputum are the most important activities engaged in by the patient with chest surgery. These activities reduce bronchotracheal secretions, prevent atelectasis, and promote adequate ventilation. While Nos. 1 and 3 are also important in preventing postop-

erative complication, airway integrity is always the first priority. No. 4 is employed for patients having herniorrhaphies.

73. (4) The rationale for turning, coughing, and deep breathing every one to two hours is to rid the lungs of the side effects of anesthesia. Inhalant anesthetics, like cigarette smoke, irritate the mucous membranes lining the bronchi, increasing mucous production. It is exceedingly important that the patient understand that these activities are important in mobilizing and removing these excess secretions. Failure to remove them may lead to atelectasis or hypostatic pneumonias. Nos. 1, 2, and 3 are all appropriate interventions.

74. (2) Mr. Chen has a space-occupying lesion, residual symptoms of pneumonia, and tachypnea. Space-occupying lesions and pneumonia tend to decrease vital capacity by reducing inspiratory capacity. In order to maintain arterial oxygen levels the respiratory rate is increased, which results in excess CO_2 excretion by the lungs (respiratory alkalosis). It is important to remember that patients can be hypoxic ($\downarrow PO_2$) but not hypercapnic ($\uparrow CO_2$—respiratory acidosis) because of the facility with which carbon dioxide passes through the respiratory membrane. No. 1 is incorrect because Mr. Chen's pathology tends to decrease, not increase, vital capacity. The total lung capacity (No. 3) is usually increased with the hyperinflation of obstructive airway disease. Even though Mr. Chen has an extensive smoking history, neither his health history nor his physical assessment findings indicate hyperinflation (chronic cough, barrel chest). No. 4 is partially correct and partially incorrect. With extensive rhonchi and wheezes one would expect a slight to moderate decrease in the forced expiratory volume in one second (FEV_1); however, Mr. Chen's respiratory rate and lack of other symptoms (lethargy, easy fatigue) tend to contradict the occurrence of respiratory acidosis.

75. (3) The purpose of the incentive spirometer is to encourage deep breathing. The patient is able to directly visualize his progress by the number and height of balls he is able to raise. After-effects of this activity may indeed be coughing up of sputum (No. 1) and arousal (No. 2) as the patient competes with himself. Incentive spirometry can be used as a rough measure of tidal volume and expiratory reserve volume (No. 4) since the patient breathes in deeply and exhales completely into the incentive spirometer.

76. (2) The primary purpose of the water-seal drainage system is to remove excess fluid and air from the pleural space, thereby speeding reinflation of the lung, reestablishing normal negative intrapleural pressure, and preventing the development of pneumothorax in the unaffected lung. Secondarily, water-seal drainage enables the nurse to monitor blood loss. Nos. 1 and 3 are incorrect since both are opposite effects of those

intended. No. 4 is incorrect because atelectasis is caused by insufficient removal of secretions from the bronchial tree.

77. (4) In a two-bottle, water-sealed drainage system the first bottle, the one proximal to the patient, collects the drainage from the chest tubes. The first bottle is attached to the second bottle by a short tube. In the second bottle there is also a long glass tube that is open to the atmospheric air at the top and submerged below the water on the bottom. It is the distance this tube is submerged below the water that determines the amount of pressure exerted on the intrapleural space. In some instances the second bottle may have a third tube attached to suction. Nos. 1 and 2 are incorrect because the first bottle is the drainage bottle. No. 3 is incorrect because, with the exception of the Pleuro-Vac system (which has a mechanism for removing specimens without interfering with the suction), the water-sealed drainage system is never opened.

78. (4) Your first nursing measure should be to mark the time and amount of drainage in the collection bottle to assure a baseline measurement for further observations. Your next measure is to secure the tubes to the bed linen (No. 3) in order to prevent kinking or unnecessary looping of the drainage tubes, which would hinder the flow of air and fluid. The milking of chest tubes (No. 1) is a matter of debate at this time. While the process of stripping or milking does assist in the removal of fibrin and clots from the chest tubes, compression of the tubes also increases intrapleural pressures by preventing the movement of air and fluid. Whether the chest tubes are milked or not will depend upon institutional or individual physician's policies. No. 2 is incorrect because the drainage system is always kept in a dependent position to maintain gravity flow of air and fluids.

79. (1) Fluid in the long tube of the suction bottle will cease to fluctuate when the tubing is plugged by fibrin or a clot and/or when negative intrapleural pressures have been reestablished and the lung has reexpanded. The likelihood of lung reexpansion on the second postoperative day is quite small. Therefore it is necessary to check the tubing for fibrin, clots, or severe kinking. If the tubing is kinked it needs to be repositioned. Milking of the tube may be ordered if fibrin or clots are suspected. No. 2 is incorrect because an air leak is indicated by bubbling in the water-sealed suction bottle. Pulmonary edema (No. 3) would be reflected by dyspnea, orthopnea, rales, and pink, frothy sputum. No. 4 is not entirely incorrect since the patient's position may be such that the chest tubes are unnecessarily looped or kinked and repositioning the patient may facilitate flow. However, it is not the best answer.

80. (2) Humidification of oxygen is extremely important

in reducing its drying effects on the mucous membranes of the bronchial tree. Humidification of oxygen is generally provided by a water nebulizer. Nos. 1, 3, and 4 are incorrect because oxygen is not highly permeable in water, thus water tends to inhibit rather than facilitate oxygen diffusion across the respiratory membrane. Humidification expands the volume of the inhaled gas but by doing so decreases the partial pressure of the gas in the alveoli. Normal alveolar partial pressures of oxygen are approximately 100 mm Hg, whereas the partial pressures of oxygen in the atmosphere are approximately 135 mm Hg.

81. (3) Maintenance of infusion rates as ordered is extremely important. In this example, you can use the following equation:

$$\frac{\text{gtts/ml of given set}}{60\,(\text{minutes/hr})} \times \text{total hourly volume} = \text{gtts/min}$$

or

$$\frac{12}{60} \times \frac{1000}{10} = \frac{1}{5} \times \frac{100}{1} = 20\,\text{gtts/min}$$

82. (1) Intermittent positive-pressure breathing (IPPB) facilitates the flow of air deep into the lungs by exerting pressures greater than atmospheric pressures (positive pressure) on inspiration. The patient needs to learn to take slow, controlled inspirations to prevent hyperventilation. Nos. 2, 3, and 4 are incorrect because negative inspiratory pressures would reduce inflow of air, positive expiratory pressures are consistent with CPAP or PEEP ventilatory systems, and pressures normally become more negative as the patient exhales.

83. (2) Arm exercises are initiated to prevent ankylosis of the shoulder. Most patients tend to splint incisional discomfort by limiting movement on the affected side. This protective mechanism may lead to "frozen shoulder" or ankylosis. Therefore, it is important to initiate movement early to maintain muscle tone and joint integrity. No. 1 is an example of wrist drop due to poor positioning of wrist joints. No. 3 is usually a normal finding, although it may occur with improper positioning with upper motor neuron lesions. Intercostal muscle spasticity (No. 4) is rare and is not due to positioning.

84. (4) Current practice precludes the clamping of the chest tubes (No. 3) or their removal from the water-sealed drainage system for any reason (No. 1). It is believed that clamping increases the risk of a tension pneumothorax because air may enter the intrapleural space during inspiration but cannot escape during expiration. Likewise, removing the chest tubes from the suction drainage system (No. 2) will result in an equalization of intrapleural pressures, with atmo-

spheric pressures thus also increasing the risk of pneumothorax. Chest tubes are not removed to facilitate transportation of the patient; they are removed only after the physician is satisfied with the degree of reexpansion.

85. (3) The basic pathology in diabetes is failure of the beta cells in the islets of Langerhans to produce insulin in sufficient quantities or at all. This results in hyperglycemia. As the maximum transport of glucose in the renal tubules is surpassed, glucose concentrations increase and an osmotic diuresis with sodium depletion ensues. Inadequate glucagon secretion by the alpha cells of the islets of Langerhans results in decreased glycogenolysis and decreased blood glucose. Hence, No. 1 is a result of diabetes mellitus and Nos. 2 and 4 are incorrect.

86. (2) The conversion of fats and proteins into a source of energy is called gluconeogenesis. Normally this phenomenon is called into play when serum glucose and liver glycogen stores are decreased. In diabetes, this process is instigated by the inability of the cells to utilize glucose. It has two adverse effects: it increases blood glucose levels by converting proteins and fats into glucose, and it increases the breakdown of fats into glycerol and fatty acids. Oxidation of fatty acids results in the formation of ketone bodies. Excessive accumulation of these products in the blood causes a form of metabolic acidosis known as ketoacidosis. Glycogenolysis (No. 1) is the conversion of glycogen to glucose. Glucosuria (No. 3) is glucose in the urine and ketogenesis (No. 4) is the process of converting fats into glycerol and fatty acids.

87. (1) Both emotional and physical stress increase the levels of circulating epinephrine. This hormone acts to increase glycogenolysis in the liver, which raises serum glucose levels and results in glucosuria. Early-morning urines (No. 2) are not usually elevated because insulin levels of the previous morning are generally sufficient to cover the evening meal. While Miss Marble's NPH insulin may need to be supplemented during her postoperative course (No. 3), generally the patient returns to his/her usual dosage during convalescence. Glomerulo-filtration (No. 4) is usually less at night because of the decrease in metabolic rate and blood pressure during sleep.

88. (2) Normal fasting serum glucose levels are 60–100 mg/100 ml of blood. Levels below 60 indicate hypoglycemia, levels above 120 mg/100 indicate hyperglycemia. Hence, Nos. 1, 3, and 4 are incorrect.

89. (1) When excessive quantities of fatty acids are oxidized, blood buffer systems may become exhausted. Ketoacidosis develops and acetone bodies are excreted in the urine. In an emergency room situation, diabetic acidosis can be recognized not only by the increased

rate and depth of respirations (Kussmaul's respirations) but by the odor of acetone on the breath. Neither osmotic diuresis (No. 2) nor failure in the sodium-hydrogen ion exchange mechanism (No. 3) causes acetonuria. In the latter case failure to excrete excess hydrogen ions would decrease urinary acids. Volatile hydrogen ions (CO_2) are excreted by the lungs; a decrease in nonvolatile hydrogen ions in the glomerular filtrate (No. 4) would move the pH of the urine toward the alkaline side.

90. (2) Miss Marble is demonstrating early signs of diabetic acidosis. Before notifying the physician (No. 1) it is necessary to collect the data, urine sugar and acetone, on which the physician will base the insulin order. The physician should also be notified of Miss Marble's vital signs and intake and output. Generally, urinary output is depressed for about 36 hours after surgery due to increased circulating levels of ADH. Given that Miss Marble has also had insensible water loss (respirations and perspiration), her assessment data strongly indicates dehydration or hypovolemia. The physician may order an increase in the amount and rate of intravenous fluids (contrary to No. 4). An antiemetic may be administered if nausea persists after blood sugar and fluid balance are rectified (No. 3).

91. (2) Miss Marble's vital signs and urine output reflect a decrease in extracellular volume secondary to osmotic diuresis. Increased ADH release decreases urinary output (No. 1). A hypo-osmolar fluid imbalance is one in which there is more water than solute in the extracellular fluid compartment (No. 3). Like circulatory overload (No. 4), symptoms of a hypo-osmolar imbalance include widened pulse pressure, increased blood pressure, distended neck veins, and respiratory rales.

92. (3) Glycogenolysis and therefore serum glucose levels are increased due to the stresses of surgery. In order to control blood glucose levels and prevent ketoacidosis, secondary to increased tissue metabolism (No. 2), regular insulin is given in doses adjusted according to the results of urine tests (rainbow or sliding scale). Regular insulin may be given alone until urine tests for glucosuria and ketonuria stabilize or as a supplement along with an intermediate-acting insulin such as NPH. No. 3, decreased insulin production, results from the extent of Miss Marble's dysfunction, not the stress of surgery. Insulin does facilitate the movement (No. 4) of potassium across the cellular membrane, thus preventing hyperkalemia, but this is not the *best* answer.

93. (2) NPH is an intermediate-acting insulin with an onset time of two hours, peak action in 6–12 hours, and a duration of action of 24 hours. Hence, Nos. 1, 3, and 4 are incorrect.

94. (3) The patient receiving NPH insulin is most likely to experience a hypoglycemic reaction in the late afternoon. Several factors may be involved, such as increased physical activity and/or inadequate dietary intake. Patient should be instructed to carry gumdrops or Lifesavers as a source of quickly absorbed carbohydrates should symptoms occur. Nos. 1, 2, and 4 are not as likely.

95. (3) Hypoglycemic or insulin reactions are the result of decreased circulatory serum glucose to the brain. This stimulates epinephrine release. Early symptoms include cold, clammy skin, nervousness, tremors, numbness of the hands or around the lips, and cardiac palpitations. Later symptoms may mimic alcoholic intoxication, such as staggering gait, slurring of words, combative behavior, or uncontrolled weeping. As hypoglycemia deepens the patient may develop convulsions and coma. Nos. 1, 2, and 4 are symptoms of ketoacidosis, which acts to depress the central nervous system.

96. (3) See rationale for question 95 above. No. 1 is incorrect in that respirations in insulin shock, while shallow, are increased. No. 2 is incorrect because the breath of the patient in insulin shock is noncontributory, not fetid. Fetid breath may occur with liver failure or poor dental hygiene. In No. 4 behavioral responses are switched, that is, confusion and lethargy are common with ketoacidosis and cold, clammy skin is consistent with insulin shock.

97. (2) The glucose tolerance test. Procedurally, the patient consumes a high-carbohydrate diet for three days before the test. All drugs that may influence the test are discontinued during this period (oral contraceptives, aspirin, steroids). On the day of the test a fasting blood sugar (No. 1) and urine are collected before the test as controls. After ingestion of a glucose load, specimens of blood and urine are collected at hourly intervals for three hours. In diabetes mellitus, glucose levels are elevated. The postprandial blood glucose (No. 3) is determined by giving the patient an oral glucose load only. Blood glucose levels are then evaluated in two hours. Usually glucose levels will return to normal during this period of time (No. 4). The tolbutamide response test may also be utilized to confirm diabetes. After fasting overnight, a baseline FBS is drawn. Intravenous tolbutamide is then given and blood samples drawn in 20–30 minutes. After this test the patient should be given orange juice and instructed to eat breakfast.

98. (3) Within three hours the patient's serum glucose levels should not only have returned to normal, but some hypoglycemia should be expected. Nos. 1, 2, and 4 are incorrect.

99. (3) A diabetic's diet is most often based on an exchange system. Foodstuffs in this system are divided into six types. Foods from within each list can be substituted for another in the same list because they have approx-

imately the same food value. Peanut butter is in the meat exchange list, as is cottage cheese, and therefore these can be substituted for one another. Cream cheese and butter (Nos. 2 and 4) are considered fats, and whole milk (No. 1) is on the milk exchange list.

100. (2) Given Miss Marble's food allowances, all these foods would be allowed except for the Coca-Cola. All concentrated sweets and regular soft drinks are contraindicated on a diabetic diet. Hence Nos. 1, 3, and 4 are incorrect.

101. (1) Emergency surgery must be performed in order to save the life of the patient, save the function of an organ or limb, remove a damaged organ or limb, or stop hemorrhage. Few emergency situations are so urgent as to require immediate response, eliminating the necessary laboratory data to evaluate the patient's physiologic response to the situation. However, true emergency situations cannot be postponed to the following surgical day. Hence Nos. 2, 3, and 4 are incorrect.

102. (4) An abdominal hysterectomy is generally the treatment of choice for uterine fibroids with excessive vaginal bleeding. If the ovaries are not pathologic there is no reason for surgical removal. A vaginal hysterectomy (No. 2) is the treatment of choice for a prolapsed uterus, and a D & C (No. 3) is primarily a diagnostic tool, not a measure to control excessive uterine bleeding. No. 1, panabdominal hysterectomy, involves the removal of the uterus, Fallopian tubes, and ovaries and is usually performed for extensive endometriosis or carcinoma.

103. (2) Few surgeries warrant immediate treatment; however, the urgency of the situation does decrease patient preparation time. Consequently, the patients' physiologic stress increases, placing greater demands on their metabolic functions and increasing the risk of complications. Emergency surgery does not compromise the use of general anesthesia. It is imperative to ascertain before an emergency surgery the time, type, and amount of the last oral intake, as gastric lavage or suctioning may be necessary to prevent aspiration during the surgery. Generally patients are NPO twelve hours before surgery. Hence, Nos. 1, 3, and 4 are incorrect.

104. (1) Anticoagulants increase bleeding time and tendency toward hemorrhage. Antihypertensives such as reserpine, hydralazine, and methyldopa potentiate the hypotensive effects of anesthetic agents, thereby creating problems with maintenance of blood pressure. Thiazide diuretics may induce potassium depletion and lead to respiratory depression during anesthesia. Nos. 2, 3, and 4 are incorrect because neither insulin, digoxin, nor vitamins and minerals potentiate the central nervous system depression due to anesthesia.

105. (3) The initial response would be to notify the physician of the critical hemoglobin (oxygen-carrying pro-

tein) level. A hemoglobin of 10 mg% is desirable for the patient, decreasing the deleterious risks of general anesthetic and hypovolemic shock. Most likely a blood transfusion will be ordered before surgery (No. 2). Your actions are then charted on the nurses' notes (No. 4) and the lab slip is attached to the chart (No. 1).

106. (3) Manipulation of abdominal contents during surgery produces inhibition of peristalsis for 24 to 48 hours. Measures to avoid potential distention could include insertion of a nasogastric tube before surgery and continuous postsurgical suction until peristalsis returns; rectal tubes can be inserted to remove excess air in lower colon; and early ambulation promotes return of gastrointestinal functioning. Auscultation of the abdomen for return of bowel sounds will be necessary in assessing the return and degree of peristalsis, at which time oral intake may be started. Abdominal massage is not recommended. Hence Nos. 1, 2, and 4 are incorrect.

107. (1) Sitting for long periods of time and/or wearing constrictive clothing tend to increase pelvic congestion. Paced and gradual ambulation aids in increasing venous return and general strength. Lifting of heavy objects and early sexual activity may injure the incision site and promote bleeding. Therefore it is important to reinforce the physician's instructions that sexual activity may be resumed within a specific period of time (usually six to eight weeks). Hence, Nos. 2, 3, and 4 are incorrect.

108. (3) Following a hysterectomy the vaginal flow is usually brownish in nature and will gradually diminish and cease. If the flow continues and is obviously red in nature, the physician must be notified. These signs could indicate a bleeding vessel. Once the uterus is removed, the patient is infertile and contraception is not necessary. Hence Nos. 1, 2, and 4 should be included in the teaching plan.

109. (3) It is not uncommon for a patient to feel that she will no longer be able to fulfill her role and needs as a woman following a hysterectomy. Verbalization of feelings allows the nurse to assess the patient's coping mechanisms and encourages the patient to deal with her emotional response. No. 3 is an open-ended question that allows the patient room to respond. No. 4 would be appropriate after the patient has aired her feelings. Nos. 1 and 2 avoid the problem initially. No. 2 may be appropriate if, after talking to the patient, you assess that the patient's responses represent a more significant or deep-seated problem.

110. (2) Second-degree burns involve both the epidermis and some of the dermis. They have a pink-red appearance and are characterized by moisture or blisters. Second-degree burns are very painful, as nerve endings remain and may be exposed to the air. A first-degree

burn involves the epidermis (No. 1). An example is sunburn: the skin is usually red and dry. In third-degree burns, subcutaneous tissue, muscle and even bone are also involved (Nos. 3 and 4). Typically, a third-degree burn is white, gray, or charred in color and is dry and leathery in appearance. Nerve endings have been destroyed so the area is painless.

111. (3) Critical burns are classified as second degree over 30% of the body and/or third degree over 10% of the body. Extensive burns involving the face, hands, and feet or those associated with respiratory injuries are also considered critical. The most frequently used method of calculating the extent of a burn is called the "rule of nines." While this method is fairly simple to apply, it is somewhat inaccurate. This is particularly true when it is applied to children, because allowances are not made for the proportional differences in head and extremity size between children and adults. Hence Nos. 1, 2, and 4 are incorrect.

112. (2) Age is important baseline data because rate of infusion of IVs to maintain appropriate quantity and specific gravity of urinary output differs; for example, 10 to 20 ml/h for infant versus 50 to 70 ml/h for adults. Weight is significant if the Evans or Brooke formulas are used for fluid replacement therapy. Both these formulas utilize both the size of the burn and the weight of the patient to calculate the amount of fluid to be replaced. Vital signs and skin turgor are both important measures of the degree or extent of hypovolemia. As dehydration develops, skin turgor becomes poor, mucous membranes dry, and the eyeballs feel soft. Likewise, the pulse may become thready and the blood pressure may decrease. Level of mentation is less helpful in this particular situation because of the fear, pain, and acute anxiety experienced by some patients. Quantity and specific gravity of urine output is an important assessment of the adequacy of fluid replacement, rather than part of the initial assessment. Hence Nos. 1, 3, and 4 are incorrect.

113. (1) The hypovolemia and shock that accompany burns greatly increase the body's stress response. Increased serum levels of norepinephrine, epinephrine, and aldosterone facilitate venous return and thus assist in maintaining cardiac output and blood pressure. The pituitary is also stimulated in the stress response to increase circulating levels of ADH (decreases water output) and cortisol. Increased levels of the latter hormone are implicated in the development of Curling's ulcer (stress ulcer), which patients of all ages and with both minor and major burns may develop. Generally, milk and antacids are used to reduce its occurrence. No. 2 is incorrect because negative ion balance occurs due to protein mobilization for healing. Patients with burns are given high-protein, high-calorie meals as well as supplemental vitamins to promote wound-heal-

ing. No. 3 is incorrect because hemolysis of red blood cells and decreased hematocrit are primarily due to the injury itself rather than to epinephrine agglutination. In thermal burns up to 40% of the red blood cell mass may be hemolyzed. Hypothermia is a problem in the postburn period but is the result of the loss of skin areas; hence No. 4 is incorrect. The patient treated by the open or exposed method of burn therapy is particularly susceptible to chilling. Increased thermostat settings and radiant heat lamps may be employed to aid in maintaining normal body temperature.

114. (2) Aldosterone secretion by the adrenal cortex is stimulated by decreases in cardiac output. Aldosterone acts to conserve sodium in the kidney tubules, passively increasing water reabsorption and improving fluid volume balance. Normally, if Mr. Noble had only a water loss, he would also be hypernatremic because of this mechanism. However, in burns the patient's hypovolemia (hemoconcentration) is due to both fluid and electrolyte loss in edema fluids as well as through the denuded areas of skin. No. 1 is not the best answer because, while ADH is being released, its action has not at this time prevented hemoconcentration. No. 3 is incorrect because very little sodium is released due to cellular disruption. Sodium is the main cation of the extracellular fluid. No. 4 is incorrect because increased serum potassium levels stimulate the release of aldosterone.

115. (1) Hyponatremia or decreased serum sodium may develop in burn patients because sodium tends to move with water into edema fluids as well as into denuded areas of skin. Nos. 2 and 4 are incorrect because both these mechanisms tend to increase sodium reabsorption by the kidney tubules. Inadequate fluid replacement (No. 3) would tend to mask hyponatremia because of hemoconcentration.

116. (2) Hyperkalemia (excesses in serum potassium) occurs in burns due to three separate mechanisms: (a) cellular injury resulting in the movement of potassium from the intracellular space into the extracellular space; (b) decreased glomerular filtration and urine output preventing excretion of increased serum potassium; and (c) inadequate tissue metabolism resulting in increased hydrogen ion formation (metabolic acidosis). In the kidney tubules hydrogen and potassium ions are exchanged for sodium ions. In metabolic acidosis more hydrogen ions are excreted than potassium ions. Exudate formation itself does not significantly affect serum potassium levels. During physical and emotional stress aldosterone levels are increased, thereby lowering serum potassium. Hyperbilirubinemia itself does not affect potassium concentration, though red blood destruction probably increases the amount of circulating potassium, as potassium is the major intracellular cation. Hence Nos. 1, 3, and 4 are incorrect.

117. (3) Potassium is transported back into the cells along with glucose. Therefore the administration of insulin and glucose will facilitate the movement of potassium back into the cell. Kayexalate is a resin that attacks and binds potassium. It may be given either orally or as an enema; however, its use would not be indicated in this case unless more conservative means were unsuccessful. Morphine sulfate and synthetic aldosterone are not indicated for the management of hyperkalemia. Hence Nos. 1, 2, and 4 are incorrect.

118. (4) The hypovolemia that occurs in the initial stage of burns is the result of fluid lost from denuded areas of skin and edema in and around the burned surface area. Edema formation is due to a shift of plasma fluids to the interstitial space. When tissues are burned, a change in the permeability of both tissue and capillary membranes occurs. This change as well as increased vasodilation result in a shift of excessively large amounts of extracellular fluid (electrolytes and proteins) into the burned area. Most of this fluid loss occurs deep in the wound, where fluid moves into the deeper tissue. Burns of highly vascular area (muscle, face) are believed to cause more severe fluid volume shifts than comparable burns to other areas of the body. Hence Nos. 1, 2, and 3 are incorrect.

119. (2) With the exception of the Evans formula, whole blood is administered to burn patients only when the hematocrit begins to manifest red blood cell loss. Several fluid formulas have been developed to serve as a guideline for fluid replacement in the burn patient. The Evans formula is the oldest and is based upon both the size of the wound and the patient's weight. Colloids (blood, dextran, plasma) and crystalloids (electrolyte solutions) are administered during the first 48 hours. The Brooke formula is quite similar except that blood is not given until the hematocrit level has fallen and the need is demonstrated. More recently developed, the Parkland formula is based on the premise that volume expansion is dependent upon the rate of infusion rather than the type of replacement. During the first 24 hours fluid volume is replaced with electrolyte solutions (Ringer's lactate) only. During the second 24 hours, dextrose and water are used to maintain fluid volume, and colloids are used only if urine output is not maintained. Hence Nos. 1, 3, and 4 are incorrect.

120. (2) Each of these measures is utilized to assess the adequacy of fluid replacement. However, in the acute burn period, hourly urine outputs and vital signs provide significant information on fluid balance. Decreased urine output, increased pulse rate, and restlessness are early signs of inadequate fluid replacement. Increases in blood pressure, pulse, respirations, and urine output are early signs of circulatory overload. Changes in daily weights provide accurate data over the long run and are extremely important in monitoring fluid volumes in patients on diuretic therapy, such as patients with congestive heart failure, cirrhosis, etc. Hence Nos. 1, 3, and 4 are incorrect.

121. (1) The diuretic stage of burns occurs 48–72 hours after injury. The fluid shift is just the opposite of the initial stage. Fluids, electrolytes, and proteins may move very rapidly from the interstitial space back into the vascular compartment. Unless renal damage has occurred, diuresis ensues, due to the increased blood volume and renal blood flow. Serum electrolytes and hematocrit are decreased due to hemodilution. If urine output is insufficient at this time, symptoms of circulatory overload and cardiac failure will occur. Hence Nos. 2, 3, and 4 are incorrect.

122. (2) Hematocrit is reduced due to hemodilution and volume overload resulting from the interstitial-to-plasma fluid shift. Erythropoietin factor is produced by the kidneys and would only be reduced if there was kidney failure. Metabolic acidosis does increase red blood cell fragility but it is not applicable in this situation. Hypoalbuminemia causes loss of oncotic pressures in the vascular compartment. The primary effect of this phenomenon is movement of fluid from the vascular compartment to the interstitial space, the outcome of which is hemoconcentration. Hence Nos. 1, 3, and 4 are incorrect.

123. (3) Patients with burns limited to an extremity are generally treated by a closed method; that is, wounds are covered with a layer of sterile, fine mesh gauze impregnated with an antibacterial agent such as mafenide 1%. Wounds are cleansed one or more times per day and dressings are reapplied using strict sterile technique. Patients treated by the closed or semi-open method do not have to be isolated. Patients treated by the open method (wounds completely exposed to the air) require strict isolation to prevent infection. The open method is usually used for minor burns, areas difficult to dress (burns of trunk, perineum), or new skin grafts. Hence Nos. 1, 2, and 4 are incorrect.

124. (2) Mafenide 1% (Sulfamylon) is a white antibacterial ointment applied once or twice daily. Besides causing pain on application, this medication is a carbonic anhydrase inhibitor that interferes with the kidney's ability to excrete hydrogen ion, and thus may cause metabolic acidosis. Patients who are treated with mafenide 1% need to have their acid-base balance monitored by blood gas determinations. Clinical signs of metabolic acidosis are increased rate and depth of respirations. Silver nitrate causes black discoloration of linens and its hypotonicity causes electrolyte imbalances. Patients treated with silver nitrate will need supplemental sodium, potassium, and chloride. Hence Nos. 1, 3, and 4 are incorrect.

125. (1) To prevent contractures, the affected limb is kept

straight (knee extension) and slightly abducted (to prevent pressure in hip joint) and the foot is supported (ankle flexion) to prevent footdrop. Nos. 2, 3, and 4 are incorrect because all or part of each response could produce a contracture.

126. (2) Desperation and panic may strike while the injury is occurring but rarely sets in during the recovery period. During the acute stage of burn recovery, anxiety is common due to the stress and pain of injury and dressing changes. Anxiety decreases the individual's ability to perceive situations realistically, which may result in an altered mental state. During the intermediate phase of burn recovery, patients may react to continued pain, changes in body image, and financial stresses with various psychologic responses ranging from withdrawal and depression to acting out anger by refusing to cooperate with medical regimen. Hence Nos. 1, 3, and 4 are incorrect.

127. (2) Body image changes are the most frequent basis for psychologic responses during the recuperative phase. This is particularly true if the patient is young or has sustained facial or neck burns. Self-esteem is also often lowered. The patient needs to be encouraged to talk about the changes he perceives between what he was and what he is now. Sessions with a psychiatric nurse specialist may be helpful. Occasionally individual and/or group therapy is indicated. Pain and immobility create problems in the acute phase of burns. Anger may be a response during each phase as the patient reacts to various real and imagined losses. Financial concerns do affect responses during the recuperative phase, but are not a significant concern for all patients. Hence Nos. 1, 3, and 4 are incorrect.

128. (3) Most erythrocyte and leukocyte breakdown occurs in the spleen. Liver functions are many and varied, including detoxification of chemicals (estrogen, adrenocorticoids, aldosterone, drugs, poisons, and heavy metals), synthesis of plasma proteins (albumin, fibrinogen, globulin) and several clotting factors (prothrombin, factor VII), storage of glycogen, iron, vitamins (A, D, E, K, and B_{12}), synthesis and secretions of bile, gluconeogenesis (glucose from amino acids and fats), and deamination of amino acids. Hence Nos. 1, 2, and 4 are incorrect.

129. (2) The primary pathophysiologic effect of decreased serum proteins is decreased plasma oncotic pressures. As plasma proteins decrease, the mechanism for holding fluid and electrolytes in the vascular compartment is lost. This results in edema formation. As blood volumes decrease, the sympathoadrenal mechanism is called into play, which increases aldosterone and ADH secretion. The increased reabsorption of sodium and water resulting from these hormones only adds to the existing edema. Blood hydrostatic pressures may be

increased secondary to venous stasis due to obstruction of the portal vein. Interstitial oncotic pressures are normally negative. Hence Nos. 1, 3, and 4 are incorrect.

130. (2) Ecchymoses occurs in cirrhosis due to decreased synthesis of clotting factors as well as decreased vitamin K storage. Furthermore, increased venous pressures due to mechanical obstruction in the liver result in increased capillary fragility. Dilatation and slow blood flow in veins also cause the formation of spider angiomas, particularly on the upper chest, palmar redness, and varicosities (esophageal and rectal are common). Hence Nos. 1, 3, and 4 are incorrect.

131. (4) Blood volumes are decreased while total body fluid is increased due to the physiologic effects of hypoproteinemia (decreased serum proteins) as discussed in answer 129. These factors plus increasing obstruction of the portal vein cause fluids, electrolytes, and serum proteins to move out of the vascular compartment and into the interstitial space. The abdomen provides a large potential space for the accumulation of these fluids. Nos. 1, 2, and 3 are all factors in the development of ascites.

132. (1) Anemia occurs in cirrhosis due to (a) erythrocyte destruction in the engorged spleen, (b) gastrointestinal blood losses, and (c) folic acid deficiencies from inadequate dietary intake. Decreased amino acid breakdown and synthesis result in increasing serum ammonia levels, which may further inhibit dietary intake. Kupffer's cells line the venous sinusoids in the liver and are primarily macrophagic. Hence Nos. 2, 3, and 4 are incorrect.

133. (2) The diet of a cirrhotic patient should provide ample protein for tissue repair, at least .5 g/lb. Some modification occurs if serum ammonia levels are elevated. Sufficient carbohydrate intake to sustain weight and prevent proteins from being utilized for energy is essential. Salt is restricted to assist in decreasing edema formation. Fluids may also be restricted to 1000 to 1500 ml/day. Vitamin supplements, particularly fat-soluble vitamins (A, D, and K) are usually prescribed because of decreased bile production for their absorption and the inability of the liver to store them successfully. Initially, if the patient has a very poor appetite, liquid protein supplements such as Sustagen may be given. Frequent small feedings may also increase intake. Hence Nos. 1, 3, and 4 are incorrect.

134. (1) Spironolactone (Aldactone) is an aldosterone inhibitor, inhibiting the effects of hyperaldosteronemia, which is common in cirrhosis. This drug safely increases sodium and water excretion but does not cause concomitant losses of potassium as do other diuretics. For this reason potassium supplements are not generally given to the patient. An example of a carbonic anhydrase inhibitor is Diamox; a thiazide is

Diuril or HydroDiuril; and an osmotic diuretic is mannitol. Hence Nos. 2, 3, and 4 are incorrect.

135. (2) Potassium chloride—see preceding rationale. Spironolactone would not contraindicate the administration of vitamin B_6, ascorbic acid, or calcium gluconate. Nos. 1, 3, and 4 are less appropriate answers.

136. (4) Frequent small meals do not visually overwhelm the patient and require less energy for ingestion. As patients with cirrhosis frequently have very poor appetites, the nurse may have to be very creative in her approaches to assure adequate nutritional intake. Hence Nos. 1, 2, and 3 are incorrect.

137. (2) After explaining the procedure to the patient, the nurse should instruct him to void. This prevents accidental nicking or perforation of the bladder during the procedure. Following bladder evacuation, vital signs are taken to establish baseline information. The patient is then positioned in a chair or high-Fowler's position in bed and the abdomen prepared. Nos. 1, 3, and 4 are later procedures.

138. (2) Hypotension and shock can occur during or after paracentesis. Fluid from the vascular compartment shifts into the abdomen to replace fluids that are withdrawn. This complication can be minimized if withdrawal of ascitic fluid is limited to 1000 ml and/or if lost fluid is replaced by administration of salt-poor albumin. To assess for this complication, vital signs are taken every 15 minutes during the procedure and afterwards till stable, then every hour for four hours. Disequilibrium (No. 1) occurs with rapid removal of wastes during renal dialysis. Hypoalbuminuria (no protein in urine) is a normal physical finding; therefore No. 3 is incorrect. Paralytic ileus (No. 4) is rarely a complication of this procedure.

139. (2) See rationale 138 above.

140. (1) The earliest clinical signs of bleeding include restlessness, pallor, tachycardia, and cooling of the skin. These symptoms occur as the result of vasoconstriction (increased sympathetic stimulation) in order to maintain venous return and cardiac output. When these mechanisms are no longer effective, the blood pressure begins to fall (No. 3). It is essential to identify bleeding early, because liver cells are very susceptible to ischemia. No. 2 represents symptoms of ketoacidosis. No. 4 may occur with increases in intracranial pressure.

141. (3) The Sengstaken-Blakemore tube is a triple-lumen tube composed of a catheter that goes to the stomach for suctioning, a lumen that ends in a gastric balloon, and a lumen that ends in an esophageal balloon. The primary purpose of this tube is to stop bleeding by applying pressure to the cardiac portion of the stomach and against the esophageal varices. The secondary purposes of this tube are: (a) to reduce blood transfusion requirements, and (b) to prevent accumulation of blood in the gastrointestinal tract. The liver is unable to detoxify the ammonia produced by protein-rich blood in the gut; the increased ammonia levels could precipitate hepatic coma. Hence Nos. 1, 2, and 4 are incorrect.

142. (2) Symptoms of severe respiratory distress indicate that the tube has dislodged and is obstructing the airway. If this occurs, scissors, kept at the bedside, should be used to cut the tube, deflating both balloons. Following deflation, the doctor should be notified in order to assess Mr. Swenson's condition and determine ongoing medical therapy. Traction on the Sengstaken tube should only be increased or decreased by the attending physician. Hence Nos. 1, 3, and 4 are incorrect.

143. (2) Ammonia is formed in the intestines by the action of intestinal bacteria on proteins. Tap water enemas may be given to remove protein-rich blood that has resulted from bleeding esophageal varices. Also, in an effort to reduce serum ammonia levels, potassium is administered because it is necessary for cerebral metabolism of ammonia. Antibiotics such as neomycin that are poorly absorbed by the intestines are also given to decrease the intestinal flora that manufacture ammonia. Since ammonia is formed during muscle contraction, active range-of-motion exercises are contraindicated. To prevent skin breakdown in a patient such as Mr. Swenson, who is jaundiced and edematous, passive exercises, turning, and frequent skin care are indicated. Hence Nos. 1, 3, and 4 are incorrect.

144. (1) Prognosis is generally poor if hepatic coma lasts longer than 24 hours. Other measures that have been utilized to decrease serum ammonia and allow for regeneration of hepatocytes include hemodialysis, exchange blood transfusions, and administration of lactalose, which, when degraded in the large bowel, decreases the pH of the feces, thus preventing formation of ammonia and promoting its excretion. Hence Nos. 2, 3, and 4 are incorrect.

145. (3) For patients having elective surgery, routine preoperative laboratory studies generally include a complete blood count, urine analysis, and prothrombin time. Some institutions also require a VDRL. The urinalysis provides information about specific gravity or the ability of the kidney to concentrate and dilute urine, the presence of albumin or pus indicating renal infection; and the presence of sugar and acetone. The CBC detects the presence of anemia, infection, allergy, and leukemia. Prothrombin time (increased) may indicate a need for preoperative vitamin K therapy.

Electrolytes (No. 1), enzymes such as SGOT (No. 2), and serum glucose (No. 4) are ordered only if the patient's history or physical condition warrants a more complete workup.

146. (4) The Trendelenburg test tests the competency of the superficial veins. The patient is asked to elevate the involved leg to empty the veins. A tourniquet is then applied lightly to occlude the superficial veins. The patient is then asked to stand, the tourniquet is removed, and the direction and degree of vein filling is observed. No. 1 is also a test of venous competence. Ordinarily, distended veins decrease markedly during walking as muscular contractions facilitate venous flow in deeper veins. No. 2 describes a phlebography, and No. 3 is a test generally used on the jugular vein when pump failure is suspected.

147. (1) Vein-strippings are done not only for advancing varicosities but also for cosmetic reasons. Vein-stripping is not done for thrombophlebitis (No. 2), though it is done for stasis ulcerations following successful healing of the ulcer. No. 3 is incorrect since lymphedema is due to blockage of lymph channels and Reynaud's disease is a syndrome that affects the arterial vasculature. No. 4 is incomplete.

148. (4) Vein-stripping is a painful and tiresome procedure and, for the patient's comfort, is almost always done under general anesthesia. Nos. 1, 2, and 3 are incorrect because local anesthesia is limited to small areas such as laceration repair. Topical anesthesia only decreases pain sensation in mucous membranes and, since the incisions for vein-stripping are made in the groin as well as the ankle, regional anesthesia would be impractical. Vein-stripping could be done using spinal anesthesia.

149. (3) Sitting in a chair is contraindicated because the pressure this position exerts behind the knees and at the hips impedes venous return and increases dependent venous pressures. Nos. 1, 2, and 4 are appropriate nursing actions. The legs of the patient with a vein-stripping are wrapped from foot to groin with elastic bandages. The patient is also usually ambulated the day of surgery to enhance venous return by way of muscle contraction.

150. (2) Elevation of the foot of the bed enhances venous return and reduces edema by utilizing the force of gravity. By reducing edema the patient is more comfortable (No. 4) and has less overall discomfort (No. 1). Raising the foot of the bed should not greatly affect arterial blood flow (No. 3).

151. (1) Elastic stockings are applied before standing up in order to prevent stagnation of blood in the lower extremities. If the patient has been standing or exercising (No. 3), he/she should sit in a chair with legs elevated for at least 15 minutes before applying the stockings. Elastic stockings should be removed regularly both to inspect and to provide skin care (No. 2). The patient should be cautioned not to sit or stand in any one position for a prolonged period of time. Stockings should fit properly and be kept wrinkle-free because when improperly used they can cause the condition (venous stasis) they are designed to prevent (No. 4).

152. (2) Changes in mentation are always significant. In a patient already in respiratory distress, decreasing mentation is an indicator of ventilatory insufficiency. These symptoms should be reported to the physician at once. Given Mrs. Arturri's depressed ventilatory excursion, increasing oxygen flow at this time would probably not relieve hypoxia, nor would increasing intravenous infusion rates and/or stimulatory efforts. Hence Nos. 1, 3, and 4 are incorrect.

153. (1) Pneumonia causes ventilation/perfusion imbalances in the lungs. In the area or areas of consolidation, both oxygen and carbon dioxide diffusion is decreased. However, if the unaffected areas of the lungs have the capacity to respond to the hypoxia with increased ventilation (tachypnea) the Pco_2 is usually decreased because carbon dioxide can diffuse across the respiratory membrane twenty times faster than oxygen. While No. 2 is also correct, it does not explain the phenomenon as well as No. 1. No. 3 is a correct statement physiologically, but does not relate to the question. No. 4 is partially true in that carbon dioxide is more permeable in water than oxygen, and this is the mechanism that allows it to diffuse twenty times faster over the respiratory membrane. However, rate and depth of respirations control movement of gases in the airways.

154. (2) The purpose of a tracheostomy is to provide more controlled ventilation and to ease removal of respiratory secretions. When long-term therapy is indicated, it reduces or prevents respiratory fatigue. A tracheostomy is done when intubation is necessary for a period greater than three to five days, when the patient is unable to handle respiratory secretions, and/or if there is upper-airway obstruction. Desired effects of improving ventilation are reduction in anxiety due to air hunger (No. 1) and improved cerebral oxygenation (No. 3). A side effect of tracheostomy is increased risk of pulmonary infection, which is not true in the case of endotracheal intubation (No. 4), though both may cause injury to mucous membranes.

155. (1) Since tracheostomy inhibits the patient from talking, it is essential to establish a mode of postoperative communication so that the patient can express her needs. The mode chosen should be communicated to the rest of the staff so that the approach to the patient is consistent. Blood work may or may not be ordered before tracheostomy, though blood gases are frequently ordered to establish baseline data in order to evaluate the effectiveness of the intervention. Inserting a Foley catheter is not a priority unless urinary output has decreased. A standard surgical prep, cleansing and shaving of the operative area, is not done before tracheostomy. However, the physician does cleanse the area with an antiseptic before performing the tracheostomy. Hence Nos. 2, 3, and 4 are incorrect.

156. (2) A recent study indicates that the most sensitive indicator of increased tracheobronchial secretions is increased or decreased systolic and diastolic blood pressure. The study indicated that increases of as little as 5 mm Hg were significant. Other indicators include increased temperature, pulse, and rate and depth of respirations (No. 1), and coarse, prolonged expiratory breath sounds (No. 3). The amount of secretions was directly related to the total number of indicators present. High-pitched, crowing inspiratory sounds are associated with upper-airway obstruction No. 4.

157. (3) Pre- and postsuctioning ventilation with 100% oxygen is important in reducing hypoxemia, which occurs when the flow of gases in the airways is obstructed by the suctioning catheter. Nos. 1 and 2 are proper nursing actions prior to suctioning the patient with an endotracheal tube rather than a tracheal tube. No. 4 is a correct nursing procedure prior to suctioning any patient; however, it does not prevent hypoxemia.

158. (3) While there is some controversy at present as to whether this procedure does in fact facilitate entry into the right and left bronchi, it is still employed in many settings. Turning the patient's head from side to side does not prevent nuchal rigidity or decrease tissue resistance, though it probably does provide passive exercise for the sternocleidomastoid and trapezius muscles. Hence Nos. 1, 2, and 4 are incorrect.

159. (2) Suction is applied only after the catheter is in place and ready for withdrawal. Applying suction intermittently as well as rotating the suction catheter assist in reducing the negative pressure effects of suctioning. Suctioning should also be limited to periods of 10 to 15 seconds. Nos. 1, 3, and 4 are incorrect because of the negative effects each of these responses would have on patient aeration.

160. (2) Cuff pressures of 20 mm Hg or less are used to maintain the position of the tracheal or endotracheal tube. The primary objective of cuff inflation is to use the smallest volume possible to create an air-tight seal without occluding the mucosa. Nos. 1, 3, and 4 are all significantly higher pressures than are desirable.

161. (2) During the early postinsertion period, the inner cannula is removed using aseptic technique every two to four hours for cleansing. If secretions are copious or very viscous, more frequent cleansing may be necessary. If the patient is receiving oxygen therapy or is on mechanical ventilation, these treatments are continued through the outer cannula. Hence Nos. 1, 3, and 4 are incorrect.

162. (4) The natural pathway of humidification, the upper respiratory tract, has been bypassed. Therefore, to prevent drying out of the mucous membranes of the bronchi as well as crusting of secretions, humidification per nebulization is provided. No. 1 is correct in that supplying humidification during oxygen therapy has become standardized, but this is not the rationale for its use. Nos. 2 and 3 are also not specific to the question, but are probably true to some extent.

163. (1) Crepitus in the neck or upper chest is a sign that the tracheal tube is no longer in place and is delivering oxygen into the interstitial or mediastinal space. This condition may severely impair ventilation of the lungs. No. 2 creates an air leak around the tracheal tube. No. 3 can cause necrosis of the trachea. No. 4 is characterized by fluid, not air, in the tissues.

164. (2) Some authorities believe that the basic psychosomatic issue underlying the development of ulcers is an unresolved dependence-independence conflict. This conflict frequently prevents the patient from accepting a dependent role even on a temporary basis. However, the unresolved dependency wish that many of these people have frequently results in irritable, angry behavior when treatments aren't exactly on time. Other psychosomatic research has linked anxiety and neurotic behavior with the occurrence of angina pectoris, repressed anger and hostility with the development of rheumatoid arthritis, and compulsive time orientation (type A personality) with onset of myocardial infarction. Hence Nos. 1, 3, and 4 are incorrect.

165. (2) Enemas and/or cathartics are not administered before an upper GI series; however, they are given after the series to aid in the elimination of the barium. Nos. 1, 3, and 4 are correct.

166. (3) Gastroscopy is an uncomfortable procedure. To mislead the patient by telling him it isn't can only increase anxiety and discomfort during the procedure. This procedure involves the passage of a long tube into the stomach with a lighted, mirrored lens that permits direct visualization of the stomach mucosa. The patient must lie quietly during insertion of the tube to prevent perforation of the esophagus. Nos. 1, 2, and 4 are nursing actions prior to gastroscopy.

167. (3) Following gastroscopy, food and fluids are withheld until the gag reflex returns (generally three to four hours) in order to prevent aspiration. The gag reflex is inactivated by either an anesthetic spray or an oral preparation gargled by the patient prior to insertion of the gastroscopy tube. Inhibition of the gag reflex facil-

itates insertion. Nos. 1 and 2 are incorrect since the period of time is too brief. No. 4 is incorrect not only because it is generally not necessary to wait six to eight hours for the gag reflex to return, but because this procedure does not precipitate an electrolyte imbalance.

168. (3) The vagus nerve stimulates both an increase in hydrochloric acid secretion and gastric motility. Vagotomy as well as decreasing hydrochloric acid secretion also alter the motility of the stomach and intestines; this may result in a sensation of fullness after meals, eructation, and abdominal distention. No. 1 is incomplete. Nos. 2 and 4 are the reverse of effects of vagal action.

169. (3) Sippy diets are rarely employed in either the medical or presurgical management of gastric ulcer patients anymore. These diets, which consisted of milk every two hours alternating with an antacid administration every two hours in between milk feeding, are no longer considered effective therapy and in some instances led to hypernatremia when the patient ingested insufficient water. Nos. 1, 2, and 4 are appropriate preoperative nursing interventions.

170. (3) Patients with high abdominal incisions are prone to atelectasis following surgery because they tend to breathe shallowly to prevent incisional pain. However, the nurse must also institute measures to prevent thrombophlebitis, wound infection, and dehiscence. Abdominal distention due to air-swallowing is unlikely because the patient has a nasogastric tube in place. Urinary retention after surgery is generally due to the effects of anesthesia on the autonomic nervous system rather than to the residual effects of anticholinergic medications. Hence Nos. 1, 2, and 4 are incorrect.

171. (2) Bloody drainage from the nasogastric tube more than twelve hours after surgery should be considered unusual and reported to the surgeon. Prolonged bleeding may be indicative of a slow bleeder, a blood dyscrasia, or problems with incisional closure. Any of these may increase blood loss and lead to shock. Nos. 1, 3, and 4 are incorrect because they are normal findings in the early postgastrectomy period.

172. (3) If resistance to instillation of irrigating fluids into the nasogastric tube occurs, fluid should not be forced through with greater pressure. Generally what has occurred is that the tube is adhering to the mucous membrane. Occasionally, withdrawing the tube slightly or rotating it slightly will resolve the problem and allow for instillation of fluids. If continued resistance occurs, the physician should be notified as it is essential to maintain the patency of the tube. Nasogastric tubes are irrigated with normal saline (No. 1) to prevent electrolyte imbalance, with minimal pressure to prevent undue stress on suture (No. 2). The inability to recover

irrigating fluids should be reported immediately to the physician (No. 4).

173. (3) Removal of gastric secretions incurs the loss of sodium, potassium, and hydrochloric acid ions. The loss of these ions may lead not only to metabolic alkalosis ($\downarrow H^+$) but also to hypokalemia. Nos. 1 and 2 are incorrect because hypernatremia and hyperkalemia indicate an excess in sodium and potassium ions. Hypoproteinemia (No. 4) occurs with liver dysfunctions and is not a side effect of nasogastric suctioning.

174. (2) The patient should be cautioned to limit the number of ice cubes he sucks on because the nasogastric suction will remove not only the increased water ingested from the melted cubes, but also essential electrolytes. Nos. 1, 3, and 4 are appropriate mouth care measures for a patient who has a nasogastric tube.

175. (2) The nasogastric tube is removed after bowel sounds have been reestablished (generally around the third day) and after the patient has passed flatus or stool. Before removal, the tube is frequently clamped for a two- to four-hour period to test the patient's tolerance. Gastric residue is measured after this period. If it is more than 100 ml, the nasogastric tube is left in place. Likewise, if the patient experiences any pain, nausea, vomiting, or distention during this period the tube is left in. If no symptoms occur and there is a minimal amount of gastric residue, the tube is removed. Hence, Nos. 1, 3, and 4 are incorrect.

176. (3) Pernicious anemia may occur following subtotal gastrectomy (when large portions of the stomach are removed) due to the loss of tissue that produces the intrinsic factor. Loss of this factor necessitates the parenteral administration of vitamin B_{12}, the extrinsic factor. No. 1 is incorrect because the extrinsic factor is found in food. Nos. 2 and 4 are incorrect because it is the loss of intrinsic factor that results in the malabsorption of vitamin B_{12}.

177. (1) Patients are ambulated as soon as possible to prevent the complications of bedrest; generally ambulation can begin as soon as 24 hours after surgery. In some instances, as when the patient is severely debilitated or has complications due to ulcer perforation, bedrest may be prolonged as in Nos. 2 and 3. If this is the case, the nurse will need to observe closely for signs of complications (atelectasis, thrombophlebitis, etc.) and institute measures to prevent them. The patient is rarely if ever gotten up immediately after awakening, as in No. 4.

178. (4) While 70% to 80% of patients having subtotal gastrectomies may experience some symptoms of dumping syndrome, it is a significant problem for only a small percentage (5–10%). The term dumping is used because the symptoms are believed to be due to the rapid emptying of the gastric contents into the small intestines. This produces gastric distention, and some authorities believe that large amounts of extracellular fluid then enter the intestines to dilute the hypertonic stomach contents. The subsequent lowering of the blood volume produces shocklike symptoms, such as weakness, diaphoresis, faintness, and palpitations. Hence Nos. 1, 2, and 3 are incorrect.

179. (3) The symptoms of dumping syndrome are most likely to occur following the ingestion of large amounts of sugars or carbohydrates. Therefore a diet that is high in protein and fats and low in carbohydrates is recommended to reduce symptomatology and to provide the patient with essential energy requirements. Nos. 2 and 4 are incorrect because they contain high carbohydrates, and No. 1 is incorrect because it does not supply sufficient protein for energy and tissue repair. High protein intake is essential after surgery and most prolonged illnesses for rebuilding tissue.

180. (1) Patients experiencing dumping syndrome should be advised to ingest liquids between meals rather than with meals. Taking fluids between meals allows for adequate hydration, reduces the amount of bulk ingested with meals, and aids in preventing rapid gastric emptying. Six small meals rather than three large meals as well as resting after eating are also measures used to prevent the occurrence of symptoms, which usually disappear over time. Hence Nos. 2, 3, and 4 are incorrect.

181. (4) Due to intestinal distention, patients with dumping syndrome have a feeling of fullness (No. 3) rather than hunger. Nos. 1 and 2 are also symptoms that occur with dumping syndrome. See answer 178 for rationale.

182. (4) Concentrated sugars and carbohydrates should be avoided by these patients. Likewise, fluid ingestion with meals or snacks should also be avoided to prevent rapid emptying of the stomach. Nos. 1, 2, and 3 are examples of high-protein, high-fat, low-carbohydrate foods.

183. (4) In response to direct questioning by the patient, the nurse needs to provide brief, accurate information. Some patients who have had gastrectomies are able to tolerate three meals a day before discharge from the hospital. However, for the majority of patients, it takes six to twelve months before their surgically reduced stomachs have stretched enough to accommodate a larger meal. No. 1 is incorrect since it is an open-ended response designed to elicit additional information. No. 2 is correct as far as it goes, but still doesn't answer the patient's question. If you don't know the answer to a patient's question, admit that you do not know but will try to get the information. No. 3 is incorrect since it gives inaccurate information.

184. (2) Blood flow to the intestines is increased following ingestion of meals in order to facilitate digestion and absorption. As a result of this circulatory shift, other organs receive less volume. This blood shift is partially responsible for feelings of sleepiness and lethargy following large meals. If a patient has a large atheromatous plaque in one of his coronary arteries, the decreased pressure and flow of blood may result in transient ischemia. Decreased pancreatic enzyme secretion results in diarrhea and steatorrhea (large amounts of fats in the stools). Air-swallowing during eating may produce an uncomfortable feeling of fullness that may be relieved by eructation (belching), but should not decrease arterial oxygenation. Likewise, a decrease in heart rate and blood pressure will decrease rather than increase myocardial oxygen consumption. Hence Nos. 1, 3, and 4 are incorrect.

185. (4) Baroreceptors in the carotid sinus and aortic arch constantly monitor and respond to variations in blood pressure. Decreased cardiac output results in a drop of blood pressure. These receptors transmit afferent signals to the cardiovascular center in the medulla. Activation of these centers results in increased vasoconstriction, heart rate, and force of cardiac contraction via adrenergic efferents in the sympathetic nervous system. Nos. 1, 2, and 3 are incorrect because vagal stimulation of the SA node decreases heart rate, arrhythmias generally produce an irregularity in heart rhythm, and Mr. Davis's vital signs and mentation do not indicate shock at this time.

186. (3) Circulatory reflexes, responding to decreases in arterial pressure, are designed to increase venous return and maintain perfusion of vital organs. This is primarily accomplished by massive vasoconstriction, which acts to decrease venous capacitance (venous pooling) and decrease renal blood flow (decreasing glomerular filtration and urine output), and by arteriolar constriction, which acts to shunt blood to major organs, such as the brain and heart. Many of the signs and symptoms seen in acutely ill patients can be related to the activation of these reflexes: cold, clammy skin, decreased peristalsis, increased heart rate, increased serum glucose, and decreased urine output. Hence Nos. 1, 2, and 4 are incorrect.

187. (4) The left coronary artery bifurcates shortly after its origin into the anterior descending and circumflex arteries. The anterior descending passes down the groove between the two ventricles and supplies the anterior portion of the left ventricle as well as part of the intraventricular septum. Occlusion of this artery produces an ECG pattern consistent with anterior MI. The circumflex branch (No. 1) passes to the left and posteriorly. It has numerous vessels that perfuse most of the left atria and the diaphragmatic and lateral walls of the left ventricle. Occlusion of this artery produces an ECG pattern consistent with inferior and lateral-wall MI. The right coronary artery (No. 2) passes around the groove between the right atria and right ventricle and enters the posterior portion of the intraventricular septum. It supplies the posterior portion of the heart, and occlusion of this artery produces a pattern consistent with true posterior MI. Occlusion of the left coronary artery (No. 3) would result in a massive MI since two-thirds of the heart's blood supply would be blocked.

188. (1) Mr. Davis's pH is within normal range (pH 7.35–7.45). Therefore even though his serum bicarbonate is reduced, indicating metabolic acidosis, his lungs have been able to excrete enough CO_2 to keep his total pH within normal range. A pH below 7.35 in this case would represent uncompensated metabolic acidosis. pCO_2 in hyperventilation is also reduced (below 40 mm Hg) but serum bicarbonates are usually normal. In alveolar hypoventilation the pCO_2 is elevated and the condition of respiratory acidosis exists. Hence Nos. 2, 3, and 4 are incorrect.

189. (3) ST segment depression occurs in the leads reciprocal to the area of injury. In Mr. Davis's case, ST depression would occur in leads II, III, and AVF. Leads I and AVL as well as some or all precordial leads (since these record the injury and necrosis in the anterior portion of the heart) would demonstrate abnormal Q waves (greater than 0.04 sec), ST segment elevation, and peaked T waves in leads V_1–V_6. Nos. 1, 2, and 4 are findings consistent with anterior MI.

190. (1) Morphine sulfate acts on subcortical brain levels not only to inhibit perception of pain and to decrease apprehension and anxiety by inducing euphoria, but also to decrease sympathetic nervous system stimulation, thereby reducing peripheral arterial resistance and increasing venous capacitance. A side effect of this last action is hypotension. No. 2 is incorrect because morphine reduces arterial resistance. No. 3 is incorrect because a second side effect of morphine is respiratory depression. No. 4 is incorrect because it describes actions directly opposite to the effects of morphine.

191. (2) Morphine strongly depresses the medullary respiratory centers. Therefore, before administering the narcotic, the nurse should assess the patient's respiratory rate and depth to prevent severe respiratory depression. Hence Nos. 1, 3, and 4 are incorrect.

192. (3) Lidocaine is the treatment of choice in this situation. Ventricular tachycardia is a serious arrhythmia. It must be treated at once because (a) it may compromise cardiac output and (b) it is considered a precursor of ventricular fibrillation. Standing coronary care unit orders generally cover the administration of lidocaine in this situation, so it is not necessary to notify the physician in order to obtain a verbal order. Oxygen flow rate is increased only if clinical signs indicate the patient is in distress, which is unlikely with a short

burst of ventricular tachycardia. Recent research data indicate that morphine sulfate may stabilize the threshold for ventricular fibrillation, but it is not the drug of choice in this situation. Hence Nos. 1, 2, and 4 are incorrect.

193. (2) Continued high grades of ventricular ectopy in this situation are an indication of increased myocardial irritability. Action needs to be taken to prevent life-threatening ventricular tachycardia or fibrillation. Procedure at this time is to initiate 2–4 mg lidocaine drip. Following the implementation of this intervention, the patient should be assessed for signs of increased myocardial ischemia (chest pain, ST segment elevation) and for cardiac decompensation (apprehension, anxiety, pulmonary rales), and the attending physician should be notified. Nos. 1, 3, and 4 are later interventions.

194. (2) While ECG changes can be utilized to identify the site, extent of changes, and acuteness of an infarct, the extent of the injury is usually approximated by the peak levels of serial enzymes (CPK, SGOT, LDH). Of these enzymes CPK–MB or CPK^2 gives the most specific information about the amount of myocardial necrosis. The duration of chest pain (No. 3) is dependent not only upon the extent of tissue ischemia but also upon other factors such as affective responses and muscle spasm. Primary ventricular fibrillation (No. 4) does not indicate the extent of infarct, but occurs due to metabolic changes in the ischemic area. Sinus tachycardia (No. 1) may result from a number of factors including emotional responses and heart failure.

195. (1) An early indication of cardiac decompensation is tachycardia. Therefore, Mr. Davis's vital signs, mentation, and pulmonary status should be assessed to rule out this complication of myocardial infarction. Other causes of tachycardia are hypovolemia, anxiety, and pain. Assessment of pain and emotional status can be determined during cognitive assessment. Any further actions, such as encouraging verbalization of feelings (No. 2), administering oxygen (No. 3), and/or decreasing the rate of the intravenous infusion (No. 4) will be determined by your assessment findings.

196. (4) Tachycardia decreases diastole, which decreases ventricular filling time and stroke volume. A significant decrease in stroke volume will result in a concomitant fall in cardiac output and tissue perfusion. Decreased cerebral perfusion and cellular hypoxia will result in signs of increased restlessness, anxiety, apprehension, and irritability. However, these symptoms only occur at very high rates or when myocardial contractility is compromised, as with myocardial infarction (No. 3). Tachycardia is the result of increased sympathetic nervous system stimulation of the heart and may result in the patient's awareness of his heart beat, thus increasing anxiety (No. 2). Likewise, in order to prime the pump, venous return is enhanced by the activation of circulatory reflexes, not depressed as in No. 1.

197. (2) While summoning the physician, you should ensure that the patient's head is elevated. A sitting position bent slightly forward is best (a bedside table with pillows can be used for the patient to rest on), as it allows for the greatest lung expansion and gravity aids in shifting fluids toward the bases of the lungs. Lowering the legs tends to decrease venous return by pooling blood in the periphery. Supplemental O_2 may be given while awaiting medical orders, but initial nursing actions should be directed toward decreasing venous return and improving ventilation (No. 4). Morphine SO_4 may only be given per physician order (No. 1), and suctioning (No. 3) at this time is not indicated.

198. (3) Mr. Davis's dyspnea is due to the inability of his left ventricle to maintain cardiac output, not to a decrease in venous return. This dysfunction causes blood to back up in the pulmonary vasculature, causing increased pulmonary pressure and exudation of fluids into the interstitial space, alveoli, and bronchioles; that is, pulmonary edema. The mechanical congestion of the lungs decreases expandability (compliance) and increases the work of breathing; that is, the patient becomes aware of his efforts at breathing (dyspnea). Pulmonary edema also decreases the pulmonary membrane available for diffusion of gases, thereby decreasing arterial oxygen and increasing the likelihood of carbon dioxide retention. Hence Nos. 1, 2, and 4 are incorrect.

199. (2) Correct procedure for applying rotating tourniquets is as follows: (a) Explain procedure to patient, letting him know limbs will be swollen and discolored during treatment. (b) Take vital signs and check each limb for peripheral pulse, color, and temperature before applying tourniquets. Cuffs should not be applied to limbs that are ischemic or infected, or that have peripheral vascular disease or intravenous lines. Vital signs are repeated every 15 to 30 minutes throughout procedure. (c) Wrap cuffs high on each extremity and inflate to a pressure slightly above the diastolic pressure. This pressure will retard venous return but will not occlude arterial blood flow. Peripheral pulses should be palpable at all times. (d) Systematically rotate cuffs. Usually no limb is compressed for more than 45 minutes at a time. Release time is usually 15 minutes. (e) Continually observe for signs of shock and pulmonary or arterial emboli. (f) Remove cuffs on one limb at a time at 15-minute intervals when treatment is discontinued. Continue to observe for any signs of recurring pulmonary edema. Hence, No. 1 is incorrect because cuff placement should be high on limb; No. 3 is incorrect because the distal pulse should not be occluded by the tourniquet; and No. 4 is incorrect because a cuff should not be placed on a limb with an intravenous line.

200. (2) Digoxin increases the force and velocity of cardiac contraction and slows the heart rate by delaying conduction through the atrioventricular node. The hemodynamic effects of its action include increased cardiac output, decreased right atrial and venous pressures, decreased left ventricular filling pressure and increased excretion of sodium and water. Epinephrine increases the force of cardiac contractions but also increases heart rate, which in this case would increase cardiac embarrassment. Furosemide (Lasix) is a rapidly acting diuretic that enhances excretion of sodium and water. However, while its use is indicated to reduce fluid volume during the acute phase of Mr. Davis's pulmonary edema, it has no known direct effects on the cardiac musculature. Hydralazine is a peripheral vasodilator utilized in hypertensive therapy. It is not indicated in this situation. Hence Nos. 1, 3, and 4 are incorrect.

201. (3) The best indicator that digoxin has been effective in strengthening cardiac contraction and increasing glomerular filtration is a decrease in heart rate (vagal effect) and increased urinary output. As a result of these drug effects cardiac output is improved, raising blood pressure and decreasing pulmonary congestion. Hence Nos. 1, 2, and 4 are only partially correct.

202. (2) Central venous pressure is a reflection of pressures in the right atrium and systemic veins. While CVP is the least sensitive indicator of left ventricular end diastolic pressures (increased with decreased ventricular compliance due to myocardial infarction and left ventricular failure), it is a safer line than a PA line. In addition it can be utilized to estimate blood volumes, obtain venous blood samples, and administer fluids. Hence, Nos. 1, 3, and 4 are incorrect.

203. (1) Normal CVP pressures are 4–10 cm of water. Lower values indicate hypovolemia and higher values reflect hypervolemia or increasing left end diastolic pressures. Hence Nos. 2, 3, and 4 are incorrect.

204. (1) Having established, by stimulating the patient, that he is unconscious and not asleep, you should immediately call for help. This may be done by dialing the operator from the patient's phone and giving the hospital code for cardiac arrest and the patient's room number to the operator or, if a phone is not available, by pulling the emergency call button. Noting the time is important baseline information for arrest procedure. Hence Nos. 2, 3, and 4 are incorrect.

205. (2) Your next action is to position the patient for possible resuscitation. Roll him on his back and remove any pillows. Hence Nos. 1, 3, and 4 are incorrect.

206. (1) Your next action is to open and clear the airway. In some instances opening the airway will be sufficient stimulus to make him resume breathing if respirations have stopped. Check pupils. Dilated pupils are an unreliable sign of hypoxia (illness history and drug therapy), but reactive pupils provide good baseline data on which to evaluate efficiency of resuscitation. Hence Nos. 2, 3, and 4 are incorrect.

207. (3) After opening airway and checking pupils, check for breathing. If patient is not breathing, give four quick breaths and then one breath every five seconds. Hence Nos. 1, 2, and 4 are incorrect.

208. (2) Check carotid pulsations for 5–10 seconds. If absent, give closed-chest massage. Maintain ratio between ventilation and compression (2:15). Tilt patient's head, give two full breaths without letting lungs deflate completely, and then resume massage. Maintain a compression rate of at least 60 per minute. Continue procedure until help arrives. (In an unmonitored arrest the priorities are airway (A), breathing (B), and circulation (C). In a monitored arrest the sequence is circulation (C), so a chest thump may be appropriate to interrupt a malignant ventricular arrhythmia.

209. (2) Life-threatening illnesses, especially those with complications resulting in periods of prolonged bedrest, provoke alterations in body image. To assist a patient experiencing altered body image, the nurse needs to ascertain how the patient viewed his body previously and how he views it now. Doing this may unleash a torrent of feeling from the patient, which may help the nurse discover ways to help him cope. Nos. 1 and 3, while acknowledging his mood, tend to cut off further response from the patient. No. 4 is too open-ended.

210. (4) Conflicts concerning discharge instructions following myocardial infarction are common. When you prepare patients for discharge, it is important to recognize that both the patient and his spouse may have several fears they have not verbalized. Allow time for and encourage verbalization of feelings. Likewise, be sure that discharge instructions are feasible for the individual's life style. If they are not, work out a plan of modification with the patient, family, and physician. Referral to a community health nurse and/or local cardiac rehabilitation support group may also facilitate the rehabilitation. Nos. 1, 2, and 3 are incorrect, as they cut off patient's and spouse's range of response and may therefore preclude obtaining pertinent data.

211. (2) Acute glomerular nephritis is an autoimmune response to an antigen produced by beta-hemolytic streptococci. Antibodies produced to fight the antigen also react against the glomerular tissue. This causes proliferation and swelling of endothelial cells in the glomerular capillary wall and results in passage of blood cells and protein into the glomerular filtrate. Acute glomerular nephritis is not the result of direct infection (Nos. 1 and 3) or of hypoxia (No. 4).

212. (2) The decreased amounts of creatinine in the urine are a reflection of the glomerular filtration rate, indicating the ability of the kidney to clear the renal blood of this substance. The filtration fraction is simply the amount of glomerular filtrate entering the tubules.

Renal blood flow is estimated by measuring renal excretion of PAH (para-aminohippuric acid). While the amount and specific gravity of urine may be determined, it is not the primary function of this laboratory test. Hence Nos. 1, 3, and 4 are incorrect.

213. (3) Protein in the glomerular filtrate increases the osmotic pressure and osmolarity of the tubular fluid, thus less water can be reabsorbed by the tubular cells and more water is lost in urine. This same principle is in effect when the transport maximum for glucose is exceeded and osmotic diuresis ensues. When protein is lost in the urine, glomerular oncotic pressures (that is, the forces holding water in the glomerular capillary) are decreased. Increased arterial pressure under normal circumstances will increase urine output. Increased amounts of circulating aldosterone increase sodium and water retention. Hence Nos. 1, 2, and 4 are incorrect.

214. (1) The kidneys secrete the erythropoietin factor, which stimulates the bone marrow to produce red blood cells. In chronic kidney disease, secretion of this factor decreases as greater portions of the kidney are destroyed by the disease process. Hypertension does not suppress bone marrow centers, as local blood flow regulators tend to compensate over the long run by supplying tissue with adequate blood flow for metabolic purposes. Unlike metabolic acidosis, metabolic alkalosis does not increase RBC fragility. Frank bleeding into the urine is uncommon in chronic renal disease. Hence Nos. 2, 3, and 4 are incorrect.

215. (1) Hyperkalemia tends to develop in renal dysfunction for two reasons: in the kidneys, more hydrogen ions than potassium ions are selectively secreted in exchange for sodium ions, and decreasing glomerular filtration and urine output tend to decrease the excretion of all electrolytes and waste products of metabolism. Potassium does not move out of the cell to balance sodium shifts in edema, nor does respiratory alkalosis affect potassium reabsorption in the kidneys. Nausea and vomiting cause hypokalemia. Hence Nos. 2, 3, and 4 are incorrect.

216. (3) Mr. Lawson's specific gravity indicates that his kidneys have lost their ability to concentrate his urine. Therefore he has a greater water loss than would normally be expected. Water loss without concomitant electrolyte loss causes the extracellular fluids to become hyperosmolar (that is, the patient is dehydrated). Hyperosmolarity of ECF causes the thirst receptors in the hypothalamus to shrink, which stimulates the thirst mechanism. Hence Nos. 1, 2, and 4 are incorrect.

217. (2) The evening before an intravenous pyelogram, the patient is administered oral cathartic (Fleets) or enemas to clean the bowel of fecal material and flatus, thereby improving visualization of the kidneys and ure-

ters. If Mr. Lawson is having difficulty maintaining fluid volume balance, an intravenous infusion may be initiated to prevent dehydration, but it is not standard (No. 4). The radiopaque dye used in this procedure is injected by a physician in the radiology department not the night before (No. 1). No. 3 is not part of IVP preparation.

218. (4) Lethargy, disorientation, and increased rate and depth of respirations are clinical manifestations of metabolic acidosis. As hydrogen ion concentration rises, the central nervous system is depressed, causing the patient to become increasingly lethargic and slower in his responses. Likewise, the lungs endeavor to compensate for a metabolic acidosis by increasing both the rate and depth of respirations. Serum bicarbonates provide an estimate of metabolic components of acid-base balance. The level of these ions is controlled by the kidney's ability to secrete hydrogen ions and actively reabsorb bicarbonate ions. Decreased levels of bicarbonate indicate metabolic acidosis, while increased levels of serum bicarbonate indicate metabolic alkalosis. Nos. 1, 2, and 3 are symptoms of alkalosis.

219. (3) Methyldopa acts to decrease blood pressure by inhibiting the formation of dopamine, thus decreasing the amount of norepinephrine that is secreted in adrenergic synapses. Decreased adrenergic stimulation results in decreased vasoconstriction, which causes peripheral vascular resistance. No. 1 is an example of the effects of hydralazine; No. 2, of guanethidine SO_4; and No. 4, of diazepam.

220. (3) The single best measure for assessing Mr. Lawson's fluid volume status is daily weight. Significant water loss must occur before there are changes in skin turgor and mucous membranes (No. 1). Similarly, blood pressure (No. 2) may not reflect changes in fluid volume status if the fluid is sequestered in the interstitial spaces (edema formation). Finally, intake and output measures are important (No. 4) but generally do not reflect insensible water losses (water lost per respiration and diaphoresis) and are not always as sensitive to decreases in urine output in chronic renal dysfunction as they are in more acute illnesses.

221. (2) The diet for patients with chronic renal failure is restricted in total amount of protein and amino acid content. Eggs and milk are generally included in the diet because they contain all the essential amino acids. Meats from animals, fish, and fowl are restricted due to their sulfur-containing, nonessential amino acids. Hence Nos. 1, 3, and 4 are incorrect.

222. (2) Mr. Lawson's increasing symptomatology is due to a decrease in the number of functioning nephrons with resultant decrease in glomerular filtration due to the extension of his disease process. Mr. Lawson has moved from the second stage of chronic kidney disease (renal

insufficiency, characterized by water diuresis and mild azotemia) to renal failure, which is characterized by acidosis, marked electrolyte imbalances, fluid retention, anemia, and increases in serum urea, uric acid, and creatinine. Hence Nos. 1, 3, and 4 are incorrect.

223. (4) Increased circulating levels of uric acid, an end product of purine metabolism, are responsible for Mr. Lawson's goutlike joint discomfort. Hyperphosphatemia does occur in the third stage of chronic kidney disease, but normally this would stimulate the parathyroid gland to increase parathormone, thus raising calcium levels and lowering phosphate. However, in chronic renal failure the kidney fails to produce a metabolite of vitamin D, which effectively reduces parathormone activity, lowering serum calcium levels. If symptoms of this electrolyte imbalance develop (such as tetany), they are related to hypocalcemia. The effect of increased serum creatinine levels is central nervous system depression. Hence Nos. 1, 2, and 3 are incorrect.

224. (1) Increased serum potassium (hyperkalemia) causes the T waves to lose their normal rounded configuration and become more pointy or peaked (the difference in shape between a mountain and a mound). ST segments are not significantly affected by this electrolyte imbalance. Hence Nos. 2, 3, and 4 are incorrect.

225. (2) Mr. Lawson's blood gases indicate that he is mildly acidotic. His pH is still within normal limits, so that between his remaining functional nephrons and his lungs, he has been able to compensate for his increase in circulating hydrogen ions. Mr. Lawson does have respiratory alkalosis, but it represents respiratory compensation rather than the primary pathologic mechanism. If respiratory alkalosis were the underlying pathology, Mr. Lawson's pH would demonstrate alkalosis (pH above 7.40). Hence Nos. 1, 3, and 4 are incorrect.

226. (1) The kidneys and the lungs regulate the bicarbonate buffer. The bicarbonate buffer system is composed of a weak acid, carbonic acid (H_2CO_3), and its salt, sodium bicarbonate ($NaHCO_3$). The respiratory system controls the volatile hydrogen ion concentration by varying the rate of carbon dioxide removal. The kidney, acting much more slowly, regulates the nonvolatile hydrogen ions by varying the removal of hydrogen ions and base bicarbonate from body fluids. The other principal buffer systems are the phosphate and proteins. Proteins are the most powerful of the three buffer systems. Hemoglobin is a protein that can act as a buffer. These latter systems are not controlled by the activity of either the lungs or the kidneys. Hence Nos. 2, 3, and 4 are incorrect.

227. (2) Symptoms of circulatory overload result from varying degrees of cardiac decompensation, with blood backing up into the pulmonary (moist rales) and sys-

temic circuits (neck vein distention, dependent edema, periorbital edema, and hepatomegaly). Symptoms of circulatory failure or hypovolemia include apprehension, soft eyeballs, flattened neck veins, shock, decreased pulse pressure, and poor skin turgor. Hence Nos. 1, 3, and 4 are incorrect.

228. (1) Kayexalate (sodium polystyrene sulfonate) is a cation-exchange resin. As it passes along the intestine or is retained in the colon after enema administration, sodium ions are partially released and replaced by potassium ions, allowing for fecal excretion of potassium ions. Kayexalate is extremely unpalatable and may be administered in syrup, chilled, mixed in the diet, and if necessary, administered directly into the stomach per nasogastric tube. Side effects of Kayexalate administration include anorexia, nausea, vomiting, constipation, hypokalemia, hypocalcemia, and sodium retention. Hence Nos. 2, 3, and 4 are incorrect.

229. (2) Furosemide is a rapidly acting diuretic with a peak action in 1–2 hours and a duration of 6–8 hours. Hence Nos. 1, 3, and 4 are incorrect.

230. (3) Before beginning the dialysis procedure, baseline information needs to be collected so that the therapy can be accurately evaluated. Baseline information will include vital signs, body temperature, weight, ECG, and electrolyte levels. If the patient does not have a Foley catheter (often by this time they do because of the need to assess hourly outputs), the patient is asked to void. Following voiding the patient is positioned in a supine or low-Fowler's position and the abdomen is prepared and draped. Nos. 1, 2, and 4 are actions subsequent to No. 3.

231. (2) The dialysate is warmed to body temperature before administration to minimize discomfort and optimize clearance of waste products. Warming the fluid tends to dilate the peritoneal vessels, increasing the amount of urea that passes through the membrane. It has little effect on the osmotic gradient (No. 1), does not prevent peritonitis, which is secondary to infection (No. 3), and does not speed infusion time (No. 4), although it does make it more comfortable.

232. (2) Generally, the dwelling time of the dialysate is 30–45 minutes, occasionally longer. The dwell time as well as the instillation and outflow times are prescribed by the physician according to the patient's needs. Ten to fifteen minutes is too short a time to allow for diffusion of waste products. Hence Nos. 1, 3, and 4 are incorrect.

233. (3) The cumulative inflow and outflow records should show an outflow equal to or in excess of the amount instilled. While the amount of excess outflow allowed is also determined by the physician, this rarely exceeds 200 ml per cycle. Occasionally, drainage is less than

expected. Nursing measures to enhance outflow include turning the patient from side to side, elevating the head of the bed (increases intraabdominal pressures), and/or gently massaging the abdomen. If the problem continues, notify the physician before initiating another cycle. She or he may attempt to clear the catheter by rotation or by probing it for fibrin clots (No. 2). Nos. 1 and 4 will not improve flow.

234. (4) Flattened neck veins in a supine position are a characteristic of hypovolemia. Indications of fluid retention include inadequate fluid drainage (greater intake than output), increased blood pressure, and signs of congestive heart failure (distended neck veins, increased dependent edema, rales, and decreased mentation). Hence Nos. 1, 2, and 3 are incorrect.

235. (3) A BUN of less than 20 mg% and serum creatinine less than 1.2 mg% would be optimal outcome measures for this patient (that is, within normal range). A serum K^+ of less than 3.5 mEq/L would be indicative of hypokalemia, a serum Na^+ above 148 mEq/L indicates hypernatremia. Quantity of urine output should increase to over 500 ml/24 hours. The abdomen should be soft and tympanic to percussion. Dullness to percussion in the abdomen is consistent with fluid excess. Hence Nos. 1, 2, and 4 are incorrect.

236. (2) Intravenous pyelogram tests both the function and patency of the kidneys. After the intravenous injection of a radiopaque dye, the size, location, and patency of the kidneys can be observed by roentgenogram, as well as the patency of the urethera and bladder as the kidneys function to excrete it. No. 1 is an example of a KUB or flat plate of the abdomen, which can reveal gross structural changes in the kidneys and urethra. Renal blood flow (No. 3) is determined by the injection of PAH (para-aminohippuric acid) and measurement of its excretion in the urine. No. 4 is an example of renal angiogram.

237. (4) Fluids are not pushed prior to this procedure; they are withheld for up to eight hours prior to testing to produce a slight dehydration that aids in concentrating the dye in the kidneys and urinary system. Nos. 1, 2, and 3 are appropriate nursing actions in the preparation of the patient for IVP.

238. (2) After arterial punctures, your nursing priority is to observe for bleeding or hematoma formation, particularly in the first four hours after the procedure. Vital signs (No. 1) are monitored as well as the peripheral pulse (No. 4) distal to the puncture site. Because of the size of the vessel, bleeding can quickly cause volume depletion and shock. The specific gravity and urinary output (No. 3) are monitored, but this is not as significant as observing the puncture site.

239. (2) Erythropoietin factor, which is produced by the kidney, stimulates the production of red blood cells. Certain tumors of the kidney tend to increase the production of this factor so that the patient develops a polycythemia. Some tumors as they enlarge also infringe on the renal blood flow (No. 1), causing hypertension via increased renin secretion. Polyuria (No. 3) is rarely associated with renal tumors; rather, it occurs due to destruction of nephrons, glomerular membranes, or hyperosmolar conditions such as diabetes mellitus. Blood loss (No. 4) does tend to increase red blood cell production by the bone marrow; however, this is a compensatory mechanism designed to restore losses and will not cause polycythemia.

240. (2) Because the flank incision in nephrectomy is directly below the diaphragm, deep breathing is painful. Additionally, there is a greater incisional pull each time the person moves than there is with abdominal surgery. Incisional pain following nephrectomy generally requires analgesic administration every 3 to 4 hours for 24 to 48 hours after surgery. Therefore turning, coughing, and deep breathing exercises should be planned to maximize the analgesic effects. Patient may be on either side as long as drainage tubes are not kinked and gravity flow is uninhibited (No. 1). A low- or semi-Fowler's position is generally more comfortable for the patient and of sufficient height to encourage gravity flow from drainage tubes (No. 3). Fluid administration is directed toward maintaining blood volume and urine output (No. 4).

241. (2) Daily weights are taken following nephrectomy. Daily increases of two or more pounds is indicative of fluid retention and should be reported to the physicians. Intake and output records may also reflect this imbalance. Increased specific gravity of urine (No. 1) indicates that the patient is underhydrated rather than overhydrated. A urinary output of 50 ml/hr (No. 3) is the desired minimum following renal surgery. Periorbital edema (No. 4) is a later sign of excess fluid retention.

242. (1) Hemorrhage may follow nephrectomy because of the difficulty in securing ligatures in the short renal artery stump. It may occur on the day of surgery or 8 to 12 days postoperatively when normal tissue sloughing occurs with healing. Dressing and urine are observed for bright red bleeding, vital signs are monitored, and the patient is continually observed for any other indications of shock. Hyperkalemia (No. 2), tetany (No. 3), and polyuria (No. 4) are not complications that commonly occur after nephrectomy.

243. (2) While nausea may occur following the administration of narcotics, if it is accompanied by the absence of bowel sounds and upper abdominal distention, gastric or small intestine dilatation should be suspected and your findings reported to the physician. Changing the patient's position (No. 1) and insertion of a rectal tube (No. 3) are not helpful if peristalsis is not present (bowel sounds). Administering morphine (No. 4) is not indicated until the source of Mr. Cloutier's discomfort is diagnosed.

244. (3) Paralytic ileus is characterized by diminished, absent, or uncoordinated bowel sounds due to inappropriate or absent autonomic nervous system (vagal) stimulation of the intestinal tract. Paralytic ileus may occur due to anesthetic interruption of autonomic outflow or hypokalemia. Edema of the intestinal mucosa (No. 1) is usually found with inflammation or ulcerative colitis. Acute dilatation of the colon (No. 2) and high tinkling bowel sounds (No. 4) are associated with large bowel obstruction.

245. (1) The Miller-Abbott tube is a double-lumen tube with one tube leading to the inflatable balloon and the other tube utilized for aspiration of intestinal contents. No. 2 is an example of a Levin tube used for gastric suction. No. 3 is an example of a Harris tube and No. 4, a Cantor tube, both utilized for intestinal decompression like the Miller-Abbott.

246. (1) Chilling of the tube before insertion assists in relieving some of the nasal discomfort. Water-soluble lubricants along with viscous Xylocaine may also be used. However, since mercury is instilled into the balloon of the Miller-Abbott tube after insertion, it is usually only lightly lubricated before insertion. The patient may be administered a sedative (No. 2) on physician's orders to reduce apprehension during insertion. Warming the tube (No. 3) has no advantages. The patient is usually positioned (No. 4) in a high-Fowler's position during insertion to aid in swallowing of the tube.

247. (2) After the tube has been inserted into the stomach, its movement into the duodenum can be facilitated by having the patient lie on his right side for two hours. After the tube has passed the pylorus (this is usually checked by X ray), placing the patient in a Fowler's position or ambulating him will help move the tube to the point of obstruction. Also during this time either the physician or nurse may advance the tube 3 to 4 inches at specified intervals (No. 1). Remaining quiet or flat in bed (Nos. 3 and 4) will not facilitate the advancement of the tube either through the pylorus or through the small intestine.

248. (4) Recognizing the patient's concern is essential both in maintaining rapport and in keeping the lines of communication open. Having done this, you can now assure the patient that one kidney is sufficient to handle renal functions. This statement can then be followed by other discharge instructions such as the need of adequate fluid intake, avoiding infections, and untoward signs that the patient needs to observe for. Hence Nos. 1, 2, and 3 are incorrect.

249. (2) An indirect hernia occurs when a loop of intestine passes through the abdominal ring and follows the course of the spermatic cord into the inguinal canal. It is most common in men, particularly those engaging in strenuous activities. No. 1 is an example of a femoral hernia; No. 3, a direct hernia; and No. 4, an umbilical hernia.

250. (3) Coughing, vigorous exercise, and straining or lifting increase intraabdominal pressures, which tend to extrude the intestines through weakened areas of the abdominal wall. Mr. Dobson's history indicates that he has all of the above. Other causes of hernia include Nos. 1, 2, and 4.

251. (2) A truss should be applied before getting out of bed or after the hernia has been reduced by lying down with the feet elevated in bed or in the bath. If the hernia cannot be reduced, the truss should not be applied (Nos. 1 and 3). While the truss is not a cure for a hernia and its use is not as common as it once was, it is far more effective in keeping a hernia reduced than is an athletic supporter (No. 4).

252. (2) Mr. Dobson's smoking history and history of chronic cough necessitate directing preoperative nursing measures toward clearing his respiratory tract of excess secretions that may lead to postoperative complications. Besides oral hygiene, postural drainage, incentive spirometers, IPPB, and mucolytic agent may be instituted or ordered before surgery. Since postoperative coughing is contraindicated with hernia repairs, removal of secretions is a priority, as is instruction in deep-breathing techniques. Nos. 1, 3, and 4 are correct and should also be included in your preoperative teaching plan.

253. (3) Since the patient has a history of chronic cough, and since hernias can be repaired with spinal anesthesia, this approach may have the least amount of risk for postoperative complications. General anesthesia (No. 1) has the greatest risk for respiratory complications after surgery. Intravenous (No. 2) and local infiltration (No. 4) would not supply the depth of anesthesia needed to complete the repair.

254. (2) Timed forced expiratory volume measures the functional ability of an individual to remove air from his lungs. Reduction in FEV_1 is usually due to airway obstruction from excess mucus. While inadequate innervation of the intercostals (No. 3) would also reduce the FEV_1, there is nothing in this case study to indicate that Mr. Dobson has neuromuscular problems. Vital capacity measures the individual's ability to move a volume of air in and out of the lungs (No. 1). Atelectasis (No. 4) is determined by X ray, clinical symptomatology, and blood gases.

255. (1) The skin preparation area for hernia repair includes the entire abdomen from just below the nipple line to the midthigh. It includes all visible pubic hair when the legs are together and should extend to the bedline on each side. No. 2 is an example of an abdominal prep when the incision is above the umbilicus. No. 3 is a lower-extremities prep for surgeries such as a femoral arterial graft. No. 4 is a perineal prep used for vaginal or rectal surgeries.

256. (2) To avoid the complication of a painful spinal headache that can last for several days, the patient is kept flat in a supine position for approximately 4–12 hours postoperatively. Headaches are believed due to the seepage of cerebral spinal fluid from the puncture site. By keeping the patient flat, cerebral spinal fluid pressures are equalized, which avoids trauma to the neurons. No. 1 is the position for patients having general anesthesia. No. 3 is incorrect because knees are flexed. No. 4 is the position for patients with head traumas.

257. (2) Since the patient is awake with a spinal anesthetic, level of consciousness and airway integrity are lower priorities than circulatory status. Patients who have had spinal anesthesia have varying degrees of hypotension due to the vasodepressor effect of the anesthetic agent on the autonomic nervous system. Reflexes will be depressed in the lower extremities because of the anesthetic and should be checked after circulatory status. However, sensory impulses remain blocked longer than motor activity, so safety measures should be instituted to prevent injury from bedding, poor positioning, or sources of heat.

258. (2) Postoperative inflammation and edema underlie the frequent occurrence of scrotal swelling after indirect hernia repair. This complication is very painful, and any movement by the patient results in discomfort. Elevating the scrotum on rolled towels or providing support with a suspensory helps to reduce edema. Ice bags facilitate pain relief. Pain medication (No. 3) may also be administered, but vigorous coughing (No. 4) is contraindicated following herniorrhaphy. No. 1 is inappropriate as this is not an emergency side effect of surgery.

259. (3) While most patients are able to rest more comfortably and even sleep after administration of a narcotic, extreme or prolonged lethargy indicates that the medication dose may be too large. The physician should be consulted for both a change of dose and/or route of administration (Nos. 1 and 2). Alternate modes of pain relief can and should be instituted if Mr. Dobson's discomfort is not severe, but not as a delaying tactic (No. 4) when the issue is the appropriateness of a specific medication dose.

260. (4) If all the secondary measures have been utilized and the patient's bladder is distended, the physician should be notified if he or she has not left a catheterization order. Occasionally drugs such as Prostigmin are ordered to stimulate bladder contractions before resorting to catheterization. Catheters should not be inserted without an order (No. 2), nor should the patient be unduly fatigued by other measures (Nos. 1 and 3). The bladder should not be allowed to become overdistended.

261. (1) Urinary retention following spinal anesthesia is due to blockage of autonomic nervous system fibers, which innervate the bladder and sensory perception. No. 2, though correct, is not as complete as No. 1. All patients secrete ADH postoperatively because of the surgical insult. However, ADH reduces the volume of urine (No. 3), as does lowered blood pressure (No. 4), but neither causes urinary retention.

262. (2) Prostigmin is an anticholinesterase. It enhances bladder tone and contraction, enabling complete emptying of the bladder. It is also used in the treatment of myasthenia gravis. Urecholine is an example of a cholinergic drug, also used to treat postoperative urinary retention. Atropine is an example of an anticholinergic drug, which would act to inhibit initiation of urination. Beta blockers such as propranolol do not affect the bladder. Hence Nos. 1, 3, and 4 are incorrect.

263. (2) Given Mr. Dobson's complaint and evidence of pink drainage, you should suspect dehiscence. Dehiscence is characterized by a gush of pinked serous drainage and a parting of the wound edges. Dehiscence generally occurs in the fifth to seventh day following surgery and occurs due to increased intraabdominal pressures from flatus, coughing, retching, or inadequate tissue support. Late hemorrhage (No. 1) would be accompanied by signs of shock such as decreased blood pressure, rapid pulse, and diaphoresis. Wound infection (No. 3) would be characterized by pain, redness, and fever. Evisceration (No. 4) occurs after dehiscence when loops of intestine escape through the opened incision.

264. (1) The patient should remain quiet in a low-Fowler's or horizontal position. He should be cautioned not to cough so as not to extrude any intestines by increasing intraabdominal pressures. The physician should be notified next. Remain with the patient, reassuring him, monitoring vital signs, and having others bring equipment such as an IV set-up, nasogastric tube, and suction equipment. The surgeon should also be notified that the patient will be returning to the operating room. The patient should be kept NPO (No. 2) in above position (No. 3) and the dressing left in place to prevent evisceration (No. 4).

265. (4) All straining and lifting should be avoided for at least three weeks to prevent undue stress on the sutures. Other less strenuous activities such as Nos. 1, 2, and 3 are appropriate, though good body mechanics should be reviewed with the patient.

266. (2) The functions of the gallbladder are to collect, concentrate, and store bile that is produced by the liver. Bile reaches the gallbladder via the hepatic duct, which later joins the cystic duct emanating from the gallbladder to form the common bile duct. The common bile duct joins the pancreatic duct, which opens into the duodenum. Contraction of the gallbladder and therefore flow of bile are stimulated by the hormone cholecystokinin, which is secreted by the duodenal mucosa when food enters the duodenum. Hence Nos. 1, 3, and 4 are incorrect.

267. (3) Fat-soluble vitamins, particularly vitamin K, are poorly absorbed in the absence of bile. Decreased absorption of vitamin K results in decreased levels of circulating prothrombin, thus reducing normal clotting levels. Peripheral neuritis occurs with vitamin B_6 deficiencies and scurvy with deficiency in vitamin C; these are water-soluble vitamins. Macrocytic anemia is consistent with a vitamin B_{12} deficiency, which may be due to lack of intrinsic factor in the stomach. Hence Nos. 1, 2, and 4 are incorrect.

268. (3) Obstruction of the bile duct will cause elevated serum and urine bilirubin (dark urine) as well as a decreased amount of urobilinogen in the feces (clay-colored stools). Bilirubin is an end product of hemoglobin breakdown. Normally it is conjugated in the liver and secreted into the intestines in the bile, where it is converted into urobilinogen and excreted in the stools. No. 1 is incorrect because biliary obstruction itself does not directly affect blood pressure. However, if the obstruction is acute and accompanied by pain, changes in blood pressure in response to increased sympathetic tone can be expected. No. 2 is incorrect because between-meal eructation is a symptom of ulcer disease. Eructation in gallbladder disease occurs after eating, particularly if large amounts of fat have been ingested. No. 4 is also incorrect. Longitudinal ridging of the fingernails is a sign seen frequently in anemia.

269. (4) While the primary use of probantheline Br in many clinical situations involving the gastrointestinal tract is to reduce gastric secretions and intestinal hypermobility, it is used in gallbladder disease because of its antispasmotic effects on the gallbladder and bile duct. No. 1 is therefore correct, but not the best choice. Nos. 2 and 3 are incorrect because probantheline Br does not reduce bile secretions nor does its calming effect on gastric motility reduce the amount of chyme entering the duodenum.

270. (3) Morphine sulfate causes spasms of the sphincter of Oddi, thereby increasing intraductal pressures and abdominal pain. Papaverine and meperidine, both synthetic opiates, as well as nitroglycerin may be administered to relieve pain associated with gallbladder disease. No. 1 is incorrect, since the effect of morphine is to increase spasms in the gallbladder. No. 2, while correct, is not the best answer. Opiates are withheld when a patient has an acute abdomen and the diagnosis is unknown or tentative. In this case, Mrs. Klein has an established history of gallbladder disease and rather specific symptomatology. No. 4 is incorrect in that while morphine does relax vascular smooth muscle, this effect does not increase bile synthesis in the liver.

271. (2) The contrast medium utilized in IV cholangiograms, like that used in intravenous pyelogram, contains iodine. It is important to ascertain before the test whether the patient is aware of any allergy to iodine. Salt water fish generally leave a high iodine content, so it is helpful to ascertain if the patient has an allergy to fish, and if so, to what kind. Nos. 3 and 4 are less specific responses that provide interesting, though not essential, data. No. 1 is helpful in planning patient teaching and may also elicit No. 2.

272. (2) Patients, if given anything by mouth, are given a low-fat meal the evening before IV cholangiogram or oral cholecystogram. Since Mrs. Klein is quite ill at this time, she may or may not be able to tolerate oral intake. However, in order to have a clear visualization of the gallbladder, the bowel is cleansed, food and fluids are withheld for six to eight hours, and the patient is informed of possible reaction to injection of the contrast medium. Hence Nos. 1, 3, and 4 are incorrect.

273. (3) Telepaque tablets are administered one at a time in five-minute intervals, one hour after eating a fat-free meal, with a minimal amount of water (usually 8 oz). Water is allowed until bedtime, but food is withheld in order to allow as much dye as possible to concentrate in the gallbladder. The next morning an initial X ray is taken, after which the patient is given a fatty meal and several more pictures are taken to observe the function of the gallbladder. Hence Nos. 1, 2, and 4 are appropriate actions.

274. (3) Heating pads are not used to relieve the abdominal discomfort of cholelithiasis and cholecystitis, since they have little effect on reducing spasms of deeper organs. Instead, antispasmotics are utilized. Nos. 1, 2, and 4 are appropriate nursing measures in the preoperative period.

275. (2) Patients with high abdominal surgeries tend to breathe shallowly after surgery in order to splint incisional discomfort. Consequently, these patients need both assistance and encouragement to deep breathe and cough. Splinting of the incisional area by the nurse helps, as well as planning deep breathing and particularly coughing times to follow the administration of a pain reliever. Nos. 1 and 3 are correct statements, but not the best answers. Patients with abdominal surgeries tend to guard against coughing, as it increases intraab-

dominal pressures and incisional discomfort. Women do tend to be thoracic breathers and need to be taught abdominal or diaphragmatic breathing in the preoperative period. No. 4 is incorrect, because N/G tubes do not inhibit deep breathing; rather, they tend to increase oral respirations, which causes drying of the oral mucous membranes.

276. (2) Sitting the patient up allows for deeper ventilation and splinting of the incisional area reduces incisional discomfort. No. 1 is also correct, but not specific enough. Generally 20–30 minutes should elapse before instituting coughing techniques following administration of an analgesic to allow for the full effects of the drug. No. 3 is incorrect unless she is in a good deal of pain; if so, she should be medicated, then coughed. No. 4 is incorrect because oral intake is withheld until bowel activity is reestablished. Secretions can be kept mobilized by frequent turning and deep breathing.

277. (1) The purpose of the T-tubes is to maintain the patency of the bile duct after surgery. Localized edema in the surgery area tends to obstruct the outflow of bile, which is continually being synthesized by the liver. A secondary effect of this procedure is that bile flow is directed away from the duodenum (No. 4). The T-tube does not directly prevent postoperative hemorrhage (No. 2) or postoperative wound infection (No. 3).

278. (4) Normally drainage from the T-tube averages 300–500 ml during the first few days after surgery and then gradually decreases; the tube is generally removed in 7–10 days. By the fourth postoperative day, flow has usually begun to decrease. Excessive drainage at this time should be reported, as it indicates possible reobstruction of the duct. Nos. 1, 2, and 3 are normal postoperative findings.

279. (2) The T-tube is clamped prior to eating to increase bile flow into the duodenum and assist in the digestion of fats. No. 1 is incorrect because the act of eating normally stimulates bile secretion, and clamping of the T-tube will not inhibit its flow except to the dependent drainage bag. No. 3 is incorrect because bile does not affect peristalsis, although inadequate bile flow can result in abdominal distention. No. 4 is also correct, though it is not the best answer. If the patient is able to tolerate clamping of the T-tube, then bile is flowing normally into the duodenum and the duct is patent.

280. (1) Following clamping of the T-tube, observe the patient for signs of abdominal distress, pain, nausea, chills, or fever. These symptoms may be due to a localized reaction to the bile, edema, or obstructed flow. Severe abdominal pain may indicate leakage of bile into the peritoneal cavity. Eructation or burping may occur after eating if bile flow was insufficient. Jaundice is a late symptom of biliary obstruction. An increased respiratory rate may occur if the patient has abdominal discomfort, pain, or nausea. Hence Nos. 2, 3, and 4 are incorrect.

281. (3) There are no specific dietary restrictions following cholecystectomy. Patients are advised, however, to avoid foods high in fats. Most patients tend to avoid these foods anyway because they are more comfortable if they do so. Generally, after about three months, patients may begin to experiment with certain foods to ascertain their tolerance to them. No. 1 is incorrect because some fat is allowed in the diet at all times. No. 2 is incorrect because fats are not limited to those classified as polyunsaturates. No. 4 is incorrect because fats are allowed in the postcholecystectomy diet to tolerance.

282. (1) Whole milk has a high fat content, so patients are generally advised to switch to low-fat or skim milk. Cottage cheese, whole-grain breads, and eggs are allowed in the postcholecystectomy diet, though eggs may be limited to four per week. Hence Nos. 2, 3, and 4 are incorrect.

283. (2) Sigmoidoscopy involves the insertion of a rigid instrument into the anus that allows direct visualization of the anal canal, rectum, and sigmoid colon. The patient is usually prepared for this procedure with enemas or rectal suppositories. No. 1 is an example of a lower GI. No. 3 describes a colonoscopy, and No. 4 describes two of the procedures that can be accomplished with a colonoscope.

284. (2) Neomycin sulfate is used preoperatively because it is poorly absorbed in the intestinal tract and acts to decrease the bacteria count in the colon. As the result of this action, postoperative infection is reduced (No. 1). Neomycin does not reduce tumor size (No. 3), nor does it directly affect peristalsis (No. 4).

285. (1) Toxic doses of neomycin may result in eighth cranial nerve damage much like that produced by streptomycin. Kidney damage may also occur, extending from milk albuminuria to elevation in blood urea nitrogen. Nausea and vomiting are common with ingestion of antibiotics, though not specific to neomycin. Erythromycin most commonly causes nausea, vomiting, and diarrhea. Anaphylactic reactions are associated most commonly with penicillin administration. Hence Nos. 2, 3, and 4 are incorrect.

286. (3) A double-barrel colostomy has two stomas that may or may not be separated by skin. The proximal loop discharges feces and the distal loop discharges mucus. The closure of this temporary colostomy usually occurs in approximately six months. No. 1 is an example of an ascending colostomy, No. 2 describes a transverse loop colostomy, and No. 4 describes a descending colostomy.

287. (2) The stomas will begin to secrete mucus within 48

hours and the proximal loop should begin to drain fecal material within 72 hours. Ileostomies (No. 1) begin to drain immediately. Nos. 3 and 4 are incorrect because peristalsis generally returns within 48 to 72 hours postoperatively.

288. (4) Colostomy irrigations should be timed as closely as possible to the patient's normal defecation pattern. Generally irrigations are begun between the fifth and seventh postoperative day. The purpose of these irrigations is to "retrain" the bowel for normal evacuation. Irrigations are least effective in establishing regular evacuations in those patients with semisoft or liquid stools and those who had prior irregular patterns of defecation. Hence, Nos. 1, 2, and 3 are incorrect.

289. (1) The purpose of the colostomy irrigation is to promote peristalsis and reestablish regular defecation patterns. Irrigations are secondarily designed to prevent constipation (No. 2) and fecal impactions, which may result in diarrhea (No. 3). As irrigations are done with tap water, they do not act to reduce intestinal flora (No. 4).

290. (1) Carbonated drinks, cabbage, sauerkraut, and nuts tend to increase flatulence, and most patients feel uncomfortable passing flatus into the colostomy bag, as it causes it to inflate. Onions, cheese, and fish may cause odorous drainage. Generally the initial diet following a colostomy is a low-fiber diet for several weeks. As the diet is increased, the individual patient can determine more accurately which foods cause constipation, diarrhea, flatus, or dyspepsia. Hence Nos. 2, 3, and 4 are incorrect.

291. (1) The basic pathophysiologic changes associated with chronic bronchitis are hypertrophy of the mucous glands lining the bronchi and the production of increased amounts of mucus (sometimes thick and difficult to expectorate) that tend to narrow airway and trap air distal to the mucus. Bronchoconstriction and edema of the bronchial walls is characteristic of asthma. Exudate in the alveoli and increasing lung stiffness are consistent with pneumonia. Hence Nos. 2, 3, and 4 are incorrect.

292. (1) A wheeze is a high-pitched, musical chest sound produced by airflow in narrowed bronchioles. It is primarily an expiratory sound and is always considered pathologic. Stridor is a high-pitched crowing sound on inspiration and is due to upper-airway obstruction such as edema, adhesions, tracheal hypertrophy, etc. Rhonchi are medium-pitched sonorous sounds produced by airflow obstruction in larger airways. Hence Nos. 2, 3, and 4 are incorrect.

293. (1) The hypochloremia (low chloride) that tends to occur with chronic obstructive lung disease is the result of both the active reabsorption of bicarbonate ions by the kidney, thus passively increasing chloride excretion, and the increasing inhibition of the reverse chloride shift in the lungs. Hemoglobin levels and serum osmolarity do not directly affect chloride concentrations. Hence Nos. 2, 3, and 4 are incorrect.

294. (2) To read blood gases, first note the pH. In this case, Mr. Collins's pH is 7.38. This pH is within the normal range (7.35 to 7.45) but is on the acidotic side. Next you need to look at the pCO_2 and $^-HCO_3$ to see which one is causing the shift to acidosis. In this case the pCO_2 is 65 (acidosis) and the $^-HCO_3$ is 32 (alkalosis). Therefore, Mr. Collins has compensated respiratory acidosis because his kidneys have been able to conserve enough bicarbonate to keep his pH within normal range. In this case a pH below 7.35 would indicate uncompensated respiratory acidosis. If Mr. Collins had compensated metabolic alkalosis, his pH would be between 7.41 and 7.45. If he had uncompensated metabolic alkalosis, his pH would be above 7.45. Hence Nos. 1, 3, and 4 are incorrect.

295. (4) Indications of respiratory distress and the increased work of breathing in this patient are characterized by the use of the accessory muscles of respiration, the sternocleidomastoid and trapezius muscles. Utilizing these muscles enables the patient to increase the size of his thorax, thus allowing air to move in. Patients with chronic bronchitis and air-trapping generally are not able to increase the depth of breathing by increasing diaphragmatic excursion. Some patients may be utilizing pursed-lip exhalations, but these help maintain open airways for the expulsion of gases. Hence Nos. 1, 2, and 3 are incorrect.

296. (1) The observed total lung capacity (TLC), functional residual capacity (FRC), and residual volume (RV) are all increased over expected values. These values indicate that Mr. Collins is hyperinflated, a common phenomenon with airway obstruction and air-trapping. Hyperventilation is characterized by an increase in PO_2 and pH. Hypercapnia is identified when pCO_2 is elevated. Hyperpnea is simply an increase in respiratory rate. Hence Nos. 2, 3, and 4 are incorrect.

297. (2) Increased lung volumes (TLC, FRC, RV) and decreased airflow—vital capacity (VC) and forced expiratory volume in one second (FEV_1)—are functional problems consistent with obstructive lung disease. In restrictive lung disease, volumes generally are decreased. Vascular lung disease has no effect on ventilatory capacity, but directly affects diffusion of gases; that is, pulmonary infarction decreases blood flow to lungs, so some alveoli that are ventilated are no longer perfused. Hence Nos. 1, 3, and 4 are incorrect.

298. (1) Treatment with bronchodilators such as isoproterenol will decrease bronchoconstriction, improving the movement of air in and out of the lungs. These pulmonary function studies indicate that Mr. Collins has

been able to increase his inspiratory capacity by 1000 ml (VC 2800–3800) and his expiratory capacity (RV decreased, FRC decreased, and FEV_1 increased). Hence Nos. 2, 3, and 4 are incorrect.

299. (4) Anatomical dead space refers to the air in the lungs that does not take part in respiration (O_2-CO_2 exchange). It is the air in the respiratory passages—the nose, trachea, bronchi, bronchioles. The anatomical dead space does not generally increase or decrease. Physiologic dead space refers to the ratio of ventilation to perfusion. Normally, there are some alveoli that may be ventilated but poorly perfused, or perfused but poorly ventilated, with blood flow to the bases of the lungs greater than to the apices. However, in pulmonary disease the mismatch between ventilation and perfusion is greatly increased, thus increasing the amount of physiologic dead space. In obstructive lung disease, with air-trapping, alveolar walls are damaged or destroyed, thus decreasing the surface area for diffusion of gases. Also hypoxia in the lungs causes constriction of the vasculature, decreasing blood flow to some ventilated alveoli. Prolonged or chronic respiratory hypoxia results in pulmonary hypertension and hypertrophy of the right ventricle (cor pulmonale). Hence Nos. 1, 2, and 3 are incorrect.

300. (2) The most important effect of intermittent positive-pressure breathing (IPPB) is increased alveolar ventilation, which decreases the occurrence of atelectasis (No. 3). It also helps to mobilize secretions (No. 1) and decrease airway resistance (No. 4) through mechanical bronchodilation.

301. (2) Theophylline relaxes bronchial smooth muscles, which helps to relieve the wheezing and coughing associated with bronchospasm. Side effects are rare, but the earliest signs of overdose are usually anorexia, nausea, and vomiting. Tachycardia, restlessness, tremors, headache, and insomnia are side effects associated with catecholamine bronchodilators such as ephedrine and isoproterenol. Hence Nos. 1, 3, and 4 are incorrect.

302. (3) Deep breathing, coughing, and pursed-lip exhalations are all techniques that the nurse can teach the patient to improve ventilation. Adequate fluid intake (No. 1) is essential for keeping sputum liquified; however, very hot and/or very cold drinks should be avoided since they may cause bronchospasm. Patients with COPD also need to be taught to avoid exposure to infections, early signs of infection, and the need to seek medical intervention promptly should symptoms occur. Nos. 2 and 4 are not indicated in this patient's therapy.

303. (3) The position that allows for the greatest amount of lung expansion is sitting up and leaning slightly forward. This position can be facilitated by allowing the patient to rest his arms on a bedside table. The position that also facilitates lung expansion, but not to the same degree, is high-Fowler's. Both the prone position and the Trendelenburg position tend to decrease full lung expansion due to increased pressure of abdominal contents on the diaphragm. Hence Nos. 1, 2, and 4 are incorrect.

304. (2) While it is not possible to make a patient stop smoking, the patient should be presented with information about methods used by other people who were successful in stopping. While most people are aware of the deleterious effects of smoking, patients need to be reminded of the relationship between smoking and their present condition. Fluid intake and nutrition need to be discussed and adapted to individual needs. Patients should be able to identify drugs, giving the name, correct dosage, timing, and potential side effects. Alcohol in moderation is not restricted (No. 1). Activities should be encouraged to tolerance (No. 4). Vocational rehabilitation should be present as an option but not emphasized (No. 3).

305. (1) The Mantoux test is injected intradermally on the polar aspect of the forearm. If correctly administered, a pale elevation similar to a mosquito bite should be apparent. Nos. 2, 3, and 4 are not used for this test.

306. (4) The Mantoux test is read in 48–72 hours. Color is observed and the injection site is palpated for induration. Reading the test in less than 48 hours may lead to inaccurate interpretation. Hence Nos. 1, 2, and 3 are incorrect.

307. (1) An induration of 10 mm or more is considered a positive reaction. The skin is generally reddened. Indurations of 5–9 mm are considered doubtful reactions. Individuals with doubtful reactions should be retested unless they have had a known contact with persons with tuberculosis. Indurations of less than 5 mm are considered negative reactions. Hence Nos. 2, 3, and 4 are incorrect.

308. (3) Proper handling of sputum is essential to allay droplet transference of bacilli in the air. Patients need to be taught to cover their nose and mouth with tissues when sneezing or coughing. Chemotherapy generally renders the patient noninfectious within days to a few weeks, usually before cultures for tubercle bacilli are negative. Until chemical isolation is established, many institutions require the patient to wear a mask when visitors are in the room or when the nurse is in attendance. Patients should be in a well-ventilated room, without air recirculation, to prevent air contamination. Hence Nos. 1, 2, and 4 are unnecessary precautions.

309. (2) Pyridoxine (vitamin B_6) 25–50 mg a day is ordered prophylactically to prevent symptoms of peripheral neuritis. Serious side effects of INH therapy are rare. Nos. 1, 3, and 4 have no effect on peripheral neuritis.

310. (3) Since tubercle bacilli multiply very slowly, and since antitubercular drugs are bacteriostatic, not bacteriocidal, the patient must continue therapy for at least two years to allow time for the body's defenses to contain the organisms. Individuals who have been inspected for tuberculosis but who do not have evidence of active disease are treated prophylactically with INH for a one-year period. Hence Nos. 1, 2, and 4 are incorrect.

311. (3) A thyroid scan utilizes the uptake of ^{131}I by the thyroid gland to determine the size, shape, and function of the gland. Also identified are areas of increased uptake (hot areas) indicating increased metabolic function as in hyperthyroidism (No. 2) and areas of decreased or no uptake (cold areas), which are associated with malignancy. Nos. 1 and 4 both describe the TSH stimulation test.

312. (1) Following an injection of the small dose of ^{131}I used in a thyroid scan, no radiation precautions are necessary. Full radiation precaution (No. 2) is utilized for radium implants. No. 3 may be employed when ^{131}I therapy is utilized to control and reduce hypersecretion by the thyroid (hyperthyroidism). No. 4 is not an example of normal radiation therapy policy.

313. (3) Surgical treatment of hyperthyroidism involves a subtotal thyroidectomy in which approximately five-sixths of the thyroid tissue is removed. While this procedure does not cure hyperthyroidism, it reduces the amount of circulating thyroid hormone by reducing the amount of functioning tissue. No. 1, complete or total thyroidectomy, is rarely done for hyperthyroidism today, but is indicated for thyroid malignancy. No. 2, removal of half of the thyroid, would leave enough functioning hyperactive tissue to prevent diminution of symptoms in the patient. No. 4 is incorrect because the patient with hyperthyroidism does not need additional thyroid hormone; he/she receives antithyroid medications such as propylthiouracil (PRU) or methimazole (Tapazole) to reduce both circulating and stored thyroid.

314. (3) To prevent undue stress on the suture line and underlying surgical repair, the patient is taught to support the back of the neck when repositioning and to avoid both hyperextension and flexion of the neck. No. 1 is incorrect because active flexion of the neck is avoided and because after a total thyroidectomy the patient will receive thyroid medications to prevent hypothyroidism and to maintain a euthyroid state. No. 2 is also incorrect due to the focus on active flexion and extension neck exercises, which would put undue stress on the suture line. No. 4 is partially correct; however, again active flexion exercises are contraindicated.

315. (4) Since the integrity of the gastrointestinal tract is not interrupted during thyroid surgery, paralytic ileus is a rare complication. However, hemorrhage (No. 1) must be continually observed for, as the thyroid itself and the surrounding tissues are highly vascular. Evidence of bleeding should be sought by observing not only the dressings but also the sheets under the patient's neck and shoulders. Respiratory obstruction (No. 2) may occur secondary to edema or laryngeal nerve damage. Tetany (No. 3) and hypocalcemia may occur secondary to transient or permanent damage to the parathyroid glands.

316. (3) Tetany caused by hypocalcemia can be assessed for by briskly tapping the facial nerve, which is located near the middle of the masseter muscle just proximal to the ear lobe (Chvostek's sign). A positive reaction occurs when there is facial-muscle contraction, which includes a twitch of the upper lip on that side. Checking urine calcium levels (No. 1) is not helpful in assessing for early signs of hypocalcemia since urine calcium levels are dependent not only on parathormone excretion but also on oral intake. No. 2 describes Homans' sign, which is utilized to determine the presence of deep vein thrombosis. No. 4 is a late sign of hypocalcemia.

317. (1) Nursing measures designed to reduce the occurrence of postthyroidectomy hemorrhage include frequent checks of the dressings and bedclothes under the patient, semi-Fowler's to prevent hyperextension of the neck, and ice packs to reduce hematoma formation and edema. No. 2 is partially correct; however, the supine position would increase edema since it prevents gravity drainage of the wound site. No. 3 is incorrect because coughing will increase stress on the sutures unless the head and neck are well supported, and moist packs tend to increase local blood flow, which in turn tends to increase edema formation in this patient. No. 4 is incorrect because flexionlike hyperextension puts increased stress on the suture line.

318. (3) Maintenance of an adequate airway is always the primary goal of nursing care. Respiratory obstruction is a very serious complication; therefore it is wise to have both an emergency tracheostomy set and suctioning apparatus available at the bedside of the patient who has had a thyroidectomy. No. 1 is also correct but not the best answer, since the onset of this complication is more gradual. With adequate nursing observation, it can be handled before it becomes life-threatening. No. 2 is incorrect because thoracentesis is utilized to remove excess fluid from the pleural space. The correct nursing strategy for the occurrence of postoperative bleeding (No. 4) is to notify the physician immediately.

319. (3) In early respiratory obstruction, the patient generally complains of a feeling of fullness or a choking sensation. Swallowing difficulties are fairly common due to tracheal irritation; however, difficulty in swallowing in conjunction with a choking sensation is indicative of airway obstruction. No. 1, hoarseness and weakness of the voice, is common and is secondary to edema of the larynx. No. 2, stridor and cyanosis, is a late sign of airway obstruction. No. 4, disorientation and combative behaviors, is indicative of severe anoxia.

320. (3) An immediate response to the choking sensation is assessment of the surgical site by examining under the dressing. If it appears edematous, loosen the dressing and have someone remain with the patient. Notify the physician (No. 4), who might order the sutures or clips to be removed. Elevating the head to a high-Fowler's position (No. 1), while the preferred position for improving ventilation of the lung, will not reduce upper-airway obstruction. No. 2 is inappropriate for this situation and may actually increase the patient's distress.

321. (2) The patient who has had thyroid surgery should be assisted in supporting the head and neck whenever their positions are changed during the first three postoperative days. Supporting the head is particularly important during early ambulation procedures, when sudden movement may result in hyperextension of the neck. Nos. 1, 3, and 4 are incorrect because none of these responses takes into account the need to prevent hyperextension of the neck.

322. (1) A freshly applied cast generates heat as moisture evaporates and cast hardens. To facilitate drying, keep it exposed to the air. Do not use plastic covers or Chux on pillows to elevate the limb, as these tend to slow drying. No. 2 is incorrect; signs of increased pressure are numbness and tingling, pain, and loss of movement. No. 3 does not take into account that discomfort and apprehension can be reduced if the patient understands what is to be expected. No. 4 is not an appropriate response to the question because it also fails to recognize the patient's cognitive needs.

323. (3) Signs of circulatory constriction include blanching (delayed capillary refill) and cyanosis, swelling of the toes, pain that is out of proportion for the type of fracture, and temperature changes. Tingling and numbness (No. 1), loss of movement (No. 2), and constant pain (No. 4) are symptoms associated with constriction or pressure on a peripheral nerve.

324. (3) Bivalving the cast involves full-length splitting of the cast on each side. The underlying padding is also cut, as blood-soaked padding shrinks and can also cause circulatory constriction. After the cast is cut, it is spread sufficiently to relieve constriction. This procedure does not disturb reduction of the bone. The cast is then reapplied (No. 1) after the swelling has gone down. No. 2 is the technique used when the cast is removed. The patient's limb (No. 4) should always be elevated following bivalving, as the underlying condition (edema and swelling) is best relieved by elevation of the limb, ice packs, and isometric exercises.

325. (4) While range-of-motion exercises of joints not enclosed in the cast are encouraged, the primary purpose of the cast is to immobilize those joints above and below the fracture. Therefore encouraging the patient to flex his right knee would be counterproductive to the aim of therapy. Nos. 1, 2, and 3 are appropriate exercises for this patient.

326. (2) It is not safe to insert any foreign object under a cast, as the skin may be broken and become infected. Scratching also disturbs the padded surface under the cast, causing it to become wrinkled, which may lead to skin irritation and breakdown. Itching under the cast can be relieved by directing air from a blower under the cast. Oral medication is not generally effective in relieving this type of skin irritation (No. 1). Rolling the cast (No. 3) while Mr. Mackey scratched would only increase the risk of skin damage. Taking the pencil from Mr. Mackey (No. 4) would deny his ability both to understand the rationale and to take responsibility for his actions.

327. (2) The three-point gait is appropriate when weight-bearing is not allowed on the affected limb. The swing-to and swing-through crutch gaits may also be used when only one leg can be utilized for weight-bearing. Nos. 1 and 3 are utilized when weight-bearing is allowed in both feet. No. 4, the tripod gait, is utilized when the patient has little or no sensation or movement (paralysis) in the lower limbs.

328. (1) In the use of crutches, all weight-bearing should be on the hands. Constant pressure in the axilla from weight-bearing can lead to damage of the brachial plexus nerves and produce crutch paralysis. Nos. 2, 3, and 4 are appropriate instructions to give to the patient preparing for crutch-walking.

329. (3) Even though Mr. Edwards will have only one eye patched after surgery, familiarization with the physical arrangement of his room and with nursing personnel will decrease the occurrence of disorientation, which affects many elderly patients. It is not necessary to keep Mr. Edwards flat in bed before or after surgery (No. 1). Patches (No. 2) are not generally applied to both eyes. Eye-drop instillations (No. 4) are part of the postoperative or predischarge teaching plan.

330. (1) Local anesthesia is used in cataract surgery not only because this surgery is a short procedure, but also because most patients are elderly, with one or more chronic diseases, which may be exacerbated by general anesthesia. Intravenous anesthesia with sodium pentothal is most frequently used when unconsciousness

is desirable for short procedures or when an anesthetic induction is desired for general anesthesia. Rectal anesthesia, while rarely used today, has been used to induce short-term anesthesia in children. Hence Nos. 2, 3, and 4 are incorrect.

331. (1) An iridectomy, or removal of a wedge from the iris, is performed with cataract removal to prevent the forward push of the aqueous humor from blocking the canal of Schlemm, which would produce a secondary glaucoma. Iridectomy does not affect pupillary dilatation (No. 2), facilitate retinal circulation (No. 3), or prevent corneal scarring (No. 4).

332. (3) Postoperatively the cataract patient may be placed in a flat or low-Fowler's position on his back or turned to the unoperated side. Turning the patient to the operative side (No. 4) or raising the head of the bed (No. 1) increases the stress on the sutures and may lead to hemorrhage. The patient may assume a prone position with the head turned to the unoperative side (No. 2), though most patients find a side-lying position more comfortable.

333. (3) Coughing, brushing the teeth, and shaving are activities that tend to increase intraocular pressures and are therefore restricted during the early postoperative period. Other activities to avoid include vomiting, bending, and stooping. Self-feeding (No. 1) is encouraged to help reduce the patient's perception of helplessness, though food should be cut for the patient to reduce exertion. Bathroom privileges (No. 2) and ambulation (No. 4) are permitted. However, constipation should be avoided, so a preoperative enema may be ordered as well as a stool softener in the postoperative period. The ambulating patient should have slip-on slippers to avoid bending or stooping.

334. (1) Patients should be informed that the cataract glasses will magnify objects; this not only causes distortions in the shape of an object but may also result in color distortions. The spatial changes that result from these lenses may cause the patient to underreach for an object or have difficulty walking and climbing stairs. Peripheral vision is decreased (No. 2), so that the patient needs to be taught to turn his head and utilize the central vision provided by the lenses. Nos. 3 and 4 are incorrect because the magnification created by these lens (up to 35%) is not similar to the size perception before the cataract formed, nor do they cause double vision.

335. (2) Epileptic seizures or convulsions are the result of excessive, simultaneous, disordered neuronal discharge in the brain. This dysrhythmic electrical discharge may be focal (Jacksonian seizure) or widely dispersed (grand mal seizures). Theories for the initiation of these convulsions vary from decreased intracellular K to decreased cerebral spinal fluid to alteration in neuronal defenses due to trauma, toxins, or inflammation. Hence Nos. 3 and 4 are incorrect, and depending upon existing potential in the individual, No. 1 may be a precipitating factor.

336. (2) Grand mal seizures are characterized by auras preceding the convulsion, loss of consciousness, loss of tonic and clonic sphincter control, and incontinence of both urine and feces. Brief, abrupt loss of consciousness with a characteristic "blank stare" is indicative of petit mal seizures. Localized twitching of facial muscles, especially of the angle of the mouth or within a finger or toe, is characteristic of a Jacksonian seizure. Focal or partial seizures usually involve only a portion of the brain and reflect the area of the brain activated by abnormal discharge (such as tonic and clonic contractions of the large muscles in an arm or leg). Hence Nos. 1, 3, and 4 are incorrect.

337. (3) Dilantin (phenytoin, diphenylhydantoin) is consistently found to be effective against most types of seizures except petit mal. Its precise action is unknown, but it appears to stabilize cell membranes by altering intracellular sodium concentrations. Plasma levels of the drug are checked frequently to avoid toxicity and to determine effective dosage. Side effects include gastritis and nervousness, and at toxic levels may cause ataxia. Phenobarbital (No. 1) and trimethadione (No. 4) are used in the control of petit mal seizures. Diazepam (No. 2) may be used as adjunct therapy in seizure disorders.

338. (2) To prevent airway obstruction, the patient's head should be turned to the side. If the patient's teeth are clenched, no effort should be made to forcibly open the mouth because the tongue may inadvertently be pushed back, obstructing the airway. If the patient's mouth is open and there is danger of his biting his tongue, a soft object may be placed between the teeth to prevent this injury. Nos. 1, 3, and 4 are all appropriate nursing actions.

339. (2) Dilantin must be injected IV slowly and in small increments to prevent vasodepression and circulatory collapse. Respiratory depression is generally associated with morphine sulfate. Adrenergic (alpha) drugs such as Levophed may cause vein and tissue necrosis and have rarely caused sudden malignant increases in blood pressure. Hence Nos. 1, 3, and 4 are incorrect.

340. (1) Glaucoma is defined as an imbalance between the rate of secretion of intraocular fluids and the rate of their absorption. Glaucoma may be acute/closed-angle (obstruction of the angle between the cornea and iris) or chronic/open-angle (obstruction occurs proximal or distal to the angle). It is characterized by increased intraocular pressures. Narrowing of the arterioles and retinal ischemia are the result of prolonged hypertension. Buckling of the retina is associated with retinal detachment. Hence Nos. 2, 3, and 4 are incorrect.

341. (3) Increased intraocular pressures tend to depress the optic disc, so that the retinal vessels that emerge from the center of the disc seem to disappear near the rim and reappear at a slightly different angle just past the rim. No. 1, blurring of the optic disc margins, occurs with palpilledema due to localized disease of the optic nerve or increased intracranial pressure. No. 2, pallor of the disc and/or white patches either in part or throughout the disc, is consistent with optic disc atrophy and may occur both with glaucoma and papilledema. No. 4 describes a scleral crescent, which is a normal ophthalmic finding.

342. (2) The normal range of intraocular pressures is 12–22 mm Hg. No. 1 is below the range of normal pressures and may occur in hypovolemia (soft eyeballs) or dehydration. No. 3 is incorrect because ocular pressures are measured in millimeters of mercury. No. 4 is incorrect because pressures above 22 mm Hg are considered elevated.

343. (3) Generally the patient with wide- or open-angle glaucoma has few complaints of intense symptomatology. The usual onset of this condition is slow, silent, and painless. However, some patients do experience prodromal symptoms such as aching and discomfort around the eye, disturbed accommodation to darkness, blurring of peripheral vision, and, less commonly, halos around lights. Any complaint of pain or increasing discomfort with radiation to the forehead and temporal area is a grave sign of a sudden increase in pressure. Hence Nos. 1, 2, and 4 are incorrect.

344. (3) In wide- or open-angle glaucoma, the obstruction to aqueous outflow is due to degenerative changes in either the trabeculum, Schlemm's canal, or the aqueous veins. Closed-angle glaucoma is characterized by obstruction of aqueous outflow due to narrowing of the angle between the anterior chamber and the root of the iris. Nos. 1, 2, and 4 are incorrect because wide- or open-angle glaucoma occurs more frequently than closed-angle, is characterized by slow, insidious, painless onset rather than the acute symptoms of closed-angle glaucoma, and is certainly familial if not hereditary. Due to this latter characteristic, family members of patients with open-angle glaucoma should be encouraged to have their intraocular pressures assessed yearly, particularly past age forty.

345. (2) Pilocarpine constricts the pupil by causing contraction of the ciliary muscles, thus widening the outflow channels and increasing aqueous flow. No. 1 is incorrect because pilocarpine is a parasympathomimetic; that is, it mimics the action of acetylcholine at cholinergic nerve endings, thus decreasing pupil size. No. 3 is incorrect in that diuretics such as Diamox, which is a carbonic anhydrase inhibitor, are used to decrease aqueous production. No. 4 does not describe the actions of any medication utilized in glaucoma therapy.

346. (1) Pilocarpine is a parasympathomimetic drug whose miotic effects act to reduce pressure and increase aqueous flow by constriction of the ciliary muscles, thus constricting the pupil and relieving congestion in the canal of Schlemm. Sympathomimetic drugs such as ephedrine are utilized in the treatment of glaucoma because they have an action similar to anticholinesterase drugs such as eserine; that is, they potentiate parasympathetic effects at cholinergic nerve endings. Beta blockers exert their main effects on heart rate. Hence Nos. 2, 3, and 4 are incorrect.

347. (2) Vigorous activities such as brushing the teeth and hair are generally discouraged during periods of acute distress. These activities tend to increase aqueous production and therefore pressures because they activate sympathetic nervous system stimulation of the vasculature. Quiet activities such as watching TV, moderate reading, self-feeding, and passive range-of-motion exercises are encouraged. Hence Nos. 1, 3, and 4 are incorrect.

348. (3) Eye drops should be instilled into the conjunctival sac to prevent medication from hitting the sensitive cornea. The patient should then be instructed to close his eye, but not squeeze shut, so that the medication can be distributed evenly over the eye. Nos. 1 and 4 are incorrect because instillation on these structures would increase corneal irritation. No. 2 is incorrect because drops instilled into the inner canthus are likely to run down the outer aspects of the nose.

349. (3) The most frequent cause of noncompliance to the medical treatment of wide- or open-angle glaucoma is the miotic effects of pilocarpine. Pupillary constriction impedes normal accommodation, making night driving difficult and hazardous, reducing the patient's ability to read for extended periods, and making participation in games with fast-moving objects impossible. No. 1 is incorrect because daytime driving is not restricted. No. 2 is incorrect because this process is painless. The fact that the process is painless and insidious may in fact increase patients' noncompliance because they do not usually experience any adverse reactions if they do not instill their eyedrops. Nausea and vomiting are rare toxic effects of pilocarpine and are usually very mild; hence No. 4 is incorrect.

350. (2) The legal definition of blindness is 20/200 or less in the better eye with corrective lenses, or when the visual field subtends an angle no greater than 20°. No. 1 is incorrect because use of corrective lenses may bring the individual's vision within normal range. No. 3 is incorrect because the individual's visual acuity is within normal range, though greatly reduced. No. 4 is incorrect because central and nasal vision is intact and therefore the individual would have a visual field greater than 20°.

351. (2) The primary dysfunction in myasthenia gravis occurs at the myoneural junction (the synapse between the end of a myelinated nerve fiber and a skeletal muscle fiber). Normally, acetylcholine is secreted by the nerve ending, which acts on the muscle fiber membrane by increasing its permeability to sodium. If sufficient sodium enters the muscle fiber membrane, an action potential is promulgated that causes the muscle fiber to contract. To enable the muscle fiber to repolarize, the acetylcholine in the synaptic junction is destroyed by cholinesterase. In myasthenia gravis, these normal impulses are blocked at the myoneural junction. No. 1 is incorrect because degeneration of the basal ganglia results in increased muscle tone, as occurs with Parkinson's disease. No. 3 is incorrect because increased stimulation of muscle fibers by anterior motor neurons would also increase muscle contractions. No. 4 is partially correct in that there does seem to be a familial tendency toward the development of myasthenia; however, if myasthenia is generalized it usually affects not only facial and mastication muscles but also ocular movement (diplopia and ptosis) as well as muscles of the neck, trunk (respirations), and limbs.

352. (1) Normally, the thymus gland atrophies in adulthood. However, patients with myasthenia gravis frequently have proliferative changes in this gland (70%). In studies involving over 1,000 patients, removal of the gland (thymectomy) resulted in remission or improvement in 75% of the patients. Nos. 2, 3, and 4 are characteristics accurately describing the occurrence and course of myasthenia gravis.

353. (3) Edrophonium (Tensilon) is a short-acting anticholinesterase compound. A positive Tensilon test (a prompt and dramatic increase in muscle strength) is consistent with the diagnosis of myasthenia gravis. No. 1 is incorrect because an exacerbation of symptoms would indicate another cause for the muscle dysfunction. No. 2 is partially correct: ptosis is relieved but so is sagging of other facial muscles. No. 4 is incorrect because the increase in muscle strength is accompanied by decreased fatigability as long as the drug continues to circulate.

354. (3) The backbone of treatment for patients with myasthenia gravis is drugs classified as anticholinesterases. These drugs increase the response of muscles to nerve impulses and improve muscle strength by inhibiting the rapid removal of acetylcholine from the myoneural junction. No. 1 is partially correct in that adrenergic drugs such as ephedrine sulfate are administered to improve muscle tone, but these drugs do not inhibit cholinesterase at the myoneural junction. Likewise, anticholinergic drugs (No. 2) such as atropine are also utilized in the treatment of myasthenia, primarily to reduce the incidence of side effects of the anticholinesterase drugs and to reverse their effect if "cholinergic crisis" occurs. Cholinergic drugs (No. 4) are not indicated in the treatment of myasthenia gravis.

355. (1) The most common side effects of pyridostigmine Br (Mestinon) and neostigmine Br (Prostigmin) include anorexia, nausea, diarrhea, and abdominal cramps. These symptoms are due to increased gastrointestinal secretions, smooth muscle contractions (peristalsis), and irritation of the gastric mucosa. No. 2 is incorrect because increased cholinergic discharge increases bladder tone and contraction, thus facilitating voiding. Nos. 3 and 4 are incorrect because the symptoms listed are consistent with increased adrenergic, not cholinergic discharge or stimulation.

356. (1) The gastric distress that occurs with these medications can be reduced by administering the drugs with milk, soda crackers, or antacids. Nos. 2, 3, and 4 are nursing actions consistent with Nos. 2, 3, and 4 in the previous question.

357. (3) In order to take full advantage of the effects of anticholinesterase drugs, they should generally be scheduled 20 to 30 minutes before eating. Nos. 1 and 2 are not totally incorrect in that these drugs generally act over a three-hour period; however, peak action occurs quickly and patients with dysphagia need time to eat, chew, and swallow during meals. Rushing at meals causes unnecessary fatigue. No. 4 may not allow enough time for the drug to take effect.

358. (2) Signs of "cholinergic crisis" include pupils constricted to < 2 mm, severe diarrhea, nausea, vomiting, hypersalivation, lacrimation, pallor, and hypotension. Bradycardia may occur but is uncommon. In severe cases, confusion progressing to coma may occur due to blockage of cerebral synapses. Nos. 1 and 3 are symptoms related to increased adrenergic discharge. No. 4 is only partially correct.

359. (1) In cholinergic crisis, all anticholinesterase drugs are withdrawn and atropine (an anticholinergic drug) is given in 2-mg doses IV every hour until signs of atropine toxicity develop (dry mouth, blurred vision, tachycardia, rash or flushing of the skin, and elevated temperature). Nos. 2, 3, and 4 are incorrect because they do not act to decrease cholinergic responses. Ephedrine is utilized in myasthenia gravis to increase muscle tone, potassium chloride is utilized to increase serum K^+ because it is believed that adequate serum potassium levels potentiate the effects of cholinergic drugs, and neostigmine Br is an anticholinesterase that acts to improve cholinergic transmission of impulses at the myoneural junction.

360. (3) Before assessing and planning any rehabilitation program, the nurse must first assess the patient's and the family's understanding of and attitudes toward myasthenia as well as their emotional response and coping abilities. Before ascertaining any further information about job stresses and/or life style, any unusual fears, misconceptions, or problems relating to the patient's condition need to be identified and dealt with. It may be necessary to utilize the skills of a psychiatric nurse specialist, health psychologist, or psychiatrist to evaluate the situation and assist in planning interventions. Hence No. 1, 2, and 4 are incorrect.

361. (2) Since the dysfunction in myasthenia gravis occurs at the myoneural junction, it is considered a lower motor neuron lesion. Upper motor neuron lesions (No. 1) involve cranial neurons and their axons in the spinal cord. Combined lesions (No. 3) generally occur with spinal injury when axons of cranial neurons are destroyed, resulting in hyperreflexia and increased muscle tone below the level of the lesion and destruction of motor neurons at the level of the injury, which in turn leads to hyporeflexia, decreased muscle tone, and muscle atrophy in those muscles normally innervated by these neurons. Myasthenia gravis (No. 4) is not an inherited disorder. Recent evidence suggests an autoimmune basis.

362. (1) The most common cause of hypothyroidism today is excess thyroid tissue destruction due to radioactive iodine therapy for hyperthyroidism. Spontaneous hypothyroidism is believed due to an autoimmune response. Several studies have revealed a high incidence of antibodies for thyroid antigen in patients with spontaneous atrophy. Other less common causes include surgical removal, Hashimoto's thyroiditis, overuse of antithyroid drugs, and pituitary tumors or insufficiency that decrease the circulating levels of TSH (thyroid-stimulating hormone). Hence Nos. 2, 3, and 4 are incorrect.

363. (3) A deficiency of thyroid hormone causes widespread metabolic changes. Alterations in fluid and electrolyte balance due to increased capillary permeability lead to fluid retention that results in edema, particularly of the eyelids, hands, and feet. The basal metabolic rate is also reduced, causing symptoms of anorexia, constipation, and intolerance to cold due to a lowered body temperature. The lowered metabolic rate also decreases cellular oxygen consumption; as a result, the heart rate, pulse pressure, and blood pressure are reduced. Reduced cerebral blood flow affects both perception and coordination and results in symptoms of lethargy, generalized weakness, and slowing of both intellectual and motor functions. Hence Nos. 1, 2, and 4 are incorrect.

364. (2) If treatment with thyroid hormone is effective, it should reflect an overall increase in metabolic rate and a decrease in fluid retention; that is, increased blood pressure, pulse rate, pulse pressure, temperature, and rate and depth of respirations. As a result of improved renal blood flow, glomerular filtration and urine output should also increase, thus reducing the weight gain due to fluid retention. Nos. 1, 3, and 4 are incorrect because each contains at least one outcome that is not consistent with improved status.

365. (1) The patient with hyperthyroidism has an increased metabolic rate due to excess serum thyroxine leading to symptoms of systolic hypertension, heat intolerance, widened pulse pressure, and emotional excitability. The diastolic blood pressure reduces due to decreased peripheral resistance. Weight loss occurs because of increased catabolism despite an increase in appetite. Hence Nos. 2, 3, and 4 are incorrect.

366. (4) Thyroglobulin (Proloid) is a purified extract of pig thyroid and is utilized in the treatment of hypothyroidism. Nos. 1, 2, and 3 are current methods for treating Graves' disease, or hyperthyroidism.

367. (2) Patients with hyperthyroidism have an increased BMR (basal metabolic rate) as well as increased T_3 and T_4. Increased serum cholesterol (No. 1), increased TSH (No. 3), and increased menstrual volume (No. 4) are findings consistent with hypothyroidism. Menstruation in hyperthyroidism is characteristically decreased in volumes. Cycle lengths may be shortened or prolonged, but eventually amenorrhea develops.

368. (1) Thyroid storm may be precipitated by a number of stresses such as infection, real or threatened loss of a loved one, or thyroid surgery undertaken before the patient was prepared adequately with antithyroid drugs. The patient's temperature may rise as high as 106 F (41 C). Likewise, other symptoms of hyperthyroidism are exaggerated, such as tachycardia, increased hypertension, tremulousness, and restlessness. Without treatment the patient progresses from delerium to coma, and death ensues as the result of congestive heart failure. Hence Nos. 2, 3, and 4 are incorrect.

369. (1) The primary pathology in Cushing's syndrome is increased serum cortisol, which acts to accelerate the rate of gluconeogenesis in the body, thus mobilizing stored fats and proteins. Serum glucose is increased, stimulating insulin secretion by the pancreas and resulting in abnormalities in fat metabolism and deposition. Weight gain is common; the torso enlarges and fat pads develop on the back of the neck and in the cheeks, giving the patient the characteristic "buffalo hump" and "moon facies." Increased epinephrine secretion is associated with pheochromocytoma. Increased aldosterone with primary aldosteronism and decreased ACTH secretion is associated with dysfunctions of the pituitary gland. Hence Nos. 2, 3, and 4 are incorrect.

370. (2) Lassitude and muscle weakness are early clinical signs of Cushing's syndrome. Catabolism from gluconeogenesis occasionally results in a marked decrease in skeletal mass; and the patient's extremities may appear wasted. No. 1 is incorrect because gluconeogenesis from excess cortisol secretion results in hyperglycemia. No. 3 is partially correct. Hypersecretion of aldosterone in Cushing's disease is rare; however, large quantities of cortisol tend to increase sodium and water retention and potassium excretion. Edema and hypokalemia occur only in severe cases. Discoloration and hyperpigmentation (No. 4) occur with adrenal insufficiency.

371. (1) Signs and symptoms of Addison's disease include hypotension, hypoglycemia, muscular weakness, fatigue, weight loss, hyperkalemia, and depression. These symptoms are primarily due to disturbances in sodium, water, and potassium imbalances that cause severe dehydration. Nos. 2 and 4 are symptoms of Cushing's syndrome. No. 3 is incorrect because hyperglycemia and weight gain are also consistent with Cushing's syndrome.

372. (1) The primary fluid and electrolyte imbalances in Addison's disease are hyponatremia, hypovolemia, and hyperkalemia. These imbalances are caused by decreased aldosterone secretion. Calcium levels are not affected by this condition (No. 4). Nos. 2 and 3 are incorrect because they occur with excessive secretion of this hormone.

373. (2) Since dehydration is a common problem in Addison's disease, close observation of the patient's hydration level is crucial. To promote optimal hydration and sodium intake, fluid intake is increased, particularly fluids containing electrolytes, such as broths, carbonated beverages, and juices. Daily weights and intake and output records are essential for monitoring fluid balance. Likewise, since the patient's ability to react to stress is decreased, maintaining a quiet environment becomes a nursing priority. Drug therapy in Addison's disease is directed toward oral replacement of adrenocorticosteroids such as cortisone, prednisone, and fludrohydrocortisone (Florinef). Hence Nos. 1, 3, and 4 are incorrect.

374. (1) Iron-deficiency anemia is characterized by a decrease in red blood cell color due to a decrease in iron (hypochromic) and an increase in immature red blood cells (microcytic). No. 2 describes the red blood cells in pernicious anemia. Nos. 3 and 4 do not describe particular conditions.

375. (1) Oral iron preparations tend to irritate the gastric mucosa, so they should be administered with or immediately after meals. Patients may complain of constipation or loose stools with oral therapy. Patient education should include the fact that stools will change color (dark green to black); that ferrous sulfate is apt to deposit on teeth and gums, so frequent oral hygiene is necessary; and that therapy will need to continue even after hemoglobin levels return to normal in order to ensure adequate iron stores in the body. Hence Nos. 2, 3, and 4 are incorrect.

376. (2) Salicylates, particularly acetylsalicylic acid (aspirin), are given in divided doses after each meal and at bedtime for their analgesic (reduced pain), antiinflammatory (reduced swelling), and antipyretic (reduced fever) effects. No. 1 is incorrect because relief of pain was already described in the question. Nos. 3 and 4 are incorrect because salicylates neither inhibit nor stimulate the autonomic nervous system synapses.

377. (2) Fever and increased pulse rates occur in rheumatoid arthritis due to the systemic inflammatory process of this dysfunction. If the fever is high or prolonged, increased fluid losses could occur due to insensible water loss (No. 1); however, the effects on body temperature would be secondary to the primary inflammatory response. While the stress response (No. 3) does increase pulse rate, it does not normally significantly affect body temperature. No. 4 is incorrect because salicylates have an antipyretic effect.

378. (1) The primary purpose of passive range-of-motion exercises is to prevent contractures and decreased range of motion. Secondarily passive range-of-motion exercises assist the nurse in evaluating functional abilities, pain tolerance, and the effectiveness of drug therapy. Hence Nos. 2, 3, and 4 are incorrect.

379. (2) In rheumatoid arthritis both the erythrocyte sedimentation rate and C-reactive protein levels are increased. Anemia is common, so hemoglobin and hematocrit are usually decreased. The Wasserman is normally negative. The platelet count is not affected either. Hence Nos. 1, 3, and 4 are incorrect.

380. (1) A hot tub bath or shower in the morning helps many patients limber up and reduces the symptoms of early-morning stiffness. Cold and ice packs are used to a lesser degree, though some patients state that cold decreases localized pain, particularly during acute attacks. Sleeping with a hot pad may cause localized injury. Some patients, however, have found electric blankets helpful in reducing early-morning stiffness. Passive ROM exercises may be helpful, but this is not the response of choice. Taking salicylates on an empty stomach may increase gastric irritation and distress. Hence Nos. 2, 3, and 4 are incorrect.

381. (3) The primary objective in giving corticosteroids is to lessen the symptoms of the disease process. Most patients initially respond well to these drugs; however, as the disease progresses, higher and higher doses are required to relieve symptoms. Nos. 1 and 2 are incorrect because corticosteroids have no curative effects, only palliative. Many of the side effects of corticosteroid

administration are due to the effects of these drugs on glucose metabolism (No. 4), such as Cushing's-like syndrome.

382. (3) Side effects of prednisone therapy mimic the manifestations of Cushing's syndrome (moon facies, abnormal fat deposits, purple striae, hyperglycemia with glucosuria, hypertension, obesity, and emotional disturbances). Side effects of other drugs utilized in the management of rheumatoid arthritis include nausea, vomiting, tinnitus, headaches, and vertigo with indomethacin (Indocin) administration, and dermatitis ranging from erythema to exfoliative dermatitis with gold salts therapy. Hence Nos. 1, 2, and 4 are incorrect.

383. (2) In preparing the patient for discharge on prednisone therapy, you should caution him to: (a) take oral preparations after meals; (b) remember that routine checks of vital signs, weight, and lab studies are critical; (c) never to stop or change the amount of medication without medical advice; and (d) store the medication in a light-resistant container. No. 1 is incorrect because prednisone, as well as other medications given in rheumatoid arthritis therapy, is irritating to the GI tract and should be taken after meals. No. 3 is incorrect because although fluid, electrolyte, and serum glucose levels need frequent evaluation while on prednisone therapy, CBCs need regular checking if the patient is on phenylbutazone (Butazolidin), oxyphenbutazone (Tandearil), or ibuprofen (Motrin) therapy. No. 4 is a precaution given to patients on hydroxychloroquine SO_4 (Plaquenil) or chloroquine (Aralen) therapy.

384. (2) Patients should not be encouraged to do exercises to the point of unusual pain, nor should pain last longer than one-half hour after exercise. If pain lasts longer than this, the exercises are too strenuous. No. 1 is incorrect because pulse and respiratory rates are affected not only by physical stress but by emotional or psychologic stress as well. Nos. 3 and 4 indicate that therapy has been effective.

385. (1) In assessing any patient's emotional responses, you should first assess the patient's ego strength, body image, and coping abilities for life situations in general. The manner in which the patient views herself will greatly affect her attitudes toward her disease and her emotional response. If the patient normally denies or represses threatening information or situations, desirable outcomes may be difficult to achieve. The evidence of recent research indicates that social supports are extremely important in maintaining health. The relationship between Mrs. Sanches and her mother should be assessed. However, if Mrs. Sanches has a strong self-image, the issues between mother and daughter should be resolvable either alone or with objective outside help. Economic status and work history, depending upon their value to Mrs. Sanches, may or may not be important determinants of her emotional response. Hence Nos. 2, 3, and 4 are incorrect.

386. (2) Patients with radioactive implants should be positioned flat in bed to prevent dislodgement of the vaginal packing. The patient may roll to the side for meals, but the upper body should not be raised more than 20°. Nos. 1, 3, and 4 are incorrect because these positions are more likely to change the position of the cobalt seeds.

387. (2) It is not necessary to isolate the patient with radioactive implants (No. 1), but to prevent undue exposure to radiation contacts, contact time should be brief and distance between the patient and family/professional maximized. Specific instructions as to the amount of time permitted with the patient and the safe distance should be posted. Nos. 3 and 4 are incorrect because the best position for the patient is supine.

388. (3) During treatment (total insertion time varies between 48–144 hours), vaginal discharge may become foul smelling due to tissue destruction; however, perineal care is generally not allowed due to the danger of dislodging the needles. Frequently, patients find this quite distressing. A douche given under low pressure following removal of the applicator helps to reduce this side effect of therapy. Bladder atony is a rare complication, diarrhea rather than constipation is more likely to occur. Sexual libido following this therapy seems more dependent on the relationship of the partners before therapy than on the therapy itself. Hence Nos. 1, 2, and 4 are incorrect.

389. (2) Local radiation is generally used under four conditions: the tumor is relatively well defined, a larger dose of radiation can be delivered than by an external source, there is a critical need to reduce involvement of other tissue, and the site is accessible for introduction of seeds or implants. As a result of cobalt implantation, diarrhea may occur due to radiation-induced toxicosis of the mucous membranes of the large bowel. Diarrhea may be painful as well as profuse and bloody. No. 1 is incorrect because the rationale for doing an implant is that the tumor is generally well defined. The effects of severe diarrhea may indeed be electrolyte imbalance (No. 3) but this is not the cause in this situation. No. 4 may indeed be occurring, but is not the basis for Mrs. Ryan's present symptoms.

390. (3) Although complete or partial amputation may result from trauma (No. 1), the majority are necessitated by arteriosclerosis obliterans. Long-standing complications of diabetes mellitus are peripheral vascular insufficiency and infections (No. 2), which increase the likelihood of amputation. Less often bone tumors (No. 4), particularly of the knee, may necessitate amputation.

391. (4) The loss of a limb is significant. The patient facing the amputation must deal with his perception of himself, incorporate the changes in body image, and be allowed to grieve. The nurse must be sensitive to the patient's stage of grieving and provide information as he asks, at a level consistent with his ability to comprehend. While the attending physician (No. 1), his family (No. 2), and the nursing staff (No. 3) may affect the patient's perception of a situation, the work of grieving is primarily personal, with movement both forward and backward as the patient progresses through the stages.

392. (3) Although Mr. Henry expresses a willingness to learn, his apprehension will limit his ability to assimilate too much. He must be told specific arm and leg exercises, including frequent repositioning onto the abdomen to prevent contracture. In the postoperative period the focus changes to crutch-walking (No. 2). Prior to discharge alternate vocational pursuits may be discussed as indicated (No. 1). Encouraging the patient to verbalize fears and concerns (No. 4) is not a specific teaching strategy but rather an intervention designed to give support as well as to identify potential problems.

393. (3) The choice of anesthesia depends upon the surgeon's choice and the patient's condition. However, while a spinal anesthetic (No. 2) may be used, the sawing of the bone can be very distressing to the patient, so usually a general anesthesia is preferred. IV regional blocks (No. 1) may not provide adequate blockage of impulses for this procedure, and again the patient is awake. Muscle relaxants (No. 4) are administered in conjunction with general anesthesia.

394. (1) Above-the-knee amputations are often necessary because of the extent of the disease. The most critical factor in determining the level of the amputation is the adequacy of the arterial blood supply. Nos. 2 and 3 describe the advantages associated with a below-the-knee (B/K) amputation. No. 4 is incorrect because a below-the-knee amputation not only heals faster than an above-the-knee amputation, but it is less painful postsurgically, less psychologically disturbing, and less prone to contractures.

395. (4) All insulin-dependent diabetics are to receive daily insulin. Hence, No. 1 is incorrect. However, the physician should write specific orders for insulin coverage on the day of surgery. The reason for this is that both the physical and psychologic stress of surgery tend to increase serum glucose levels via glycogenolysis and the patient's usual insulin may be insufficient (No. 2). Frequently, a rainbow coverage of regular insulin is ordered to supplement or temporarily replace daily doses of NPH or other longer-acting insulins. The patient is not given fluids (No. 3) before surgery, particularly if a general anesthetic is to be administered.

396. (1) To reduce bleeding and edema the stump is elevated for the first 24 hours; however, after 24 hours hip flexion contracture may occur with prolonged elevation. No. 2 is incorrect because this procedure is used for open amputation. No. 3 is a procedure used with a below-the-knee amputation to prevent contractures in the knee joint. No. 4 is a standard postoperative procedure initiated by the surgeon in the OR to facilitate shrinkage of the stump and to prevent edema.

397. (2) The most common complication occurring in the postoperative period is pulmonary embolus. This is a particularly significant problem in elderly patients with a history of vascular insufficiency. Therefore, an antiembolism stocking is applied to the unaffected limb and early physiotherapy and ambulation with a walker is encouraged. These measures will also prevent thrombophlebitis (No. 4), which tends to occur with long bedrest. Hemorrhage and shock (No. 1) are always a potential problem after any surgery. To assess for this problem any bright red drainage on the stump dressing should be outlined so that the rate of bleeding can be determined. Disseminated intravascular clotting (No. 3) is a problem associated with prolonged shock.

398. (4) The day following surgery the patient with an above-the-knee (AK) amputation is turned on his or her abdomen for a short period. Thereafter he or she is turned to the prone position at least three times daily. While in this position the patient should practice push-up exercises that strengthen arm and shoulder muscles, thereby facilitating both transfer procedures and preparation for crutch-walking. Later the patient is taught to lift buttocks and stump off the bed while in a supine position, an exercise that develops abdominal muscles necessary for stabilizing the pelvis when the patient stoops or bends (No. 3). Hyperextension of the thigh and stump (No. 2) is encouraged for patients with below-the-knee amputations only. Patients with AK amputations may only perform this exercise on medical orders, as it tends to put undue stress on the suture line. Sandbags or blanket rolls are used after this surgery to prevent outward rotation of the stump; hence No. 1 is incorrect.

399. (3) Phantom limb pain or sensation is an unpleasant complication that sometimes follows amputation. This phenomenon is not completely understood but is believed to result from afferent nerve fibers (sensory) severed during surgery. The pain in the limb may be identical to that perceived by the patient before surgery. The patient needs to be aware of the nature of this discomfort. Sometimes the sensation will disappear if the patient looks at the stump and recalls that the limb has been amputated. In cases where discomfort persists, alcohol may be injected into the nerve ends for temporary relief, the nerve endings may be removed, or on rare occasions reamputation may be required. Nos. 1 and 2 are incorrect because they negate the patient's perceptions of discomfort and avoid the issue. No. 4 is also incorrect because an explanation of the phenomenon and other palliative measures should precede the administration of a narcotic.

400. (4) After the stump has healed, an elastic bandage is applied to it to produce·shrinkage and a conical shape. It is a compression dressing, with maximal compression at the distal end of the stump and minimal compression at the proximal end. The stump is wrapped with a clean bandage each day and rewrapped four times each day to maintain compression. Elevation of the stump after the first 24 hours is always contraindicated because of the risk of flexion contracture in the hip (No. 1). Pushing the stump against a hard surface (No. 2) will facilitate toughening the skin for weight-bearing once the prosthesis is applied, but does not facilitate reduction in size and shaping of the stump. Warm, moist soaks (No. 3) may be applied to reduce phantom pain discomfort, but are not applicable to this situation.

ANNOTATED BIBLIOGRAPHY

Beland, I., and Passos, J.: Clinical nursing, ed. 3, New York, 1975, Macmillan Publishing Co.
This text uses a conceptual approach with emphasis placed on understanding pathophysiologic and psychosocial relationships. The holistic approach promotes the understanding and synthesis of the many factors affecting the patient's response to health and illness and to medical and nursing interventions. This is an excellent reference for the more experienced practitioner.

Brunner, L., and Suddarth, D.: Textbook of medical-surgical nursing, ed. 3, Philadelphia, 1975, J. B. Lippincott Company.
This comprehensive text focuses on assessment and priority-setting in nursing management of patient problems. The text includes a number of tables that outline procedures, therapies, and complications. Frequent illustrations also aid understanding. The book presents a great deal of information in a fairly concise, readable format.

Holloway, N.: Nursing the critically ill adult, Menlo Park, Ca., 1979, Addison-Wesley Publishing Co.
A recipient of the American Journal of Nursing Book of the Year Award, this book contains a wealth of data for those interested in critical care nursing.

Jones, D. A., Dunbar, C. F., and Jirovec, M. M.: Medical-surgical nursing, New York, 1978, McGraw-Hill Book Co.
This concisely written, highly informative text reflects the changing scope of the nurse's role in health care. Nursing

is explored according to the levels of nursing care. First-level nursing care focuses on the identification of populations susceptible to specific health problems. Second-level nursing focuses on the maintenance of individuals with health problems in the community. Third-level care discusses acute health problems of patients in the hospital, and fourth-level care, the rehabilitation process in the hospital and community setting.

LeMaitre, G., and Finnegan, J.: The patient in surgery, ed. 3, Philadelphia, 1975, W. B. Saunders Co.

This text presents an in-depth guide to the biologic and psychosocial assessment of the surgical patient. Specific surgeries are presented in a case study outline format that includes aspects of the patient's health history, physical findings, preparation for surgery, the surgical procedure with attendant hazards, and postoperative care. Study questions are supplied to further enhance learning.

Luckman, J., and Sorenson, K.: Medical-surgical nursing: a psychophysiologic approach, ed. 2, Philadelphia, 1980, W. B. Saunders Co.

This text offers an in-depth presentation of current medical-surgical nursing practice as well as a discussion of basic behavioral and physiologic concepts. A wide range of specific health problems are presented, and the components of the nursing process are consistently related to underlying psychophysiologic principles. The authors have included unit objectives and varied learning activities to facilitate mastery of the material and to enhance learning. Referencing is extensive.

Moidel, H., Giblin, E., and Wagner, B.: Nursing care of the patient with medical-surgical disorders, ed. 2, New York, 1976, McGraw-Hill Book Co.

A well-written, easily read text that focuses on the nursing process and provides consistent rationales for nursing interventions. Frequent diagrams, tables, and illustrations facilitate comprehension of the material presented.

Phipps, W. J., Long, B. C., and Woods, N. F.: Medical-surgical nursing, St. Louis, 1979, The C. V. Mosby Company.

This book presents a concise, in-depth presentation of the concepts and processes inherent in nursing. The initial three units provide a firm theoretical base for nursing practice, and the last portion of the text presents material associated with medical-surgical nursing in a fairly traditional manner. Throughout the text, the emphasis is on assisting the patient to improve his or her health status either through direct physical care by the nurse or through the use of emotional and social supports. Health-teaching is directed toward providing the patient with information necessary for self-care. The authors also provide evaluation criteria for each specific care problem.

Shafer, K., Sawyer, J., McCluskey, A., Beck, E., and Phipps, W. J.: Medical-surgical nursing, ed. 6, St. Louis, 1975, The C. V. Mosby Company.

A nursing textbook classic, this edition focuses on the assessment and understanding of physiologic disturbances and approaches nursing interventions in terms of goals and objectives. The format allows for the rapid review of common patient problems and nursing care.

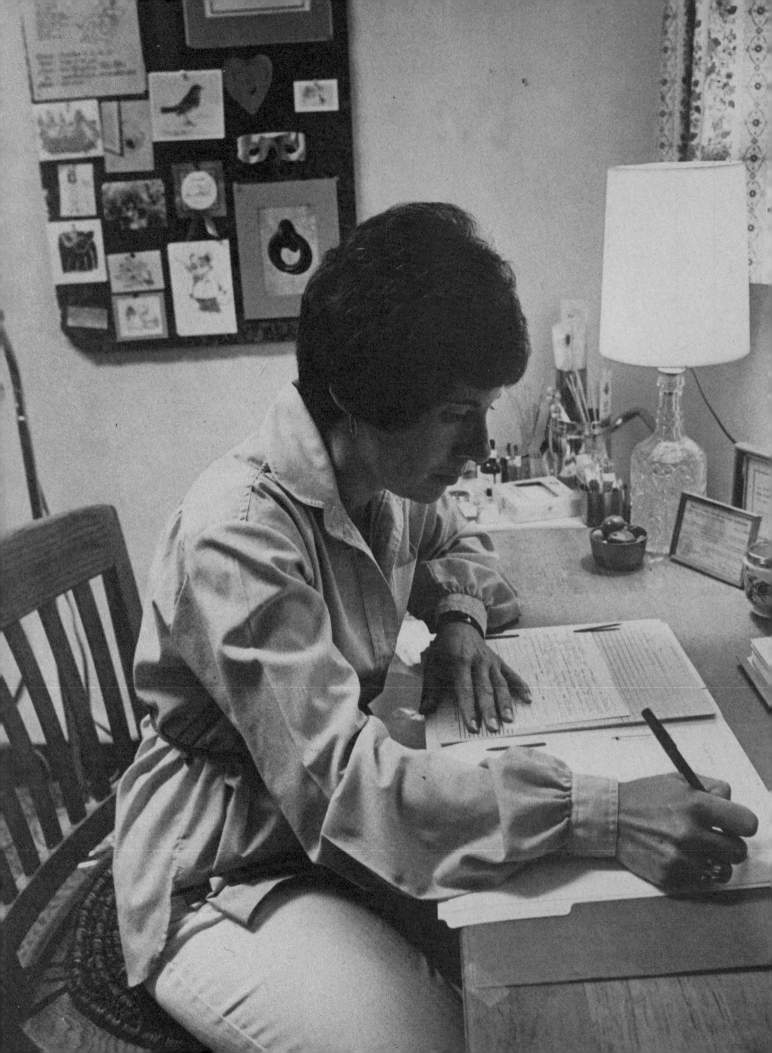

Unit 6 / ETHICAL AND LEGAL ASPECTS OF NURSING

Introduction

The RN licensure examination includes questions that test your knowledge of nursing trends and the scope of nursing practice based on codes of ethics (standards of practice) and legal considerations. The concepts of management and accountability tested in the exam are covered in this unit. The purpose of this unit is to provide a frame of reference for determining the actions for which a nurse is legally and ethically accountable in patient management situations. Applications of ethical and legal considerations are given in two settings: intensive care of the acutely ill neonate and psychiatric care.

Sally Lagerquist
Judy Massong

NURSING ETHICS

Nursing ethics involve rules and principles to guide right conduct in terms of moral duty and obligation, designed to protect the rights of human beings. In nursing, ethical codes provide professional standards and formal guidelines for nursing activities to protect both the nurse and the patient.

1. **Code of ethics**—serves as a frame of reference when judging priorities or possible courses of action.
   A. *Purpose:*
   1. To provide a basis for regulating relationships between nurse, patient, coworkers, society, and profession.
   2. To provide a standard for excluding unscrupulous nursing practitioners and for defending nurses unjustly accused.
   3. To serve as a basis for nursing curricula.
   4. To orient new nurses and the public to ethical professional conduct.

ANA CODE FOR NURSES*

1. The nurse provides services with respect for human dignity and the uniqueness of the client unrestricted by considerations of social or economic status, personal attributes, or the nature of health problems.

Illness is a universal phenomenon; therefore the need for nursing is also universal. Because nursing is required by the broad spectrum of people who make up society, the nurse should be free of value judgments about "good people and bad people"; it is necessary to accept each person, as well as the person's attitudes, customs, and beliefs. In this way nurses can best provide support to people of varied backgrounds.

2. The nurse safeguards the client's right to privacy by judiciously protecting information of a confidential nature.

It is clearly the nurse's responsibility to keep confidential any information received from the patient, only conveying details about illness or the physical, social, or personal situation of the patient to other per-

*American Nurses' Association. 1976. *Code for nurses with interpretive statements*. Kansas City, Missouri: American Nurses' Association. Reprinted with permission.

sons who are also professionally concerned directly with the patient's care.

In some instances, the nurse may be required to provide testimony in a court. In these instances, the court will advise the nurse as to what is admissible and to what the nurse must testify.

Because people can be seriously harmed and embarrassed by a breach in confidence of the nurse, all nurses must use good professional judgment in what they say, being sure that it is stated to the correct person and that what is conveyed could be of value in promoting the health of the patient. The basis of this ethical principle is also found in the law.

3. The nurse acts to safeguard the client and the public when health care and safety are affected by the incompetent, unethical, or illegal practice of any person.

Nurses themselves are responsible for maintaining their own competence, updating their knowledge and skills as it is appropriate. Not to do so would imply that a nurse could not provide as high a standard of practice as the profession considers necessary.

4. The nurse assumes responsibility and accountability for individual nursing judgments and actions.

The nurse has a responsibility to report to the appropriate authority or to the professional association any conduct of other nurses or physicians that endangers patients. The priority of the nurse is the patient, patient safety, and patient care.

5. The nurse maintains competence in nursing.

Maintaining competence in nursing practice is essential; nurses must keep abreast of new developments to ensure the best standards of patient care. An essential quality of the nurse is a zest for continued study, since knowledge and skills for nursing need to be continually updated. The nurse who pursues knowledge independently is undoubtedly more effective in practice than one who does not.

6. The nurse exercises informed judgment and uses individual competence and qualifications as criteria in seeking consultation, accepting responsibilities, and delegating nursing activities to others.

Nurses need to recognize their own areas of competence and incompetence; they have a right to refuse to carry out responsibilities that they consider unethical. Policies of agencies and the law assist the nurse as to what practices are considered to be within the nurse's area of responsibility. In addition, if a nurse is not familiar with some nursing activity, it is the nurse's right to explain this and to refuse to carry it out.

7. The nurse participates in activities that contribute to the ongoing development of the profession's body of knowledge.

Increasingly, nurses are becoming involved in research activities as individual practitioners and as employees of hospitals and community health agencies. Nurses themselves are conducting research into nursing practice as well as are a variety of health personnel such as physicians and biochemists.

The nurse who plans to participate should first make sure that the patient understands and agrees to be part of the research; second, the nurse should make sure that the research proposed has the approval of the agency research committee or the appropriate approving authority of the agency.

8. The nurse participates in the profession's efforts to implement and improve standards of nursing.

Peer review and established nursing standards assist in improving nursing. The nurse has a responsibility to participate in these activities as well as to participate in educational programs.

Standards for practice must always change as the health care system changes. The professional nurse has a responsibility to assist in making these changes and implementing them.

9. The nurse participates in the profession's efforts to establish and maintain conditions of employment conducive to high quality nursing care.

Each nurse, acting through the professional organization, needs to be concerned with the economic and general welfare of the members of the profession. These are important factors in both recruiting nursing students and in retaining nurses in the work force. Through the nursing association, nurses assist in the establishment of employment practices and in bargaining for economic and general benefits.

10. The nurse participates in the profession's effort to protect the public from misinformation and misrepresentation and to maintain the integrity of nursing.

Nurses are generally held in respect by members of the public, who have confidence in their knowledge and their advice. Often when a nurse speaks, it is assumed that the opinion given is the opinion of all nurses. For example, to advertise or recommend a product might be harmful or misleading to the public. The nurse appears to have knowledge that the partic-

ular product is better than others on the market; this may not be true because that knowledge is usually beyond the nurse's qualifications and authority.

11. The nurse collaborates with members of the health professions and other citizens in promoting community and national efforts to meet the health needs of the public.

A professional nurse, with specialized knowledge and skills, has a responsibility to contribute in such a manner as to assist people to meet the health needs of the community. Citizens are increasingly concerned and becoming involved in planning health care. A nurse can offer such a group information that would be pertinent and helpful. Nurses also have a responsibility to act on committees with other health members and other professionals such as teachers and social workers in meeting the health problems of the people in the community.

2. Conflicts and problems

A. *Personal values versus professional duty*—nurses have the right to refuse to participate in those areas of nursing practice that are against their personal values, as long as a patient's welfare is not jeopardized. Example: therapeutic abortions.

B. *Nurse versus agency*—conflict may arise regarding whether or not to give out needed information to patient or to follow agency policy, which does not allow it. Example: an emotionally upset teenager asks nurse about how to get an abortion, a discussion which is against agency policy.

C. *Nurse versus colleagues*—conflict may arise when determining whether to ignore or report others' behavior. Examples: you see another nurse steal medications; you know that a peer is giving a false reason when requesting time off; or you observe an intoxicated colleague.

D. *Nurse versus patient/family*—conflict may stem from knowledge of confidential information. Should you tell? Example: patient or family member relates a vital secret to the nurse.

E. *Conflicting responsibilities*—to whom is the nurse primarily responsible when needs of the agency and the patient differ? Example: MD asks nurse not to list all supplies used for patient care, as patient cannot afford to pay the bill.

3. Trends in nursing practice

A. Overall characteristics:
1. Some trends are subtle and slow to emerge; others are obvious and quick.

2. Trends may conflict; some will prevail, others get modified by social forces.

B. Trends:

1. *Broadened focus of care*—from care of ill to care of sick and healthy, from individual to care of family. Focus on prevention of illness, promotion of optimum level of health, holism.

2. *Increasing scientific base*—in bio-social-physical sciences, not mere reliance on intuition, experience and observation.

3. *Increasingly complex technical skills* and use of *technologically advanced equipment* such as monitors and computers.

4. *Increased independence* in use of judgement, such as teaching nutrition in pregnancy and providing primary prenatal care.

5. *New roles,* such as *nurse clinician,* require advanced skills in a particular area of practice. Examples: psychiatric nurse consults with staff about problems; *primary care* nurse takes medical histories and does physical assessment; one nurse coordinates 24-hour care during hospital stay; *independent nurse practitioner* has own office in community where patients come for care.

6. *Community nursing services* rather than hospital-based; needs of the healthy are served as well as those of the ill.

7. *Development of nursing standards* to reflect specific nursing functions and activities.

   a. Assure *safe* standard of care to patients and families.

   b. Provide criteria to measure *excellence* and *effectiveness* of care.

C. ANA Standards of Nursing Practice:

STANDARDS OF NURSING*

1. The collection of data about the health status of the client/patient is systematic and continuous. The data are accessible, communicated, and recorded.

2. Nursing diagnoses are derived from health status data.

3. The plan of nursing care includes goals derived from the nursing diagnoses.

4. The plan of nursing care includes priorities and the prescribed nursing approaches or measures to achieve the goals derived from the nursing diagnoses.

5. Nursing actions provide for client/patient participation in health promotion, maintenance, and restoration.

6. The nursing actions assist the client/patient to maximize his health capabilities.

7. The client/patient's progress or lack of progress toward goal achievement is determined by the client/patient and the nurse.

8. The client/patient's progress or lack of progress toward goal achievement directs reassessment, reordering of priorities, new goal setting, and revision of the plan of nursing care.

D. Four levels of nursing practice:

1. *Promotion of health* to increase level of wellness. Example: provide dietary information to reduce risks of coronaries.

2. *Prevention of illness or injury*. Example: immunizations.

3. *Restoration of health*. Example: teach how to change dressing, care for wound.

4. *Consolation of dying*—assist person to attain peaceful death.

E. Five components of nursing care:

1. *Nursing-care activities*—assist with basic needs, give medications and treatments; observe response and adaptation to illness and treatments; teach self-care; guide rehabilitation activities for daily living.

2. *Coordination of total patient care*—all health team members should work together toward common goals.

3. *Continuity of care*—when transfer location of care.

4. *Evaluation of care*—flexibility and responsiveness to changing needs: patients' reactions and perceptions of their needs.

5. *Delegate responsibility and direct nursing care provided by others*—based on particular patient/family needs and skills of other nursing personnel.

F. *Three main nursing roles* in relation to care of patients and their families. The emphasis of each role varies with the situation, with adaptation of skills and modes of care as necessary.

1. *Therapeutic role* (instrumental). Function: work toward "cure" in acute setting.

2. *Caring role* (expressive). Function: provide support through human relations, show concern, demonstrate acceptance of differences.

3. *Socializing role*. Function: offer distractions and respite from focus on illness.

---

*From American Nurses' Association. 1973. *Standards of nursing practice.* Kansas City, Missouri. Reprinted with permission. (Rationale for the above *Standards of nursing practice* are available from the ANA.)

NURSING ORGANIZATIONS

1. International Council of Nurses (ICN)

A. *Purpose:* to provide a medium through which national nursing associations can work together, share common interests. Formed in 1899.

B. *Functions:*
1. Serves as representatives of and spokespersons for nurses at international level.
2. Promotes organization of national nurses' associations.
3. Assists national organizations to develop and improve services for public health practice of nursing and social/economic welfare of nurses.

2. World Health Organization (WHO)—special intergovernmental agency of the UN, formed in 1948.

A. *Purpose:* to bring all people to the highest possible level of health.

B. *Functions:* provides assistance in the form of education, training, improving health standards, fighting disease, and reducing water pollution in member countries.

3. American Nurses' Association (ANA)—national professional association in the US, composed of the nurses' associations of the 50 states, Guam, Virgin Islands, Puerto Rico, and Washington, D.C.

A. *Purpose:* to foster high standards of nursing practice and promote the education and welfare of nurses.

B. *Functions:* officially represents professional nurses in this country and internationally; defines practice of nursing; lobbies and promotes legislation affecting nurses' welfare and practice.

4. National League for Nursing (NLN)—composed of both individuals and agencies.

A. *Purpose:* to foster the development and improvement of all nursing services and nursing education.

B. *Functions:*
1. Provides educational workshops.
2. Assists in recruitment for nursing programs.
3. Provides testing service for both RN and LPN (LVN) licensure.

LEGAL ASPECTS OF NURSING

1. Definition of terms

A. *Common law:* accumulation of law as a result of judicial court decisions.

B. *Civil law* (private law): law that derives from legislative codes and deals with relations between private parties.

C. *Public law:* concerns relationships between an individual and the state. The thrust of public law is to attain what are deemed valid public goals, such as reporting child abuse.

D. *Criminal law:* concerns actions against the safety and welfare of the public, such as robbery. It is part of the public law.

2. Nursing licensure—mandatory licensure required in order to practice nursing.

A. *Nurse Practice Act:* each state has one to protect nurses' professional capacity, to legally control nursing through licensing, and to define standards of professional nursing.

B. *American Nurses' Association (1980):* "The practice of nursing means the performance for compensation of professional services requiring substantial specialized knowledge of the biological, physical, behavioral, psychological, and sociological sciences and of nursing theory as the basis for assessment, diagnosis, planning, intervention, and evaluation in the promotion and maintenance of health; the casefinding and management of illness, injury, or infirmity; the restoration of optimum function; or the achievement of a dignified death. Nursing practice includes but is not limited to administration, teaching, counseling, supervision, delegation, and evaluation of practice and execution of the medical regimen, including the administration of medications and treatments prescribed by any person authorized by state law to prescribe. Each registered nurse is directly accountable and responsible to the consumer for the quality of nursing care rendered."[*]

C. *Revoking a license:* Board of Examiners in each state in the US and each province in Canada has the power to revoke licenses for just cause, such as incompetence in nursing practice, conviction of crime, drug addiction, obtaining license through fraud, or hiding criminal history.

3. Crimes and torts

A. *Crime:* an act committed in violation of societal law and punishable by fine or imprisonment. A crime does not have to be intended (as in giving a client an accidental overdose that proves to be lethal).
1. *Felonies:* crimes of a serious nature (such as mur-

---

[*]American Nurses' Association. 1980. *The nursing practice act: suggested state legislation.* Kansas City, Missouri: American Nurses' Association. Reprinted with permission of the American Nurses' Association.

der) punishable by imprisonment of greater than 6 months.

2. *Misdemeanors:* crimes of a less serious nature (such as shoplifting), usually punishable by fines or short prison term or both.

B. *Tort:* a wrong committed by one individual against another or another's property. Fraud, negligence and malpractice are torts (such as losing a client's hearing aid or bathing him in water that burns him).

1. *Fraud:* misrepresentation of fact with intentions for it to be acted upon by another person (such as falsifying college transcripts when applying for a graduate nursing program).

2. *Negligence:* "Omission to do something that a reasonable person, guided by those *ordinary* considerations which ordinarily regulate human affairs would *do*, or doing something which a reasonable and prudent person would *not* do" (Creighton, 1975, p. 119). Types of negligent acts:

   a. Sponge counts: incorrect counts or failure to count.
   b. Burns: heating pads, solutions, steam vaporizers.
   c. Falls: siderails left down, baby left unattended.
   d. Failure to observe and take appropriate action—forget to take vital signs and check dressing in a newly postoperative patient.
   e. Wrong medicine, wrong dose and concentration, wrong route, wrong patient.
   f. Mistaken identity—wrong patient for surgery.
   g. Failure to communicate—ignore, forget, fail to report complaints of patient or family.
   h. Loss of or damage to patient's property—dentures, jewelry, money.

3. *Malpractice:* part of the law of negligence as applied to the *professional* person; any professional misconduct, unreasonable lack of skill, or lack of fidelity in professional duties, such as accidentally giving wrong medication or forgetting to give correct medication. Proof of intent to do harm is not required in acts of commission or omission.

4. *Invasion of privacy*—compromising a person's right to withhold self and own life from public scrutiny. Implications for nursing—avoid unnecessary discussion of patient's medical condition; patient has a right to refuse to participate in clinical teaching; obtain consent prior to teaching conference.

5. *Libel and slander*—wrongful action of communication that damages person's reputation by print, writing, or pictures (libel), or by spoken word using false words (slander). Implications for nursing—make comments about patient only to another health team member caring for that patient.

6. *Privileged communications*—Information relating to condition and treatment of patient requires confidentiality and protection against invasion of privacy.

7. *Assault and battery*—violating a person's right to refuse physical contact with another.
   A. Definitions:
      1. Assault—the attempt to touch another or the threat to do so.
      2. Battery—physical harm through willful touching of person or clothing.
   B. Implications for nursing—need to obtain consent to treat, with special provisions when patients are under age, unconscious, or mentally ill.

8. *Good Samaritan Act*—protects health practitioners against malpractice claims resulting from assistance provided at scene of an emergency (unless there was willful wrongdoing) as long as the level of care provided is the same as any other reasonably prudent person would give under similar circumstances.

9. *Nurses' responsibilities to the law*
   A. A nurse is liable for nursing acts, even if directed to do something by an MD.
   B. A nurse is not responsible for the negligence of the employer (hospital).
   C. A nurse is responsible for refusing to carry out an order for an activity believed to be injurious to the patient.
   D. A nurse cannot legally diagnose illness or prescribe treatment for a patient. (This is the MD's responsibility.)
   E. A nurse is legally responsible when participating in a criminal act (such as assisting with criminal abortions or taking medications for own use from patient's supply).
   F. A nurse should reveal patient's confidential information only to appropriate health care team members.
   G. A nurse is responsible for explaining nursing activities but not for commenting on medical activities in a way that may distress the patient or the MD.

H. A nurse is responsible to recognize and protect the rights of patients to refuse treatment or medication, and to report their concerns and refusals to the MD or appropriate agency people.

I. A nurse needs to respect the dignity of each patient and family.

QUESTIONS MOST FREQUENTLY ASKED BY NURSES ABOUT NURSING AND THE LAW

1. Taking orders

A. *Should I accept verbal phone orders from an MD?* Generally, no. Specifically, follow your hospital's by-laws, regulations, and policies regarding this. Failure to follow the hospital's rules could be considered negligence.

B. *Should I follow an MD's orders if (a) I know it is wrong, or (b) I disagree with his judgement?* Regarding (a)—No, if you think a reasonably prudent nurse would not follow it; but first inform the MD and record your decision. Report it to your supervisor. Regarding (b)—Yes, because the law does not allow you to substitute your nursing judgement for a doctor's medical judgement. Do record that you questioned the order, and that the doctor confirmed it before you carried it out.

C. *What can I do if the MD delegates a task to me for which I am not prepared?* Inform the MD of your lack of education and experience in performing the task. Refuse to do it. If you inform him or her and still carry out the task, both you and the MD could be considered negligent if the patient is harmed by it. If you do not tell the MD and carry out the task, you are solely liable.

2. Obtaining patient's consent for medical and surgical procedures

A. *Is a nurse responsible for getting a consent for medical/surgical treatment?* Obtaining consent requires explaining the procedure and risks involved, which is the MD's responsibility. A nurse may accept responsibility for *witnessing* a consent. This carries with it little legal liability other than obtaining the correct signature and describing the patient's condition at time of signing.

3. Patient's records

A. *What should be written in the nurse's notes?* All facts and information regarding a person's condition, treatment, care, progress, and response to illness and treatment. Purpose of record: factual documentation of care given to meet legal standards; used to refute unwarranted claims of negligence or malpractice.

B. *How should data be recorded?* Entries should:
1. State time given.
2. Be written and signed by caregiver or supervisor who observed action.
3. Follow chronological sequence.
4. Be accurate, precise, and clear.
5. Be legible.
6. Use universal abbreviations.

4. Confidential information

A. *If called on the witness stand in court, do I have to reveal confidential information?* It depends on your state, as each state has its own laws pertaining to this. Consult a lawyer. Inform the judge and ask for specific directions before relating in court information that was given to you within a confidential, professional relationship.

B. *Am I justified in refusing (on the basis of "invasion of privacy") to give information about the patient to another health agency to which a patient is being transferred?* No. You are responsible for providing continuity of care when the patient is moved from one facility to another. Necessary and adequate information should be transferred, to serve as a source of accurate and necessary information and as necessary communication between appropriate professional health care workers. The patient's consent for this exchange of information should be obtained. Circumstances under which confidential information can be released include:
1. By authorization and consent of the patient.
2. By order of the court.
3. By statutory mandate, as in reporting cases of child abuse or communicable diseases.

5. Liability for mistakes—yours and others.

A. *Is the hospital or the nurse liable for mistakes made by the nurse while following orders?* Both the hospital and the nurse can be sued for damage if a mistake made by the nurse injures the patient. The nurse is responsible for her own actions. The hospital would be vicariously liable.

B. *Who is responsible if a nursing student or another staff nurse makes a mistake. The supervisor? The instructor?* Ordinarily the instructor and/or supervisor would not be responsible unless the court thought the instructor and/or supervisor was negligent in supervising or in assigning a task beyond the capability of the person in question. No one is responsible for another's negligence unless he or she contributed to or participated in that negligence. Each person is personally liable for his or her own negligent actions and failure to act as a reasonably prudent nurse.

C. *Are you responsible for injury to a patient by a staff member who was observed (but not reported) by you to be intoxicated while giving care?* Yes, you may be responsible. You have a duty to take reasonable action to prevent a patient's injury.

6. Good Samaritan Act

A. *For what would I be liable if I voluntarily stopped to give care at the scene of an accident?* You would be protected under the Good Samaritan Act and required to live up to reasonable and prudent nursing standards in those specific circumstances. You would not be treated by the law as if you were performing under professional standards of properly sterile conditions, with proper technical equipment.

7. Leaving against medical advice (AMA)

A. *Would I or the hospital be liable if a patient left "AMA," refusing to sign the appropriate hospital forms?* None of the involved parties would ordinarily be liable in this case as long as (a) the medical risks were explained, recorded, and witnessed, and (b) the patient is a competent adult. The law permits patients to make decisions that may not be in their own best health interest. You cannot interfere with the right and exercise of the decision to accept or reject treatment.

8. Restraints

A. *Can I put restraints on a patient who is combative even if there is no order for this?* Only in an emergency, for a limited time, for the limited purpose of protecting the patient from injury, not for convenience of personnel. Notify attending MD immediately. Consult with another staff member, obtain patient's consent if possible, document facts and reasons, get coworker to witness the record. Apply restraints properly, check frequently to ensure they do not impair circulation, cause pressure sores, or other injury. Remove restraints at the first opportunity, and use them only as a last resort after other reasonable means have not been effective. Restraints of any degree may constitute false imprisonment. Freedom from unlawful restraint is a basic human right protected by law.

9. Wills

A. *What do I do when a patient asks me to be a witness to her or his will?* There is no legal obligation to participate as a witness but a moral and ethical obligation to do so. You should not, however, help draw up a will, as this could be considered practicing law without a license. You would be witnessing that (a) the patient is signing the document as her or his last will and testament; (b) at that time, to the best of your knowledge, the patient (testator) was of sound mind, was lucid, and understood what she or he was doing (that is, she or he must not be under the influence of drugs or alcohol or otherwise unable to know what she or he is doing); and (c) the testator was under no overt coercion as far as you could tell, but was acting freely, willingly, and under her or his own impetus.

10. Disciplinary action

A. *For what reasons may the RN license be suspended or revoked?*
   1. Obtaining license by fraud (omission of information, false information).
   2. Negligence and incompetence.
   3. Substance abuse.
   4. Conviction of crime (state or federal).
   5. Practicing medicine without a license.
   6. Practicing nursing without a license (expired, suspended).
   7. Allowing unlicensed person to practice nursing or medicine.
   8. Giving patient care while under the influence of alcohol or other drugs.
   9. Habitually using drugs.
   10. Discriminatory and prejudicial practices in giving patient care (pertaining to race, color, sex, age, or ethnic origin).

B. *What could happen to me if I am proven guilty of professional misconduct?*
   1. License may be revoked.
   2. License may be suspended.
   3. Behavior may be censured and reprimanded.
   4. You may be placed on probation.

C. *Who has the authority to carry out any of the above penalties?* The State Board of Registered Nursing that granted your license.

D. *I am the head nurse. One of my nurses aides has a history of failing to appear to work and not giving notice of or reason for absence. How should I handle this?* An employee has the right to know hospital policies, what is expected of an employee, and what will happen if an employee does not meet the expectations stated in his or her job description or in hospital policies and procedures. As a head nurse, you need to document behavior factually, clearly, and concisely, as well as any discussion and decision about future course of action. The employee needs the chance to read and sign it. The head nurse then sends a copy to her or his supervisor.

11. Floating

A. *Is a nurse hired to work in psychiatry obligated to cover in ICU when the latter is understaffed?* The issue is the hiring contract (implied or expressed). The contract is a composite of the mutual understanding by involved parties of rights and responsibilities, any written documents, and hospital policies. If the nurse was hired as a psychiatric nurse, he or she could legally refuse to go to the ICU. If the hospital intends to float personnel, such a policy should be clearly stated during the hiring process. Also at this time the employer should determine the employee's education, skills, and experience. On the other hand, if emergency staffing problems exist, a nurse should go to the ICU regardless of personal preference.

12. Dispensing medication

A. *Can a nurse legally remove a drug from a pharmacy when the pharmacy is closed (during the night) if the MD insists that the nurse go to the pharmacy to get the specifically prescribed medication immediately?* Within the legal boundaries of the Pharmacy Act, a nurse may remove one dose of a particular drug from the pharmacy for a particular patient during an unanticipated emergency within a limited time and availability of resources. However, the hospital should have a written policy for the nurse to follow and should authorize a specific person to use the services of the pharmacy under certain circumstances.

13. Illegible orders

A. *What should I do if I cannot decipher the MD's handwriting when she or he persists in leaving illegible orders?* Talk to the MD regarding the dangers of your giving the wrong amount of the wrong medication via the wrong route at the wrong time. If that does not help, follow appropriate channels. Do not follow an order you cannot read. You will be liable for following orders you thought were written.

14. Heroic measures

A. *The wife of a terminally ill patient approaches me*

with the request that heroic measures not be used on her husband. She has not discussed this with him but knows that he feels the same way. Can I act on this request? No. The patient is the only one who can legally make this decision as long as he or she is mentally competent.

15. Medication

A. *An MD orders pain medication prn for a patient. The patient asks for the medication, but when I question her she says the pain "isn't so bad." If in my judgement the patient's pain is not severe, am I legally covered if I give half of the pain medication dosage ordered by the MD?* A nurse cannot substitute his or her judgement for the MD's. If you alter the amount of medication prescribed by the MD without a specific order to do so, you may be liable for practicing medicine without a license.

16. Malfunctioning equipment

A. *At the end of shift report the nurse going off duty tells me that the tracheal suctioning machine is malfunctioning and describes how she got it to work. Should I plan to use the machine in the evening shift and follow her suggestions about how to make it work?* Do not plan to use equipment that you know is not functioning properly. You could be held liable since you could reasonably foresee that proper functioning of equipment would be needed for your patient. You have been put on notice that there are defects. Report this to the supervisor or person responsible for maintaining equipment in proper working order.

ETHICAL AND LEGAL CONSIDERATIONS IN INTENSIVE CARE OF THE ACUTELY ILL NEONATE

1. Responsibilities of the health agency

A. Provide an NICU or transfer to another hospital.

B. Personnel—adequate number trained in neonate diseases, special treatment, and equipment.

C. Equipment—adequate supply on hand, functioning properly (especially temperature regulator in incubator, oxygen analyzer, blood-gas machine).

2. Dying infants

A. Decision regarding resuscitation in cardiac arrest, with brain damage from cerebral anoxia. It is difficult to predict the effect of anoxia in infancy on the child's later life.

B. Decision to continue supportive measures.

C. Issue of euthanasia, such as in severe myelomeningocele at birth.

1. Active euthanasia (giving overdose).

2. Passive euthanasia (not placing on respirator).

3. Extended role of nurse in NICU—may raise issues of nursing practice versus medical practice, as when a nurse draws blood samples for blood-gas determinations without prior order. To be legally covered:

A. The nurse must be trained to perform specialized functions.

B. The functions must be written into the nurse's job description.

4. Issue of negligence—such as cross-contamination in nursery.

5. Issue of malpractice—such as assigning care of critically ill infant on respirator to untrained student or aide.

A. May be liable for inaccurate bilirubin studies for neonatal jaundice; may be legally responsible if brain damage occurs in absence of accurate laboratory tests.

B. May be liable for brain damage in infant due to respiratory or cardiac distress. Nurse needs to make sure that there are frequent blood-gas determinations to ensure adequate oxygen to prevent brain damage. Nurse also needs to make sure that the infant is not receiving too high a concentration of oxygen, which may lead to retrolental fibroplasia.

LEGAL ASPECTS OF PSYCHIATRIC CARE

1. Four sets of criteria to determine criminal responsibility at time of alleged offense

A. *M'Naghten Rule* (1832)—a person is not guilty if:

1. Person did not know the *nature and quality* of the act.

2. Person could not distinguish right from wrong— if person did not know what he or she was doing, person did not know it was wrong.

B. *The Irresistible Test* (used together with M'Naghten Rule)—person knows right from wrong, but:

1. Driven by *impulse* to commit criminal acts regardless of consequences.

2. Lacked premeditation in sudden violent behavior.

C. *American Law Institute's Test:*

1. Not responsible for criminal act if person lacks

capacity to "appreciate" the wrongfulness of it or to "conform" conduct to requirements of law.

2. Excludes "an abnormality manifested only by repeated criminal or antisocial conduct"—namely, psychopathology.

D. *Durham Test* (Product Rule—1954):

1. Accused not criminally responsible if act was a "product of mental disease."

2. Types of admissions

A. *Voluntary:* person, parent, or legal guardian applies for admission; person agrees to receive treatment and to follow hospital rules; civil rights are retained.

B. *Involuntary:* process and criteria vary among states (Figure 6–1).

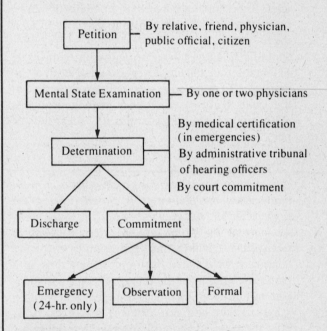

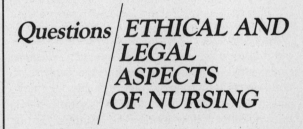

FIGURE 6–1. Typical procedure for involuntary commitment.

Questions / ETHICAL AND LEGAL ASPECTS OF NURSING

(Answer blanks are provided at the back of this book.)

1. An ambiguous order was written by a physician. The nurse, familiar only with the injectible form of the medication and unaware of the elixir form, believed the order incorrect. She/he should:

1. Ask the two physicians who are currently on the ward whether she should give the medication as she understood the order.
2. Ask her head nurse if the order is correct.
3. Call the physician who ordered the medication.
4. Contact the nursing supervisor about the problem.

2. A female patient had been receiving a drug by injection over a number of weeks. As the patient's clinical symptoms changed, the physician wrote an order on the patient's order sheet changing the mode of administration from injection to oral. When the nurse on the unit, who had been off duty for several days, was preparing to give the medication to the patient by injection, the patient objected and referred the nurse to the physician's new orders. The nurse should:
1. Go back to the order sheet and check for the order.
2. Talk with the nurse who had taken care of this particular patient while she had been off duty.
3. Talk with the head nurse about the advisability of using oral rather than injectible medications.
4. Check the order sheet for the changed order and then speak with the attending physician concerning the changed order.

3. A nurse had been caring for a female patient whose vital signs had previously been unstable. The nurse had not had a coffee break or a lunch break all day. By 2 P.M. the patient had been stable for a number of hours. The physician in charge had seen the patient and had told the nurse that the patient appeared "much improved." The nurse should:
1. Leave for her/his lunch break.
2. Forego his/her lunch break because of the patient's previous unstable condition.
3. Arrange to eat lunch in the patient's room.
4. Discuss the situation with the nurse in charge of the unit and determine who should cover the patient while the staff nurse is at lunch.

4. In hospital X, whenever there are patients in the recovery room two nurses are usually present. The hospital policy expects the nurses to take their breaks before patients arrive from surgery. On this particular day, there are two nurses on duty and two patients in the recovery room who have had minor surgeries performed that morning. Nurse A had not had a coffee break that morning. Nurse A should:
1. Stay because hospital policy expects there to be two nurses in attendance while there are patients in the recovery room.
2. Leave for coffee break because there are only two patients in the recovery room and one nurse can handle two patients quite easily.
3. Talk with the nursing supervisor and secure permission from him/her.
4. Leave to get coffee and come right back.

5. While driving down the freeway, nurse B spots an overturned car with the driver lying next to the car. Which

of the following best describes what nurse B can do without being held liable?
1. She may drive on without stopping, or stop and render emergency first aid.
2. She may stop, start to render aid, and then leave.
3. She must stop at the scene of an accident and render first aid.
4. She may stop and render aid, but if she performs a medical act, she may be charged with the illegal practice of medicine.

6. Your patient is terminally ill and has asked you to witness his will. Which of the following statements is true?
1. As a nurse, you have a legal obligation to act as a witness to a will.
2. As a nurse, you should help the patient draw up his will.
3. As a nurse, you should make sure that the patient is of sound mind, is lucid (not under the influence of drugs or alcohol), and understands what he is doing.
4. Only lawyers or family members can act as a witness to a will. If the nurse acts as a witness, the will may automatically be declared invalid.

7. Your patient has just returned from the recovery room. He is complaining of pain that is not "too severe" and has requested pain medication. You noted that the patient had been given pain medication in the recovery room. Which of the following statements indicates the best action to take?
1. Administer the dosage the physician had ordered on a prn basis.
2. Consult the physician and let him know that the patient is requesting medication for pain that is "not too severe."
3. Give half of the pain medication dosage ordered as prn by the physician.
4. Chart that the patient was complaining of pain but that it was "not too severe."

8. As a nurse, if I am being sued for malpractice, which of the following will occur?
1. My license will be revoked or suspended *automatically*.
2. I will automatically be put on probation until the matter is cleared up.
3. I will automatically be charged with a crime.
4. The State Board of Registered Nurses would be notified of the suit and, depending on the offense and outcome of the suit, it may hold a hearing to determine the status of the license.

9. A nurse's license will be revoked or she/he will be put on probation for which of the following?
1. The nurse lost a malpractice suit.
2. The nurse was found guilty of practicing while under the influence of drugs or alcohol.
3. The nurse was accused of negligence.
4. The nurse gave the wrong medication.

10. If a nurse applies restraints on her patient, she *may* be held liable by the patient for restraint of freedom of movement (false imprisonment) if:
    1. She does not immediately obtain an order from the physician.
    2. She does so after other means to subdue the patient have failed.
    3. She tries but does not obtain the patient's consent.
    4. She applies restraints for the convenience of the personnel.

11. The nurse has been working with a terminally ill male patient for weeks. The patient is lucid. His wife pleads with the nurse not to use heroic measures on her husband but to let him die "with dignity." The nurse should:
    1. Tell the wife that she needs to talk with the attending physician, patient (if possible), and other significant people about her concerns.
    2. Act on the wife's request.
    3. Ignore the wife's request and proceed with her care.
    4. Tell the wife that to do as she had requested would be equivalent to murdering the patient.

12. The surgical unit has not been busy all day. The head nurse and a few of the senior staff nurses are talking near the desk. You, as a new nurse, answer the telephone so that the other nurses may continue their conversation. Dr. D is on the line and would like you to take a telephone order. He states that the order is important. You do not know Dr. D or the patient to whom he is referring very well. As a new nurse, your best response would be:
    1. To take the telephone order.
    2. To refuse to take the order.
    3. To ask the head nurse or one of the other senior staff nurses to take the order.
    4. To ask the physician to call back and you will take the telephone order after you have read the hospital policy manual.

13. Which of the following statements concerning consent is *false*?
    1. If an informed consent is not obtained from the patient, the nurse, doctor, and/or hospital may be liable for assault.
    2. One need only obtain a general consent to treatment.
    3. In an emergency a nurse may do what she can to save life and limb, even in cases in which she has no consent.
    4. Consent may be given by conduct as well as expressed words.

14. Nurse A gave a patient the wrong medication. The patient was seriously injured. The patient sued. Who will most likely be held liable?
    1. The nurse.
    2. No one, because it was just an accident.

3. The hospital.
4. The nurse and the hospital.

15. The supervisor of the cardiovascular unit was responsible for checking the staffing patterns. She assigned nurse B to work on the unit because nurse B had had numerous years of experience on that particular unit. That evening, nurse B made a treatment error and a patient was injured. Who is liable?
    1. Nurse B.
    2. Nurse B and the supervisor.
    3. Nurse B and the hospital.
    4. Nurse B, the supervisor, and the hospital.

16. Nurse A noticed that nurse B was intoxicated while giving care. However, nurse A did not report this fact to her supervisor. That same day, nurse B made a medication error and a patient was injured. Who *may be* held responsible?
    1. Nurse B (the one intoxicated).
    2. Nurse A, nurse B, and the hospital.
    3. Nurse A (the one who did not report nurse B).
    4. Nurse B (the one intoxicated) and the hospital.

17. A graduate nurse who was new to the unit was caring for an elderly gentleman. The physician on call ordered a treatment that the nurse had not heard of. She should:
    1. Inform the physician of her lack of education and experience and refuse to do the treatment without supervision.
    2. Inform the physician of her lack of education and experience, and then proceed to perform the treatment.
    3. Refuse to perform the treatment.
    4. Carry out the treatment as best she can.

18. Which of the following is *not* true about informed consent?
    1. Obtaining consent is the responsibility of the physician.
    2. A nurse may accept responsibility for witnessing a consent form.
    3. A physician subjects himself/herself to liability if he/she withholds any facts that are necessary to form the basis of an intelligent consent.
    4. If a nurse witnesses a consent for surgery, the nurse is, in effect, indicating that the patient is "informed."

19. You are a staff nurse coming on shift. The *day* nurse has just told you that the suction equipment in Mr. Clay's room is not working properly. Since you will be working with Mr. Clay, you should do which of the following?
    1. Follow the *day* nurse's suggestions on how to get the malfunctioning equipment to work.
    2. Continue to use the malfunctioning machine, hoping that it will function for your shift.
    3. Ask your supervisor to show you how to work with the malfunctioning equipment.

4. Replace the equipment or report it to whomever is responsible for maintaining equipment in proper working condition.

20. Duncan Green is a competent adult who has refused treatment and wishes to leave AMA (against medical advice). Mr. Green has also refused to sign any of the appropriate AMA forms. All of the following statements are true except:
    1. The physician and/or hospital is always liable for any injury that might occur as a result of the patient's decision to leave AMA.
    2. The law usually permits competent, adult patients to make decisions that may not be in their own best health interest.
    3. Even if the patient is a competent adult, the law may interfere with the patient's decision to refuse medical treatment if the patient has small children that need to be taken care of.
    4. The physician might be held liable if it can be proven that the patient did not receive sufficient information about risks involved with leaving AMA.

21. Nurse A, the only Spanish-speaking emergency room nurse, admitted a six-year-old child. The child's mother explained in Spanish that she had removed two ticks from the child the previous day. The child was now running a very high temperature and had a rash on his abdomen. Nurse A reported her information to the emergency room physician, who did not speak Spanish. The nurse failed to tell the doctor about the ticks. The physician diagnosed the child as having measles. Over the course of the day, the child's health deteriorated until he died. Who is liable?
    1. Nurse A.
    2. Nurse A and the physician.
    3. Nurse A and the hospital.
    4. Physician.

22. Nurse B was on weekend call for the operating room. Late Saturday night, the nursing supervisor called nurse B to tell her that they were expecting an emergency appendectomy within the hour. While gowning the surgeon, nurse B smelled alcohol on the doctor's breath. Nurse B mentioned this to the anesthesiologist, who also admitted smelling alcohol on the surgeon. Both the nurse and the anesthesiologist felt the surgeon was somewhat unstable on his feet. However, neither the nurse nor the other doctor said anything. If the patient had been injured during the surgery, who would have been liable?
    1. Nurse B, anesthesiologist, surgeon, and hospital.
    2. Nurse B and surgeon.
    3. Surgeon and hospital.
    4. Hospital, surgeon, and anesthesiologist.

23. A child about eleven months old was brought by her mother to a hospital for examination, diagnosis, and treatment. The child was seen by a nurse and physician.

At the time the child was suffering from a comminuted spiral fracture of the right tibia and fibula that gave the appearance of having been caused by twisting. The child also had numerous bruises and burns on her body. In addition, she had a nondepressed linear fracture of the skull in the process of healing. When approached, the child demonstrated fear and apprehension. The mother had no explanation for the child's wounds. No further X rays were taken, and the child was released to the mother without report to concerned agencies. One month later the child was brought in again by the mother and was seen by a different physician. The second physician correctly diagnosed the battered-child syndrome and filed the proper reports. The child was placed in a foster home and the foster home filed suit. Who may be liable?
    1. First nurse, first doctor, and hospital.
    2. First doctor.
    3. No one.
    4. First nurse.

24. While getting a patient ready for surgery, nurse A removed the patient's dentures. The nurse wrapped the dentures in a towel so as not to break them and left them on the bedside stand. While the nurse was out of the room, two nurses' aides stripped the bed and threw all the linen, including the towel, in the laundry hamper. Upon returning from surgery, the patient requested her dentures. However, the nurse and nursing aides were unable to find them. Who is liable?
    1. The nurse.
    2. The nurse and the hospital.
    3. The nurse and nursing aides.
    4. The nurse, nursing aides, and hospital.

25. A teenage girl who had complained of dizziness the previous day wanted to take a shower. The physician gave his permission for the patient to shower with assistance. The nurse started to get the girl out of bed and over to the shower. The nurse questioned the patient about her dizziness. The girl replied that she was not dizzy. The mother then said that she would watch her daughter in the shower and help her back to bed. The nurse then left the room. While the nurse was out, the patient fainted getting back into bed. The patient injured her head. Who is liable?
    1. The nurse.
    2. The doctor, nurse, and hospital.
    3. The nurse and the hospital.
    4. No one is liable.

26. What does the Durham Test state about the accused?
    1. It states the same as the M'Naghten rule.
    2. Accused is not criminally responsible if his act was the product of mental disease.
    3. Accused is not criminally responsible if his act was a result of impulsiveness.
    4. Accused is not criminally responsible if he does not appreciate the wrongfulness of his act.

27. What does voluntary admission require of the individual?
    1. The individual must ask to be admitted to a psychiatric hospital and must agree to abide by its rules.
    2. The request for hospitalization needs to originate with the individual to be admitted.
    3. The individual needs to make written application to a hospital, agree to treatment, and agree to abide by the rules.
    4. The individual needs to be responsible for the hospital bill.

28. Standards of Practice for Psychiatric Mental Health Nursing have been developed by:
    1. A joint commission of psychiatric nurses and psychiatrists.
    2. Psychiatric nurses who are members of the American Nurses' Association.
    3. A panel of representative psychiatric nurses in the United States.
    4. The Division on Psychiatric and Mental Health Nursing Practice of the American Nurses' Association.

29. The Standards of Practice for Psychiatric Mental Health Nursing are organized around:
    1. Different models of treatment.
    2. Rights of the clients.
    3. The nursing process.
    4. Legal aspects of treatment.

30. The Community Mental Health Centers Amendments of 1975, Title III of Public Law 94–63:
    1. Cut the flow of funds to Community Mental Health Centers and set forth general guidelines for service.
    2. Extended the flow of funds to Community Mental Health Centers and set forth specific guidelines for service.
    3. Cut the flow of funds to Community Mental Health Centers and set forth specific guidelines for service.
    4. Extended the flow of funds to Community Mental Health Centers and set forth general guidelines for service.

31. Congress, in the Mental Health Centers Act of 1974, also stated that it wanted to:
    1. Increase federal operation funds to centers and have centers under federal support.
    2. Provide funding on a declining basis at the federal level and encourage the goal of independence from federal support.
    3. Provide funding on a declining basis at the federal level but maintain federal control.
    4. Get out of the community mental health business.

32. The principal recommendation of the Report of the President's Commission on Mental Health, 1978, was:
    1. The federal government should get out of mental health.
    2. The government should upgrade the old federal grant program for community mental health to encourage the creation of necessary services where they are inadequate and to increase the flexibility of communities planning a comprehensive network of services.
    3. Community mental health programs should strictly adhere to the provision of specific services to all communities.
    4. A new federal grant program should be established for community mental health to encourage the creation of necessary services where they are inadequate and to increase the flexibility of communities planning a comprehensive network of services.

33. In order for nurses to control their own profession, they need to demonstrate:
    1. Expertise in implementing client care levels already determined by law.
    2. The ability to participate in the drafting of health care laws that directly reflect client care levels.
    3. The ability to participate in the drafting of laws at all levels and in all areas of health care.
    4. Neutrality by ignoring political power, thus being free from political influence in giving health care.

34. The ICN's Code for Nurses, "Ethical Concepts Applied to Nursing," approved by the Council of Nurse Representatives in 1973, states that:
    1. The professional body of nurses of a particular country carries the responsibility for nursing practice and for maintaining competence.
    2. The hospital employing the nurse carries the responsibility for nursing practice and for maintaining competence.
    3. The laws of the country in which the nurse works carry the responsibility for nursing practice and for maintaining competence.
    4. The individual nurse carries personal responsibility for nursing practice and for maintaining her competence by continual learning.

35. The National Health Planning and Resource Development Act of 1974 allows:
    1. Physicians the largest representation on local and state health care boards that make decisions about health care.
    2. Hospital administrators the largest representation on local and state health care boards that make decisions about health care.
    3. The consumer the largest representation on local and state health care boards that make health care decisions.
    4. Health professionals as a group the largest representation on local and state health care boards that make health care decisions.

Answers— Rationale / ETHICAL AND LEGAL ASPECTS OF NURSING

1. (3) The nurse would be negligent for any untoward effects of the drug if she/he failed to contact the physician who ordered the drug before the nurse administered it. In *Norton* v. *Argonaut Insurance Co.,* [144 So. 2nd 249 (La. Ct. App. 1962)], the court stated that it was the responsibility of the nurse to clarify the order with the physician involved.

2. (4) While No. 1 is a correct answer, No. 4 is the best because the nurse would validate the changed order and learn the physician's rationale for the change. In *Larrimore* v. *Homeopathic Hospital Association,* [54 Del. 449, 181 A. 2d 573 (1962)], the court found that the nurse who went ahead and gave the medication was negligent. The courts went on to say that the jury could find the nurse negligent by applying ordinary common sense to establish the applicable standard of care.

3. (4) The nurse would come back to her patient revitalized after having her lunch break, and the patient would be covered the whole time the nurse is away. In deciding that the nurse would not be negligent to leave such a patient, the court would emphasize that the question of liability should be determined in light of the circumstances as they existed at the time. When the nurse left the patient, it was not foreseeable that an increased risk to the patient would result. On the contrary, the patient would be looked after, and the nurse could take care of her own needs, too. *Child* v. *Vancouver General Hospital,* [71 W. W. R. 656 (1979)].

4. (1) In a court of law, hospital policy may be used to set the standard of care by which the nurses' actions are judged. Since the hospital policy states that two nurses must be in attendance while patients are in the recovery room, both the nurse who left (Nos. 2 and 4) and the supervisor who authorized the nurse's absence (No. 3) would be held liable for any untoward effect on the patient. *Laidlaw* v. *Lions Gate Hospital,* [70 W.W.R. 727 (1969)].

5. (1) The court has stated that no one is obliged by law to assist a stranger, even if he/she can do so by a word and without the slightest danger to him/herself. Hence, No. 3 is incorrect. But once one has undertaken to give assistance, the law imposes on him/her a duty of care toward the person assisted. Hence, No. 2 is incorrect. The court also states that under emergency circumstances a nurse, like any other person, may perform a medical act to preserve life and limb. Either law or custom exempts such actions from coming within the medical practice acts. This, then, would rule out No. 4.

6. (3) Anyone can act as a witness. No. 1 is incorrect because a nurse has no legal obligation to participate as a witness, only a moral and ethical obligation. No. 2 would also be incorrect because only a lawyer or the patient him/herself can draw up a will. If the nurse draws up the will, she/he could be charged with practicing law without a license. If a nurse does act as a witness, he/she should determine that the patient is of sound mind or the will could be declared invalid—not because the nurse acted as a witness (No. 4), but because the patient was not of sound mind.

7. (2) The physician should be notified of the patient's complaints, and the new orders should be established. This is what the courts would consider prudent under the circumstances and what a reasonable nurse should do. No. 1 would not be the best choice because the patient had already been given pain medication in the recovery room, and another full dose might be too much. Without further information, this is a very dangerous choice, and the nurse would be held liable for any untoward effects. No. 3 would also be incorrect because a nurse cannot substitute her/his judgement for the physician's without consulting the physician first. If a nurse alters the amount prescribed without an order from the physician, the nurse could be charged with practicing medicine without a license. No. 4 is incomplete. A nurse must chart the patient's complaints, but must also indicate what was done about them.

8. (4) Only the State Board of Registered Nurses has the authority to revoke or suspend a license. This can occur only after the nurse has been given a fair hearing before an impartial hearing body. Hence, Nos. 1, 2, and 3 are incorrect, because they assume a penalty should be made before the State Board is notified.

9. (2) All state Practice Acts list "guilty of practicing while under the influence of drugs or alcohol" as a reason for revocation of a license or for putting a nurse on probation. Nos. 1, 3, and 4 may cause the nurse to lose her license; however, other circumstances would have to be considered first, such as the frequency with which these had occurred.

10. (4) Freedom from unlawful restraint is a basic human right. Restraints of any type may constitute false imprisonment. False imprisonment is an actionable tort for which a nurse may be held liable by a patient. The patient may have an actionable case of false imprisonment if the restraints were applied for staff convenience only. Most likely the nurse would not be held liable for false imprisonment even if she/he does not immediately obtain an order from the physician for the restraints. However, No. 1 is not the *best* choice.

Restraints should be used only in emergency situations, for a limited time, for the limited purpose of protecting the patient, and not for the convenience of the staff. Even though the patient's consent (No. 3) is not usually obtainable under the circumstances, the nurse should try in order to avoid being held liable for false imprisonment. However, these restraints should only be applied as a last resort (No. 2).

11. (1) This type of case is an example of the most difficult medical/ethical/legal questions today. The answers are ambiguous at best. However, in this case No. 1 would be best since neither the nurse (No. 3), the wife (No. 2), nor the doctor can make that decision as long as the patient is a competent adult. No. 4 is incorrect because the nurse's values should not supersede the wife's concerns for her husband's welfare.

12. (3) Get a senior nurse who knows the policies, the patient, and the doctor. Generally speaking, a nurse should not accept telephone orders. However, if it is necessary to take one, follow the hospital's policy regarding telephone orders. Failure to follow hospital policy could be considered negligence. In this case, the nurse was new and did not know the hospital's policy concerning telephone orders. The nurse was also unfamiliar with the doctor and the patient. Therefore the nurse should not take the order unless (a) no one else is available and (b) it is an emergency situation. Nos. 1 and 2 are both incomplete, as they do not take into account the mitigating circumstances described above. Since the doctor has said that the order is important, the nurse should not delay the doctor while she/he reads the manual. Hence, No. 4 is incorrect.

13. (2) *Assault* is the unjustifiable attempt to touch another person or the threat to do so in such circumstances as to cause the other reasonably to believe that it will be carried out. The lack of informed consent is an important part of the meaning of assault. Consent is a defense to an action for assault. However, if the treatment or procedure goes beyond the patient's consent (as it probably would if consent was only to "general" treatment, as in No. 2), the nurse, the doctor, and/or the hospital may be liable. Hence, No. 1 is a true statement. In an emergency situation in which the nurse is trying to save the patient's life, if the patient does not or cannot consent to treatment, the nurse usually will not be held to have assaulted the patient. Hence, No. 3 is also a true statement. Consent may be given by conduct as well as by expressed words, as in No. 4. For example, in a case in which a person held up his arm to be vaccinated, the court said he had consented. However, it is best to get the consent in writing, specifically outlining the treatment or procedure to be performed. The consent will most likely be deemed invalid, however, if the patient is a child, is mentally incompetent, or is intoxicated.

14. (4) *Both* you and the hospital can be sued for damages if a mistake you make injures the patient. The nurse is always responsible for his/her own actions. The hospital, as the employer, will be vicariously liable under the *respondeat superior doctrine*—the employer is liable for the negligent conduct of its nurses when the act was committed within the scope of employment. Nos. 1 and 3 are incomplete; No. 2 is incorrect.

15. (3) The hospital is *always* initially held liable under the theory of *respondeat superior*—vicarious liability of the employer. Nos. 2 and 4 are incorrect because the supervisor would *not* be responsible unless the court thought that the supervisor was negligent in supervising or assigning a task beyond the capabilities of another. In this case, nurse B had had numerous years of experience on the cardiovascular unit. Without further data, the supervisor would not have been negligent for assigning nurse B to the cardiovascular unit. No. 1 is incomplete.

16. (2) This answer includes all parties: the hospital, nurse A, and nurse B. The hospital, as the employer, might be held liable under the theory of respondeat superior—vicarious liability. Nurse B would be held responsible, since each nurse is personally liable for his or her own negligent actions. Nurse A might also be held responsible, since every nurse is obligated to act so that patients are safe from injury. In this case, nurse A knew of B's intoxicated state. Nurse A did not act as a *reasonably prudent nurse* when she failed to inform a supervisor. Nos. 1, 3, and 4 are incomplete.

17. (1) If you inform the physician and still carry out the treatment (No. 2), both you and the physician could be held liable if the patient is negligently harmed. The nurse would be liable because she did not act as a reasonably prudent nurse, and the physician would be liable because he knew of the nurse's lack of knowledge and did not step in to protect the patient. If the nurse does not tell the physician and still carries out the treatment (No. 4), she would be solely liable. The nurse should not refuse to perform the treatment (No. 3) unless she has no supervision.

18. (4) The nurse who witnesses a consent for surgery or other procedure is witnessing only that the signature is that of the purported person and that the person's condition is as indicated at the time of signing. The nurse is not witnessing that the patient is "informed." Nos. 1, 2, and 3 are all true statements.

19. (4) As a nurse, you should *not* plan to use equipment that you know is malfunctioning. You could be held liable since you were on notice and could reasonably foresee that properly functioning equipment would be needed by your patient. Hence, Nos. 1, 2, and 3 are incorrect.

20. (1) This is the only clearly false option. Neither the physician nor the hospital would ordinarily be liable if (a) the medical risk is explained and a full report concerning the incident is documented; and (b) the patient is a competent adult. The court does not usually interfere with one's right to refuse treatment, as in No. 2. However, the court will closely scrutinize a situation in which the patient's refusal to accept treatment results in death or in the patient's inability to care for children. If the children might be left wards of the court, the court may force the patient to accept treatment, as in No. 3. Hence, Nos. 2, 3, and 4 are incorrect.

21. (3) The court in *John Ramsey, Jr. et al.* v. *Physicians Memorial Hospital, Inc. et al.* stated: " . . . evidence supported finding that the failure of nurse to notify physician of patient history involving removal of ticks from one of the children constituted a violation of her duties as a nurse, and failure to relate the information to the physician was the contributing proximate cause of death of the child." The hospital is *also* held liable under the doctrine of respondeat superior for the negligent conduct of its nurses when committed within the scope of their employment. Hence, No. 1 is incomplete, because it doesn't include the hospital. The physician would most likely *not* be held liable because of the language barrier and the nurse's clear failure to communicate. Hence, Nos. 2 and 4 are incorrect.

22. (1) Both nurses and doctors are under a duty to protect the safety of their patients. In this case, the patient's safety was potentially jeopardized, yet neither the anesthesiologist nor the nurse reported the situation. Therefore, if something had happened to the patient during surgery, the court could have made a good argument to say that all were negligent. Hence, Nos. 2, 3, and 4 are incomplete. When a nurse encounters a situation as described here, what can she do? First, for her own safety, the nurse should prepare a summary of the incidents. The nurse might also consult with nurse colleagues who have worked with the physician, as they could confirm or deny the problem and possibly offer support. Second, the nurse should report the incident to her supervisor and director of nursing, who have a liaison with the surgical/medical staff. If the action is not pursued successfully, the nurse can bring the problem to the attention of the hospital administrator. Again, if no action is forthcoming, the nurse may seek out a board member who might be sensitive to the situation. In any case, these are difficult situations a nurse may find him/herself in. There is no easy solution.

23. (1) Most state statutes provide that every hospital to which any person is brought who is suffering from any injuries inflicted by another must report the fact immediately to the local law enforcement authorities. Most state statutes also impose the same duty on other health care professionals, school officials and teachers, child care supervisors, and social workers. Hence, Nos. 2 and 4 are incomplete; No. 3 is incorrect. From *Landeros* v. *Flood* as well as other cases, it seems clear that the responsibility of professional people—doctors, nurses, and others who must deal with injured children—includes the duty to report suspicious evidence to the proper authorities.

24. (2) However, it could be argued that No. 1 is correct. The nurse's liability for the negligent loss of or damage to a patient's property is based on her duty as a person, trained or untrained, to act as a reasonable and ordinary, prudent person. In this case, the nurse put the dentures in a towel without a label. She might reasonably expect that aides would be stripping the linen after the patient left for surgery. Therefore, her act was not that of an ordinary prudent person. The nurse would be liable. Since the nurse is liable, the hospital, as her employer, *might* also be held liable. This would be for court determination. Since the aides had no knowledge of the dentures, and they were acting reasonably, they would not be liable for the lost dentures. Hence, Nos. 3 and 4 are incorrect.

25. (4) While No. 4 is best, this is a very close case. When family members help with a hospitalized patient, liability becomes complicated. Where members of the nursing team offer to assist patients in bathing, feeding, etc., and an apparently capable family member prefers to assist the patient, this is usually acceptable and neither the hospital nor the health care team is liable. Thus, Nos. 1, 2, and 3 can be eliminated as correct choices. However, the nurse should never assume that the presence of a family member obviates her helping the client.

26. (2) The Durham Test says that a person is not criminally responsible if the act was a product of mental disease. No. 1 is incorrect because the M'Naghten rule states that a person is insane if he cannot determine right from wrong. No. 3 is wrong because it is *not* what the Durham Test states. No. 4 is wrong because it is an interpretation of the M'Naghten rule.

27. (3) The request must be in writing. Nos. 1 and 2 are true, but incomplete. No. 4 has nothing to do with voluntary admission.

28. (4) This division of the ANA sets the standards. Therefore, No. 1 cannot be correct. Nos. 2 and 3 are also incorrect, although they may be part of No. 4.

29. (3) Nos. 1, 2, and 4 may be referred to in the standards, but the standards were organized around the nursing process.

30. (2) The Amendments extended the flow of funds and set forth specific guidelines for service. No. 1 is incorrect because it did not cut funds or set general guide-

lines. No. 3 is incorrect because it did not cut funds. No. 4 is incorrect because it did not set general guidelines.

31. (2) Congress intended to provide funding on a declining basis and to encourage independence from federal support. No. 1 is incorrect because Congress does not want centers under continual federal support. No. 3 is incorrect because it did not want to maintain federal control. No. 4 is incorrect because, although Congress wanted declining funding and control, it remains interested in community mental health centers.

32. (4) This was the principal recommendation. No. 1 is incorrect. No. 3 is incorrect because they want flexibility in services. No. 2 is incorrect because they did not want to upgrade the old grant, they wanted to provide a new one.

33. (3) Nurses, for control and better health care, should be active at all levels and in all areas of health care. No. 1 passively carries out others' ideas. No. 2 is too limited in scope. No. 4 is also passive, with an additional loss of control.

34. (4) This is what the document states. Other choices do not give the individual nurse primary responsibility.

35. (3) The Act states that the boards must consist of 60% *consumers* who are not affiliated with any health professional group. Hence, Nos. 1, 2, and 4 are incorrect.

SUGGESTED REFERENCES

American Nurses' Association: Code for nurses, Kansas City, Missouri, 1976.

American Nurses' Association: Standards of nursing practice, Kansas City, Missouri, 1973.

Bullough, B.: "Influences on role expansion," *American Journal of Nursing,* 76(9):1476–1481, September 1976.

Creighton, H.: Law every nurse should know, Philadelphia, 1975, W. B. Saunders Co.

International Council of Nurses: ICN code for nurses: ethical concepts applied to nursing, Geneva, 1973.

National Commission for the Study of Nursing and Nursing Education: "Summary report and recommendations," in Jerome Lysaught: Action in nursing: progress in professional purpose, New York, 1974, McGraw-Hill Book Co.

Somers, A.: Health care in transition: directions for the future, Chicago, 1971, Hospital Research and Educational Trust.

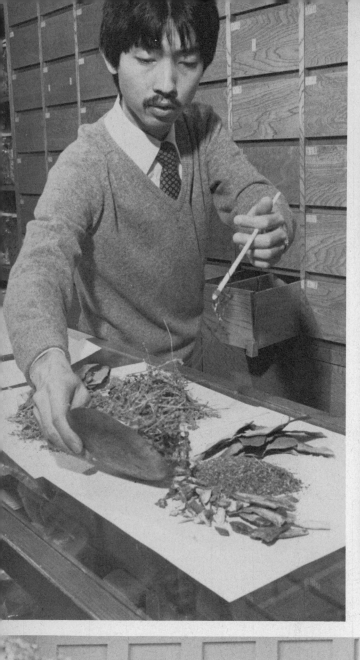
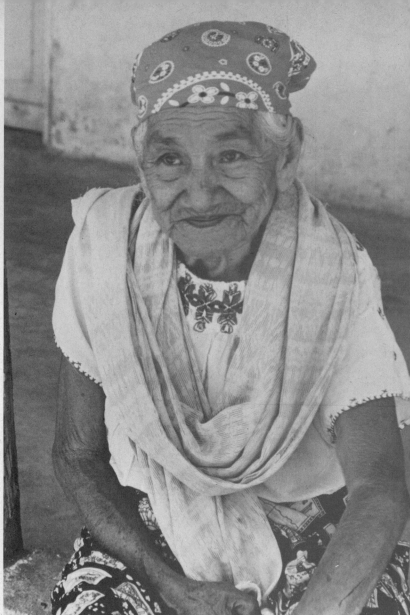
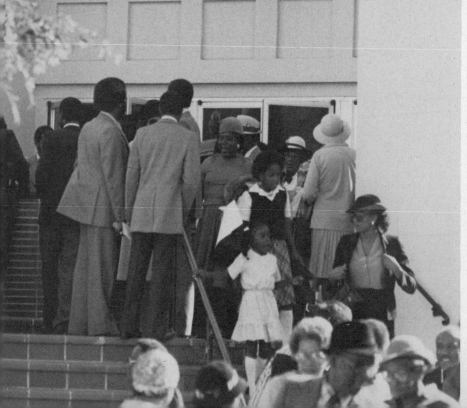
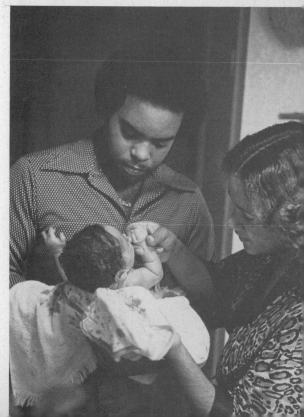

Unit 7 / CULTURAL DIVERSITY IN NURSING PRACTICE

In a society of many cultures, such as ours, it is imperative to develop a sensitivity to the cultural aspects of client care. Such a sensitivity can only be fostered by a committed openness to diversity and willingness to learn about the background, values, beliefs, particular health concerns of various groups. Although no single book—much less a short outline—can hope to provide all the information needed for a full cultural awareness, it is hoped that the facts presented here, and the suggested references at the end of the unit, will provide the student with a useful starting point.

Sally Lagerquist

It is important to recognize the specific values, beliefs, and problems of different ethnic groups that relate to health and illness. This section will highlight a few examples to point out the importance of cultural factors in assessing actual problems and needs and in planning for health care. However, it is not meant to be all-inclusive of such variations. (For an outline of cultural food patterns, refer to Table 3–14 in Unit 3, p. 197.)

CONSIDERATIONS FOR HEALTH CARE

1. *General considerations for physical health care—*based on unique health needs.
A. Assessing *physical differences*.
   1. Newborn:
      a. Mongolian spots—normal in Black, Asian, and Native American.
      b. Head configuration—related to maternal/fetal cephalopelvic proportion differences.
   2. Preschool: for example, *earwax type*—dry earwax in Native Americans and Asians; wet earwax in Blacks and Whites.
   3. Differential growth and development scores; for example, when compared with White norms, Blacks generally have higher scores, Asians generally have lower scores.
   4. Certain muscles may be absent in some groups of people; for example, peroneus tertius in foot, palmaris longus in wrist.
   5. Bony protuberances (mandibular and palatine) may occur in some groups of people and not in others.
   6. Variation in teeth: some groups of people may have peg teeth, extra teeth, natal teeth.
   7. Tongues: some may be characteristically fissured; others "scrotal"; still others "geographic."
   8. Different patterns of superficial veins on anterior chest of pregnant women in some groups.
B. Variation in *susceptibility* to disease:
   1. Tuberculosis—urban Jews most resistant; Blacks and Native Americans most susceptible.
   2. Duodenal ulcers—more prevalent in blood type O.
   3. Cancer of the stomach—more prevalent in blood type O.
   4. Venous thromboembolic disease in women—less prevalent in blood type O.
   5. Sickle cell anemia—most common in Blacks (1 in 400), Mediterranean people, and those whose ancestors lived in malaria-plagued areas.
   6. Overgrowth of connective tissue components—keloid formation in Blacks; also Blacks have greater incidence of Burkitt's lymphoma, multiple myeloma, systemic lupus erythematosus, increased tendency toward endomyocardial fibrosis after myocardial infarct.
   7. Eye problems—color blindness in East Indians; myopia in Chinese.
   8. Gout—high incidence among Puerto Ricans and Filipinos.
   9. Hypertension—higher among Filipino males, Blacks, and Jews.
   10. Lactase deficiency—more prevalent among Blacks and Asians.
   11. Acatalasia—mostly found among Japanese, Koreans, and Chinese.
   12. Coccidioidomycosis—more common among Blacks and Filipinos.
   13. Sarcoidosis—ten times more prevalent among Blacks.
   14. Cystic fibrosis—high incidence in White population.
   15. Cleft lip—1:1,000 in Whites; 1:500 in Japanese; 1:200 in Blacks.
   16. Congenital hip dysplasia—less incidence in Asians (who carry infants in hip straddle position); high incidence in Navajo Indians (who use swaddling and cradle boards).
C. Variations in *body size and shape:*
   1. Eyelids—epicanthic folds; skin droop over cartilage plate over eye.
   2. Ears—free, floppy, or attached.
   3. Noses—size and shape correlate with ancestral homeland; for example, cold regions produced small noses (for example, Asians, Aleutians); dry areas produced high bridges (for example, Iranians, Native Americans); moist, warm climates produced broad flat noses (for example, Blacks).
   4. Tooth size—largest among Australian Aborigines, who also have four extra molars; large size also in Asians, Blacks.
D. Variations in *blood group:*
   1. American Indians generally have blood type O, and no type B.
   2. Japanese and Chinese have almost equal rates of A, B, and O, but little AB.
   3. American Blacks and Whites have the same percentage of type A and O.
   4. Rh negative is most often found among Whites, much rarer in other groups, and nonexistent among Eskimos.
   5. Twinning (dizygote) is highest among Blacks (up

to 4% of births); 2% in Whites, and ½% in Asians. It is also related to the age of the mother.

2. General considerations for mental health care

A. Therapies need to include *extended* families as opposed to individuals or nuclear families.

B. Cultural and racial as well as individual components must be considered when assessing precipitating or predisposing causes of illness.

C. Values may conflict; for example, individualism versus concern for family or social interactions; self-actualization versus survival needs.

D. Some ethnic groups *do not value or possess* qualities required for some psychiatric therapies, such as verbal skills, introspection, ability to delay gratification, ability to discuss personal problems with strangers.

E. Therapy resources *may not be accessible or considered useful or relevant* for members of some ethnic groups.

F. Common feelings and behavior patterns may be shared by many minority groups:
1. Feelings of *inferiority and inadequacy,* often a result of prejudice and racism.
2. *Incompetent* behavior as an outcome of feeling inferior and inadequate.
3. *Suppressed anger,* resulting in displaced hostility and paranoid ideas.
4. *Withholding and withdrawal;* not comfortable with sharing feelings or experiences.
5. *Selective inattention;* may block out or deny frustration or insults.
6. *Overcompensation* in some areas to make up for denied opportunities in other areas.

3. Social considerations in health assessment

A. Language barriers.

B. Food habits—important implications for hospital food, special diets, instructions about meal planning.

C. Perceptions of illness may include:
1. Punishment for sin.
2. Work of malevolent persons or evil spirits.

D. Behavior during illness may stem from perception of cause of illness.
1. May refuse medication if sickness is taken to indicate the need to atone.
2. May practice bargaining or atonement rituals.
3. May do penance by fasting.

E. Variations in time orientation:
1. May be more oriented to the here and now than to the future.

2. Implication: need *short-range* nursing goals.

F. Differences in concept of family:
1. Involves *extended* family.
2. Some family needs may take priority over individual's health needs.

G. Male/female norms vary in some cultures.
1. Men must be strong, stoic, without crying or complaining, always in control of emotions such as fear.
2. Women value modesty; that is, some cultures do not allow inspection by strange men, including physicians.

H. Pain perception—varies from one culture to another.

EXAMPLES OF HEALTH BELIEFS, PRACTICES, PROBLEMS

1. Native Americans (American Indians)

A. *Health beliefs and practices:*
1. Imbalance between ill person and natural/supernatural forces; for example, bad thoughts, wishes can cause illness.
2. Sacred foods, curative and preventive rituals by medicine men.

B. *Death or loss:*
1. No belief in hereafter, but will join the dead.
2. Quality of here and now more important than longevity.
3. Can accept death; little worry about how, when, why.

C. *Eye contact:*
1. Direct eye contact seen as disrespectful.
2. May take away other's soul.

D. *Kinship:* important for family, relatives, friends to congregate for long periods near patient.

E. *Time:*
1. Casual, not controlled by clock.
2. May be directed by other factors, for example, sun or season.

F. *Health problems:*
1. High suicide, homicide, alcoholism rate.
2. Increasing emotional problems in children.
3. Otitis media a major problem.
4. Nutritional deficiencies.
5. Infant illness and death during first year higher than among Whites.
6. Lead poisoning from sniffing leaded gasoline on reservations.

2. Blacks

A. *Health problems:*

1. Tuberculosis three times greater than among Whites.
2. High incidence of hypertension.
3. Uterine cancer twice as common as in Whites.
4. Sickle cell anemia disease—1 in 400; 1 in 12 carry the trait.
5. Malnutrition.
6. Very high rates of violent death, murder, accidental death.

3. Latinos
A. *Health beliefs:*
1. *Mal de ojo*—headaches, fever, fatigue, prostration caused by the evil eye.
2. *Empacho*—in children, produces abdominal swelling.
3. *Susto*—emotional illness with insomnia, restlessness, nervousness.
4. *Espanto*—fright caused by supernatural spirits or events.
5. *Coraje*—rage, hyperactivity, yelling and screaming.
6. Chronic illness—have offended God and are being punished.
7. Health means: being free of pain, being obese rather than thin.
8. Hospital is a place to die.
9. Illness is a family affair.
10. Very modest about bathing; defecating and urinating are very personal and don't like to answer questions about it.
B. *Diet:*
1. Specific foods help good health (tea from French orange); other foods can produce poor health (rice and coffee in the evening).
2. Herbs, hot and cold foods used to treat hot and cold problems.

4. Asians
A. *Health beliefs:*
1. Yin and yang regulate health and treatment.
   a. Increased yin results in nervous, digestive disorders.
   b. Increased yang results in dehydration, fever, irritability.
2. Treat hot illness with cold foods and vice versa.
3. Hospital is a place to die.
4. Blood is not replaceable—may refuse blood transfusion.
5. One dose herbal medicine is enough, may refuse multiple doses of Western medicine.
6. Believe in acupuncture.

B. *Health problems:*
1. Eye problems.
2. Dental caries.
3. Malnutrition.
4. Tuberculosis.

5. Jews
A. *Health beliefs* based on Talmudic laws.
1. Abortion—mandatory to save a mother's life, regardless of fetal age.
2. Contraception allowed.
3. Death—euthanasia is prohibited; death means absence of spontaneous respirations; autopsies not allowed unless they will help another patient.
4. Dietary—many Jews follow *kosher* dietary regulations.
   a. Meat and dairy products cannot be combined in cooking or eaten in the same meal. Separate dishes and cooking utensils required for meat and dairy products.
   b. Shellfish not allowed, only fish with scales and fins.
   c. Meat allowed only from animals with cloven hoofs who chew their cud, slaughtered according to ritual under rabbinical supervision.
B. *Health problems:*
1. Diabetes mellitus.
2. Buerger's disease.
3. Tay-Sachs disease.
4. Obesity.
5. Ulcerative colitis.

SUGGESTED REFERENCES

American Nurses' Association: "Unique needs of ethnic minority clients in a multiracial society: a biological, psycho-social, socio-cultural perspective," in Affirmative action: toward quality nursing care for a multiracial society, Kansas City, Missouri, 1976.

Brink, P., ed.: Transcultural nursing: a book of readings, Englewood Cliffs, New Jersey, 1976, Prentice-Hall, Inc.

Campbell, T., and Chang, B.: "Health care of the Chinese in America," *Nursing Outlook*, 21(4):245–249, April 1973.

Comer, J. P., and Poussaint, A.: Black child care: how to bring up a healthy black child in America: a guide to emotional and psychological development, New York, 1975, Simon and Schuster, Inc.

Gonzales, H. H.: "Health care needs of the Mexican American," in Ethnicity and health care, New York, 1976, National League for Nursing.

Henderson, G., and Primeaux, M., eds.: Transcultural health care, Menlo Park, Calif., 1981, Addison-Wesley Publishing Co.

Leininger, M., ed.: "Humanism, health and cultural values," in Health care dimensions, Philadelphia, 1974, F. A. Davis Co.

Martin, B.: "Ethnicity and health care: Afro-Americans," in Ethnicity and health care, New York, 1976, National League for Nursing.

Nursing Clinics of North America: Symposium on cultural and biological diversity and health care, 12(1):5–86, March 1977.

Primeaux, M.: "Caring for the American Indian patient," *American Journal of Nursing,* 76(1):91–94, January 1977.

Rotkovich, R.: "The Jewish heritage," in Ethnicity and health care, New York, 1976, National League for Nursing.

Spratlen, L. P.: "Introducing ethnic-cultural factors in models of nursing: some mental health care applications," *Journal of Nursing Education,* 15:2, March 1976.

Wang, R.: "Chinese-Americans and health care," in Ethnicity and health care, New York, 1976, National League for Nursing.

Wood, R.: "The American and health," in Ethnicity and health care, New York, 1976, National League for Nursing.

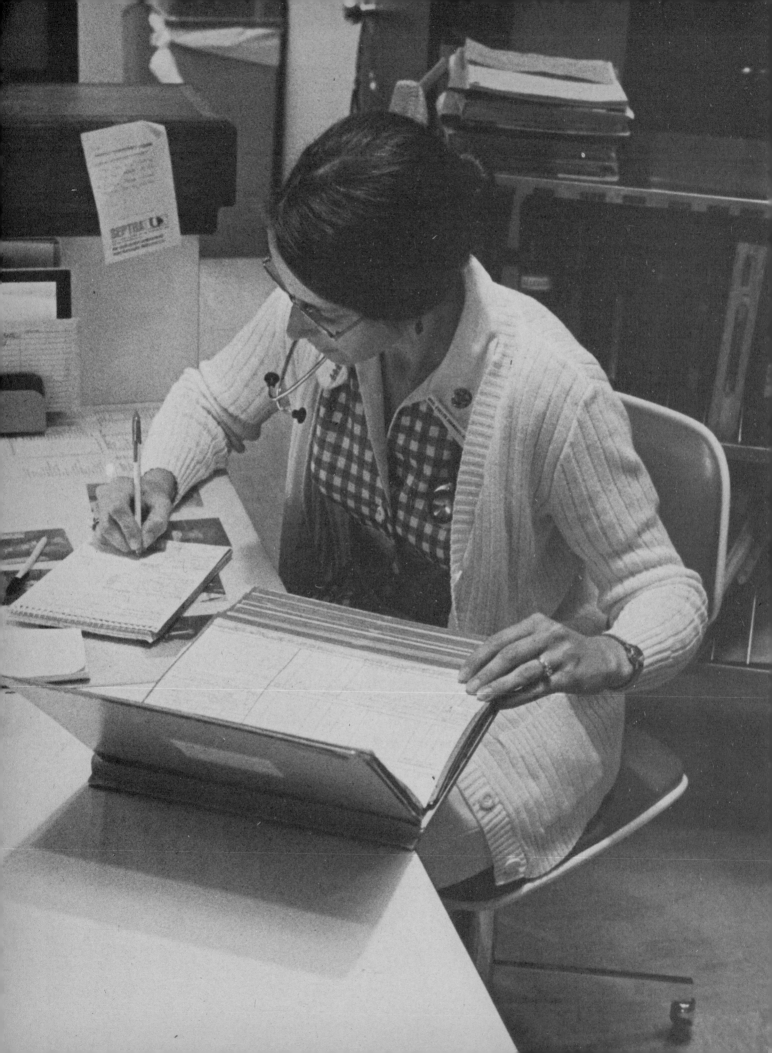

Appendices

Appendix A / DIETS

NUTRITION DURING PREGNANCY AND LACTATION

1. **Milk group**—important for calcium, protein of high biologic value, and other vitamins and minerals.
   Pregnancy—three to four servings.
   Lactation—four servings.
   Count as one serving—1 cup milk; ½ cup undiluted evaporated milk; ¼ cup dry milk; 1¼ cups cottage cheese; 1½ cups cheddar or Swiss cheese; or 1½ cups ice cream.

2. **Meat group**—important for protein, iron, and many B vitamins.
   Pregnancy—three to four servings.
   Lactation—three servings.
   Count as one serving (12–14 g protein)—2 oz lean meat, fish, or poultry; 2 eggs; 2 frankfurters; 4 tbsp peanut butter; or 1 cup cooked dry beans, dry peas, or lentils.

3. **Vegetable and fruit group**—vitamins and minerals (especially A and C) and roughage.
   Pregnancy—four to five servings.
   Lactation—five servings.
   Count as one serving—½ medium grapefruit; 1 medium apple, banana, or orange; ¾ cup fruit juice.
   Good sources (vitamin C)—citruses, cantaloupe, mango, papaya, strawberries, broccoli, and green and red chili peppers.
   Fair sources (vitamin C)—tomatoes, honeydew melon, asparagus tips, raw cabbage, collards, kale, mustard greens, potatoes (white and sweet), spinach, and turnip greens.
   Good sources (vitamin A)—dark green or deep yellow vegetables and a few fruits (apricots, broccoli, pumpkin, sweet potato, spinach, cantaloupe, carrots, and winter squash).
   Good sources of folic acid—dark green foliage-type vegetables.

4. **Bread and cereal group**—good for thiamine, iron, niacin, and other vitamins and minerals.
   Pregnancy—four to five servings.
   Lactation—four to five servings.
   Count as one serving—1 slice bread, 1 oz ready-to-eat cereal, ½ to ¾ cup cooked cereal, cornmeal, grits, macaroni, noodles, rice, or spaghetti.

SPECIAL PEDIATRIC DIETS

1. **Low-carbohydrate diet**—avoid cream sauces and soups.
   A. For obesity; reducing.
   B. For diabetics—controlled amounts of carbohydrates, fats, and proteins.
   C. For epilepsy—ketogenic: low-carbohydrate, high-fat.

2. **Gluten-free diet**—elimination of all foods made from wheat and rye, used for celiac disease.

3. **High-protein diet**—lean meat, cheese, and green vegetables.
   A. Infectious hepatitis.
   B. Malabsorption (for example, ulcerative colitis).
   C. Malnutrition.

D. Patients with extensive burns.

E. Nephrotic syndrome (may also be on low-sodium diet).

F. Acute leukemia (combined with high-calorie and soft-food diets).

G. Neoplastic disease.

4. *Low-protein diet*—eggs, fruit (apples, applesauce), and vegetables (carrots, potatoes).

A. Usually accompanied by high-carbohydrate diet and normal fats and calories.

B. Acute nephritis.

C. Uremia.

D. Anuria.

E. Renal failure.

5. *Low-sodium diet*—avoid canned vegetables and fruits.

A. Acute nephritis.

B. Nephrotic syndrome.

C. Congestive heart failure.

6. *High-roughage, high-residue diet*—raw vegetables and fruit.

A. Constipation.

B. Long-term immobilization.

7. *Inborn-errors-of-metabolism diets*—based on specific disease or condition, as ordered.

COMMON THERAPEUTIC DIETS *

1. Clear-liquid diet

Purpose: Relieve thirst and help maintain fluid balance.

Use: Postsurgically and following acute vomiting or diarrhea.

Food allowed: Carbonated beverages, coffee (caffeinated and decaffeinated), tea, fruit-flavored drinks, fruit juices, clear flavored gelatins, broth, consommé, sugar, and hard candy.

Foods avoided: Milk and milk products, fruit juices with pulp, and fruit.

Sample menu

Breakfast	Lunch	Dinner
¾ c cranberry juice	1 c apple juice	1 c orange drink
½ c broth	¾ c bouillon	¾ c consommé
½ c lime Jello	½ c cherry Jello	½ c lemon Jello
2 tsp sugar	1 tsp sugar	2 sticks hard candy
Coffee or tea	Coffee or tea	Coffee or tea

Between-meal nourishment: ¾ c gingerale or Seven-Up.

2. Full-liquid diet

Purpose: Provide an adequately nutritious diet for patients who cannot chew or who are too ill to do so.

Use: Acute infection with fever, gastrointestinal upsets, after surgery as a progression from *clear liquids.*

Foods allowed: Clear liquids, milk drinks, cooked cereals, custards, ice cream, sherbets, eggnog, all fruit juices, vegetable juices, creamed vegetable soups, mashed potatoes, mild cheese sauce or puréed meat, and seasonings.

Foods avoided: Nuts, seeds, coconut, fruit, jam, and marmalade.

---

*Clear-liquid, full-liquid, soft, sodium-restricted, renal, high-protein, high-carbohydrate, purine-restricted, bland, and low-fat, cholesterol-restricted diets were reprinted by permission from *Recent Advances in Therapeutic Diets,* Second Edition, by Staff of the Department of Nutrition, The University of Iowa © 1973 by the Iowa State University Press, Ames, Iowa.

Sample menu: Diet offered in six feedings or more.

Breakfast	Lunch	Dinner
½ c strained orange juice	¾ c cream of tomato soup	¾ c broth
½ c strained oatmeal with butter, hot milk, sugar	½ c apricot nectar	¾ c eggnog
	1 scoop vanilla ice cream	½ c strawberry Jello with whipped cream
1 c milk	1 c milk	
Coffee or tea with cream and sugar	Coffee or tea with cream and sugar	1 c milk
		Coffee or tea with sugar

Midmorning snack	Midafternoon snack	Evening snack
½ c egg custard	Vanilla milkshake	1 c hot chocolate

3. Soft diet

Purpose: Provide adequate nutrition for those who have trouble chewing.

Use: Patients with no teeth or ill-fitting dentures; transition from full-liquid to general diet; and for those who cannot tolerate highly seasoned, fried, or raw foods following acute infections or gastrointestinal disturbances, such as gastric ulcer or cholelithiasis.

Foods allowed: Very tender minced, ground, baked, broiled, roasted, stewed, or creamed beef, lamb, veal, liver, poultry, or fish; crisp bacon or sweetbreads; cooked vegetables; pasta; all fruit juices; soft raw fruits; soft breads and cereals; all desserts that are soft; and cheeses.

Foods avoided: Coarse whole-grain cereals and breads; nuts; raisins; coconut; fruits with small seeds; fried foods; high-fat gravies or sauces; spicy salad dressings; pickled meat, fish, or poultry; strong cheeses; brown or wild rice; raw vegetables as well as lima beans and corn; spices such as horseradish, mustard, and catsup; and popcorn.

Sample menu

Breakfast	Lunch	Dinner
Orange sections	1 c tomato bouillon	Grapefruit sections
1 egg, soft-boiled	1 biscuit	3 oz beef patty
½ c oatmeal	3 oz roast chicken	¼ c beef broth gravy
1 slice toast	½ c green beans	¼ c cooked carrots
1 tsp butter	½ c buttered rice	Baked potato, without skin, buttered
1 c milk	1 slice angel-food cake	1 dinner roll
2 tsp sugar	1 c milk	1 tsp butter
Coffee or tea	Coffee or tea with sugar	1 slice custard pie
		Coffee or tea

4. Sodium-restricted diet

Purpose: Reduce sodium content in the tissues and promote excretion of water.

Use: Congestive heart failure, hypertension, renal disease, cirrhosis, toxemia of pregnancy, and cortisone therapy.

Modifications: Mildly restrictive 2-g sodium diet to extremely restricted 200-mg sodium diet.

Foods avoided: Table salt; all commercial soups including bouillon; gravy, catsup, mustard, meat sauces, soy sauce, buttermilk, ice cream, sherbet, sodas, beet greens, carrots, celery, chard, sauerkraut, spinach, all canned vegetables, frozen peas, all baked products containing salt, baking powder or baking soda, potato chips, popcorn, fresh or canned shell fish, all cheeses, smoked or commercially prepared meats, salted butter or margarine, bacon, olives, and commercially prepared salad dressings.

Sample menu: 500 mg strict salt-restricted diet—milk or milk drinks limited to two cups per day.

Breakfast
½ c frozen orange juice
½ c farina
1 egg, soft-boiled
1 slice toast, enriched unsalted
  bread
1 tsp unsalted butter
1 tbsp peach jelly
1 c milk
Coffee or tea with sugar

Lunch
Saladbowl: lettuce, endive, raw
  cauliflower, green pepper,
  tomato wedges, sliced chicken
  strips
1 tbsp 1000 Island dressing,
  unsalted
1 roll, unsalted
1 tsp butter, unsalted
1 peach, fresh and sliced

Dinner
Roast beef, 4 oz
1 baked potato
2 tsp chive butter
½ c fresh peas and mushrooms
1 roll and butter, unsalted
½ banana, sliced
1 c milk
Coffee or tea with sugar

5. Renal diet

Purpose: Control protein, potassium, sodium, and fluid levels in body.

Use: Acute and chronic renal failure, hemodialysis.

Food allowed: High-biologic proteins such as meat, fowl, fish, cheese, and dairy products—range between 20 and 60 mg per day. Potassium is usually limited to 40 mEq per day. Vegetables such as cabbage, cucumber, and peas are lowest in potassium. Sodium is restricted to 500 mg per day. See sodium-restricted diet. Fluid intake is restricted to the daily urine volume plus 500 ml, which represents insensible water loss. Fluid intake measures water in fruit, vegetables, milk, and meat.

Food avoided: Cereals, bread, macaroni, noodles, spaghetti, avocados, kidney beans, potato chips, raw fruit, yams, soybeans, nuts, gingerbread, apricots, bananas, figs, grapefruit, oranges, percolated coffee, Coca-Cola, Orange Crush, Gatorade, and breakfast drinks such as Tang or Awake.

Sample menu: Contains 60 g protein, 60 mEq potassium, 35 mEq sodium, and 1000 ml fluid.

Breakfast
½ c peach nectar
1 egg, soft-cooked
1 slice toast, white, enriched,
  unsalted
2 tsp butter, unsalted
1 tbsp grape jelly
2 tsp sugar
1 c Sanka

Lunch
1 oz chicken unsalted
½ c green beans, unsalted,
  drained
1 slice bread, unsalted, white,
  enriched
3 tsp butter, unsalted
1 tbsp grape jelly
½ small banana
¾ c Kool-Aid

Dinner
2 oz roast beef, sirloin
½ c cubed white potato,
  drained, unsalted
2 halves canned pears, drained
¾ c tossed lettuce salad
2 tbsp oil & vinegar dressing
2 tsp butter, unsalted
1 tsp sugar
1 c tea

Midmorning snack
1 c puffed wheat
½ c milk
1 tsp sugar
1 small apple

Midafternoon snack
½ c unsalted gelatin
10 vanilla wafers

Evening snack
1 slice bread, enriched,
  unsalted, white
1 oz turkey, unsalted
2 tsp butter, unsalted
½ c gingerale
2 tsp sugar

6. High-protein, high-carbohydrate diet

Purpose: Corrects large protein losses and raises the level of blood albumin. May be modified to include low-fat, low-sodium, and low-cholesterol diets.

Use: Burns, hepatitis, cirrhosis, pregnancy, hyperthyroidism, mononucleosis, protein deficiency due to poor eating habits, geriatric patients with poor food intake, nephritis, nephrosis, and liver and gallbladder disorders.

Foods allowed: General diet with added protein. In adults, high-protein diets usually contain 135 to 150 g protein.

Foods avoided: Restrictions are dependent on added modifications to the diet. These modifications are determined by the patient's condition.

Sample menu

Breakfast
½ c apple juice
¾ c Cream of Wheat
2 eggs, scrambled
1 slice whole-wheat toast
2 tsp butter
1 tbsp grape jelly
1 c milk
2 tsp sugar
Coffee or tea

Midmorning snack
1 c milk

Lunch
3 oz grilled hamburger on bun
½ sliced tomato on lettuce
¼ c cottage cheese
2 tsp butter
1 slice angel-food cake
1 scoop strawberry ice cream
Coffee, tea, or milk

Midafternoon snack
½ c egg custard

Dinner
6 oz club steak
½ c mashed potatoes
½ c buttered carrots
½ c coleslaw
1 dinner roll
2 tsp butter
½ c sherbet
4 vanilla wafers
1 c milk
Coffee or tea

Evening snack
Vanilla milkshake

7. Purine-restricted diet
Purpose: Designed to reduce the amount of consumed uric acid–producing foods.
Use: High–uric acid retention, uric acid renal stones, and gout.
Foods allowed: General diet plus two to three quarts of liquid daily.
Foods avoided: Cheese containing spices or nuts, fried eggs, meat, liver, seafood, lentils, dried peas and beans, broth, bouillon, gravies, oatmeal and whole wheats, pasta, noodles, and alcoholic beverages. Limited quantities meat, fish, and seafood allowed.

Sample menu

Breakfast
½ c orange juice
½ c corn flakes
2 eggs, soft-boiled
2 slices toast, white
2 tbsp butter
2 tbsp apple butter
1 c milk, nonfat
Coffee or tea

Midmorning snack
1 c milk, nonfat

Lunch
1 c tomato soup
Sandwich:
  2 oz chicken
  2 slices white bread
  1 tbsp mayonnaise
½ c lime Jello
Coffee or tea

Midafternoon snack
1 c milk, nonfat
2 brownies without nuts

Dinner
3 oz Swiss steak
1 baked potato
½ c string beans
2 rolls
2 tbsp butter
½ c strawberry parfait
Coffee or tea

Evening snack
1 c hot chocolate, made with
  nonfat milk

8. Bland diet
Purpose: Provision of a diet low in fiber, roughage, mechanical irritants, and chemical stimulants.
Use: Ulcers (gastric and duodenal), gastritis, hyperchlorhydria, functional GI disorders, gastric atony, diarrhea, spastic constipation, biliary indigestion, and hiatus hernia.
Foods allowed: Varied to meet individual needs and food tolerances.
Foods avoided: Fried foods including eggs, meat, fish, and seafood; cheese with added nuts or spices; commercially prepared luncheon meats; cured meats such as ham; gravies and sauces; raw vegetables; potato skins; fruit juices with pulp; figs; raisins; fresh fruits; whole wheats; rye bread; bran cereals; rich pastries; pies; chocolate; jams with seeds; nuts; seasoned dressings; regular coffee; strong tea; cocoa; alcoholic and carbonated beverages; and pepper.

Sample menu

Breakfast	*Lunch*	*Dinner*
½ c applesauce	1 c creamed tomato soup	6 oz white fish, broiled
1 egg, poached	Sandwich:	½ c mashed potatoes
1 slice white toast	3 oz cheese	½ c green peas
1 tsp butter	2 slices white bread	1 dinner roll
1 tsp grape jelly	1 tbsp mayonnaise	1 tsp butter
1 c whole milk	½ c sherbet	½ c vanilla ice cream
Coffee, decaffeinated	Coffee, decaffeinated	Weak tea or decaffeinated coffee
1 tsp sugar		1 tsp sugar

Midmorning snack	*Midafternoon snack*	*Evening snack*
1 c buttermilk	1 vanilla milkshake	1 egg custard

9. Low-fat, cholesterol-restricted diet

Purpose: Reduce hyperlipemia, provide dietary treatment for malabsorption syndromes, and patients having acute intolerance for fats.

Use: Hyperlipidemia, atherosclerosis, pancreatitis, cystic fibrosis, sprue, gastrectomy, and massive resection of the small intestine.

Foods allowed: Nonfat milk; low-carbohydrate, low-fat vegetables; most fruits; breads; pastas; cornmeal; lean meats; unsaturated fats such as corn oil; desserts made without whole milk; and unsweetened carbonated beverages.

Foods avoided: Whole milk and whole-milk or cream products, avocados, olives, commercially prepared baked goods as donuts and muffins, poultry skin, highly marbled meats, shellfish, fish canned in oil, nuts, coconut, commercially prepared meats, butter, ordinary margarines, olive oil, lard, pudding made with whole milk, ice cream, candies with chocolate, cream, sauces, gravies, and commercially fried foods.

Sample menu

Breakfast	*Lunch*	*Dinner*
½ grapefruit	Sandwich:	4 oz lamb chops (2)
¾ c puffed wheat	2 slices whole wheat bread	1 baked potato
1 tsp sugar	2 oz sliced chicken	1 tsp safflower margarine
1 slice white toast	2 tsp mayonnaise	½ c cooked carrots
2 tsp safflower margarine	½ c coleslaw	¾ c tossed lettuce salad
2 tsp jelly	1 small banana	Lemon wedge
1 c skimmed milk	Coffee or tea	½ c fruit sherbet
Coffee or tea		Coffee or tea

10. Diabetic diet

Purpose: Control the progression of diabetes mellitus.

Use: Diabetes mellitus.

Foods allowed: Foods are divided into groups from which exchanges can be made. Coffee, tea, broth, bouillon, spices, and flavorings can be used as desired. Vegetable A exchanges, one cup, contain mostly green vegetables, while vegetable B exchanges, one-half cup, contain the remaining vegetables. The amounts of the remaining exchanges depend on the food selected. Fruit exchanges are fruits without sugar or syrup. Meat, fat, and milk exchanges. The number of exchanges allowed from each group is dependent on the total number of calories allowed.

Foods avoided: Concentrated sweets or regular soft drinks.

Sample menu

Breakfast	*Lunch*	*Dinner*
½ c orange juice	1 hamburger with bun	1 c tossed green salad
1 poached egg	2 oz broiled meat	4 oz roast lamb
1 slice toast	1 sliced tomato	½ c rice
⅔ c corn flakes	2 tsp mayonnaise	½ c cabbage
1 tsp margarine	1 tsp mustard	2 tbsp French dressing
1 slice crisp bacon	2 small carrots	1 tsp margarine
1 c milk, nonfat	1 medium apple	Diet gelatin with ½ c
Black coffee or tea	Tab	fruit cocktail
		Black coffee or tea

Bedtime: 1 c nonfat milk
2 graham crackers

Sample food exchange lists for diabetic diet*

Daily menu guide—1500 calories

	Breakfast	*Lunch*	*Dinner*
Carbohydrate 150 g	1 fruit exchange (List 3)	2 meat exchanges (List 5)	2 meat exchanges (List 5)
	2 bread exchanges (List 4)	2 bread exchanges (List 4)	1½ bread exchanges (List 4)
Protein 70 g	1 meat exchange (List 5)	Vegetable(s) as desired (List 1)	Vegetable(s) as desired (List 1)
Fat 70 g	1 milk exchange (List 7)	1 fruit exchange (List 3)	1 vegetable exchange (List 2)
	2 fat exchanges (List 6)	1 milk exchange (List 7)	1 fruit exchange (List 3)
	Coffee or tea (any amount)	1 fat exchange (List 6)	½ milk exchange (List 7)
		Coffee or tea (any amount)	1 fat exchange (List 6)
			Coffee or tea (any amount)

List 1 allowed as desired**

Seasonings: Cinnamon, celery salt, garlic, garlic salt, lemon, mustard, mint, nutmeg, parsley, pepper, saccharin and other sugarless sweeteners, spices, vanilla, and vinegar.

Other foods: Coffee or tea (without sugar or cream), fat-free broth, bouillon, unflavored gelatin, rennet tablets, sour or dill pickles, cranberries (without sugar), rhubarb (without sugar).

Vegetables: Group A—insignificant carbohydrate or calories. You may eat as much as desired of raw vegetables. If cooked vegetable is eaten, limit amount to 1 cup.

Asparagus	Cabbage
Broccoli	Cauliflower
Brussels sprouts	Celery

Chicory	Okra
Cucumbers	Peppers, green or red
Eggplant	
Escarole	Radishes
Greens: beet, chard, collard, dandelion, kale, mustard, spinach, turnip	Sauerkraut
	String beans
	Summer squash
Lettuce	Tomatoes
Mushrooms	Watercress

List 2 vegetable exchanges

Each portion supplies approximately 7 g of carbohydrate and 2 g of protein, or 36 calories.

Vegetables: Group B—One serving equals ½ cup, or 100 g.

Beets	Pumpkin
Carrots	Rutabagas
Onions	Squash, winter
Peas, green	Turnips

*Courtesy of Eli Lilly Company.
**Need not be measured.

List 3 fruit exchanges*

Each portion supplies approximately 10 g of carbohydrate, or 40 calories.

	Household Measurement	Weight of Portion
Apple	1 small (2-inch diam)	80 g
Applesauce	½ c	100 g
Apricots, fresh	2 med	100 g
Apricots, dried	4 halves	20 g
Banana	½ small	50 g
Berries	1 c	150 g
Blueberries	⅔ c	100 g
Cantaloupe	¼ (6-inch diam)	200 g
Cherries	10 large	75 g
Dates	2	15 g
Figs, fresh	2 large	50 g
Figs, dried	1 small	15 g
Grapefruit	½ small	125 g
Grapefruit juice	½ c	100 g
Grapes	12	75 g
Grape juice	¼ c	60 g
Honeydew melon	⅛ (7-inch)	150 g
Mango	½ small	70 g
Orange	1 small	100 g
Orange juice	½ c	100 g
Papaya	⅓ med	100 g
Peach	1 med	100 g
Pear	1 small	100 g
Pineapple	½ c	80 g
Pineapple juice	⅓ c	80 g
Plums	2 med	100 g
Prunes, dried	2	25 g
Raisins	2 tbsp	15 g
Tangerine	1 large	100 g
Watermelon	1 c	175 g

List 4 bread exchanges

Each portion supplies approximately 15 g of carbohydrate and 2 g of protein, or 68 calories.

	Household Measurement	Weight of Portion
Bread	1 slice	25 g
Biscuit, roll	1 (2-inch diam)	35 g
Muffin	1 (2-inch diam)	35 g
Cornbread	1½-inch cube	35 g
Flour	2½ tbsp	20 g
Cereal, cooked	½ c	100 g
Cereal, dry (flakes or puffed)	¾ c	20 g
Rice or grits, cooked	½ c	100 g
Spaghetti, noodles, etc.	½ c	100 g
Crackers, graham	2	20 g
Crackers, oyster	20 (½ c)	20 g
Crackers, saltine	5	20 g
Crackers, soda	3	20 g
Crackers, round	6–8	20 g
Vegetables		
Beans (lima, navy, etc.), dry, cooked	½ c	90 g
Peas (split peas, etc.), dry, cooked	½ c	90 g
Baked beans, no pork	¼ c	50 g
Corn	⅓ c	80 g
Parsnips	⅔ c	125 g
Potato, white, baked or boiled	1 (2-inch diam)	100 g
Potatoes, white, mashed	½ c	100 g
Potatoes, sweet, or yams	¼ c	50 g
Sponge cake, plain	1½-inch cube	25 g
Ice cream (omit 2 fat exchanges)	½ c	70 g

List 5 meat exchanges

Each portion supplies approximately 7 g of protein and 5 g of fat, or 73 calories (30 g equal 1 oz).

	Household Measurement	Weight of Portion
Meat and poultry (beef, lamb, pork, liver, chicken, etc.) (med. fat)	1 slice (3 × 2 × ⅛ inch)	30 g
Cold cuts	1 slice (4½-inch sq. ⅛-inch thick)	45 g
Frankfurter	1 (8–9 per lb.)	50 g
Codfish, mackerel, etc.	1 slice (2 × 2 × 1-inch)	30 g
Salmon, tuna, crab	¼ c	30 g
Oysters, shrimp, clams	5 small	45 g
Sardines	3 med	30 g
Cheese, cheddar, American	1 slice (3½ × 1½ × ¼-inch)	30 g
Cheese, cottage	¼ c	45 g
Egg	1	50 g
Peanut butter	2 tbsp	30 g

Limit peanut butter to one exchange per day unless allowance is made for carbohydrate in the diet plan.

---

*Fresh, dried, or canned without sugar.

List 6 fat exchanges

Each portion supplies approximately 5 g of fat, or 45 calories.

	Household Measurement	Weight of Portion
Butter or margarine	1 tsp	5 g
Bacon, crisp	1 slice	10 g
Cream, light	2 tbsp	30 g
Cream, heavy	1 tbsp	15 g
Cream cheese	1 tbsp	15 g
French dressing	1 tbsp	15 g
Mayonnaise	1 tsp	5 g
Oil or cooking fat	1 tsp	5 g
Nuts	6 small	10 g
Olives	5 small	50 g
Avocado	1/8 (4-inch diam)	25 g

List 7 milk exchanges

Each portion supplies approximately 12 g of carbohydrate, 8 g of protein, and 10 g of fat, or 170 calories.

	Household Measurement	Weight of Portion
Milk, whole	1 c	240 g
Milk, evaporated	1/2 c	120 g
Milk, powdered*	1/4 c	35 g
Buttermilk*	1 c	240 g

*Add two fat exchanges if milk is fat-free.

11. Acid and alkaline ash diet

Purpose: To furnish a well-balanced diet in which the total acid ash is greater than the total alkaline ash each day.
Use: Retard the formation of renal calculi. The type of diet chosen is dependent on laboratory analysis of the stones.

Acid and alkaline ash food groups

Acid ash
Meat
Whole grains
Eggs
Cheese
Cranberries
Prunes
Plums

Alkaline ash
Milk
Vegetables
Fruit (except cranberries, prunes, and plums)

Neutral
Sugars
Fats
Beverages (coffee and tea)

Foods allowed: You may eat all you want of the following foods:

1. Breads: any, preferably whole grain; crackers, rolls.
2. Cereals: any, preferably whole grain.
3. Desserts: angel food or sunshine cake; cookies made without baking powder or soda; cornstarch pudding, cranberry desserts, custards, gelatin desserts, ice cream, sherbet, plum or prune desserts; rice or tapioca pudding.
4. Fats: any, as butter, margarine, salad dressings, Crisco; Spry, lard, salad oils, olive oil, etc.
5. Fruits: cranberries, plums, prunes.
6. Meat, egg, cheese: any meat, fish or fowl, two servings daily; at least one egg daily.
7. Potato substitutes: corn, hominy, lentils, macaroni, noodles, rice, spaghetti, vermicelli.
8. Soup: broth as desired; other soups from foods allowed.
9. Sweets: cranberry or plum jelly; sugar, plain sugar candy.
10. Miscellaneous: cream sauce, gravy, peanut butter, peanuts, popcorn, salt, spices, vinegar, walnuts.

Restricted foods: Do not eat any more than the amount allowed each day.

1. Milk: 1 pint daily (may be used in other ways than as beverage).
2. Cream: 1/3 cup or less daily.
3. Fruits: one serving of fruit daily (in addition to the prunes, plums, and cranberries); certain fruits listed below are not allowed at any time.
4. Vegetables including potato: two servings daily; certain vegetables listed below are not allowed at any time.

Foods avoided:

1. Carbonated beverages, as ginger ale, Coca-Cola, root beer.
2. Cakes or cookies made with baking powder or soda.
3. Fruits: dried apricots, bananas, dates, figs, raisins, rhubarb.
4. Vegetables: dried beans, beet greens, dandelion greens, carrots, chard, lima beans.
5. Sweets; chocolate or other candies than those listed above; syrups.
6. Miscellaneous: other nuts, olives, pickles.

Sample menu

Breakfast	*Lunch*	*Dinner*
Grapefruit	Creamed chicken	Broth
Wheatena	Steamed rice	Roast beef, gravy
Scrambled eggs	Green beans	Buttered noodles
Toast, butter, plum jam	Stewed prunes	Sliced tomato
Coffee, cream, sugar	Bread, butter	Mayonnaise
	Milk	Vanilla ice cream
		Bread, butter

FOOD LIST FOR READY REFERENCE IN MENU PLANNING

1. High-cholesterol foods—based on portions of 100 g.

Beef	70 mg
Butter	250 mg
Cheese	60–120 mg
Egg yolks	1500 mg
Fish	70 mg
Ice cream	45 mg
Kidney	375 mg
Liver	300 mg
Margarines, vegetable	0 mg
Milk, whole	11 mg
Milk, skim	3 mg
Pork	70 mg
Veal	90 mg

2. High-sodium foods—over 500 mg/100 g portion.

Bacon, cured	1021 mg
Bacon, Canadian	2555 mg
Baking powder	8220 mg
Beef, corned, cooked	1740 mg
Beef, corned, canned	540 mg
Beef, dried, cooked, creamed	716 mg
Biscuits, baking powder	626 mg
Bouillon cubes	24,000 mg
Bran, added sugar and malt	1060 mg
Bran flake with thiamine	925 mg
Bran flakes with raisins	800 mg
Breads	
Wheat	529 mg
French	580 mg
Rye	557 mg
White	507 mg
Whole wheat	527 mg
Butter	987 mg
Cheese	
Cheddar	700 mg
Parmesan	734 mg
Swiss	710 mg
Pasteurized American	1136 mg
Pasteurized American spread	1625 mg
Cocoa	525 mg
Cookies, gingersnaps	571 mg
Corn flakes	1005 mg
Cornbread	950 mg
Crackers	
Graham	670 mg
Saltines	1100 mg
Margarine	987 mg
Milk, dry, skim	532 mg
Mustard	
Brown	1307 mg
Yellow	1252 mg
Oat products	1267 mg
Olives	
Green	2400 mg
Ripe	803 mg
Peanut butter	607 mg
Pickles, dill	1428 mg
Popcorn with oil and salt	1940 mg
Salad dressing	
Blue and Roquefort	1094 mg
French	1370 mg
Thousand Island	700 mg

RECOMMENDED DAILY DIETARY ALLOWANCES[a]

	Age (years)	Weight (kg)	Weight (lbs)	Height (cm)	Height (in)	Energy (kcal)[b]	Protein (g)	Fat-soluble vitamins Vitamin A activity (RE)[c]	(IU)	Vitamin D (IU)	Vitamin E activity[e] (IU)
Infants	0.0–0.5	6	14	60	24	kg × 117	kg × 2.2	420[d]	1,400	400	4
	0.5–1.0	9	20	71	28	kg × 108	kg × 2.0	400	2,000	400	5
Children	1–3	13	28	86	34	1,300	23	400	2,000	400	7
	4–6	20	44	110	44	1,800	30	500	2,500	400	9
	7–10	30	66	135	54	2,400	36	700	3,300	400	10
Men	11–14	44	97	158	63	2,800	44	1,000	5,000	400	12
	15–18	61	134	172	69	3,000	54	1,000	5,000	400	15
	19–22	67	147	172	69	3,000	54	1,000	5,000	400	15
	23–50	70	154	172	69	2,700	56	1,000	5,000		15
	51 +	70	154	172	69	2,400	56	1,000	5,000		15
Women	11–14	44	97	155	62	2,400	44	800	4,000	400	12
	15–18	54	119	162	65	2,100	48	800	4,000	400	12
	19–22	58	128	162	65	2,100	46	800	4,000	400	12
	23–50	58	128	162	65	2,000	46	800	4,000		12
	51 +	58	128	162	65	1,800	46	800	4,000		12
Pregnant						+300	+30	1,000	5,000	400	15
Lactating						+500	+20	1,200	6,000	400	15

[a]Reproduced with permission of the Food and Nutrition Board, National Academy of Sciences—National Research Council Recommended Daily Dietary Allowances, Revised 1974. The allowances are intended to provide for individual variations among most normal persons as they live in the United States under usual environmental stresses. Diets should be based on a variety of common foods in order to provide other nutrients for which human requirements have been less well defined.

[b]Kilojoules (kJ) = 4.2 × kcal.

[c]Retinol equivalents.

[d]Assumed to be all as retinol in milk during the first six months of life. All subsequent intakes are assumed to be half as retinol and half as β-carotene when calculated from international units. As retinol equivalents, three fourths are as retinol and one fourth as β-carotene.

Sausages
Bologna .... 1300 mg
Frankfurters .... 1100 mg
Soy sauce .... 7325 mg
Tomato catsup .... 1042 mg
Tuna, in oil .... 800 mg

3. High-potassium foods—more than 400 mg/100 g.
Almonds .... 773 mg
Bacon, Canadian .... 432 mg
Baking powder, low-sodium .... 10,948 mg
Beans, white .... 416 mg
Beans, lima .... 422 mg
Beef, hamburger .... 450 mg

Bran with sugar and malt .... 1070 mg
Cake
Fruitcake .... 496 mg
Gingerbread .... 454 mg
Cashew nuts .... 464 mg
Chicken, light meat .... 411 mg
Cocoa .... 800 mg
Coffee, instant .... 3256 mg
Cookies, gingersnaps .... 462 mg
Dates .... 648 mg
Garlic loaves .... 529 mg
Milk
Dry, skim .... 1745 mg
Powdered .... 720 mg

Water-soluble vitamins							Minerals					
Ascorbic acid (mg)	Folacin[f] (µg)	Niacin[g] (mg)	Ribo-flavin (mg)	Thiamin (mg)	Vitamin B_6 (mg)	Vitamin B_{12} (µg)	Calcium (mg)	Phos-phorus (mg)	Iodine (µg)	Iron (mg)	Magne-sium (mg)	Zinc (mg)
35	50	5	0.4	0.3	0.3	0.3	360	240	35	10	60	3
35	50	8	0.6	0.5	0.4	0.3	540	400	45	15	70	5
40	100	9	0.8	0.7	0.6	1.0	800	800	60	15	150	10
40	200	12	1.1	0.9	0.9	1.5	800	800	80	10	200	10
40	300	16	1.2	1.2	1.2	2.0	800	800	110	10	250	10
45	400	18	1.5	1.4	1.6	3.0	1,200	1,200	130	18	350	15
45	400	20	1.8	1.5	2.0	3.0	1,200	1,200	150	18	400	15
45	400	20	1.8	1.5	2.0	3.0	800	800	140	10	350	15
45	400	18	1.6	1.4	2.0	3.0	800	800	130	10	350	15
45	400	16	1.5	1.2	2.0	3.0	800	800	110	10	350	15
45	400	16	1.3	1.2	1.6	3.0	1,200	1,200	115	18	300	15
45	400	14	1.4	1.1	2.0	3.0	1,200	1,200	115	18	300	15
45	400	14	1.4	1.1	2.0	3.0	800	800	100	18	300	15
45	400	13	1.2	1.0	2.0	3.0	800	800	100	18	300	15
45	400	12	1.1	1.0	2.0	3.0	800	800	80	10	300	15
60	800	+2	+0.3	+0.3	2.5	4.0	1,200	1,200	125	18+[b]	450	20
80	600	+4	+0.5	+0.3	2.5	4.0	1,200	1,200	150	18	450	25

[e]Total vitamin E activity, estimated to be 80% as α-tocopherol and 20% other tocopherols.

[f]The folacin allowances refer to dietary sources as determined by *Lactobacillus casei* assay. Pure forms of folacin may be effective in doses less than one fourth of the recommended dietary allowance.

[g]Although allowances are expressed as niacin, it is recognized that on the average 1 mg of niacin is derived from each 60 mg of dietary tryptophan.

[b]This increased requirement cannot be met by ordinary diets; therefore, the use of supplemental iron is recommended.

Peanuts, roasted .... 701 mg
Peanut butter .... 670 mg
Peas .... 1005 mg
Pecans .... 603 mg
Potatoes, boiled in skin .... 407 mg
Scallops .... 476 mg
Tea, instant .... 4530 mg
Tomato puree .... 426 mg
Turkey, light meat .... 411 mg
Veal .... 500 mg
Walnuts, black .... 460 mg
Yeast, brewers .... 1894 mg

4. Foods high in B vitamins

Thiamine	Riboflavin	Niacin
Pork	Liver	Liver
Dried beans	Poultry	Fish
Dried peas	Beef	Poultry

Liver	Oysters	Peanut butter
Lamb	Tongue	Lamb
Veal	Fish	Veal
Nuts	Cottage cheese	Beef
Peas	Veal	Pork

5. Foods high in vitamin C

Oranges	Grapefruit	Broccoli
Strawberries	Tomato	Melon
Dark-green, leafy vegetables	Cabbage	Liver
Potato		

6. Foods high in iron, calcium, and residue

Iron	Calcium	Residue
Breads	Milk	Whole-grain
Brown	Dry	cereals

NUTRIENTS FOR HEALTH

Nutrients are chemical substances obtained from foods during digestion. They are needed to build and maintain body cells, regulate body processes, and supply energy.

About 50 nutrients, including water, are needed daily for optimum health. If one obtains the proper amount of the 10 "leader" nutrients in the daily diet, the other 40 or so nutrients will likely be consumed in amounts sufficient to meet body needs.

Nutrient	Important sources of nutrient	Provide energy
Protein	Meat, Poultry, Fish Dried Beans and Peas Egg Cheese Milk	Supplies 4 Calories per gram.
Carbohydrate	Cereal Potatoes Dried Beans Corn Bread Sugar	Supplies 4 Calories per gram. Major source of energy for central nervous system.
Fat	Shortening, Oil Butter, Margarine Salad Dressing Sausages	Supplies 9 Calories per gram.
Vitamin A (Retinol)	Liver Carrots Sweet Potatoes Greens Butter, Margarine	
Vitamin C (Ascorbic Acid)	Broccoli Orange Grapefruit Papaya Mango Strawberries	
Thiamin (B_1)	Lean Pork Nuts Fortified Cereal Products	Aids in utilization of energy.
Riboflavin (B_2)	Liver Milk Yogurt Cottage Cheese	Aids in utilization of energy.
Niacin	Liver Meat, Poultry, Fish Peanuts Fortified Cereal Products	Aids in utilization of energy.

One's diet should include a variety of foods because no *single* food supplies all the 50 nutrients, and because many nutrients work together.

When a nutrient is added or a nutritional claim is made, nutrition labeling regulations require listing the 10 leader nutrients on food packages. These nutrients appear in the chart below with food sources and some major physiological functions.

Some major physiologic functions	
Build and maintain body cells	*Regulate body processes*
Constitutes part of the structure of every cell, such as muscle, blood, and bone; supports growth and maintains healthy body cells.	Constitutes part of enzymes, some hormones and body fluids, and antibodies that increase resistance to infection.
Supplies energy so protein can be used for growth and maintenance of body cells.	Unrefined products supply fiber—complex carbohydrates in fruits, vegetables, and whole grains—for regular elimination. Assists in fat utilization.
Constitutes part of the structure of every cell. Supplies essential fatty acids.	Provides and carries fat-soluble vitamins (A, D, E, and K).
Assists formation and maintenance of skin and mucous membranes that line body cavities and tracts, such as nasal passages and intestinal tract, thus increasing resistance to infection.	Functions in visual processes and forms visual purple, thus promoting healthy eye tissues and eye adaptation in dim light.
Forms cementing substances, such as collagen, that hold body cells together, thus strengthening blood vessels, hastening healing of wounds and bones, and increasing resistance to infection.	Aids utilization of iron.
	Functions as part of a coenzyme to promote the utilization of carbohydrate. Promotes normal appetite. Contributes to normal functioning of nervous system.
	Functions as part of a coenzyme in the production of energy within body cells. Promotes healthy skin, eyes, and clear vision.
	Functions as part of a coenzyme in fat synthesis, tissue respiration, and utilization of carbohydrate. Promotes healthy skin, nerves, and digestive tract. Aids digestion and fosters normal appetite.

(Continued)

NUTRIENTS FOR HEALTH   (Continued)

Nutrient	Important sources of nutrient	Provide energy
Calcium	Milk, Yogurt Cheese Sardines and Salmon with Bones Collard, Kale, Mustard, and Turnip Greens	
Iron	Enriched Farina Prune Juice Liver Dried Beans and Peas Red Meat	Aids in utilization of energy.

Source: National Dairy Council, Guide to good eating, 1977.

Foods high in iron, calcium, and residue, cont.

Corn
Ginger
Fish
  Tuna
Poultry
Organ meats
Whole-grain
  cereals
Shellfish
Egg yolk
Fruits
  Apples
  Berries
Dried fruits
  Dates
  Prunes
  Apricots
  Peaches
  Raisins
Vegetables
  Dark-green,
    leafy
  Potatoes
  Tomatoes
  Rhubarb
  Squash
Molasses
Dried beans
  and peas
Peanut butter
Brown sugar
Noodles
Rice

Skim
Whole
Evaporated
Buttermilk
Cheese
  American
  Swiss
  Hard
  Kale
  Turnip greens
  Mustard greens
  Collards

Oatmeal
Bran
Shredded Wheat
Breads
  Whole wheat
  Cracked wheat
  Rye
  Bran muffins
Vegetables
  Lettuce
  Spinach
  Swiss chard
  Carrots, raw
  Celery, raw
  Corn
  Cauliflower
  Eggplant
  Sauerkraut
  Cabbage
Fruits
  Bananas
  Figs
  Apricots
  Oranges

7. Foods to be used in low-protein and low-carbohydrate diets

Protein*
Milk
  Buttermilk
  Evaporated,
    reconstituted
  Low-sodium
  Skim and dry
Meat
  Chicken
  Lamb
  Turkey
  Beef
  Veal
Fish
  Sole
  Flounder
  Haddock
  Perch
Cheese
  Cheddar
  American
  Swiss
  Cottage
Eggs
Fruits
  Apples
  Grapes

Carbohydrates
All meats
Cheese
  Hard
  Soft
  Cottage
Eggs
Shell fish
  Osyters
  Shrimp
Fats
  Bacon
  Butter
  French dressing
  Salad oil
  Mayonnaise
  Margarine
Vegetables
  Asparagus
  Green beans
  Beet greens
  Broccoli
  Brussels sprouts
  Cabbage
  Celery
  Cauliflower
  Cucumber

*These proteins are allowed in various amounts on controlled-protein diets for renal decompensation.

Some major physiologic functions	
Build and maintain body cells	*Regulate body processes*
Combines with other minerals within a protein framework to give structure and strength to bones and teeth.	Assists in blood clotting. Functions in normal muscle contraction and relaxation, and normal nerve transmission.
Combines with protein to form hemoglobin, the red substance in blood that carries oxygen to and carbon dioxide from the cells. Preventings nutritional anemia and its accompanying fatigue. Increases resistance to infection.	Functions as part of enzymes involved in tissue respiration.

*Protein**	*Carbohydrates*		*Protein**	*Carbohydrates*
Pears	Lettuce		Cereals	Strawberries
Pineapple	Green pepper		Cornflakes	Cantaloupe
Vegetables	Spinach		Puffed rice	Lemons
Cabbage	Squash		Puffed wheat	Rhubarb
Cucumber	Tomatoes		Farina	
Lettuce	Fruits		Rolled oats	
Tomato	Avocados			

Appendix B / INTRAVENOUS THERAPY

INTRAVENOUS THERAPY

1. Infusion systems

A. Plastic bag:
  1. Contains no vacuum—needs no air to replace fluid as it flows from container.
  2. Medication can be added with syringe and needle through a resealable latex port.
     a. During infusion, administration set should be completely clamped before medications are added.
     b. Prevents undiluted, and perhaps toxic, dose from entering administration set.

B. Closed system:
  1. Requires partial vacuum—however, only filtered air enters container.
  2. Medication may be added during infusion through air vent in administration set.
     a. Care must be utilized to maintain sterility during procedure.
     b. Medications also may be added through a solid rubber stopper prior to infusion.

C. Open system:
  1. Requires partial vacuum—air is not filtered.
  2. Medications are added into an outlet port before sterile latex disk is removed.
     a. Vacuum check—latex disk should be depressed; if not, sterility will be questionable.
     b. During infusion—medications added through designated area on rubber after infusion set is clamped.
     c. Agitate and mix thoroughly before beginning administration.

D. Administration sets:
  1. Standard—deliver 10 to 25 drops/ml.

2. Pediatric or mini-drop sets—deliver 50 to 60 drops/ml.
3. Controlled-volume sets—permit accurate infusion of measured volumes of fluids.
    a. Particularly valuable when piggybacked into primary infusion.
    b. Solutions containing drugs can then be administered intermittently.
4. Y-type administration sets—allow for simultaneous or alternate infusion of two fluids.
    a. May contain filter and pressure unit for blood transfusions.
    b. Air embolism significant hazard with this type of administration set.
5. Positive-pressure sets—designed for rapid infusion of replacement fluids.
    a. In emergency, built-in pressure chamber increases rate of blood administration.
    b. Pump chamber must be filled at all times to avoid air embolism.
    c. Application of positive pressure to infusion fluids is responsibility of physician.
6. Infusion pumps—utilized to deliver small volumes of fluid or doses of high-potency drugs.
    a. Used primarily in neonatal, pediatric, and adult intensive-care units.
    b. Have increased the safety of parenteral therapy and reduced nursing time.

2. Fluid administration

A. Factors influencing rate:
1. Patient's size.
2. Patient's physical condition.
3. Age of patient.
4. Type of fluid.
5. Patient's tolerance to fluid.

B. Flow rates for parenteral infusions can be computed using the following formula:

$$\frac{gtt/ml \text{ of given set}}{60 \text{ (minutes in hours)}} \times \text{total hourly volume}$$
$$= gtt/minute$$

If 1000 ml are to be infused in an eight-hour period and the administration set delivers 15 gtt/ml, the gtt/minute is 31.2 gtt/minute.

$$\frac{15}{60} \times 125 = \frac{1}{4} \times 125 = 31.2 \, gtt/minute$$

C. Generally the type of fluid administration set determines its rate of flow.

1. Fluid administration sets—approximately 15 gtt/minute.
2. Blood administration sets—approximately 10 gtt/minute.
3. Pediatric administration sets—approximately 60 gtt/minute.
4. Always check information on the administration set box to determine the number of gtt/ml before calculating; varies with manufacturer.

D. Factors influencing flow rates:
1. Gravity—a change in the height of the infusion bottle will increase or decrease the rate of flow; for example, raising the bottle higher will increase the rate of flow and vice versa.
2. Blood clot in needle—stopping the infusion for any reason or an increase in venous pressure may result in partial or total obstruction of needle by clot.
    a. Delay in changing infusion bottle.
    b. Blood pressure cuff on or restraints on or above infusion needle.
    c. Patient lying on arm in which infusion is being made.
3. Change in needle position—against or away from vein wall.
4. Venous spasm—due to cold blood or irritating solution.
5. Plugged vent—causes infusion to stop.

3. Complications of intravenous therapy

A. Local complications:
1. *Thrombophlebitis*—inflammation and thrombosis of vein.
    a. *Assessment*—pain, redness, swelling, and heat along the length of the vein.
    b. Contributing factors—
        (1) *Length* of infusion—infusions in place over 24–48 hours most frequent factor.
        (2) Infusion *fluid*—hypertonic glucose, drug additives, or solutions with pH significantly different from plasma.
        (3) Infusion *site*—venous injury can occur due to motion of needles.
        (4) *Technique*—maintenance of aseptic technique during venipuncture is essential.
    c. *Preventive nursing measures*—
        (1) Do not use veins in lower extremities.
        (2) If irritating solution is to be infused, use vein with ample blood volume.
        (3) Avoid infusion sites over joints.
        (4) Tape needles securely to avoid motion.

2. *Infiltration*—dislodgement of the needle with fluid flowing into surrounding tissue.
   a. Signs and symptoms—edema of infusion site.
   b. *Nursing measures*—
      (1) If edema is present, the presence of blood return in adapter with negative pressure (lowering of IV bottle below infusion site) does not mean infusion is still entering vein.
      (2) Confirm infiltration by applying a tourniquet proximal to infusion site, restricting venous flow; if infusion continues, extravasation is evident, and the needle should be removed immediately.

B. Systemic complications:
   1. *Infections*—occur when pathogens are introduced into the blood stream.
      a. *Assessment*—chills, fever, general malaise, headache, backache, nausea, and vomiting.
      b. *Immediate nursing measures*—
         (1) Terminate infusion.
         (2) Take vital signs.
         (3) Notify physician.
         (4) Send solution to lab for culture.
      c. *Preventive nursing measures*—
         (1) Utilize aseptic venipuncture technique.
         (2) Inspect fluids for cloudiness or extra matter.
         (3) Use open solutions within 24 hours.
         (4) Change administration sets every 24 hours.
         (5) Avoid irrigating plugged cannulas.
   2. *Pulmonary embolism*—substance, usually blood clot, enters pulmonary circulation and obstructs pulmonary artery.
      a. *Assessment*—dyspnea, orthopnea, and signs of circulatory and cardiac collapse.
      b. *Preventive nursing measures*—
         (1) Infuse blood or plasma through adequate filters.
         (2) Avoid venipuncture in lower extremities, as these veins are prone to trauma and thrombosis formation.
         (3) Restart infusions that have become clogged—do not irrigate.
         (4) Be sure all drugs are completely dissolved before adding to infusions.
   3. *Air embolism*—usually a complication of blood infused under pressure; it is a complication that

may occur with any infusion—small, tenacious bubbles of air block pulmonary capillaries.
   a. *Assessment*—cyanosis; hypotension; weak, rapid pulse; increased CVP; and loss of consciousness.
   b. *Immediate nursing measures*—
      (1) Place patient on left side with head down (prevents air from entering pulmonary circulation).
      (2) Administer oxygen.
      (3) Notify physician.
   c. *Preventive nursing measures*—
      (1) Avoid allowing infusion bottles to run dry; pay particular vigilance to infusions in which the extremity is elevated above the heart or that are flowing through CVP catheter—the negative pressures in these veins facilitate air entering circulation.
      (2) Closely observe infusions utilizing Y-type administration set; if one container empties, it becomes a source of air.
         (a) Avoid running fluids simultaneously if possible.
         (b) Check valves and microfilters.
   4. *Circulatory overload*—rapid infusion of fluids may result in increased venous pressure, cardiac embarrassment, and pulmonary edema (a hazard particularly for the elderly with decreased cardiac and renal reserves).
      a. *Assessment*—dyspnea, orthopnea, hypotension, tachycardia, decreased pulse pressure, distended neck veins, cough, and frothy, bloody sputum.
      b. *Immediate nursing measures*—
         (1) Reduce infusion rate to minimal.
         (2) Sit patient in upright position.
         (3) Administer oxygen if indicated.
         (4) Notify physician.
      c. *Preventive nursing measures*—
         (1) Maintain infusions at prescribed rate of flow.
         (2) Do not apply positive pressure to increase flow rate.
         (3) Discard solutions not infused in 24-hour period—do not add to next day's solutions or try to catch up.

4. Fluid and electrolyte therapy
A. Types of therapy:
   1. Maintenance therapy—provides water, electro-

TRANSFUSION WITH BLOOD OR BLOOD PRODUCTS

Blood or blood product	Indications	Actions
Whole blood	1. Acute hemorrhage. 2. Hypovolemic shock.	1. Restores blood volume. 2. Raises hemoglobin count and, therefore, oxygen-carrying capacity.
Red blood cells, packed	1. Acute anemia with hypoxia. 2. Aplastic anemia. 3. Bone marrow failure due to malignancy. 4. Patients who need red blood cells but not volume.	1. Raises hemoglobin count.
Red blood cells, frozen	1. See *Red blood cells, packed.* 2. Patients sensitized by previous transfusions.	See *Red blood cells, packed.*
White blood cells (leukocytes)	Currently being used in severe leukopenia with infection (research still being done).	Elevates leukocyte count.
Platelet concentrate	1. Severe deficiency. 2. Bleeding thrombocytopenic patients with platelet counts below 10,000.	1. Elevates platelet count. 2. Aids hemostasis by facilitating clot formation.
Single-donor fresh plasma	1. Clotting deficiency—concentrates not available or deficiency not fully diagnosed. 2. Shock.	1. Elevates level of clotting factors. 2. Expands blood pressure.

Shelf life	*Side effects*	*Nursing implications*
21 days.	1. Hemolytic reaction. 2. Fluid overload. 3. Febrile reaction. 4. Pyogenic reaction. 5. Allergic reaction.	1. See surgical complications for complete discussion of nursing responsiblities. 2. Protocol for checking blood before transfusion is begun varies with each institution; however, at least two people must verify that the unit of blood has been cross-matched for a specific patient.
1. 21 days in original container. 2. 24 hours if container is opened.	See *Whole blood.*	See *Whole blood.*
1. In frozen state, three years. 2. Thawed state, 24 hours.	1. Less likely to cause antigen reaction. 2. Decreased possibility of transmitting hepatitis.	See *Red blood cells, packed.*
Must be given when collected.	1. Elevated temperature. 2. Graft versus host disease.	1. Careful monitoring of temperature. 2. Must be given as soon as collected.
48 hours.	1. Fever. 2. Chills. 3. Hives. 4. Development of antibodies that will destroy platelets in future transfusions. *Contraindications* 1. Idiopathic thrombocytopenic purpura. 2. Disseminated intravascular coagulopathy.	Monitor temperature.
Given within six hours of collection.	1. Side effects rare. 2. Congestive heart failure. 3. Possible hepatitis.	Use sterile, pyrogen-free filters.

(Continued)

TRANSFUSION WITH BLOOD OR BLOOD PRODUCTS   *(Continued)*

Blood or blood product	Indications	Actions
Plasma removed from whole blood (up to five days after expiration date, which is 21 days)	1. Shock due to loss of plasma. 2. Burns. 3. Peritoneal injury. 4. Hemorrhage. 5. While awaiting blood cross-match.	Expands blood volume.
Freeze-dried plasma	See *Plasma removed from whole blood.*	Expands blood volume.
Single-donor fresh-frozen plasma	1. See *single-donor fresh plasma.* 2. Inherited or acquired disorders of coagulation. 3. Presurgical hemophiliac.	1. Increases level of deficient clotting factor. 2. Facilitates hemostasis.
Cryoprecipitate concentrate (factor VIII— antihemophilic factor)	For hemophilia patients. 1. Prevention. 2. Preoperatively. 3. During bleeding episodes.	Facilitates control of bleeding by elevating level of factor VIII.
Superconcentrate of factor VIII, lyophilized	See *Cryoprecipitate concentrate.*	See *Cryoprecipitate concentrate.*
Factor II, VII, IX, and X compiled	Specific deficiencies.	1. Elevates serum level. 2. Facilitates hemostasis. 3. Allows surgery.
Fibrinogen (factor I)	Fibrinogen deficiency.	1. Elevates serum level. 2. 2 g equal to 12 units of whole blood.
Albumin or salt-poor albumin	1. Shock due to hemorrhage, trauma, infection, surgery, or burns. 2. Treatment of cerebral edema. 3. Low-serum protein levels.	Restores vascular volume by elevating oncotic pressure.
Plasma protein factor	See *Albumin.*	See *Albumin.*

Shelf life	Side effects	Nursing implications
Three years.	See *Single-donor fresh plasma.*	See *Single-donor fresh plasma.*
Seven years.	See *Single-donor fresh plasma.*	Must be reconstituted with sterile water before use.
1. Six months without preservative. 2. Twelve months with preservatives. 3. Thawed just before use.	See *Single-donor fresh plasma.*	1. Freezing preserves various clotting factors, especially V and VIII. 2. Increasing temperature causes destruction of factor VIII. 3. Notify blood bank to thaw about 30 minutes before administration. 4. Give immediately.
3–12 months.	Rare.	.55 ml cryoprecipitate concentrate has same effect on serum level as 1600 ml of fresh frozen plasma.
Manufacturer's dating.	Rare.	Commercially prepared.
Manufacturer's dating.	Hepatitis.	Commercially prepared.
Five years—give within one hour after reconstitution.	Increased risk of hepatitis since the hepatitis virus combines with fibrinogen during fractionation.	1. Reconstitute with sterile water. 2. *Do not* warm fibrinogen or use hot water to reconstitute. 3. *Do not* shake. 4. Must be given with a filter.
Three to five years.	None; these are heat-treated products.	Commercially prepared.
Three to five years.	Minimal risk.	Commercially prepared.

(Continued)

TRANSFUSION WITH BLOOD OR BLOOD PRODUCTS (Continued)		
Blood or blood product	Indications	Actions
Dextran	Hypovolemic shock.	Expands intravascular volume by elevating oncotic pressure.

lytes, glucose, vitamins, and, in some instances, protein to meet daily requirements.

2. Restoration of deficits—in addition to maintenance therapy, fluid and electrolytes are added to replace previous losses.

3. Replacement therapy—infusions to replace current losses in fluid and electrolytes.

B. Types of intravenous fluids:

1. Isotonic solutions—fluids that approximate the osmolality (290 mOsm/liter) of normal blood plasma.

   a. Sodium chloride (0.9%)—normal saline
      (1) Indications—
          (a) Extracellular fluid replacement when Cl^- loss is equal to or greater than Na^+ loss.
          (b) Treatment of metabolic alkalosis.
          (c) Na^+ depletion.
          (d) Initiating and terminating blood transfusions.
      (2) Possible side effects—
          (a) Hypernatremia.
          (b) Acidosis.
          (c) Hypokalemia.
          (d) Circulatory overload.

   b. 5% dextrose in water (5% D/W).
      (1) Provides calories for energy, sparing body protein and development of ketosis from fat breakdown.
          (a) 3.75 calories are provided per gram of glucose.
          (b) USP standards require use of monohydrated glucose, so only 91% is actually glucose.
          (c) 5% D/W yields 170.6 calories; 5% D/W means 5 g glucose/liter.
              $50 \times 3.75 = 187.5$ calories
              $0.91 \times 187.5 = 170.6$ calories
      (2) Indications—
          (a) Dehydration.
          (b) Hypernatremia.
          (c) Drug administration.
      (3) Possible side effects—
          (a) Hypokalemia.
          (b) Osmotic diuresis—dehydration.
          (c) Transient hyperinsulinism.
          (d) Water intoxication.

   c. 5% dextrose in normal saline.
      (1) Prevents ketone formation and loss of potassium and intracellular water.
      (2) Indications—
          (a) Hypovolemic shock—temporary measure.
          (b) Burns.
          (c) Acute adrenocortical insufficiency.
      (3) Same side effects as normal saline.

   d. Isotonic multiple-electrolyte fluids—utilized for replacement therapy; ionic composition approximates blood plasma.
      (1) Types—Plasmanate, Polysol, lactated Ringer's.
      (2) Indicated in vomiting, diarrhea, excessive diuresis, and burns.
      (3) Possible side effect—circulatory overload.
      (4) Lactated Ringer's is contraindicated in severe metabolic acidosis and/or alkalosis and liver disease.
      (5) Same side effects as normal saline.

2. Hypertonic solutions—fluids with an osmolality much higher than 290 mOsm ($+50$ mOsm); increase osmotic pressure of blood plasma thereby drawing fluid from the cells.

   a. 10% dextrose in normal saline.
      (1) Administered in large vein to dilute and prevent venous trauma.
      (2) Utilized for nutrition and to replenish Na^+ and Cl^-.
      (3) Possible side effects—
          (a) Hypernatremia (excess Na^+).

Shelf life	Side effects	Nursing implications
Some will last indefinitely.	1. Rare allergic reaction. 2. Patients with heart or kidney disease susceptible to heart failure or pulmonary edema.	Commercially prepared.

(b) Acidosis (excess Cl^-).

(c) Circulatory overload.

  b. 3% and 5% sodium chloride solutions.

    (1) Slow administration essential to prevent overload (100 ml/hour).

    (2) Indicated in water intoxication and severe sodium depletion.

3. Hypotonic solution—fluids whose osmolality is significantly less than blood plasma (-50 mOsm); these fluids lower plasma osmotic pressures causing fluid to enter cells.

  a. 0.45% sodium chloride—utilized for replacement when requirement for Na^+ use is questionable.

  b. 2.5% dextrose in 0.45% saline, 5% dextrose in 0.45% saline, and 5% dextrose in 0.2% saline—these are all hydrating fluids.

    (1) Indications—

      (a) Fluid replacement when some Na^+ replacement is also necessary.

      (b) Encourage diuresis in patients who are dehydrated.

      (c) Evaluate kidney status before instituting electrolyte infusions.

    (2) Possible side effects—

      (a) Hypernatremia.

      (b) Circulatory overload.

      (c) Use with caution in edematous patients with cardiac, renal, or hepatic disease.

      (d) After adequate renal function is established, appropriate electrolytes should be given to avoid hypokalemia.

4. Alkalizing agents—fluids used in the treatment of metabolic acidosis.

  a. 1/6 M lactate.

    (1) Administration—rate usually not more than 300 ml/hour.

    (2) Side effects—observe carefully for signs of alkalosis.

  b. Sodium bicarbonate.

    (1) Indications—

      (a) Replace excessive loss of bicarbonate ion.

      (b) Emergency treatment of life-threatening acidosis.

    (2) Administration—

      (a) Depends on patient's weight, condition, and carbon dioxide level.

      (b) Usual dose is 500 ml of a 1.5% solution (89 mEq).

    (3) Side effects—

      (a) Alkalosis.

      (b) Hypocalcemic tetany.

      (c) Rapid infusion may induce cellular acidity and death.

5. Acidifying solutions—fluids used in treatment of metabolic alkalosis.

  a. Types—

    (1) Normal saline (see *Isotonic solutions*).

    (2) Ammonium chloride.

  b. Administration—dosage depends on patient's condition and serum lab values.

  c. Side effects—

    (1) Hepatic encephalopathy in presence of decreased liver function, since ammonium is metabolized by liver.

    (2) Toxic effects of irregular respirations, twitching, and bradycardia.

    (3) Contraindicated with renal failure.

6. Blood and blood products.

  a. Indications—

    (1) Maintenance of blood volume.

    (2) Supply red blood cells to maintain oxygen-carrying capacity.

    (3) Supply clotting factors to maintain coagulation properties.

    (4) Exchange transfusion.

ELECTROLYTE DISTURBANCES

Disturbance	Symptoms	Etiology	Nursing assessment and implications
Hypervolemia (increase in sodium and water)	Dyspnea Edema Jugular vein distention Weight gain	Over-hydration Excessive intake Congestive heart failure (CHF)	Maintain fluid and sodium restrictions Monitor intake and output Weigh daily Administer diuretics
Hypovolemia (decreased sodium and water)	Thirst Weakness Elevated hematocrit Rapid weak pulse Decreased urine output	Acute hemorrhage Diuretics Decreased intake Gastric suctioning	Replace losses Monitor intake and output Weigh daily
Hypernatremia	Thirst Oliguria Anuria Elevated temperature	Excessive intake of salt Excessive loss of water	Administer hypotonic solutions, as ordered
Hyponatremia	Headache Apprehension Abdominal cramps Oliguria	Extended submersion in fresh water Water intoxication	Administration of sodium containing solutions
Hyperkalemia	Weakness Flaccid paralysis Cardiac arrhythmias Nausea	Kidney disease Burns Acidosis	Administration of calcium, glucose, insulin, cation-exchange resins, and polystyrene sodium sulfonate (Kayexalate) as ordered
Hypokalemia	ECG changes Malaise Anorexia Vomiting	Diuretics Gastric suction Fistulas Alkalosis	Administration of potassium replacements
Hypermagnesemia	Muscle weakness Hyperventilation Hypotension	Overuse of antacids Renal insufficiency Epsom salt enemas Severe dehydration	Emergency—administration of 10% calcium gluconate solution treats underlying problem
Hypomagnesemia	Tremors Hyperactive reflexes Positive Chvostek Convulsions	Rare Severe renal disease Stress	Administration of magnesium sulfate, as ordered
Hypercalcemia	Hypotonicity of muscles Decreased neuromuscular irritability	Hyperthyroidism Hyperparathyroidism Thiazide diuretics Bone tumors	Administration of steroids and parenteral normal saline, as ordered Restrict calcium intake
Hypocalcemia	Carpopedal spasms Tetany Chvostek Positive	Parathyroid hormone Deficiency Peritonitis	Administration of calcium or vitamin D, as ordered

(5) Prime oxygenating pump.

C. *Nursing responsibilities:*
1. Awareness of imbalance and appropriate therapy.
2. Reporting pertinent observations.
3. Knowledgeable regarding clinical parameters to be assessed—
    a. Vital signs.
    b. Weight.
    c. Intake and output.
    d. Skin texture and elasticity.
    e. Peripheral veins.
    f. Central venous pressure.
    g. Pulmonary artery pressure.
    h. Laboratory values.

HYPERALIMENTATION—TOTAL PARENTERAL NUTRITION

1. Indications
A. Negative nitrogen balance
B. Conditions that interfere with protein ingestion, digestion, and absorption
C. May be used up to six months to maintain nutritional requirements—average daily volume 3300 ml/day

2. Types of solutions
A. Hydrolyzed protein (Hyprotigen, Amigen)
B. Synthetic amino acids (Freamine)
C. Usual components
1. 5% amino acid
2. 10% to 25% glucose
3. Multivitamins
4. Electrolytes
D. Supplements may be added as needed
1. Fructose
2. Alcohol
3. Fat emulsions

4. Minerals—iron, copper, calcium
5. Trace elements—iodine, zinc, magnesium
6. Vitamins—A, C, and B
7. Androgen hormone therapy
8. Additional electrolytes

3. Administration
A. Dosage
1. Dependent on patient's clinical status
2. One liter q5–6h
3. Solution should be mixed under laminar flow hoods—usually done by pharmacist
4. Solution should be stored in refrigerator after mixing
    a. Solution expires in 24 hours if refrigerated
    b. Solution expires in 12 hours once removed from refrigerator
5. Incompatible with antibiotics
6. Keep flow rate constant—do not adjust rate to "catch up" IV.
B. Routes
1. Must be given through large veins, such as subclavian
2. Confirmation of catheter placement by X ray before infusion begins.
C. Side effects
1. Hyperosmolar coma
2. Hyperglycemia
3. Septicemia
4. Thrombosis and sclerosis of vein
D. Nursing implications
1. In-line filter should always be used
2. Aseptic occlusive dressing should be changed at least every 48 hours
3. Clinitest and Acitest q4h, with sliding-scale urine coverage
4. The catheter is to be utilized for *nothing* except hyperalimentation—if the catheter has been used for CVP readings or to draw blood, hyperalimentation *must* be discontinued

Appendix C/DIAGNOSTIC TESTS

LABORATORY VALUES*

Blood Values

1. **Hematocrit**—the volume of packed red blood cells per 100 ml of blood.
   A. Men—45% (38% to 54%).
   B. Women—40% (36% to 47%).
   C. *Increase*—polycythemia, dehydration.
   D. *Decrease*—anemia.

2. **Hemoglobin**—measures the oxygen-carrying pigment of the red blood cells.
   A. Men—14–16 g/100 ml.
   B. Women—12–16 g/100 ml.
   C. *Increase and decrease*—See *Hematocrit*.

3. **Red blood count (RBC)**
   A. Men—5.0 (4.5–6.0) × 10^6/cu mm.
   B. Women—4.5 (4.3–5.5) × 10^6/cu mm.
   C. *Increase*—polycythemia vera, leukemia.
   D. Secondary—chronic obstructive lung disease, cyanotic congenital heart, diseases with hypoxemia.

4. **Red blood cell indices**
   A. Mean cell volume (MCV)—80–94 (cuµ).
      1. *Increase*—macrocytic anemia.
      3. *Decrease*—microcytic anemia.
   B. Mean cell hemoglobin (MCH)—27–32 µg/cell.
      1. *Increase*—macrocytic anemia.
      2. *Decrease*—microcytic anemia.
   C. Mean cell hemoglobin concentration (MCHC)—33% to 38%.
      1. *Decrease*—severe hypochromic anemia.

5. **White blood count (WBC)**
   A. Normal value—4500–11,000/cu mm.
   B. *Mild to moderate increase*—infections, mainly bacterial; severe sepsis in the elderly.
   C. *Marked increase*—severe sepsis.

*Among the sources used to compile this information were Tilkian, S. M., and Conover, M. H.: Clinical implications of laboratory test, St. Louis, 1975, The C. V. Mosby Co.; Widmann, F. K.: Goodale's clinical interpretation of laboratory tests, ed. 7, Philadelphia, 1973, F. A. Davis Company; and The Lippincott manual of nursing practice, Philadelphia, 1974, J. B. Lippincott Company.

6. **WBC differential**
   A. Neutrophils—1800–7000 cu mm.
      1. *Increase*—bacterial infections, inflammations, tumors, physical and emotional stress, drugs.
      2. *Decrease*—acute viral infections, anorexia nervosa, primary and secondary splenic neutropenia, drug-induced, and alcoholic ingestion.
   B. Eosinophils—50–300/cu mm, or 1% to 3%.
      1. *Increase*—allergic disorders, parasitic infestation, eosinophilic leukemia.
      2. *Decrease*—acute and chronic stress, excess ACTH, cortisone, and epinephrine, and endocrine disorders.
   C. Basophils—0–100/cu mm, or 0% to 1%.
      1. *Increase*—myeloproliferative disease.
      2. *Decrease*—anaphylactic reaction, hyperthyroidism, radiation therapy, acute and chronic infections, ovulation, pregnancy, and aging.
   D. Lymphocytes—1000–4000/cu mm.
      1. *Increase*—chronic lymphocytic leukemia, infectious mononucleosis, whooping cough, acute lymphocytosis, viral infections with eczemas, and chronic bacterial infections.

7. **Platelets**—200,000–500,000/cu mm.
   A. *Increase*—polycythemia, splenectomy status, essential thrombocytosis.
   B. *Absence*—thrombocytopenia.

8. **Prothrombin time**
   A. Sensitive to deficiencies of the procoagulants—Factor I (fibrinogen factor), Factor II (prothrombin factor), Factor V (labile factor), Factor VII (stable factor), and Factor X (Stuart factor).
   B. *Increase*—hepatic disease, anticoagulant therapy, malabsorption, and defibrination syndrome.

9. **Partial thromboplastin**
   A. Time 35–50 seconds.
   B. Measures deficiencies in stage II of coagulation—deficiency of Factors VIII, IX, and X.

10. **Bleeding time**
    A. 30 seconds to 6 minutes.
    B. Prolonged in hemorrhagic purpura and in chloroform poisoning.

11. **Sedimentation rate**—speed at which RBCs settle in uncoagulated blood.
A. Men—0–9 mm/hour.
B. Women—0–20 mm/hour.
C. A nonspecific screening test; normal value rules out significant inflammatory disease.

Blood Chemistry

1. **Alkaline phosphatase, total serum**
A. Adults:
   1. 1.4–4.1 units/100 ml (Bodansky method).
   2. 4–13 units/100 ml (King-Armstrong method).
   3. 20–48 IU/ml.
B. *Increase*—early obstructive jaundice, Paget's disease of bone, Ca with bone metastasis, cholangiolitic hepatitis, cirrhosis, hyperparathyroidism, and osteomalacia.

2. **Amylase**—60–160 units/ml.
A. *Increase*—acute pancreatitis, mumps, duodenal ulcer, and carcinoma of the head of the pancreas.
B. *Decrease*—chronic pancreatitis, cirrhosis, acute alcoholism, and toxemias of pregnancy.

3. **Ascorbic acid, serum**—0.4–1.5 mg/100 ml.
A. *Decrease*—rheumatic fever, collagen diseases, renal and hepatic disease, and congestive heart failure.

4. **Bilirubin, serum**
A. Direct—0–0.3 mg/100 ml.
B. Indirect—0.1–1.0 mg/100 ml.
C. Total—0.1–1.2 mg/100 ml.
D. *Increase*—low-grade hemolytic diseases, massive hemolysis, cirrhosis, obstructive liver disease, hepatitis, cholangitis, and carcinoma or calculus of lower biliary tract.

5. **Sulfobromophthalein (Bromsulphalein) (BSP)**
A. Less than 6% retention after 45 minutes.
B. *Increase*—acute hepatic disease.

6. **Cephalin flocculation**
A. No precipitate.
B. *Increase*—severe liver disease, malaria, and infectious mononucleosis.

7. **Calcium, serum**—9–11.5 mg/100 ml or 4.5–5.7 mEq/liter.
A. *Increase*—hyperparathyroidism, sarcoidosis, multiple myeloma, malignancies with bone metastases, milk-alkali syndrome, hyperthyroidism, bone fractures, Paget's disease of the bone.
B. *Decrease*—hypoparathyroidism, osteomalacia, rickets, acute pancreatitis, pregnancy, diuretics, respiratory alkalosis.

8. **Carbon dioxide combining power**—50–65 vol % or 24–30 mEq/liter.
A. *Increase*—alkali ingestion, serum alkalosis, and intracellular acidosis, vomiting, hypoventilation.
B. *Decrease*—uremia, diabetic ketoacidosis, lactic acidosis, renal tubular necrosis, hyperventilation, diarrhea.

9. **Chloride, serum (as Cl)**—95–106 mEq/liter or 355–376 mg/100 ml.
A. *Increase*—renal tubular acidosis and inappropriate IV or tube feedings; hyperventilation, diabetes insipidus, uremia.
B. *Decrease*—spironolactone and chronic obstructive lung disease, CHF, hypoventilation, pyloric obstruction, vomiting, salt depletion.

10. **Cholesterol (total serum)**—110–300 mg/100 ml.
A. Increase—liver disease with biliary obstruction and nephrotic stage of glomerulonephritis, familial.
B. Decrease—malnutrition, extensive liver disease, and hyperthyroidism.

11. **Creatinine, serum**—0.6–1.2 mg/100 ml.
A. *Increase*—kidney disease with greater than 50% nephron destruction.

12. **Creatine phosphokinase (CPK)**
A. Men—55–170 U/liter.
B. Women—30–135 U/liter.
C. *Increase*—muscular dystrophy, myocardial infarction, dissecting aortic aneurysms, heavy exercise or surgical procedures with damage to skeletal muscles, CVAs, salicylate poisoning, and acute alcohol ingestion.

13. **Fatty acids, serum**—250–390 mg/100 ml.
A. *Increase*—diabetes mellitus, anemia, nephrosis, and hypothyroidism.
B. *Decrease*—hyperthyroidism.

14. **Fibrinogen, serum**—0.2–0.4 g/100 ml.
A. *Increase*—pneumonia, acute infections, and nephrosis.
B. *Decrease*—cirrhosis, toxic liver necrosis, anemia, and typhoid fever.

15. Blood glucose (fasting)—80–120 mg/100 ml.

A. *Increase*—acute stress, pheochromocytoma, Cushing's syndrome, hyperthyroidism, acute and chronic pancreatitis, diabetes mellitus, and ketoacidosis.

B. *Decrease*—pancreatic islet cell tumor, pituitary hypofunction, Addison's disease, extensive liver disease, and reactive hypoglycemia.

16. Iodine, protein-bound, serum (PBI)—4–8 μg/100 ml.

A. *Increase*—hyperthyroidism.

B. *Decrease*—hypothyroidism.

17. Iron-binding capacity—250–450 μg/100 ml.

A. *Increase*—iron-deficiency anemia.

B. *Decrease*—chronic infections.

18. Lactic dehydrogenase (LDH)

A. 80–120 Wacker units.

B. 150–450 Wroblewski units.

C. 71–207 IU/liter.

D. *Increase*—myocardial infarction, pernicious anemia, chronic viral hepatitis, pneumonia, pulmonary emboli, CVA, and renal tissue destruction.

19. Lipids, total, serum—400–1000 mg/100 ml.

A. *Increase*—hypothyroidism, diabetes, nephrosis, and glomerulonephritis.

B. *Decrease*—hyperthyroidism.

20. Phosphatase, alkaline, serum

A. King-Armstrong method—8–14 units/1000 ml.

B. Bodansky method—1–4 units/100 ml.

C. *Increase*—rickets, liver disease, and hyperparathyroidism.

21. Phosphorus, inorganic, serum—1.8–2.6 mEq/liter or 3.0–4.5 mg/100 ml.

A. *Increase*—chronic glomerular disease, hypoparathyroidism, milk-alkali syndrome, and sarcoidosis.

B. *Decrease*—hyperparathyroidism, rickets, osteomalacia, renal tubular acidosis, and malabsorption syndrome.

22. Potassium, serum—3.5–5.0 mEq/liter.

A. *Increase*—diabetic ketosis, renal failure and Addison's disease.

B. *Decrease*—thiazide diuretics, Cushing's syndrome, cirrhosis with ascites, hyperaldosteronism, steroid therapy, malignant hypertension, poor dietary habits, chronic diarrhea, diaphoresis, renal tubular necrosis, malabsorption syndrome, vomiting.

23. Protein, serum—albumin/globulin

A. Total—6.0–7.8 g/100 ml.

B. Albumin—3.2–4.5 g/100 ml.

C. Globulin—2.3–3.5 g/100 ml.

D. *Decrease*—chronic liver disease and myeloproliferative diseases.

24. Sodium, serum—138–144 mEq/liter.

A. *Increase*—increased intake, either orally or IV; CNS disease or damage.

B. *Decrease*—Addison's disease, sodium-losing nephropathy, vomiting, diarrhea, fistulas, tube drainage, burns, renal insufficiency with acidosis, starvation with acidosis, paracentesis, thoracentesis, ascites, congestive heart failure, hypothermia, and diabetic hyperglycemia.

25. T₃ uptake—25% to 38%.

A. *Increase*—hyperthyroidism and TBG deficiency.

B. *Decrease*—hypothyroidism, pregnancy, and TBG excess.

26. Thyroxin—5–11 μg/100 ml.

A. *Increase*—hyperthyroidism, pregnancy, and TBG excess.

B. *Decrease*—hypothyroidism and TBG deficiency.

27. Serum glutamic oxaloacetic transaminase (SGOT)—up to 40 units/100 ml.

A. *Increase*—hepatitis, severe liver necrosis, myocardial infarction, cirrhosis, skeletal muscle disease, pulmonary infarction, shock, thyrotoxicosis, burns, infection, GI hemorrhage, and excessive protein catabolism.

B. Decrease—increased fluid intake, hepatic failure.

28. Urea nitrogen, serum (BUN)—10–18 mg/100 ml.

A. Increase—acute or chronic renal failure, congestive heart failure, and obstructive uropathy.

29. Uric acid, serum

A. Men—2.1–7.8 mg/100 ml.

B. Women—2.0–6.4 mg/100 ml.

C. *Increase*—gout, chronic renal failure, starvation, and diuretic therapy.

30. Vitamin B₁₂—300–1000 pg/ml.

A. *Increase*—hepatic cellular damage and myeloproliferative disorders.

B. *Decrease*—alcoholism, vegetarianism, total or partial gastrectomy, sprue and celiac disease, and fish tapeworm infestation.

31. **Zinc**—55–150 µg/100 ml.
A. *Increase*—hyperthermia.
B. *Decrease*—alcoholic cirrhosis, leukemia, and pernicious anemia.

Blood Gases

1. **pH, serum**—7.35–7.45.
A. *Increase*—metabolic alkalosis-alkali ingestion and respiratory alkalosis-hyperventilation.
B. *Decrease*—metabolic acidosis-ketoacidosis, shock and respiratory acidosis-alveolar hypoventilation.

2. **Oxygen pressure (PO$_2$), whole blood, arterial**—95–100 mm Hg.
A. *Increase*—oxygen administration in the absence of severe lung disease.
B. *Decrease*—chronic obstructive lung disease, severe pneumonias, pulmonary embolism, pulmonary edema, and respiratory muscle disease.

3. **Carbon dioxide pressure (PCO$_2$), whole blood, arterial**—35–45 mm Hg (mean is 40).
A. *Increase*—alveolar hypoventilation, loss of H^+ through nasogastric suctioning or vomiting.
B. *Decrease*—hyperventilation.

Urinalysis

1. **pH**—4.8–8.0.
A. *Increase*—metabolic alkalosis.
B. *Decrease*—intracellular acidosis due to potassium depletion.

2. **Specific gravity**—1.015–1.025.
A. *Decrease*—distal renal tubular disease, polycystic kidney disease, and diabetes insipidus.

3. **Glucose**—negative.
A. *Increase*—diabetes mellitus.

4. **Protein—negative.**
A. *Increase*—nephrosis, glomerulonephritis, and lupus erythematosus.

5. **Casts**—negative.
A. *Increase*—nephrosis, glomerulonephritis, and lupus erythematosus.

6. **Red blood cells**—negative.
A. *Increase*—renal calculi, hemorrhagic cystitis, and tumors of the kidney.

7. **White blood cells**—negative.
A. *Increase*—inflammation of the kidneys, ureters, or bladder.

8. **Color**—normal: yellow.
A. Red to reddish brown—hematuria.
B. Brown to brownish grey—bilirubinuria and urobilinuria.
C. Tea-colored—possible obstructive jaundice.

9. **Sodium**—80–180 mEq/24 hours.
A. *Increase*—salt-wasting renal disease.
B. *Decrease*—congestive heart failure and primary aldosteronism.

10. **Chloride**—110–250 mEq/24 hours.
A. *Increase*—chronic obstructive lung disease.
B. *Decrease*—metabolic alkalosis.

11. **Potassium**—40–80 mEq/24 hours.
A. *Increase*—osmotic diuresis.
B. *Decrease*—renal failure.

12. **Creatinine clearance**—1.0–1.6 g/24 hours.
A. *Decrease*—renal disease.

13. **Creatine**—1–2 g/24 hours.
A. *Increase*—typhoid fever, salmonella, and tetanus.
B. *Decrease*—muscular atrophy, anemia, and leukemia.

14. **Hydroxycorticosteroids**—2–10 mg/24 hours.
A. *Increase*—Cushing's disease.
B. *Decrease*—Addison's disease.

15. **Ketosteroids**
A. Male—1–22 mg/24 hours.
B. Female—6–16 mg/24 hours.
C. *Increase*—hirsutism and adrenal hyperplasia.
D. *Decrease*—thyrotoxicosis, Addison's disease, and myxedema.

16. **Catecholamines (VMA)**
A. Epinephrine—10 mg/24 hours.
B. Norepinephrine: 100 mg/24 hours.
   1. *Increase*—pheochromocytoma.

Urine Tests

1. **Schilling test**
A. One-third of absorbed Vitamin B$_{12}$ should appear in urine.

B. *Decrease*—gastrointestinal malabsorption and pernicious anemia.

2. *Phenolphthalein (PSP)*

A. At least 25% excreted in 15 minutes, 40% in 30 minutes, and 60% in 120 minutes.
B. *Decrease*—renal disease, low in nephritis; pyelonephritis; and congestive heart failure.

COMMON PROCEDURES

1. **Noninvasive diagnostic procedures**—those procedures that provide an indirect assessment of organ size, shape, and/or function; these procedures are considered safe, are easily reproducible, need less complex equipment for recording, and generally do not require the written consent of the patient and/or guardian.

A. General *nursing responsibilities* in noninvasive techniques:
   1. Reduce patient's anxieties and provide emotional support by—
      a. Explaining the purpose and procedure of test.
      b. Answering questions regarding safety of the procedure as indicated.
      c. Remaining with patient during procedure when possible.
   2. Utilize procedures in the collection of specimens that avoid contamination and facilitate diagnosis—clean-catch urines and sputum specimens after deep breathing and coughing, for example.

B. Graphic studies of the heart and brain:
   1. *Electrocardiogram*—graphic record of the electrical activity generated by the heart during depolarization and repolarization; utilized to diagnose abnormal cardiac rhythms and coronary heart disease.
   2. *Ballistocardiogram*—graphic record of body movements that occur as the result of the force of the heart beat; utilized to measure cardiac output, strength of myocardial contraction, aortic elasticity and presence of coronary artery disease, mitral stenosis, or chronic constrictive pericarditis.
   3. *Phonocardiogram*—graphic record of heart sounds; utilized to keep a permanent record of the patient's heart sounds before and after cardiac surgery.
   4. *Electroencephalogram*—graphic record of the electrical potentials generated by the physio-

logic activity of the brain; utilized to detect surface lesions or tumors of the brain and presence of epilepsy.
   5. *Echoencephalogram*—beam of pulsed ultrasound is passed through the head and returning echoes are graphically recorded; detects shifts in cerebral midline structures caused by subdural hematomas, intracerebral hemorrhage, and tumors.

C. Roentgenologic studies (X ray):
   1. *Chest*—utilized to determine the size, contour, and position of the heart; the size, location, and nature of pulmonary lesions; disorders of thoracic bones or soft tissue; diaphragmatic contour and excursion; pleural thickening or effusions; and gross changes in the caliber or distribution of the pulmonary vasculature.
   2. *Kidney, ureter, and bladder (KUB)*—determine size, shape, and position of kidneys, ureters, and bladder.
   3. *Mammography*—examination of the breast with or without the injection of radiopaque dye into the ducts of the mammary gland.
   4. *Skull*—outline configuration and density of brain tissues and vascular markings; utilized to determine the size and location of intracranial calcifications, tumors, abscesses, or vascular lesions.

D. Roentgenologic studies (fluoroscopy)—require the ingestion or injection of a radiopaque substance to visualize the target organ.
   1. Additional *nursing responsibilities* include:
      a. Administration of enemas or cathartics prior to or following the procedure.
      b. Keeping the patient NPO 6 to 12 hours prior to examination.
      c. Ascertaining patient's history of allergies or allergic reactions.
      d. Observing for allergic reactions to dye following procedure.
      e. Providing fluid and food following procedure to counteract dehydration.
   2. Common fluoroscopic examinations:
      a. *Upper GI*—ingestion of barium sulfate, a white, chalky, radiopaque substance followed by fluoroscopic and X-ray examination; utilized to determine—
         (1) Patency and caliber of esophagus; may also detect esophageal varices.
         (2) Mobility and thickness of gastric walls, presence of ulcer craters, filling defects due to tumors, pressures from

outside the stomach, and patency of pyloric valve.

(3) Rate of passage in small bowel and presence of structural abnormalities.

b. *Lower GI*—rectal instillation of barium sulfate followed by fluoroscopic and X-ray examination; determines the contour and mobility of the colon and the presence of any space-occupying tumors.

c. *Cholecystogram*—ingestion of organic iodine dye Telepaque (iopanoic acid) followed in 12 hours by X-ray visualization; gallbladder disease is indicated with poor or no visualization of the bladder; accurate only if gastrointestinal and liver function is intact.

d. *Cholangiogram*—intravenous injection of a radiopaque dye followed by fluoroscopic and X-ray examination of the bile ducts; failure of the dye to pass certain points in the bile duct pinpoints obstruction.

e. *Intravenous pyelography (IVP)*—injection of a radiopaque dye followed by fluoroscopic and X-ray films of kidneys and urinary tract; identifies lesions in kidneys and ureters and provides rough estimate of kidney function.

f. *Cystogram*—instillation of radiopaque medium into the bladder through a catheter; utilized to visualize bladder wall and evaluate ureterovesical valves for reflux.

E. Pulmonary function studies (see Table 5–5):
1. Ventilatory studies—utilization of a spirometer to determine how well the lung is ventilating.
   a. *Vital capacity (VC)*—largest amount of air that can be expelled after a maximal inspiration.
      (1) Normally 4000 to 5000 ml.
      (2) Decreased in restrictive lung disease.
      (3) May be normal, slightly increased, or decreased in chronic obstructive lung disease.
   b. *Forced expiratory volume (FEV$_T$)*—percentage of vital capacity that can be forcibly expired in one, two, or three seconds.
      (1) Normally 81% to 83% in one second, 90% to 94% in two seconds, and 95% to 97% in three seconds.
      (2) Decreased values indicate expiratory airway obstruction.
   c. *Maximum breathing capacity (MBC)*—maximal amount of air that can be breathed in and out in one minute with maximal rates and depths of respiration.
      (1) Best overall measurement of ventilatory ability.
      (2) Reduced in restrictive and chronic obstructive lung disease.
2. Diffusion studies—measure the rate of exchange of gases across alveolar membrane.
   a. Carbon monoxide single-breath, rebreathing, and steady-state techniques—utilized because of special affinity of hemoglobin for carbon monoxide; decreased when fluid is present in alveoli or when alveolar membranes are thick or fibrosed.

F. Sputum studies:
1. Gross sputum evaluations—collection of sputum samples to ascertain quantity, consistency, color, and odor.
2. *Sputum smear*—sputum is smeared thinly on a slide so that it can be studied microscopically; determines cytologic changes (malignant cell) or presence of pathogenic bacteria such as tubercle bacilli.
3. *Sputum culture*—sputum samples are implanted or inoculated into special media; used to diagnose pulmonary infections.
4. *Gastric lavage or analysis*—insertion of a nasogastric tube into the stomach to siphon out swallowed pulmonary secretions; detects organisms causing pulmonary infections; especially useful for detecting tubercle bacilli.

G. Examination of gastric contents:
1. Gastric analysis—aspiration of the contents of the fasting stomach for analysis of free and total acid.
   a. Gastric acidity is generally *increased* in presence of duodenal ulcer.
   b. Gastric acidity is usually *decreased* in pernicious anemia and in cancer of the stomach.
2. Stool specimens—examined for amount, consistency, color, character, and melena; utilized to determine presence of urobilinogen, fat, nitrogen, parasites, and other substances.

2. *Invasive diagnostic procedures*—procedures that directly record the size, shape, or function of an organ and that are often complex, expensive, or require the utilization of highly trained personnel; these procedures may result in morbidity and occasionally mortality of the patient and therefore

require the written consent of the patient or guardian.

A. *General nursing responsibilities:*
1. Prior to procedure, institute measures to provide for patient's safety and emotional comfort.
   a. Have patient sign permit for procedure.
   b. Ascertain and report any patient history of allergy or allergic reactions.
   c. Explain procedure briefly and accurately advise patient of any possible sensations, such as flushing or a warm feeling, as when a contrast medium is injected.
   d. Keep patient NPO 6 to 12 hours before procedure if anesthesia is to be used.
   e. Allow patient to verbalize concerns and note attitude toward procedure.
   f. Administer preprocedure sedative, as ordered.
   g. If procedure done at bedside—
      (1) Remain with patient, offering frequent reassurance.
      (2) Assist with optional positioning of patient.
      (3) Observe for indications of complications—shock, pain, or dyspnea.
2. Following procedure institute measures to avoid complications and promote physical and emotional comfort.
   a. Observe and record vital signs.
   b. Check injection cutdown or biopsy sites for bleeding, infection, tenderness, or thrombosis.
      (1) Report untoward reactions to physician.
      (2) Apply warm compresses to ease discomfort, as ordered.
   c. Encourage relaxation by allowing patient to discuss experience and to verbalize feelings.

B. Procedures used in evaluating cardiovascular system:
1. *Angiocardiography*—intravenous injection of a radiopaque solution or dye for the purpose of studying its circulation through the patient's heart, lungs, and great vessels; used to check the competency of heart valves, diagnose congenital septal defects, detect occlusions of coronary arteries, confirm suspected diagnoses, and study heart function and structure prior to cardiac surgery.
2. *Cardiac catheterization*—insertion of a radiopaque catheter into a vein to study the heart and great vessels.
   a. *Right-heart catheterization*—catheter is inserted through a cutdown in the antecubital vein into the superior vena cava and through the right atrium, ventricle, and into the pulmonary artery.
   b. *Left-heart catheterization*—catheter may be passed retrograde to the left ventricle through the brachial or femoral artery; it can be passed into the left atrium after right-heart catheterization by means of a special needle that punctures the septa; or it may be passed directly into the left ventricle by means of a posterior or anterior chest puncture.
   c. Cardiac catheterizations are utilized to—
      (1) Confirm diagnosis of heart disease and determine the extent of the disease.
      (2) Determine the existence and extent of congenital abnormalities.
      (3) Measure pressures in the heart chambers and great vessels.
      (4) Obtain estimate of cardiac output.
      (5) Obtain blood samples to measure oxygen content and determine presence of cardiac shunts.
   d. *Specific nursing interventions*—
      (1) Preprocedure patient teaching:
         (a) Fatigue due to lying still for three or more hours is a common complaint.
         (b) Some fluttery sensations may be felt—occurs as catheter is passed backwards into the left ventricle.
         (c) Flushed warm feeling may occur when contrast medium is injected.
      (2) Postprocedure observations:
         (a) Monitor ECG pattern for arrhythmias.
         (b) Check extremities for color and temperature and peripheral pulses (femoral and dorsalis pedis) for quality.
3. *Angiography (arteriography)*—injection of a contrast medium into the arteries to study the vascular tree; utilized to determine obstructions or narrowing of peripheral arteries.

C. Procedures used in evaluating the respiratory system:
1. Pulmonary circulation studies—utilized to

determine regional distribution of pulmonary blood flow.

  a. *Lung scan*—injection of radioactive isotope into the body, followed by lung scintiscan, which produces a graphic record of gamma rays emitted by the isotope in lung tissues; determines lung perfusion when space-occupying lesions or pulmonary emboli and infarction are suspected.

  b. *Pulmonary angiography*—X-ray visualization of the pulmonary vasculature after the injection of a radiopaque contrast medium; used to evaluate pulmonary disorders such as pulmonary embolism, lung tumors, aneurysms, and changes in the pulmonary vasculature due to such conditions as emphysema or congenital defects.

2. *Bronchoscopy*—introduction of a special lighted instrument (bronchoscope) into the trachea and bronchi; used to inspect the tracheobronchial tree for pathologic changes, remove tissue for cytologic and bacteriologic studies, remove foreign bodies or mucus plugs causing airway obstruction, assess functional residual capacity of diseased lung, and apply chemotherapeutic agents.

  a. *Prebronchoscopy nursing actions*—
    (1) Oral hygiene.
    (2) Postural drainage if indicated.

  b. *Postbronchoscopy nursing actions*—
    (1) Instruct patient not to swallow oral secretions but to let saliva run from side of mouth.
    (2) Save expectorated sputum for laboratory analysis and observe for frank bleeding.
    (3) NPO until gag reflex returns.
    (4) Observe for subcutaneous emphysema and dyspnea.
    (5) Apply ice collar to reduce throat discomfort.

3. *Thoracentesis*—needle puncture through the chest wall and into the pleura to remove fluid and, occasionally, air from the pleural space.

  a. *Nursing responsibilities* prior to thoracentesis—
    (1) Position patient in high-Fowler's position or sitting up on edge of bed with feet supported on chair—facilitates accumulation of fluid in the base of the chest.
    (2) If patient is unable to sit up—turn on unaffected side.
    (3) Evaluate continually for signs of shock, pain, cyanosis, increased respiratory rate, and pallor.

D. Procedures used in evaluating the renal system:

1. *Renal angiograms*—small catheter is inserted into the femoral artery and passed into the aorta or renal artery, radiopaque fluid is instilled, and serial films are taken.

  a. Utilized to diagnose renal hypertension and pheochromocytoma and to differentiate renal cysts from renal tumors.

  b. Postangiogram *nursing actions* include checking pedal pulse for signs of decreased circulation.

2. *Cystoscopy*—visualization of bladder, urethra, and prostatic urethra by insertion of a tubular, lighted, telescopic lens (cystoscope) through the urinary meatus.

  a. Utilized to directly inspect the bladder, collect urine from the renal pelvis, obtain biopsies from bladder and urethra, remove calculi, and treat lesions in the bladder, urethra, and prostate.

  b. *Nursing actions* following procedure include—
    (1) Observing for urinary retention.
    (2) Warm sitz baths to relieve discomfort.

3. *Renal biopsy*—needle aspiration of tissue from the kidney for the purpose of microscopic examination.

E. Procedures used in evaluating the digestive system:

1. *Celiac angiography, hepatoportography, splenoportography, and umbilical venography*—injection of a contrast medium into the portal vein or related vessel to determine patency of vessels supplying target organ or to detect lesions in the organs that distort the vasculature.

2. *Esophagoscopy and gastroscopy*—visualization of the esophagus, the stomach, and sometimes the duodenum by means of a lighted tube inserted through the mouth.

3. *Proctoscopy*—visualization of rectum and colon by means of a lighted tube inserted through the anus.

4. *Peritoneoscopy*—direct visualization of the liver and peritoneum by means of a peritoneoscope inserted through an abdominal stab wound.

5. *Liver biopsy*—needle aspiration of tissue for the purpose of microscopic examination; utilized to

determine tissue changes, to facilitate diagnosis, and to provide information regarding a disease course.

6. *Paracentesis*—needle aspiration of fluid from the peritoneal cavity to relieve excess fluid accumulation or for diagnostic studies.
   a. Specific *nursing actions* prior to paracentesis—
      (1) Have patient void—prevents possible injury to bladder during procedure.
      (2) Position patient—sitting up on side of bed with feet supported by chair.
      (3) Check vital signs and peripheral circulation frequently throughout procedure.
      (4) Observe for signs of hypovolemic shock—may occur due to fluid shift from vascular compartment following removal of protein-rich ascitic fluid.
   b. Specific *nursing actions* following paracentesis—
      (1) Apply pressure to injection site and cover with sterile dressing.
      (2) Measure and record amount and color of ascitic fluid and send specimens to lab for diagnostic studies.

F. Procedures used in evaluating the reproductive system in women:
   1. *Culdoscopy*—operative procedure in which a culdoscope is inserted into the posterior vaginal cul-de-sac; utilized to visualize the uterus, fallopian tubes, broad ligaments, and peritoneal contents.
   2. *Hysterosalpingography*—X-ray examination of the uterus and fallopian tubes following insertion of a radiopaque dye into the uterine cavity; determines patency of fallopian tubes and detects pathology in uterine cavity.
   3. *Breast biopsy*—needle aspiration or incisional removal of breast tissue for microscopic examination; utilized to differentiate between benign tumors, cysts, and malignant tumors in the breast tissue.
   4. *Cervical biopsy and cauterization*—removal of cervical tissue for microscopic examination and cautery to control bleeding or obtain additional tissue samples.

G. Procedures evaluating the neuroendocrine system:
   1. *Radioactive iodine uptake test (iodine 131 uptake)*—ingestion of a tracer dose of ^{131}I followed in 24 hours by a scan of the thyroid for amount of radioactivity emitted.
      a. High uptake indicates hyperthyroidism.
      b. Low uptake indicates hypothyroidism.
   2. *Eight-hour intravenous ACTH test*—administration of 25 units of ACTH in 500 ml of saline over an eight-hour period.
      a. Utilized to determine function of adrenal cortex.
      b. 24-hour urine specimens are collected before and after administration for measurement of 17-ketosteroids and 17-hydroxycorticosteroids.
      c. In Addison's disease, urinary output of steroids does not increase following administration of ACTH; normally steroid excretion increases three- to fivefold following ACTH stimulation.
      d. In Cushing's syndrome, hyperactivity of the adrenal cortex increases the urine output of steroids tenfold in the second urine specimen.
   3. *Cerebral angiography*—fluoroscopic visualization of the brain vasculature after injection of a contrast medium into the carotid or vertebral arteries; utilized to localize lesions (tumors, abscesses, intracranial hemorrhages, and occlusions) that are large enough to distort cerebral vascular blood flow.
   4. Air studies:
      a. *Pneumoencephalogram*—withdrawal of CSF and injection of air or oxygen into the spinal subarachnoid space by means of a lumbar puncture; used to visualize the ventricles and subarachnoid spaces of the brain; may also be used to relieve intractable headache or to diagnose degenerative cerebral atrophy and massive tumors.
      b. *Ventriculogram*—withdrawal of CSF and injection of air or oxygen directly into the lateral ventricles through a needle thrust through the brain and into the ventricle; utilized to visualize the patency of the ventricular system, localize brain tumors, and detect cerebral anomalies such as atrophy.
      c. Specific *nursing responsibilities* following air studies—
         (1) Position patient flat in bed for at least 12 hours.
         (2) Observe for signs of increased intracranial pressure, shock, prolonged headache, or vomiting.
         (3) Turn from side to side every two hours

to hasten passage of air from ventricles.
    (4) Apply ice cap to head intermittently.
5. *Myelogram*—through a lumbar-puncture needle, a contrast medium is injected into the subarachnoid space of the spinal column to visualize the spinal cord; utilized to detect herniated or ruptured intervertebral disks, tumors, or cysts that compress or distort spinal cord.
6. *Brain scan*—intravenous injection of a radioactive substance followed by a scan for emission of radioactivity.

    a. Increased radioactivity at site of pathology.
    b. Utilized to detect brain tumors, abscesses, hematomas, and arteriovenous malformations.
7. *Lumbar puncture*—puncture of the lumbar subarachnoid space of the spinal cord with a needle to withdraw samples of cerebrospinal fluid (CSF); utilized to determine intracranial pressures, to evaluate CSF for infections, and to determine presence of hemorrhage.

Appendix D/DRUGS

TABLE OF COMMON DRUGS

Drug and dosage	Use	Action
1. ADRENERGIC DRUGS		
a. Epinephrine (Adrenalin), Isoproterenol (Isuprel) HCl, levarterenol bitartrate (Levophed), and metaraminol (Aramine)	Stokes-Adams disease, cardiac arrest, paroxysmal atrial tachycardia, neurogenic hypotension and shock, cardiogenic shock following MI, and circulatory collapse	Increases rate and strength of heart beat and causes arterial and venous constriction
b. Epinephrine—inhalation of 0.3 mg; isoproterenol SO_4—inhalation of 0.125 mg	Acute and chronic asthmatic states, pulmonary emphysema, and chronic bronchitis and bronchiectasis	Stimulates beta II receptors in smooth muscle of bronchi, resulting in relaxation and dilatation of bronchi
2. ADRENOCORTICAL STEROIDS		
a. Cortisone acetate—po or IM, 20–100 mg qd in single or divided doses	Adrenocortical insufficiency, rheumatoid arthritis, allergic diseases and reactions, ulcerative colitis, and nephrosis	Anti-inflammatory effect of unknown action, promotes fat storage and utilization of glucose during stress, and increases K^+ and Ca^{++} excretion and Na^+ retention.
b. Desoxycorticosterone acetate (hydrocortisone)—IM, 1–5 mg	Addison's disease, extensive burns, surgical shock, and adrenal surgery	Promotes reabsorption of sodium and restores plasma volume, BP, and electrolyte balance in adrenal cortical insufficiency
c. Dexamethasone (Decadron)—po, 0.5–5 mg qd; IM or IV, 4–20 mg qd	Addison's disease, allergic reactions, leukemia, Hodgkin's disease, iritis, dermatitis, and rheumatoid arthritis	Anti-inflammatory effect and less sodium and water retention
d. Prednisone—po, 2.5–15 mg qd	Rheumatoid arthritis and cancer therapy	Anti-inflammatory effect of unknown action and decreased sodium and water retention
3. ANALGESICS		
a. Aspirin or acetylsalicylic acid—po or R, 0.3–0.6 g	Minor aches and pains, fever of colds and influenza, rheumatic fever, rheumatoid arthritis, and anticoagulant therapy	Selectively depresses subcortical levels of CNS
b. Meperidine HCl (Demerol)—po or IM, 50–100 mg q3–4h	Pain due to trauma or surgery and allay apprehension prior to surgery	Acts on CNS to produce analgesia, sedation, euphoria, and respiratory depression

Assessment: side effects	*Nursing implications*
Palpitations, pallor, headache, hypertension, anxiety, insomnia, dilated pupils, nausea, vomiting, and glycosuria	Constant monitoring of blood pressure, pulse, and CVP; check infusion site frequently for signs of leakage and infiltration—will cause tissue sloughing
see Epinephrine	Teach patient to use nebulizer properly; patient's lips should be held tightly around mouth piece before medicated mist is released
Moon facies, hirsutism, thinning of skin and striae, hypertension, menstrual irregularities, glaucoma, delayed healing, psychoses	Administer oral preparation pc and with snack at bedtime; administer deep IM into gluteal muscle (never deltoid—causes cutaneous atrophy); monitor vital signs; observe for euphoria, depression, and mania; promote skin care and activity to tolerance; salt-restricted diet, high in protein and KCl supplement; protect from injury
Edema, hypertension, pulmonary congestion, and hypokalemia	Adjust dietary salt with blood pressure readings, monitor vital signs, and weigh daily
see Cortisone acetate	Contraindicated in tuberculosis; *see Cortisone acetate for nursing care*
Insomnia and gastric distress	*see Cortisone acetate*
Erosive gastritis with bleeding, coryza, urticaria, nausea, vomiting, tinnitus, impaired hearing, and respiratory alkalosis	Administer with food or pc; observe for nasal, oral, or subcutaneous bleeding; push fluids; check Hct, Hb, and prothrombin times frequently
Palpitations, bradycardia, hypotension, nausea, vomiting, syncope, sweating, tremors, and convulsions	Check respiratory rate and depth before giving drug; administer IM, as subcutaneous administration is painful and can cause local irritation

(Continued)

TABLE OF COMMON DRUGS *(Continued)*

Drug and dosage	Use	Action
3. ANALGESICS (Continued)		
	Maternal use: Maternal relaxation may (a) slow labor or (b) speed up labor	Depresses CNS: maternal and fetal; allays apprehension, po peak action: 1–2 hours; IM peak action: first hour
c. Morphine SO_4—po, 8–20 mg; subq 8–15 mg; IV, 4–8 mg	Control pain and relieve fear, apprehension, and restlessness as in pulmonary edema	Depresses CNS reception of pain and ability to interpret stimuli; depresses respiratory center in medulla
	Maternal use: preeclampsia-eclampsia, uterine dysfunction, and pain relief	Increases cerebral blood flow, provides antihypertensive action, and CNS depressant
d. Pantopium (Pantopon)—po, subq, or IM, 5–20 mg	*Maternal use:* control pain and relieve fear and apprehension	Enhances sedative-analgesic effects of narcotics—used in place of morphine
e. Alphaprodine HCl (Nisentil)—subq, 40–60 g	*Maternal use:* control pain, especially during labor	Synthetic narcotic similar to meperidine (Demerol) HCl, subq peak action 1–2 hours, IV peak action first hour
f. Codeine—po or subq, 15–60 mg (gr ¼ to 1)	*Maternal use:* control pain; may be used during puerperium	Nonsynthetic narcotic analgesic
g. Oxycodone HCl (Percodan)—po, 3–20 mg; subq, 5 mg	*Maternal use:* control pain; may be used during puerperium; five to six times more potent than codeine	Less potent and addicting than morphine; for moderate pain: episiotomy, and "after pains"; peak action 1 hour
4. ANTACIDS		
a. Aluminum hydroxide gel (Amphojel)—po, 5–10 ml q2–4h or 1h pc	Gastric acidity, peptic ulcer, and phosphatic urinary calculi	Buffers HCl in gastric juices without interfering with electrolyte balance
b. Calcium carbonate (Titralac, Ducon)—po, 1–2 g taken with H_2O pc and hs	Peptic ulcer and chronic gastritis	Reduces hyperacidity
c. Aluminum hydroxide and magnesium trisilicate (Gelusil)—po, 5–30 ml pc and hs	Peptic acid gastritis, heartburn, and esophagitis	Neutralizes and absorbs excess acid
d. Magnesium and aluminum hydroxides (Maalox suspension)—po, 5–30 ml pc and hs	Gastric hyperacidity, peptic ulcer, and heartburn	Neutralizes and binds acids
5. ANTIARRHYTHMICS		
a. Quinidine SO_4—po, 0.2–0.6 g q2h loading dose for 5 doses maintenance dose: 400–1000 mg tid-qid	Atrial fibrillation, PAT, ventricular tachycardia, and PVCs	Lengthens conduction time in atria and ventricles and blocks vagal stimulation of heart

Assessment: side effects	Nursing implications
As above; also, can depress fetus	Monitor maternal vital signs, contractions, progress of labor, and response to drug; monitor FHR; if delivery occurs during peak action, prepare to give narcotic antagonist to mother and/or neonate
Nausea, vomiting, flushing, confusion, urticaria, depressed rate and depth of respirations, and decreased blood pressure	Check rate and depth of respirations before administering drug; observe for gas pains and abdominal distention; smaller doses for aged; monitor vital signs; observe for postural hypotension
Respiratory and circulatory depression in mother and neonate, may depress contractions	Observe for level of sedation, respirations, arousability, and deep-tendon reflexes; give narcotic antagonist as necessary; check I & O, urinary retention possible
Addictive, may depress fetus	*see Meperidine HCl*
Addictive; may depress fetus, especially if used with barbiturate; respiratory depression; dizziness; sweating; nausea; vomiting; and restlessness	*see Meperidine HCl*
Of little use during labor; allergic response	Note patient's response to the medication
see Morphine SO₄	Administer per order and observe for effect
Constipation and fecal impaction	Shake well before administering; encourage fluids to prevent impaction and milk-alkali syndrome
None known	
Diarrhea and hypermagnesemia	Avoid prolonged administration to patients with renal insufficiency
Constipation and fecal impaction	Encourage fluid intake; contraindicated for debilitated patients or those with renal insufficiency
Nausea, vomiting, diarrhea, vertigo, tremor, headache, abdominal cramps, AV block, and cardiac arrest	Count pulse before administering; report changes in rate quality or rhythm; give drug with food; monitor BP daily

(Continued)

TABLE OF COMMON DRUGS   (Continued)

Drug and dosage	Use	Action
5. ANTIARRHYTHMICS (Continued)		
b. Procain amide HCl (Pronestyl)—po, IM 500–1000 mg 4–6 times qd; IV, 1 g	Atrial and ventricular arrhythmias, PVCs, overdose of digitalis, and general anesthesia	Depresses myocardium and lengthens conduction time between atria and ventricles
c. Lidocaine HCl—IV or 50–100 mg bolus	Ventricular tachycardia, and PVCs	Depresses myocardial response to abnormally generated impulses
6. ANTIBIOTICS		
a. Dia-mer-sulfonamides (Sulfonamides duplex), sulfisoxazole (Gantrisin), sulfamethizole (Thiosulfil), and sulfisomidine (Elkosin)	Acute, chronic, and recurrent urinary tract infections	Bacteriostatic and bactericidal
b. Penicillin—Penicillin G, Penicillin G Potassium, and Penicillin G Procaine	*Streptococcus, Staphylococcus, Pneumococcus, Gonococcus,* and *Treponema pallidum*	Primarily bactericidal
c. Tetracyclines: chlortetracycline (Aureomycin), doxycyline (Vibramycin hyclate), oxytetracycline (Terramycin), and tetracycline HCl (Sumycin)	Wide spectrum antibiotic	Primarily bacteriostatic
7. ANTICHOLINERGICS		
a. Atropine SO_4—0.3–1.2 mg po, subq, IM, or IV; ophthalmic 0.5%–1% up to 6 times qd	Peptic ulcer, spasms of GI tract, Stokes-Adams syndrome, and control excessive secretions during surgery	Blocks parasympathomimetic effects of acetylcholine on effector organs
b. Tincture of belladonna—0.3–0.6 ml tid	Hypermobility of stomach and bowel, biliary and renal colic, and prostatitis	Blocks parasympathomimetic effects of acetylcholine
c. Propantheline bromide (Pro-Banthine)—po, 15 mg qid; IM or IV, 30 mg	Decreases hypertonicity and hypersecretion of GI tract, ulcerative colitis, and peptic ulcer	Blocks neural transmission at ganglia of autonomic nervous system and at parasympathetic effector organs
8. ANTICOAGULANTS		
a. Heparin—initial dose: 30,000 units	Acute thromboembolic emergencies	Prevents thrombin formation
b. Warfarin sodium (Coumadin)—initial dose: po, 40–60 mg; po, 20–30 mg elderly; maintenance dose: po, 5–10 mg qd	Venous thrombosis, atrial fibrillation with embolization, and pulmonary emboli myocardial infarction	Depresses liver synthesis of prothrombin and factors VII, IX, and X

Assessment: side effects	Nursing implications
Polyarthralgia, fever, chills, urticaria, nausea, vomiting, psychoses, and rapid decrease in BP	Check pulse rate before administering; monitor heart action during IV administration
Drowsiness, dizziness, nervousness, confusion, and paresthesias	Check apical and radial pulses for deficits; observe for signs of toxicity; monitor ECG for prolongation of PR interval
Nausea, vomiting, oliguria, anuria, anemia, leukopenia, dizziness, jaundice, and skin rashes	Maintenance of blood levels very important; encourage fluids to prevent crystal formation in kidney tubules—push up to 3000 ml/day
Dermatitis and delayed or immediate anaphylaxis	Outpatients should be observed for 20 minutes postinjection; hospitalized patients should be observed at frequent intervals for 20 minutes after injection
GI upsets as diarrhea, nausea, and vomiting; sore throat; black hairy tongue; glossitis; and inflammatory lesions in anogenital region	Phototoxic reactions have been reported; patients should be advised to stay out of direct sunlight and medication should not be given with milk or snacks, as food interferes with absorption of tetracyclines
Dry mouth, dysphagic rash, skin flushing, urinary retention; *Contraindications:* glaucoma and paralytic ileus	Observe for postural hypotension in ambulating patients; administer cautiously in aged; and monitor vital signs for pulse and respiratory rate changes
Dry mouth, thirst, dilated pupils, skin flushing, elevated temperature, and delirium	Administer 30 to 60 minutes before meals; observe for side effects; Physostigmine salicylate is antidote
Nausea, gastric fullness, constipation, and mydriasis	Give before meals; observe urinary output to avoid retention, particularly in elderly; mouth care pc will relieve dryness; and contraindicated in presence of glaucoma
Hematuria, bleeding gums, and ecchymosis	Observe clotting times—should be between 20–30 minutes; heparin antagonist is protamine sulfate
Minor or major hemorrhage, alopecia, fever, nausea, diarrhea, and dermatitis	Drug effects last three to four days; antagonist is vitamin K

(Continued)

742   APPENDICES

TABLE OF COMMON DRUGS   (*Continued*)

Drug and dosage	Use	Action
9. ANTICONVULSANTS		
a. Phenytoin, or diphenylhydantoin (Dilantin) SO_4—po, 30–100 mg 3–4 times qd; IM, 100–200 mg 3–4 times qd; IV, 150–250 mg	Psychomotor epilepsy, convulsive seizures, and ventricular arrhythmias	Depresses motor cortex by preventing spread of abnormal electrical impulses
b. Valium (diazepam)—po, 2–10 mg bid-qid; IM or IV, 5–10 mg	All types of seizures	Induces calming effect on limbic system, thalamus, and hypothalamus
c. Magnesium sulfate.		
10. ANTIDIARRHEALS		
a. Paregoric or camphorated opium tincture—5–10 ml q2h, not more than qid	Diarrhea	Acts directly on intestinal smooth muscle to increase tone and decrease propulsive peristalsis
b. Kaolin with pectin (Kaopectate)—adults: po, 60–120 ml after each BM; children: over 12, po, 60 ml; 6–12, po, 30–60 ml; 3–6, po, 15–30 ml after each BM	Diarrhea	Reported to absorb irritants and soothe intestinal muscle; usefulness of mixture supported by tradition rather than controlled studies
c. Diphenoxylate HCl with atropine sulfate (Lomotil)—po, 5–10 mg tid-qid	Diarrhea	Increases intestinal tone and decreases propulsive peristalsis
11. ANTIEMETICS		
a. Trimethobenzamide HCl (Tigan)—25 mg qid, po, IM, R	Prevention and treatment of nausea and vomiting	Suppresses chemoreceptors in the trigger zone located in the medulla oblongata
b. Prochlorperazine dimaleate (Compazine)—5–30 mg qid po, IM, R	Control of nausea, vomiting and retching	Suppresses chemoreceptors in trigger zone and diminishes some motor activity
12. ANTIHISTAMINES		
a. Diphenhydramine HCl (Benadryl)—po, 25–50 mg tid-qid; IM or IV, 10–50 mg q4–6h	Allergic and pyrogenic reactions to blood transfusions and penicillin; motion sickness; radiation sickness; hay fever; and Parkinson's disease	Inhibits action of histamine on receptor cells and decreases action of acetylcholine

Assessment: side effects	Nursing implications
Nervousness, ataxia, gastric distress, nystagmus, slurred speech, hallucinations, and gingival hyperplasia	Give with meals or pc; frequent and diligent mouth care; advise patient that urine may turn pink to red-brown; teach patient signs of adverse reactions
Drowsiness, ataxia, and paradoxical increase in excitability of CNS	IV may cause phlebitis; inject IM deeply into tissue; give IV injection very slowly, as respiratory arrest can occur
Occasional nausea; prolonged use may produce dependence	Contains approximately 1.6 mg morphine or 16 mg opium and is subject to Federal Narcotics Regulations; administer with partial glass of water to facilitate passage into stomach; observe number and consistency of stools—discontinue drug as soon as diarrhea is controlled; keep in tight, light-resistant bottles
Granuloma of the stomach	Do not administer for more than two days, in presence of fever, or to children less than 3 years of age
Rash, drowsiness, dizziness, depression, abdominal distention, headache, blurred vision, and nausea	May potentiate action of barbiturates, opiates, and other depressants; closely observe patients receiving these drugs and administer narcotic antagonists such as levallorphan (Lorfan) tartrate, naloxone HCl (Narcan), and nalorphine (Nalline) HCl as ordered; administer cautiously to patients with hepatic dysfunction—may precipitate hepatic coma
Drowsiness, vertigo, diarrhea, headache, hypotension, jaundice, blurred vision, and rigid muscles	Inject deeply into a large muscle to prevent escape of solution; can cause edema, pain, and burning
Drowsiness, orthostatic hypotension, palpitations, blurred vision, diplopia, and headache	Use cautiously in children, pregnant women, and patients with liver disease
Sedation, dizziness, inability to concentrate, headache, anorexia, dermatitis, nausea, diplopia, and insomnia	Avoid use in newborn or premature infants and patients with glaucoma; supervise ambulation; caution against driving or operating mechanical devices that require alertness

(Continued)

TABLE OF COMMON DRUGS   (Continued)

Drug and dosage	Use	Action
12. ANTIHISTAMINES *(Continued)*		
b. Chlorpheniramine maleate (Chlor-Trimeton)—po, 2–4 mg tid-qid; subq, IM, or IV, 10–20 mg	Asthma, hay fever, serum reactions, and anaphylaxis	Inhibits action of histamine
c. Tripelennamine HCl (Pyribenzamine)—po, 25–50 mg bid-qid; IV or IM, 25 mg	Asthma, hay fever, pruritus, and motion sickness	Inhibits histamine and promotes sedation
13. ANTIHYPERLIPEMIAS		
a. Cholestyramine resin (Questran)—po, 4 g packet tid ac	Reduction of blood cholesterol	Binds bile acids in the intestine and prevents their reabsorption, thus reducing serum cholesterol 10%–20%
b. Clofibrate (Atromid-S)—po, 500 mg qid	Endogenous hyperlipemias	Inhibits hepatic synthesis of triglycerides, phospholipids, and cholesterol; also decreases platelet adhesiveness and displaces various plasma proteins
14. ANTIHYPERTENSIVES		
a. Reserpine (Serpasil)—po, 0.25 mg qd	Mild and moderate hypertension	Depletes catecholamines and decreases peripheral vasoconstriction, heart rate, and BP
	Maternal use: preeclampsia-eclampsia	CNS depressant, tranquilizer, sedation is major effect; decreases neural transmission to nerves; decreases tone in blood vessels
b. Guanethidine SO$_4$ (Ismelin)—po, 10–150 mg qd in divided doses	Severe to moderately severe hypertension	Blocks norepinephrine at postganglionic synapses
c. Methyldopa (Aldomet)—po, 500 mg–2 g qd in divided doses	Severe to moderately severe hypertension	Inhibits formation of dopamine, a precursor of norepinephrine
d. Hydralazine HCl (Apresoline)—po, 10–50 mg qid	Moderate hypertension	Dilates peripheral blood vessels
	Maternal use: preeclampsia-eclampsia	Relaxes peripheral blood vessels (opens vascular bed—physiologic dehydration)
e. Pentolinium (Ansolysen) tartrate—po, 60–600 mg qd in divided doses	Malignant hypertension, and hypertensive crisis	Blocks sympathetic stimulation at ganglion; dilates peripheral vasculature; very potent

Assessment: side effects	Nursing implications
Nausea, gastritis, diarrhea, headache, dryness of mouth and nose, nervousness, and irritability	Parenteral administration may drop blood pressure; administer slowly, observing for side effects; caution patient about drowsiness
Dry mouth, vertigo, headache, nervousness, frequency, and blood dyscrasia	Blurred vision and drowsiness; caution patient about driving or handling mechanical equipment that requires alertness
Mild nausea and constipation; occasionally epigastric distress and diarrhea	Administer vitamin A, D, and K (fat-soluble vitamins) to supplement deficiencies due to decreased absorption; give drugs such as digitalis, chlorothiazide, thyroid, iron, or warfarin sodium one hour before or four hours after cholestyramine resin (Questran) (drug may also absorb other drugs given concomitantly)
Urticaria, stomatitis, pruritus, leukopenia, nausea, elevation of SGOT and SGPT activity, and weight gain	Contraindicated in pregnancy, lactation, renal and hepatic impairment, and in children; administer reduced dose of warfarin (Coumadin) sodium and monitor prothrombin times of patients on anticoagulant therapy
Depression, nasal stuffiness, increased gastric secretions, rash, and pruritus	Watch for signs of mental depression; closely monitor pulse rates of patients also receiving digitalis
Low level of toxicity; nasal stuffiness; weight gain; diarrhea; allergic reactions—dry mouth, itching, skin eruptions	Siderails up; must not stand up without assistance; observe carefully; and monitor B/P
Orthostatic hypotension, diarrhea, and inhibition of ejaculation	Postural hypotension is marked in the morning and is accentuated by hot weather, alcohol, and exercise; teach to rise slowly.
Initial drowsiness, depression with feelings of unreality, edema, jaundice, and dry mouth	Contraindicated in active and chronic liver disease; encourage not to drive car if drowsy
Palpitations, tachycardia, angina pectoris, tremors, and depression	Encourage moderation in exercise and identification of stressful stimuli
Headache, heart palpitation, gastric irritation, coronary insufficiency, edema, chills, fever, and severe depression	Siderails up; must not stand up without assistance; may be given with diuretics; observe carefully; IM route only; and monitor BP
Orthostatic hypotension, diarrhea, and inhibition of ejaculation	Teach to rise slowly

(Continued)

TABLE OF COMMON DRUGS *(Continued)*

Drug and dosage	*Use*	*Action*
15. ANTILACTOGENICS		
a. Diethylstilbestrol (DES)—po or IM, 0.2–5.0 mg qd; vaginal supp 0.1–0.5 mg hs	*Maternal use:* synthetic estrogen to control postpartum breast engorgement, menopausal symptoms, and osteoporosis pain of mammary carcinoma	Functions as natural estrogen in its effect on pituitary, ovaries, myometrium, endometrium, and other tissues
b. Deladumone (testosterone enanthate and estradiol valerate)—IM, 200 mg xI	*Maternal use:* suppresses lactation; prevents breast engorgement when given immediately after delivery	Depresses production of lactogenic hormone by posterior pituitary
c. Testosterone cypionate—IM, 100 mg	*Maternal use:* suppresses lactation; treatment for breast engorgement; palliative therapy for breast cancer and menopausal symptoms	*see Deladumone*
16. BRONCHODILATORS		
a. Aminophylline—po, 250 mg, bid-qid; R, 250–500 mg; IV, 250–500 mg over 10–20 min	Rapid relief of bronchospasm; asthma; and pulmonary edema	Relaxes smooth muscles and increases cardiac contractility; interferes with reabsorption of Na^+ and Cl^- in proximal tubules
b. Ephedrine SO_4—po, subq, or IM, 25 mg tid-qid	Asthma, allergies, bradycardia, and nasal decongestant	Relaxes hypertonic muscles in bronchioles and GI tract
c. Isoproterenol HCl (Isuprel)—inhalation of 1:100 or 1:200 sol	Mild to moderately severe asthma attack, bronchitis, and pulmonary emphysema	Relaxes hypertonic bronchioles
17. CARDIAC GLYCOSIDES		
a. Digitoxin—digitalizing dose: po, 1.2–1.5 mg; IM or IV, 1.2 mg; maintenance dose: po, 1.2 mg qd	Congestive heart failure, atrial fibrillation and flutter, and supraventricular tachycardia	Increases force of cardiac contractility, slows heart rate, decreases right atrial pressures, and promotes diuresis
b. Digoxin—digitalizing dose: po, 1.5–3.0 mg; IM or IV, 0.75–1 mg; maintenance dose: po, 0.25–0.75 mg qd	*see Digitoxin for Use, Action, Side effects, and Nursing implications*	
c. Lanatoside C (Cedilanid)—digitalizing dose: po, 6 mg; maintenance dose: po, 1 mg qd	*see Digitoxin for Use, Action, Side effects, and Nursing implications*	
d. Deslanoside (Cedilanid D)—digitalizing dose: IV or IM, 1.2–1.8 mg	*see Digitoxin for Use, Action, Side effects, and Nursing implications*	
e. Ouabain—digitalizing dose: IV or IM, 0.25–0.5 mg	*See Digitoxin for Use, Action, Side effects, and Nursing implications*	
f. Digitalis	*Maternal use:* cardiac decompensation	Increases force (efficiency) of cardiac contractions; promotes diuresis; indicated by signs-symptoms of cardiac failure

Assessment: side effects	Nursing implications
Anorexia, nausea, vomiting, diarrhea, dizziness, and fainting—many side effects with long-term usage	Administer as ordered; observe for side effects; never give if woman is pregnant—predisposes to vaginal cancer in female offspring at puberty
Rare, following one dose; masculinization and electrolyte imbalance following long-term therapy	Administer as ordered; observe for side effects
see Deladumone	Administer as ordered; observe for side effects
Nausea, vomiting, cardiac arrhythmias, intestinal bleeding, insomnia, and restlessness	Give oral with or after meals; monitor vital signs for changes in BP and pulse; and weigh daily
Wakefulness, nervousness, dizziness, palpitations, and hypertension	Monitor vital signs; avoid giving dose near bed time; check urine output in older adults
Nervousness, tachycardia, hypertension, and insomnia	Monitor vital signs before and after treatment; teach patient how to use nebulizer
Arrhythmias; nausea; vomiting; anorexia; malaise; color vision, yellow or blue	Hold medication if pulse rate less than 60 or over 120; encourage juices high in potassium, such as orange juice; and observe for signs of electrolyte depletion, apathy, disorientation, and anorexia
Symptoms of toxicity: slow pulse, nausea, headache, and malaise	Observe for toxicity; observe for improvement in symptoms

(Continued)

TABLE OF COMMON DRUGS *(Continued)*

Drug and dosage	Use	Action
18. CHOLINERGIC DRUGS		
a. Bethanechol Cl (Urecholine)—po, 5–30 mg; subq, 2.5–5 mg; neostigmine Br (Prostigmin)—po, 10–30 mg; IM or subq, 0.25–1 mg	Postoperative abdominal atony and distention; for bladder atony or for bringing on micturition; postsurgical or postpartum urinary retention	Increased tone and motility of GI musculature; increased bladder tone and decreased sphincter tone
19. CHOLINERGIC MIOTICS		
a. Pilocarpine HCl—0.1 ml of 0.5%–4% sol; 1–6 times qd; physostigmine salicylate (Eserine)—0.1 ml of 0.25–1% sol not more than qid	Wide-angle glaucoma	Contraction of the sphincter muscle of iris resulting in miosis
20. CNS STIMULANTS		
a. Amphetamine SO_4—po, 5–10 mg od-tid; IM or IV, 10–30 mg	Mild depressive states, childhood neuroses, narcolepsy, postencephalitic parkinsonism, and obesity control	Raises blood pressure, decreases sense of fatigue, and elevation of mood
b. Pentylenetetrazol (Metrazol)—IV, 5 ml of 10% sol; po, 200 mg tid	Overdose of barbiturates	Respiratory stimulation
21. DIURETICS		
a. Thiazides (Diuril, HydroDiuril, and Esidrix)—po, 0.5–1 g qd.	Edema, congestive heart failure, Na^+ retention in steroid therapy, hypertension	Inhibits sodium chloride and water reabsorption in the proximal tubules of the kidneys
	Maternal use: preeclampsia-eclampsia	Decrease fluid retention, eliminate Na^+, control BP, and no acidosis
b. Spironolactone (Aldactone)—po, 25 mg bid-qid	Cirrhosis of liver and when other diuretics are ineffective	Inhibits effects of aldosterone in distal tubules of kidney
c. Furosemide (Lasix)—po, 40–80 mg qd in divided doses	Edema and associated heart failure, cirrhosis, renal disease, nephrotic syndrome, and hypertension	Inhibits Na^+ and water reabsorption in ascending Loop of Henle and distal renal tubule
d. Ethacrynic acid (Edecrin)—po, 50–200 mg qd in divided doses	Pulmonary edema, ascites, edema of congestive heart failure	Inhibits the reabsorption of Na^+ in the ascending Loop of Henle
e. Meralluride (Mercuhydrin)—IM, 1–2 ml; mercaptomerin (Thiomerin)—IM, 1–2 ml; mercurophylline (Mercuzanthin)—IM, 1–2 ml	Acute edematous states	Enhances sodium excretion in proximal renal tubules

Assessment: side effects	Nursing implications
Heartburn, belching, abdominal cramps, diarrhea, nausea, and vomiting, incontinence, profuse sweating, and salivation	Warn patient of some discomforting side effects; have urinal or bedpan close at hand and answer calls quickly; atropine SO_4 is the antidote for cholinergic drugs
Browache, headache, ocular pain, blurring and dimness of vision, allergic conjunctivitis, nausea, vomiting, and profuse sweating	Let patient know that initially the medication may be irritating; teach proper technique for instilling eye drops—all equipment for instilling eye drops should be kept sterile, discard cloudy solutions
Restlessness, dizziness, tremors, insomnia, increased libido, suicidal and homicidal tendency, palpitations, and angina pain	Avoid administering drug after 4 PM; dependence on drug may develop; and contraindicated with MAO inhibitors, hyperthyroidism, and psychotic states
Convulsion and vomiting	Observe for hypoxia, muscular twitching, and convulsions
Hypokalemia, nausea, vomiting, diarrhea, dizziness, and paresthesias; may accentuate diabetes	Watch for muscle weakness; give well-diluted potassium chloride supplement; monitor urine for changes in S and A
All diuretics must be used with caution since they produce fluid-electrolyte imbalance in mother-fetus; may cause allergic reaction	Weigh daily, accurate I & O, assess edema, and replace electrolytes per order; less electrolyte imbalance with proper precautions (replace K^+ with orange juice, banana, etc.)
Headache, lethargy, diarrhea, ataxia, skin rash, gynecomastia	Potassium-sparing drug; *do not* give supplemental KCl; monitor for signs of electrolyte imbalance
Dermatitis, pruritus, paresthesia, blurring of vision, postural hypotension, nausea, vomiting, and diarrhea	Assess for weakness, lethargy, leg cramps, anorexia; peak action in 1 to 2 hours; duration 6 to 8 hours; do not give at bed time; supplementary KCl indicated; may induce digitalis toxicity
Nausea, vomiting, diarrhea, hypokalemia, hypotension, gout, dehydration, deafness, and metabolic acidosis	Assess for dehydration—skin turgor, neck veins; hypotension; KCl supplement
Metabolic alkalosis due to hypochloremia or bone marrow depression	Closely observe urine output—mercurial salts may cause tubular necrosis and renal failure; watch for signs of chloride depletion—apathy, somnolence, weakness, and disorientation

(Continued)

TABLE OF COMMON DRUGS *(Continued)*

Drug and dosage	Use	Action
21. DIURETICS *(Continued)*		
f. Osmotic diuretic 30% urea, 10% invert sugar, 20% mannitol	Cerebral edema	Hypertonic solution that kidney tubules cannot reabsorb and thus causes obligatory water loss
g. Acetazolamide (Diamox)	*Maternal use:* preeclampsia-eclampsia	Potent diuretic; produces acidosis; self-limiting effect
h. Ammonium Cl	*Maternal use:* preeclampsia-eclampsia	Promotes Na^+ excretion; may lead to acidosis; self-limiting effect
22. ENZYMES		
a. Chymotrypsin (Chymar)—po, 50,000–100,000 U qid; IM 0.5–1.0 ml qd	Inflammatory edema, hematomas from traumatic injuries	Accelerates healing by removing fibrinlike material which blocks capillaries and lymphatics
b. Pancreatin N.F.—po, 0.5–1.0 g	Pancreatic deficiencies, sprue, chronic pancreatitis, and cystic fibrosis	Contains pancreatic enzyme, amylase, lipase, and trypsin needed for amino acid digestion
23. EXPECTORANTS		
a. Ammonium Cl—po, 300 mg	Stimulate secretory activity of respiratory tract; diuretic	NH_4 ions cause gastric irritation, which reflexly stimulates respiratory tract secretions
b. Ipecac—po, 0.5–1 ml, for cough; po, 15–30 ml for emesis	Bronchitis, bronchiectasis, emergency emetic for poison ingestion	*see Ammonium Cl*
c. Potassium iodide—po, 300 mg tid-qid	Bronchial asthma, bronchitis, actinomycosis, blastomycosis, and sporotrichosis	Reduces viscosity of bronchial secretions by stimulating flow of respiratory tract fluids
d. Terpin hydrate—po 5–10 ml q3–4h	Bronchitis, emphysema	Liquifies bronchial secretions
24. HORMONES		
a. Testosterone—po, 5–10 mg qd; IM 25 mg bid	Replacement therapy in hypogonadism, eunuchism, climacteric impotence, and advanced cancer of breast	Promotes Na^+ and H_2O retention, primary and secondary male sex characteristics; counteracts excessive amounts of estrogen
b. Progesterone—subq or IM, 5–30 mg qd; subling, 10–25 mg	*Maternal use:* amenorrhea, dysmenorrhea, endometriosis, and habitual abortion	Converts endometrium into secreting structure, prevents ovulation, stimulates growth of mammary tissue
c. Estradiol—po, 0.2–0.5 mg od-tid; IM, 0.5–1.5 mg bid-tid	*Maternal use:* menopausal symptoms, osteoporosis, hypogenitalism, sexual infantilism, postpartum breast engorgement	Inhibits release of pituitary gonadotropins; promotes growth of female genital tissues
d. Methallenestril (Vallestril), estrogen—po, 0.2–5 mg qd	*Maternal use:* similar to DES and Tace; advantage: ease of administration and cost	Antilactogenic; suppresses production of lactogenic hormone from posterior pituitary

Assessment: side effects	Nursing implications
Electrolyte depletion symptomatology—lassitude, apathy, decreased urinary output, and mental confusion; may be fetotoxic	Weigh daily; I & O; assess edema; give early in day to allow sleep at night; observe for side effects; replace electrolytes as ordered
see Acetazolamide	see Acetazolamide
Pain, local edema, urticaria, allergic reactions	Institute hypersensitivity test before administration
None, used for differences in normal enzymes	Administer with meals
Nausea, vomiting, and bradycardia	Monitor respirations; keep IV record to avoid dehydration and metabolic acidosis
Violent emesis, tachycardia, decreased BP, and dyspnea	Contraindicated in liver and renal disease; if given for emesis, follow dose with as much water as patient will drink
Sore mouth, throat, conjunctivitis, headache, mental depression, ataxia, fever, and sexual impotence	Administer diluted in milk or juice to decrease gastric irritation; observe for side effects and teach patient signs
Nausea, vomiting, and gastric irritation	Administer undiluted; push fluids
Nausea; dyspepsia; masculinization; hypercalcemia; menstrual irregularities; renal calculi; and Na^+, K^+, and H_2O retention	Observe for edema; weigh daily; I & O; push fluids for bedridden patients to prevent renal calculi
Nausea, vomiting, dizziness, edema, headache, protein metabolism	Administer deep IM and rotate sites; weigh daily to ascertain fluid retention
Anorexia, nausea, vomiting, diarrhea, fluid retention, and mental depression	Weigh daily; encourage frequent physical check-ups
see Diethylstilbestrol, under Antilactogenics; rare with dosage given for antilactogenic effect	Administer as ordered; observe for side effects

(Continued)

TABLE OF COMMON DRUGS *(Continued)*

Drug and dosage	Use	Action
24. HORMONES *(Continued)*		
e. Chlorotrianisene (Tace), estrogen—po, 12–50 mg qd	*Maternal use:* suppresses lactation	*see Methallenestril*
f. Medroxyprogesterone (Provera)—po, 2.5–10 mg tabs	*Maternal use:* For amenorrhea, functional uterine bleeding, and threatened abortion and dysmenorrhea	Similar to progesterone but can be taken orally
g. Hydroxyprogesterone caproate (Delalutin)—IM, 250 mg/2 ml q4 wks	*Maternal use:* For menstrual disorders and ovarian and uterine dysfunction	Synthetic derivative of progesterone but has a longer duration of action if given by parenteral route
h. Menotropins (Pergonal)—IM, 9–12 days, followed by 1 10,000 U HCG	*Maternal use:* purified preparation of gonadotropic hormones extracted from urine of postmenopausal women; treatment of secondary anovulation	Induces ovulation
25. NARCOTIC ANTAGONISTS		
a. Levallorphan (Lorfan) tartrate	*Maternal use:* reverses respiratory depression in mother and/or neonate	Weak narcotic that competes with strong narcotics for CNS receptor sites; relieves narcotic-induced respiratory depression without altering analgesic effect; may be given with a narcotic; does *not* relieve depression from other drugs or causes
b. Nalorphine (Nalline) HCl	*See Levallorphan;* for treatment of narcotic addiction, refer to pharmacology text	*see Levallorphan tartrate*
c. Naloxone (Narcan) HCl	*Maternal use:* reverses respiratory depression in mother and/or neonate	Reverses respiratory depression of morphine SO_4, meperidine HCl, and methadone HCl; does not cause respiratory depression, sedation, or analgesia itself
26. SEDATIVES AND HYPNOTICS		
a. Chloral hydrate—po, 250 mg tid; hypnotic: po, 0.5–1.0 g; R supp, 0.3–0.9 g	Sedation for elderly; delirium tremens, pruritus, mania, and barbiturate and alcohol withdrawal	Depresses sensorimotor areas of cerebral cortex
b. Phenobarbital Na—sedative: po, 20–30 mg tid; hypnotic: po, 100–300 mg; IV or IM, 100–200 mg butabarbital Na (Butisol); pentobarbital Na (Nembutal); and secobarbital Na (Seconal)	Preoperative sedation; emergency control of convulsions; petit mal epilepsy	Depresses central nervous system, promoting drowsiness
c. Chlordiazepoxide (Librium) HCl—po, 5–10 mg; IM or IV, 50–100 mg	Psychoneuroses, preoperative apprehension, chronic alcoholism, and anxiety	CNS depressant resulting in mild sedation, appetite stimulant, and anticonvulsant

Assessment: side effects	Nursing implications
Breast engorgement is common; side effects rare after one course of treatment	Administer as ordered; observe for side effects; initiate other measures for breast engorgement.
Drowsiness	Administer as ordered; teach patient regarding self-administration
Requires priming with estrogen; GI symptoms, headache, and allergy	Administer as ordered; observe for effect
Abortions occur in 25%; failure rate 55% to 80% of patients	Assist in collection of urine to assess estrogen levels; counsel regarding couple's need to have daily intercourse from day of HCG injection until ovulation
May cause respiratory depression if narcosis is due to causes other than a stronger narcotic	Note time, type of narcotic, dosage mother received, administer to mother or neonate, as ordered follow with other resuscitation prn
see Levallorphan tartrate	see Levallorphan tartrate
No known side effects	see Levallorphan tartrate
Nausea, vomiting gastritis; pinpoint pupils; delirium; rash; decreased BP, pulse, respirations, and temperature; hepatic damage	Caution—should not be taken in combination with alcohol; dependency is possible
Cough, hiccups, restlessness, pain, hangover, and CNS and circulatory depression	Observe for hypotension during IV administration; put up side rails on bed of older patients; observe for increased tolerance
Ataxia, fatigue, blurred vision, diplopia, lethargy, nightmares, and confusion	Ensure anxiety relief by allowing patient to verbalize feelings; advise patient to avoid driving and alcoholic beverages

(Continued)

TABLE OF COMMON DRUGS *(Continued)*

Drug and dosage	Use	Action
26. SEDATIVES AND HYPNOTICS *(Continued)*		
d. Hydroxyzine pamoate (Vistaril)—po, 25–100 mg qid	*see Chlordiazepoxide;* antiemetic in postoperative conditions	CNS relaxant with sedative effect on limbic system and thalamus
e. Meprobamate (Equanil, Miltown)—400 mg tid-qid	Anxiety, stress, and petit mal epilepsy	*see Hydroxyzine pamoate*
27. UTERINE CONTRACTANTS		
a. Oxytocin (Pitocin, Syntocinon)—IM, 0.3–1 ml; IV, 1 ml (10 U) in 1000 ml sol	Synthetic pituitrin of posterior pituitary; stimulates rhythmic contractions of uterus	(a) To induce labor, (b) to augment contractions, and (c) to prevent or control postpartum atony; and antidiuretic effect
b. Methylergonovine maleate (Methergine)—po, 0.2 mg; IV, (gr 1/320)	Primarily for control of postpartum hemorrhage	Stimulates stronger and longer contractions than Ergotrate
c. Ergonovine maleate (Ergotrate)—po, 0.2 mg (gr 1/320)	Rapid sustained action for control of postabortal or postpartum hemorrhage; promotes involution	Stimulates uterine contractions of three or more hours
28. VASODILATORS		
Nitroglycerin—subling, 0.3–0.6 mg prn	Angina pectoris	Directly relaxes smooth muscle, dilating blood vessels; lowers peripheral vascular resistance; and increases blood flow
b. Cyclandelate (Cyclospasmol)—po, 100–200 mg qid with meals and hs	Thrombophlebitis, intermittent claudication, frostbite, Raynaud's disease, and peripheral arteriosclerosis	Acts directly on smooth vascular muscle to relax it and enhance blood flow
c. Erythrityl tetranitrate (Cardilate)—po, 10 mg tid	Long-term treatment of angina pectoris	Acts directly to relax smooth muscle of coronary muscular; slow onset; long duration

Assessment: side effects	*Nursing implications*
Drowsiness, headache, itching, dry mouth, and tremor	Give deep IM only; potentiates action of warfarin (Coumadin) sodium, narcotics, and barbiturates
Voracious appetite, dryness of mouth, and ataxia	Older patients prone to drowsiness and hypotension, observe for jaundice
Avoid when (a) cervix is unripe, (b) CPD, (c) abruptio placentae, and (d) cardiovascular disease; tetanic contractions; FHR deceleration; uterine rupture; and cardiac arrhythmias	Monitor FHR, and contractions, maternal BP, and pulse; under physician's supervision, monitor and record IV, dosage in IV, and I & O (see discussion of water intoxication) postpartum: this oxytocic is drug of choice in presence of hypertension
Nausea, vomiting, transient hypertension, dizziness, and tachycardia	Do not give if mother is hypertensive; do not use if solution is discolored; and *do not use in labor*
Nausea and vomiting; occasional transient hypertension, especially if given IV	Store in cool place; monitor maternal BP and pulse; and *do not use in labor*
Faintness, throbbing headache, vomiting, flushing, hypotension, and visual disturbances	Instruct patient to sit or lie down when taking drug to reduce hypotensive effect; may take one to three doses at 5-minute intervals to relieve pain; up to ten per day may be allowed; if headache occurs instruct patient to expel tablet as soon as pain relief occurs; keep drug at bedside and on person; watch expiration dates and replace as needed—tablets lose potency with continued exposure to air and humidity; alcohol ingestion soon after taking nitroglycerine may produce shocklike syndrome due to sharp drop in blood pressure; advise patient not to smoke as nicotine has vasoconstrictive effect
Faintness, flushing, and hypotension	Administer with meals to reduce gastrointestinal symptoms or give with antacid; contraindicated in pregnancy, glaucoma, obliterative coronary artery disease or cerebrovascular disease, and in patients with bleeding tendencies
Faintness, dizziness, headache, hypotension, and skin flushing	Protect drug from light and exposure, as this reduces potency; *see Nitroglycerin*

CHEMOTHERAPY

Agent	Use	Action
ANTIMETABOLITES Cytosine arabinoside 6-Mercaptopurine Methotrexate	Acute leukemia	Inhibits DNA synthesis; metabolized by liver and excreted by kidneys
CORTICOSTEROIDS Prednisone Cortisone acetate Hydrocortisone	Leukemia, hypercalcemia, anemia, and reduction of CNS edema	*see Adrenocortical steroids*
ALKALATING AGENTS (Chlorambucil Cyclophosphamide)	Chronic leukemia, Hodgkin's disease, and lymphomas	Alter property of DNAs, nucleic acid, preventing mitosis
NATURAL PRODUCTS Doxorubicin hydrochloride Dactinomycin or actinomycin D (antibiotic) Vinblastine SO_4 Vincristine SO_4 Daunomycin (Daunorubicin) (antibiotic) BCG (Bacille Calmette-Guérin)	Sarcomas, Wilm's tumor, acute leukemia, lymphomas, neuroblastoma, and rhabdomyosarcoma	Proposed mechanism for action— inhibition of RNA and DNA
MISCELLANEOUS AGENTS Hydroxyurea Procarbazine HCl	Chronic leukemia, Hodgkin's disease, and sarcomas	Inhibits DNA synthesis; crosses blood-brain barrier, metabolized by liver, and excreted by kidneys

Side effects	*Nursing implications*
Causes nausea, vomiting, diarrhea, GI ulcers, stomatitis, photosensitivity, and alopecia	Antiemetics, good oral hygiene, bland diet, and way of coping with no hair (caps or wigs)
No acute toxicity; increased appetite, fluid retention; long-term effects include moon face, striae, trunk obesity, purpura, osteoporesis, muscle weakness, and psychosis; and possible hypertension, infection due to immunosuppression, gastric bleeding, and ulcers	Prepare patient and family for body changes and possible effects on behavior; avoid exposure to infection; avoid aspirin; and give medication with food or beverage to minimize gastric irritation
Nausea, vomiting, dermatitis, leukopenia, thrombocytopenia, and fever	Watch for signs and symptoms of infection and administer antiemetic
Nausea, vomiting, fever, stomatitis, anorexia, acne, alopecia, bone marrow depression, malaise, and diarrhea or neurotoxia with constipation and urinary retention	Good oral hygiene, bland diet, attractive meals in social atmosphere, antiemetic, and prepare child and parents for resulting hair loss
Nausea, vomiting, bone marrow depression, alopecia, rash, pruritus, GI toxicity	Antiemetic, bland diet, observe for infection, and prepare for loss of hair

COMPARISON CHART OF MAJOR SUBSTANCES USED FOR MIND ALTERATION

Official name of drug or chemical	*Slang name(s)*	*Usual single adult dose*	*Duration of action (hours)*	*Method of taking*	*Legitimate medical uses (present and projected)*	*Potential for psychological dependence**	*Potential for tolerance leading to increased dosage)*
Alcohol Whisky, gin, beer, wine	Booze, Hooch, Suds	1½ oz. gin or whiskey, 12 oz. beer	2–4	Swallowing liquid	Rare. Sometimes used as a sedative (for tension)	High	Yes
Caffeine Coffee, tea, Coca-Cola, No-Doz, APC	Java	1–2 cups, 1 bottle, 5 mg	2–4	Swallowing liquid	Mild stimulant. Treatment of some forms of coma	Moderate	Yes
Nicotine (and coal tar) Cigarettes, cigars	Fags, nails	1–2 cigarettes	1–2	Smoking (inhalation)	None (used as an insecticide)	High	Yes
Sedatives Alcohol—see above	Downers					High	Yes
Barbiturates Amytal Nembutal Seconal Phenobarbital	Barbs, blue devils, yellow jackets, dolls, red devils, phennies, goofers	50–100 mg	4	Swallowing pills or capsules	Treatment of insomnia and tension Induction of anesthesia		
Doriden (Glutethimids)		500 mg					
Chloral hydrate		500 mg					
Miltown, Equanil (Meprobamate)		400 mg					

Potential for physical dependence	Overall potential for abuse and toxicity**	Reasons drug is sought by users (drug effects and social factors)	Usual short-term effects (psychological, pharmacological, social)	Usual long-term effects (psychological, pharmacological, social)	Form of legal regulation and control††
Yes	High	To relax. To escape from tensions, problems and inhibitions. To get "high" (euphoria). Seeking manhood or rebelling (particularly those under 21). Social custom and conformity. Massive advertising and promotion. Ready availability.	CNS depressant. Relaxation (sedation). Euphoria. Drowsiness. Impaired judgment, reaction time, coordination and emotional control. Frequent aggressive behavior and driving accidents.	Diversion of energy and money from more creative and productive pursuits. Habituation. Possible obesity with chronic excessive use. Irreversible damage to brain and liver, addiction with severe withdrawal illness (D.T.s) with heavy use. Many deaths.	Available and advertised without limitation in many forms with only minimal regulation by age (21 or 18), hours of sale, location, taxation, ban on bootlegging and driving laws. Some "black market" for those under age and those evading taxes. Minimal penalties.
No	Very Minimal	For a "pick-up" or stimulation. "Taking a break." Social custom and low cost. Advertising. Ready availability.	CNS stimulant. Increased alertness. Reduction of fatigue.	Sometimes insomnia, restlessness, or gastric irritation. Habituation.	Available and advertised without limit with no regulation for children or adults.
No	High	For a "pick-up" or stimulation. "Taking a break." Social custom. Advertising. Ready availability.	CNS stimulant. Relaxation (or distraction) from the process of smoking.	Lung (and other) cancer, heart and blood vessel disease, cough, etc. Higher infant mortality. Many deaths. Habituation. Diversion of energy and money. Air pollution. Fire.	Available and advertised without limit with only minimal regulation by age, taxation, and labeling of packages.
Yes	High	To relax or sleep. To get "high" (euphoria). Widely prescribed by physicians, both for specific and nonspecific complaints. General climate encouraging taking pills for everything.	CNS depressants. Sleep induction. Relaxation (sedation). Sometimes euphoria. Drowsiness. Impaired judgment, reaction time, coordination and emotional control. Relief of anxiety/tension. Muscle relaxation.	Irritability, weight loss, addiction with severe withdrawal illness (like D.T.s). Diversion of energy and money. Habituation, addiction.	Available in large amounts by ordinary medical prescription which can be repeatedly refilled or can be obtained from more than one physician. Widely advertised and "detailed" to M.D.s and pharmacists. Other manufacture, sale or possession prohibited under federal drug abuse and similar state (dangerous) drug laws. Moderate penalties. Widespread illicit traffic.

(Continued)

COMPARISON CHART OF MAJOR SUBSTANCES USED FOR MIND ALTERATION (Continued)

Official name of drug or chemical	Slang name(s)	Usual single adult dose	Duration of action (hours)	Method of taking	Legitimate medical uses (present and projected)	Potential for psychological dependence*	Potential for tolerance leading to increased dosage)
Stimulants	Uppers					High	Yes
Caffeine—see above							
Nicotine—see above							
Amphetamines	Pep pills, wake-ups	2.5–15.0 mg	4	Swallowing pills, capsules or injecting in vein	Treatment of obesity, narcolepsy, fatigue, depression		
Benzedrine	Bennies, cartwheels						
Methedrine	Crystal, speed, meth						
Dexedrine	Dexies or Xmas trees (spansules)						
Preludin		25 mg					
Cocaine	Coke, snow	Variable		Sniffing or injecting	Anesthesia of the eye and throat		
Tranquilizers						Minimal	No
Librium (Chlordiaze-poxide)		5–25 mg	4–6	Swallowing pills or capsules	Treatment of anxiety, tension, alcoholism, neurosis, psychosis, psychosomatic disorders, and vomiting		
Phenothiazines							
Thorazine		10–50 mg					
Compazine		5–10 mg					
Stelazine		2–5 mg					
Reserpine (Rouwolfia)		.1–.25 mg					
Marijuana or Cannabis†	Pot, grass, tea, weed, stuff, hash, joint, reefers	Variable—1 cigarette or pipe, or 1 drink or cake (India)	4	Smoking (inhalation) Swallowing	Treatment of depression, tension, loss of appetite and high blood pressure	Moderate	No

Potential for physical dependence	Overall potential for abuse and toxicity**	Reasons drug is sought by users (drug effects and social factors)	Usual short-term effects (psychological, pharmacological, social)	Usual long-term effects (psychological, pharmacological, social)	Form of legal regulation and control††
No	High	For stimulation and relief of fatigue. To get "high" (euphoria). General climate encouraging taking pills for everything.	CNS stimulants. Increased alertness, reduction of fatigue, loss of appetite, insomnia, often euphoria.	Restlessness, irritability, weight loss, toxic psychosis (mainly paranoid). Diversion of energy and money. Habituation. Extreme irritability, toxic psychosis.	Amphetamines, same as Sedatives above. Cocaine, same as Narcotics below.
No	Minimal	Medical (including psychiatric) treatment of anxiety or tension states, alcoholism, psychoses, and other disorders.	Selective CNS depressants. Relaxation, relief of anxiety/tension. Suppression of hallucinations or delusions, improved functioning.	Sometimes drowsiness, dryness of mouth, blurring of vision, skin rash, tremor. Occasionally jaundice, agranulocytosis, or death.	Same as Sedatives above, except not usually included under the special federal or state drug laws. Negligible illicit traffic.
No	Minimal to Moderate	To get "high" (euphoria). As an escape. To relax. To socialize. To conform to various subcultures whigh sanction its use. For rebellion. Attraction of behavior labeled as deviant. Availability.	Relaxation, euphoria, increased appetite, some alteration of time perception, possible impairment of judgment and coordination. Mixed CNS depressant-stimulant.	Usually none. Possible diversion of energy and money. Habituation. Occasional acute panic reactions.	Unavailable (although permissible) for ordinary medical prescription. Possession, sale, and cultivation prohibited by state and federal narcotic or marijuana laws. Special penalties. Widespread illicit traffic.

(Continued)

COMPARISON CHART OF MAJOR SUBSTANCES USED FOR MIND ALTERATION   (Continued)

Official name of drug or chemical	Slang name(s)	Usual single adult dose	Duration of action (hours)	Method of taking	Legitimate medical uses (present and projected)	Potential for psychological dependence*	Potential for tolerance leading to increased dosage)
Narcotics (opiates, analgesics)						High	Yes
Opium	Op	10–12 "pipes" (Asia)	4	Smoking (inhalation)	Treatment of severe pain, diarrhea, and cough		
Heroin	Horse, H, smack, shit, junk	Variable—bag or paper w. 5–10 percent heroin		Injecting in muscle or vein			
Morphine		10–15 mg	4–6	Swallowing or injection			
Codeine		15–30 mg					
Percodan		1 tablet					
Demerol		50–100 mg					
Methadone	Dolly	2.5–40 mg					
Cough syrups (Cheracol, Hycodan, Romilar, etc.)		2–4 oz. (for euphoria)					
LSD	Acid, sugar cubes, trip	150 μg	10–12	Swallowing liquid, capsule, pill (or sugar cube)	Experimental study of mind and brain function. Enhancement of creativity and problem solving. Treatment of alcoholism, mental illness, and the dying person. (Chemical warfare)	Minimal	Yes (rare)
Psilocybin	Mushrooms	25 mg	6–8				
S.T.P.		6 mg					
D.M.T.							
Mescaline (peyote)	Cactus	350 mg	12–14	Smoking and chewing plant			
Antidepressants							
Ritalin		5–10 mg	4–6	Swallowing pills or capsules	Treatment of moderate to severe depression	Minimal	No
Dibenzazepine (Tofranil, Elavil)		25 mg, 10 mg					
MAO inhibitors (Nardil, Parnate)		10 mg, 15 mg					

Potential for physical dependence	Overall potential for abuse and toxicity**	Reasons drug is sought by users (drug effects and social factors)	Usual short-term effects (psychological, pharmacological, social)	Usual long-term effects (psychological, pharmacological, social)	Form of legal regulation and control††
Yes	High	To get "high" (euphoria). As an escape. To avoid withdrawal symptoms. As a substitute for aggressive and sexual drives which cause anxiety. To conform to various sub-cultures which sanction use. For rebellion.	CNS depressants. Sedation, euphoria, relief of pain, impaired intellectual functioning and coordination.	Constipation, loss of appetite and weight, temporary impotency or sterility. Habituation, addiction with unpleasant and painful withdrawal illness.	Available (except heroin) by special (narcotics) medical prescriptions. Some available by ordinary prescription or over-the-counter. Other manufacture, sale or possession prohibited under state and federal narcotics laws. Severe penalties. Extensive illicit traffic.
No	Moderate	Curiosity created by recent widespread publicity. Seeking for meaning and consciousness—expansion. Rebellion. Attraction of behavior recently labeled as deviant. Availability.	Production of visual imagery, increased sensory awareness, anxiety, nausea, impaired coordination; sometimes consciousness-expansion.	Usually none. Sometimes precipitates or intensifies an already existing psychosis; more commonly can produce a panic reaction.	Available only to a few medical researchers (or to members of the Native American Church). Other manufacture, sale or possession prohibited by state, dangerous drug or federal drug abuse laws. Moderate penalties. Extensive illicit traffic.
No	Minimal	Medical (including psychiatric) treatment of depression.	Relief of depression (elevation of mood), stimulation.	Basically the same as Tranquilizers above.	Same as Tranquilizers above.

(Continued)

COMPARISON CHART OF MAJOR SUBSTANCES USED FOR MIND ALTERATION   *(Continued)*

Official name of drug or chemical	Slang name(s)	Usual single adult dose	Duration of action (hours)	Method of taking	Legitimate medical uses (present and projected)	Potential for psycho-logical de-pendence*	Potential for tolerance leading to increased dosage)
Miscellaneous						Minimal to moderate	Not known
Glue, gasoline & solvents		Variable	2	Inhalation	None except for anti-histamines used for allergy and amyl nitrite for fainting		
Amyl nitrite		1–2 ampules					
Antihistamines		25–50 mg		Swallowing			
Nutmeg		Variable					
Nonprescription "sedatives" (Compoz)							
Catnip							
Nitrous oxide							

*The term "habituation" has sometimes been used to refer to psychological dependence and the term "addiction" to refer to the combination of tolerance and an abstinence (withdrawal) syndrome. Drug abuse (dependency) properly involves (excessive, often compulsive) use of a drug to an extent that it damages an individual's health or social or vocational adjustment, or is otherwise specifically harmful to society. ·

**Always to be considered in evaluating the effects of these drugs are the amount consumed, purity, frequency, time interval since ingestion, food in the stomach, combinations with other drugs, and most importantly, the personality or character of the individual taking it and the setting or context in which it is taken. The determinations made in this chart are based upon the evidence with human use of these drugs rather than upon related artificial experimental situations, animal research, or political (propagandistic) statements.

Potential for physical dependence	Overall potential for abuse and toxicity**	Reasons drug is sought by users (drug effects and social factors)	Usual short-term effects (psychological, pharmacological, social)	Usual long-term effects (psychological, pharmacological, social)	Form of legal regulation and control††
No	Moderate to High	Curiosity. To get "high" (euphoria). Thrill seeking. Ready availability.	When used for mind-alteration generally produces a "high" (euphoria) with impaired coordination and judgment.	Variable—some of the substances can seriously damage the liver or kidney and some produce hallucinations.	Generally easily available. Some require prescriptions. In several states glue banned for those under 21.

†Hashish or charas is a more concentrated form of the active ingredient THC (tetrahydrocannabinol) and is consumed in smaller doses analogical to vodka-beer ratios.

††Only scattered, inadequate health, educational or rehabilitation programs (usually prison hospitals) exist for narcotics addicts and alcoholics (usually outpatient clinics) with nothing for the others except sometimes prison.

Appendix E / OXYGEN THERAPY

1. Purpose—to relieve hypoxia and provide adequate tissue oxygenation.

2. Clinical indications
A. Shock.
B. Cardiac disorders—myocardial infarction and congestive heart failure.
C. Respiratory depression, insufficiency, or failure.
D. Anemia.
E. Supportive therapy for unconscious patients.

3. Precautions
A. Patients with chronic obstructive pulmonary disease should receive low flow rates of oxygen to prevent inhibition of hypoxic respiratory drive.
B. Excessive amounts of oxygen for prolonged periods of time will cause retrolental fibroplasia and blindness in premature infants.
C. Oxygen delivered without humidification will result in drying and irritation of respiratory mucosa, decreased ciliary action, and thickening of respiratory secretions.
D. Oxygen supports combustion, and fire is a potential hazard during its administration.
   1. Ground electrical equipment.
   2. Prohibit smoking.
   3. Institute measures to decrease static electricity.
E. High flow rates of oxygen per ventilator or cuffed tracheostomy and endotracheal tubes can produce signs of oxygen toxicity in 24 to 48 hours.
   1. Cough, sore throat, decreased vital capacity, and substernal discomfort.
   2. Pulmonary manifestations due to:
      a. Atelectasis.
      b. Exudation of protein fluids into alveoli.
      c. Damage to pulmonary capillaries.
      d. Interstitial hemorrhage.

4. Oxygen administration
A. Oxygen is dispensed from cylinder or piped-in system.
B. Methods of delivering oxygen:
   1. Nasal catheter—
      a. Effective and comfortable.
      b. Delivers 30% to 40% oxygen at flow rates of 6–8 liters/minute.
      c. Can produce excoriation of nares.
   2. Nasal prongs—
      a. Comfortable, simple, and allows patient to move about in bed.
      b. Delivers 30% to 40% oxygen at flow rates of 6–8 liters/minute.
      c. Difficult to keep in position unless patient is alert and cooperative.
   3. Face tent—
      a. Well tolerated, provides means for supplying extra humidity.
      b. Delivers 30% to 55% oxygen at flow rates of 4–8 liters/minute.
   4. Venturi mask—
      a. Mask allows for accurate deliverance of prescribed concentration of oxygen.
      b. Delivers 25% to 35% oxygen at flow rates of 4–8 liters/minute.
   5. Face mask—
      a. Poorly tolerated—utilized for short periods of time.
      b. Delivers 35% to 65% oxygen at flow rates of 6–12 liters/minute.
      c. Significant rebreathing of carbon dioxide at low oxygen flow rates.
      d. Hot—may produce pressure sores around nose and mouth.
   6. T-piece—
      a. Provides humidification and enriched oxygen mixtures to tracheostomy or ET tube.
      b. Delivers 40% to 60% oxygen at flow rates of 4–12 liters/minute.

5. Ventilators
A. Indications:
   1. Hypoventilation.
   2. Hypoxia.
   3. Counteract pulmonary edema by changing pressure gradient.
   4. Decrease work of breathing.
B. Contraindications:
   1. Tuberculosis—may rupture tubercular bleb.
   2. Hypovolemia—increased intrathoracic pressures decrease venous return.
   3. Air trapping—increased because adequate exhalation is not allowed.

C. Complications:
 1. Decreased blood pressure.
 2. Atelectasis.
 3. Infection.
 4. Oxygen toxicity.
 5. Difficulties weaning.
 6. Gastric dilatation.
D. Types of ventilators:
 1. Oscillating or rocking bed.
   a. Indirectly aids respirations by using weight and gravity of abdominal contents to change position of diaphragm.
   b. Used for patients with paralytic disease and as an aid in weaning.
 2. Iron lung and chest respirators.
   a. Driven by motors that create negative pressure within tank or shell and thus allow air to enter patient's lungs.
   b. Utilized for patients with neuromuscular disease.
 3. Intermittent positive-pressure breathing.
   a. Produces pressures greater than atmospheric pressures, intermittently.
   b. Improves tidal volume and minute volume and aids in overcoming respiratory insufficiency.
   c. Produces more uniform distribution of alveolar aeration and reduces work of breathing.
   d. Utilized to deliver both oxygen and medications to patients during treatment and rehabilitative pulmonary therapy.
   e. Contraindicated in pneumothorax, active tuberculosis, and history of recent hemoptysis.
 4. Pressure-preset ventilators.

   a. Bird—Mark VII.
    (1) Pressure-cycled, pneumatic-powered.
    (2) When preset pressure is reached, valve closes, terminating inspiration.
    (3) Flow rate, sensitivity, and pressure limit all adjustable.
    (4) Adjustable flow rate allows for increasing tidal volume.
    (5) Disadvantage—changes in compliance or airway resistance can affect oxygen concentration and tidal volume.
   b. Bennett—PR II.
    (1) Positive-pressure-cycled, time-cycled, flow-sensitive.
    (2) May be triggered by patient's inspiration or controlled by pressure or time setting.
    (3) Oxygen delivery variable, so frequent monitoring is *essential*.

6. *Volume respirators*
A. Emerson:
 1. Delivers preset tidal volume.
 2. Oxygen concentration adjusted by lighter flow being fed into machine.
 3. No alarms—malfunctions can go undetected.
 4. Has a sigh mechanism but no positive end-expiration pressure (PEEP), which maintains lung inflation.
 5. Utilized for patients with decreased compliance (stiff lungs).
B. Bennett—MA-1 and Ohio 560.
 1. Similar function and capabilities to Emerson.
 2. Sophisticated alarm system.
 3. Excellent humidification systems.
 4. PEEP capabilities.

Appendix F / POSITIONING THE PATIENT

SUMMARY OF USUAL POSITIONING FOR SPECIFIC SURGICAL CONDITIONS

Surgical condition	Key points about positioning	Rationales
Unconscious patient	Turn on side with head lowered—"coma" position	Important to let secretions drain out by gravity. Must prevent aspiration
Respiratory distress	Orthopnea position usually desirable	Allows for maximum expansion of lungs
Lobectomy	Do not put in Trendelenburg position	Pushes abdominal contents against diaphragm May cause respiratory embarrassment
Pneumonectomy	Turn only toward operative side for short periods	Gives unaffected lung room for full expansion Prevents mediastinal shift In case of bleeding there will not be drainage into the unaffected bronchi
Flail chest	Position on affected side	Reduces the instability of the chest wall that is causing the paradoxical respiratory movements
Coronary surgery	May be ordered flat on back for 24 hours	Important to prevent possible hypotension which may occur if head of bed raised
Ileo-femoral bypass surgery for arterial insufficiency	Do not elevate legs Avoid hip flexion—walk or stand but do not sit	Arterial flow is helped by gravity Flexion of the hip compresses the vessels of the extremity
Vein strippings Vein ligations	Keep legs elevated Do not stand or sit for long periods	Prevent venous stasis Prevents venous pooling
Ruptured appendix	Keep in Fowler's position—not flat in bed	Keeps infection from spreading upward in the peritoneal cavity
Gastric resection	Lie down after meals	May be useful in preventing the dumping syndrome
Hiatal hernia (before repaired)	Head of bed elevated on shock blocks	Prevents esophageal irritation from gastric regurgitation
Mastectomy	Do not abduct arm first few days Elevate hand and arm higher than shoulder	Puts tension on suture line Prevents lymphedema
Radium implantation in cervix	Bedrest—usually may elevate head to 30°	Must keep radium insert positioned correctly

Surgical condition	Key points about positioning	Rationales
Retinal detachment	Affected area toward bed—complete bed rest No sudden movements of head—may use sand bags to prevent turning	Gravity may help retina fall in place Any increase in intraocular pressure may further dislodge retina Necessary to cover both eyes to reduce ocular movements
Cast on extremity	Keep extremity elevated	Prevents edema
Patient in straight traction	Check specific orders about how much head may be elevated	Body is used as the countertraction—this must not be less than the pull of the traction
Patient in balanced suspension traction	May have more freedom to move about than patient in straight traction.	In balanced suspension additional weights supply countertraction.
Hip prosthesis	Keep affected leg in abduction (splint or pillow between legs) Avoid adduction, external rotation and flexion of the hip	If affected leg is flexed, allowed to adduct and internally rotate. The head of the femur may be displaced from the socket.
Amputation of a lower extremity	No pillows under stump after first 24 hours Turn patient prone several times a day	Prevents flexion deformity of the limb
Laminectomy	Log roll (if fusion done may be in a cast)	Prevents any bending of the spine
Craniotomy	Head elevated	Prevents collection of fluid in surgical area which might contribute to increased intracranial pressure
Burns (extensive)	Usually flat for first 24 hours	Potential problem is hypovolemia which will be more symptomatic in a sitting position

Source: Jane Vincent Corbett, University of San Francisco. Used by permission.

Appendix G / PATIENTS' RIGHTS*

A PATIENT'S BILL OF RIGHTS

1. The patient has the right to considerate and respectful care.

According to this right, a patient is entitled to an acceptable standard of care and to consideration during the provision of that care. Included is the right of the patient to an explanation about what is happening, the why and the when, and the opportunity to participate in the planning whenever this is feasible. It has been advocated by the Department of Health, Education, and Welfare in the United States that health institutions establish the mechanisms whereby patients' grievances can be heard and investigated.

A trend that follows in this general area is that of the **patient advocate,** *a role assumed by nurses in some settings. The patient advocate represents the patient and works on the patient's behalf. Frequently nurses function as patient advocates in situations in which they arrange, for example, for the services of another community agency. However, in some settings a specific health professional is designated the patient's advocate by title and function. This person serves as an educational consultant for patients and for staff. Explanations can often assist a patient to accept some particular treatment to which, for example, she has previously objected. When a patient complains that the hospital has lost his clothing, or that a nurse intentionally hurt him, then the patient advocate represents the patient in investigating the claims and coming to some solution. Sometimes a patient advocate can assist the administration of an agency to change policies that patients find objectionable and that the agency can amend.*

2. The patient has the right to obtain from his physician complete current information concerning his diagnosis, treatment, and prognosis, in terms the patient can be reasonably expected to understand. When it is not medically advisable to give such information to the patient, the information should be made available to an appropriate person in his behalf. He has the right to know by name the physician responsible for coordinating his care.

By this statement the patient has a right to understand the diagnosis, treatment, and prognosis. This means that the patient needs to have an understanding of some medical terminology such as prognosis in order that what the patient learns has meaning. Just as patients have a right to accurate information about their health, they also have a right not to be informed if it is considered that the information would have negative effects upon them, such as an acute depressive reaction or an acute anxiety reaction. The physician is responsible for making this decision and informing the appropriate member of the family if it is indicated.

3. The patient has the right to receive from his physician information necessary to give informed consent prior to the start of any procedure and/or treatment. Except in emergencies, such information for informed consent should include but not necessarily be limited to the specific procedure and/or treatment, the medically significant risks involved, and the probable duration of incapacitation. Where medically significant alternatives for care or treatment exist, or when the patient requests information concerning medical alternatives, the patient has the right to such information. The patient also has the right to know the name of the person responsible for the procedures and/or treatment.

Consent is a free, rational act that presupposes knowledge about the thing to which consent is given by a person who is legally capable of consent. Informed consent includes:

1. *Explanation of the condition.*
2. *Explanation of the procedures to be used and the consequences.*
3. *Description of alternative treatments or procedures.*

*American Hospital Association. 1973. A patient's bill of rights. *Nursing Outlook.* 21:82 and 24:29. Reprinted with the permission of the American Hospital Association. Italicized comments from Kozier, B. and Erb, G. L. 1979. *Fundamentals of nursing.* Addison-Wesley.

4. *Description of the benefits to be expected (not assured).*

5. *Answers to the patient's inquiries.*

6. *Understanding that the patient has not been coerced to agree and may withdraw if he changes his mind.*

Patients have the right to an informed consent, that is, the right to consent to any treatment or procedures, after being fully informed. Patients also have a right to know, to question, and to understand therapies such as medications they are receiving. They have a right to a specific answer to questions. This is a relatively recent change based upon changes in both the common and the statutory laws. Consumers at one time felt that they were at the mercy of health professionals and that they had no right to ask questions or to ask for explanations about what they did not understand. These responsibilities belong to the physician; however, frequently they will be delegated to the nurse in both the hospital and the community settings.

Patients also have the right to know the name of the physician who is coordinating care. A number of physicians often look after one patient in some medical centers, and the patient sees several physicians in the course of a hospital day, often none of whom are the patient's own general practitioner. The reasons for this are probably twofold: the education programs for physicians that are conducted in many large centers and the trend toward specialization in medical practice. As a result, the patient can be confused by the number of faces and really not know who is primarily responsible for care and its coordination.

4.   The patient has the right to refuse treatment to the extent permitted by law and to be informed of the medical consequences of his action.

Patients can change their minds and refuse a treatment and/or procedure. They may do this in writing, verbally, or both. If the patient tells the nurse that he or she refuses a treatment, the nurse has two responsibilities, (a) not to go ahead with the treatment and (b) to inform the hospital or agency authorities and the patient's physician. It then becomes the physician's responsibility to explain to the patient the medical consequences of this decision.

5.   The patient has the right to every consideration of his privacy concerning his own medical care program. Case discussion, consultation, examination, and treatment are confidential and should be conducted discreetly. Those not directly involved in his care must have the permission of the patient to be present.

Patients have the right to be examined or seen by only those essential to their care or therapy. Others must obtain permission from the patient. Although it is the physician's responsibility to obtain this consent, it is also often delegated to nurses. For example, for an examination by an intern or medical student or for a consultation by a consulting physician, the nurse needs to ensure that the patient has given consent before the examination or consultation. If the patient has not done so freely, the nurse must report this to the hospital authorities and to the physician.

The right to privacy has many facets. Individuals differ in their needs for privacy and in the violations or exposures that threaten these needs. Some request the restriction of visitors. Some need to be alone and withdraw while expressing feelings such as when crying. Most, however, like their bodies covered from exposure and prefer private enclosures for bathing or toileting. Participation in research or educational endeavors may or may not be of concern to patients. Nonetheless, such participation requires verbal or written consent. Even after death the right for privacy persists. The right to not be observed, exposed, or touched by the unauthorized or to not receive an autopsy are examples. Rights of privacy after death move to the surviving relatives.

6.   The patient has the right to expect that all communications and records pertaining to his care should be treated as confidential.

This right presents several challenges to the nurse's discretion and judgment. Receiving confidential information is a straightforward matter, but how to handle this information is less so. A certain amount of this information must be communicated to other health workers to provide continuity in the patient's care. The patient needs to know how the information will be handled and what information needs to be shared with others. The degree of the patient's illness and the type of information influence the nurse's decisions. In some situations the patient may object.

It is legally recognized that the patient's record is the property of the health agency, but nine states allow patients access to the information in the record.

7.   The patient has the right to expect that within its capacity a hospital must take reasonable response to the request of a patient for services. The hospital must provide evaluation, service, and/or referral as indicated

by the urgency of the case. When medically permissible, a patient may be transferred to another facility only after he has received complete information and explanation concerning the needs for and alternatives to such a transfer. The institution to which the patient is transferred must first have accepted the patient for transfer.

8.   The patient has the right to obtain information as to any relationship of his hospital to other health care and educational institutions insofar as his care is concerned. The patient has the right to obtain information as to the existence of any professional relationships among individuals, by name, who are treating him.

Rights 7 and 8 refer chiefly to the responses of hospitals and to referrals to other health agencies. In the latter instance, the patient is provided with the right to information about the relationships of the hospital with educational institutions such as universities and other health-care agencies, such as privately owned hospitals. In addition, the patient has the right to know whether the owner of a private hospital is related to the physician in the institute to which the patient is being transferred.

9.   The patient has the right to be advised if the hospital proposes to engage in or perform human experimentation affecting his care or treatment. The patient has the right to refuse to participate in such research projects.

Nurses are often involved in research conducted with the participation of patients. In 1966, the US Department of Health, Education, and Welfare articulated a series of regulations in regard to experimentation. These regulations include:

1. *Voluntary, specific consent to participate in the research, with a clear explanation of the experiment, including possible dangers.*

2. *Complete freedom to refuse on the part of the patient.*

3. *The qualifications of the researcher and the researcher's responsibilities.*

4. *The relationship between the value of the research and its political values.*

Furthermore, the American Nurses' Association and the Canadian Nurses' Association have published guidelines for nurses who participate in research projects. These are designed to protect both the patient and the nurse.

10.   The patient has the right to expect reasonable continuity of care. He has the right to know in advance what appointment times and physicians are available and where. The patient has the right to expect that the hospital will provide a mechanism whereby he is informed by his physician or a delegate of the physician of the patient's continuing health.

Consumers of health care are also demanding a reasonable standard in the continuity of care. They are asking that while in hospital, they be adequately informed in order to maintain a program of health care after discharge. Teaching the patient and family appropriate health care often becomes the nurse's responsibility.

11.   The patient has the right to examine and receive an explanation of his bill regardless of source of payment.

Many agencies provide detailed documentation of costs of services and supplies. Nurses may or may not be involved in recording some of these, such as the number and kinds of dressings or the type and quantity of medication. In some situations it may be the nurse's responsibility to offer the explanation of the bill or certain aspects of it.

12.   The patient has the right to know what hospital rules and regulations apply to his conduct as a patient.

Rules, regulations, and policies of the hospital that are of concern to the patient need to be explained. Some agencies distribute information pamphlets to patients that include regulations about smoking and visiting and information about the availability of televisions, telephones, cafeteria services, and chaplain services. The nurse is frequently the person who receives questions about these matters. It is the nurse who also is responsible for informing patients about special regulations such as no smoking in rooms where oxygen is being administered.

DECLARATION ON THE RIGHTS OF DISABLED PERSONS *

1. The term "disabled person" means any person unable to ensure by himself or herself wholly or partly the necessities of a normal individual and/or social life, as a result of a deficiency, either congenital or not, in his or her physical or mental capabilities.

2. Disabled persons shall enjoy all the rights set forth in this Declaration. These rights shall be granted to all disabled persons without any exception whatsoever and without distinction or discrimination on the basis of race, colour, sex, language, religion, political or other opinions, national or social origin, state of wealth, birth or any other situation applying either to the disabled person himself or herself or to his or her family.

3. Disabled persons have the inherent right to respect for their human dignity. Disabled persons, whatever the origin, nature, and seriousness of their handicaps and disabilities, have the same fundamental rights as their fellow-citizens of the same age, which implies first and foremost the right to enjoy a decent life, as normal and full as possible.

4. Disabled persons have the same civil and political rights as other human beings; article 7 of the Declaration of the Rights of Mentally Retarded Persons applies to any possible limitation or suppression of those rights for mentally disabled persons.

5. Disabled persons are entitled to the measures designed to enable them to become as self-reliant as possible.

6. Disabled persons have the right to medical, psychological and functional treatment, including prosthetic and orthetic appliances, to medical and social rehabilitation, education, vocational education, training and rehabilitation, aid, counselling, placement services and other services which will enable them to develop their capabilities and skills to the maximum and will hasten the process of their social integration or reintegration.

7. Disabled persons have the right to economic and social security and to a decent level of living. They have the right, according to their capabilities, to secure and retain employment or to engage in a useful, productive and remunerative occupation and to join trade unions.

8. Disabled persons are entitled to have their special needs taken into consideration at all stages of economic and social planning.

9. Disabled persons have the right to live with their families or with foster parents and to participate in all social, creative or recreational activities. No disabled person shall be subjected, as far as his or her residence is concerned, to differential treatment other than that required by his or her condition or by the improvement which he or she may derive therefrom. If the stay of a disabled person in a specialized establishment is indispensable, the environment and living conditions therein shall be as close as possible to those of the normal life of a person of his or her age.

10. Disabled persons shall be protected against all exploitation, all regulations and all treatment of a discriminatory, abusive and degrading nature.

11. Disabled persons shall be able to avail themselves of qualified legal aid when such aid proves indispensable for the protection of their persons or property. If judicial proceedings are instituted against them, the legal procedures applied shall take their physical and mental condition fully into account.

12. Organizations of disabled persons may be usefully consulted in all matters regarding the rights of disabled persons.

13. Disabled persons, their families and communities shall be fully informed, by all appropriate means, of the rights contained in this Declaration.

THE DYING PERSON'S BILL OF RIGHTS *

I have the right to be treated as a living human being until I die.

I have the right to maintain a sense of hopefulness, however changing its focus may be.

---

*Adopted by the General Assembly of the United Nations, December, 1975.

I have the right to be cared for by those who can maintain a sense of hopefulness, however changing this might be.

I have the right to express my feelings and emotions about my approaching death in my own way.

I have the right to participate in decisions concerning my care.

I have the right to expect continuing medical and nursing attention even though "cure" goals must be changed to "comfort" goals.

I have the right not to die alone.

I have the right to be free from pain.

I have the right to have my questions answered honestly.

I have the right not to be deceived.

I have the right to have help from and for my family in accepting my death.

I have the right to die in peace and dignity.

I have the right to retain my individuality and not be judged for my decisions which may be contrary to beliefs of others.

I have the right to discuss and enlarge my religious and/or spiritual experiences, whatever these may mean to others.

I have the right to expect that the sanctity of the human body will be respected after death.

I have the right to be cared for by caring, sensitive, knowledgeable people who will attempt to understand my needs and will be able to gain some satisfaction in helping me face my death.

DECLARATION ON THE RIGHTS OF MENTALLY RETARDED PERSONS*

1. The mentally retarded person has, to the maximum degree of feasibility, the same rights as other human beings.

2. The mentally retarded person has a right to proper medical care and physical therapy and to such education, training, rehabilitation and guidance as will enable him to develop his ability and maximum potential.

3. The mentally retarded person has a right to economic security and to a decent standard of living. He has a right to perform productive work or to engage in any meaningful occupation to the fullest possible extent of his capabilities.

4. Whenever possible, the mentally retarded person should live with his own family or with foster parents and participate in different forms of community life. The family with which he lives should receive assistance. If care in an institution becomes necessary, it should be provided in surroundings and other circumstances as close as possible to those of normal life.

5. The mentally retarded person has a right to a qualified guardian when this is required to protect his personal well-being and interests.

6. The mentally retarded person has a right to protection from exploitation, abuse and degrading treatment. If prosecuted for any offense, he shall have a right to due process of law with full recognition being given to his degree of mental responsibility.

7. Whenever mentally retarded persons are unable, because of the severity of their handicap, to exercise all their rights in a meaningful way or it should become necessary to restrict or deny some or all of these rights, the procedure used for that restriction or denial of rights must contain proper legal safeguards against every form of abuse. This procedure must be based on an evaluation of the social capability of the mentally retarded person by qualified experts and must be subject to periodic review and to the right of appeal to higher authorities.

THE PREGNANT PATIENT'S BILL OF RIGHTS*

1. The Pregnant Patient has the right, prior to the administration of any drug or procedure, to be informed by the health professional caring for her of

---

*Adopted by the United Nations, December, 1971.

*From Doris B. Haire, author, and the International Childbirth Education Association, Publisher.

any potential direct or indirect effects, risks or hazards to herself or her unborn or newborn infant which may result from the use of a drug or procedure prescribed for or administered to her during pregnancy, labor, birth or lactation.

2. The Pregnant Patient has the right, prior to the proposed therapy, to be informed, not only of the benefits, risks and hazards of the proposed therapy but also of known alternative therapy such as available childbirth education classes which could help to prepare the Pregnant Patient physically and mentally to cope with the discomfort or stress of pregnancy and the experience of childbirth, thereby reducing or eliminating her need for drugs and obstetric intervention. She should be offered such information early in her pregnancy in order that she may make a reasoned decision.

3. The Pregnant Patient has the right, prior to the administration of any drug, to be informed by the health professional who is prescribing or administering the drug to her that any drug which she receives during pregnancy, labor and birth, no matter how or when the drug is taken or administered may adversely affect her unborn baby, directly or indirectly, and that there is no drug or chemical which has been proven safe for the unborn child.

4. The Pregnant Patient has the right if cesarean section is anticipated, to be informed prior to the administration of any drug, and preferably prior to her hospitalization, that minimizing her and in turn, her baby's intake of nonessential preoperative medicine will benefit her baby.

5. The Pregnant Patient has the right, prior to the administration of a drug or procedure, to be informed of the areas of uncertainty if there is no properly controlled follow-up research which has established the safety of the drug or procedure with regard to its direct and/or indirect effects on the physiological, mental and neurological development of the child exposed, via the mother, to the drug or procedure during pregnancy, labor, birth or lactation (this would apply to virtually all drugs and the vast majority of obstetric procedures).

6. The Pregnant Patient has the right, prior to the administration of any drug, to be informed of the brand name and generic name of the drug in order that she may advise the health professional of any past adverse reaction to the drug.

7. The Pregnant Patient has the right to determine for herself, without pressure from her attendant, whether she will accept the risks inherent in the proposed therapy or refuse a drug or procedure.

8. The Pregnant Patient has the right to know the name and qualifications of the individual administering a medication or procedure to her during labor or birth.

9. The Pregnant Patient has the right to be informed, prior to the administration of any procedure, whether that procedure is being administered to her for her or her baby's benefit (medically indicated) or as an elective procedure (for convenience, teaching purposes or research).

10. The Pregnant Patient has the right to be accompanied during the stress of labor and birth by someone she cares for, and to whom she looks for emotional comfort and encouragement.

11. The Pregnant Patient has the right after appropriate medical consultation to choose a position for labor and for birth which is least stressful to her baby and to herself.

12. The Obstetric Patient has the right to have her baby cared for at her bedside if her baby is normal, and to feed her baby according to her baby's needs rather than according to the hospital regimen.

13. The Obstetric Patient has the right to be informed in writing of the name of the person who actually delivered her baby and the professional qualifications of that person. This information should also be on the birth certificate.

14. The Obstetric Patient has the right to be informed if there is any known or indicated aspect of her or her baby's care or condition which may cause her or her baby later difficulty or problems.

15. The Obstetric Patient has the right to have her and her baby's hospital medical records complete, accurate and legible and to have their records, including Nurses' Notes, retained by the hospital until the child reaches at least the age of majority, or alternatively, to have the records offered to her before they are destroyed.

16. The Obstetric Patient, both during and after her hospital stay, has the right to have access to her complete hospital medical records, including Nurses' Notes, and to receive a copy upon payment of a reasonable fee and without incurring the expense of retaining an attorney.

It is the obstetric patient and her baby, not the health professional, who must sustain any trauma or injury resulting from the use of a drug or obstetric procedure. The observation of the rights listed above will not only permit the obstetric patient to participate in the decisions involving her and her baby's health care, but will help to protect the health professional and the hospital against litigation arising from resentment or misunderstanding on the part of the mother.

MENTAL PATIENT'S BILL OF RIGHTS*

MENTAL PATIENTS' LIBERATION PROJECT

1. The mental patient is a human being and is entitled to be treated as such with as much decency and respect as is accorded to any other human being.

2. The mental patient is an American citizen and is entitled to every right established by the Declaration of Independence and guaranteed by the Constitution of the United States of America.

3. The mental patient has the right to the integrity of his or her own mind and body.

4. Treatment and medication can be administered only with his or her consent and, in the event he or she gives consent, he or she has the right to demand to know all relevant information regarding said treatment and/or medication.

5. The mental patient has the right to have access to his or her own legal and medical counsel.

6. The mental patient has the right to refuse to work in a mental hospital and/or to choose what work he or she shall do and the right to receive the minimum wage for such work as is set by the state labor laws.

7. The mental patient has the right to decent medical attention when he or she feels it is necessary, just as any other human being has that right.

8. The mental patient has the right to uncensored communication by phone, letter, and in person with whomever he or she wishes and at any time he or she wishes.

9. The mental patient has the right not to be treated like a criminal; not to be locked up against his or her will; not to be committed involuntarily; not to be fingerprinted or "mugged" (photographed).

10. The mental patient has the right to decent living conditions. He or she is paying for it and the taxpayers are paying for it.

11. The mental patient has the right to retain his or her own personal property. No one has the right to confiscate what legally belongs to him or her, no matter what reason is given. That is commonly known as theft.

12. The mental patient has the right to bring grievance against those who have mistreated him or her and the right to counsel and a court hearing, and is entitled to protection by the law against retaliation.

13. The mental patient has the right to refuse to be a guinea pig for experimental drugs and treatments and to refuse to be used as learning material for students. He or she has the right to demand reimbursement if so used.

14. The mental patient has the right not to have his or her character questioned or defamed.

15. The mental patient has the right to request an alternative to legal commitment or incarceration in a mental hospital.

---

*Adapted from the Mental Patients' Liberation Project, New York, N.Y.

Appendix H | REGIONAL AND STATE BOARDS OF NURSING AND PRACTICAL NURSING

Board of Nursing
One/East Bldg.
Suite 203
500 Eastern Blvd.
Montgomery, AL 36109

Board of Nursing
142 East 3rd Ave.
Anchorage, AK 99501

Board of Nursing
Westmark Bldg.
Suite 308
4120 W. Markham St.
Little Rock, AR 72205

Board of Registered Nursing
1020 N St.
Sacramento, CA 95814

Board of Nursing
115 State Services Bldg.
1525 Sherman St.
Denver, CO 80203

Board of Examiners for Nursing
79 Elm St.
Rm 101
Hartford, CT 06115

Board of Nursing
Cooper Bldg.
Rm 234
Dover, DE 19901

Nurses' Examining Bd.
614 H Street N.W.
Rm 112
Washington, DC 20001

Board of Nursing
111 Coast Line Drive E.
Suite 540
Jacksonville, FL 32202

Board of Nursing
166 Pryor St. S.W.
Atlanta, GA 30303

Board of Nursing
PO Box 3469
Honolulu, HI 96801

Board of Nursing
413 W. Idaho St.
Rm 203
Boise, ID 83702

Nursing Committee
Department of Registration and Education
Third Floor
628 East Adams St.
Springfield, IL 62786

Director
Department of Registration and Education
17th Floor
55 East Jackson Blvd.
Chicago, IL 60604

Board of Nurses' Registration and Nursing Education
700 North High School Rd.
Indianapolis, IN 46224

Board of Nursing
State Office Building
300 4th St.
Des Moines, IA 50219

Board of Nursing
PO Box 19235
Topeka, KS 66619

Board of Nursing
6100 Dutchmans Lane
Louisville, KY 40205

Board of Nursing
295 Water St.
Augusta, ME 04330

Board of Examiners of Nurses
201 West Preston St.
Baltimore, MD 21201

Board of Registration in Nursing
1509 Leverett Saltonstall
100 Cambridge St.
Boston, MA 02202

Board of Nursing
905 Southland
PO Box 30018
Lansing, MI 48909

Board of Nursing
717 Delaware St. S.E.
Minneapolis, MN 55414

Board of Nursing
135 Bounds St.
Suite 101
Jackson, MS 39206

Board of Nursing
PO Box 656
Jefferson City, MO 65101

Board of Nurses
Lalonde Bldg.
Helena, MT 59601

Board of Nursing
State House Station
PO Box 95065
Lincoln, NB 68509

Board of Nursing
1201 Terminal Way
Suite 203
Reno, NV 89502

Board of Nursing
Education and Nurse Registration
105 Loudon Road
Concord, NH 03301

New Jersey
Board of Nursing
1100 Raymond Boulevard
Rm 319
Newark, NJ 07102

Board of Nursing
2340 Menaul N.E.
Suite 112
Albuquerque, NM 87107

Board of Nursing
State Education Dept.
Cultural Education Center
Albany, NY 12230

Board of Nursing
PO Box 2129
Raleigh, NC 27602

Board of Nursing
420 North 4th St.
Bismarck, ND 58505

Board of Nursing Education and Nurse Registration
65 S. Front St.
Columbus, OH 43215

Board of Nurse Registration and Nursing Education
Suite 400
Northgate Complex
4030 North Lincoln Blvd.
Oklahoma City, OK 73105

Board of Nursing
574 State Office Bldg.
1400 S.W. 5th Avenue
Portland, OR 97201

Board of Nurse Examiners
PO Box 2649
Harrisburg, PA 17120

Board of Nurse Registration & Nursing Education
104 Health Dept. Bldg.
75 Davis St.
Providence, RI 02908

Board of Nursing
1777 St. Julian Place
Suite 102
Columbia, SC 29204

Board of Nursing
304 S. Phillips Ave.
Suite 205
Sioux Falls, SD 57102

Board of Nursing
R.S. Gass State Office Bldg.
Ben Allen Rd.
Nashville, TN 37216

Board of Nurse Examiners
510 South Congress
Suite 216
Austin, TX 78704

Board of Nursing
330 East 4th South St.
Salt Lake City, UT 84111

Board of Nursing
Division of Registration and Licensing
10 Baldwin St.
Montpelier, VT 05602

Board of Nursing
Seaboard Bldg. Ste. 453
3600 West Broad St.
Richmond, VA 23230

Board of Nurse Examiners
PO Box 1442
Charlotte Amalie
St. Thomas
Virgin Islands 00801

Board of Nursing
Division of Professional Licensing
PO Box 9649
Olympia, WA 98504

Board of Examiners for Registered Nurses
Embleton Bldg.
Suite 309
922 Quarrier St.
Charleston, WV 25301

Dept. of Regulation and Licensing
Division of Nurses
1400 E. Washington Ave.
Madison, WI 53702

Board of Nursing
Hathaway Building
2300 Capitol Ave.
Cheyenne, WY 82002

Appendix I / CRITICAL REQUIREMENTS FOR SAFE-EFFECTIVE NURSING PRACTICE: SUMMARY OUTLINE OF CATEGORY STRUCTURE

I. Exercises Professional Prerogatives Based on Clinical Judgment
   A. Adapts care to individual patient needs
   B. Fulfills responsibility to patient and others despite difficulty
   C. Challenges inappropriate orders and decisions by medical and other professional staff
   D. Acts as patient advocate in obtaining appropriate medical, psychiatric, or other help
   E. Analyzes and adjusts own or staff reactions in order to maintain therapeutic relationship with patient

II. Promotes Patient's Ability to Cope with Immediate, Long-Range, or Potential Health-Related Change
   A. Provides health care instruction or information to patient, family, or significant others
   B. Encourages patient or family to make decision about accepting care or adhering to treatment regime
   C. Helps patient recognize and deal with psychological stress
   D. Avoids creating or increasing anxiety or stress
   E. Conveys and invites acceptance, respect, and trust
   F. Facilitates relationship of family, staff, or significant others with patient
   G. Stimulates, remotivates patient, or enables him to achieve self-care and independence

III. Helps Maintain Patient Comfort and Normal Body Functions
   A. Keeps patient clean and comfortable
   B. Helps patient maintain or regain normal body functions

IV. Takes Precautionary and Preventive Measures in Giving Patient Care
   A. Prevents infection
   B. Protects skin and mucous membranes from injurious materials
   C. Uses positioning or exercise to prevent injury or the complications of immobility
   D. Avoids using injurious technique in administering and managing intrusive or other potentially traumatic treatments
   E. Protects patient from falls or other contact injuries
   F. Maintains surveillance of patient's activities
   G. Reduces or removes environmental hazards

V. Checks, Compares, Verifies, Monitors, and Follows Up Medication and Treatment Processes
   A. Checks correctness, condition, and safety of medication being prepared
   B. Ensures that correct medication or care is given to the right patient and that patient takes or receives it
   C. Adheres to schedule in giving medication, treatment, or test
   D. Administers medication by correct route, rate, or mode
   E. Checks patient's readiness for medication, treatment, surgery, or other care
   F. Checks to ensure that tests or measurements are done correctly
   G. Monitors ongoing infusions and inhalations
   H. Checks for and interprets effect of medication, treatment, or care, and takes corrective action if necessary

VI. Interprets Symptom Complex and Intervenes Appropriately
   A. Checks patient's condition or status
   B. Remains objective, further investigates, or verifies patient's complaint or problem

From Jacobs, A. M., et al. *Critical requirements for safe/effective nursing practice*. Published by the Council of State Boards of Nursing, American Nurses' Association. Reprinted with permission of the American Nurses' Association.

C. Uses alarms and signals on automatic equipment as adjunct to personal assessment

D. Observes and correctly assesses signs of anxiety or behavioral stress

E. Observes and correctly assesses physical signs, symptoms, or findings, and intervenes appropriately

F. Correctly assesses severity or priority of patient's condition, and gives or obtains necessary care

VII. Responds to Emergencies
   A. Anticipates need for crisis care
   B. Takes instant, correct action in emergency situations
   C. Maintains calm and efficient approach under pressure
   D. Assumes leadership role in crisis situation when necessary

VIII. Obtains, Records, and Exchanges Information in Behalf of the Patient
   A. Checks data sources for orders and other information about patient
   B. Obtains information from patient and family
   C. Transcribes or records information on chart, Kardex, or other information system
   D. Exchanges information with nursing staff and other departments
   E. Exchanges information with medical staff

IX. Utilizes Patient Care Planning
   A. Develops and modifies patient care plan
   B. Implements patient care plan

X. Teaches and Supervises Other Staff
   A. Teaches correct principles, procedures, and techniques of patient care
   B. Supervises and checks the work of staff for whom she is responsible

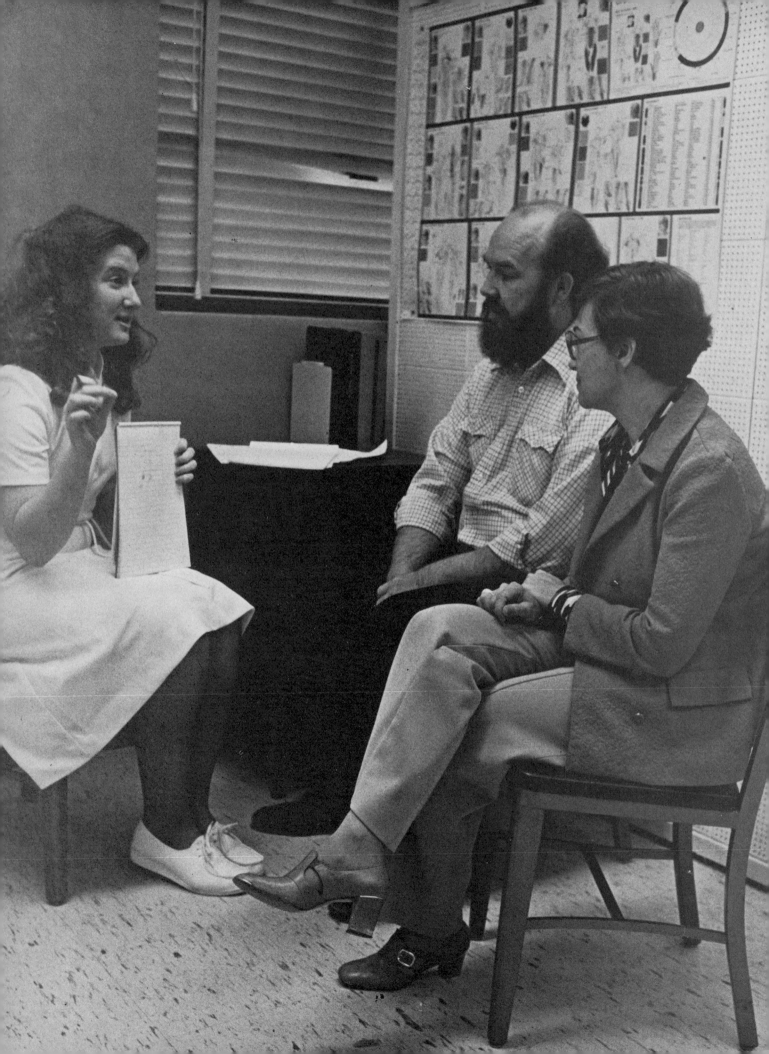

Comprehensive Integrated Case Studies

CASE STUDY 1

Charlie is a 14-year-old male who lives in the inner city with his mother (age 32), his father (age 35), his sister (age 12), and his brother (age 15). Charlie's mother is white and his father is black. His parents were married about 15 years ago. His father is a mechanical engineer, and his mother is a real estate agent.

Three weeks ago a janitor discovered Charlie setting fires in the locker room of his school. Charlie's parents were called because this was the fifth such incident in the past eight months. The school counselor suggested that Charlie's family seek professional counseling and that they consider inpatient placement for Charlie. Charlie's parents decided that this would probably be best for everyone in the family.

Charlie was placed in a private inpatient mental hospital on a coed adolescent unit with 16 other patients. During the initial weeks of family therapy, the therapist attempted to ascertain background information relevant to the family system's dynamics. Some of the significant data she collected appear below.

- The parents are an interracial couple that had to move to a different state early in their marriage because residents in their former area snubbed and ridiculed them.
- The couple married when the wife was 17 years old and the husband was 20. The wife was three months pregnant at the time.
- The husband is a compulsive worker. He works a minimum of a six days per week, averaging nine to ten hours each day.
- The wife has always been unhappy with her husband's working hours. They argue at least three or four times a week. The wife admits drinking two or three alcoholic beverages every day.

- Generally the wife is the primary caretaker of the children. In fact she states that she cannot remember her husband ever changing a single diaper, giving a bath, or disciplining any of the children.
- The parents perceive their children as follows. Charlie's brother and sister never caused any problems. All the children have been generally healthy throughout their lives. However, Charlie has always been a problem child. He has set fires since age 6, and this past year he ran away twice. His school grades have always been poor (Cs and Ds) in all subjects. In fact, he is truant from school at least four days each month.

QUESTIONS

1. As an adolescent, Charlie best characterizes his life stage by:
   1. Developing a sense of trust in others and in his environment.
   2. Finalizing his goals and plans for the future.
   3. Striving to attain independence and identity.
   4. Resolving inner conflicts and turmoil.

2. During the adolescent period the most important tasks for Charlie to complete include all of the following, *except:*
   1. Developing an individualized personality.
   2. Attaining an adequate defense mechanism.
   3. Establishing an ego identity.
   4. Refining and stabilizing the superego.

3. According to Freudian theory, Charlie may reexperience conflicts that occurred during which of the following periods of development?
   1. Oedipal.
   2. Latent.

3. Anal.

4. Phallic.

4. Charlie's parents have labeled him a problem child. Like many adolescents, Charlie may use all of the following defense mechanisms to cope with family pressure, *except:*
   1. Regression.
   2. Withdrawal.
   3. Denial.
   4. Conversion.

5. Although Charlie may be experiencing some degree of anxiety disorder or schizophrenic disorder, it may be difficult to diagnose because:
   1. Adolescents are usually reluctant to verbalize their feelings.
   2. Adolescents lack trust in others and usually withdraw from the situation.
   3. Adolescents are usually superficial in developing relationships with others.
   4. Normal adolescent behaviors often parallel those seen in some forms of mental illness.

6. In order to assess Charlie's relationship with his parents, the nurse would expect all of the following statements from Charlie, *except:*
   1. "They don't love me."
   2. "They are always checking up on me."
   3. "They treat me like a baby."
   4. "They don't understand me."

7. Charlie may exhibit all of the following behaviors, *except:*
   1. Aggression.
   2. Altruism.
   3. Homosexuality.
   4. Hypochondriasis.

8. To establish a relationship with Charlie, the nurse needs to consider all of the following facts, *except:*
   1. Boys in early adolescence feel threatened by female authority figures.
   2. Enforced inactivity deprives the adolescent of a major avenue for relieving frustration.
   3. Impulse control is a major problem for males.
   4. Fear and ambivalence will usually dissipate with the passage of time.

9. Charlie is experiencing several biologic and psychosocial changes at this time. Which of the following behaviors would you expect to see?
   1. An increase in imaginative thinking.
   2. An increased ability to learn by rote.
   3. An increase in academic achievement.
   4. An increased ability to cope with frustration.

10. During adolescence, Charlie needs all of the following, *except:*
    1. External control on his behavior by adults.
    2. Limit-setting based on fear and reprimands.

3. Adult role models for identification.

4. Stable relationships and interactions.

11. Charlie's arson attempts may exhibit which of the following behaviors?
    1. Acting out.
    2. Depression.
    3. Paranoia.
    4. Mania.

12. Charlie is diagnosed as exhibiting symptoms of an adjustment reaction to adolescence. Which of the following factors would be the *least* relevant contributor to these symptoms?
    1. Charlie's successful performance of tasks and resolution of life problems in earlier developmental periods.
    2. Charlie's mother as the primary disciplinary figure within the household.
    3. Charlie's parents' arguing three to four times per week.
    4. Charlie's parents' marrying at an early age.

13. Charlie may exhibit his depression differently from an adult. An adolescent who is depressed is most likely to exhibit which of the following behaviors?
    1. Withdrawal.
    2. Apathy.
    3. Violence.
    4. Regression.

Charlie's stay in the psychiatric hospital is punctuated by frequent outbursts of maladaptive behavior.

14. After his admission to the hospital, Charlie started hitting other clients and even struck a nurse. In assessing Charlie's behavior, the nurse should consider which of the following facts to be *most* relevant?
    1. Hitting others makes Charlie feel satisfied because he is in control of the situation.
    2. Hitting others provides Charlie with an escape from his feelings of hopelessness.
    3. Hitting others is Charlie's mechanism for alleviating anxiety.
    4. Hitting others allows Charlie to instill fear in others.

15. After Charlie has been hospitalized in the psychiatric institution for several days, he is introduced to the other adolescents in group therapy. The *most* significant factor the nurse should consider in initiating group therapy is that:
    1. Confrontation could lead to elopement.
    2. Charlie may refuse to verbalize.
    3. Group members may ignore Charlie.
    4. Charlie may act out during group therapy.

16. Charlie has been attending group therapy twice a week for three weeks. He is still fairly quiet during group therapy and speaks only when questioned. The nurse should assume that:

1. Charlie feels comfortable within the group.
2. Charlie is threatened by the group.
3. Charlie does not feel the need to verbalize.
4. Charlie is progressing as expected.

17. Charlie is becoming increasingly combative. He hits other clients as well as the nursing staff at least once or twice each day. All of the following are appropriate nursing goals, *except:*
    1. Helping Charlie develop impulse control.
    2. Helping Charlie manage his feelings appropriately.
    3. Helping Charlie learn socially acceptable behavior.
    4. Helping Charlie internalize his feelings.

18. By the time Charlie has been hospitalized three months, he has become apathetic and withdrawn. He sits in his room at least three to four hours each day. When he is requested to sit in the recreation room, he generally sits alone and stares into space. The most appropriate nursing intervention would include:
    1. Selecting a group activity for Charlie to participate in.
    2. Stimulating self-growth by providing challenging activities for Charlie.
    3. Allowing Charlie to spend at least three hours a day in his room for inner reflection.
    4. Encouraging staff members to sit with Charlie during group activities until he socializes voluntarily.

19. During the fourth month of hospitalization Charlie begins mutilating his forearms with lighted cigarettes and scratching his wrists with thumbtacks and staples he finds on the unit. All of the following are appropriate nursing interventions, *except:*
    1. Supervising Charlie closely.
    2. Avoiding confrontations with Charlie regarding his behavior.
    3. Removing all items that could be used for destructive purposes.
    4. Assisting Charlie to increase his self-esteem.

20. Charlie has developed a homosexual relationship with a 16-year-old named Rich. In assessing this behavior, the nurse should *primarily:*
    1. Avoid confronting Charlie about his attention-getting behavior.
    2. Validate Charlie's rationale for establishing the relationship.
    3. Explore Charlie's thoughts, feelings, and attitudes.
    4. Enforce limits on interactions between Rich and Charlie.

During Charlie's hospitalization his father continues to work eight to ten hours a day; his mother, however, is extremely upset. She has increased her consumption of alcoholic beverages to four to six drinks per day. She gets angry with the other children very quickly, cries spontaneously several times every day, and complains of headaches constantly.

21. In assessing Charlie's mother's behavior, the nurse should identify that she is experiencing what level of anxiety at this time?

1. Mild to moderate.
2. Moderate to severe.
3. Severe to panic.
4. Panic to overwhelming.

22. In planning care for Charlie's mother, the nurse would consider all of the following appropriate nursing interventions, *except:*
    1. Stimulating her to work at a concrete task.
    2. Encouraging her to cry.
    3. Providing her with someone to talk to.
    4. Isolating her from stimuli.

23. The most important nursing intervention in planning care for Charlie's mother would include:
    1. Referring her to an alcohol rehabilitation program.
    2. Identifying how she has coped with anxiety in the past.
    3. Arranging for inpatient hospitalization.
    4. Requesting a prescription for an antidepressant.

After Charlie has been in the hospital about five months, his mother takes an overdose of sleeping pills and alcohol. She is brought to the emergency room in an ambulance called by a neighbor, who discovered her unconscious on the living room sofa. Upon admission, she is unconscious. Her vital signs are TPR 98–60–10, BP 90/50. Her reflexes are dull.

24. The emergency room nurse's initial response should include which of the following?
    1. Administering a central nervous system stimulant.
    2. Paging the resident on call.
    3. Maintaining a patent airway.
    4. Assessing her neurologic signs.

25. Charlie's mother is hospitalized. In planning nursing care for a suicidal client, all of the following are appropriate nursing actions, *except:*
    1. Searching personal effects for toxic agents.
    2. Removing straps from clothing.
    3. Placing the client in small groups for observation.
    4. Removing sharp objects from the environment.

26. As Charlie's mother has a history of alcohol abuse, the nurse should be aware that she is most likely to exhibit which of the following in the first 72 hours following admission to the hospital?
    1. Withdrawal delirium.
    2. Suspiciousness.
    3. Mood swings.
    4. The use of coping mechanisms such as reaction formation.

27. The *least* appropriate nursing intervention for a client experiencing withdrawal delirium would be:
    1. Reinforcing time, place, and person.
    2. Providing consistent and concrete answers to questions.
    3. Administering ordered vitamins and glucose.
    4. Applying and maintaining physical restraints.

28. During Charlie's mother's twenty-first day of hospitalization, she begins to verbalize more and has interacted with one other patient on the inpatient psychiatric unit. The nurse should realize that this increase in her energy level may indicate that:
   1. She needs less individual attention.
   2. She needs more individual attention.
   3. She needs a decrease in her antidepressant medications.
   4. She is presently motivated to get well.

After Charlie's mother's release from the hospital, the entire family resumes attending family therapy once a week, and the parents begin individual and marital counseling.

29. One of the primary goals of therapy with this family system is to provide:
   1. A forum in which familial conflicts can be verbalized.
   2. Individual therapy for each family member.
   3. Treatment for the identified problem child.
   4. Crisis intervention for the family system.

30. Charlie's parents are a biracial couple. They are very reluctant to discuss this issue during family therapy sessions or even during marital counseling sessions. The nurse therapist's best response to this hesitancy would be to:
   1. Confront the couple's resistance to discussing the issue.
   2. Avoid the issue unless the couple raise it.
   3. Encourage a trusting relationship between the therapist and the couple.
   4. Refer the couple to individual psychotherapy.

31. Charlie's father is assessed as having an obsessive-compulsive personality. Which of the following behaviors would you *least* expect him to exhibit?
   1. Working 50- to 60-hour weeks.
   2. Smoking two packs of cigarettes a day.
   3. Showing flexibility in decision-making.
   4. Exhibiting a low level of concentration.

32. Charlie's father does not remember ever seeing his wife take an alcoholic drink. He also states that he has never seen his wife drunk or tipsy. Given the fact that his wife has admitted to drinking at least two or three drinks each day, what coping mechanism is Charlie's father using?
   1. Projection.
   2. Denial.
   3. Repression.
   4. Sublimation.

33. Charlie's mother is diagnosed as having an affective disorder. What drug is usually administered in treating these disorders?
   1. Lithium.
   2. Librium.
   3. Prolixin.
   4. Mellaril.

34. When administering lithium to a client with an affective disorder, the nurse must consider all of the following, *except:*
   1. If the patient's urinary output decreases significantly, diuretics should be ordered.
   2. The patient needs to be given a complete physical examination prior to administering the drug.
   3. If the patient experiences nausea, vomiting, and muscle weakness, the dosage may need regulating.
   4. If the patient exhibits symptoms of mania during the first ten days of receiving the drug, Haldol may also be administered.

Charlie has now been hospitalized eight months. Two days ago he was granted permission to walk across the hospital grounds to various activities without a staff escort. This afternoon he argued with the recreational therapist and disappeared from the hospital. The hospital security staff was notified of Charlie's disappearance; they found him walking about a mile from the hospital grounds.

35. In planning care for Charlie after this incident, the nurse would consider which of the following factors most significant?
   1. Charlie's need to be reprimanded for his deviant behavior.
   2. Charlie's need to be medicated to calm him down.
   3. Charlie's need to be listened to in order to identify his feelings.
   4. Charlie's need to understand the consequences of his actions.

After Charlie has been in the hospital a year and a half, the professional staff at the psychiatric hospital considers discharging him.

36. In planning Charlie's discharge, which of the following factors would the nurse consider most important?
   1. Charlie's thoughts and feelings about his discharge.
   2. Charlie's parents' thoughts and feelings about his discharge.
   3. Charlie's therapist's thoughts and feelings about his discharge.
   4. Charlie's sister's and brother's thoughts and feelings about his discharge.

37. Charlie asks the nurse whether he must tell other people that he has been in a mental hospital. The most appropriate response the nurse could make would be:
   1. "Yes, especially to all future school officials."
   2. "Yes, especially to all prospective employers."
   3. "No, this is an individual decision."
   4. "No, there is no specific requirement."

38. Charlie's parents have decided that they would rather have Charlie placed outside of the home when he is discharged from the hospital. The most appropriate response the nurse could make would include:
   1. Asking Charlie's parents to reassess their feelings about this decision.

2. Suggesting that Charlie's parents discuss this decision with the entire family.

3. Referring Charlie's parents to a social worker to assist in finding an alternative placement.

4. Assisting Charlie's parents in finding an appropriate discharge placement.

39. Charlie is referred to a social worker for discharge placement. All of the following may be appropriate placements, *except:*
   1. Foster-care family.
   2. Inpatient psychiatric hospital.
   3. Group home.
   4. Juvenile care home.

40. Charlie has been living in a group home for the past two months. He has asked permission to visit a friend in the psychiatric hospital. The nurse should:
   1. Allow him to visit.
   2. Assess his motives.
   3. Ask his parents' permission.
   4. Consult with the hospital staff.

ANSWERS/RATIONALE

1. (3) The adolescent is striving to attain a sense of independence and identity. Trust (No. 1) is usually developed during infancy and matures as the individual develops. Goals and plans (No. 2) are made during the adolescent period, but they are rarely finalized realistically until late adulthood. Inner conflicts (No. 4) are rarely resolved and usually heightened during this period.

2. (4) The superego may never be completely refined or stabilized. Some individuals may achieve an optimal level of function some time in late adulthood; however, rarely will the superego become stabilized during adolescence. As stated in No. 1, the individual does strive to develop an independent and unique personality during adolescence. In order to maintain a steady state of functioning, the adolescent must learn to use defense mechanisms (No. 2) in an appropriate manner. Developing a positive ego identity (No. 3) is one of the major goals of adolescence.

3. (1) In order for adolescents to achieve an optimal level of development, they must resolve the inner conflicts involving identification that occur during the Oedipal phase. Thus Nos. 2, 3, and 4 are incorrect.

4. (4) Conversion is a process whereby repressed instinctual tendencies are expressed or converted through sensory or motor manifestations, such as paralysis of a limb or blindness, that have no organic basis. Adolescents will generally regress, withdraw, or deny (Nos. 1, 2, and 3) that a certain situation or problem exists.

5. (4) Adolescents tend to oscillate between periods of high energy and moods and those of low energy and moods. In several hours they can swing from a very depressed to a manic level of functioning. Most adolescents are initially reluctant to share their feelings with others (No. 1). They want to avoid feelings of embarrassment, rejection, shame, etc. Adolescents may also be reluctant to trust others right away (No. 2); however, whether they are generally willing to share their feelings openly or not depends on many individual factors such as maturity, personality, and independence. Nevertheless, many meaningful and intimate relationships may develop during adolescence (No. 3).

6. (1) Although many adolescents may feel that their parents are too strict, harsh, or untrusting, they are usually subconsciously, if not consciously, aware that their parents love them. However, the struggle for freedom from parental control usually initiates the statements made in Nos. 2, 3, and 4.

7. (2) Altruistic concern for the welfare of others is normally not a basic characteristic of adolescents. Adolescents still need to focus on themselves to a degree. They perform tasks in the interest of gaining something for themselves (e.g., they might clean the garage so that they can use the car for the evening). Frustration, a normal characteristic of adolescence, usually leads to aggression (No. 1). Adolescents may display and experiment with homosexual tendencies (No. 3), and they may exhibit hypochondriasis (No. 4) in order to gain attention or meet needs; for example, they might feign illness in order to miss school or to avoid tasks they are unsure they can master.

8. (4) The passage of time will not help Charlie cope effectively with his feelings of fear and ambivalence. These feelings are a normal part of the maturation process, and only with effective limit-setting and psychologic support will the adolescent's ability to cope be strengthened. In early adolescence boys generally are intolerant of female authority figures (No. 1). They perceive these females as a threat to their emerging masculine identity. Adolescents need physical activity to alleviate tension (No. 2). Males in general have problems dealing with impulse control (No. 3) and need consistent limits set on their behaviors.

9. (1) Adolescents are preoccupied with their changing bodies, their relationships, and their fantasies. Although they have difficulty with rote learning (No. 2), they have an increased potential for imaginative thinking. During this period they are less able to concentrate on their academic work (No. 3), which leads to increased feelings of frustration that are usually *not* accompanied by an increased ability to cope (No. 4).

10. (2) Limits do need to be set, but they should be based on mutual respect rather than fear. Adult (or external) controls on behavior (No. 1) are essential and must be consistent. Role models serve to stimulate the identifi-

cation process (No. 3) both consciously and unconsciously. Stable relationships (No. 4) are essential if the adolescent is to mature and to develop a sense of trust.

11. (1) Acting out is the expression through behavior (rather than through words) of emotions that occur when the client relives or reproduces the feelings, wishes, or conflicts that are operating unconsciously. Charlie may be feeling frustrated, angry, ambivalent, etc., for numerous reasons, such as conflict between himself and his parents, a reaction to his parents' intramarital conflicts, sibling rivalry, or frustration due to poor self-esteem.

12. (4) The fact that Charlie's parents married at an early age may be significant in terms of how they relate to each other as well as to their children; however, Nos. 1, 2, and 3 are all *more* relevant in terms of assessing Charlie's personal needs at this time: his successes and failures in maturing through each stage of development, his need for a male role model to ensure adequate progression through the identification process, and the anxiety and ambivalence generated by his parents' arguments, which cause him to doubt his parents' feelings for each other as well as their feelings for him.

13. (3) Hostility and aggression are considered the underlying factors in the psychogenesis and psychodynamics of depression. The adolescent is in a stage of development where he experiences extensive anger due to frustration. The adolescent has a greater energy level because of the increased libidinal energy available in his system. In order to expend this energy, many adolescents act out their feelings of depression in violent ways rather than become withdrawn, apathetic, or regressive (Nos. 1, 2, and 4).

14. (2) Hitting others provides Charlie with an outlet for his feelings of hopelessness and despair. Although this behavior may not make him feel happy or satisfied, it does provide a defense against feeling unhappy. Nos. 1, 3, and 4 are not primary motivations of this behavior.

15. (1) If a confrontation develops too soon, Charlie may feel threatened and run away from the hospital. Although Nos. 2, 3, and 4 are all true, they have less significant consequences. Charlie's refusal to verbalize is expected only initially because he probably will not trust the group members at first. The other group members may also feel threatened by a new member and may not trust him. Acting out is a coping mechanism that Charlie uses to mask his fear of a new situation or his sense of being threatened.

16. (4) Since Charlie has only attended six sessions of group therapy, it is expected that he would only speak when questioned. He is probably still unsure of his own feelings and is in the preinteraction phase of trusting other group members. Nos. 1, 2, and 3 are probably not true at this point.

17. (4) It is important for the angry client to express his feelings overtly. Internalizing them would cause increased feelings of frustration and anxiety and would therefore be counterproductive. Nos. 1, 2, and 3 are all appropriate goals.

18. (4) Charlie initially needs to be forced to socialize. He must be stimulated by the staff to participate in minimally demanding group activities (No. 1). Allowing him a minimum of three hours in his room (No. 3) will probably stimulate an increase in isolation and withdrawal. Perhaps the nurse could establish a behavior modification program involving a trade-off of 15 minutes in his room for every 45 minutes spent socializing and interacting with others. If activities are too challenging (No. 2), Charlie may become frustrated and feel incompetent, which would lead to a decrease in self-esteem.

19. (2) Confrontation could help Charlie identify the inappropriateness of mutilation and other destructive behaviors as attention-getting devices. Nos. 1, 3, and 4 are all appropriate interventions.

20. (3) Charlie's thoughts, feelings, and attitudes toward sexual relationships need to be explored in order to assess his level of maturity in deciding his sexual preference. Confrontation (No. 1) could help Charlie identify his use of homosexual behavior as an attention-seeking device. Validation of his rationale for seeking homosexual relationships (No. 2) may be identified more appropriately through exploring his thoughts, feelings, and attitudes regarding his sexual orientation. Enforcing limits on his relationships (No. 4) will only make him angry and is in any case an invasion of his right to privacy and freedom of choice. As long as neither Charlie nor Rich is forcing himself on the other, their relationship should not be interfered with. However, if it is determined that for some appropriate reason this relationship is detrimental to either individual's optimal level of functioning, then limits should be set.

21. (2) Levels of anxiety cannot be identified absolutely. The nurse must assess all behaviors and look at the interrelationships to determine on what level the client is functioning at this time. Clients experiencing a moderate to severe level of anxiety generally exhibit physical symptoms such as crying, headaches, pounding heart, gastric discomfort, and muscular tension. They usually have a reduced ability to perceive and communicate. Nos. 1, 3, and 4 are less likely.

22. (4) Isolation may lead to withdrawal and depression. Charlie's mother needs positive reinforcement and reassurance to increase her self-esteem. Isolation may also lead to an increase in her drinking and depression. Based on the symptoms Charlie's mother is exhibiting, involving her in simple, concrete tasks may help her feel useful (No. 1). Crying helps her alleviate anxiety through the physical expression of her feelings (No. 2). Encour-

aging the verbalization of her feelings (No. 3) will demonstrate that someone cares for her enough to listen, and may decrease her anxiety level.

23. (2) Past coping mechanisms are important in assessing the client's ability to return to a steady state of functioning. Strengths and weaknesses in the client's ability to rationally assess and cope with her feelings need to be explored. Referrals may need to be made (No. 1), but an initial assessment of the client needs to be completed first. Inpatient hospitalization may be needed (No. 3); however, the assessment of her ability to cope with the situation may assist in identifying whether hospitalization is needed. Obtaining a prescription for an antidepressant at this time may prove to be detrimental (No. 4). Even if she does not decide to overdose, medication without psychologic support is generally ineffective.

24. (3) The first priority with any unconscious client is to maintain a patent airway. The nurse would need a physician's order to administer any medication or stimulant (No. 1), which may not be appropriate in this situation. The emergency room nurse would see that the attending resident was paged (No. 2), but this task could be delegated while the nurse administered primary care. Monitoring neurologic signs (No. 4) is also essential but can be done after ensuring that the client can breathe.

25. (3) The client should be placed under one-to-one, not group, observation to ensure effective protection against suicidal behaviors. Nos. 1, 2, and 4 are all appropriate actions.

26. (1) Individuals who have used alcohol habitually over an extended time period usually exhibit symptoms of withdrawal delirium when the alcohol intake is severely decreased or curtailed. Nos. 2, 3, and 4 are less likely reactions.

27. (4) The psychologic effect of being restrained can be severe. Therefore any form of restraint should be applied as a last resort. Isolating the patient from other patients during the initial adjustment period would serve to decrease stimuli and possibly prevent the need for restraints. Nos. 1, 2, and 3 are all appropriate interventions.

28. (2) An increase in Charlie's mother's energy level may provide her with enough motivation to make another suicide attempt. Generally, depressed patients do not kill themselves because their energy level is very low. Therefore the one-to-one relationship needs to be maintained and stressed at this time. Nos. 1, 3, and 4 are dangerous assumptions at this time.

29. (1) Family therapy should promote the expression of feelings. Intragroup dynamics of the family system should be assessed, and appropriate coping strategies identified. The objectives of family therapy are not primarily to provide individual therapy for each family member (No. 2). If a family member needs one-to-one therapy, individual therapy is usually provided in conjunction with, but at a separate time from, family therapy sessions. The identified client is treated in individual and family therapy sessions (No. 3). However, the primary focus of family therapy is not just treatment of this particular individual. Crisis intervention may be one aspect of family therapy (No. 4), but it is not necessarily the primary goal in this case. Crisis intervention may be used initially to assist in returning the family system to a steady state of functioning.

30. (3) Establishing trust between the therapist and the couple is essential to facilitate effective therapy and possible resolution of the marital and familial conflicts. Confrontation (No. 1) may prove very threatening in this situation, and the couple may leave therapy to avoid feelings of anxiety. Avoidance (No. 2) is nontherapeutic in this situation because it does not help resolve the conflict. A referral may be appropriate (No. 4); however, the nurse should initially use all her therapeutic techniques in assisting the couple to identify relevant issues and possibly to resolve conflicts before making a referral.

31. (3) Most obsessive-compulsive individuals are highly inflexible and resist change because change stimulates anxiety and they are unable to cope with stress. Nos. 1, 2, and 4 are all likely behaviors.

32. (2) Denial is the failure to acknowledge the existence of an affect, experience, idea, or memory. The person blocks from conscious awareness that which is painful, anxiety-provoking, or threatening. Charlie's father may perceive that his behavior contributes to his wife's use of alcohol, and he may use denial to avoid facing feelings of guilt. Projection (No. 1) is the attribution of one's feelings, impulses, thoughts, and wishes to others or to the environment. Repression (No. 3) is an unconscious mechanism used to avoid painful experiences, unacceptable thoughts and impulses, and disagreeable memories by "forgetting." Sublimation (No. 4) is the transformation of psychic energy associated with unacceptable sexual or aggressive behaviors into socially acceptable outlets.

33. (1) Lithium is used to treat affective disorders. Mellaril (No. 4) is a major tranquilizer used to treat schizophrenia. Mellaril has been used to treat the manic phase of bipolic affective disorders, but it is not the primary drug. Prolixin (No. 3) is a long-acting psychotropic used primarily to treat schizophrenia. It can be administered biweekly in an injection for a long-term effect. Librium (No. 2) is a minor tranquilizer used to relieve the mild or moderate anxiety usually associated with affective and somatoform disorders.

34. (1) Lithium is excreted through the kidneys. Consequently, the kidneys must function adequately to avoid lithium toxicity. Diuretics should not be given concur-

rently with lithium because they may potentiate sodium and fluid depletion, which may lead to lithium toxicity. Haldol (No. 4) is a major tranquilizer that is sometimes administered simultaneously with lithium during the first week to ten days to control manic symptoms. Nausea, vomiting, and muscle weakness (No. 3) are all possible side effects of lithium. They indicate a need for close observation and regulation of the drug if they disrupt the person's level of functioning. Every patient should be screened prior to the administration of any medication (No. 2). However, since lithium is a drug that is taken over a long period of time, blood levels must be consistently regulated and physical examinations routinely scheduled (i.e., physical exams every three months initially, then every six months once the patient appears to be regulated).

35. (3) Charlie is probably very frightened and angry. He needs to feel that his side will be considered if he is to cope effectively with these feelings and with his behavior. Nos. 1, 2, and 4 are all staff-oriented and provide little psychologic support for Charlie as an individual striving for independence.

36. (1) Charlie's thoughts and feelings about plans for his discharge are essential. It is Charlie who must be able to identify and implement effective coping mechanisms. He must be able to seek assistance as needed and to realize when he is no longer able to cope effectively.

37. (3) Although there are several forms that elicit disclosure of this information, there is no law that mandates disclosure (No. 4). Charlie has to make this decision independently. The nurse should provide therapeutic support for whatever he decides. Nos. 1 and 2 are not true statements.

38. (2) Although Charlie's parents may perceive this as a parental decision, it is important for Charlie's sister and brother to be included in the decision-making process because the entire family system will be affected by this change. Asking the parents to reassess their feelings (No. 1) may help them evaluate the situation, but it avoids facing the issue as a family decision. A referral may be appropriate (Nos. 3 and 4); however, all parties involved in the decision must be listened to before making a referral or searching for an alternative placement.

39. (2) Long-term inpatient hospitalization would be inappropriate in Charlie's case. He has already been hospitalized for an extended period of time. In order to resocialize him to function effectively in society, he needs a structured and familylike environment, not a hospital or psychiatric institution. Nos. 1, 3, and 4 are all appropriate placements.

40. (2) Charlie may have valid reasons for wanting to visit his friend, but allowing him to visit without assessing his motives (No. 1) may prove detrimental to Charlie, his friend, and the staff. Charlie's parents (No. 3) essen-

tially relinquished their decision-making authority by allowing Charlie to become a ward of the State. The hospital staff would have to be consulted prior to Charlie's visit, regardless of his motive. However, No. 4 is too vague in that it does not specify what issues would be covered in the consultation.

CASE STUDY 2

Lauren is a 28-year-old white female who suspects that she is about three months pregnant. She has scheduled an appointment within the next week to see her physician for a complete physical examination.

Lauren has been married half a year to a transit-bus driver named Justin, age 32, who has had the same job for the past six years. Lauren has worked as an administrative assistant for the bus company for nearly seven years. Her hours are from 9:00 A.M. to 5:00 P.M., Monday to Friday, whereas Justin rotates through three different shifts every month.

Lauren and Justin live in a one-bedroom apartment just outside the city limits. Lauren's pregnancy was unexpected and unplanned, and the couple have not yet decided whether they really want to have any children at all.

Lauren is the eldest of three children. She has a 26-year-old brother and a 10-year-old sister, both of whom have Down's syndrome. Her parents are both alive and healthy.

Justin is an only child. His father died of a myocardial infarction at age 35, when Justin was 15. His mother was recently diagnosed as extremely hypertensive, with a blood pressure of 180/90–100.

QUESTIONS

1. In assessing Lauren's reasons for suspecting she may be three months pregnant, the most relevant question for the nurse to ask would be:
   1. Are you currently taking oral contraceptives?
   2. When was your last menstrual period?
   3. How much weight have you gained?
   4. Have you ever been pregnant before?

2. If the first day of Lauren's LMP was July 10, 1981, what is her EDC?
   1. April 17, 1982.
   2. May 30, 1982.
   3. March 14, 1982.
   4. June 1, 1982.

3. Given that Lauren is three months pregnant, what symptoms would she be exhibiting at this time?

1. Quickening.
2. Amenorrhea.
3. Positive HCG test.
4. Nausea and vomiting.

4. How often during the second trimester should Lauren be examined?
   1. Once a week.
   2. Once every two weeks.
   3. Every other month.
   4. Once a month.

5. If this is Lauren's second pregnancy but the first did not reach viability, what would her parity be?
   1. 1001.
   2. 0010.
   3. 0100.
   4. 0101.

6. In health-teaching Lauren and Justin about the pregnancy, the nurse should tell them that all of the following are positive signs, *except*:
   1. Fetal heart sounds.
   2. Positive pregnancy tests.
   3. Fetal movements felt by examiner.
   4. Outline of fetal skeleton seen on an X ray.

7. In performing Lauren's prenatal assessment, the nurse should implement all of the following screening tests during each visit, *except*:
   1. A blood test for an increase in glucose.
   2. Urine screening for albumin.
   3. Assessment of Lauren's weight gain.
   4. Screening of Lauren's blood pressure.

8. Lauren and Justin have expressed some concern over having an unplanned baby at this time. Which of the following questions would be the most appropriate to ask the couple to assess their feelings?
   1. What do you plan to do about this pregnancy?
   2. Do you want to schedule an abortion?
   3. Would you like to schedule an appointment to see a counselor?
   4. What are your feelings regarding this pregnancy?

Lauren has expressed anxiety over the fact that her brother and sister have Down's syndrome, and she asks the nurse what this involves.

9. In health-teaching Lauren about Down's, the nurse should tell her all of the following, *except*:
   1. Down's syndrome is an abnormality that can result from an extra chromosome.
   2. Down's syndrome is only seen in children born to older women.
   3. Down's syndrome can be diagnosed in utero.
   4. Down's syndrome is a form of mental retardation.

10. In assessing an infant with Down's syndrome, the nurse should expect all of the following, *except*:
    1. The infant's physiognomy resembles that of an Asian.

2. Mental development seldom reaches beyond that of the average child of 5–7 years.
3. It will have little resistance to infection.
4. Special education assures adequate development.

During Lauren's thirtieth week of pregnancy she is diagnosed as having preeclampsia. Questions 11–17 concern this situation.

11. In planning Lauren's care during this period, the nurse should consider all of the following, *except*:
    1. Keeping stimuli such as light and noise at a minimum level.
    2. Monitoring Lauren's weight qd.
    3. Approximating Lauren's intake and output.
    4. Assessing Lauren for signs and symptoms of labor.

12. The nurse observes Lauren having a convulsion. The nurse's primary action should be to:
    1. Maintain a patent airway.
    2. Observe for bowel or bladder evacuation.
    3. Administer cardiac pulmonary resuscitation.
    4. Maintain a safe environment.

13. Lauren verbalizes concern about the possibility of having to remain hospitalized for the next eight weeks because of her preeclampsia. The *most* therapeutic response the nurse could make would be:
    1. It may not be that bad if you keep busy.
    2. Tell me how you are feeling.
    3. I'll sit with you a while.
    4. Maybe you should tell your doctor how you are feeling.

14. Lauren and Justin express anxiety about having limited insurance coverage. The *most* appropriate nursing intervention would be to:
    1. Refer the couple to social services for possible assistance.
    2. Initiate a family-counseling referral.
    3. Provide supportive counseling.
    4. Assess the couple's needs through discussion.

15. Lauren and Justin are concerned about what effect preeclampsia may have on the fetus. In health-teaching the couple about the signs and symptoms of fetal distress, the nurse should consider all of the following, *except*:
    1. Persistent bradycardia of 100 or less per minute.
    2. Persistent tachycardia of 160 or more per minute.
    3. Passage of meconium.
    4. Low blood glucose.

16. To assess the health status of the fetus, an amniocentesis may be performed for the purposes of all of the following, *except*:
    1. Diagnosis of fetal jeopardy.
    2. Assessment of fetal maturity.
    3. Diagnosis of sickle cell anemia.
    4. Assessment of placental function.

17. The nurse's role in assisting with implementing the amniocentesis includes all of the following, *except:*
    1. Informing the woman about the risks involved.
    2. Reinforcing what the procedure will encompass.
    3. Assisting with sonography to locate the placenta.
    4. Monitoring the fetal heart rate.

18. Lauren is concerned about her weight gain of 15 pounds in week 29 of pregnancy. The nurse assessing Lauren should identify that she is primarily concerned about:
    1. The baby's nutritional status.
    2. Her own body image.
    3. Her need to diet.
    4. Her need to gain more weight.

19. As Lauren remains essentially healthy, the nurse's health-teaching about safeguards to maintain throughout pregnancy should advise Lauren to:
    1. Stop working by week 32 of gestation.
    2. Wear comfortable clothes.
    3. Avoid alcoholic beverages.
    4. Eat a minimum of three full meals each day.

20. During week 31 of gestation Justin verbalizes feelings of being rejected and left out. He asks the nurse how he should cope with these feelings. The most therapeutic response would be:
    1. "Just think, this will all be over soon."
    2. "Things can't be all that bad."
    3. "Let's talk about how you are feeling."
    4. "You should consider how Lauren is feeling."

21. The couple presently live in a one-bedroom apartment approximately a quarter of a mile outside the city limits. In assessing this situation and implementing care, the nurse should:
    1. Arrange for Justin and Lauren to see a social worker to discuss moving.
    2. Assess how the couple perceive their housing needs.
    3. Refer the couple to a public health nurse for follow-up.
    4. Look for apartments in the paper and share the information with Lauren and Justin.

Lauren and Justin ask the nurse about the possibility of participating in natural childbirth classes.

22. In health-teaching the couple about natural childbirth, the nurse should *first:*
    1. Evaluate the couple's knowledge of childbirth techniques.
    2. Assess the couple's level of readiness to learn.
    3. Consult a childbirth nurse practitioner regarding what to tell the couple.
    4. Refer the couple to a LaMaze childbirth class.

23. Although the LaMaze and Grantly Dick–Read methods of childbirth have several theoretical differences, they both agree with all of the following, *except:*
    1. If the couple comprehends the physiology of the contractions and of labor tension, then fear is reduced.

2. Conditioned responses are necessary in order to shift focus away from the pain.
3. Breathing techniques may assist in decreasing the tension.
4. Health-teaching involving both the male and female is essential.

When Lauren is 32 weeks pregnant, she comes into the emergency room complaining of constant pain across her lower abdomen and back and of intermittent, dark vaginal bleeding.

24. In assessing Lauren's condition, the nurse should suspect that she is experiencing:
    1. Eclampsia.
    2. Abruptio placentae.
    3. Placenta previa.
    4. Normal labor.

25. Lauren is diagnosed as having abruptio placentae. The nurse should now keep all of the following in mind, *except:*
    1. Lauren is unlikely to go into shock because she is not bleeding excessively.
    2. The fetus may be in fetal distress because it is exhibiting hyperactivity.
    3. Lauren is probably very anxious, so she should be informed of what is happening in concrete and specific language.
    4. Lauren and Justin should be informed that the baby will probably be delivered by cesarean surgery.

During Lauren's tenth week of pregnancy she experiences hyperemesis gravidarum.

26. Signs and symptoms the nurse should assess include all of the following, *except:*
    1. Weight loss.
    2. Edema.
    3. Hiccups.
    4. Anorexia.

27. Lauren continues to experience symptoms of hyperemesis gravidarum in her fifteenth week of pregnancy. She is hospitalized for treatment. All of the following are appropriate nursing interventions, *except:*
    1. Assessing for acetone breath.
    2. Maintaining client on NPO status for the first 24 hours.
    3. Monitoring I & O carefully.
    4. Restricting all visitors except her mate.

In week 41 of Lauren's pregnancy, she enters the hospital in active labor (i.e., contractions are every 10 minutes). Her water broke approximately 45 minutes prior to admission. Questions 28–30 concern this situation.

28. The nurse's primary intervention would be to:
    1. Health-teach the couple the stages of labor.
    2. Prepare Lauren for delivery.
    3. Assess the couple's level of preparation.
    4. Reassure the couple and to answer any questions.

29. Lauren is in the transitional phase of the first stage of labor. During this time the nurse would expect Lauren to be:
    1. Irritable.
    2. Excited.
    3. Euphoric.
    4. Serious.

30. Immediately before Lauren goes into the delivery room, Justin expresses anxiety about going in with her. The most appropriate response the nurse could make would be:
    1. "Many people find it scary the first time."
    2. "You'll do fine, don't worry."
    3. "Think of Lauren. How will she feel if you don't go in?"
    4. "Once you get in there you'll forget all about being afraid."

31. After Lauren delivers, the infant's condition is assessed. His respirations do not establish readily, he is slightly cyanotic, and there is some muscle flaccidity. The most appropriate nursing action would be to:
    1. Initiate CPR immediately.
    2. Clear airway and administer oxygen.
    3. Reassure the parents.
    4. Check Lauren's chart for her last medication (drug, time, and amount).

32. Lauren has decided to breastfeed. The nurse's health-teaching should instruct Lauren that all of the following statements are true, *except:*
    1. Rest and relaxation are essential.
    2. An adequate diet is important.
    3. Larger breasts produce more milk.
    4. Birth control is necessary throughout breastfeeding.

33. In planning Lauren's discharge care, the nurse would initiate health-teaching including all of the following factual information, *except:*
    1. Lauren should wash her breasts with warm water and pat dry.
    2. Lauren should expect the vaginal discharge to become pinkish in color by day 5 or 6.
    3. Lauren may experience afterpains for the first couple of days following discharge.
    4. Lauren's milk may not come in until the third or fourth day postpartum.

34. Lauren and Justin express concern about when they can resume intercourse. After validating the information with Lauren's physician, the nurse would inform the couple that:
    1. Generally it's a good idea to wait until after the sixth-week-postpartum check-up.
    2. If there are no unforeseen problems, three weeks is usually the recommended waiting time.
    3. The couple may have sex as soon as they arrive home from the hospital, as long as Lauren feels up to it.
    4. The couple should wait until Lauren ceases to breast-feed.

35. Justin comes in with Lauren and their new son for the sixth-week-postpartum visit. He expresses concern about Lauren's strange behavior. He states that she is listless and apathetic and doesn't eat much. What would be the nurse's most appropriate response?
    1. Inform him that many women experience some degree of depression after the birth of a baby.
    2. A psychiatric referral should be made to assist Lauren in coping with this crisis.
    3. Notify the physician of Justin's concern and ask the physician to prescribe an antidepressant for Lauren.
    4. Suggest that Justin be patient, since these symptoms will dissipate.

36. After the baby is 6 months old, Justin and Lauren bring him in for a physical examination. As all his immunizations are up to date, what should he receive today?
    1. DTP and TOPV.
    2. TOPV.
    3. DTP.
    4. MMR.

37. When the baby is 18 months old, Justin is dismissed from work and Lauren returns to work. Justin refuses to seek employment or to watch the baby. The most appropriate nursing response would be to:
    1. Suggest that the couple seek marital counseling.
    2. Recommend individual therapy for Justin.
    3. Provide crisis intervention.
    4. Assess the couple's level of functioning.

Justin is diagnosed as being moderately hypertensive.

38. In assessing Justin's BP, the nurse most likely finds that his resting diastolic pressure is:
    1. Between 110 and 120 mm Hg.
    2. Between 90 and 110 mm Hg.
    3. Between 120 and 140 mm Hg.
    4. Between 100 and 115 mm Hg.

39. Justin is eventually hospitalized with a BP of 170/100, difficulty breathing, dizziness, and weakness. The nurse establishing his care should consider all of the following, *except:*
    1. Ensuring that a different nurse take care of Justin each day to prevent hospital fatigue.
    2. Reducing situations that create and increase physical stress.
    3. Identifying any misconceptions Justin may have regarding hypertension.
    4. Stressing the importance of reporting even minor symptoms to the physician.

40. In planning discharge care for Justin after his treatment for hypertension, the nurse should consider all of the following, *except:*
    1. Medication scheduling and side effects.
    2. Dietary restrictions.
    3. Importance of not smoking.
    4. Sexual activity restrictions.

ANSWERS/RATIONALE

1. (2) The date of Lauren's last period is the most relevant question to ask in performing the initial assessment because it will assist the nurse in making a preliminary determination of possible pregnancy. Whether Lauren is presently taking oral contraceptives (No. 1) may be relevant, but it would be more pertinent to assess generally what type of birth control the couple may be using and if they have been using it effectively. How much weight she has gained and whether she has been pregnant before (Nos. 3 and 4) are relevant to performing the assessment, but not essential to determining whether she is pregnant at the present time.

2. (1) According to Nägele's rule of LMP + 7 days − 3 months + 1 year, the calculations would be: 7/10/81 − 3 months = 4/10/81, + 7 days = 4/17/81, + 1 year = 4/17/82. Nägele's rule assumes that the woman has a 28-day cycle and that pregnancy occurred on the fourteenth day. If Lauren's cycle is longer or shorter than 28 days, appropriate adjustments must be made. Only about 4–5% of women deliver on EDC plus or minus seven days.

3. (3) This is one of the most accurate indicators of pregnancy. Quickening (No. 1) usually does not occur until the sixteenth week of gestation. Not all women have amenorrhea (No. 2), especially during the first trimester. Nausea and vomiting (No. 4) are not necessarily experienced by all women.

4. (4) If there are no complications, prenatal examinations should be scheduled once a month for the first 32 weeks. After week 32 examinations should be performed every 2 weeks (No. 2). Beginning week 36, exams are performed weekly until delivery (No. 1). No. 3 allows too much time to elapse and may lead to increased complications.

5. (2) The formula for determining parity is: first—number of full-term births; second—number of premature births; third—number of abortions; and fourth—number of living children. *Hint:* the slogan "full power and light" may assist you in remembering how to determine parity.

6. (2) Positive pregnancy tests (except the bioassay test for the beta subunit of HCG, which is accurate) are considered among the *probable* signs of pregnancy. Nos. 1, 3, and 4 are all positive signs.

7. (1) Testing Lauren's blood does not need to be done every visit. However, blood tests should be done during the initial prenatal visit and, barring any complications, sometime around week 32 of gestation. Nos. 2, 3, and 4 should all be performed during each visit to assess overall functioning of the system.

8. (4) The most therapeutic and open-ended response is to focus on *feelings*. No. 1 puts stress on the couple to make a decision that they may not be ready to make at this time. No. 2 presents a very limited alternative without assessing the couple's feelings. No. 3 is an appropriate response but does not provide for adequate *nursing* intervention. It is the nurse's role to provide a comprehensive assessment, and referrals should be made only when, in the nurse's professional judgment, she or he is unable to work through the situation.

9. (2) One form of Down's syndrome, trisomy 21, is associated with maternal age (over 35); however, another form of the syndrome, mosaicism, occurs in children born to women of any age.

10. (4) Although many of these children are trainable using copying techniques repeatedly and consistently reinforced, others are not trainable and may never exceed the mental age of 5–7 years (No. 2).

11. (3) Lauren's intake and output must be carefully monitored throughout the entire day. Accuracy is paramount. Reduction of stimuli is important to assist in maintaining a stable BP and in avoiding overstimulation of her CNS. Lauren should be weighed at least once a day (if not more often) to assess fluid loss or retention. Evaluating whether she is in labor or not is important in order to assess the health status of the fetus and mother (No. 4). Nos. 1 and 2 are also appropriate actions.

12. (1) The primary nursing action would be to maintain a patent airway to ensure O_2 for the woman and fetus. CPR (No. 3) may be needed if Lauren progresses into cardiac arrest. However, in implementing CPR, maintaining a patent airway is the foremost priority. Providing a safe environment (No. 4) is an important second priority. Observing bowel and bladder functioning (No. 2) may also be important to a thorough assessment of the convulsions but is of less priority than providing a patent airway or ensuring safety.

13. (2) This response is open ended and will elicit the most information. No. 1 merely provides false reassurance. No. 3 may be a therapeutic response, but it is a short-term intervention unless the nurse consistently sits with Lauren for a while every day. If possible, the same nurse should be assigned to Lauren each day. Referring Lauren to her doctor (No. 4) is an inappropriate nursing intervention because the nurse can work in conjunction with the physician to provide psychologic support.

14. (4) An effective assessment of the couple's needs is obtained through discussing the couple's own perceptions of those needs. Nos. 1, 2, and 3 may be appropriate actions once a thorough assessment is complete, but should never precede discussion with the couple.

15. (4) Hypoglycemia may occur, but it is usually not a top priority when teaching the couple about intrauterine

fetal distress. A decrease in blood glucose is usually assessed after birth.

16. (3) It would be difficult to diagnose sickle cell anemia in utero. Also, the risk to the fetus in performing the amniocentesis would outweigh the value of diagnosing sickle cell disease in utero. Nos. 1, 2, and 4 are all appropriate.

17. (1) Obtaining consent and informing the woman about the risks involved are legally the physician's role. The nurse's role is to reinforce the physician's teaching and to validate that the information has been given to the patient.

18. (2) Throughout pregnancy, especially after the second trimester, most women express anxiety over their change in body image. The nurse must be aware of the need to provide positive reinforcement and encouragement in order to facilitate and maintain Lauren's self-esteem. No. 1 is inappropriate because during this stage of pregnancy the mother is very self-focused. Most women realize that dieting during pregnancy (No. 3) is contraindicated unless prescribed by a physician. No. 4 is of no concern to the pregnant woman because she is gaining plenty of weight.

19. (2) The least restrictive safeguard is No. 2. Each individual's situation must be assessed prior to suggesting the other safeguards. Many women feel up to working until the day of delivery and continue to work as long as their physician approves (No. 1). Admonishment is not needed if woman does not drink (No. 3). No. 4 would depend on the woman's or her fetus's needs.

20. (3) This is the most open-ended response, allowing Justin to feel important enough to be listened to. Encouraging him to verbalize his feelings at this time may initiate a trusting relationship between the nurse and the clients and may serve to strengthen the couple's relationship. Nos. 1, 2, and 4 neither encourage Justin to talk nor validate his feelings.

21. (2) Validating the clients' perceptions of their own needs is most important. Referrals can always be initiated if the couple desire to resolve the issue in this manner (Nos. 1 and 3). No. 4 is incorrect because the nurse should allow the couple to make this decision themselves.

22. (1) In evaluating their present knowledge of childbirth techniques, the nurse will be able to set up a more efficient and effective program of learning for the couple. They may have already investigated resources and may need more validating than primary health-teaching. The next goal would be to meet the couple at their level of readiness (No. 2) in order to ensure optimal learning. The nurse may consult or refer to a specialist in the area (No. 3) if unsure of the information. No. 4 may be inappropriate if the couple desire an alternative method or do not think that LaMaze is effective.

23. (2) Conditioned responses are used primarily in the LaMaze technique, which emphasizes the use of a focal point and a coach throughout the labor process. The Read method tends to emphasize the importance of decreasing the fear of the unknown through adequate health-teaching. Nos. 1, 3, and 4 are common to both methods.

24. (2) Lauren is experiencing symptoms of abruptio placentae. The nurse must assess the situation as efficiently as possible and implement care immediately because of the danger to the mother and the fetus. In eclampsia (No. 1) the signs and symptoms usually include an increased BP, edema, weight gain, and oliguria (diminished urinary output). If the condition is not rapidly treated, convulsions and coma will probably ensue. Pain is a key symptom of abruptio placentae but usually not a symptom of placenta previa (No. 3). This would not be considered normal labor (No. 4) because she is only 32 weeks pregnant, and she is experiencing pain and bleeding.

25. (1) A woman experiencing abruptio placentae is at risk for shock even when the observed amount of bleeding is minimal. Shock is usually more profound than the amount of bleeding suggests. Nos. 2, 3, and 4 are all true.

26. (2) In most instances women exhibit signs of starvation and dehydration because of the lack of fluid intake, and persistent vomiting. Nos. 1, 3, and 4 are all signs and symptoms of hyperemesis gravidarum.

27. (4) Lauren's husband should also be restricted from visiting because he may be a contributing factor in increasing her anxiety. Nos. 1, 2, and 3 are all appropriate interventions.

28. (4) In this case the nurse's calm, assured manner would be most therapeutic. It would serve to decrease the couple's anxiety and to facilitate an effective admission and delivery. Health-teaching the stages of labor (No. 1) at this time would be inappropriate because the couple's anxiety level would probably interfere with effective learning. However, reinforcing any previously learned material and answering questions may be useful. No. 2 is inappropriate because although Lauren is in active labor, she is not ready to deliver at this time. Assessing the couple's level of preparation (No. 3) would be done in conjunction with answering questions. It would be more important to assess their level of readiness rather than preparation at this point in time.

29. (1) Lauren is more apt to become irritable, uncooperative, and discouraged during the transitional phase. Excitement and euphoria (Nos. 2 and 3) are associated with the latent phase; seriousness (No. 4), with the active phase.

30. (1) Providing reassurance that it's normal for most people to fear the unknown may bolster Justin's confidence. If more time were available you would try to explore his fears and provide emotional support. No. 2 is inappropriate because it provides false reassurance, which may merely increase his anxiety. No. 3 may stimulate feelings of guilt. No. 4 may not necessarily be true and may provide false reassurance.

31. (2) Providing and maintaining a patent airway and administering oxygen immediately are essential in order to establish regular respirations. CPR (No. 1) may not be necessary if respirations are adequately established. Reassuring the parents (No. 3) is not appropriate now. No one can accurately predict the outcome at this point. Checking the mother's chart for type of drug, amount, and time given (No. 4) is more appropriately the job of a second staff member in attendance. The neonate may be a candidate for Narcan.

32. (3) The actual size of the breasts is not as important as the amount of glandular tissue, because it is not the adipose tissue but the secreting tissues of the mammary gland that produce the milk. Diet and rest (Nos. 1 and 2) are essential to promoting lactation. A nursing mother may ovulate and could become pregnant while lactating (No. 4).

33. (3) Afterpains are generally experienced by multiparas within the first few days postpartum. Nos. 1, 2, and 4 are all correct information.

34. (2) All physicians and/or institutions have their own guidelines. However, three weeks is generally appropriate if the lochea has decreased and becomes fairly clear in color, and if there are no other problems. No. 3 is too soon, and Nos. 1 and 4 are longer than is usually necessary.

35. (1) Many women experience some feeling of slight to moderate depression. Sleep deprivation and an inadequate support system may contribute to the "blues." However, if the behaviors become severe (i.e., persistent over a long period of time and increasingly exaggerated), professional help should be initiated (No. 2). No. 3 is inappropriate because a physician's referral may not be necessary and because it is not the nurse's job to ask the physician to prescribe antidepressants. Lauren may not even need any medication. Justin should be informed that patience, understanding, and help with housework and care of the infant may assist in decreasing some of Lauren's anxiety (No. 4).

36. (3) The immunization schedule is as follows:

2 months	DTP and TOPV.
4 months	DTP and TOPV.
6 months	DTP.
1–12 years	Measles and TB tests.
18 months	Rubella and mumps, or
12–15 months	Can give measles, mumps, and rubella (MMR) combined.
4–6 years	DTP and TOPV.
14–16 years	TB yearly now, every 10 years thereafter.

37. (4) An initial assessment of the couple's biologic, psychologic, and social levels of functioning is essential in order to determine the type of intervention required. No. 1 is inappropriate because the couple may not need or desire counseling. No. 2 is incorrect because Justin may not consider individual therapy either necessary or helpful. Although some form of crisis intervention may be needed (No. 3), it should not be initiated until the nurse has assessed the couple's level of functioning.

38. (2) The client with mild hypertension usually has a blood pressure of between 90 and 100 mm Hg. BPs of 110–120 mm Hg (No. 1) are considered moderately hypertensive; those of 120–140 mm Hg (No. 3), severely hypertensive. BPs of 100–115 (No. 4) cross over two levels of hypertension; persons with these BPs would probably be considered to have a mild-to-moderate level of hypertension.

39. (1) It is most important to provide consistency in assigning nurses to care for the person with hypertension in order to minimize stress and provide constant and consistent reinforcement of care and health-teaching. No. 4 is important in that it will ensure appropriate regulation of treatment. Nos. 2 and 3 are also appropriate nursing actions.

40. (4) There are generally no limitations on sexual activities merely due to a patient's hypertension. Unless these restrictions are warranted because of an individual's specific condition, they are considered irrelevant when teaching the average hypertensive client.

CASE STUDY 3

Mr. and Mrs. Franco are in their early thirties. They are both of Spanish descent. They have one daughter, Carmen, age 6, and Mrs. Franco recently gave birth to identical twins José and Carlos, age 3 months. José and Carlos were born at 8 months' gestation. José weighed 4 lb 6 oz and Carlos weighed 4 lb 10 oz. Their birth was otherwise unremarkable, and they were both discharged after three and a half weeks' hospitalization. At discharge each weighed about 5 lb.

Mrs. Franco had no complications following the vaginal delivery of her twins. She remained hospitalized for one week following delivery in order to rest and begin nursing the infants. Breastfeeding was initiated after the boys were one week old, and it has been successful so far.

Mrs. Franco is a homemaker. She has never held a full-time job. Before she married Mr. Franco 10 years ago, she worked as a waitress part time and lived at home with her parents. Mr. Franco is a freelance carpenter and works regularly except in periods of extremely cold weather. Carmen is in the first grade at the neighborhood school.

Mr. and Mrs. Franco arrive in the emergency room at 4:00 A.M. with their son José. On admission, Mrs. Franco tells the nurse that she had just finished nursing Carlos when she went over to check José because he seemed extremely quiet. Upon approaching the crib she noticed he was not moving. She placed her hand on his chest and discovered that he was not breathing. She called out in panic, and her husband ran to the nursery. Mr. Franco grabbed José and shook him to try to make him breathe. José did not respond, so the Francos called a neighbor to stay with Carmen and Carlos while they brought José to the emergency room. José was taken from his parents and examined. He never regained consciousness and was pronounced dead at 5:00 A.M.

QUESTIONS

1. When interviewing the Francos, the nurse needs to be primarily concerned with:
   1. Assessing the infant's physiologic status.
   2. Validating any precipitating factors.
   3. Evaluating the couple's emotional status.
   4. Health-teaching the couple about the infant's condition.

2. In assessing what may have contributed to José's condition, the nurse should suspect that he probably died of:
   1. SIDS.
   2. Child abuse.
   3. Pneumonia.
   4. Suffocation.

3. When the physician pronounces José dead after performing an examination, the person responsible for informing the Francos is:
   1. The social worker.
   2. The attending physician.
   3. The emergency room nurse.
   4. The hospital minister.

4. When working with families that have lost a child to SIDS, the nurse should know that the primary etiology of this syndrome is:
   1. Cardiac arrhythmias.
   2. Suffocation.
   3. Unknown.
   4. Depression of respirations.

5. The parents of SIDS infants usually express many emotions. The nurse should anticipate that they will most likely exhibit which of the following symptoms initially?
   1. Depression.
   2. Anger.
   3. Apathy.
   4. Guilt.

6. The nurse needs to know that SIDS usually occurs:
   1. Between two and four months after birth.
   2. Within three weeks of birth.
   3. More than six months after birth.
   4. Between six and nine months after birth.

7. Sudden infant death occurs more frequently when which of the following factors is involved?
   1. Low birthweight.
   2. Multiple births.
   3. Middle-class family.
   4. Familial history of the syndrome.

8. The Francos ask the nurse what they could have done to prevent the death of their son. The most appropriate response would be:
   1. "There is nothing anyone could have done."
   2. "You did everything possible."
   3. "Feeding him only small amounts of breastmilk during the night could have helped."
   4. "Stimulating him periodically throughout the night could have helped."

9. Mrs. Franco insists on seeing José before leaving the hospital. The most therapeutic nursing action includes:
   1. Arranging for her to see her son.
   2. Discussing this with the family's priest.
   3. Informing Mr. Franco that seeing José would be detrimental to his wife's health.
   4. Telling the Francos that hospital policy forbids her seeing José.

10. Mrs. Franco sits quietly in the waiting room. She is rocking back and forth, mumbling, "No, that's not possible." In assessing her behavior, the nurse needs to be aware that she is exhibiting:
    1. Anger.
    2. Apathy.
    3. Depression.
    4. Denial.

11. Mrs. Franco becomes hysterical. She begins to cry uncontrollably. Mr. Franco asks the nurse to "do something." The most appropriate intervention would include:
    1. Providing the Francos with privacy.
    2. Obtaining an order for a tranquilizer.
    3. Sitting quietly with the couple.
    4. Asking Mrs. Franco to calm down.

12. The most appropriate plan for immediate follow-up care for the Franco family would include:
    1. Referring the family to a psychotherapist.

2. Arranging for the social worker to visit the family.
3. Assessing the family's need for follow-up care.
4. Asking the family to identify their needs.

13. The nurse working with an SIDS family should:
1. Be knowledgeable about various theories of psychotherapy.
2. Have extensive experience working with dying patients.
3. Be able to identify personal feelings about death.
4. Be able to suppress personal feelings about death.

14. The most therapeutic form of intervention for the family who has lost a child to SIDS would include:
1. Psychotherapy for individual family members.
2. Talking with other SIDS families.
3. Family therapy.
4. Home visits by the public health nurse.

15. Although the extended family of an SIDS infant may have good intentions, they often use which of the following coping mechanisms?
1. Projection.
2. Anger.
3. Sublimation.
4. Suppression.

Several weeks after the funeral, Mrs. Franco tells the public health nurse that she is experiencing difficulty producing enough breastmilk to satisfy Carlos.

16. The most appropriate response for the nurse to make would be:
1. "You probably have a virus and should see a doctor right away."
2. "Carlos is probably reacting to the loss of his brother and not sucking long enough to stimulate an adequate supply."
3. "Milk production may decrease with an increase in stress."
4. "The lactation ducts may be occluded."

17. When teaching Mrs. Franco about a decrease in milk production, the nurse should:
1. Recommend weaning the baby onto formula.
2. Assess Mrs. Franco's feelings about nursing.
3. Refer Mrs. Franco to the La Leche League.
4. Suggest supplemental feedings of glucose water.

The Francos are concerned about their daughter's reaction to José's death. They approach the nurse with a number of questions.

18. When teaching the Francos about death and dying, the nurse should inform them that:
1. It is important to focus their daughter's attention on some useful activity she enjoys.
2. It is imperative to tell their daughter everything that happened.
3. It is important to talk with their daughter on a level she can comprehend.

4. It is imperative to keep their daughter from discussing José's death with her playmates.

19. The Francos ask the nurse what they should tell Carmen about José's death if she asks where he is. The most therapeutic response would include:
1. Assessing what this family system believes occurs after death.
2. Advising them to tell her that José has gone to heaven.
3. Assessing what the family thinks is appropriate.
4. Advising them to tell her that José is sleeping.

20. When working with a 6-year-old who has lost a sibling, the nurse should expect:
1. Withdrawal.
2. Guilt.
3. Depression.
4. Anger.

The physician suggests that the Francos bring Carlos in for an examination.

21. The Francos ask the nurse why Carlos needs to be examined. The most appropriate response would be:
1. "Twins are more susceptible to death due to SIDS."
2. "The physician wants to ensure that Carlos is perfectly healthy."
3. "The physician wants to determine whether Carlos is susceptible to SIDS."
4. "It is important that Carlos be examined in order to prevent SIDS from occurring again."

Carlos is screened and diagnosed as being susceptible to extended periods of apnea. The physician suggests placing Carlos on an apnea monitor at home. Questions 22–25 concern this situation.

22. The Francos ask the nurse what the monitor will do. The most appropriate response would be:
1. "It will stimulate his breathing."
2. "It will monitor his vital signs."
3. "It will sound an alarm if he stops breathing."
4. "It will maintain his respirations."

23. The Francos agree to place Carlos on the monitor. When teaching the parents about the monitor, the nurse should emphasize all of the following factors, *except:*
1. Responding to the monitor's alarm immediately.
2. Initiating CPR if the infant is not breathing.
3. Remaining in the infant's room throughout the night.
4. Contacting the emergency room following any attack.

24. When teaching the parents to provide CPR for an infant, it is important to stress:
1. Applying systematic pressure to the chest with the heel of the hand.
2. Compressing the chest at a rate of 90–100 compressions per minute.
3. Placing the resuscitator's mouth over the infant's mouth to ensure an adequate seal.

4. Keeping the infant uncovered to prevent a spiking in temperature and an increased demand for oxygen.

25. The nurse working with a family that is using an apnea monitor should know that the monitor's most problematic side effect is:
   1. The alarm sounds if the infant moves around the crib.
   2. The parents may become overprotective.
   3. The infant may experience a developmental lag.
   4. The monitor is generally unreliable.

26. About eight months after José's death, Mrs. Franco expresses a desire to become pregnant. Mr. Franco does not want another child. The nurse working with the couple should:
   1. Refer the couple to a marital therapist.
   2. Assist both individuals to identify their feelings and needs.
   3. Inform Mrs. Franco that she is trying to replace her lost infant.
   4. Suggest that Mrs. Franco undergo a gynecologic examination.

The Francos tell the nurse at the well-child clinic that Carmen has been a "tyrant" for the past eight months.

27. The nurse should suspect that Carmen is acting out because:
   1. She is neglected.
   2. She misses her brother.
   3. She feels confused.
   4. She is experiencing growing pains.

28. Which of the following tools would be the most appropriate method to evaluate a 6-year-old child's level of anxiety?
   1. Denver Developmental Screening Test.
   2. Rorschach ink blots.
   3. Thematic Apperception Test.
   4. IQ Test.

29. In health-teaching a parent about the normal growth and development of a 6-year-old, the nurse needs to know that the child is primarily concerned with:
   1. Developing trust.
   2. Demonstrating autonomy.
   3. Exhibiting initiative.
   4. Attaining an identity.

30. During which period of life do children begin to imitate adult behavior and desire to share in adult activities?
   1. Autonomy *vs* shame and doubt.
   2. Initiative *vs* guilt.
   3. Identity *vs* identity diffusion.
   4. Trust *vs* mistrust.

About a year after José's death, Carlos began experiencing several mild seizures. His mother states that his last seizure occurred early this morning. He was conscious throughout the seizure. His eyes rolled back, and he was unresponsive to

her voice for about 45 seconds. Immediately following this incident he began crying. She called the physician, who asked her to describe the symptoms and to bring Carlos to his office as soon as possible.

31. Which of the following factors would most likely contribute to Mrs. Franco's high stress level at this time?
   1. Being Spanish-speaking.
   2. Losing José.
   3. Observing the seizure.
   4. Being over 30 years old.

32. The nurse should inform the parents that the primary goal of intervention during a seizure is:
   1. To protect the child from injury.
   2. To control the seizure activity.
   3. To monitor all vital signs closely.
   4. To provide CPR to ensure adequate oxygenation.

33. The parents need to be able to evaluate the seizure accurately. They should be taught to observe the seizure and note all of the following characteristics, *except:*
   1. Duration.
   2. Intensity.
   3. Type.
   4. Scope.

34. When a child is experiencing a seizure, which of the following actions is contraindicated?
   1. Padding the crib sides.
   2. Placing a tongue depressor on the night stand.
   3. Having oxygen available at the bedside.
   4. Having suction equipment available.

35. In providing care for the child experiencing a febrile seizure, the nurse should:
   1. Give the child an alcohol sponge bath.
   2. Administer 5 cc Tylenol stat.
   3. Sponge the child with tepid water.
   4. Keep the child well covered.

Carlos is diagnosed as having epilepsy when he is 2½ years old.

36. The nurse should expect Carlos to exhibit all of the following symptoms, *except:*
   1. An aura before a grand mal seizure.
   2. Muscular rigidity.
   3. Defecation due to contracture of the abdominal muscles.
   4. A decrease in respiratory functioning.

37. The nurse health-teaching the parents of an epileptic child should stress that all of the following are goals of prolonged treatment, *except:*
   1. Curing the disease.
   2. Providing emotional support for the family.
   3. Controlling the convulsions.
   4. Teaching the child and the family to accept the epilepsy.

38. Which of the following drugs may be used to control epileptic convulsions without causing excessive drowsiness?
1. Phenobarbital.
2. Thorazine.
3. Dilantin.
4. Mysoline.

39. One of the most frequent side effects of Dilantin involves:
1. Respiratory depression.
2. Hypertrophy of the gums.
3. Fluid retention.
4. Hypotension.

40. In health-teaching the family about epilepsy, the nurse needs to emphasize the importance of:
1. Keeping the child's condition a family secret.
2. Pushing fluids in order to facilitate hydration.
3. Restraining the child to prevent injury.
4. Providing the child with a Medic Alert tag.

ANSWERS/RATIONALE

1. (3) In order to facilitate effective communication and ensure accurate data collection, the nurse needs to identify the couple's overall level of functioning and ability to cope with the situation. No. 1 would be performed by another nurse and/or the attending physician. One nurse needs to be assigned to care primarily for the parents in this situation. No. 2 may be done in conjunction with No. 3. However, it is essential to identify the couple's level of functioning in order to assess their ability to discuss the situation. No. 4 is inappropriate because the couple is functioning at a panic level of anxiety and learning abilities are impaired.

2. (1) The most appropriate cause of death would be *sudden infant death syndrome* (SIDS) because there are no clear indications that the infant died of abuse, pneumonia, or suffocation. There was no evidence of illness prior to death, i.e., no history of a virus, cold, or difficult breathing. Hence Nos. 2, 3, and 4 are incorrect.

3. (2) Although the health team may work together to provide support for the family system, it is the physician's primary responsibility to inform the family of the death of their child. Nos. 1, 3, and 4 may provide emotional support. (However, it is important to identify what religion the family practices and whether they desire to see a priest, minister, rabbi, or other religious leader.)

4. (3) Although there are many theories, including suffocation caused by an enlarged thymus and abnormalities in the respiratory center, no etiology has been clearly identified. Nos. 1, 2, and 4 involve several of the theories that have been identified, but none is definitely the primary cause.

5. (4) Initially most parents feel very guilty because they think they could have prevented the death ("If only we had checked on the infant more.") or could have done something differently. Nos. 1 and 2 will usually occur after the initial shock diminishes. No. 3 may occur if the parents are not assisted in coping with their feelings and instead proceed to withdraw.

6. (1) SIDS usually occurs within the first year of life. The peak time appears to be from two to four months of age. It rarely occurs before three weeks (No. 2) or after eight months (No. 4), and even six months is comparatively unusual (Nos. 3 and 4).

7. (1) SIDS occurs more frequently in low-birthweight infants and in the lower socioeconomic groups (No. 3). There is no validated data to support Nos. 2 and 4. However, if one identical twin dies of SIDS, there seems to be a greater risk that the other will exhibit prolonged periods of apnea.

8. (1) This is the most accurate statement, and it also provides reassurance. No one knows of any cure or intervention for SIDS at this time. Many theorists believe that stimulating the infant during periods of apnea may prevent death, but this is by no means certain. No. 2 may be perceived as false reassurance. It is important that health professionals identify that nothing could have been done to save their son at the time he was discovered. No. 3 is inaccurate because there is no clear evidence to demonstrate that small feedings would prevent this condition. There is no evidence to support No. 4 as an effective preventive action.

9. (1) This is a health-team decision that needs to be supported by the hospital administration in order to assist the family in working through the grieving process. No. 2 may be a violation of the family's privacy. The priest's input may be considered if the family requests it. No. 3 is an inappropriate assumption that would need further validation. No. 4 should not be standard policy in any hospital today. It is essential for many families to see the deceased in order to work through their grief.

10. (4) Mrs. Franco is in a phase of shock and disbelief, or denial. She is unable to cope with the stress or to acknowledge reality. Nos. 1 and 3 may occur once she is able to acknowledge José's death. No. 2 is often seen with withdrawal and depression.

11. (3) It is essential that the nurse be readily available to provide physiologic, sociologic, and psychologic support when needed. The husband has requested assistance; therefore, although privacy is important, remaining with the couple to provide support and guidance is paramount (No. 1). No. 2 may not be appropriate unless sitting with the couple does not decrease her anxiety. No. 4 will probably be ineffective. Furthermore, she may need to feel that it is okay to express her feelings, and the nurse should encourage her to be as open as possible.

12. (3) Immediately following a death, the nurse must assess and validate the family's needs for follow-up care. It is important to look at their past ability to cope with stress, how effective these coping mechanisms were, and so forth. However, initially the family will be unable to communicate their feelings and perceptions due to their high level of anxiety. No. 1 may be necessary if the family is unable to cope effectively with their anxiety. No. 2 would depend on the individual family's needs. No. 4 may be appropriate once the family is able to communicate their feelings and needs.

13. (3) It is important for all health team members to be in touch with their feelings about death and dying in order to help the family work through *their* feelings. Nos. 1 and 2 may help the nurse teach the family to express their feelings, but No. 3 is still primary. No. 4 is inappropriate because suppression may lead to avoidance and to the ineffective resolution of feelings.

14. (2) Talking with other SIDS families has proven highly effective for many families because they can share a common crisis, feelings of guilt, a loss, etc. Nos. 1 and 3 depend on the individual family's needs. No. 4 may be performed in conjunction with No. 2.

15. (1) Projection is the blaming of someone or something else for situations over which one has no control. In this case extended family members may feel guilty or angry over the death of their grandchild and project this guilt or anger onto the parents of the deceased infant. No. 2 is not a defense mechanism but is considered a contributing factor to several defense mechanisms (introjection, displacement, projection, etc.). No. 3 is the channeling of unacceptable impulses into acceptable modes of expression, such as displacing sexual energy by delving into art or music. No. 4 is the deliberate blocking of information from the conscious mind.

16. (3) Many times the physiologic response to stress may be a decrease in milk production. This may rectify itself over time, provided the anxiety is controlled. However, as long as the system is under prolonged, intense stress, the milk supply will probably remain diminished. Nos. 1 and 4 are inaccurate statements unless substantiated by physiologic evidence. Carlos is probably too young to react physiologically to his brother's death (No. 2). However, it is possible that he is experiencing some emotional trauma in response both to the increase in familial tension and to no longer hearing or seeing his brother.

17. (2) Any recommendation must be based on an assessment of Mrs. Franco. This will ensure that her needs are met at an appropriate level and may prevent unnecessary stress and feelings of guilt at a later time. No. 1 may be appropriate if she thinks she would rather wean or if the combination of breastfeeding and supplemental feeding proves inadequate for the infant or mother. No. 3 may

be appropriate, especially if there is a mother there who has experienced a similar loss. However, this referral should be initiated only after assessing and validating the need and appropriateness with the patient and with La Leche League. No. 4 may be appropriate after No. 2. However, the supplemental feedings will need to be validated with a physician, and they will probably consist of some type of formula rather than glucose water.

18. (3) In order to meet their daughter's needs, it is important to talk with her at a level she can understand and at her level of readiness. Nos. 1 and 4 foster denial and avoidance. No. 2 may not be appropriate in that it could overwhelm the child.

19. (1) The nurse must first assess the family's beliefs. No. 2 may go against these beliefs. No. 3 is inappropriate in this case because the family is seeking assistance from the nurse. No. 4 should be avoided not only because it is untrue, but also because it teaches the child to deny death.

20. (2) Many times siblings subconsciously wish they had never had a baby brother or sister. If the sibling dies the child feels very guilty, as if he or she wished this would happen or caused the sibling's disappearance. Nos. 1 and 3 are usually exhibited when the child cannot cope with the guilt feelings. No. 4 may arise once the child comprehends the situation and the child's guilt feelings surface. Emotional support and reinforcement that the child did not cause his sibling's death are important.

21. (3) A variety of tests are used to identify an infant's susceptibility to SIDS, including apnea-screening, respiratory status test, examining the thymus for enlargement, etc.; but there is no definitive method to prevent SIDS (No. 4). However, monitors are available that alert parents to possible apneic spells. No. 1 may induce fear unnecessarily. There may be a greater risk that the surviving twin of an SIDS victim will exhibit prolonged periods of apnea, but this does not necessarily lead to death. No. 2 is correct but less specific than No. 3.

22. (3) The apnea monitor will sound an alarm during any periods of apnea to warn the parents or caretakers. Although the alarm may startle the infant and stimulate breathing, it should not be relied upon for this function (No. 1). The monitor screens his respirations (and pulse, with some monitors) but not his temperature (No. 2). It will not *maintain* his respirations (No. 4).

23. (3) This defeats the purpose of having the alarm. Nos. 1, 2, and 4 are all appropriate actions. Many hospitals also have SIDS centers, and the parents are instructed to call this center when any problems occur.

24. (2) This is the rate for infants. The rate for small children is 80 compressions per minute. For infants pressure should be evenly applied with the fingers over the middle third of the sternum (No. 1). In order to form a

seal the resuscitator should place his or her mouth over the mouth *and* nose of the infant (No. 3). The infant should be covered to prevent heat loss, to diminish the need for oxygen, and to assist in controlling shock (No. 4).

25. (2) Many parents become "slaves" to the monitor and the infant. No. 1 should only occur if the electrodes are not properly placed. The monitor should have very little effect on the infant's developmental level, provided it is used appropriately and the child is environmentally stimulated (No. 3). Most apnea monitors are reliable if working and properly used (No. 4).

26. (2) The nurse can establish a therapeutic relationship with the couple and assist them to identify and express their needs. No. 1 may be necessary if the nurse cannot help the couple resolve their conflicts. No. 3 may be an inappropriate assumption. No. 4 may be necessary if the couple decide to have another child.

27. (3) Most children who lose a sibling feel overwhelmed and confused. No. 1 is an unvalidated inference. No. 2, missing her brother, is one aspect of the confusion she may be experiencing. No. 4 is an inaccurate statement with no professional rationale to support it.

28. (3) The TAT is used to diagnose a child's general anxiety or behavior problems. No. 1 is usually used for infants and preschoolers. No. 2 may be used with children, but the TAT has proven more effective in diagnosing anxiety. No. 4 is not used to evaluate anxiety, but to establish intelligence levels. IQ tests are usually more accurate after ages 9 or 10.

29. (3) From ages 3 to 6 children want to learn to do things independently. From ages 6 to 12 children develop a strong sense of duty and are concerned with becoming a success and being recognized as a success by their peers and parents. No. 1 is usually seen during infancy, No. 2 during the toddler years, and No. 4 at the beginning of adolescence.

30. (2) During the preschool years, ages 3 to 6, children have an active imagination. They begin to explore their environment and to imitate adult role models. No. 1 is usually seen during the toddler years and is characterized by a "holding on and letting go" phenomenon. No. 3 is demonstrated during adolescence and is characterized by the individual's asking "What will this mean to me?" Self-esteem is developing very rapidly during this period. No. 4 is seen during infancy, when the infant attempts to obtain the satisfaction of basic needs such as warmth, love, food, etc.

31. (2) Every time Carlos has a seizure probably reminds Mrs. Franco of her other son's death. Her ethnic heritage is not responsible for her level of stress at this time (No. 1). No. 3 would probably be more significant if this were the first seizure Carlos experienced. No. 4 is in itself irrelevant.

32. (1) Preventing injury is the first priority. No. 2 is impossible once the seizure has started. Respirations may be observed and the pulse taken if the child is amenable to touch. The temperature should never be taken during seizure activity because of the danger of injuring the child with the thermometer (No. 3). No. 4 may not be appropriate during seizures unless respiratory or cardiac failure occurs.

33. (3) It is not necessary for the parents to be able to identify a specific type of seizure, such as petit mal, Jacksonian, grand mal, etc., but they should be able to tell the nurse how long the seizure lasted (No. 1), whether the child remained conscious (No. 2), and what parts of the body were involved (No. 4).

34. (2) Use of a tongue depressor is no longer recommended due to the inherent danger of injury to the tongue and of aspirating part of the depressor. An airway may be inserted if necessary to provide adequate oxygenation. No. 1 may be used if absolutely necessary. However, the nurse needs to remember that padding decreases the visual field, which may make the child feel isolated and may stimulate withdrawal. Nos. 3 and 4 are appropriate in order to facilitate emergency care when needed.

35. (3) Moist cloths should be used to decrease the child's temperature gradually. Alcohol is usually contraindicated (unless specifically ordered) because isopropyl alcohol is absorbed by inhalation and may lead to a coma if the room is not adequately ventilated (No. 1). Alcohol may also decrease the temperature suddenly, causing a disequilibrium within the system that may lead to physiologic shock. No. 2 may only be given if ordered, and the dose depends upon the weight of the child. The child should be dressed in as few clothes as possible in a comfortable environment in order to keep the temperature as low as possible (No. 4). The child does need to be observed closely for chills that may be caused by a decrease in temperature.

36. (1) Most children do not experience an aura before a grand mal seizure. The older child may experience a headache, digestive upsets, irritability, or lethargy before a grand mal seizure. Nos. 2, 3, and 4 may all be exhibited by young children, older children, and adults.

37. (1) There is no known cure for epilepsy at this time. Nos. 2, 3, and 4 are appropriate objectives of prolonged therapy.

38. (3) Dilantin is an effective anticonvulsant that does not produce excessive drowsiness. Phenobarbital, a barbiturate, effectively controls grand mal seizures but does produce drowsiness (No. 1). No. 2 is a major tranquilizer used to treat depression. No. 4 is given to control grand mal and psychomotor seizures but may cause drowsiness and ataxia.

39. (2) This hypertrophy is usually nonhemorrhagenic and painless. Respiratory and circulatory depression rarely occur as a result of Dilantin administration (No. 1). Nos. 3 and 4 are not identified side effects of Dilantin.

40. (4) A Medic Alert tag is essential in order to notify others that the child is an epileptic who may need assistance. No. 1 is nontherapeutic because it makes the child feel inferior and ashamed. Many times a fluid overload seems to stimulate seizures (No. 2). A slight state of dehydration may assist in controlling seizures in some cases. Restraining the child may cause unintentional injury to the system (No. 3).

CASE STUDY 4

Laura, a three-year-old black female, is the youngest of four children. She has two brothers, John and Justin, age 10 and 11 respectively, and one sister, Ann, age 4. Laura's family lives in Washington, D.C., in a three-bedroom apartment. Laura attends day care five days a week from 7:30 A.M. to 5:30 P.M. Her mother, age 40, works for a volunteer bureau; her father, age 41, is a construction worker.

Laura was playing in the basement of the apartment complex with her brother John when she found a glass container and drank the liquid. She immediately began to cry and scream in pain. She vomited the liquid and some gastric juices. John grabbed her and carried her upstairs to the apartment. Her mother called an ambulance, and she and Laura proceeded to the local hospital's emergency room (ER).

When they arrived at the ER the clerk secretary greeted Laura and her mother at the desk. Laura's mother was obviously upset. She was talking very rapidly and wringing her hands, tears were in her eyes, and her voice trembled. Laura was crying hysterically; her mouth and lips were inflamed, edematous, and chapped. The clerk called Ms. Fenner, the RN on duty, who immediately realized that Laura was in a great deal of pain and that both Laura and her mother were quite scared.

Ms. Fenner introduced herself and began the admission procedure at once. In her initial assessment she identified that Laura had swallowed approximately 1 oz of liquid lye, which caused inflammatory first- and second-degree burns over the entire oral cavity and outer and inner lips, possible burning of the pharynx, esophagus, and larynx (since Laura had regurgitated and vomited some of the lye), and psychologic shock. She contacted the physician on duty, the X-ray team, and other relevant health team members to begin instituting immediate medical care.

QUESTIONS

1. What would be the most therapeutic nursing response to Laura's mother's high level of anxiety?
   1. "I've seen cases like this before. Everything will be just fine."
   2. "You have nothing to worry about. These things just happen sometimes."
   3. "Now tell me how this all happened."
   4. "I know you're worried, so I'll sit with you while Laura is being examined."

2. Since Laura has experienced severe burning of the oral cavity and possibly of the esophagus, pharynx, and larynx, the primary nursing intervention would be:
   1. Observing for symptoms of shock.
   2. Checking airway for signs of obstruction.
   3. Maintaining adequate hydration by offering Laura small amounts of clear liquid.
   4. Initiating intravenous therapy immediately.

3. Laura is taken into the emergency treatment room while her mother waits in the lounge. Laura appears extremely anxious and scared. She is crying continuously. What is the most appropriate nursing response?
   1. "Don't cry, little girl. Everything will be okay."
   2. "I know you're afraid. We have a lot of patients who hurt themselves this way."
   3. "I know you're afraid. I'm here."
   4. "Your mommy is right outside, so don't cry."

The attending physician decides that immediate admission to the hospital is necessary for Laura.

4. In making the necessary arrangements, the nurse identifies that Laura's family has no hospitalization insurance. The most appropriate nursing intervention would be:
   1. Referring the family to the social worker on duty for follow-up care.
   2. Discussing possible referrals that may be initiated.
   3. Discussing alternative hospitals that would be less expensive.
   4. Discussing the care Laura will receive.

5. Laura is scheduled to undergo dilation of the pharynx the first morning following her admission to the hospital. When teaching Laura about the procedure, the nurse realizes that all of the following are relevant, *except:*
   1. Laura's age.
   2. Laura's level of comprehension.
   3. Laura's present state of anxiety.
   4. Laura's level of readiness.

6. In observing Laura during the first two days after admission, the nurse notices that her temperature increased from 99 F to 104 F and that her respirations were irregular and shallow. The primary nursing intervention would be:
   1. Administering 5 cc Tylenol elixir stat.

2. Notifying the attending physician.
3. Giving Laura a tepid-water sponge bath.
4. Calling Laura's family immediately.

After being dilated, Laura begins to hemorrhage internally. She is taken to surgery immediately. Upon her return to the floor, whole blood is ordered for her.

7. The nurse planning to administer the blood should know that, after removing it from the refrigerator, the blood should be transfused within:
   1. Six hours.
   2. Two hours.
   3. Four hours.
   4. One hour.

8. While observing Laura throughout the blood transfusion, the nurse should be alert to all of the following as possible signs of a transfusion reaction, *except:*
   1. Shortness of breath.
   2. Pain in the lower back.
   3. Polyuria.
   4. Hematuria.

Laura has been in the hospital one week. She has failed to talk with anyone, including her family. She sits in the corner of her crib crying and rocking back and forth.

9. The most important nursing intervention would be:
   1. Establishing a one-to-one relationship with Laura to assure continuity.
   2. Assigning different staff to work with her each day to ensure variety.
   3. Ignoring Laura's behavior because it probably will subside within a couple of days.
   4. Referring Laura for a complete psychiatric evaluation to provide effective care.

While Laura is hospitalized she is screened for lead poisoning. Questions 10–15 concern this situation.

10. All of the following are possible sources of lead poisoning, *except:*
    1. Inhaling the dust from destruction of old slum housing.
    2. Ingesting paint chips from old buildings.
    3. Drinking water that runs through lead pipes.
    4. Eating fruit that has been contaminated with insect spray.

11. In observing the child for signs and symptoms of lead poisoning, the nurse should be alert to which of the following?
    1. Decreased intracranial pressure.
    2. Dehydration.
    3. Cerebral edema.
    4. Myocardial ischemia.

12. In the treatment of lead poisoning, all of the following are the most commonly used medications, *except:*
    1. EDTA (ethylenediamino tetraacetate).

2. BAL (British anti-lewisite).
3. Tetracycline.
4. Penicillamine.

13. The most common route for eliminating lead from the body is through:
    1. The skin.
    2. The kidneys.
    3. The lungs.
    4. The bowels.

14. When assessing a child receiving BAL, the nurse needs to be alert to which of the following side effects?
    1. Hypotension.
    2. Bradycardia.
    3. Vomiting.
    4. Hyperreflexia.

15. When assessing the child receiving atropine, opiates, or calcium salts, the nurse must be aware that the child is probably being treated for which of the following conditions?
    1. Lead colic.
    2. Severe encephalopathy.
    3. Peripheral neuritis.
    4. Muscular incoordination.

16. The nurse planning care for a hospitalized child needs to consider all of the following, *except:*
    1. The child may exhibit loss of recently acquired developmental skills.
    2. The child may initially withdraw from the immediate environment.
    3. The child may exhibit symptoms of being afraid of the nurse.
    4. The child may initially panic and cry constantly.

17. Laura is scheduled for discharge at the end of five weeks. In planning her discharge care, the nurse would do which of the following?
    1. Refer Laura's family to a social worker for follow-up care and discharge planning.
    2. Discuss with the family their need for referral and assistance.
    3. Reassure Laura's family that she received optimal care.
    4. Initiate a referral for family therapy for Laura's family.

A few days before Laura is discharged, her brother Justin falls from a tree and fractures his left femur. He is admitted to a hospital five miles down the road from Laura's hospital.

18. When assessing Laura and Justin's family at this time, the nurse would identify that they were functioning at what level of stress?
    1. Mild to moderate anxiety.
    2. Moderate to severe anxiety.
    3. Severe to panic anxiety.
    4. Panic to traumatic anxiety.

19. While preparing Justin's leg for casting, the nurse must ensure that Justin's leg is not cut. This precaution is designed to prevent:
1. Phlebitis.
2. Osteomyelitis.
3. Hemorrhage.
4. Itching.

20. While checking Justin's cast using the blanching test, the nurse would do which of the following?
1. Compress one of his left toenails.
2. Press on the bottom of his left foot.
3. Compress both a left and a right toenail.
4. Apply cold water to his left foot.

21. All of the following may be symptoms of circulatory impairment in Justin's left leg, *except:*
1. Inflammation.
2. Coldness.
3. Cyanosis.
4. Edema.

22. To facilitate the proper drying of Justin's cast, the nurse should do all of the following, *except:*
1. Leave the cast exposed to air.
2. Ensure that Justin remains in one position.
3. Place Justin on a bedboard.
4. Handle the cast with the palms of the hands.

23. The nurse should promote Justin's comfort while the cast is drying by:
1. Covering with a blanket the parts of his body not casted.
2. Administering pain medication every four hours.
3. Using a cradle to hold the blanket over the cast.
4. Opening the windows to allow fresh air to circulate.

24. When teaching Justin about the care of his cast, the nurse should consider which of the following factors most important?
1. Justin's level of physiologic development.
2. Justin's level of maturity and readiness to learn.
3. Justin's cognitive level of functioning.
4. Justin's chronologic age.

25. When teaching Justin how to care for his cast at home, the nurse should emphasize:
1. The need to wash the cast off at least once a day to avoid malodors.
2. The importance of keeping the cast elevated at all times.
3. The need to avoid scratching under the cast.
4. The importance of rotating his leg within the cast to maintain adequate range of motion.

26. To assess Justin's susceptibility to excoriation of the skin, the nurse should consider all of the following, *except:*
1. Observing for the presence of objects inside the cast.
2. Providing adequate padding around the bony prominences.

3. Removing pedaling from the cast edges.
4. Observing for indentations made by pressure on the wet cast.

27. In planning care for Justin, the nurse should consider all of the following developmental factors, *except:*
1. Justin will probably be able to respond appropriately to the limitations and requests of the nurse.
2. Justin will probably fear permanent harm to his body due to his fracture.
3. Justin will probably experience separation anxiety due to his isolation from friends.
4. Justin will probably enjoy sharing a room with other children.

28. The nurse would do which of the following to assess Justin's adjustment to hospitalization?
1. Allow Justin to interact with other children and encourage him to verbalize his feelings.
2. Assign various staff members to care for Justin in order to facilitate his verbalization.
3. Encourage Justin to draw pictures, and discuss these drawings with him.
4. Sit with Justin for at least 45 minutes each day to allow him to verbalize.

29. One of the most important factors the nurse needs to consider in planning care for Justin is:
1. His need to have stringent limits set.
2. His need for flexible limits.
3. His need for very few limits.
4. His need for autonomy.

During his fourth day of hospitalization, Justin begins to harass the younger children and disobey the nurse's instructions. Questions 30 and 31 concern this situation.

30. The most appropriate response the nurse could make would be:
1. "You are a bad boy."
2. "You may not hurt the younger children."
3. "You have to do as I say."
4. "I'm going to tell your mother about this behavior."

31. The nurse should handle Justin's aggressive outbursts through which of the following nursing actions?
1. Planning for isolated play to allow time for inner reflection.
2. Encouraging release of tension through verbalization of his feelings.
3. Offering constructive play activities periodically throughout the day.
4. Requesting medications to calm the child and promote quiet behavior.

32. In implementing care for Justin during the first 48 hours, the nurse should consider which of the following activities *most* appropriate?
1. Bathing Justin each morning.
2. Planning Justin's menu.

3. Allowing Justin to clean up the playroom.

4. Encouraging Justin to read to other children.

33. During Justin's fifth day of hospitalization he experiences epistaxis. The most appropriate nursing intervention would include:

1. Having Justin blow his nose forcefully.
2. Laying Justin in a prone position.
3. Tightening Justin's collar.
4. Applying ice over the bridge of Justin's nose.

After Justin is discharged from the hospital, he begins to experience rectal itching and spotty bleeding in the rectal area. Justin's mother contacts the public health nurse, who makes a home visit.

34. The nurse suspects that Justin is experiencing signs and symptoms of which of the following conditions?

1. Hemorrhoids.
2. Impetigo.
3. Pediculosis.
4. Pinworms.

35. In health-teaching Justin's mother about the treatment of pinworms, the nurse would consider which of the following the top priority?

1. Treatment is focused primarily on Justin because he is the carrier.
2. Reinfection may be prevented if Justin remains outside the hospital.
3. Treatment is directed at the entire family.
4. Reinfection may occur if Justin has contact with any animal that is a carrier.

36. When a child is diagnosed as having pinworms, the primary nursing action should be health-teaching the family about the importance of adequate:

1. Nutrition.
2. Cleanliness.
3. Rest.
4. Recreation.

During a routine visit to the health department for a physical examination, the public health nurse discovers that John, Laura's 10-year-old brother, has never been screened for sickle cell anemia.

37. If both of John's parents are diagnosed as carriers, what are John's chances of actually having sickle cell anemia?

1. 1:4.
2. 2:4.
3. 3:4.
4. 0:4.

38. The nurse would inform individuals diagnosed as having sickle cell anemia that they should avoid which of the following activities?

1. Flying in small aircraft.
2. Playing basketball.
3. Water skiing.
4. Swimming in the ocean.

39. When health-teaching the parents of a child with sickle cell anemia, the nurse should inform them that sickle cell anemia may be difficult to diagnose accurately because:

1. The disease mimics other conditions such as rheumatic fever, syphilis, and tuberculosis.
2. Testing procedures have not been adequately established to identify the disease.
3. The disease comes and goes, making an accurate diagnosis difficult.
4. The disease cannot be accurately diagnosed unless the child is in crisis.

40. One of the primary preventive measures the nurse should teach the parents of a child with sickle cell anemia is:

1. The need for the child to avoid physical activity.
2. The need for the child to consume large quantities of liquids each day.
3. The need for the child to restrict his or her nutritional intake of fruits and vegetables.
4. The need for the child to avoid producing children in the future.

ANSWERS/RATIONALE

1. (4) The nurse should focus on how the client feels without implying blame. Since Laura's mother is experiencing a panic level of anxiety, it is imperative that she be calmed down and encouraged to ventilate her feelings at her level of readiness. It is important to be supportive, nonthreatening, and empathic to facilitate a decrease in anxiety. Nos. 1 and 2 are nontherapeutic because they foster false reassurance. No. 3 is inappropriate because Laura's mother is experiencing a panic level of anxiety and will probably be unable to verbalize what occurred.

2. (2) Adequate oxygenation is foremost in importance. The primary intervention should be to ensure a patent airway, followed by observation for signs and symptoms of shock (No. 1). Liquids would be contraindicated (No. 3) because of Laura's burns and possible shock. A medical order would be needed to initiate intravenous therapy (No. 4).

3. (3) It is essential to reassure Laura in a manner compatible with her levels of readiness and anxiety. Nos. 1 and 2 merely provide false reassurance. No. 4 may stimulate an increase in anxiety by drawing attention to the mother's absence from the room.

4. (2) The nurse must realize that various alternatives are available within each community to assist in paying medical expenses. Referrals may include the public health nurse, a medical assistant worker, a social worker, etc. Although it is most important that Laura receive optimal care, in reality these bills may initiate a familial crisis that could possibly be avoided. The nurse should be capable of making some referrals before having to contact a social worker (No. 1). No. 3 is inappropriate because Laura is already hospitalized in this facility and the family does not need the additional stress of seeking other health care agencies. No. 4 should be done in conjunction with initiating referrals; however, relieving the crisis is essential.

5. (1) Age is less relevant in terms of identifying Laura's level of readiness and willingness to learn and understand. It is more important to meet the client's needs at this time at her level of comprehension and state of anxiety. Many times age does not positively correlate with the individual's level of comprehension. Nos. 2, 3, and 4 are all relevant.

6. (2) It is important to notify the physician immediately of the behaviors observed. There were no standing orders for Nos. 1 and 3. Notification of the family may be relevant (No. 4), but Laura's symptoms need to be treated first.

7. (3) Refrigerating blood assists in delaying the growth of bacteria. The blood must be administered within four hours, but not so rapidly that the client experiences overload. Hence Nos. 1, 2, and 4 are incorrect.

8. (3) Signs and symptoms of a transfusion reaction usually include hematuria, oliguria, anuria, shortness of breath, and pain in the lower back and legs. Polyuria is not a normal sign.

9. (1) Laura is probably experiencing severe separation anxiety and exhibiting symptoms of acute depression and detachment. The family and Laura need reassurance that this behavior is probably temporary as long as appropriate intervention is implemented. A consistent one-to-one relationship will establish trust and demonstrate empathy. No. 2 would promote an increase in anxiety stemming from feelings of uncertainty. No. 3 may stimulate increased anxiety and progressive withdrawal. No. 4 may not be necessary as long as empathy and support are provided.

10. (4) There is no direct evidence that ingesting insect spray has the same effect on the body as ingesting lead paint or other lead-based substances such as those in Nos. 1, 2, and 3.

11. (3) The child experiencing symptoms of lead poisoning may exhibit cerebral edema, an increase in intracranial pressure, seizures, coma, and death if the condition is not treated. Hence Nos. 1, 2, and 4 are incorrect.

12. (3) EDTA (No. 1) forms a nonionized chelate with lead, which is excreted in the urine. BAL (No. 2) is used in combination with EDTA to increase excretion of lead in the urine. Penicillamine (No. 4) is also used to facilitate the deleading process.

13. (2) Lead is excreted primarily through the eliminative subsystem of the kidneys. Hence Nos. 1, 3, and 4 are incorrect.

14. (3) Side effects of British anti-lewisite (BAL) include hypertension, tachycardia, and vomiting. Nos. 1, 2, and 4 are not normal side effects.

15. (1) Atropine, opiates, and calcium salts are all antispasmodics used to treat lead colic. Hence Nos. 2, 3, and 4 are incorrect.

16. (2) Children generally display separation anxiety by initially crying and overtly protesting the situation (No. 4), not by withdrawing. Hospitalized children generally regress and may lose those skills acquired recently (No. 1). Children are generally afraid of strangers (No. 3). Moreover, a child being treated for lead poisoning will probably exhibit an intense fear of nurses because they administer many intramuscular injections.

17. (2) The family needs to be allowed some choice in the decision-making process at this time. Their input is essential in assisting the family to returning to a steady state of functioning. Referral to a social worker (No. 1) may not be necessary. Reassurance alone (No. 3) does not meet the family's needs. Therapy (No. 4) may not be necessary for this family.

18. (2) The family has an extensive amount of stress to cope with at this time. With two hospitalized children in two different hospitals, the family would appear to be functioning at the moderate to severe level of anxiety. However, if the family system's coping mechanisms do not serve to balance the stress, they may progress to a panic level of anxiety.

19. (2) Any laceration could become infected by normal skin bacteria (e.g., Staphylococcus aureus) and cause contamination of bone fragments during the casting procedure, especially when pins are inserted.

20. (3) The blanching test measures circulatory effectiveness by briefly compressing a toenail and then quickly releasing the pressure. This compression should be performed on both left and right toenails to compare the speed of color return in the uncasted and casted extremities.

21. (1) The general symptoms of circulatory impairment include pallor, coldness, cynanosis, and edema, but not inflammation.

22. (2) It is an important preventive measure to rotate Justin's body position at least once every two hours to promote adequate circulation to all parts of the body. The cast should be handled with the palms of the hands to avoid applying pressure and making indentations with the fingers (No. 4). Nos. 1 and 3 both help the cast dry properly.

23. (1) Justin may be losing body heat through evaporation,

therefore he will probably feel cold and clammy. Covering the body can minimize the loss of body heat. Pain medication (No. 2) can only be administered if ordered and probably will only be necessary during the first 12–15 hours the cast is drying. A cradle should *not* be used to cover the cast (No. 3) because it will slow the drying process. Justin will probably be cold due to lost body heat, therefore the opening of windows and doors is contraindicated (No. 4).

24. (2) Justin's maturity and readiness to learn are paramount considerations in assessing the appropriate level of instruction for him. His level of physiologic development may be inconsistent with his ability to learn (No. 1). His cognitive skills may not be consistent with his level of readiness to learn (No. 3). For example, an intelligent child may be functioning at a high level intellectually, but may not be mature enough to assimilate certain information. A child's age (No. 4) is not as significant as his overall level of maturity and readiness to learn. Chronologic age can be misleading in many instances because a child may function at a higher or lower level, depending on his environmental stimulation, intelligence, maturity, etc.

25. (3) Scratching under the cast may cause abrasions and lacerations that may lead to infections. No. 1 is contraindicated because the cast must be kept as dry as possible at all times. Showers or baths need to be taken with a plastic bag covering the cast. The cast need not be elevated (No. 2) unless the physician orders it for a certain amount of time each day. If the cast is loose enough to allow for rotation of the leg (No. 4), then it needs replacing because the cast's function is to immobilize the leg to allow time for the bones to heal.

26. (3) The pedaling should be applied and maintained on the cast to prevent skin breakdown and possible infection. Nos. 1, 2, and 4 are all appropriate considerations.

27. (4) Justin, at age eleven, will probably experience anxiety over his lack of privacy because many preadolescents are self-conscious about the bodily changes accompanying puberty. It is important for his privacy to be respected as much as possible. Putting children of similar ages in the same room when possible can be helpful. Nos. 1, 2, and 3 are all likely.

28. (1) Many times children express themselves better in a group than alone with a nurse. Assigning a variety of staff to care for a child (No. 2) may increase his lack of trust and stimulate an increase in his anxiety level. If a child trusts the staff or a certain staff member, drawings could possibly be used to explore the child's feelings (No. 3). However, initially the use of drawings may be threatening. Preadolescents tend to feel that they must draw well in order to share their drawings with others. Also the nurse must avoid attempting to analyze any drawings. Drawings are best used to assist the client in exploring what the drawing may mean to him. Initially, sitting with Justin for 45 minutes each day may be threatening to him (No. 4). The nurse must meet the child at his level of readiness to develop a trusting relationship.

29. (2) A preadolescent needs realistic and flexible limits set for him. Justin is a dependent human being striving to achieve some degree of autonomy. The nurse must use caution in setting limits for the child while at the same time not allowing him too much control. Stringent limits (No. 1) are inappropriate because they threaten the child's self-concept and interfere with his need to assert some control over his life. Nos. 3 and 4 are inappropriate because the preadolescent still needs some guidance in formulating his self-concept and life goals.

30. (2) Limits need to be set clearly and unambiguously. No. 1 is inappropriate because value judgements should be avoided when setting limits on a child's behavior. Nos. 3 and 4 are merely threats; they do not specify why Justin's behavior is inappropriate. Love should not be withheld for misbehavior. Limits must be firmly set without resorting to threats.

31. (3) The best nursing intervention for handling aggression is preventing it. Appropriate activities such as clay-modeling or a bedside punching ball facilitate a release in tension. Children generally do not enjoy solitary play at the preadolescent stage (No. 1). In fact many times isolation may lead to frustration, an increase in anxiety, and aggression. Many 11-year-old children are unable to express their aggressive feelings verbally (No. 2). Medication should be avoided unless absolutely necessary. In this case, medication is not warranted (No. 4).

32. (4) Reading to other children may be an appropriate activity for Justin if he feels comfortable reading. No. 3 is inappropriate because Justin is incapable of moving around extensively during the first few days of hospitalization. Justin should be allowed to select his own menu with some guidance (No. 2). Justin may need assistance bathing himself; however, he should be encouraged to perform as much of his own care as feasible (No. 1).

33. (4) Ice may facilitate vasoconstriction, thereby decreasing the bleeding. Clothes should be loosened around the collar to decrease the pressure in this area (No. 3). Justin should be placed in a semierect position to allow blood to flow downward and out of the nasal passages instead of toward the back of the throat, which could possibly obstruct the airway (No. 2). Blowing the nose (No. 1) is contraindicated in that it may stimulate an increase in bleeding.

34. (4) In children these signs and symptoms would be most indicative of pinworms or of oxyuriasis (parasitic infection) caused by pinworms. Hemorrhoids (No. 1) are rarely found in preadolescents. The first symptoms of impetigo (No. 2) usually involve lesions that are erythematous papules, followed by superficial vesicles

containing fluid. These vesicles become purulent, and an area of erythema develops around each one. Eventually the pustule ruptures and crusts develop. This condition is seen more during infancy because of an infant's low resistance to bacteria. Pediculosis, or lice (No. 3), come in several types, the most common of which is head lice. Severe itching of the scalp causes scratching, leading to excoriation with serous, purulent, or sanguineous exudation. Crusts form and hair is usually matted. Lice may be found on other parts of the body (such as in pubic hair), but in children they are usually found on the scalp.

35. (3) To assure that all possible carriers are freed from infection and to prevent reinfection, it is essential that all the individuals Justin comes in contact with be treated. Treating Justin alone (No. 1) would be fruitless because he would probably be reinfected by one of his family members. It is probable that Justin became infected through contact with someone in the hospital; however, he has probably infected other individuals at home, so merely remaining outside the hospital would not prevent reinfection (No. 2). No. 4 is an inappropriate response because pinworm contamination is due to human-to-human contact with an infectious individual.

36. (2) Because pinworms are transmitted when an organism enters the body through the oral cavity, cleanliness is essential for this family system. Nutrition is always important (No. 1); however, no dietary changes will prevent or cure pinworms. Rest and recreation (Nos. 3 and 4) are important in health maintenance, but they cannot in themselves prevent or cure pinworms.

37. (1) When two carriers have children, the odds are as follows. One child in four will inherit all normal hemoglobin (AA) and be free of the disease. Two children in four will inherit both hemoglobin A and hemoglobin S (AS), thereby becoming carriers of the trait like their parents. One child in four will inherit all sickling hemoglobin (SS), thereby becoming a victim of sickle cell anemia. *Note:* Just because a family has four children does not necessarily mean the odds will always be distributed equally. A one-in-four chance occurs with every pregnancy if both parents are carriers.

38. (1) Under reduced oxygen tension the abnormal hemoglobin (S) sickles, and these malformed cells clump together, obstructing the capillaries and causing what is known as a sickle cell crisis, which leads to anoxia within the body system. Flying in an unpressurized plane would decrease the oxygen supply and possibly cause a sickle cell crisis. Nos. 2, 3, and 4 are all appropriate sports for individuals with sickle cell anemia as long as they do not overexert themselves and rapidly decrease the oxygen supply in their systems.

39. (1) Sickle cell anemia involves vascular occlusion similar to many other diseases, such as thalassemia, tuber-culosis, osteomyelitis, rheumatic fever, and syphilis; therefore an accurate diagnosis is sometimes very difficult to make. Testing procedures have been updated and greatly improved within the past ten years (No. 2). The disease never goes away (No. 3), but individuals do function without constantly being in crisis. An accurate diagnosis of sickle cell anemia is not dependent on the child's being in crisis. If the sickling is not readily seen on a smear, a drop of blood can be placed on a slide and sealed off from oxygen by petroleum jelly, and sickling may occur within 1 to 24 hours at room temperature. There is also a test tube test that is faster than 24 hours.

40. (2) Dehydration stimulates sickling of cells; therefore adequate hydration is essential to maintaining an optimal level of functioning. The child should not have to avoid all physical activity (No. 1), but this activity needs to be monitored and tailored to fit each individual's needs. The child's nutritional intake of fruits and vegetables (No. 3) needs to be encouraged. An adequate diet is necessary to promote an optimal level of health, especially for these individuals. If the child is fortunate enough to live through child-bearing age, No. 4 is a decision each individual must make. However, the risk involved for a female with sickle cell anemia is extreme. Even if she is capable of becoming pregnant and enduring labor, she may still lose her life at any time throughout her pregnancy.

CASE STUDY 5

Juanita is a 33-year-old Spanish-speaking female who arrived in the labor room complaining of severe cramping and excessive bleeding. Juanita is presently eight months (36 weeks) pregnant with her first child. She has never been pregnant before, even though she and her husband Tyronne have been trying for the past 8 years.

Juanita's pregnancy has so far been unremarkable. She was in her fourth month when she first suspected she was pregnant because her breasts were tender and slightly enlarged. She had missed several menstrual periods as well, although it was not unusual for her to go two to three months without a period.

Juanita received adequate prenatal care as scheduled. She was very conscientious about restricting her intake of salt and alcohol. She had even stopped smoking after finding out that she was pregnant. Before she stopped she had smoked about three-fourths of a pack of cigarettes a day and several marijuana joints every weekend. Her husband is a heavy cigarette and joint smoker. Neither Juanita nor Tyronne drinks more than three to four beers a month and a social cocktail every once in a while. They believe that too much alcohol is unhealthy and that marijuana is safer. Although Juanita has not smoked a joint since the day she found out she was pregnant, she has attended several parties where drugs were present and people were smoking joints and cigarettes. Tyronne still smokes cigarettes and joints as usual.

Juanita complained that the cramping and bleeding started about a half hour before her arrival at the hospital. The initial assessment of Juanita's status showed that she was approximately 4 cm dilated, her membranes were intact, and contractions were coming about every 4 to 6 minutes. Her husband was with her throughout the admission process and appeared to be very anxious and concerned.

QUESTIONS

1. The nurse considers the information regarding smoking cigarettes and marijuana essential because it is well established that these activities may lead to:
   1. Retarded infants.
   2. Low-birthweight infants.
   3. Deformed infants.
   4. Malnourished infants.

2. Tyronne expresses some concern over Juanita's previous smoking habits. The nurse should inform Tyronne that:
   1. Although Juanita no longer smokes, she was exposed to cigarette and marijuana smoke, which could affect her pregnancy.
   2. Juanita is assured of a healthy infant because she stopped smoking as soon as she knew she was pregnant.
   3. The early labor is probably due to Juanita's smoking marijuana.
   4. Alcohol is considered much safer than marijuana.

3. The nurse in assessing Juanita should identify that she is in what stage of active labor at this time?
   1. First.
   2. Second.
   3. Third.
   4. Fourth.

4. In observing women in the latent phase of the first stage, the nurse would expect to see which of the following behaviors?
   1. Tendency to hyperventilate.
   2. Euphoria, excitement, and talkativeness.
   3. Fairly quiet and introverted behavior.
   4. Irritability and crying.

5. The nurse should recognize that which of the following procedures may be contraindicated upon Juanita's arrival in the labor room?

   1. Initiating intravenous therapy.
   2. Taking her blood pressure.
   3. Examining her vaginal canal.
   4. Monitoring FHR.

6. Juanita's membranes are ruptured by the attending physician. The nurse should expect the amniotic fluid to:
   1. Be clear in color.
   2. Have a slightly pungent odor.
   3. Have a thick consistency.
   4. Turn litmus paper blue.

7. During the first stage of labor, maternal and fetal vital signs need to be closely monitored. The best time to observe maternal vital signs is:
   1. Immediately before a contraction.
   2. Between contractions.
   3. Immediately after a contraction.
   4. Any time the mother feels totally comfortable.

8. Juanita's physician orders a soapsuds enema. The most appropriate nursing action would be to:
   1. Administer the enema as soon as possible.
   2. Recheck the order for the type of enema.
   3. Refuse to administer the enema because this is a premature labor.
   4. Ask the physician to check the fetal position prior to giving the enema.

9. When Juanita is in labor, the nurse would ask her to do all of the following tasks, *except:*
   1. Empty her bladder.
   2. Lie on her back to facilitate adequate ventilation.
   3. Not bear down until she enters the second stage.
   4. Breathe slowly and evenly.

10. If the nurse observes the discharge of green amniotic fluid, she should realize this may indicate:
    1. Rh or ABO incompatibility.
    2. Fetal distress occurred approximately 36 hours ago.
    3. Recent or current hypoxia.
    4. Abruptio placentae has occurred.

11. Juanita requests a sip of water after being in labor for two hours in the hospital. The most appropriate nursing action would be:
    1. Checking the physician's orders.
    2. Giving her a small sip of water.
    3. Offering her ice chips.
    4. Telling her she cannot have fluids at this time.

After Juanita has been in labor for four hours in the hospital, her cervix is assessed to be 5 cm. Her vital signs are 99–100–30. BP = 132/90. FHR = 180 and difficult to auscultate with the monitor and fetal scope. The fetus is now positioned in a transverse position. Juanita and Tyronne are quickly informed of the gravity of the situation.

12. The primary priority of the nurse at this time would be:
    1. To obtain an operation permit.

2. To attempt to alleviate Tyronne and Juanita's anxiety.

3. To monitor maternal and fetal vital signs closely.

4. To provide emotional and physiologic support.

13. Tyronne tells the nurse that he and Juanita had counted on his being in the delivery room throughout their baby's birth. The most therapeutic response would be to:
    1. Refer him to the attending physician for permission to attend the birth.
    2. Assess whether he has attended childbirth education classes.
    3. Check with the attending physician and relay the response to Tyronne.
    4. Tell Tyronne to dress and meet you in the delivery room.

14. Juanita and Tyronne are informed that a cesarean delivery will be performed immediately. The couple inquire whether Juanita must be put to sleep. The most appropriate nursing response would be to:
    1. Refer the couple to the anesthesiologist.
    2. Ask the attending physician to explain the procedure to the couple.
    3. Tell the couple that she probably will receive general anesthesia.
    4. Inform the couple that most women who have a cesarean delivery receive spinal anesthesia.

15. The attending physician and anesthesiologist decide to administer spinal anesthesia. However, the amount of anesthesia used will be as minimal as possible because spinal anesthesia:
    1. Produces severe fetal depression.
    2. Causes maternal hypotension.
    3. Rapidly crosses the placenta.
    4. Depresses maternal respirations.

16. In assessing Juanita following the administration of the spinal anesthesia, the nurse should realize that if she can wiggle her toes:
    1. The effect of the spinal anesthesia has dissipated.
    2. She may still become hypotensive.
    3. This behavior is essentially meaningless.
    4. She is prone to hypertension.

17. Juanita is moved into the delivery room. Tyronne enters the delivery room and appears somewhat anxious. The nurse should ask Tyronne:
    1. "How are you feeling?"
    2. "Are you feeling up to this?"
    3. "Would you rather wait outside?"
    4. "Can I get you anything?"

18. Tyronne asks the nurse whether he will see any gore or blood during the operation. The most realistic response would be:
    1. "I'm not sure."
    2. "It depends on the technique the physician uses."

3. "Probably not, because a drape keeps the operation from view by both you and Juanita."

4. "Yes, blood and tissue will be all over the table."

19. Juanita expresses some concern over feeling the incision and experiencing pain. The most appropriate response would be:
    1. "You will feel nothing at all."
    2. "You may feel some pressure in the area the incision is made."
    3. "You may feel slight pain when the incision is made."
    4. "If you feel any pain, it is only your imagination."

20. Juanita questions the nurse about the type of incision the physician will use in her operation. The nurse should realize that Juanita's primary concern involves the possibility of:
    1. Infection.
    2. Bleeding.
    3. Scarring.
    4. Rupture.

Juanita undergoes the operation without complications. However, the neonate's apgar score at one minute is one and at five minutes is four. Oxygen is administered to the neonate immediately. The pediatrician notes that the neonate has a cleft lip and palate that is obstructing adequate ventilation. The infant's birthweight is 2500 g (5.5 lb), and it is a boy.

21. An apgar score of 4 at five minutes indicates that the neonate's condition is:
    1. Excellent.
    2. Good.
    3. Fair.
    4. Poor.

22. The nurse assisting with the care of this newborn should realize the primary goal is to:
    1. Establish an airway.
    2. Maintain an adequate temperature.
    3. Reassure the parents.
    4. Monitor the infant's vital signs.

23. While providing care for the newborn the nurse must also be aware of the parents' feelings. Both Juanita and Tyronne appear stunned. However, they are still in touch with reality and are asking appropriate questions focusing on the newborn's condition. The couple is functioning at what level of anxiety at this time?
    1. Mild to moderate.
    2. Moderate to severe.
    3. Severe to panic.
    4. Panic.

The neonate's respirations are established. He is placed in an incubator and transferred immediately to the high-risk neonatal nursery. The couple is informed that the baby's condition is serious but stable. Juanita is transferred to the recovery room.

24. Tyronne requests permission to see his wife and baby immediately. The most appropriate nursing response would be to:
   1. Obtain permission for him to see Juanita.
   2. Inform him that they both need their rest.
   3. Refer him to Juanita's physician.
   4. Allow him to go see the infant.

25. During the delivery Juanita was administered a dose of Deladumone OB. This drug is given:
   1. To decrease bleeding.
   2. To prohibit lactation.
   3. To stimulate uterine contractions.
   4. To prevent depression.

26. In implementing care for Juanita, the nurse needs to be aware of the signs and symptoms of internal hemorrhage, which include:
   1. Decrease in pulse, increase in BP and respirations.
   2. Increase in pulse and respiration, decrease in BP.
   3. Increase in pulse, respiration, and BP.
   4. No change in pulse, decrease in BP, and increase in respirations.

27. Juanita should be maintained in which of the following positions immediately following delivery?
   1. Prone.
   2. Semi-Fowler's.
   3. Supine.
   4. Trendelenburg.

Part of the nurse's role is to provide psychologic and emotional support to the parents, especially after the birth of an abnormal or unhealthy infant. In this case the nurse realizes that Juanita and Tyronne will have many different feelings to work through in the future.

28. The nurse should expect Juanita and Tyronne's initial reactions to include:
   1. Depression.
   2. Apathy.
   3. Withdrawal.
   4. Anger.

29. In providing emotional support for the couple, the nurse should realize that they will probably first want to:
   1. Talk with other couples who have experienced the same circumstances.
   2. Be left alone, unless they seek out someone to talk to.
   3. Need reassurance and emotional support.
   4. Avoid discussing the situation at this time.

30. Juanita and Tyronne ask to see their son. The most appropriate nursing action would encompass:
   1. Assessing and analyzing the couple's level of readiness.
   2. Arranging for the couple to see and hold their son immediately.
   3. Health-teaching the couple what to expect.

   4. Preparing the couple for what to expect while making the arrangements for visitation.

31. Juanita's initial reaction to seeing her son in the neonatal nursery is to cry and tremble slightly. The most appropriate nursing intervention would be to:
   1. Remove her from the area immediately.
   2. Monitor her for vital signs.
   3. Allow her to cry.
   4. Ask her what she is feeling.

32. Initially Juanita is reluctant to touch or hold her son. The nurse should realize that this reluctance may be due to all of the following, *except:*
   1. Juanita has overreacted to the situation.
   2. Juanita is fearful of hurting the baby.
   3. Juanita has not accepted the baby.
   4. Juanita dislikes the baby's appearance.

33. Juanita and Tyronne may use which of the following defense mechanisms in attempting to cope with their anxiety?
   1. Fixation.
   2. Projection.
   3. Conversion.
   4. Sublimation.

34. Juanita and Tyronne are experiencing a reactive depression. The primary difference between a reactive depression and an endogenous depression is that in a reactive depression:
   1. There is substantial weight loss, usually over 10 lb.
   2. The individual does not respond to environmental stimuli.
   3. The individual generally feels worse as the day progresses.
   4. The precipitating event is usually difficult to identify.

The couple is now aware that their son has a unilateral cleft of the lip and palate. They are anxious to have surgery performed to repair the deformities.

35. The most appropriate response to the couple's request for surgery would be to:
   1. Reinforce what the physicians have told the parents.
   2. Inform the couple that the lip may be repaired when their son is 2 to 3 months old and the palate repaired at eighteen months.
   3. Refer the couple to the surgeon.
   4. Tell the couple that surgery may be performed when their son weighs at least 10 lb.

36. When teaching Juanita and Tyronne about the cleft lip and palate, the nurse would need to be aware that:
   1. Cleft lip occurs most frequently in girls.
   2. Cleft palate occurs most frequently in boys.
   3. Cleft lip and palate almost always occur simultaneously.
   4. Cleft lip and palate are both influenced by hereditary factors.

37. In assessing the neonate born with a cleft palate, the nurse needs to be aware that all of the following are problems associated with cleft palate, *except:*
1. Increased incidences of otitis media.
2. Feeding difficulties.
3. Distortion in body image.
4. Possible mild mental retardation.

38. When teaching the parents about the care of their son with a cleft lip and palate, the nurse should inform them that:
1. It is important to use a nipple with large holes in order to make sucking easier.
2. The infant will have difficulty feeding because he cannot create a vacuum in his mouth.
3. The infant should be given small amounts of formula while being maintained in a supine position to facilitate feeding.
4. It is important to isolate the infant from others to prevent possible infection.

39. Juanita and Tyronne's son undergoes an operation for the repair of the cleft lip when he is three months old. In providing nursing care for the infant, the nurse should:
1. Place the infant in a prone position to facilitate drainage.
2. Avoid moving the infant too much in order to keep from dislodging the Logan bar.
3. Cleanse the suture area frequently in order to prevent scarring.
4. Encourage the infant to cry in order to promote adequate lung aeration.

40. The couple express some concern about caring for the infant. Tyronne is especially worried about paying excessive hospital bills because his insurance has set limits. The most appropriate nursing action would be to:
1. Refer the couple to a social worker.
2. Validate the couple's perceived needs.
3. Discuss alternatives with the couple.
4. Implement health-teaching regarding the physical care of the infant.

ANSWERS/RATIONALE

1. (2) The one factor that has been highly correlated to smoking cigarettes and grass has been low birthweight. Nos. 1, 3, and 4 have not been highly correlated.

2. (1) This is the most appropriate and honest response. However, it is essential to answer the question clearly without stimulating unnecessary fear. There is no way to guarantee the birth of a healthy infant (No. 2). Furthermore, Juanita smoked throughout the first trimester, the period of organogenesis when the conceptus is most susceptible to teratogenic effects. No. 3 is an inaccurate statement because there is no way to validate this absolutely. There are no definitive data to support No. 4.

3. (1) The first stage is the stage of the cervix. Juanita is only 4 cm dilated with contractions occurring every 4–6 minutes, and she is alert. Hence Nos. 2, 3, and 4 are incorrect.

4. (2) Euphoria, excitement, and talkativeness are all seen initially when the woman is fairly energetic and anxious to have labor begin. No. 1 usually occurs during the midactive phase. Nos. 3 and 4 usually occur in the transitional or deceleration period of the active phase of the first stage.

5. (3) Examining her vaginal canal is contraindicated initially because of the history of bleeding prior to her admission to the hospital. No. 1 is imperative in order to have a line available for any ordered medications or fluids. Nos. 2 and 4 are essential in order to establish baseline data and to monitor the mother's and infant's status.

6. (4) Amniotic fluid is alkaline, which makes litmus paper turn blue. The fluid is usually milky or opaque with small white flecks (No. 1). No offensive odor is usually apparent (No. 2). Most fluid has a thin consistency (No. 3).

7. (2) Contractions may affect the pulse, BP, and respiratory rate. If possible, take vital signs between contractions. Nos. 1 and 3 are incorrect because immediately prior to a contraction the mother is usually very excited and apprehensive; after a contraction she may feel more comfortable, but her vital signs may be altered due to the contraction itself. If the nurse waits for the mother to feel totally comfortable she may never be able to assess the maternal vital signs (No. 4).

8. (3) Enemas are not administered when there is vaginal bleeding or premature labor or when the fetus is in an abnormal presentation or position. Hence No. 1 is a nursing error. No. 2 would be appropriate if there had been no vaginal bleeding or premature labor. Soapsuds enemas are contraindicated because they are potentially dangerous due to their physiologic incompatibility with the lower gastrointestinal tract. The fetal position does need to be assessed prior to administering an enema. Notify the physician immediately (No. 4).

9. (2) The woman in labor is instructed to lie on her side to promote relaxation, to prevent supine hypotension, and to facilitate anterior rotation of the fetal head. Nos. 1, 3, and 4 are appropriate actions. A full bladder may impede progress or result in trauma to the bladder. Bearing down prior to the second stage is fruitless and serves only to expend energy and possibly to damage the cervical opening. Slow, even breathing promotes adequate ventilation for the maternal and fetal systems and controls some anxiety.

10. (3) Green fluid is usually seen when the fetus is in distress and hypoxic. Nos. 1 and 2 may result in a yellow fluid. No. 4 usually results in a port wine–colored fluid.

11. (1) Fluid orders vary among hospitals, physicians, and childbirth methods. Since Juanita is in premature labor and bleeding, the orders will probably maintain her NPO with an IV. Nos. 2, 3, and 4 are contraindicated based on Juanita's condition at this time.

12. (4) This is the most appropriate response because it attempts to provide total intervention for all parties involved. No. 1 is essentially the physician's role. It would be almost impossible to alleviate the couple's anxiety at this time (No. 2). The most appropriate intervention is to assist the couple to cope with their anxiety as effectively as possible. No. 3 is essential, but it neglects the psychologic needs of the clients.

13. (3) Depending on the hospital, this is a physician's decision, especially in cases where the fetus as well as the mother may be in danger. Time may not permit No. 1 to occur. Some hospitals and/or physicians require childbirth classes as a prerequisite to attending the delivery (No. 2). Others do not require it. No. 4 is an inappropriate nursing action without a physician's approval.

14. (2) This response allows the couple to become informed without infringing upon the physician's role. The physician can then decide to inform the couple of the procedure to be used himself or to have the anesthesiologist inform them. Time is limited and the physician may decide to inform the couple himself (No. 1). Nos. 3 and 4 are not the nurse's decisions to make.

15. (2) Hypotension is even more severe when there has been bleeding. One of the advantages of spinal anesthesia is that it causes very little fetal depression (No. 1). If administered properly, very little anesthesia should cross the placenta (No. 3). No. 4 is irrelevant unless the mother has an adverse reaction to the anesthesia.

16. (2) Wiggling the toes indicates that the motor block caused by the spinal is wearing off. However, the autonomic block is still present, and the woman may experience hypotension. The autonomic block is still present even though the effects of the anesthesia are wearing off (No. 1). Hence Nos. 3 and 4 are incorrect.

17. (1) This is an open-ended question that allows Tyronne to identify what his needs are at this time. No. 2 is too threatening. No. 3 assumes he cannot tolerate the situation, which is unfair. No. 4 is unrealistic because the nurse has many responsibilities at this time. In addition, Tyronne would have to leave the room anyway to drink or take anything.

18. (3) In most cesareans a drape is used and one can see very little gore or blood. No. 1 is not accurate; the nurse needs to find out what the procedure usually involves.

In almost all hospitals a drape of some type is used (No. 2). No. 4 is not true.

19. (2) The effect of the anesthesia will be closely checked prior to making the incision, and the level of anesthesia will be monitored throughout the procedure. Many times the woman complains of tightness or pressure in the area the physician is working (No. 1). No significant pain should be felt as long as the anesthesia is closely monitored and maintained (No. 3). No. 4 is inappropriate because it makes her feel that she should not complain about pain even if she actually does feel it.

20. (3) Usually with a transverse lie the classical or longitudinal incision is used, and the woman is concerned about her body image. Nos. 1, 2, and 4 may be concerns, but they are not usually primary in the patient's mind.

21. (3) An apgar score of 4–6 indicates the infant is in fair condition. "Excellent" is not a category in the apgar score (No. 1). "Good" is a score of 7–10 (No. 2). "Poor" is a score of 0–3 (No. 4).

22. (1) Ensuring adequate oxygenation of the infant's system is the number-one priority in order to sustain life. Nos. 2, 3, and 4 are all appropriate secondary goals.

23. (2) The couple is able to perceive events and communicate their concerns, although there is overt tension present. No. 1 is usually indicated by restlessness and increased alertness. No. 3 is indicated by an increase in physical symptoms (headaches, nausea, dizziness, etc.) and only details are perceived. No. 4 is indicated by an inability to communicate or function.

24. (1) It is important for the couple to be able to rely on each other at this time. They need time to communicate and to begin to cope with their feelings. As long as Juanita's vital signs are stable, it may be most therapeutic to allow Tyronne into the recovery room. No. 2 isolates the husband from all significant others. No. 3 evades the problem and does not alleviate any anxiety. No. 4 is a physician's decision, and the infant is probably still being worked up and treated at this time.

25. (2) This drug is a combination of testosterone enanthate and estradiol valerate, which function as a lactosuppressant. Nos. 1, 3, and 4 are all inaccurate.

26. (2) These signs indicate the possibility of bleeding and impending hypovolemic shock. However, a decrease in BP may be due to the type of anesthetic given. Nos. 1, 3, and 4 are all errors because as the system becomes overtaxed, the pulse and respiration generally increase in an attempt to provide adequate circulation and oxygen to the system.

27. (3) To decrease the possibility of headaches, nausea, vomiting, dizziness, etc., following spinal anesthesia, the woman should be kept flat on her back. Hence Nos. 1, 2, and 4 are inaccurate (No. 1, positioning on the abdo-

men; No. 2, slightly sitting; No. 4, head downward and feet upward).

28. (4) This couple is experiencing an actual loss and will probably exhibit many of the same symptoms as a person who has lost someone to death. Nos. 1, 2, and 3 will most likely occur at some later time.

29. (3) Initially this couple will be unable to make appropriate decisions regarding their own needs. They need tender support, empathy, and reassurance in order to assist them in coping with this stress. No. 1 may be appropriate at a later time. No. 2 is incorrect because this couple is probably incapable of seeking out someone to talk to or to listen. They need guidance. If left alone, they may isolate themselves, withdraw, and become depressed. Avoidance is nontherapeutic; the problems must be faced eventually (No. 4).

30. (4) It is essential that the couple be prepared for what they will see. However, it is equally as important for them to be able to see, touch, and hold their son as soon as possible to begin the attachment process. No. 1 merely delays the couple's seeing their son. The nurse continuously assesses the parents' readiness while caring for the infant. Juanita and Tyronne *do* need some preparation prior to seeing their son (No. 2). Teaching without immediate parent-child contact can increase the parents' anxiety (No. 3).

31. (3) Crying is an appropriate, expected, and natural response. Nos. 1, 2, and 4 all invade the woman's need for privacy at this time.

32. (1) Juanita's reaction is normal at this time. Nos. 2, 3, and 4 are all usual feelings expressed when a deformed child is born.

33. (2) Both Juanita and Tyronne will probably attempt to place the blame for their son's deformities on someone or something else, such as "inadequate prenatal care," "bad counseling," or "God's wish." No. 1 involves a state in which personality development is arrested in one or more aspects at a level short of maturity. No. 3 involves unconsciously translating psychic problems into physical symptoms. No. 4 involves channeling a destructive or instinctual impulse that is socially unacceptable into a socially acceptable behavior, such as coping with anger by participating in sports that require the release of a lot of energy.

34. (3) This is characteristic of a reactive depression. The individual experiencing an endogenous depression usually feels worse in the morning but better as the day progresses. There is usually a weight loss of less than 10 lb (No. 1). The individual usually responds to environmental stimuli (No. 2). The precipitating event is usually an identifiable stressor, such as the birth of an unhealthy baby (No. 4).

35. (1) This is the most appropriate response congruent with the nurse's role. No. 2 is the physician's role. The nurse should accurately reinforce the information the physician gives the couple. In addition, the information is incomplete in that the initial repair of the palate may begin as early as six months or as late as two years, depending on the condition of the infant. No. 3 avoids answering the couple's question and may stimulate an increase in anxiety. No. 4 is the physician's role.

36. (4) The exact cause of the failure of the embryonic structures of the face to form a union is unclear. However, there is a significant familial pattern, and a hereditary factor is involved. Cleft palate is seen more frequently in girls, whereas cleft lip is seen more frequently in boys (Nos. 1 and 2). Although cleft lip and palate sometimes do occur together, in many cases they occur independently (No. 3).

37. (4) There is no correlation between cleft lip and palate and increased occurrence of mental retardation. However, the parents must be counseled to treat the child as normally as possible in order to prevent environmental delays. Nos. 1, 2, and 3 are all common problems associated with cleft palate.

38. (2) The nurse must meet the parents at their level of readiness while at the same time providing them with enough information to allow them to care adequately for the infant. Sucking needs to be avoided in an infant with a cleft palate because of the possibility of aspiration and because he will not be allowed to suck postoperatively (No. 1). A special nipple or feeder is helpful, such as Lamb's nipple or Brecht feeder. The infant should be fed in an upright position to decrease the likelihood of aspiration (No. 3). The infant needs to be isolated only from those individuals with infectious diseases such as colds or chicken pox. The infant should be treated as normally as possible in order to stimulate growth and development (No. 4).

39. (3) The prevention of scarring is essential. All crusts should be cleaned away as gently as possible, and the area should be cleansed frequently in order to prevent infection. The infant should be placed on his back or side and minimally restrained to prevent him from turning onto his face. The side position is preferred in order to prevent the aspiration of mucus or the regurgitation of milk (No. 1). The infant needs to be repositioned frequently to lessen the danger of hypostatic pneumonia (No. 2). Crying should be minimized as much as possible to avoid unnecessary strain on the suture line (No. 4).

40. (2) It is important to assess and validate the couple's perceived needs in order to plan care effectively. The couple may need a social worker as well as a public health nurse, speech pathologist, audiologist, etc. Therefore it is essential to make an accurate and continuous assessment of the family's needs (No. 1). Alternatives

may be more appropriately identified after performing a total assessment (No. 3). Health-teaching is necessary, but it must be based on an assessment and validation of the family's needs as well as of their level of readiness (No. 4).

CASE STUDY 6

David is a 16-year-old white Jewish male. He is currently in the eleventh grade because he skipped a grade when he was 12. He attends a private school and was doing exceptionally well until six months ago, when he was arrested for drunk driving and his license was temporarily suspended.

After his arrest, David was released into the custody of his parents. They were very upset and placed him on house restriction for several months. He was not allowed to use the car for any reason and had to come home immediately after school each day until his father felt he had been adequately reprimanded.

Finally, after two months of being grounded, David was allowed to participate in social activities after school, but he was still not allowed to drive the family cars. David was extremely unhappy about this restriction, and he began staying out until 2:00–3:00 A.M. several nights a week.

Yesterday when David's mother was cleaning his room she found some pills and some things that looked like cigarettes. She decided this would upset her husband, so she talked with David alone when he returned home. David accused his mother of being "nosy" and of "invading his privacy," and he stormed out of the house. He didn't explain what the pills or cigarettes were or why they were in his drawer under his shirts.

David's mother became frightened when he did not return home by 1:00 A.M., so she called her husband, who was away on a business trip. He told her not to worry, as David would probably be home soon. In any case, her husband promised to return home within the next few days.

About 4:00 A.M. David's mother received a call from University Hospital's emergency room informing her that her son had just been brought there by the police. She was asked to come to the hospital immediately. Upon her arrival, she was informed that her son was found on school property running around in the nude with several other students.

On admission to the emergency room, David's vital signs were T = 97.6, P = 100, R = 16, and BP = 90/60. He was not in touch with reality and appeared to be hallucinating. He was admitted and sent to the adult medical/surgical unit because the adolescent unit was full.

QUESTIONS

1. The nurse who admits David to the unit should be primarily concerned with:
   1. Providing a general orientation to the unit.
   2. Maintaining a quiet environment.
   3. Taking precautions against seizures.
   4. Taking vital signs every four hours.

2. Since David is not in touch with reality, the most appropriate nursing intervention would be to:
   1. Maintain a safe environment.
   2. Establish a trusting relationship.
   3. Orient David to time, place, and person.
   4. Isolate David from other clients.

3. David tells the nurse that he sees big white ants crawling all over the wall. The most appropriate nursing response would be:
   1. "Tell me where they are, and I'll kill them for you."
   2. "You must be seeing things."
   3. Silence.
   4. "I don't see any ants; however, I can see that you are afraid."

4. David constantly asks the nurse to bring him french fries and a piece of apple pie. The nurse should realize that David is probably:
   1. Starving.
   2. Hallucinating.
   3. Disoriented.
   4. Playing a game.

5. The nurse assessing a drug abuser would expect to find which of the following characteristics?
   1. A very assertive individual.
   2. A very dependent individual.
   3. A very mature individual.
   4. A very aggressive individual.

6. The nurse would expect to find drug abuse least prevalent in:
   1. An upper socioeconomic family.
   2. An elderly individual.
   3. A lower socioeconomic family.
   4. An adolescent.

7. The physician identifies that David has recently taken lysergic acid diethylamide. The nurse should be aware that on the street this drug is called:
   1. Angel dust.
   2. Smack.
   3. LSD.
   4. Coke.

8. The nurse working with drug abusers needs to know that all of the following are hallucinogenic agents, *except:*
   1. Lysergic acid diethylamide.
   2. Heroin.
   3. Marijuana.
   4. Mescaline.

9. One of the most drastic side effects of LSD is:
   1. CNS depression.
   2. Possible flashbacks.
   3. Physiologic dependence.
   4. Septicemia.

10. The nurse who is well-informed about drug abuse would know that all of the following are labels describing heroin, *except:*
    1. "Scag."
    2. "Thing."
    3. "Mexican mud."
    4. "Bean."

11. People addicted to heroin are usually treated with which of the following?
    1. Methadone.
    2. Antabuse.
    3. Phenobarbital.
    4. Thorazine.

David's mother is very upset. She is in the waiting room crying uncontrollably. Questions 12–14 concern this situation.

12. The most appropriate nursing action would be to:
    1. Provide privacy for her.
    2. Ask the physician to order Valium for her.
    3. Contact her husband.
    4. Offer to sit with her.

13. The nurse assessing David's mother would expect her initial reaction to David's illness and hospitalization to be:
    1. Anger.
    2. Denial.
    3. Acceptance.
    4. Shock.

14. David's mother asks the nurse what caused her son to take drugs. The most therapeutic response would be:
    1. "David probably wanted to be like his peers."
    2. "Inappropriate limits were probably set on David's behavior."
    3. "It involves many factors."
    4. "David felt isolated and unloved."

15. The most important aspect of David's treatment is:
    1. Teaching him about the hazards of taking drugs.
    2. Informing him that using drugs is illegal.
    3. Encouraging him to want to change his behavior.
    4. Assisting him to develop alternative coping mechanisms.

16. In planning David's initial care, the nurse should:
    1. Be very direct with him.
    2. Allow him to make all the decisions about his care.
    3. Help him to feel secure to prevent anxiety.
    4. Encourage him to begin to depend on others.

David's father returns home the afternoon after David's admission to the hospital. His initial response to his wife was, "I always knew you were too easy on him. You see what giving him his way has done!"

17. In analyzing David's father's response, the nurse should realize that he is using the defense mechanism known as:
    1. Guilt.
    2. Sublimation.
    3. Projection.
    4. Displacement.

18. David's mother asks the nurse if she would talk with David's father when he arrives at the hospital. She says that she is afraid what he might say to David. The most appropriate nursing intervention would be to:
    1. Inform David's mother that you think she and her husband can work through this problem themselves.
    2. Refer David's mother to the hospital social worker.
    3. Agree to talk with David's mother and father together.
    4. Suggest that father and son work things out.

As David's hospitalization continues, the nurse must be able to handle a variety of behavior problems.

19. In implementing care for David, which of the following actions would be the *least* appropriate?
    1. Allowing David to select some of the food he wants to eat.
    2. Restricting his activity level.
    3. Encouraging friends to visit.
    4. Closely monitoring his behavior.

20. David asks the nurse, "Have you ever used drugs?" The most appropriate nursing response would be:
    1. "Yes, once I tried grass."
    2. "Why do you want to know?"
    3. "It's not appropriate for me to discuss my personal life with you."
    4. "No."

21. David's girlfriend comes to visit him in the hospital. The nurse suspects that they may become intimate. What is the most appropriate nursing intervention?
    1. Don't allow his girlfriend to visit.
    2. Inform the couple that "necking" is prohibited.
    3. Provide privacy from staff and patients.
    4. Allow visitation with supervision.

22. David's friend John brought him a marijuana cigarette. The nurse found the cigarette under David's pillow. The most appropriate nursing action would be to:
    1. Ignore the situation.
    2. Inform the police.

3. Discuss the incident with his parents.

4. Confront David.

23. David asks the nurse not to tell anyone that he was smoking a marijuana joint in his room and promises that he'll never do it again. The nurse should realize that David is *mostly*:

1. Being sincere and wanting to change.

2. Seeking attention.

3. Being manipulative.

4. Trying to avoid punishment.

24. The nurse working with drug abusers should know that the inappropriate use of drugs is a primary cause of accidental death among people aged:

1. 10 to 15 years.

2. 15 to 35 years.

3. 36 to 60 years.

4. 60 to 78 years.

25. The nurse can expect a higher incidence of drug abuse among:

1. Teachers.

2. Social workers.

3. Lawyers.

4. Physicians.

26. The most therapeutic nursing intervention when working with manipulative clients is to:

1. Make decisions for them.

2. Assist them to identify alternative behaviors.

3. Set stringent limits.

4. Confront them publicly.

27. When assessing the client who has been abusing amphetamines, the nurse would expect to see which of the following symptoms?

1. Bradycardia.

2. Increased irritability.

3. Hypotension.

4. Constipation.

28. When planning to teach a client about the side effects of amphetamines, the nurse should emphasize that:

1. Withdrawal from these drugs usually causes death.

2. The body develops a tolerance to these drugs.

3. An overdose of these drugs induces sleepiness.

4. Physiologic dependence may develop.

29. David has a friend who takes Seconal whenever he feels "too stressed," such as whenever he has an exam or feels too pressured, which happens at least four or five times a week. The nurse should be aware that Seconal can cause which of the following?

1. Tachycardia.

2. Hypertension.

3. Assaultive behavior.

4. Increased respirations.

30. David asks the nurse whether marijuana is addictive. The most appropriate response would be:

1. "It is addictive."

2. "It causes a psychologic dependence."

3. "It is not addictive."

4. "It is physiologically addictive."

David feels very isolated from his peer group because he has been placed on an adult medical floor.

31. In planning care for David, which of the following would be most effective?

1. Assisting him to develop a working relationship with his 51-year-old roommate.

2. Encouraging his friends to visit frequently.

3. Asking him what he enjoys doing.

4. Establishing a one-to-one relationship with him.

32. What recreational activities would be most appropriate?

1. A television to watch in his room.

2. Schoolwork that can be brought to the hospital.

3. A board game such as checkers or backgammon.

4. Various novels David says he wants to read.

After David has been hospitalized eight days, his father discusses his condition with the physician. The physician indicates that an inpatient, short-term drug treatment program would probably be best for David at this time. David's father becomes very hostile and states, "My son is no addict and he isn't going to be put away in any crazy house."

33. To assess David's father's reaction to the physician's recommendation, the nurse should realize that David's father is:

1. Expressing anger about the incompetent treatment he thinks David is receiving.

2. Denying that David is a drug abuser.

3. Projecting the blame onto someone else.

4. Looking for the best possible treatment for his son.

Later in the evening following the discussion with David's physician, David's father begins experiencing severe abdominal cramping and vomits a moderate amount of blood. His wife drives him to the emergency room immediately.

34. Upon David's father's arrival at the emergency room, the nurse's primary concern should be:

1. Observing for signs and symptoms of shock.

2. Paging the physician on call immediately.

3. Filling out the appropriate assessment tool.

4. Administering CPR immediately.

35. During the first 24–48 hours after admission, the most appropriate diet for David's father is likely to be:

1. NPO.

2. Clear liquids.

3. A soft, bland diet.

4. Skim or regular milk.

36. The physician suspects David's father has a peptic ulcer. The nurse should expect the physician to order which of the following diets after the first 48–72 hours?

1. Small feedings of bland food.

2. Frequent feedings of clear liquids.
3. A regular diet given frequently in small amounts.
4. NPO.

37. A person with a peptic ulcer who is on a bland diet may lack which of the following essential nutrients?
1. Vitamin C.
2. Carbohydrates.
3. Protein.
4. Vitamin A.

38. The nurse caring for David's father at this time should:
1. Plan care so he can receive at least eight hours of uninterrupted sleep each night.
2. Monitor his vital signs every two hours.
3. Make sure that he takes his antispasmodic agents at regular intervals.
4. Provide milk for him every two to three hours.

39. David's father is given belladonna to suppress the secretion of gastric juices and to delay gastric emptying. The nurse should be aware that a common side effect of belladonna is:
1. Depressed respirations.
2. Constricted pupils.
3. Excessive thirst.
4. Bradycardia.

40. David's father becomes very demanding and hostile with the nursing staff. The most appropriate nursing intervention would be to:
1. Limit contact to decrease confrontations.
2. Establish a working relationship with him.
3. Set limits on his behavior.
4. Rotate staff assignments to alleviate stress.

ANSWERS/RATIONALE

1. (3) Clients who abuse drugs react in various ways depending on the amount and type of drug taken, the combination of drugs, and individual factors such as overall general health, age, etc. However, seizures are common shortly after the ingestion of drugs such as narcotics or stimulants. Seizures may also accompany the withdrawal from drugs. No. 1 is inappropriate because the client is not even in touch with reality. Nos. 2 and 4 are secondary but important. However, vital signs should be taken as soon as possible to establish a baseline and retaken at least every 1–2 hours thereafter until the patient is stable.

2. (1) It is of paramount importance to prevent the client from hurting himself and others. No. 2 cannot be done at this time because the client is unable to communicate effectively. No. 3 may be attempted once David is able to communicate. No. 4 is important initially to prevent him from harming his parents as well as to protect him

from overstimulation, but this is just one aspect of No. 1.

3. (4) This response does not contradict the client's perceptions, is honest, and shows empathy. No. 1 humors the client and is dishonest and nontherapeutic. No. 2 makes fun of the client. No. 3 avoids the situation and makes the client feel that the nurse does not care about him.

4. (3) David is disoriented to time, place, and person. He needs constant monitoring and comprehensive support. He may be physiologically hungry; however, since he is confused, this is difficult to validate (No. 1). He may be hallucinating, but this information merely indicates that he is disoriented (No. 2). No. 4 is unlikely because he does not appear to be in touch with reality.

5. (2) Drug abusers tend to be excessively dependent and passive, become easily frustrated, and cannot cope with anxiety. Nos. 1, 3, and 4 are unusual in drug abusers because they are unable to externalize their feelings and fears or to cope effectively with stress.

6. (2) Although drug abuse may be found at every age level, the elderly seem least likely to abuse substances. This is probably due to generational differences in cultural norms and morals. (It was thought to be "weak" or "sick" to rely on drugs to escape problems.) However, many times the elderly use alcohol as an escape mechanism. Drug abuse is found among all socioeconomic classes (Nos. 1 and 3). The reasons for abuse vary from individual to individual, depending on their particular needs. Many adolescents use drugs to escape reality, cope with stress, identify with their peers, etc. (No. 4).

7. (3) It is imperative that the nurse be familiar with the street jargon for drugs in order to understand what the client is saying. Angel dust is PCP (No. 1). Smack is heroin (No. 2). Coke is cocaine (No. 4).

8. (2) Heroin is a narcotic that usually does not cause hallucinations but produces a change in perceptions, or "a high calming effect." Nos. 1 and 4 are commonly known to cause hallucinations. No. 3 may increase distortions in perception and has been known to cause hallucinations with high levels of ingestion.

9. (2) The individual may begin to experience a "high" and hallucinations without warning or recent ingestion of the drug. The stimulus for these flashbacks has not been well delineated. CNS stimulation is usually exhibited (No. 1). LSD is psychologically, not physiologically, addicting (No. 3). No. 4 is usually a side effect of drugs that are taken intravenously, such as heroin.

10. (4) "Bean" describes the hallucinogen mescaline. Nos. 1, 2, and 3 all describe heroin. Other terms describing heroin include: Chinese red, brown, smack, junk, and Big H.

11. (1) Methadone is the drug most often used to treat heroin addiction because it is long-acting (24–36 hours) and effectively controls withdrawal symptoms. Note: methadyl acetate is another medication used to treat heroin addiction, and its duration is 48–60 hours. No. 2 is used to treat alcoholism; however, it can minimally suppress the withdrawal symptoms of heroin addicts. No. 3 is a sedative-hypnotic. No. 4 is a major tranquilizer.

12. (4) Acknowledging her presence and discomfort is most important in order to provide emotional support. Privacy is important if she requests it (No. 1). However, assuming that she wants to be isolated may cause feelings of rejection and loneliness. An assessment of her overall level of functioning and coping abilities needs to be performed first (No. 2). It is also the doctor's decision to give medication. No. 3 may be appropriate if she wants him to be contacted. This decision needs to be discussed with David's mother.

13. (4) In addition to the shock of the immediate crisis, David's mother probably never accepted the fact that her son was extensively involved with drugs. No. 1 will take time to develop as she takes in the implications of the situation. No. 2 is part of the shock process. No. 3 is unrealistic at this time.

14. (3) There are no definite answers, as there are many possible causes of drug abuse. Many times not even the abuser can tell you why he began using drugs. Nos. 1 and 4 may both be contributing factors, but the nurse lacks validation. No. 2 is an unvalidated assumption that would need to be explored further.

15. (3) The treatment of drug abuse is only effective if the client is motivated to make changes in his style and pattern of living. Nos. 1, 2, and 4 are all significant components to be incorporated in health-teaching, but David must first be motivated to learn.

16. (1) Straightforward, direct communication is needed to keep David from manipulating his care. The nurse needs to be honest and to set very firm limits. No. 2 is inappropriate because an adolescent drug abuser tends to be very manipulative. However, allowing him to assist in the decision-making process is essential. Too much security will foster dependence (No. 3). He needs to identify and begin to cope with his anxiety, although anxiety generally cannot be eliminated entirely. Drug abusers are characteristically very dependent individuals (No. 4).

17. (3) He is essentially blaming the situation on David's mother because he is unable to cope effectively with his feelings at this time. No. 1 is usually not a defense mechanism because it does not help a person cope with anxiety or other feelings. Sublimation involves rechanneling a destructive or instinctual impulse that is socially unacceptable into an acceptable outlet, such as channeling anger into sports (No. 2). No. 4 involves transferring emotion from an unacceptable mode of expression to a more acceptable one (e.g., "drinking yourself under the table because your wife is dying)."

18. (3) By agreeing to talk with David's parents, the nurse can provide psychologic support and further assess and validate the family's needs. No. 1 lacks empathy and makes David's mother feel rejected. No. 2 may be an appropriate action after doing further assessment. If after further assessment and discussion with the physician and social worker the health team thinks No. 4 is appropriate, then this suggestion should be made. However, at this time it is inappropriate.

19. (3) Encouraging his friends to visit is inappropriate because they may bring him drugs or encourage him to act out by leaving the hospital or taking drugs. Visitation should not be completely curtailed but very closely monitored. No. 1 allows the client to feel he has some control over his care, which is especially important during adolescence. No. 4 allows the nurse to monitor his care more closely. Because he was brought in by the police, stringent observational requirements may be required. No. 2 helps him regain strength and decreases stimuli in the immediate environment.

20. (3) The client may perceive this as avoidance, but it is more important to be direct and honest, especially in light of the manipulative behaviors of drug abusers and adolescents. Nos. 1 and 4 are inappropriate because they provide information about the nurse's personal life that is irrelevant to the maintenance of a therapeutic relationship. No. 2 plays into his manipulation.

21. (4) Although the nurse suspects that this behavior may occur, she has no valid concern unless the couple's behavior becomes inappropriate. The nurse needs to realize that kissing is a normal part of adolescence. Some privacy may be provided; however, periodic supervision is warranted because David is a drug abuser and an adolescent. However, David still needs companionship (No. 1). He also needs to feel trusted in order to develop into an independent and mature person. No. 2 serves only to highlight mistrust, and the couple may already feel that intimacy is inappropriate in this setting. Privacy is needed with some supervision in order to promote responsible behavior (No. 3).

22. (4) Being direct with David about this issue is extremely important because the incident violates hospital policy, the law, his treatment, and his parents' rules. David should be directly confronted and the incident discussed with him and the medical staff. The health team will decide whether it is in the client's best interest to inform his parents and/or the police. Avoidance will merely perpetuate the situation (No. 1). Nos. 2 and 3 are health team decisions.

23. (3) Attempting to control the situation and do as he pleases is most likely his primary goal in light of his history of drug abuse. Bending the rules for a severe violation of hospital policy, his treatment, and the law is not justified. For No. 1 to be correct, the nurse would need further evidence of the client's desire to change, such as overt, consistent changes in his pattern of behavior, open verbalization of his feelings, etc. Nos. 2 and 4 are aspects of manipulation.

24. (2) Drug abuse is found throughout adolescence and through middle age. As societal pressures increase (economic concerns, peer pressure, occupational problems), the use of drugs increases. Nos. 1, 3, and 4 are inappropriate because even though drug abuse is on the rise in elementary and middle schools, it still has not surpassed the use in age group No. 2. Individuals in age group No. 4 tend to use alcohol as an escape rather than drugs.

25. (4) Physicians have easy access to drugs and the high-powered stress of their occupation increases the tendency to use drugs such as amphetamines to increase their energy level. Also, their need to alleviate anxiety is important. Statistics indicate professions Nos. 1, 2, and 3 have a lower tendency to abuse drugs because they have less of an opportunity to obtain them, legally or illegally.

26. (2) Many times manipulative clients are not aware of any other mechanisms for fulfilling their needs. Health-teaching them to identify manipulative behaviors may help them avoid manipulating and eventually adopt more appropriate means for meeting their needs. The clients should be involved in the decision-making process (No. 1). Limits must be realistically established (No. 3). Public confrontation may only exacerbate the power struggle (No. 4).

27. (2) Although in moderation these drugs produce a feeling of well-being and alertness, an overdose of amphetamines *causes* an increase in tension and irritability. An increase in the heart rate and blood flow is exhibited, as these drugs stimulate the release of norepinephrine (Nos. 1 and 3). Diarrhea (not constipation) is a common side effect (No. 4).

28. (2) There is no physiologic dependence, but the person has to increase the dose to receive the same effect because the body develops a tolerance. Withdrawal usually leads to severe exhaustion (No. 1). Overdoses induce hyperactivity within the system (No. 3). Psychologic, not physiologic, dependence develops from increased tolerance (No. 4).

29. (3) Seconal, a barbiturate, causes a depression of the CNS, so its effects usually include bradycardia, hypotension and depressed respiration. With large dosages of Seconal there may be an increase in anger *or* a deep sleep, depending on the individual's reaction. Hence Nos. 1, 2, and 4 are incorrect.

30. (2) There is a physical tolerance, but the dependence is purely psychologic. Nos. 1 and 3 are imprecise, and No. 4 is incorrect, because this drug is not physically addictive.

31. (3) This allows David some control over his care and makes him feel that the staff is interested in meeting his needs. No. 1 is inappropriate unless they have common interest. Frequent visits should initially be discouraged to avoid the possibility of David's receiving drugs from the outside. No. 4 may be appropriate; however, it is not as important as allowing David some control over his own care.

32. (4) Provide activities David enjoys. No. 1 does not promote intellectual stimulation and may disturb his roommate. Furthermore, the nurse has not validated whether David enjoys watching television. No. 2 is not a recreational activity. The nurse does not yet know whether David enjoys these games, and they both require a suitable partner (No. 3).

33. (2) He is attempting to cope with his anxiety by denying reality. He may also be angry (No. 1), but his behavior and verbalization indicate denial. Through the use of denial he is displacing the blame, so denial is the most appropriate answer (No. 3). He is unable to think clearly enough to seek any type of intervention (No. 4); he is reacting rather than problem-solving.

34. (1) Because the patient has experienced some gastric bleeding he should be observed closely for symptoms of shock. No. 2 is secondary to closely monitoring the patient's vital signs for symptoms of shock. No. 3 may be done when the patient and his family are under less stress. No. 4 is not indicated at this time because the patient is not experiencing cardiac or respiratory failure.

35. (4) Skim or regular milk is given initially every one to two hours to relieve the client's symptoms by neutralizing the free hydrochloric acid in the stomach. No. 1 is inappropriate because it will increase the amount of hydrochloric acid, thereby aggravating the symptoms. No. 2 may not neutralize the hydrochloric acid. No. 3 is inappropriate because the client may not be able to tolerate solid food at this time.

36. (1) Bland feedings should be given in small amounts on a frequent basis to neutralize the hydrochloric acid and to prevent overload. No. 4 would promote the production of free acid in the stomach and increase the symptoms. No. 2 may not control the amount of acid in the stomach, would be monotonous, and may lack all the necessary nutrients. No. 3 may overload the system.

37. (1) The client should be given diluted orange juice to ensure an adequate supply of ascorbic acid (vitamin C). Nos. 2, 3, and 4 can be easily obtained by a variety of foods in the bland diet.

38. (4) Milk prevents the accumulation of gastric juice throughout the night. Prevention of pain is essential, and milk will help prevent pain if given at the appropriate times. No. 1 will allow an accumulation of gastric acid and will increase pain. No. 2 is not necessary unless indicated by symptoms of shock. The emphasis should be on regular and appropriate feedings rather than on antacid or antispasmodic agents (No. 3).

39. (3) Belladonna is an anticholinergic that causes dryness of the mouth and throat, which leads to excessive thirst and possibly to difficulty swallowing. Anticholinergic drugs usually cause an increase in pulse and respirations (Nos. 1 and 4) and dilated pupils (No. 2).

40. (2) By establishing a therapeutic relationship, the nurse can tactfully establish limits while providing empathy and physical nursing care. No. 1 stimulates anxiety and increases feelings of hostility and rejection. No. 3 can be tactfully incorporated into a therapeutic relationship. No. 4 encourages avoidance and hostile feelings between the staff and the patient.

A STEP FURTHER:

A Cross Reference to Nursing Behaviors Addressed in Units 2, 3, 4, and 5 Questions

---

Note: italicized numbers refer to questions that address more than one nursing behavior.

Unit 2 / MENTAL HEALTH NURSING AND COPING BEHAVIORS

Assessment
15, 16, 17, 18, 19, 20, 21, *22*, 23, *24*, *25*, *26*, 31, 32, 36, *37*, 39, *40*, 42, 43, *45*, 47, *51*, *53*, 55, 56, 60, *61*, 62, 63, 69, *72*, 73, 74, 75, *76*, 77, 78, *82*, *85*, 87, *91*, *92*, *93*, 94, 96, 98, 99, 100, *111*, *112*, 113, 114, 115, 116, 120, 129, 133, 134, 135, 136, 137, 139, 145, 147, *153*, 155, 160, 164, 166, 168, 171, 172, 173, 174, 175, 176, 177, 179, 183, 184, 187

Analysis
2, 5, 7, 8, *9*, *14*, 22, *24*, 25, *26*, 27, *34*, 35, *38*, *40*, 44, *45*, *48*, *49*, *50*, *51*, *52*, *53*, 54, 58, *65*, 69, *70*, *71*, *79*, *80*, 81, *83*, 84, *85*, *89*, *95*, *97*, *118*, 126, *127*, 144, 146, 149, 150, *153*, *154*, 156, 157, 161, *163*, 167, 169, 170, 190, 193

Planning
6, *10*, 13, *27*, 29, 33, 35, *37*, 46, *49*, *51*, *52*, *54*, 57, *61*, *65*, 66, 67, *71*, *72*, 77, *80*, 86, 88, 90, *91*, *92*, *93*, 103, 104, 105, 106, 107, 108, 109, 110, *111*, *112*, 119, 121, 123, 124, 125, *127*, 131, 138, 140, 158, 162, *163*, 178, 182, 185

Implementation
1, *2*, 3, 4, *6*, 7, 8, *9*, *10*, 11, 12, *14*, 28, 30, *34*, *38*, 41, *48*, *50*, *58*, 59, 68, *70*, *83*, *89*, *95*, *97*, 101, 117, *118*, 128, 130, 141, 143, 148, 151, 152, 159, 180, 188, 189, 191, 194

Evaluation
76, 132, 142, *171*, 192

Unit 3 / NURSING CARE DURING THE REPRODUCTIVE YEARS

Assessment
1, 2, 3, 4, 5, 6, 7, 10, 15, 26, 45, 46, 72, 122, 125, 130, 134, 135, 162, 163, 165, 166, 167, 170, 171, 180, 202, 206, 207, 208, 209, 210, 212, 216, 219, 221, 223, 224, 225, 226, 229, 230, 231, 232

Analysis
8, 9, 12, 13, 14, 19, 21, 22, 28, 29, 30, 31, 35, 36, 37, 38, 39, 40, 41, 48, 49, 55, 57, 60, 63, 64, 65, 69, 71, 75, 90, 91, 94, 104, 105, 113, 114, 120, 122, *129*, 139, 144, 148, 151, 152, 157, 158, 160, 174, 175, 177, 178, 182, 183, 184, 185, 190, 193, 199, 215

Planning
8, 17, 23, 103, 112, 124, 126, 146, 154, 156, 188, 191, 192, 200

Implementation
16, 24, 25, 32, 42, 47, 50, 54, 56, *73*, 74, 80, 83, 88, 93, 95, 97, 107, 115, 118, 119, 121, 127, 128, *129*, 131, 132, 133, 138, 140, 142, 143, 147, 149, 150, 153, 159, 161, 169, 172, 186, 194, 195, 197, 198, 201, 203, 217, 227

Evaluation
18, 51, 53, 58, 59, 62, 66, 67, 68, *73*, 76, 77, 78, 84, 92, 96, 101, 102, 110, 117, 136, 137, 141, 145, 173, 179, 181, 187, 189, 204, 205, 211, 213, 214, 218

Unit 4 / NURSING CARE OF CHILDREN AND FAMILIES

Assessment

1, 2, 3, 8, 10, 15, 17, 23, 25, 26, 27, 28, 30, 31, 36, 46, 47, 49, 52, 58, 61, 67, 75, 80, 86, 95, 96, 99, 109, 114, 121, 125, 136, 137, 142, 144, 146, 148, 153, 154, 159, 161, 169, 190, 191

Analysis

5, 6, 9, 11, 20, 21, 22, 29, 37, 38, 42, 43, 48, 50, 51, 53, 54, 55, 56, 59, 63, 64, 68, 69, 72, 73, 76, 81, 82, 83, 84, 92, 97, 98, 100, 103, 122, 129, 143, 149, 150, 160, 162, 163, *164*, 165, 166, 173, 182, 183, 184, 185, *188*, 189, 192, 193, 194, 195

Planning

4, 16, 19, 32, 34, 44, 45, 57, 60, 62, 65, 71, 74, 89, 90, 91, 93, 94, 111, 113, 115, 128, 135, 140, 175, 176, 177, 178

Implementation

7, 12, 13, 14, 18, 24, 33, 35, *39*, 40, 41, 66, 77, 79, 85, 87, 88, 101, 102, 104, 105, 106, 107, 108, 110, *112*, 116, 118, 120, 126, 127, 130, 131, 134, 138, 139, 151, 155, 156, 157, *164*, 167, 168, 170, 171, 172, 174, 179, 180, 186, 187, *188*

Evaluation

39, 70, 78, *112*, 117, 119, 123, 124, 132, 133, 141, 145, 147, 152, 158, 181

Unit 5 / NURSING CARE OF THE ACUTELY OR CHRONICALLY ILL ADULT

Assessment

1, 2, 7, 8, 13, 16, 17, 23, 24, 37, 38, 51, 55, 68, 69, 71, 85, 88, 89, 97, 98, 103, 104, 105, 110, 112, 114, 122, 128, 131, 144, 145, 146, 153, 163, 164, 185, 186, *188, 189*, 194, 198, 202, 203, 211, 212, 218, *225*, 236, 244, 249, 257, *258*, 263, 266, 267, 268, 278, 280, 283, *291*, 292, 295, 311, 313, 319, 323, 330, 331, 335, 336, 340, 342, 343, 350, 351, 358, 360, 362, 363, 365, 368, 369, *371*, 374, 379, *389*, 390

Analysis

3, 14, 15, 25, 36, 39, 40, 47, 52, 56, *60*, 65, *74*, 86, 87, 90, 91, 92, 96, 102, 109, 111, 113, 115, 118, 121, 127, 129, 130, 132, 136, 147, 152, 155, 156, 168, 178, 181, 184, 187, *188, 189*, 196, 197, 213, 214, 215, 216, 222, 223, *225*, 226, 239, 250, *252*, 253, 254, 261, 270, *291*, 293, 294, 296, 297, 299, 300, 310, 315, 326, 341, 344, 352, 361, 367, *371*, 377, 385, *386, 389*, 391, 394, *395, 398, 399*

Planning

4, 6, 10, 26, 30, 33, 54, 57, 59, 62, 63, 67, 70, 72, 73, *74*, 78, 81, 82, 84, 93, 94, 101, 106, 108, 116, 117, 119, 124, 125, 126, 133, 135, 137, 138, 149, 154, 157, 161, 165, 166, 167, 169, 170, 173, 176, 177, 182, 200, 217, 221, 230, 231, 237, 238, 240, 242, 246, *252*, 256, *258*, 265, 271, 272, 274, 275, *286*, 288, 290, 302, *303*, 312, 318, 325, 327, 328, 329, 332, 338, 347, 355, 357, 359, 373, 378, 380, *381, 386*, 387, 388, 392, *395*

Implementation

5, 9, 11, 18, 19, 20, 21, 27, 28, 29, 31, 32, 34, 35, 42, 43, 44, 45, 46, 48, 49, 50, 53, 58, *60*, 61, 64, 66, 75, 76, 77, 80, 83, 99, 100, 107, 123, 134, 139, 141, 143, 148, 150, 151, 158, 159, 160, 172, 174, 179, 180, 183, 190, 191, 199, 204, 205, 206, 207, 208, 209, 219, 228, 229, 232, 233, 245, 247, 248, 251, 255, 259, 262, 269, 273, 277, 279, 281, 282, 284, 285, *286*, 289, 301, 304, 305, 308, 309, 314, 317, 321, 322, 324, 333, 334, 337, 339, 345, 346, 348, 354, 356, 366, 375, 376, *381*, 382, 383, 393, 396, *398*, 399, 400

Evaluation

12, 22, 41, 79, 95, 120, 140, 142, 162, 171, 175, 192, 193, 201, 210, 220, 224, 227, 234, 235, 241, 243, 260, 264, 276, 287, *303*, 306, 307, 316, 320, 349, 353, 364, 370, 372, 384, 397

Index

Unit 2

When marking the answer sheet, blacken only one circle for each question. Blacken the circle *completely*. Do *NOT* use X's or check marks. If you decide to change your answer, erase your original answer *thoroughly*. If you do not, your new answer may be scored incorrectly. You *MUST* use a No. 2 pencil to mark your answers.

	1	2	3	4
1	○	○	○	○
2	○	○	○	○
3	○	○	○	○
4	○	○	○	○
5	○	○	○	○
6	○	○	○	○
7	○	○	○	○
8	○	○	○	○
9	○	○	○	○
10	○	○	○	○

	1	2	3	4
11	○	○	○	○
12	○	○	○	○
13	○	○	○	○
14	○	○	○	○
15	○	○	○	○
16	○	○	○	○
17	○	○	○	○
18	○	○	○	○
19	○	○	○	○
20	○	○	○	○

	1	2	3	4
21	○	○	○	○
22	○	○	○	○
23	○	○	○	○
24	○	○	○	○
25	○	○	○	○
26	○	○	○	○
27	○	○	○	○
28	○	○	○	○
29	○	○	○	○
30	○	○	○	○

	1	2	3	4
31	○	○	○	○
32	○	○	○	○
33	○	○	○	○
34	○	○	○	○
35	○	○	○	○
36	○	○	○	○
37	○	○	○	○
38	○	○	○	○
39	○	○	○	○
40	○	○	○	○

	1	2	3	4
41	○	○	○	○
42	○	○	○	○
43	○	○	○	○
44	○	○	○	○
45	○	○	○	○
46	○	○	○	○
47	○	○	○	○
48	○	○	○	○
49	○	○	○	○
50	○	○	○	○

	1	2	3	4
51	○	○	○	○
52	○	○	○	○
53	○	○	○	○
54	○	○	○	○
55	○	○	○	○
56	○	○	○	○
57	○	○	○	○
58	○	○	○	○
59	○	○	○	○
60	○	○	○	○

	1	2	3	4
61	○	○	○	○
62	○	○	○	○
63	○	○	○	○
64	○	○	○	○
65	○	○	○	○
66	○	○	○	○
67	○	○	○	○
68	○	○	○	○
69	○	○	○	○
70	○	○	○	○

	1	2	3	4
71	○	○	○	○
72	○	○	○	○
73	○	○	○	○
74	○	○	○	○
75	○	○	○	○
76	○	○	○	○
77	○	○	○	○
78	○	○	○	○
79	○	○	○	○
80	○	○	○	○

Unit 2

When marking the answer sheet, blacken only one circle for each question. Blacken the circle *completely*. Do *NOT* use X's or check marks. If you decide to change your answer, erase your original answer *thoroughly*. If you do not, your new answer may be scored incorrectly. You *MUST* use a No. 2 pencil to mark your answers.

	1	2	3	4
81	○	○	○	○
82	○	○	○	○
83	○	○	○	○
84	○	○	○	○
85	○	○	○	○
86	○	○	○	○
87	○	○	○	○
88	○	○	○	○
89	○	○	○	○
90	○	○	○	○

	1	2	3	4
91	○	○	○	○
92	○	○	○	○
93	○	○	○	○
94	○	○	○	○
95	○	○	○	○
96	○	○	○	○
97	○	○	○	○
98	○	○	○	○
99	○	○	○	○
100	○	○	○	○

	1	2	3	4
101	○	○	○	○
102	○	○	○	○
103	○	○	○	○
104	○	○	○	○
105	○	○	○	○
106	○	○	○	○
107	○	○	○	○
108	○	○	○	○
109	○	○	○	○
110	○	○	○	○

	1	2	3	4
111	○	○	○	○
112	○	○	○	○
113	○	○	○	○
114	○	○	○	○
115	○	○	○	○
116	○	○	○	○
117	○	○	○	○
118	○	○	○	○
119	○	○	○	○
120	○	○	○	○

	1	2	3	4
121	○	○	○	○
122	○	○	○	○
123	○	○	○	○
124	○	○	○	○
125	○	○	○	○
126	○	○	○	○
127	○	○	○	○
128	○	○	○	○
129	○	○	○	○
130	○	○	○	○

	1	2	3	4
131	○	○	○	○
132	○	○	○	○
133	○	○	○	○
134	○	○	○	○
135	○	○	○	○
136	○	○	○	○
137	○	○	○	○
138	○	○	○	○
139	○	○	○	○
140	○	○	○	○

	1	2	3	4
141	○	○	○	○
142	○	○	○	○
143	○	○	○	○
144	○	○	○	○
145	○	○	○	○
146	○	○	○	○
147	○	○	○	○
148	○	○	○	○
149	○	○	○	○
150	○	○	○	○

	1	2	3	4
151	○	○	○	○
152	○	○	○	○
153	○	○	○	○
154	○	○	○	○
155	○	○	○	○
156	○	○	○	○
157	○	○	○	○
158	○	○	○	○
159	○	○	○	○
160	○	○	○	○

Unit 2 and 3

Unit 2

	1	2	3	4
161	○	○	○	○
162	○	○	○	○
163	○	○	○	○
164	○	○	○	○
165	○	○	○	○
166	○	○	○	○
167	○	○	○	○
168	○	○	○	○
169	○	○	○	○
170	○	○	○	○

	1	2	3	4
171	○	○	○	○
172	○	○	○	○
173	○	○	○	○
174	○	○	○	○
175	○	○	○	○
176	○	○	○	○
177	○	○	○	○
178	○	○	○	○
179	○	○	○	○
180	○	○	○	○

	1	2	3	4
181	○	○	○	○
182	○	○	○	○
183	○	○	○	○
184	○	○	○	○
185	○	○	○	○
186	○	○	○	○
187	○	○	○	○
188	○	○	○	○
189	○	○	○	○
190	○	○	○	○

	1	2	3	4
191	○	○	○	○
192	○	○	○	○
193	○	○	○	○
194	○	○	○	○

Unit 3

	1	2	3	4
1	○	○	○	○
2	○	○	○	○
3	○	○	○	○
4	○	○	○	○
5	○	○	○	○
6	○	○	○	○
7	○	○	○	○
8	○	○	○	○
9	○	○	○	○
10	○	○	○	○

	1	2	3	4
11	○	○	○	○
12	○	○	○	○
13	○	○	○	○
14	○	○	○	○
15	○	○	○	○
16	○	○	○	○
17	○	○	○	○
18	○	○	○	○
19	○	○	○	○
20	○	○	○	○

	1	2	3	4
21	○	○	○	○
22	○	○	○	○
23	○	○	○	○
24	○	○	○	○
25	○	○	○	○
26	○	○	○	○
27	○	○	○	○
28	○	○	○	○
29	○	○	○	○
30	○	○	○	○

	1	2	3	4
31	○	○	○	○
32	○	○	○	○
33	○	○	○	○
34	○	○	○	○
35	○	○	○	○
36	○	○	○	○
37	○	○	○	○
38	○	○	○	○
39	○	○	○	○
40	○	○	○	○

Unit 3

Unit 3

When marking the answer sheet, blacken only one circle for each question. Blacken the circle *completely*. Do *NOT* use X's or check marks. If you decide to change your answer, erase your original answer *thoroughly*. If you do not, your new answer may be scored incorrectly. You *MUST* use a No. 2 pencil to mark your answers.

	1	2	3	4
41	○	○	○	○
42	○	○	○	○
43	○	○	○	○
44	○	○	○	○
45	○	○	○	○
46	○	○	○	○
47	○	○	○	○
48	○	○	○	○
49	○	○	○	○
50	○	○	○	○

	1	2	3	4
51	○	○	○	○
52	○	○	○	○
53	○	○	○	○
54	○	○	○	○
55	○	○	○	○
56	○	○	○	○
57	○	○	○	○
58	○	○	○	○
59	○	○	○	○
60	○	○	○	○

	1	2	3	4
61	○	○	○	○
62	○	○	○	○
63	○	○	○	○
64	○	○	○	○
65	○	○	○	○
66	○	○	○	○
67	○	○	○	○
68	○	○	○	○
69	○	○	○	○
70	○	○	○	○

	1	2	3	4
71	○	○	○	○
72	○	○	○	○
73	○	○	○	○
74	○	○	○	○
75	○	○	○	○
76	○	○	○	○
77	○	○	○	○
78	○	○	○	○
79	○	○	○	○
80	○	○	○	○

	1	2	3	4
81	○	○	○	○
82	○	○	○	○
83	○	○	○	○
84	○	○	○	○
85	○	○	○	○
86	○	○	○	○
87	○	○	○	○
88	○	○	○	○
89	○	○	○	○
90	○	○	○	○

	1	2	3	4
91	○	○	○	○
92	○	○	○	○
93	○	○	○	○
94	○	○	○	○
95	○	○	○	○
96	○	○	○	○
97	○	○	○	○
98	○	○	○	○
99	○	○	○	○
100	○	○	○	○

	1	2	3	4
101	○	○	○	○
102	○	○	○	○
103	○	○	○	○
104	○	○	○	○
105	○	○	○	○
106	○	○	○	○
107	○	○	○	○
108	○	○	○	○
109	○	○	○	○
110	○	○	○	○

	1	2	3	4
111	○	○	○	○
112	○	○	○	○
113	○	○	○	○
114	○	○	○	○
115	○	○	○	○
116	○	○	○	○
117	○	○	○	○
118	○	○	○	○
119	○	○	○	○
120	○	○	○	○

Unit 3

	1	2	3	4
121	○	○	○	○
122	○	○	○	○
123	○	○	○	○
124	○	○	○	○
125	○	○	○	○
126	○	○	○	○
127	○	○	○	○
128	○	○	○	○
129	○	○	○	○
130	○	○	○	○

	1	2	3	4
131	○	○	○	○
132	○	○	○	○
133	○	○	○	○
134	○	○	○	○
135	○	○	○	○
136	○	○	○	○
137	○	○	○	○
138	○	○	○	○
139	○	○	○	○
140	○	○	○	○

	1	2	3	4
141	○	○	○	○
142	○	○	○	○
143	○	○	○	○
144	○	○	○	○
145	○	○	○	○
146	○	○	○	○
147	○	○	○	○
148	○	○	○	○
149	○	○	○	○
150	○	○	○	○

	1	2	3	4
151	○	○	○	○
152	○	○	○	○
153	○	○	○	○
154	○	○	○	○
155	○	○	○	○
156	○	○	○	○
157	○	○	○	○
158	○	○	○	○
159	○	○	○	○
160	○	○	○	○

	1	2	3	4
161	○	○	○	○
162	○	○	○	○
163	○	○	○	○
164	○	○	○	○
165	○	○	○	○
166	○	○	○	○
167	○	○	○	○
168	○	○	○	○
169	○	○	○	○
170	○	○	○	○

	1	2	3	4
171	○	○	○	○
172	○	○	○	○
173	○	○	○	○
174	○	○	○	○
175	○	○	○	○
176	○	○	○	○
177	○	○	○	○
178	○	○	○	○
179	○	○	○	○
180	○	○	○	○

	1	2	3	4
181	○	○	○	○
182	○	○	○	○
183	○	○	○	○
184	○	○	○	○
185	○	○	○	○
186	○	○	○	○
187	○	○	○	○
188	○	○	○	○
189	○	○	○	○
190	○	○	○	○

	1	2	3	4
191	○	○	○	○
192	○	○	○	○
193	○	○	○	○
194	○	○	○	○
195	○	○	○	○
196	○	○	○	○
197	○	○	○	○
198	○	○	○	○
199	○	○	○	○
200	○	○	○	○

Unit 3

	1	2	3	4
201	○	○	○	○
202	○	○	○	○
203	○	○	○	○
204	○	○	○	○
205	○	○	○	○
206	○	○	○	○
207	○	○	○	○
208	○	○	○	○
209	○	○	○	○
210	○	○	○	○

	1	2	3	4
211	○	○	○	○
212	○	○	○	○
213	○	○	○	○
214	○	○	○	○
215	○	○	○	○
216	○	○	○	○
217	○	○	○	○
218	○	○	○	○
219	○	○	○	○
220	○	○	○	○

	1	2	3	4
221	○	○	○	○
222	○	○	○	○
223	○	○	○	○
224	○	○	○	○
225	○	○	○	○
226	○	○	○	○
227	○	○	○	○
228	○	○	○	○
229	○	○	○	○
230	○	○	○	○

	1	2	3	4
231	○	○	○	○
232	○	○	○	○

Unit 4

	1	2	3	4
1	○	○	○	○
2	○	○	○	○
3	○	○	○	○
4	○	○	○	○
5	○	○	○	○
6	○	○	○	○
7	○	○	○	○
8	○	○	○	○
9	○	○	○	○
10	○	○	○	○

	1	2	3	4
11	○	○	○	○
12	○	○	○	○
13	○	○	○	○
14	○	○	○	○
15	○	○	○	○
16	○	○	○	○
17	○	○	○	○
18	○	○	○	○
19	○	○	○	○
20	○	○	○	○

	1	2	3	4
21	○	○	○	○
22	○	○	○	○
23	○	○	○	○
24	○	○	○	○
25	○	○	○	○
26	○	○	○	○
27	○	○	○	○
28	○	○	○	○
29	○	○	○	○
30	○	○	○	○

	1	2	3	4
31	○	○	○	○
32	○	○	○	○
33	○	○	○	○
34	○	○	○	○
35	○	○	○	○
36	○	○	○	○
37	○	○	○	○
38	○	○	○	○
39	○	○	○	○
40	○	○	○	○

Unit 4

incorrect marks

correct mark

When marking the answer sheet, blacken only one circle for each question. Blacken the circle *completely*. Do *NOT* use X's or check marks. If you decide to change your answer, erase your original answer *thoroughly*. If you do not, your new answer may be scored incorrectly. You *MUST* use a No. 2 pencil to mark your answers.

	1	2	3	4
41	○	○	○	○
42	○	○	○	○
43	○	○	○	○
44	○	○	○	○
45	○	○	○	○
46	○	○	○	○
47	○	○	○	○
48	○	○	○	○
49	○	○	○	○
50	○	○	○	○

	1	2	3	4
51	○	○	○	○
52	○	○	○	○
53	○	○	○	○
54	○	○	○	○
55	○	○	○	○
56	○	○	○	○
57	○	○	○	○
58	○	○	○	○
59	○	○	○	○
60	○	○	○	○

	1	2	3	4
61	○	○	○	○
62	○	○	○	○
63	○	○	○	○
64	○	○	○	○
65	○	○	○	○
66	○	○	○	○
67	○	○	○	○
68	○	○	○	○
69	○	○	○	○
70	○	○	○	○

	1	2	3	4
71	○	○	○	○
72	○	○	○	○
73	○	○	○	○
74	○	○	○	○
75	○	○	○	○
76	○	○	○	○
77	○	○	○	○
78	○	○	○	○
79	○	○	○	○
80	○	○	○	○

	1	2	3	4
81	○	○	○	○
82	○	○	○	○
83	○	○	○	○
84	○	○	○	○
85	○	○	○	○
86	○	○	○	○
87	○	○	○	○
88	○	○	○	○
89	○	○	○	○
90	○	○	○	○

	1	2	3	4
91	○	○	○	○
92	○	○	○	○
93	○	○	○	○
94	○	○	○	○
95	○	○	○	○
96	○	○	○	○
97	○	○	○	○
98	○	○	○	○
99	○	○	○	○
100	○	○	○	○

	1	2	3	4
101	○	○	○	○
102	○	○	○	○
103	○	○	○	○
104	○	○	○	○
105	○	○	○	○
106	○	○	○	○
107	○	○	○	○
108	○	○	○	○
109	○	○	○	○
110	○	○	○	○

	1	2	3	4
111	○	○	○	○
112	○	○	○	○
113	○	○	○	○
114	○	○	○	○
115	○	○	○	○
116	○	○	○	○
117	○	○	○	○
118	○	○	○	○
119	○	○	○	○
120	○	○	○	○

Unit 4

incorrect marks ◐ ⊗ ⊘

correct mark ●

When marking the answer sheet, blacken only one circle for each question. Blacken the circle *completely*. Do *NOT* use X's or check marks. If you decide to change your answer, erase your original answer *thoroughly*. If you do not, your new answer may be scored incorrectly. You *MUST* use a No. 2 pencil to mark your answers.

Unit 5

Unit 5

When marking the answer sheet, blacken only one circle for each question. Blacken the circle *completely*. Do *NOT* use X's or check marks. If you decide to change your answer, erase your original answer *thoroughly*. If you do not, your new answer may be scored incorrectly. You *MUST* use a No. 2 pencil to mark your answers.

	1	2	3	4
1	○	○	○	○
2	○	○	○	○
3	○	○	○	○
4	○	○	○	○
5	○	○	○	○
6	○	○	○	○
7	○	○	○	○
8	○	○	○	○
9	○	○	○	○
10	○	○	○	○

	1	2	3	4
11	○	○	○	○
12	○	○	○	○
13	○	○	○	○
14	○	○	○	○
15	○	○	○	○
16	○	○	○	○
17	○	○	○	○
18	○	○	○	○
19	○	○	○	○
20	○	○	○	○

	1	2	3	4
21	○	○	○	○
22	○	○	○	○
23	○	○	○	○
24	○	○	○	○
25	○	○	○	○
26	○	○	○	○
27	○	○	○	○
28	○	○	○	○
29	○	○	○	○
30	○	○	○	○

	1	2	3	4
31	○	○	○	○
32	○	○	○	○
33	○	○	○	○
34	○	○	○	○
35	○	○	○	○
36	○	○	○	○
37	○	○	○	○
38	○	○	○	○
39	○	○	○	○
40	○	○	○	○

	1	2	3	4
41	○	○	○	○
42	○	○	○	○
43	○	○	○	○
44	○	○	○	○
45	○	○	○	○
46	○	○	○	○
47	○	○	○	○
48	○	○	○	○
49	○	○	○	○
50	○	○	○	○

	1	2	3	4
51	○	○	○	○
52	○	○	○	○
53	○	○	○	○
54	○	○	○	○
55	○	○	○	○
56	○	○	○	○
57	○	○	○	○
58	○	○	○	○
59	○	○	○	○
60	○	○	○	○

	1	2	3	4
61	○	○	○	○
62	○	○	○	○
63	○	○	○	○
64	○	○	○	○
65	○	○	○	○
66	○	○	○	○
67	○	○	○	○
68	○	○	○	○
69	○	○	○	○
70	○	○	○	○

	1	2	3	4
71	○	○	○	○
72	○	○	○	○
73	○	○	○	○
74	○	○	○	○
75	○	○	○	○
76	○	○	○	○
77	○	○	○	○
78	○	○	○	○
79	○	○	○	○
80	○	○	○	○

Unit 5

Unit 5

incorrect marks ◍ ⊗ ⊘

correct mark ●

When marking the answer sheet, blacken only one circle for each question. Blacken the circle *completely*. Do *NOT* use X's or check marks. If you decide to change your answer, erase your original answer *thoroughly*. If you do not, your new answer may be scored incorrectly. You *MUST* use a No. 2 pencil to mark your answers.

	1	2	3	4
81	○	○	○	○
82	○	○	○	○
83	○	○	○	○
84	○	○	○	○
85	○	○	○	○
86	○	○	○	○
87	○	○	○	○
88	○	○	○	○
89	○	○	○	○
90	○	○	○	○

	1	2	3	4
91	○	○	○	○
92	○	○	○	○
93	○	○	○	○
94	○	○	○	○
95	○	○	○	○
96	○	○	○	○
97	○	○	○	○
98	○	○	○	○
99	○	○	○	○
100	○	○	○	○

	1	2	3	4
101	○	○	○	○
102	○	○	○	○
103	○	○	○	○
104	○	○	○	○
105	○	○	○	○
106	○	○	○	○
107	○	○	○	○
108	○	○	○	○
109	○	○	○	○
110	○	○	○	○

	1	2	3	4
111	○	○	○	○
112	○	○	○	○
113	○	○	○	○
114	○	○	○	○
115	○	○	○	○
116	○	○	○	○
117	○	○	○	○
118	○	○	○	○
119	○	○	○	○
120	○	○	○	○

	1	2	3	4
121	○	○	○	○
122	○	○	○	○
123	○	○	○	○
124	○	○	○	○
125	○	○	○	○
126	○	○	○	○
127	○	○	○	○
128	○	○	○	○
129	○	○	○	○
130	○	○	○	○

	1	2	3	4
131	○	○	○	○
132	○	○	○	○
133	○	○	○	○
134	○	○	○	○
135	○	○	○	○
136	○	○	○	○
137	○	○	○	○
138	○	○	○	○
139	○	○	○	○
140	○	○	○	○

	1	2	3	4
141	○	○	○	○
142	○	○	○	○
143	○	○	○	○
144	○	○	○	○
145	○	○	○	○
146	○	○	○	○
147	○	○	○	○
148	○	○	○	○
149	○	○	○	○
150	○	○	○	○

	1	2	3	4
151	○	○	○	○
152	○	○	○	○
153	○	○	○	○
154	○	○	○	○
155	○	○	○	○
156	○	○	○	○
157	○	○	○	○
158	○	○	○	○
159	○	○	○	○
160	○	○	○	○

Unit 5

Unit 5

incorrect marks ◐ ○ ⊗ ⊘

correct mark ●

When marking the answer sheet, blacken only one circle for each question. Blacken the circle *completely*. Do *NOT* use X's or check marks. If you decide to change your answer, erase your original answer *thoroughly*. If you do not, your new answer may be scored incorrectly. You *MUST* use a No. 2 pencil to mark your answers.

	1	2	3	4
161	○	○	○	○
162	○	○	○	○
163	○	○	○	○
164	○	○	○	○
165	○	○	○	○
166	○	○	○	○
167	○	○	○	○
168	○	○	○	○
169	○	○	○	○
170	○	○	○	○

	1	2	3	4
171	○	○	○	○
172	○	○	○	○
173	○	○	○	○
174	○	○	○	○
175	○	○	○	○
176	○	○	○	○
177	○	○	○	○
178	○	○	○	○
179	○	○	○	○
180	○	○	○	○

	1	2	3	4
181	○	○	○	○
182	○	○	○	○
183	○	○	○	○
184	○	○	○	○
185	○	○	○	○
186	○	○	○	○
187	○	○	○	○
188	○	○	○	○
189	○	○	○	○
190	○	○	○	○

	1	2	3	4
191	○	○	○	○
192	○	○	○	○
193	○	○	○	○
194	○	○	○	○
195	○	○	○	○
196	○	○	○	○
197	○	○	○	○
198	○	○	○	○
199	○	○	○	○
200	○	○	○	○

	1	2	3	4
201	○	○	○	○
202	○	○	○	○
203	○	○	○	○
204	○	○	○	○
205	○	○	○	○
206	○	○	○	○
207	○	○	○	○
208	○	○	○	○
209	○	○	○	○
210	○	○	○	○

	1	2	3	4
211	○	○	○	○
212	○	○	○	○
213	○	○	○	○
214	○	○	○	○
215	○	○	○	○
216	○	○	○	○
217	○	○	○	○
218	○	○	○	○
219	○	○	○	○
220	○	○	○	○

	1	2	3	4
221	○	○	○	○
222	○	○	○	○
223	○	○	○	○
224	○	○	○	○
225	○	○	○	○
226	○	○	○	○
227	○	○	○	○
228	○	○	○	○
229	○	○	○	○
230	○	○	○	○

	1	2	3	4
231	○	○	○	○
232	○	○	○	○
233	○	○	○	○
234	○	○	○	○
235	○	○	○	○
236	○	○	○	○
237	○	○	○	○
238	○	○	○	○
239	○	○	○	○
240	○	○	○	○

Unit 5

Unit 5

When marking the answer sheet, blacken only one circle for each question. Blacken the circle *completely*. Do *NOT* use X's or check marks. If you decide to change your answer, erase your original answer *thoroughly*. If you do not, your new answer may be scored incorrectly. You *MUST* use a No. 2 pencil to mark your answers.

	1	2	3	4
241	○	○	○	○
242	○	○	○	○
243	○	○	○	○
244	○	○	○	○
245	○	○	○	○
246	○	○	○	○
247	○	○	○	○
248	○	○	○	○
249	○	○	○	○
250	○	○	○	○

	1	2	3	4
251	○	○	○	○
252	○	○	○	○
253	○	○	○	○
254	○	○	○	○
255	○	○	○	○
256	○	○	○	○
257	○	○	○	○
258	○	○	○	○
259	○	○	○	○
260	○	○	○	○

	1	2	3	4
261	○	○	○	○
262	○	○	○	○
263	○	○	○	○
264	○	○	○	○
265	○	○	○	○
266	○	○	○	○
267	○	○	○	○
268	○	○	○	○
269	○	○	○	○
270	○	○	○	○

	1	2	3	4
271	○	○	○	○
272	○	○	○	○
273	○	○	○	○
274	○	○	○	○
275	○	○	○	○
276	○	○	○	○
277	○	○	○	○
278	○	○	○	○
279	○	○	○	○
280	○	○	○	○

	1	2	3	4
281	○	○	○	○
282	○	○	○	○
283	○	○	○	○
284	○	○	○	○
285	○	○	○	○
286	○	○	○	○
287	○	○	○	○
288	○	○	○	○
289	○	○	○	○
290	○	○	○	○

	1	2	3	4
291	○	○	○	○
292	○	○	○	○
293	○	○	○	○
294	○	○	○	○
295	○	○	○	○
296	○	○	○	○
297	○	○	○	○
298	○	○	○	○
299	○	○	○	○
300	○	○	○	○

	1	2	3	4
301	○	○	○	○
302	○	○	○	○
303	○	○	○	○
304	○	○	○	○
305	○	○	○	○
306	○	○	○	○
307	○	○	○	○
308	○	○	○	○
309	○	○	○	○
310	○	○	○	○

	1	2	3	4
311	○	○	○	○
312	○	○	○	○
313	○	○	○	○
314	○	○	○	○
315	○	○	○	○
316	○	○	○	○
317	○	○	○	○
318	○	○	○	○
319	○	○	○	○
320	○	○	○	○

Unit 5

When marking the answer sheet, blacken only one circle for each question. Blacken the circle *completely.* Do *NOT* use X's or check marks. If you decide to change your answer, erase your original answer *thoroughly.* If you do not, your new answer may be scored incorrectly. You *MUST* use a No. 2 pencil to mark your answers.

	1	2	3	4
321	○	○	○	○
322	○	○	○	○
323	○	○	○	○
324	○	○	○	○
325	○	○	○	○
326	○	○	○	○
327	○	○	○	○
328	○	○	○	○
329	○	○	○	○
330	○	○	○	○

	1	2	3	4
331	○	○	○	○
332	○	○	○	○
333	○	○	○	○
334	○	○	○	○
335	○	○	○	○
336	○	○	○	○
337	○	○	○	○
338	○	○	○	○
339	○	○	○	○
340	○	○	○	○

	1	2	3	4
341	○	○	○	○
342	○	○	○	○
343	○	○	○	○
344	○	○	○	○
345	○	○	○	○
346	○	○	○	○
347	○	○	○	○
348	○	○	○	○
349	○	○	○	○
350	○	○	○	○

	1	2	3	4
351	○	○	○	○
352	○	○	○	○
353	○	○	○	○
354	○	○	○	○
355	○	○	○	○
356	○	○	○	○
357	○	○	○	○
358	○	○	○	○
359	○	○	○	○
360	○	○	○	○

	1	2	3	4
361	○	○	○	○
362	○	○	○	○
363	○	○	○	○
364	○	○	○	○
365	○	○	○	○
366	○	○	○	○
367	○	○	○	○
368	○	○	○	○
369	○	○	○	○
370	○	○	○	○

	1	2	3	4
371	○	○	○	○
372	○	○	○	○
373	○	○	○	○
374	○	○	○	○
375	○	○	○	○
376	○	○	○	○
377	○	○	○	○
378	○	○	○	○
379	○	○	○	○
380	○	○	○	○

	1	2	3	4
381	○	○	○	○
382	○	○	○	○
383	○	○	○	○
384	○	○	○	○
385	○	○	○	○
386	○	○	○	○
387	○	○	○	○
388	○	○	○	○
389	○	○	○	○
390	○	○	○	○

	1	2	3	4
391	○	○	○	○
392	○	○	○	○
393	○	○	○	○
394	○	○	○	○
395	○	○	○	○
396	○	○	○	○
397	○	○	○	○
398	○	○	○	○
399	○	○	○	○
400	○	○	○	○

Unit 6

	1	2	3	4
1	○	○	○	○
2	○	○	○	○
3	○	○	○	○
4	○	○	○	○
5	○	○	○	○
6	○	○	○	○
7	○	○	○	○
8	○	○	○	○
9	○	○	○	○
10	○	○	○	○

	1	2	3	4
11	○	○	○	○
12	○	○	○	○
13	○	○	○	○
14	○	○	○	○
15	○	○	○	○
16	○	○	○	○
17	○	○	○	○
18	○	○	○	○
19	○	○	○	○
20	○	○	○	○

	1	2	3	4
21	○	○	○	○
22	○	○	○	○
23	○	○	○	○
24	○	○	○	○
25	○	○	○	○
26	○	○	○	○
27	○	○	○	○
28	○	○	○	○
29	○	○	○	○
30	○	○	○	○

	1	2	3	4
31	○	○	○	○
32	○	○	○	○
33	○	○	○	○
34	○	○	○	○
35	○	○	○	○

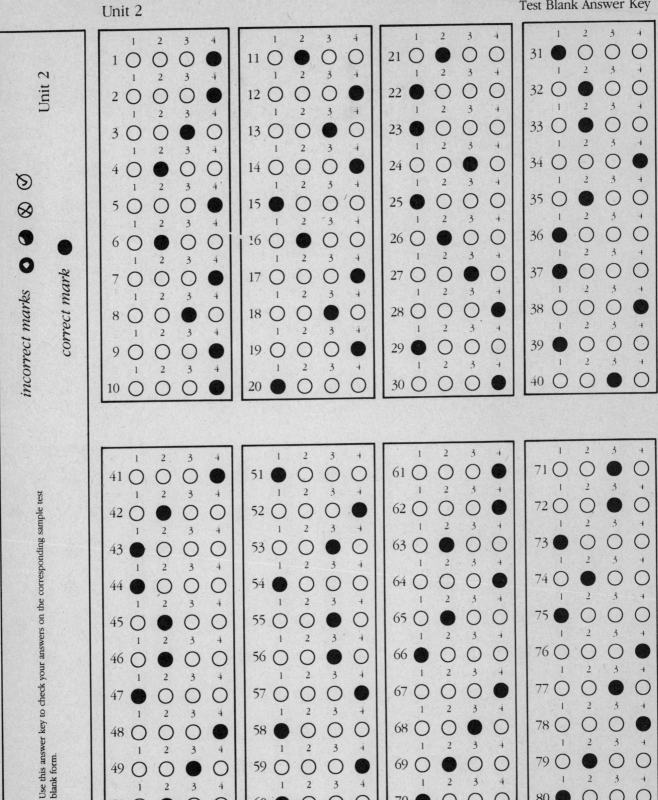

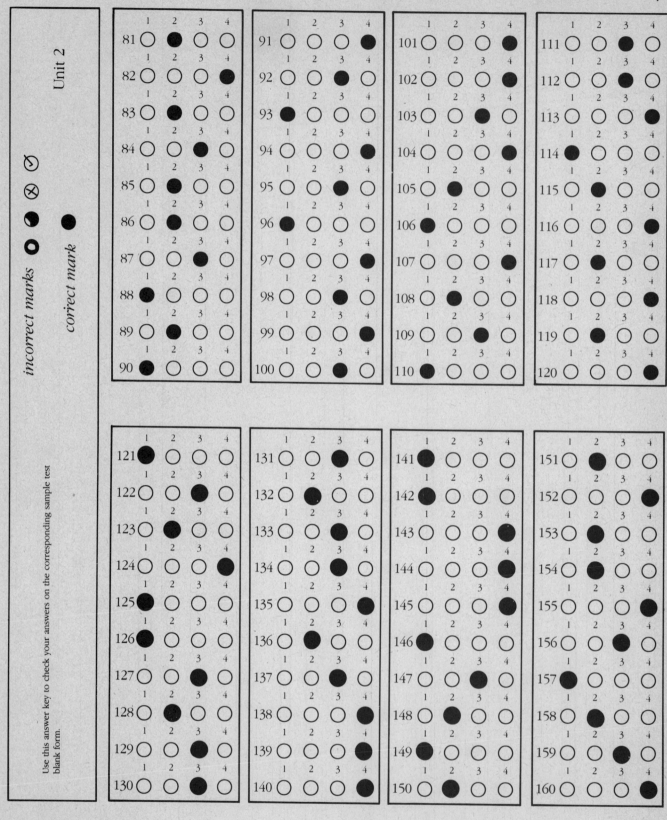

Unit 2

Unit 2 and 3

incorrect marks

correct mark

Use this answer key to check your answers on the corresponding sample test blank form.

Unit 3

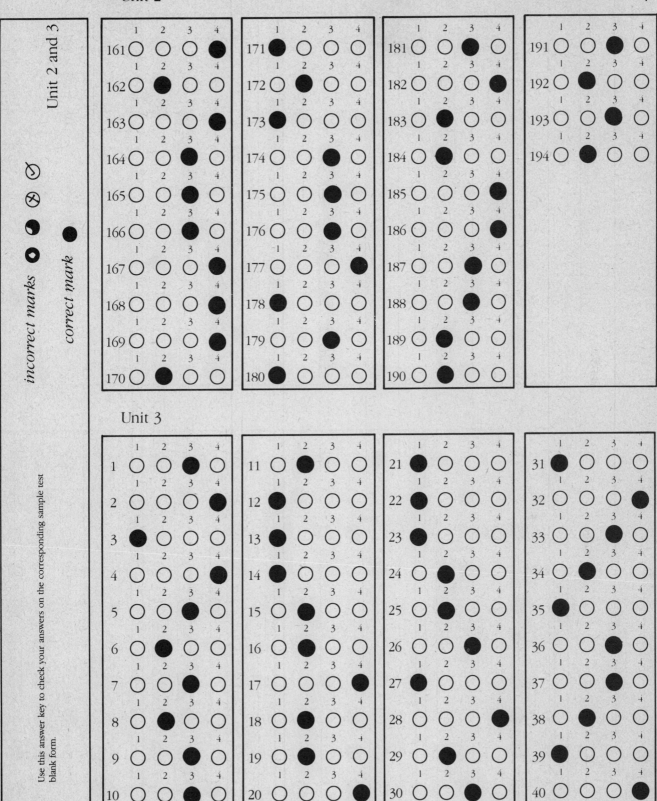

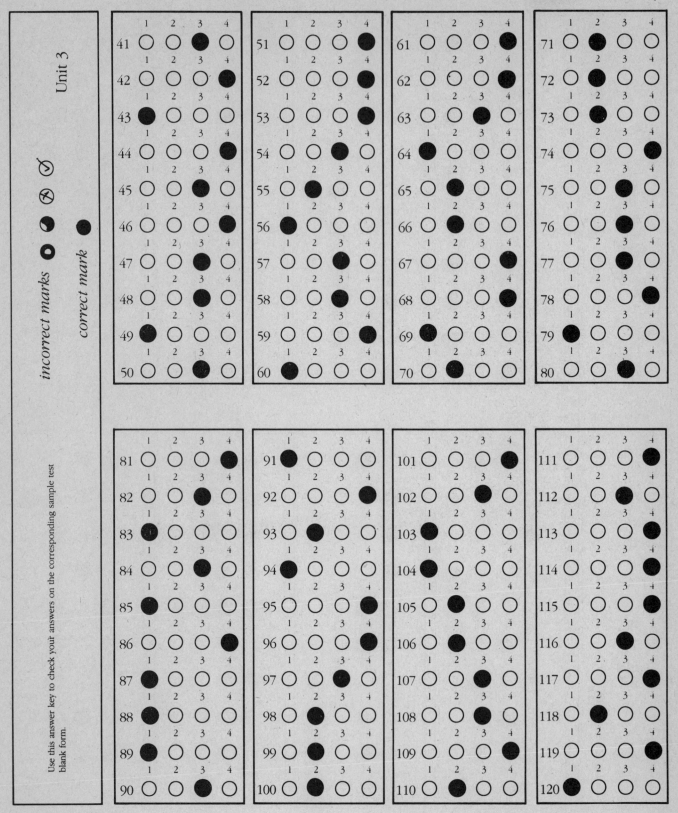

Unit 3   Test Blank Answer Key

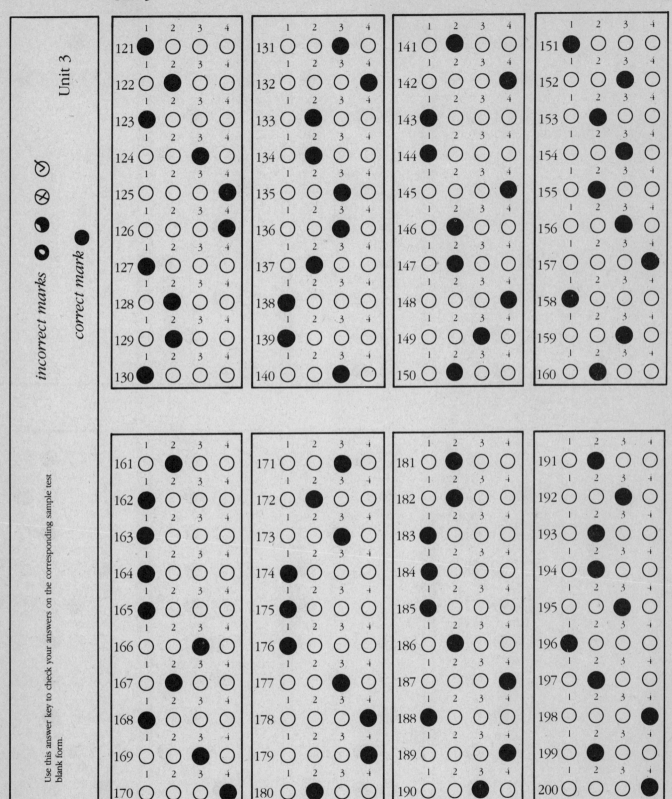

Unit 3

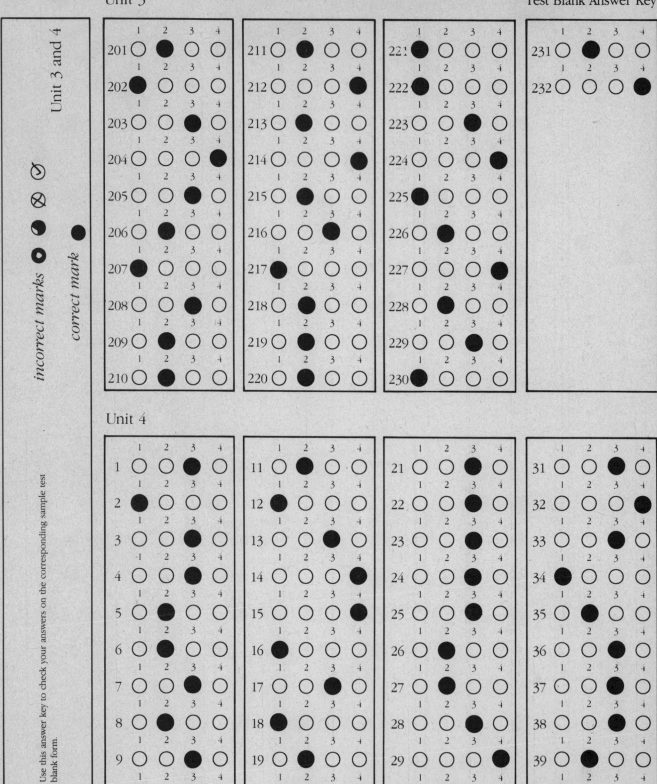

Unit 4

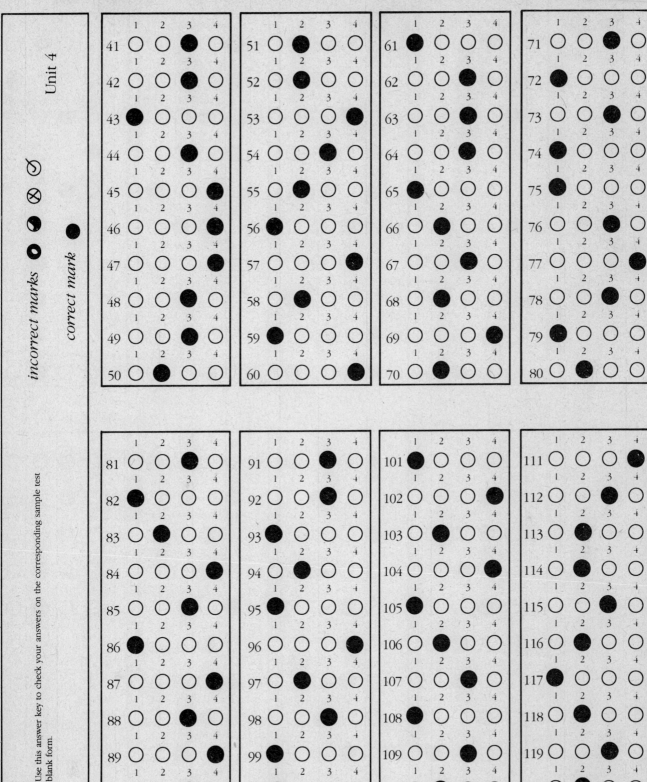

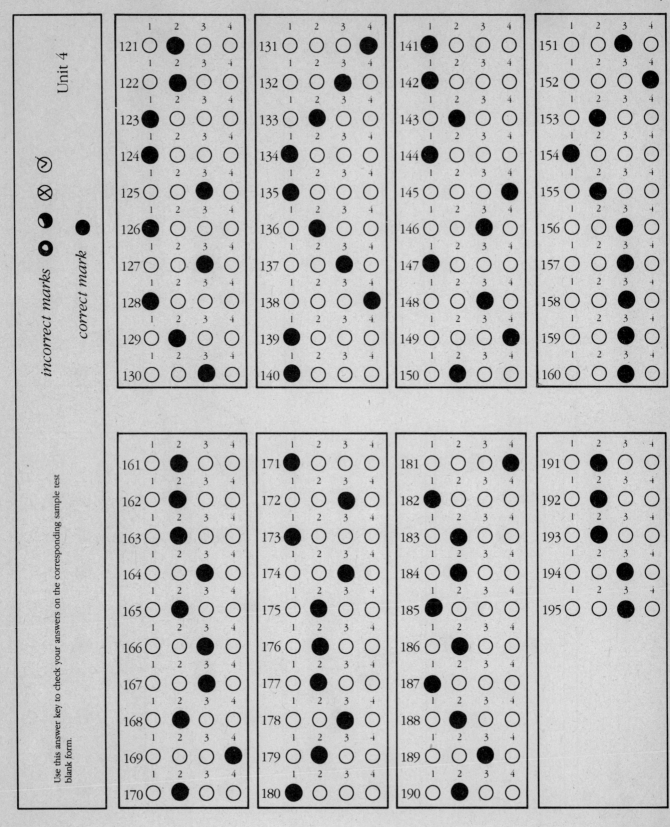

incorrect marks

correct mark

Unit 4

Use this answer key to check your answers on the corresponding sample test blank form.

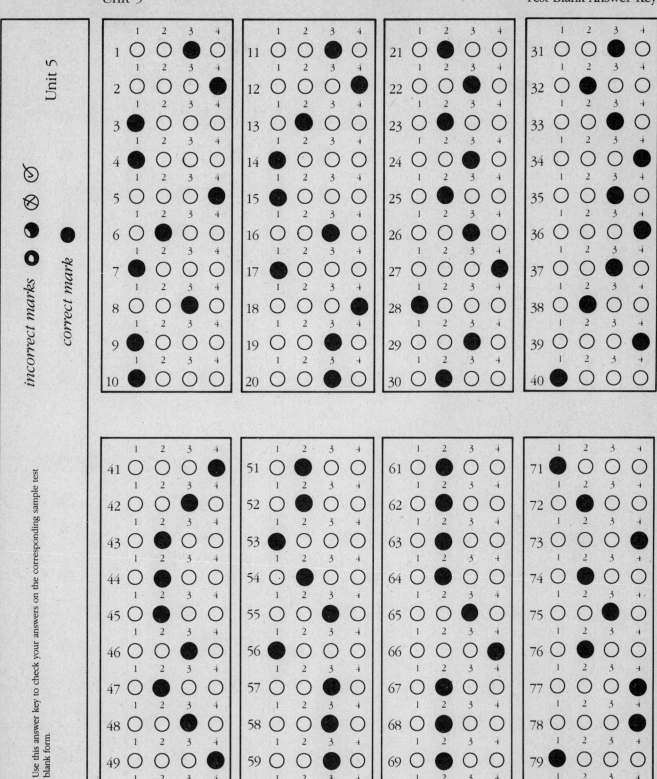

Unit 5

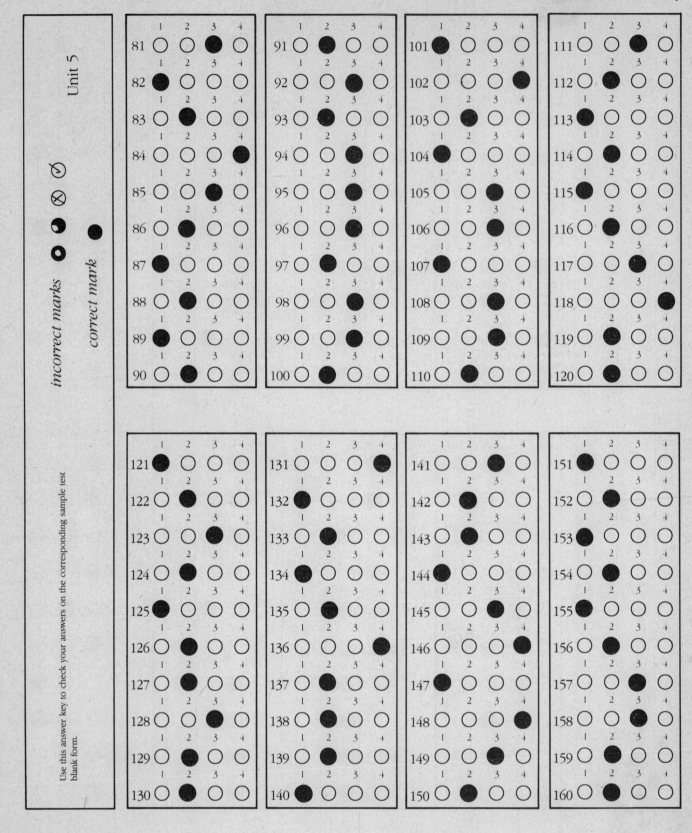

Unit 5

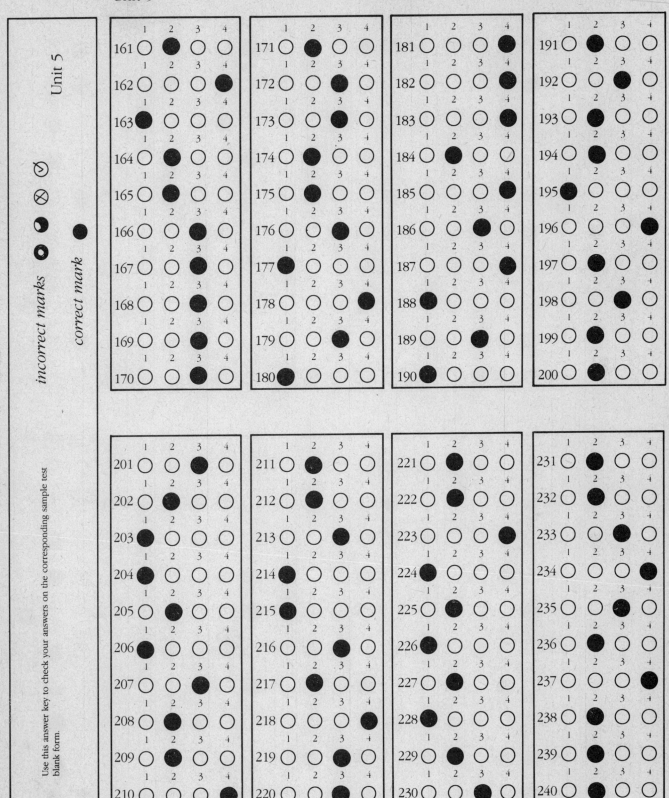

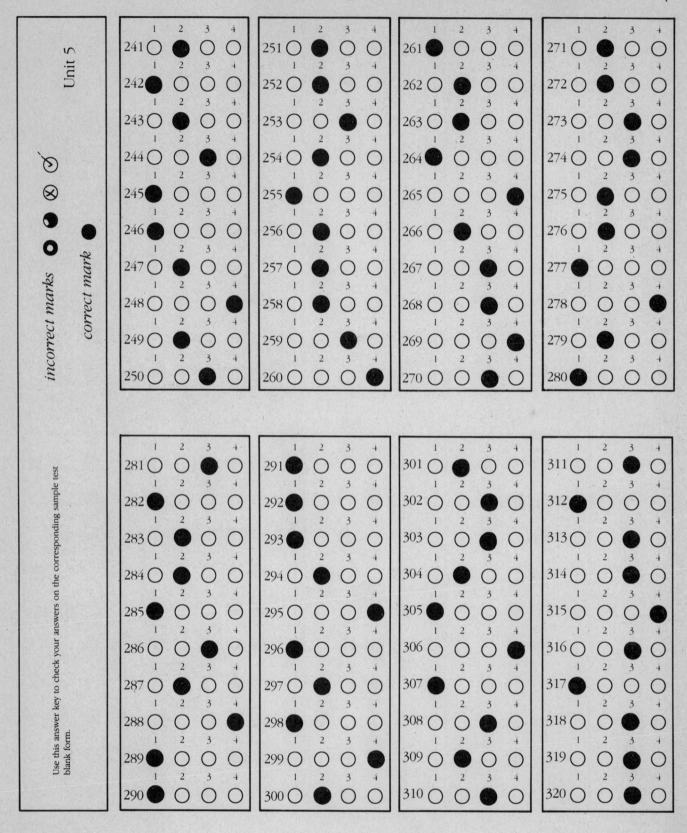

Unit 5

incorrect marks

correct mark

Use this answer key to check your answers on the corresponding sample test blank form.

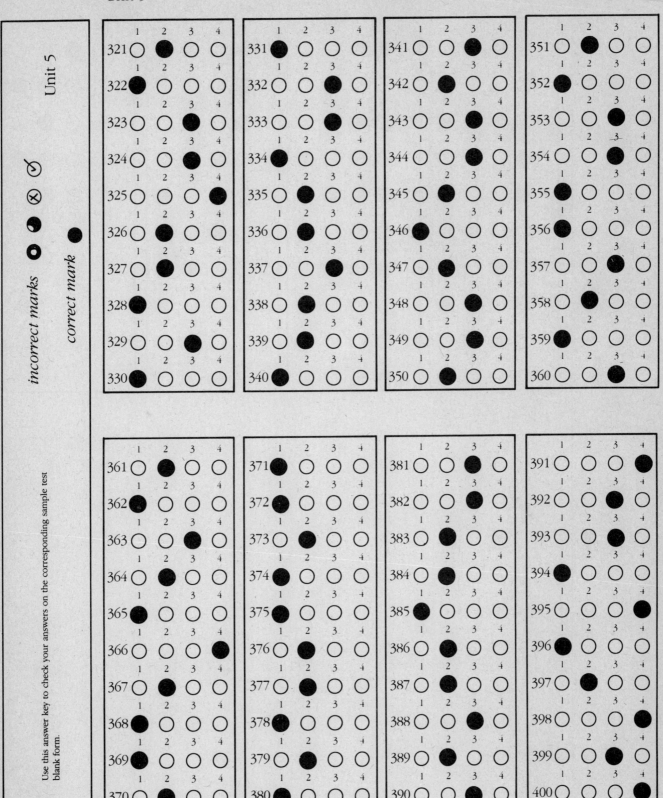

Unit 5

incorrect marks

correct mark

Use this answer key to check your answers on the corresponding sample test blank form.

Unit 6

incorrect marks ⦿ ⊗ ⊘

correct mark ●

Use this answer key to check your answers on the corresponding sample test blank form.

	1	2	3	4
1	○	○	●	○
2	○	○	○	●
3	○	○	○	●
4	●	○	○	○
5	●	○	○	○
6	○	○	●	○
7	○	●	○	○
8	○	○	○	●
9	○	●	○	○
10	○	○	○	●

	1	2	3	4
11	●	○	○	○
12	○	○	●	○
13	○	●	○	○
14	○	○	○	●
15	○	○	●	○
16	○	●	○	○
17	●	○	○	○
18	○	○	○	●
19	○	○	○	●
20	●	○	○	○

	1	2	3	4
21	○	○	●	○
22	●	○	○	○
23	●	○	○	○
24	○	●	○	○
25	○	○	○	●
26	○	●	○	○
27	○	○	●	○
28	○	○	○	●
29	○	○	●	○
30	○	●	○	○

	1	2	3	4
31	○	●	○	○
32	○	○	○	●
33	○	○	●	○
34	○	○	○	●
35	○	○	●	○

To the owner of this book:

We hope that you have enjoyed Addison-Wesley's Nursing Examination Review. Only through the comments of people who have used the book can we learn how to make it a better book for future readers.

1. Why did you purchase *Addison-Wesley's Nursing Examination Review?*

   _____

   _____

2. What did you like *most* about this book? _____

   _____

   _____

3. What did you like *least* about this book? _____

   _____

   _____

4. When did you or will you take the R.N. Licensure Exam? _____

   _____

5. When did you purchase *Addison-Wesley's Nursing Examination Review?*

   _____

6. If you have already taken the exam, do you think *Addison-Wesley's Nursing Examination Review* helped you to take the test confidently? Why or why not? _____

   _____

   _____

7. Did you participate in a review course? _____ If yes, which one? _____

   _____

8. In the space below or in a separate letter, please let us know what other comments about the book you'd like to make. We'd be delighted to hear from you. _____

   _____

   _____

   _____

   _____

(Optional)

Your name: _____ Date: _____

May we quote you in our advertising? _____ Yes

_____ No

We thank you for your participation.

Sincerely,

Sally L. Lagerquist

(fold here)

(fold here)

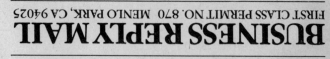

Menlo Park, CA 94025
2727 Sand Hill Road
Medical/Nursing Division
ADDISON-WESLEY PUBLISHING COMPANY, INC.

Postage will be paid by Addressee:

FIRST CLASS PERMIT NO. 870 MENLO PARK, CA 94025
BUSINESS REPLY MAIL

No Postage
Necessary
if Mailed in the
United States

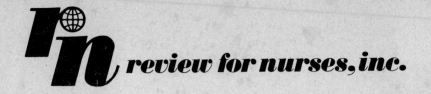

review for nurses, inc.

Five Day Review Courses

are conducted before every R.N. Licensure Exam by Review for Nurses, Inc. of San Francisco, and are given at many convenient locations throughout the U.S.

The course coordinator is Sally Lagerquist, R.N., M.S., editor/author of this review book, which is used extensively throughout the review courses.

In addition to a complete review of nursing content, the courses give practice in answering exam questions, introduce test-taking techniques, and present anxiety reduction exercises.

For information on the courses and their locations, schedules, and fees, write or call:

review for nurses, inc.

P.O. Box 16115
San Francisco, CA 94116
(415) 731-0833

Send me complete information

I am interested in reviews in:

_____ East   _____ Midwest

_____ South   _____ West

I will be taking the R.N. National Council Licensure Exam (mo./yr.) _____

Name _____ Phone (____) _____

Current address _____

City/state _____ Zip _____

Nursing school _____